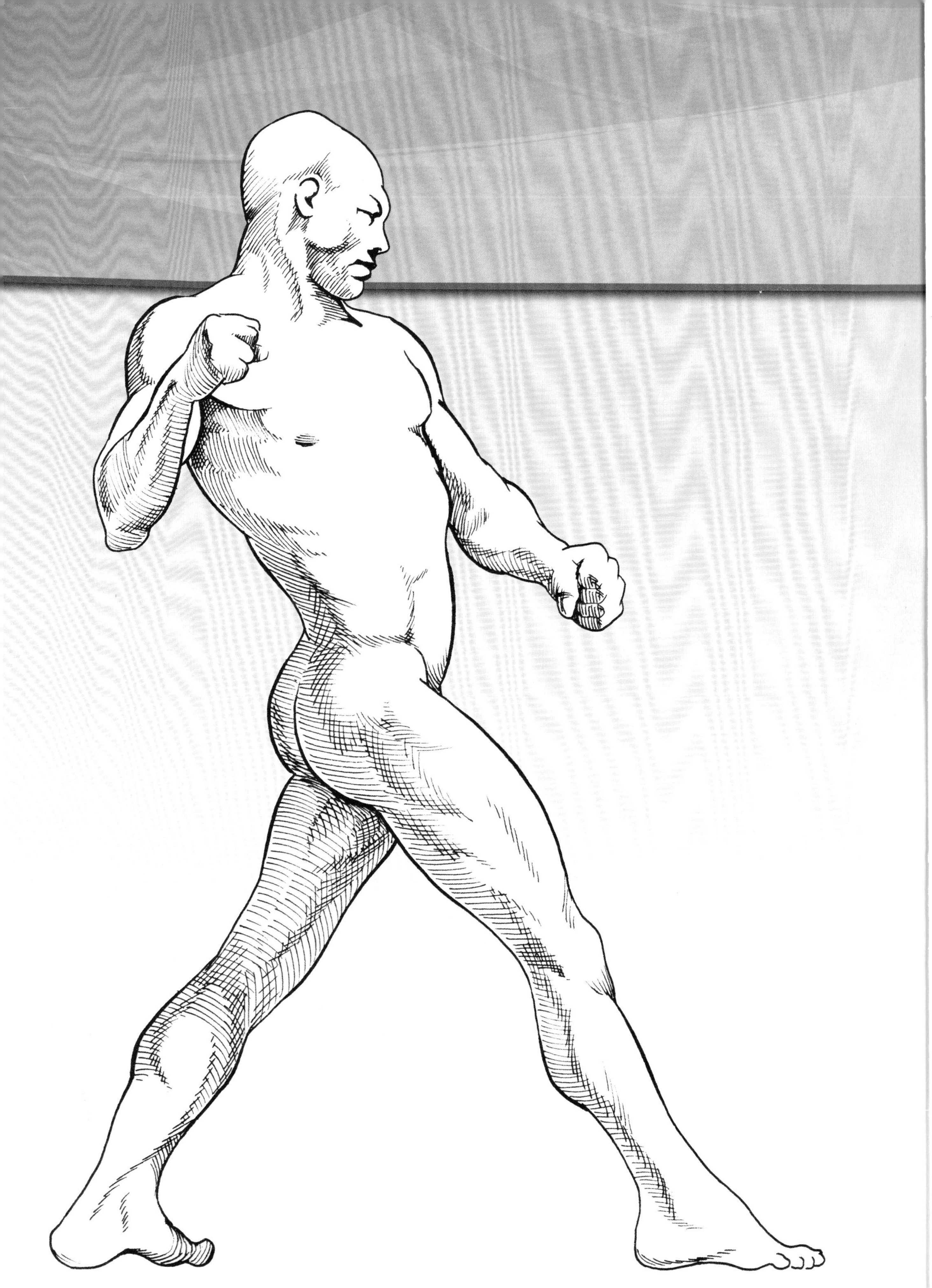

W9-AFS-472

Anatomic Exposures in Vascular Surgery

THIRD EDITION

THIRD EDITION

Anatomic Exposures in Vascular Surgery

Gary G. Wind, M.D., F.A.C.S.

Professor of Surgery
Department of Surgery
Uniformed Services University of the Health Sciences
Director of Art and Education, Vesalius.com
Bethesda, Maryland

R. James Valentine, M.D., F.A.C.S.

Professor and Chairman
Division of Vascular and Endovascular Surgery
Executive Vice Chairman, Department of Surgery
Alvin Baldwin, Jr. Chair in Surgery
University of Texas Southwestern Medical Center
Dallas, Texas

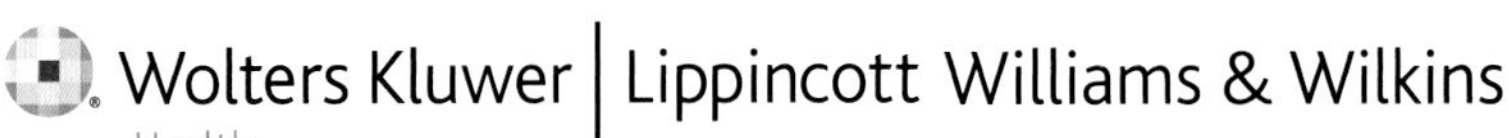
Wolters Kluwer | Lippincott Williams & Wilkins
Health

Philadelphia • Baltimore • New York • London
Buenos Aires • Hong Kong • Sydney • Tokyo

Acquisitions Editor: Brian Brown
Product Manager: Brendan Huffman
Production Project Manager: Priscilla Crater
Senior Manufacturing Manager: Benjamin Rivera
Marketing Manager: Lisa Lawrence
Design Coordinator: Stephen Druding
Production Service: S4Carlisle Publishing Services

Published by LIPPINCOTT WILLIAMS & WILKINS a WOLTERS KLUWER business

Two Commerce Square
2001 Market Street
Philadelphia, PA 19103 USA
LWW.com

Printed in China

Library of Congress Cataloging-in-Publication Data

Wind, Gary G.
Anatomic exposures in vascular surgery / Gary G. Wind, R. James Valentine; illustrated by Gary G. Wind. — 3rd ed.
p. ; cm.
Rev. ed. of: Anatomic exposures in vascular surgery / R. James Valentine, Gary G. Wind.
Includes bibliographical references and index.
ISBN 978-1-4511-8472-3 (alk. paper) — ISBN 1-4511-8472-7 (alk. paper)
I. Valentine, R. James, 1954- II. Valentine, R. James, 1954- Anatomic exposures in vascular surgery. III. Title.
[DNLM: 1. Blood Vessels—anatomy & histology—Atlases. 2. Vascular Surgical Procedures—Atlases. WG 17]

611′.13—dc23

2012036861

To purchase additional copies of this book, call our customer service department at (800) 638-3030 or fax orders to (301) 223-2320. International customers should call (301) 223-2300.

Visit Lippincott Williams & Wilkins on the Internet: at LWW.com. Lippincott Williams & Wilkins customer service representatives are available from 8:30 am to 6 pm, EST.

10 9 8 7 6 5 4 3 2 1

To our wives
Marilyn Gail Wind and Tracy Williams Valentine
for their patience and support

CONTRIBUTORS

Forearm Fasciotomy:

Jeffrey A. Marchessault, MD
Adjunct Faculty, Lincoln Memorial University-DeBusk College of Osteopathic Medicine, Harrogate TN
Associated Orthopaedics of Kingsport, TN

Vascular Exposure of the Lumbar Spine:

David Whittaker, MD, FACS
CDR, MC, USN
Chief, Vascular Surgery
Walter Reed National Military Medical Center
Bethesda, MD

Leo Daab, MD
Fellow, Vascular Surgery
Walter Reed National Military Medical Center
Bethesda, MD

CONTENTS

FOREWORD FROM THE FIRST EDITION

The illustrations are the strong point of this excellent book. These have been drawn from the perspective of a surgeon who clearly knows what is seen during a surgical operation. An anatomist illustrates the anatomy as seen in the dissecting room. Drs. Gary Wind and R. James Valentine have given us outstanding drawings of what a surgeon will see in the operating room.

Dr. Wind is experienced in the use of a microcomputer to create three-dimensional reconstructions of anatomy. These unusual visual images and models provide different concepts of conventional anatomic views. The knowledge gained from this study of many regions of the body has been used to provide the unusual and very informative illustrations that fill this book. In a standard illustration, it appears that the vertebral artery travels only a short distance before it enters the foramen in the transverse process of the sixth cervical vertebra. A surgeon who has operated on this artery at this point knows that there is a length of several centimeters before it enters the bony foramen. This book is filled with similar useful information, which has been uncovered by Dr. Wind's special anatomical reconstructions. The text is clear and concise and there is a good bibliography after each chapter. This text has obviously been written by those who know what is of importance to a clinician.

Of special interest are two sections, the introduction on embryology and the last section on vascular variation. Such variations have always been a challenge for surgeons. Embryology demonstrates the possible explanations for these variations, and the final chapter on anatomic variations will help the surgeon to expect and identify the unexpected should he or she encounter them.

This is an anatomic book written by surgeons, but the objective has not been to describe surgical procedures. It has been to describe and illustrate the anatomic relationships of blood vessels. The result is a book of great value, not only to vascular surgeons but also to anatomists, because it throws new light on an old subject—gross anatomy.

Charles G. Rob, M.D., F.R.C.S., F.A.C.S†
Professor of Surgery
Uniformed Services University of
the Health Sciences
Bethesda, Maryland

†Dr. Charles Rob passed away in 2001. He was a preeminent pioneer of vascular surgery and one of the last of the surgical giants. The force of his personality was always evident beneath his impeccable gentlemanly persona. He will be missed by us and by the surgical world as a whole.

Gary G. Wind, M.D.
R. James Valentine, M.D.

PREFACE TO THE FIRST EDITION

> Dispel from your mind the thought that an understanding of the human body in every aspect of its structure can be given in words; for the more thoroughly you describe, the more you will confuse. . . I advise you not to trouble with words unless you are speaking to blind men.
>
> —Leonardo da Vinci

Understanding the anatomy of the blood vessels is a highly visual enterprise, given the complex ramification of the vascular tree through all the tissue planes of the body. This book is designed to convey the clinical anatomy of the blood vessels through extensive new illustrations with a minimum of words. The focus is on a concise, clear presentation of key anatomic relationships necessary to understand the vascular pattern in all areas of the body. The chapters are divided into anatomic overview and surgical approach sections.

As a monograph, this book has the advantage of a uniform concept and presentation sometimes lacking in multiauthor works. At the same time, as the work progressed we were privileged to have the advice and criticism of the eminent surgeons listed as consulting editors. The visualization of the anatomy was aided by original fresh cadaver dissection for each body region. The clinical insights are based on both experience and a thorough review of current and historical references.

The literature of a relatively young specialty such as vascular surgery naturally grows by accretion as new procedures are devised and perfected. The surgical anatomy associated with the procedures is described in variable detail in the original papers and is then condensed in surgical texts and atlases. There comes a time in this evolutionary process when a comprehensive treatment of the anatomic context of vascular surgery is beneficial. It is the purpose of this book to provide a detailed and practical guide for exposing and manipulating blood vessels with minimal trauma to the surrounding structures and to the vessels themselves.

The format of the book is designed to provide a unified, integrated concept of anatomic approaches to blood vessels. The anatomy is described in the context of the latest techniques and is organized by body region. The same anatomic descriptions should be equally applicable to new procedures as they arise. The text is intended to describe clinically relevant anatomy as concisely as possible without getting bogged down in trivial and esoteric points. The reader is credited with sufficient anatomic knowledge to be comfortable with the level of presentation and with the intellectual curiosity to look up details that pique his or her interest. Illustrations showing surgical approaches depict ideal exposure, and laparotomy pads, which would normally be present to protect wound edges, are omitted for purposes of clarity and orientation. Clinical references are listed at the end of each chapter, and anatomic references are listed at the end of the book. We hope that in this way to bring crisp clarity and unity to the anatomy of vascular surgery.

PREFACE TO THE THIRD EDITION

The last two decades have witnessed a surge of interest in catheter-based vascular intervention, with a corresponding decrease in the number of open vascular procedures currently being performed. As the clinical experience with open vascular exposure declines, we believe that there is an enduring need for a comprehensive text that features vascular anatomy from a surgical point of view. The original purpose of this book has not changed—it is intended to be a detailed and practical guide for exposing blood vessels with minimal trauma to surrounding structures. The volume of recent literature regarding novel exposure techniques and refined indications for specific approaches has provided the impetus for a third edition.

Based on favorable response to the previous editions, we have maintained an emphasis on clinical anatomy, focusing on detailed illustrations rather than extensive written descriptions. A key feature of this book is that all of the illustrations were drawn by a single artist, who is also a surgeon and anatomist. This uniformity has allowed inclusion of more detail in each illustration for maximal educational benefit. A major enhancement in this third edition is the use of full color for the anatomic illustrations, giving a greater appreciation of three-dimensional relationships. The procedural text and clinical references have been updated to reflect current concepts. New sections on forearm compartment syndrome/fasciotomy and vascular exposure of the lumbar spine have been added. In addition, references to web-based three-dimensional anatomy resources have been included.

As before, chapters are divided into anatomic overview and surgical exposure sections. The text is written from a surgeon's point of view, using practical descriptions based on key anatomic relationships. Trivial and esoteric details have been avoided. Related clinical discussion is based on a thorough review of the modern literature.

Perhaps, the most important point to be made about this book is that it is intended to have lasting applicability. Human anatomy will not change in the foreseeable future. Vascular procedures may wax and wane in popularity, but exposure techniques remain a standard part of any present or future operation.

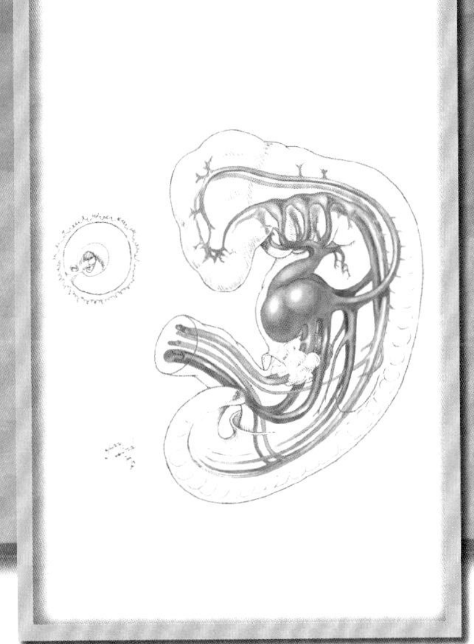

INTRODUCTION Embryology of the Arteries and Veins

Development of the Blood Vessels

Overview

Between the third and eighth week of embryonic gestation (measured in postovulatory days), the blood vessels form and evolve into an approximation of the definitive human circulatory pattern. Toward the end of the third week, primitive circulation begins, propelled by the newly fused heart. Rapid changes in the fourth week set the stage for extensive remodeling that extends through the second and final month of the embryonic period. Development at the cephalad end of the embryo proceeds more rapidly than at the caudal end as the arteries and veins change and interact with the growing thoracoabdominal organs, parietes, and extremities. The incredibly complex bioarchitectural development and reorganization take place while the embryo is between 3 mm and 3 cm in size (crown-to-rump length; Fig. 1). The next significant change in the vascular pattern occurs at birth.

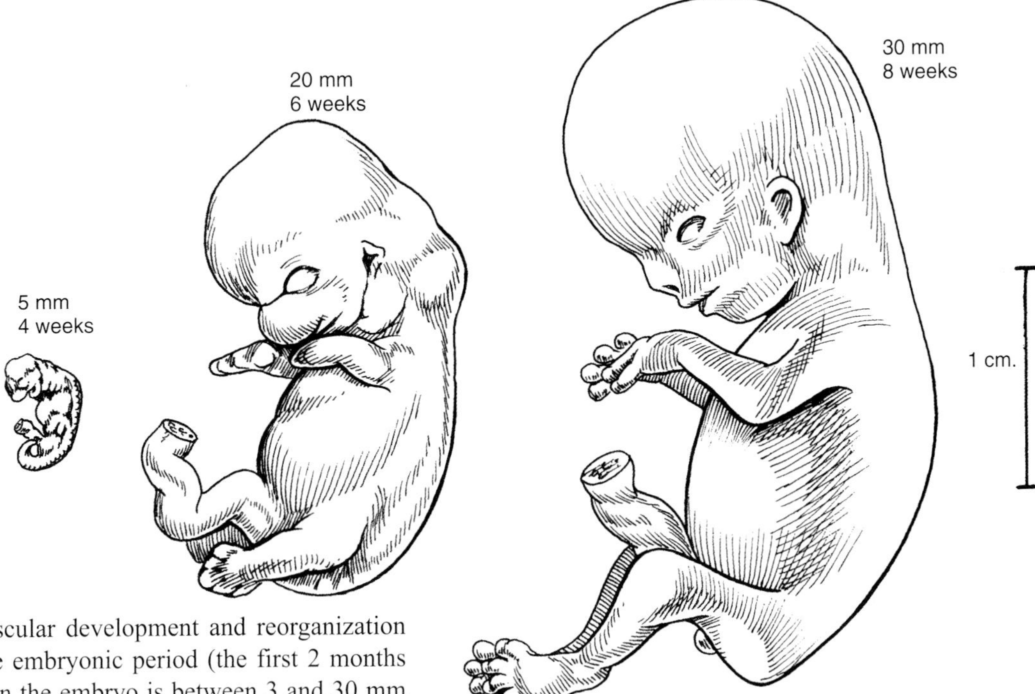

Fig. 1 Rapid vascular development and reorganization takes place in the embryonic period (the first 2 months of gestation) when the embryo is between 3 and 30 mm in crown-to-rump length. The basic pattern of definitive vessels is established by the end of this period.

Understanding the changes that take place in the evolution of the adult vascular system provides a logical framework in which to conceptualize the many variations and anomalies that one will encounter in vascular surgery.

Primordial Vessels and the Inception of Circulation

At the inception of circulation, the embryo appears as a polypoid excrescence within the chorionic vesicle (Fig. 2). The pedicle constitutes the body stalk. The head of the polyp is subtly bilobed, with the groove separating the two lobes reflecting the margins of the embryonic disk within. The dome above the 3-mm embryonic plate is the amnion, and the pendant bleb is the yolk sac.

Between these mirror-image domes, the elongating 2-mm embryonic disk rolls its lateral edges up to begin the closure of the neural groove, and the first somites appear at midbody (Fig. 3). The lining cells of mesenchymal clefts that have developed independently until this time begin to interconnect and form two pairs of longitudinal channels, one medial and one lateral. The medial channels attach to the ends of the paired heart tubes at the cephalad end of the embryo, forming the primitive aortas, which extend into distal vitelline arterial networks. The lateral set attaches to the caudal ends of the heart tubes and will become the vitelline and umbilical veins.

Within a few days, the heart has fused and begun peristaltic pulsations that propel blood through the vitelline circuits. The vitelline circulation provides nutrients from the rapidly regressing mammalian yolk sac for only a brief time before this function is assumed by the precociously maturing chorion. The umbilical vessels, extending from the vitelline complexes through the body stalk and then to the chorion, become dominant.

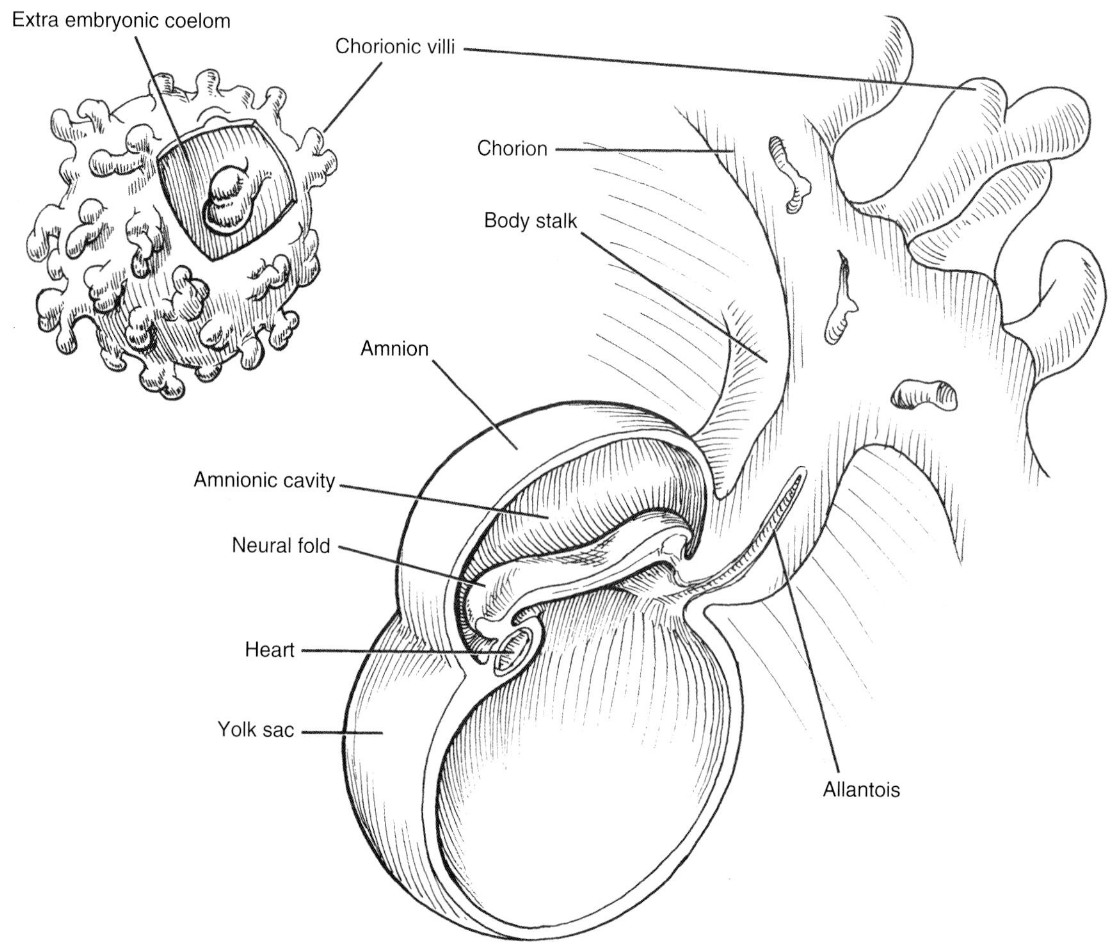

Fig. 2 At the onset of angiogenesis, the embryonic plate lies in a polypoid excrescence within the chorionic vesicle.

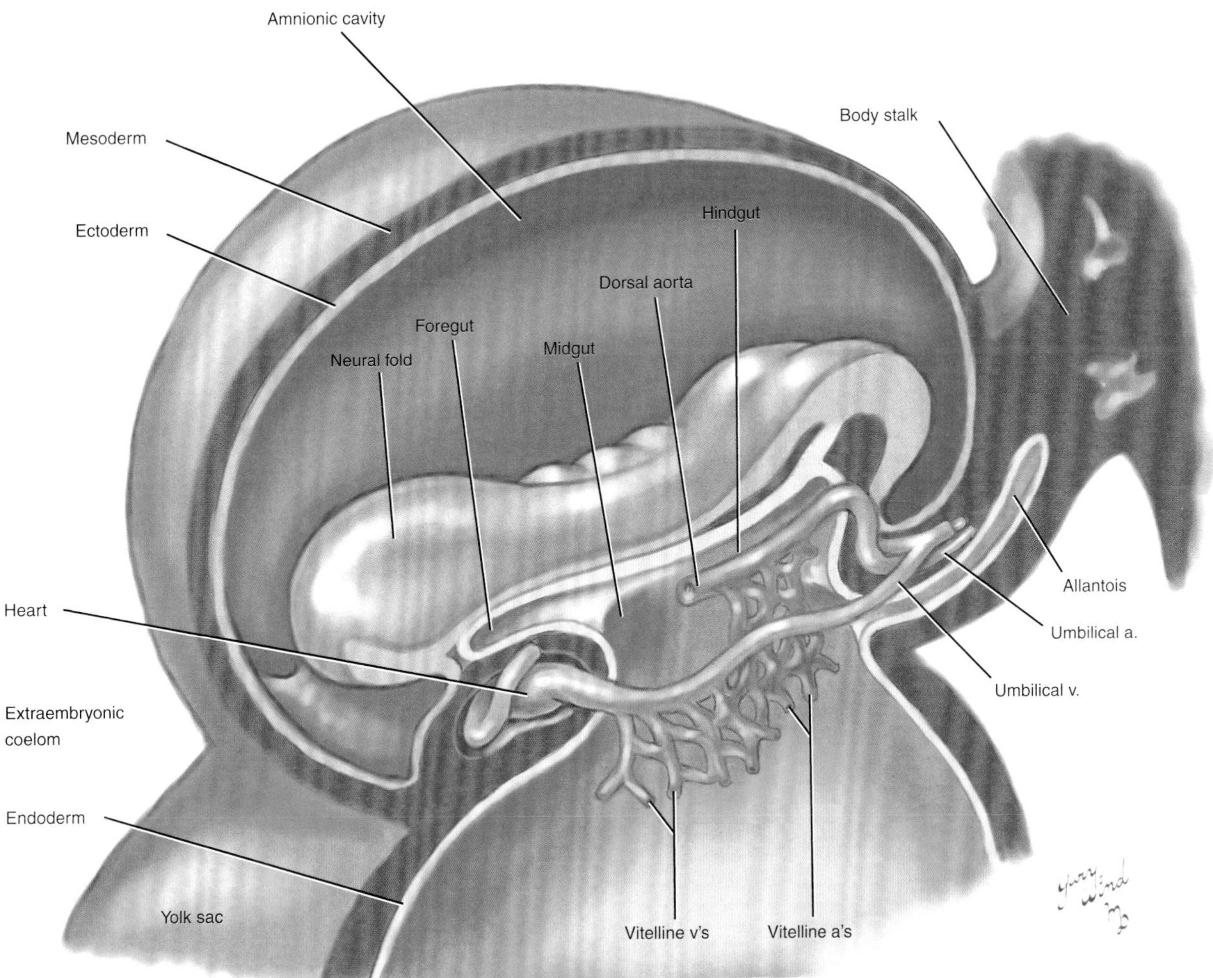

Fig. 3 The first two sets of primitive vessels attach to the ends of the newly fused heart tube.

During the fourth week, the embryo attains a length of 4 to 5 mm, develops a full complement of somites, and begins a series of changes in vascular morphology (Fig. 4). The paired aortas fuse for much of their length and develop numerous dorsal, lateral, and ventral branches. A series of five additional pairs of arterial arches pass laterally around the pharynx between the developing branchial outpouchings, connecting the cephalad apex of the heart to the remaining unfused dorsal aortas. The cephalad arches regress as fast as caudal arches are added, and the six arches undergo evolutionary changes during weeks 5 to 7 (see below). The multiple vitelline arteries regress, leaving three that will become the celiac, superior mesenteric, and inferior mesenteric arteries. Paired pre- and postcardinal veins form in the body wall and attach via common cardinal veins to the caudal horns of the heart, now known as the sinus venosus.

By the end of 4 weeks, four limb buds are evident, with the cephalad set more advanced. The remnants of the vitelline veins are forming sinusoids in the developing liver and coalescing to form the portal venous system. The subsequent simultaneous developments in the arterial and venous systems of the trunk and extremities merit separate description, keeping in mind the parallel time course of these events.

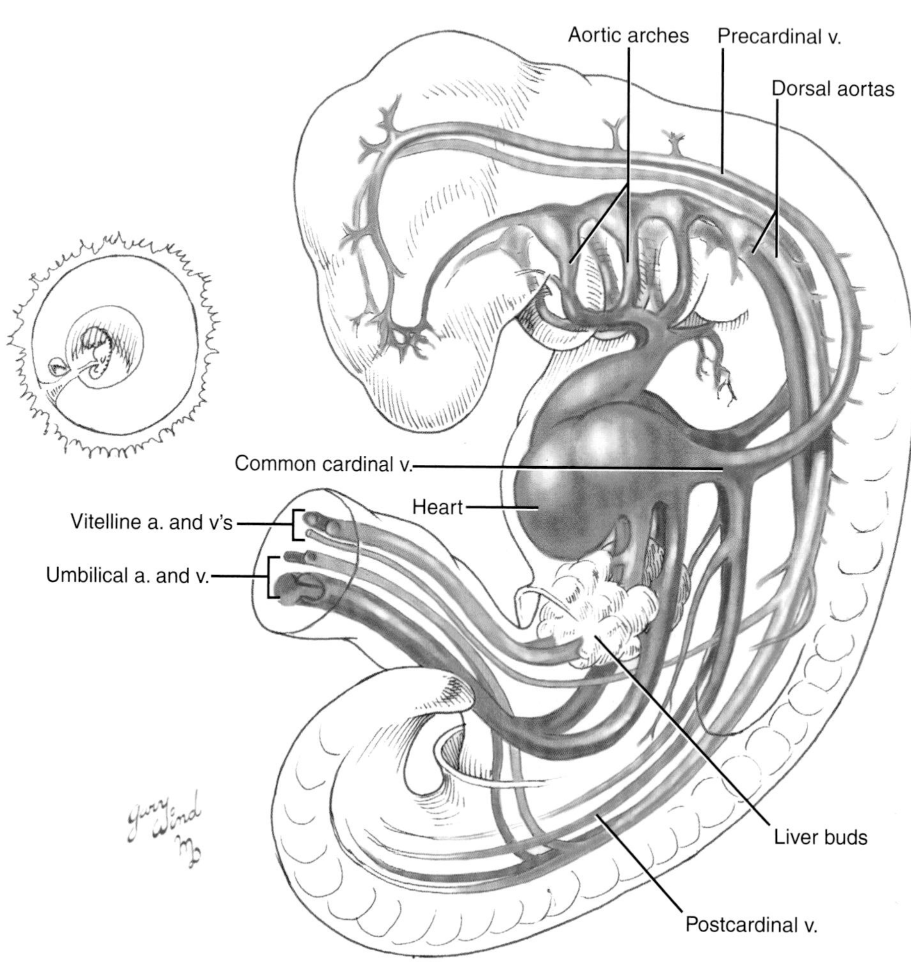

Fig. 4 In the 4-week embryo, aortic fusion has begun, arches are forming, the umbilical vessels are well defined, and the cardinal veins are formed, laying the foundations for the rapid changes of the second month.

Aortic Arches

Six sets of aortic arches have penetrated the cores of successive branchial arches, and the first, second, and rudimentary fifth have largely regressed by the beginning of the fifth week when the embryo is 6 mm in length (Fig. 5). The dorsal aortas persist at the level of the first two arches, retaining their connection to the third arch to form the internal carotid arteries. The external carotid arteries arise as new branches of the aortic sac and by differential growth migrate distally onto the third arches (Fig. 6). The roots of the third arches, therefore, become the common carotid arteries. The external carotid arteries follow the muscles derived from the first two branchial arches in their migration to the face and head.

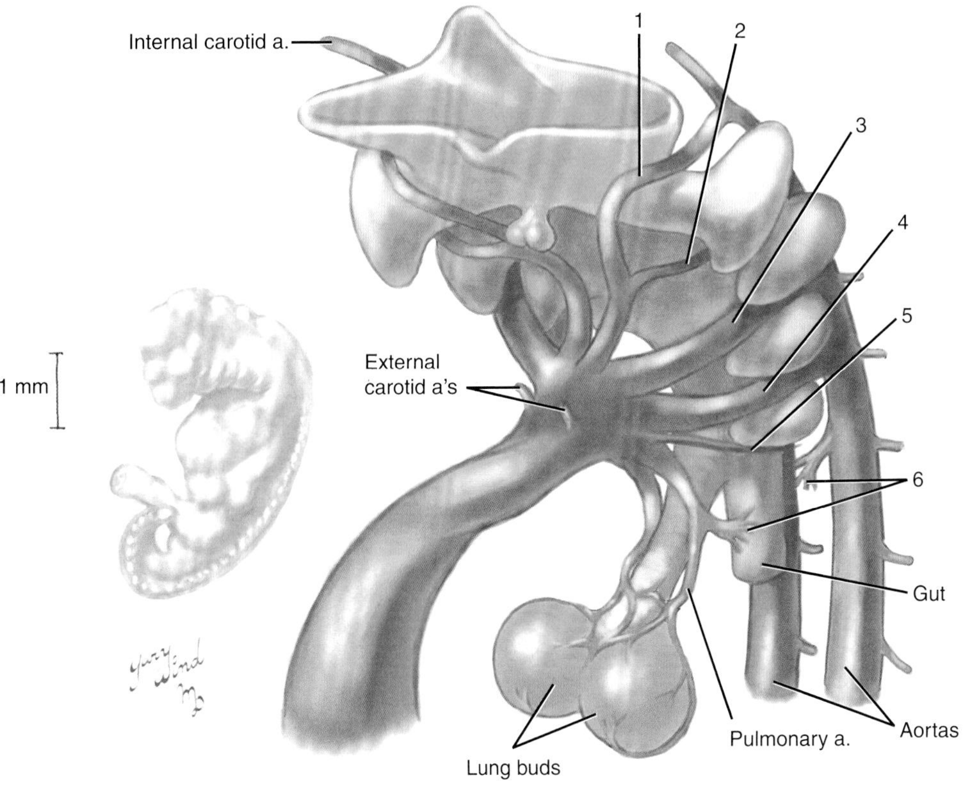

Fig. 5 The aortic arches evolve in a cephalad to caudad progression.

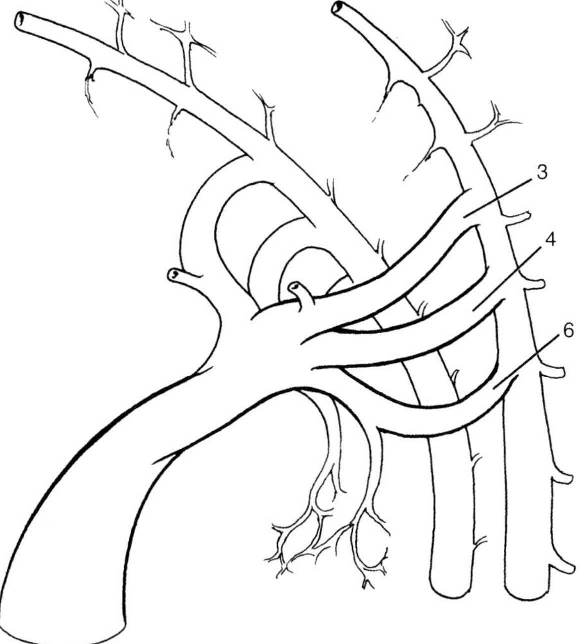

Fig. 6 The internal carotid arteries are left as cephalad dorsal aorta remnants after resorption of the first two arches and are fed by the third arches.

The fourth arches both persist, the left as the adult aortic arch and the right as the root of the right subclavian artery (Fig. 7). The subclavian arteries arise initially as outgrowths of the terminal paired aortas just proximal to their union. The resorption of the right aorta between the subclavian artery and the fused trunk isolates the right subclavian artery.

The sixth (pulmonary) arches grow from the dorsal aortas to meet the developing pulmonary arteries that extend from the aortic sac to the lung buds. The right sixth arch disappears while the left becomes the ductus arteriosus (later the ligamentum arteriosum). During weeks 5 through 7, when these arch changes are taking place, the truncus and aortic sac of the heart are separating into aortic and pulmonary stems.

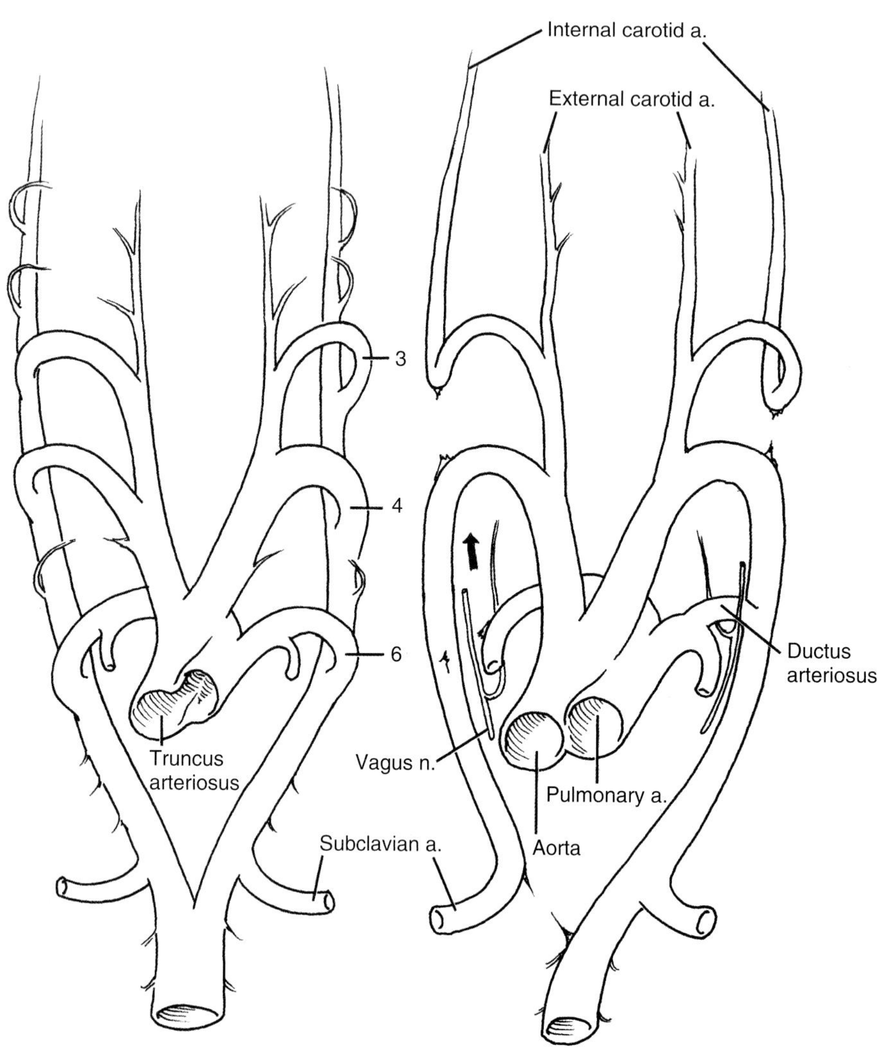

Fig. 7 Selective resorption of the remaining arches results in a definitive aortic and pulmonary pattern.

The Dorsal Aorta

While the arches are reforming at the cephalad end of the embryo, the dorsal aorta is elaborating dorsal, lateral, and ventral branches (Fig. 8). These consist of serial intersegmental branches to the body wall and extremities, genitourinary branches in the nephrotome region, and ventral visceral branches.

The dorsal branches divide into dorsal and ventral rami. The dorsal rami in the cervical region

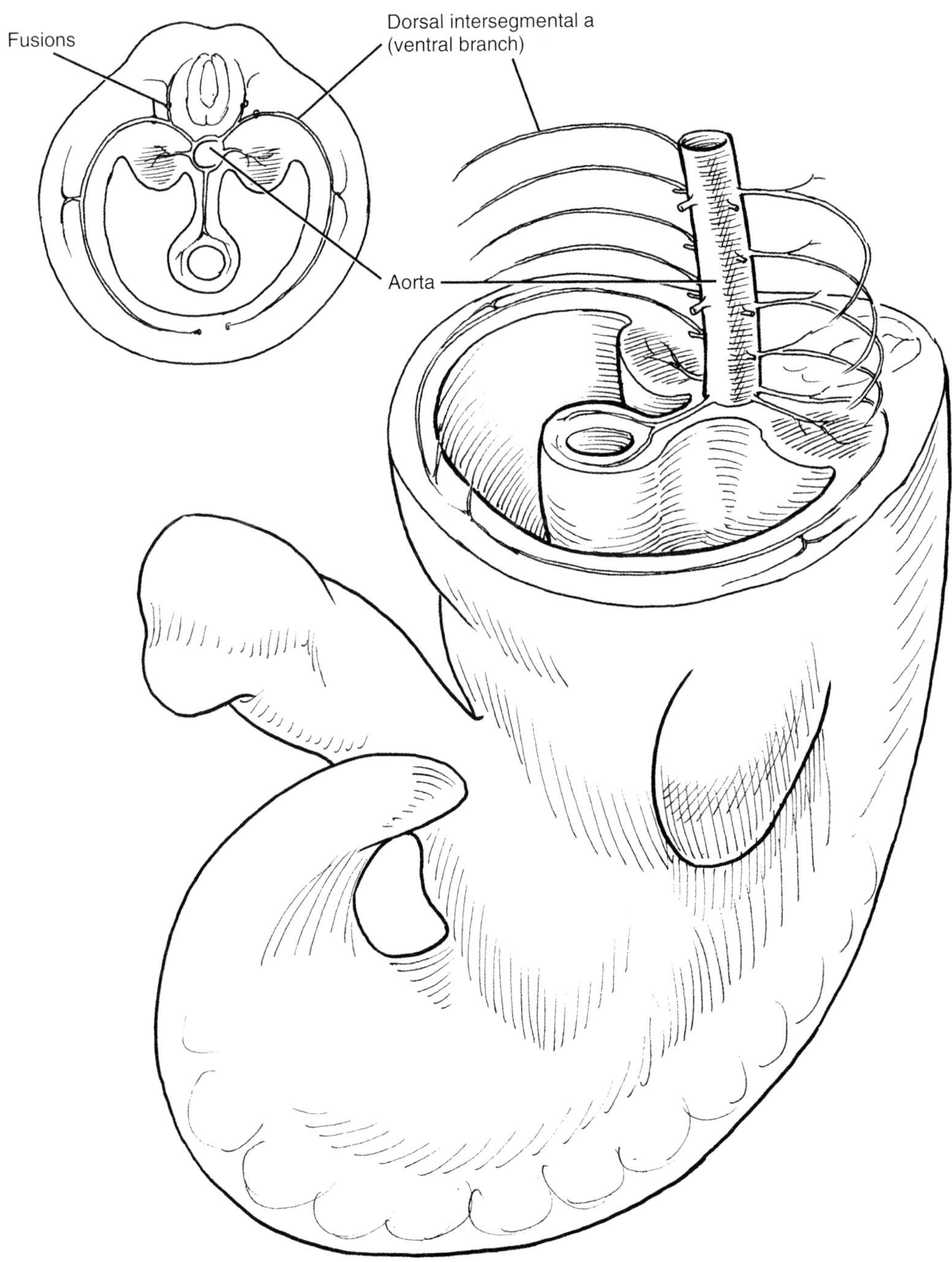

Fig. 8 The fused dorsal aorta elaborates segmental dorsal and lateral branches and retains single ventral visceral branches descended from the vitelline arteries.

form longitudinal fusions that persist when all but the most caudal segmental dorsal ramus resorb, leaving the vertebral arteries (Fig. 9). The vertebral artery and subclavian artery have a common origin from the seventh cervical intersegmental artery. The ventral rami constitute the intercostal and lumbar arteries. Two longitudinal precostal fusions similar to the dorsal branch fusions form the thyrocervical trunks cephalad to the subclavian arteries and the costocervical trunks caudal to the subclavian arteries. The axial vessels of the limb buds are also derived from dorsal intersegmental branches.

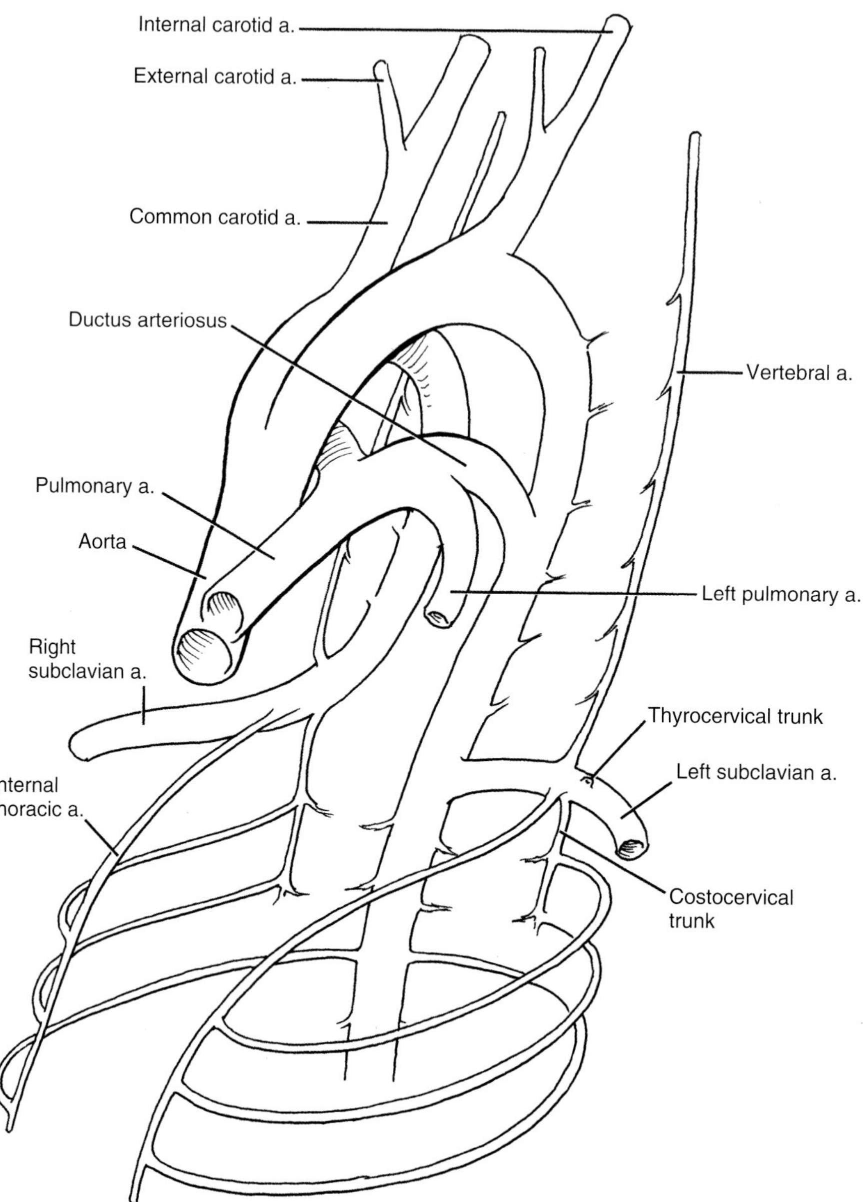

Fig. 9 Longitudinal fusion of the cervical and upper thoracic dorsal branches results in the vertebral arteries and costocervical trunks.

Multiple lateral branches extend to the nephrotome region supplying the mesonephros, gonads, metanephros, and adrenal glands (Fig. 10). As the mesonephros involutes, the number of branches also decreases, leaving the renal, adrenal, and internal gonadal vessels. The phrenic arteries are also definitive lateral branches.

The ventral branches of the aorta are derivatives of the paired vitelline arteries that become single when the aortas fuse. As the yolk sac regresses, the number of vessels decreases. Near the end of the fifth week, when the embryo is 8 mm in length, the celiac, superior mesenteric, and inferior mesenteric arteries are left. In addition, the original continuity of the umbilical arteries with the vitelline system is lost, and the umbilical arteries connect to an adjacent dorsal intersegmental branch that becomes the common iliac artery (see below and Fig. 14).

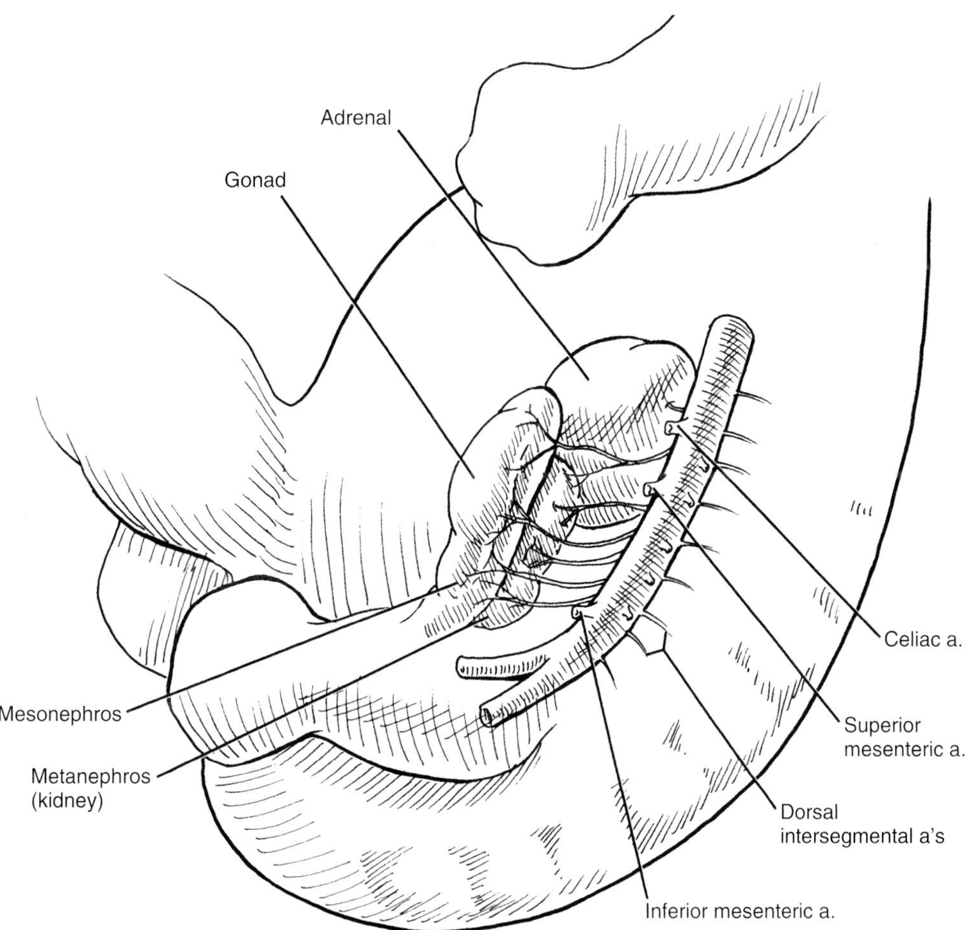

Fig. 10 Lateral branches in the nephrotome region supply the gonadal ridge, the mesonephros, and metanephros (definitive kidney).

The Extremities

The limb buds arise in the 3- to 4-mm embryo, with the upper extremities developing more precociously (Fig. 11). The base of the buds spans several segments, and the diffuse initial capillary plexus of the bud is fed by several dorsal intersegmental arteries (Fig. 12). One stem assumes a dominant position, and the others regress. The veins also form a dominant channel, which takes the form of a marginal vessel lying under the apical growth ridge of the primitive limb paddle.

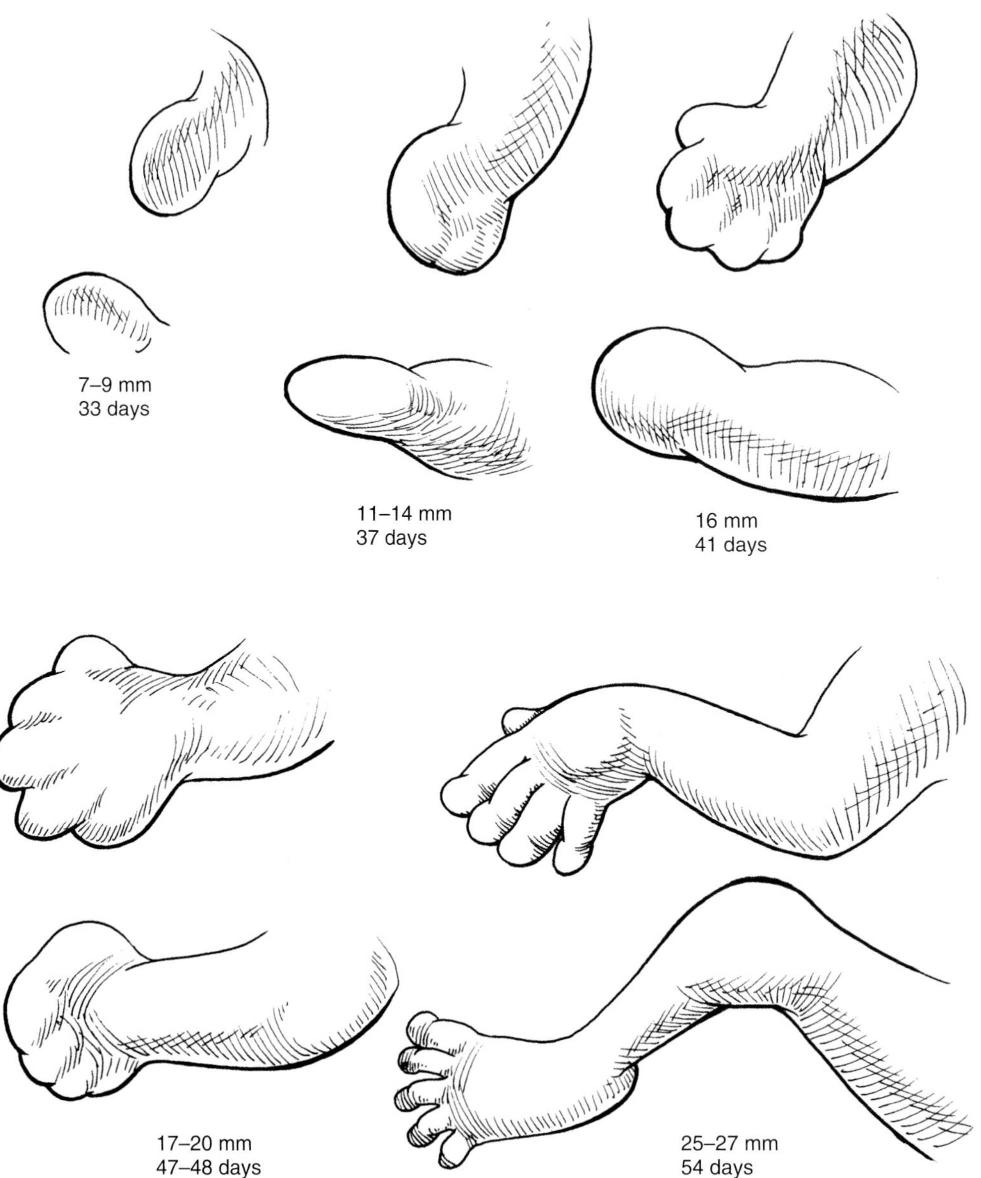

Fig. 11 The upper extremity leads the lower extremity in developmental maturity.

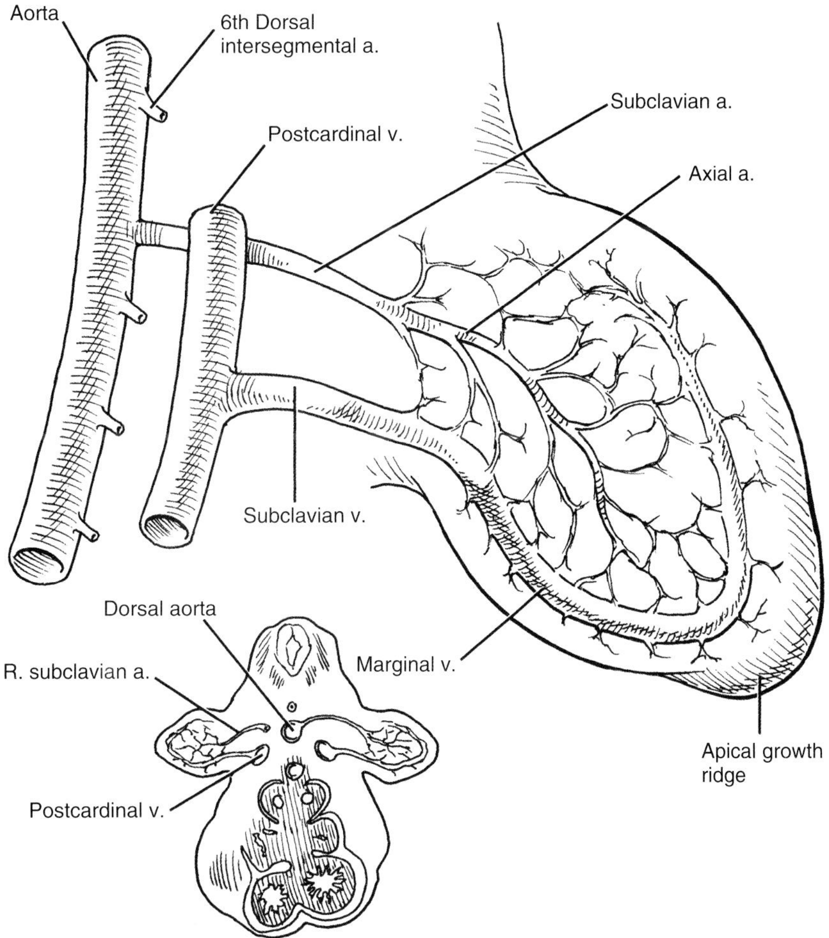

Fig. 12 The primitive axial arteries of the limbs are connected by a fine vascular mesh to a substantial marginal vein that drains initially into the postcardinal veins.

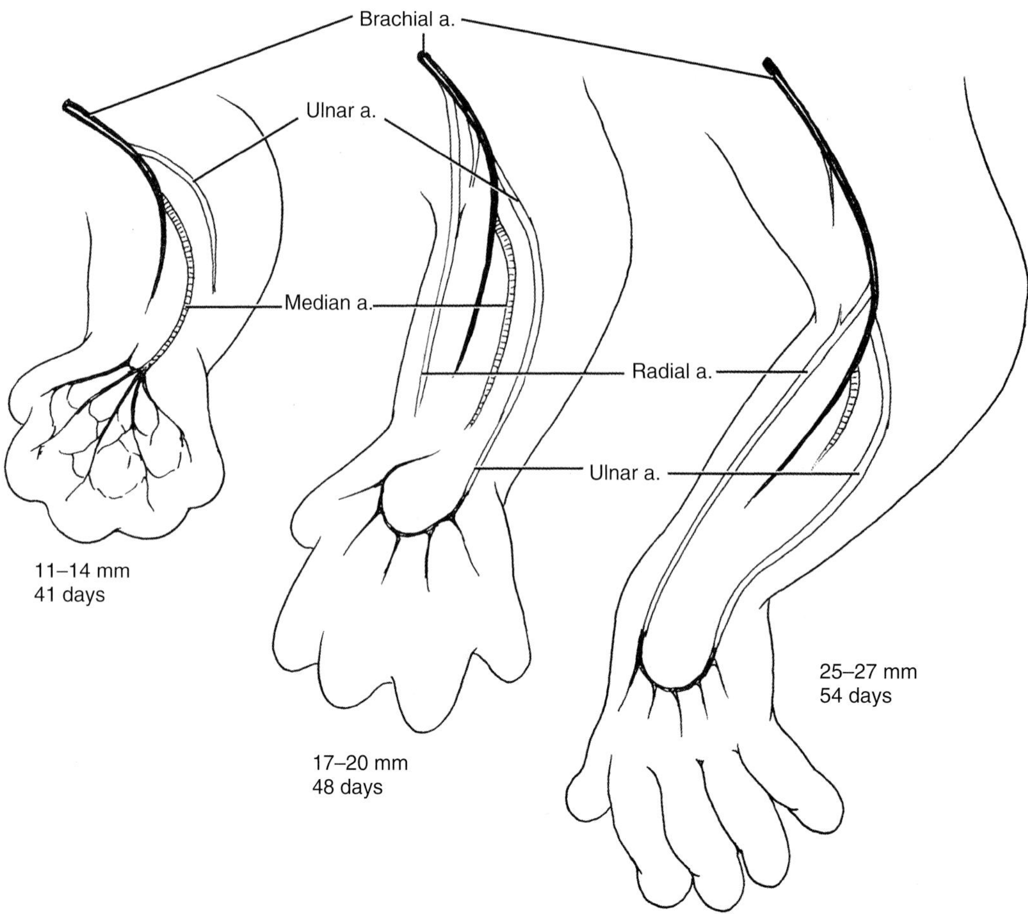

Fig. 13 Radial and ulnar arteries branch from the axial vessel and replace an intermediary median artery to supply the forearm and vascular arcade of the hand.

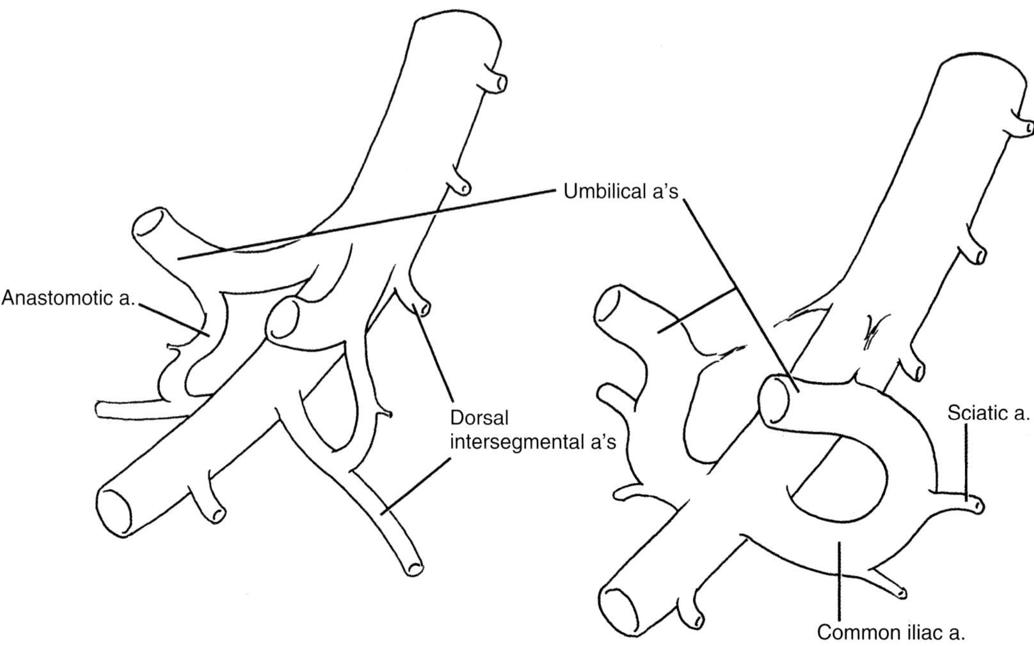

Fig. 14 The umbilical arteries shift their bases to dorsal intersegmental roots in the fourth week.

The subclavian artery, which arose in concert with the changes in the aortic arches, forms the axial artery of the upper extremity in the 5-mm, 4-week embryo. This original axis persists as the brachial and interosseous arteries of the arm and forearm (Fig. 13). The brachial artery gives rise to three branches to the vessels of the hand: the median, ulnar, and radial arteries. The median artery regresses, leaving the other two. Because of the relatively caudal initial position of the upper extremity buds, the venous arch first drains into the postcardinal vein. The cranial margin of the venous arch regresses, and the caudal margin remains as the basilic, axillary, and subclavian veins. By this stage, differential growth has shifted the drainage of the subclavian into the precardinal region.

In the fourth week, the umbilical arteries anastomose with adjacent dorsal intersegmental aortic branches (Fig. 14). This secondary connection quickly becomes dominant, and the original aortic connection is lost. The new dorsal roots of the umbilical arteries are destined to become the common and internal iliac arteries. These root vessels give rise to the primitive axial vessels of the lower extremities, sciatic arteries, and external iliac arteries.

The sciatic arteries arise from the new dorsal roots of the umbilical arteries in the 9-mm, 5-week embryo. The external iliac arteries arise from the same vessel segment as the sciatic, and the two vessels interconnect, selectively resorb, and branch to form the definitive arteries of the lower extremities (Fig. 15). The anterior and posterior tibial vessels are derived from the popliteal remnant of the sciatic artery and from the femoral artery, respectively.

The marginal vein in the lower extremity forms later than in the upper extremity, commensurate with the caudal developmental lag. As in the upper extremity, the cephalad or tibial connection of the marginal vein regresses, leaving the fibular branch. The latter interconnects with the great saphenous vein, which arises independently of the postcardinal vein. The two vessels give rise to the definitive venous drainage of the leg.

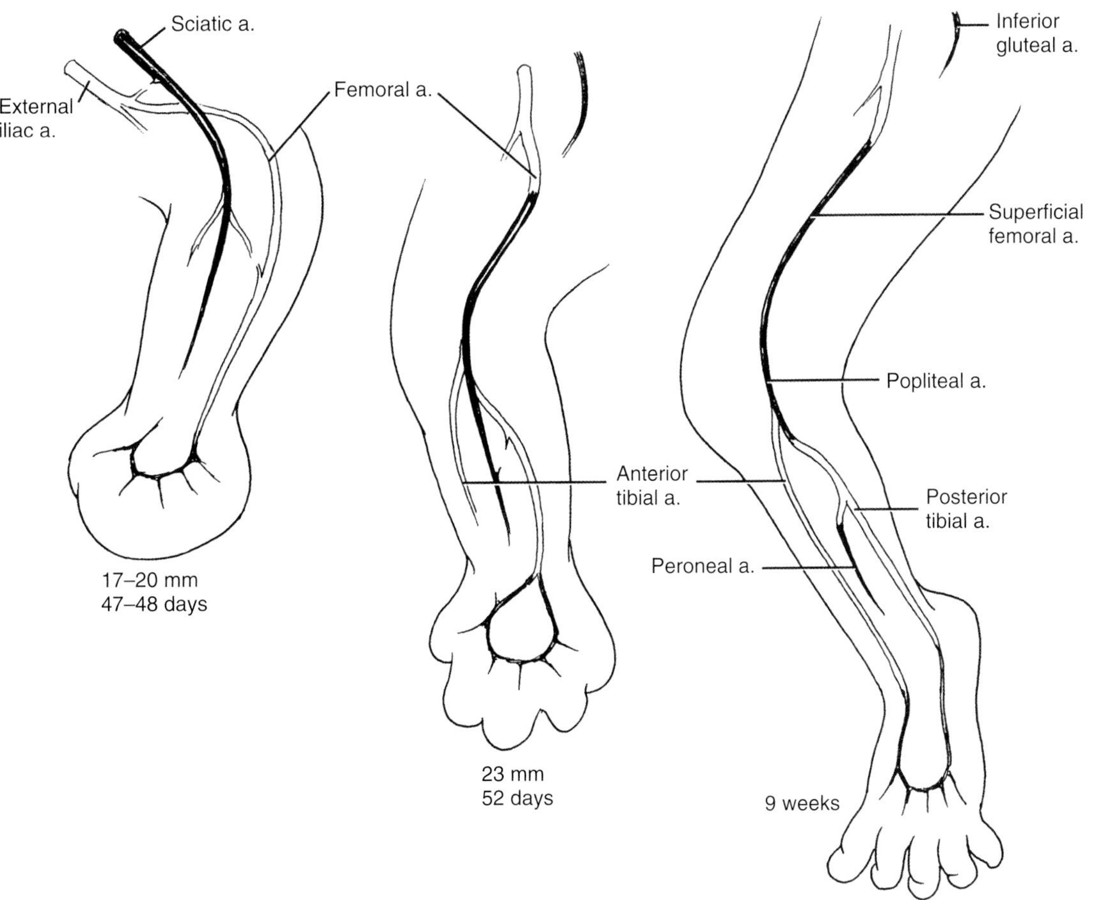

Fig. 15 The axial sciatic artery of the leg and the external iliac trunk interact to form the mature vascular pattern of the lower extremity.

The establishment of the final vascular pattern of the lower extremity lags behind that of the upper extremity, being completed in the third month, whereas the upper extremity has a mature pattern by the end of the eighth week. The middle sacral artery is the remnant of the dorsal aorta distal to the iliac arteries.

The Veins

In the third week, when the embryo is 3 mm long and the neural tube begins to close, three sets of paired veins become established (Fig. 16). The earliest are the vitelline veins from the yolk sac, then the umbilical veins from the chorion, followed by the cardinal veins draining the body proper. Venous developmental changes are more complex than arterial, involving additions, deletions, interconnection, position, and flow changes.

The vitelline veins pass from the yolk sac through the septum transversarum to enter the sinus venosus alongside the foregut. In their course through the septum transversarum, they interweave with the ingrowth of liver buds and become hepatic sinusoids (Fig. 17). Part of the sinusoidal system contributes to the ductus venosus (see below), and the suprahepatic branches on the right become the hepatic veins. The infrahepatic vitelline veins are paired by 4 weeks (5 mm) and lie on each side of the duodenum. Through cross-anastomosis and partial resorption of the vitelline veins, the portal vein is formed with a serpentine route around the duodenum. The superior mesenteric vein is a replacement of the vitelline veins connecting to the portal vein. Cephalad to the liver, the left vitelline vein and the left horn of the sinus venosus disappear.

The umbilical veins initially pass from the body stalk through the lateral body walls on each

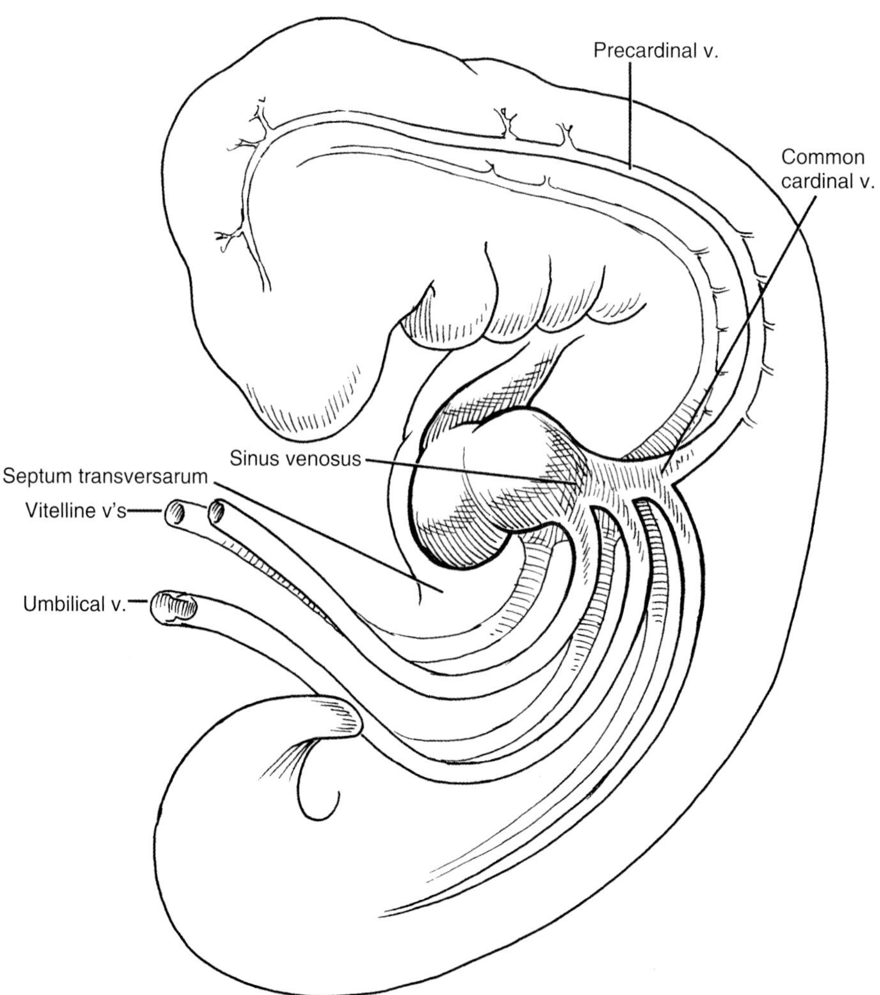

Fig. 16 Three pairs of veins give rise to the definitive venous pattern of the body.

side of the liver mass to reach the sinus venosus. As the liver expands, vascular connections between the umbilical veins and the hepatic sinusoids are established. Flow is progressively channeled through more direct pathways to the heart until the ductus venosus is established. By 4½ weeks, all the umbilical vein blood in the 6-mm embryo flows through the liver. The entire right umbilical vein and the proximal extrahepatic portion of the left umbilical vein regress, leaving only the left umbilical vein. The remaining vein shifts toward the midline and lies in the free edge of the falciform ligament.

The paired pre and postcardinal veins established in the 5-mm embryo at 4 weeks of age undergo a series of changes leading to the mature venous drainage pattern of the body. The precardinal veins mature into the veins of the superior vena caval drainage basin, and the postcardinal veins, supplemented by two sets of parallel channels, become the inferior vena caval system of the lower body.

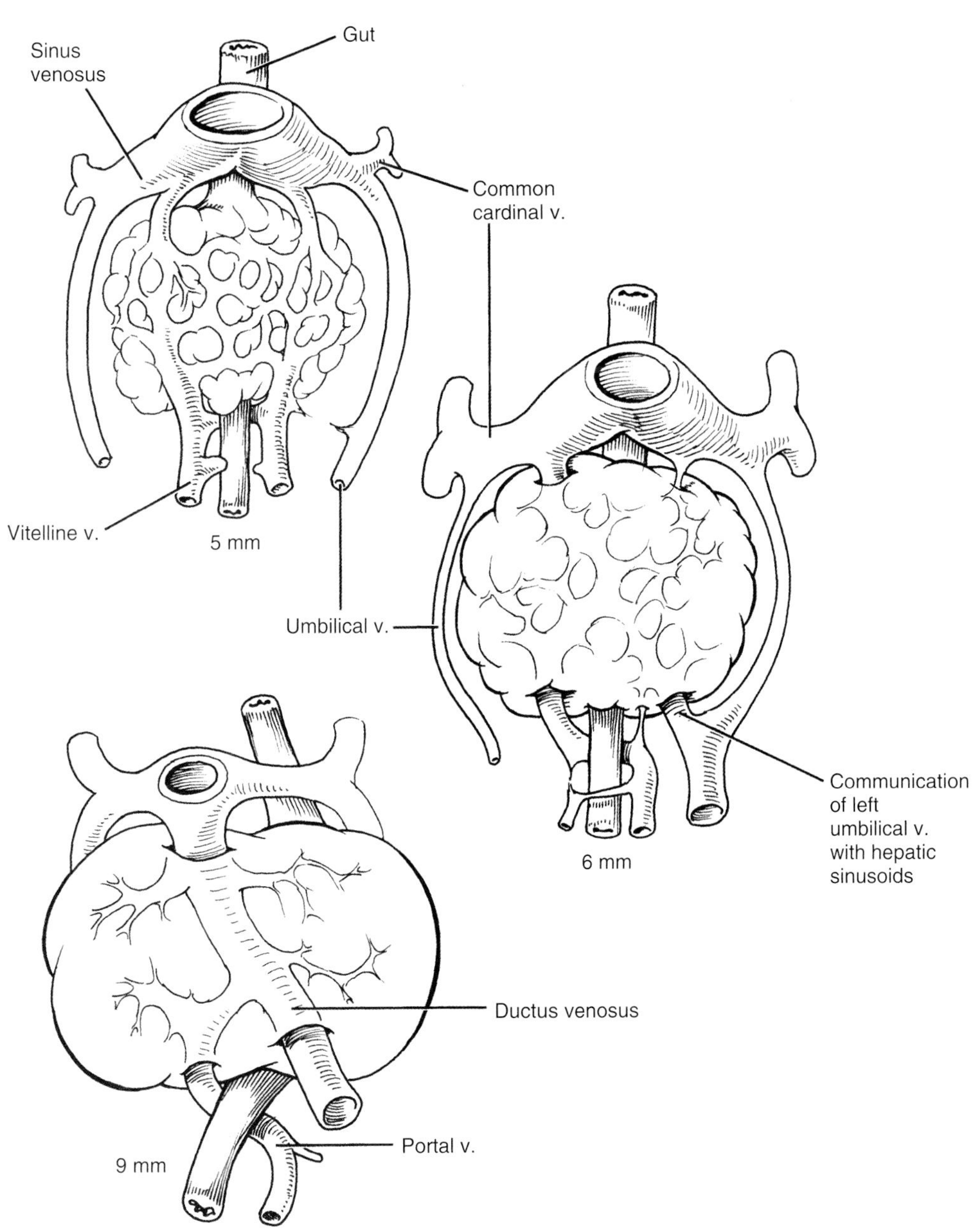

Fig. 17 The vitelline veins interdigitate with the developing liver buds to become hepatic sinusoids. The left umbilical vein connects secondarily to the intrahepatic plexus, and the major ductus venosus channel is established.

During the eighth week, an oblique venous channel connects the precardinal veins lying ventrolateral to the brain (Fig. 18). The root of the left precardinal regresses, leaving the root of the right as the superior vena cava and the cross-connection as the left brachiocephalic vein. The cephalad portions of the precardinal veins become the internal jugular veins. External jugular and subclavian veins develop independently and attach to the precardinal veins. The segment of right precardinal vein between the right subclavian and left brachiocephalic vein becomes the right brachiocephalic vein.

The evolution of the caudal venous system is not quite as straightforward. During the second month of embryonic life, the postcardinal veins are supplemented by the subcardinal and supracardinal veins, successively. As the sets of veins partially regress in the order that they appeared, multiple interconnections lead to the mature vascular pattern.

The postcardinal veins lie dorsal to the mesonephroi, which they drain along with the legs and body wall (Fig. 19). The distal ends of the postcardinals interconnect early, before the postcardinal trunks regress along with the mesonephroi. This distal connection at the level of the leg vein entry will become the left common iliac vein (Fig. 20). The root of the azygous vein is the only other remnant of the postcardinal veins.

The subcardinal veins arise after the postcardinal veins, but while the latter are still in place, and lie ventromedial to the mesonephroi. Interconnections through the mesonephroi occur between the subcardinal and postcardinal veins. A central subcardinal anastomosis arises that is destined to become the stem of the left renal vein. The subcardinal veins quickly lose their cephalad connection with the postcardinals, and the right subcardinal connects with a caudal extension of the hepatic veins, forming the future subhepatic, suprarenal portion of the inferior vena cava. The adrenal

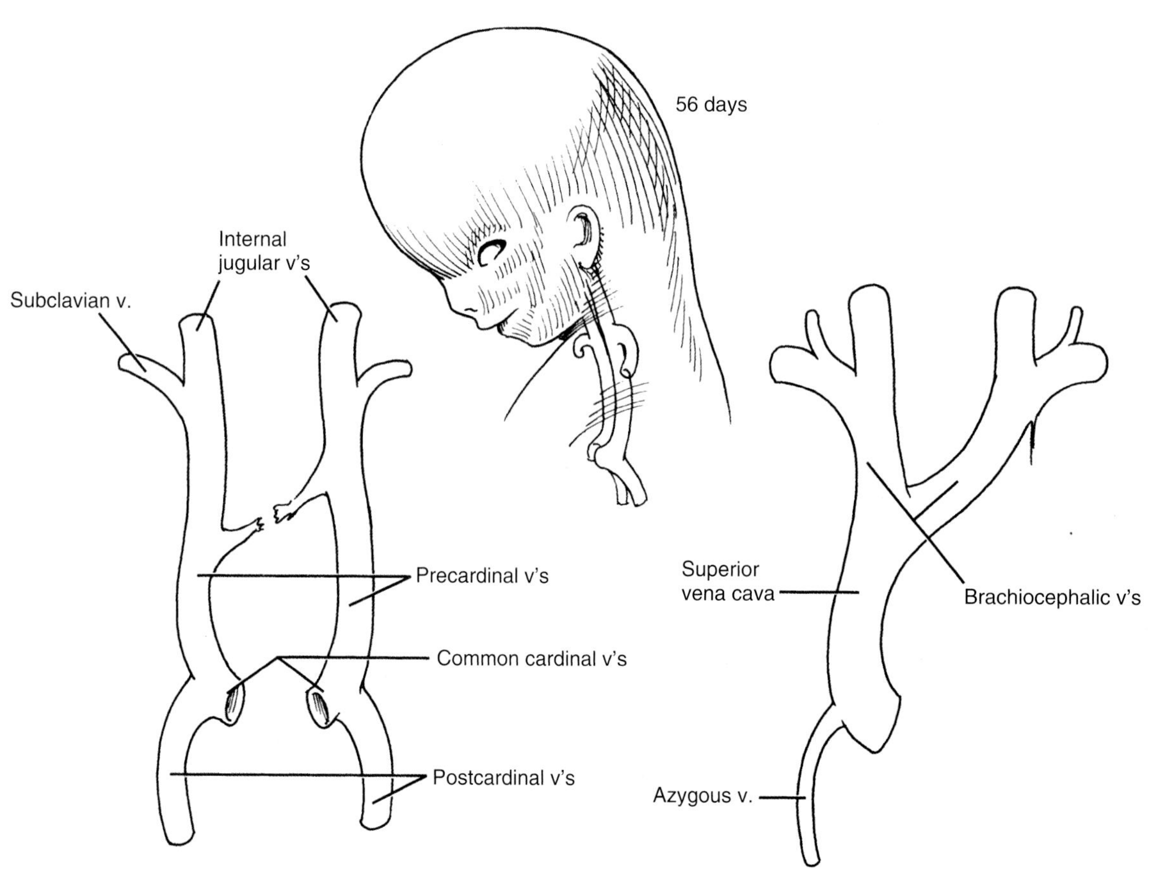

Fig. 18 A diagonal branch connects the precardinal veins in the eighth week, forming the left brachiocephalic vein.

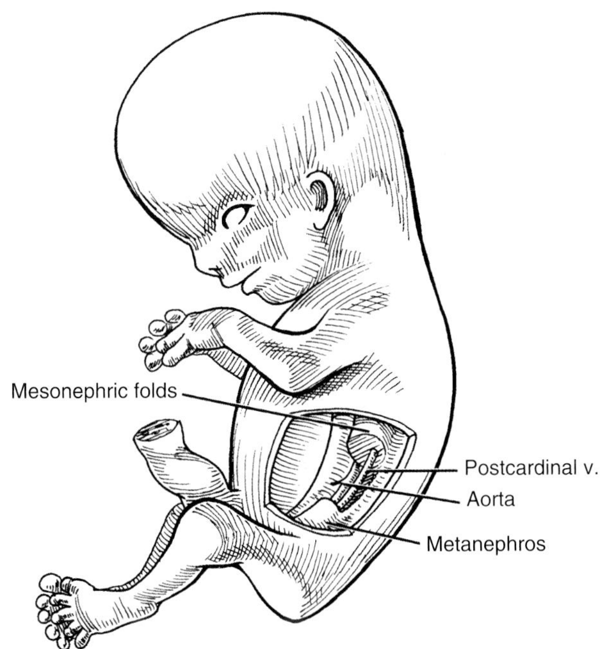

Fig. 19 The postcardinal veins lie in the dorsal substance of the mesonephric ridges, shown here in a 4-week embryo.

and gonadal veins are remnants of the subcardinal veins.

The supracardinal veins appear last and lie dorsomedial to the postcardinal veins. As the kidneys develop and assume their final position, the supracardinal veins anastomose with the subcardinal veins at the level of the developing renal veins, forming a portion of the left renal vein. The connection on the right becomes the continuation of the inferior vena cava below the renal veins, leading into the persistent caudal portion of the right supracardinal vein. The latter connects to the persistent early cross-connection of the postcardinal veins that will constitute the iliac confluence. The disconnected cephalad portions of the supracardinal veins cross-connect, forming the azygous and hemiazygous veins. The intercostal and lumbar veins that initially drain into the postcardinal veins ultimately drain into the derivatives of the supracardinal veins. Thus, the cephalad body wall branches drain into the azygous system, and the lower lumbar veins drain into the distal inferior vena cava.

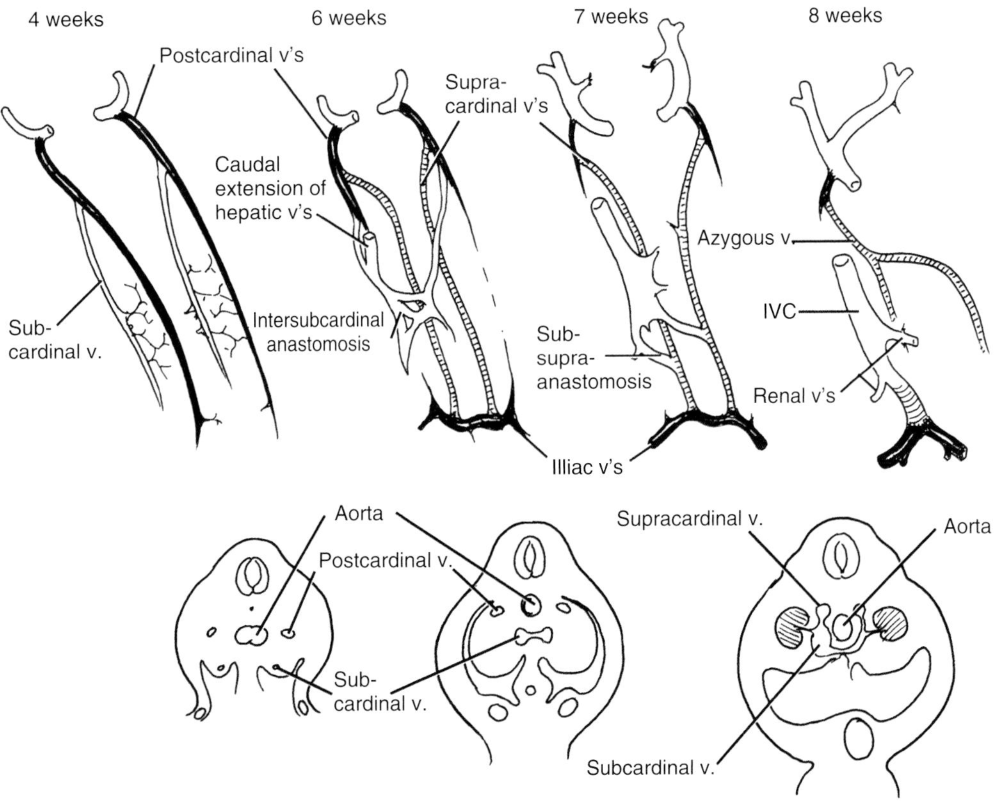

Fig. 20 Complex interactions between the postcardinal veins and their subcardinal and supracardinal derivatives result in the definitive venous drainage of the lower part of the body.

Fetal Circulation and Birth

During the remaining 7 months of gestation, the fetal period, oxygen-rich blood from the umbilical vein passes through the liver, mostly via the ductus venosus (Fig. 21). It is mixed in the heart with desaturated, waste-laden blood from the fetal body. Flow dynamics and preferential shunting through the foramen ovale and ductus arteriosus favor oxygen delivery to the cephalad end of the body. Contaminated blood returns to the placenta from the descending aorta via the common iliac to internal iliac to umbilical artery route.

At birth, the pulmonary vascular circuit suddenly fills, returning larger volumes of blood to the left atrium at the same time as the umbilical circulation ceases. The result is a reversal in right and left atrial pressures, closing the foramen ovale and ending the interatrial shunt. The ductus arteriosus is closed by muscular contraction and ultimately fibroses along with the ductus venosus and umbilical vessels.

The vestiges of the specialized fetal circulatory channels are the ligamentum arteriosum, ligamentum venosum, and round ligament of the liver in the chest and upper abdomen and the medial umbilical ligaments on the inner surface of the lower abdominal wall.

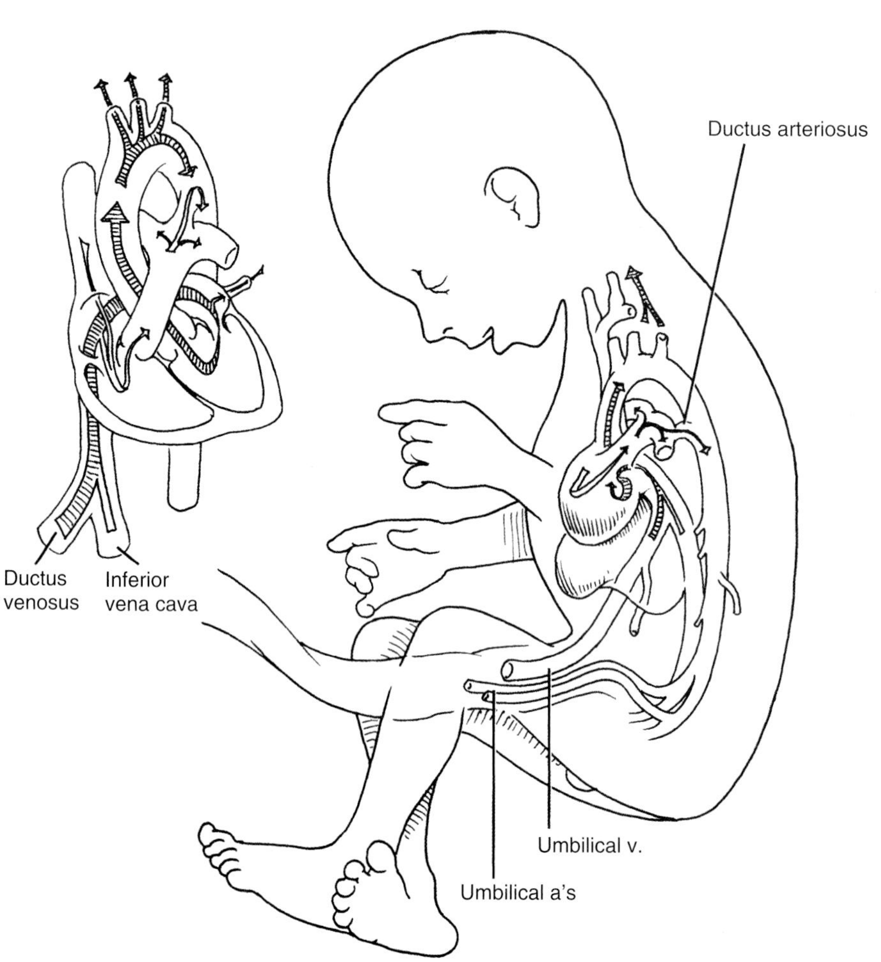

Fig. 21 The fetal circulation is dominated by preferential flow of oxygenated umbilical blood across the foramen ovale and to the head and body via the aorta. Caval and pulmonary admixture occurs directly in the inferior vena cava and atria and secondarily via the ductus arteriosus.

Bibliography

1. O'Rahilly R, Muller F. *Developmental Stages in Human Embryos.* Washington, DC: Carnegie Institution of Washington, DC;1987. Publication 637.
2. Arey LB. *Developmental Anatomy.* Philadelphia, PA: WB Saunders; 1963.
3. Gray SW, Skandalakis JE. *Embryology for Surgeons.* Philadelphia, PA: WB Saunders; 1991.
4. Moore KL. *The Developing Human.* Philadelphia, PA: WB Saunders; 2008.
5. Sadler TW. *Langman's Medical Embryology.* Baltimore, MD: Lippincott Williams & Wilkins; 2009.
6. Stewart JS, Kincaid OW, Edwards JE. *An Atlas of Vascular Rings and Related Malformations of the Aortic Arch System.* Springfield, IL: Charles C Thomas; 1964.
7. Senior HD. Development of the arteries of the human lower extremity. *Am J Anat.* 1919;25:55–95.
8. Seyfer AE, Wind G, Martin R. Study of upper extremity growth and development using human embryos and computer reconstructed models. *J Hand Surg.* 1989;14A:927–932.

EXTRACRANIAL CIRCULATION OF THE HEAD AND NECK

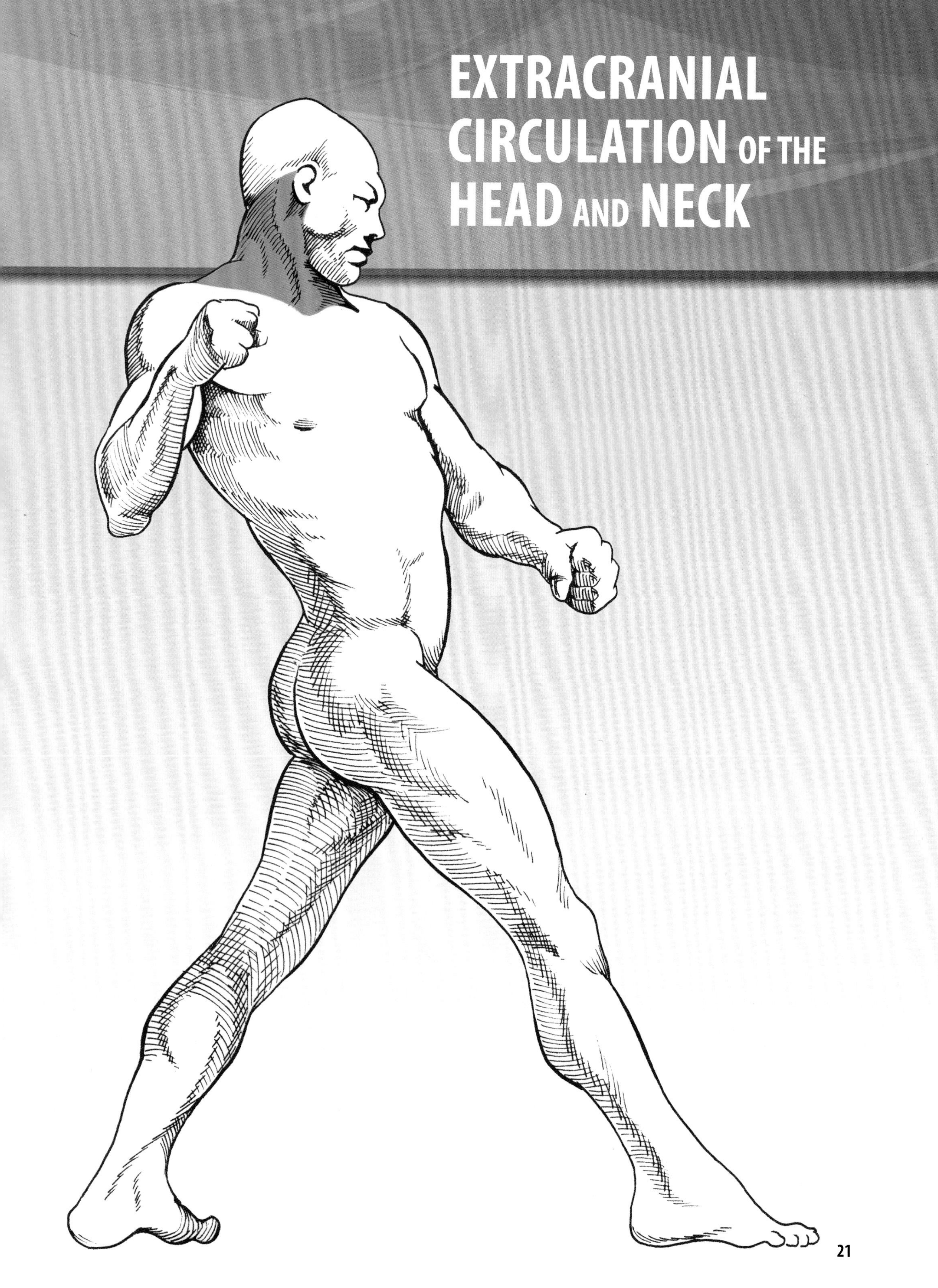

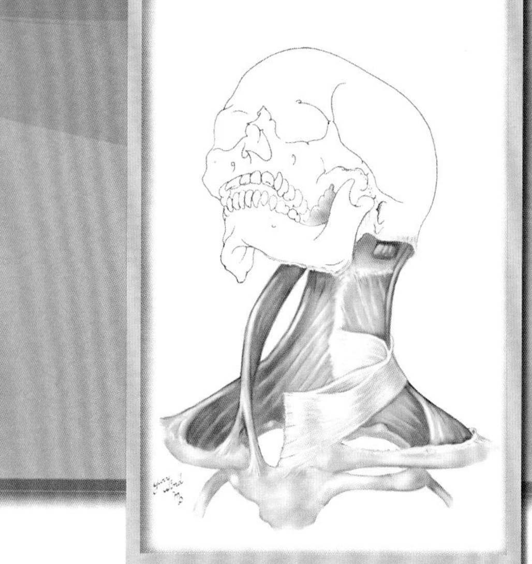

Carotid Arteries

1

Surgical Anatomy of the Neck

In the neck, nature has ingeniously compacted an intricate complex of vital structures and enfolded them on three sides with muscle and bone. It is possible to master this daunting array of anatomy if one conceptualizes the neck in a systematic way. There is a central visceral column containing the digestive and respiratory passages and the thyroid gland (Fig. 1-1). Posteriorly, the visceral compartment is bounded by the main structural element of the neck, the cervical spine, and its supporting struts of muscle. On either side of the visceral cylinder, the large, axial neurovascular structures of the neck pass between the head and the superior thoracic aperture enclosed in the loose, areolar carotid sheath. Wrapped around these central neck elements, like the spiral sheath of an electrical cable, are the strong, flat trapezius and sternocleidomastoid muscles. In the context of these structural groupings, it is now possible to make some sense of the fascial layers of the neck.

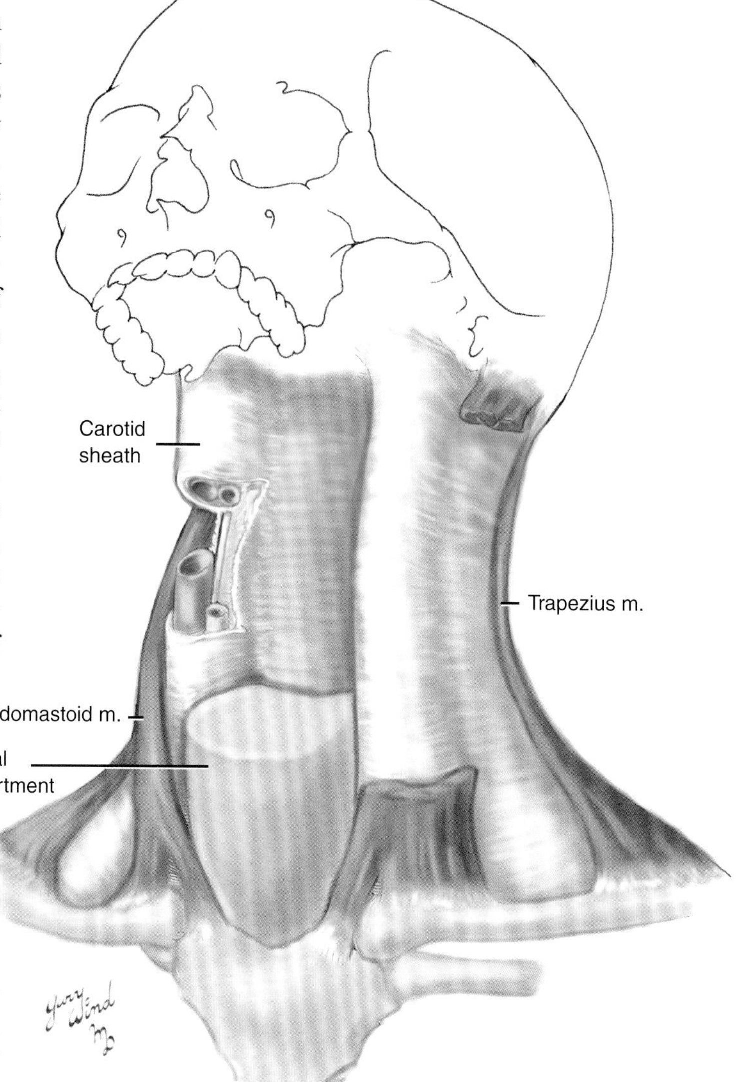

Fig. 1-1 The three major components of the neck consist of a structural column of muscle and bone, a central visceral column, and paired fascicles containing major neurovascular structures.

The Prevertebral Fascia

The supple cervical spine is surrounded by a central group of muscles attached to the ribs, to the base of the skull, and to adjacent vertebrae (Fig. 1-2). These include small intrinsic muscles and powerful erector spinae muscles posteriorly, the small longus colli and longus capitis muscles anteriorly, and the levator scapulae and scalene muscles laterally. This paraspinal grouping is wrapped in a discrete fibrous layer called the prevertebral fascia. Anteriorly, this fascia runs from the base of the skull down the vertebral bodies to blend with the anterior longitudinal ligament of the thoracic spine. Posteriorly, it attaches along a midline seam to the ligamentum nuchae of the cervical spinous processes. The prevertebral fascia covers the origins of the cervical nerves and the phrenic nerve arising from them. At the base of the neck, the prevertebral fascia takes a more complex form. Fanning out laterally, it covers the roots of the brachial plexus and the subclavian artery and forms a neurovascular wrap called the axillary sheath. The visceral components of the neck lie along the center of this delta-shaped anterior sheet of prevertebral fascia.

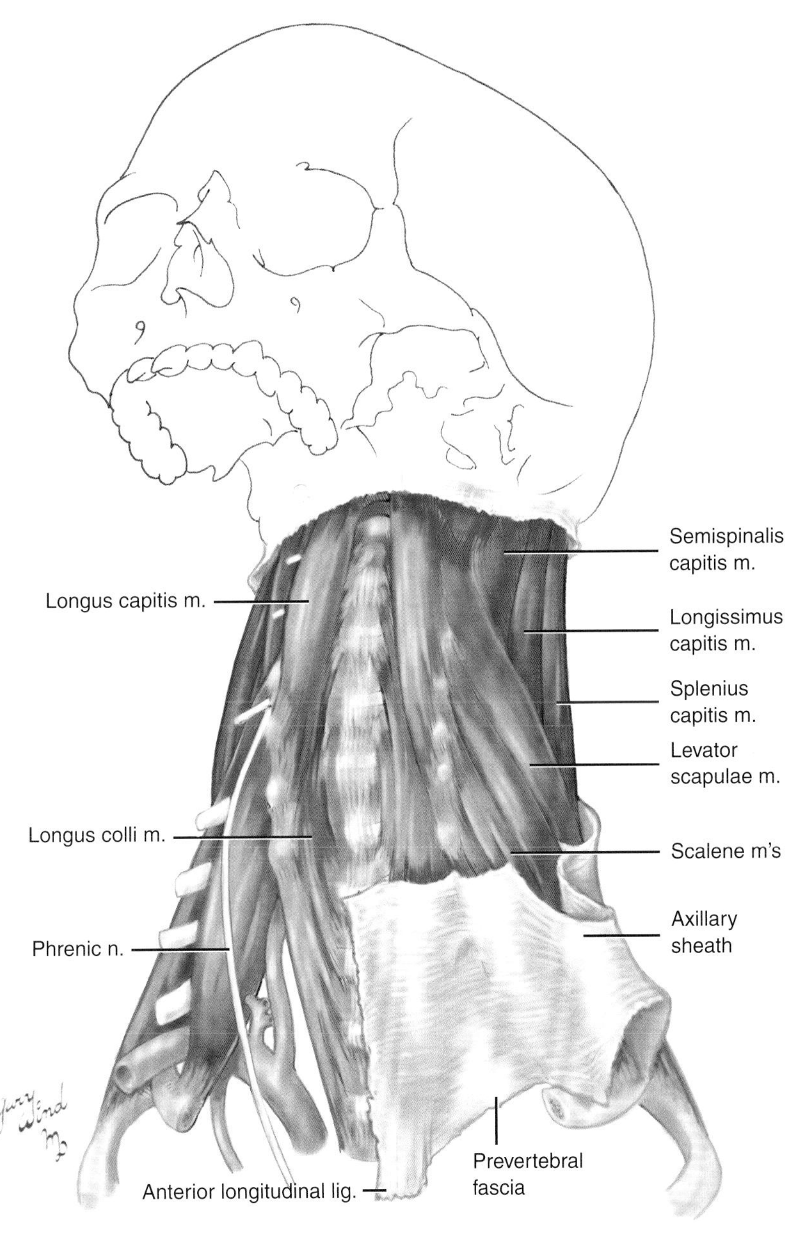

Fig. 1-2 The musculoskeletal pillar of the neck is wrapped in the prevertebral fascia that extends into the shoulder as the axillary sheath.

The Visceral Fascia

In the central neck, the roughly cylindrical visceral compartment is surrounded by a thin layer of fascia called pretracheal fascia in front and buccopharyngeal fascia behind (Fig. 1-3). The strap muscles are also enclosed within the lamellae of this layer. The portion of visceral fascia around the strap muscles has also been called the middle cervical fascia. The plane between the buccopharyngeal fascia and the prevertebral fascia is a highway for spread of air and GI contents between neck and mediastinum after esophageal injury. A variable midline adhesion between the two fascial layers may limit spread of abnormal contents to some extent.

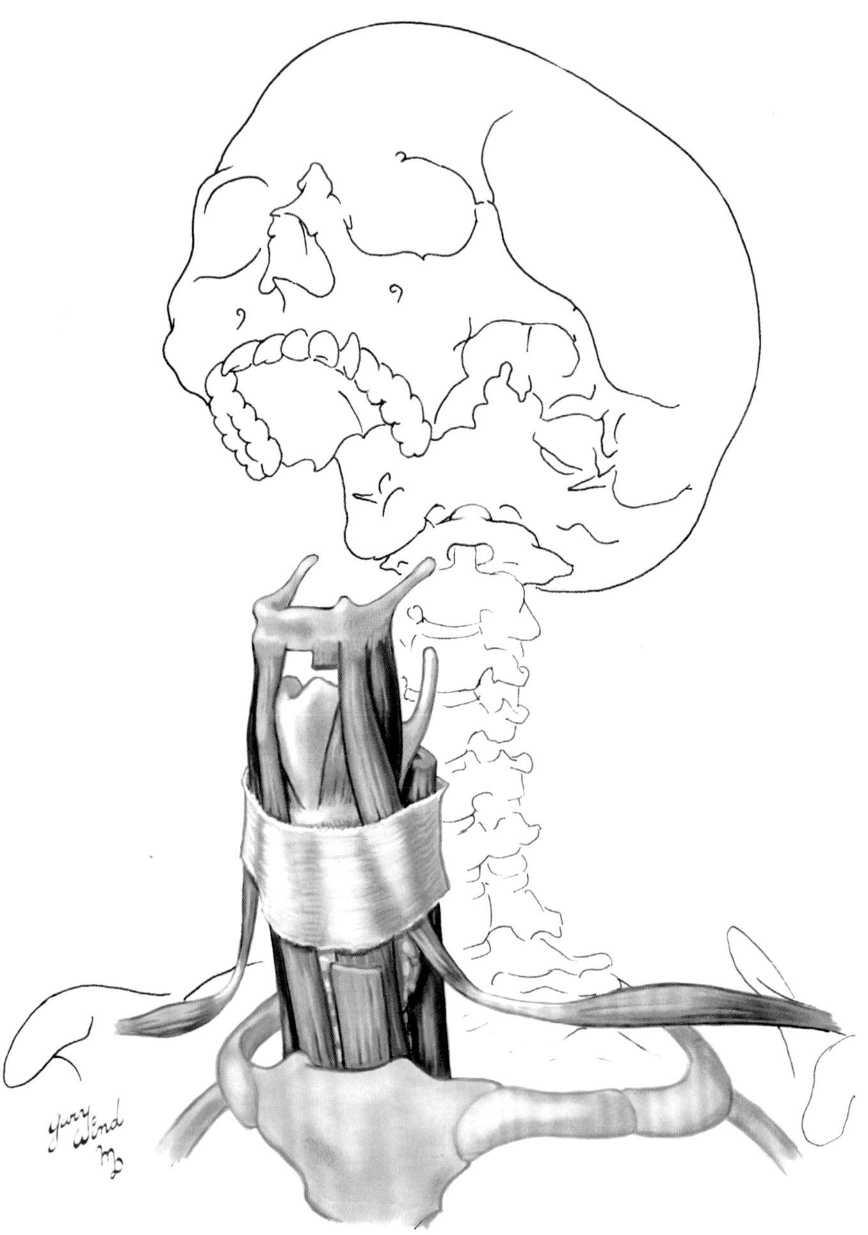

Fig. 1-3 The visceral compartment is surrounded by its own fascial layer. The portion immediately apposed to the trachea is called pretracheal fascia. The fascia around the strap muscles is sometimes called the middle layer of deep cervical fascia.

The Investing Fascia

Wrapping the neck into a neat bundle is the best defined and most superficial layer of the deep fascia, the investing fascia (Fig. 1-4). It attaches to the ligamentum nuchae in the posterior midline and splits to invest the trapezius and sternocleidomastoid muscles within its laminae. The investing fascia forms a complete sheath, with its upper margin skirting the posterior base of the skull, the zygomatic arch, and the lower border of the mandible. The lower margin attaches to sternum, clavicle, acromion, and the spine of the scapula. The parotid and submaxillary glands are also enclosed within layers of this fascia.

The flat sternocleidomastoid muscles form the final, lateral boundary of the space containing the carotid sheath.

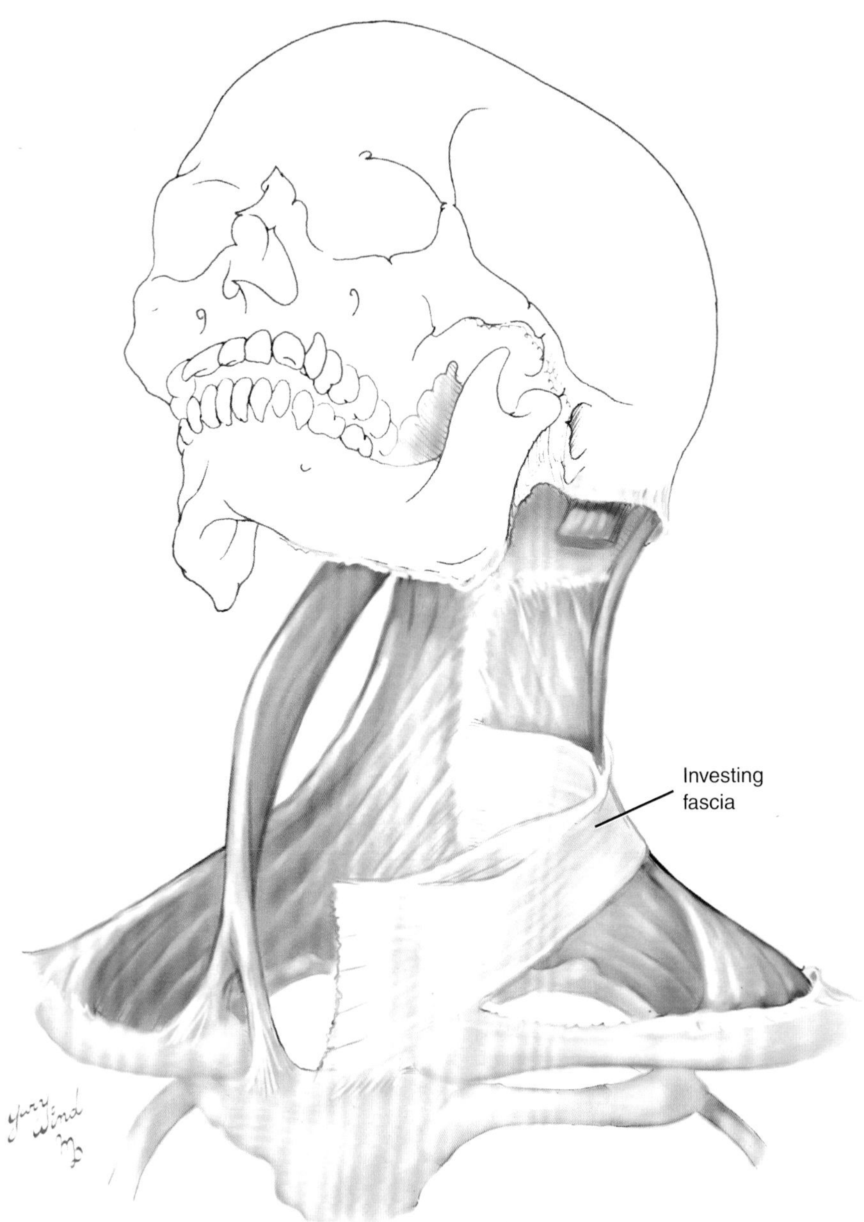

Fig. 1-4 The broad sternocleidomastoid and trapezius muscles are enclosed in the most superficial layer of the deep cervical fascia, which is also called the investing fascia.

The Carotid Sheath

The carotid sheath is best thought of as an aggregation of connective tissue filling a long cleft with a triangular cross section. The boundaries of this cleft consist of the visceral compartment medially, the prevertebral fascia posteriorly, and the sternocleidomastoid muscle anterolaterally (Fig. 1-5). The sheath is not a discrete fascial sheet like the investing fascia. It surrounds the carotid artery, the internal jugular vein, and the vagus nerve. Because of the amorphous nature of this "sheath," a path to any of the enclosed structures can be dissected with minimal disturbance to the adjacent structures.

Two additional neural structures are associated with the carotid sheath. The cervical sympathetic chain is superficially embedded in the most posterior fibers of the carotid sheath. The ansa cervicalis, providing motor innervation to the strap muscles, is slung within the anterior fibers of the sheath.

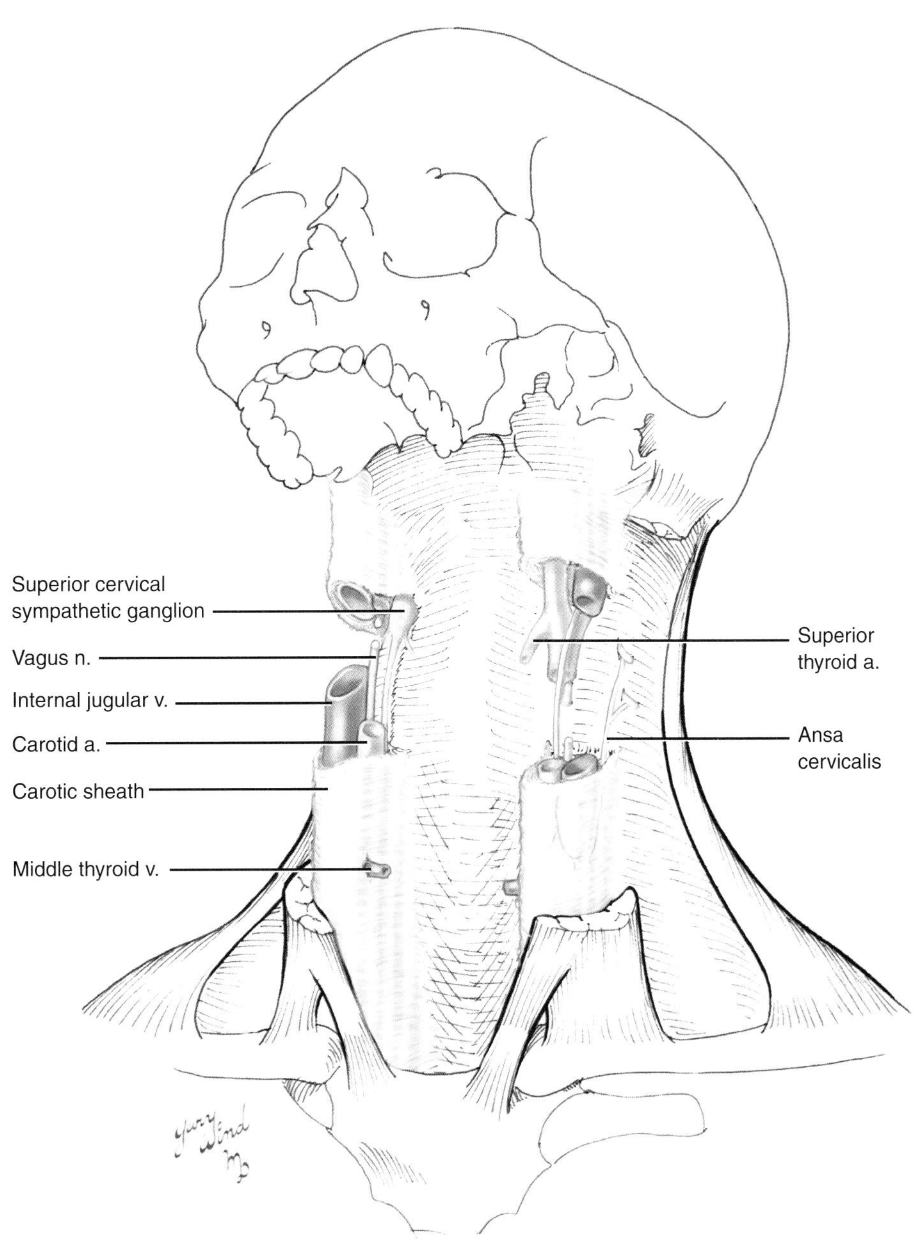

Fig. 1-5 The carotid sheath is a loose network of fascia containing the carotid arteries, the internal jugular veins, and the vagus nerves.

The Superficial Fascia

The superficial fascia of the neck contains two flat sheets of muscle, the platysma (Fig. 1-6). These muscles represent the remnant of the more extensive panniculus carnosus of other mammals with which they shake their coats. The muscles of facial expression are specialized modifications of this layer.

Cutaneous nerves and superficial veins lie in the well-defined cleavage plane between the platysma and the investing fascia. A cross section of the neck at the level of the thyroid cartilage (Fig. 1-7) demonstrates the relationships of these and the other fascia-bound anatomic groupings. With this background, the remainder of the chapter focuses on the carotid artery and its relationship to surrounding structures.

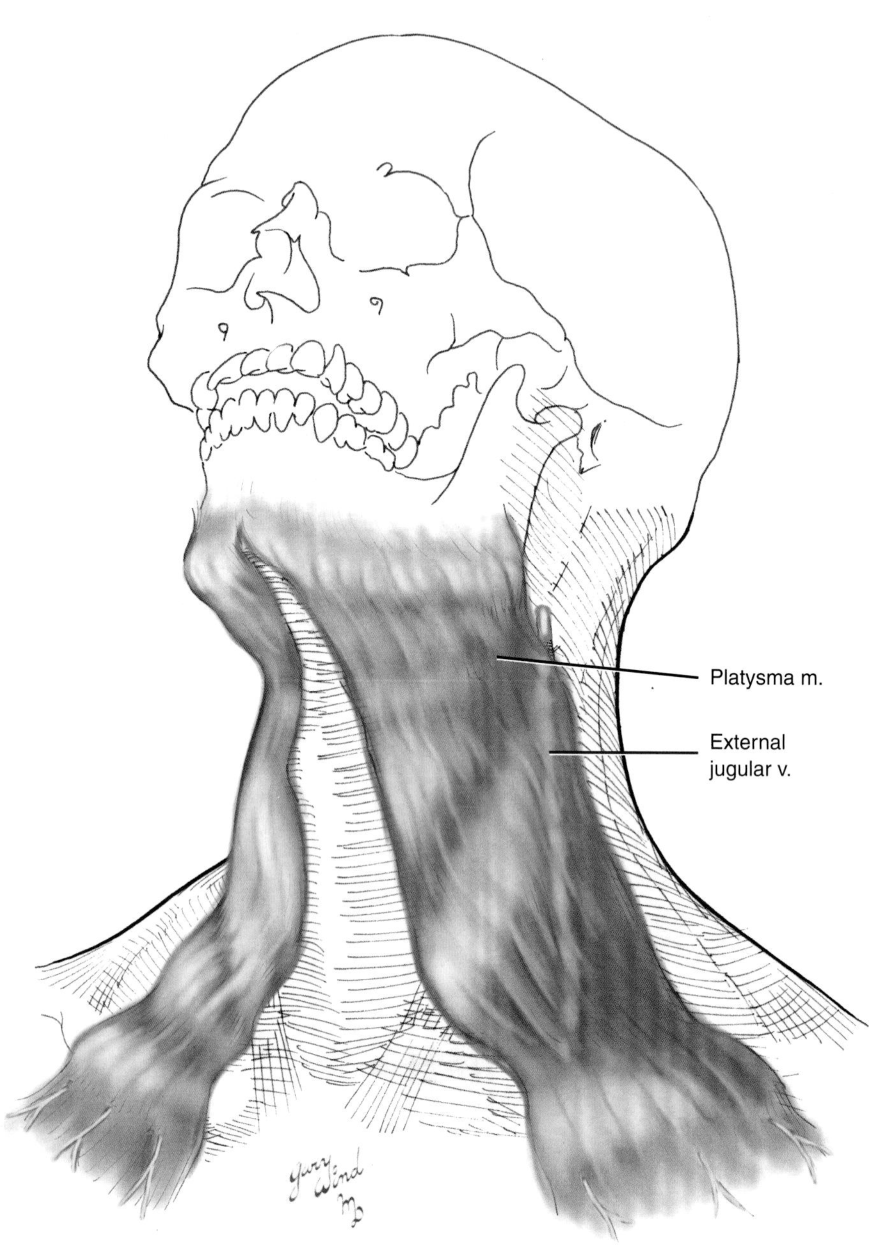

Fig. 1-6 The platysma muscle lies in the superficial fascial layer and lends substance to this plane for purposes of surgical dissection.

A normally positioned carotid bifurcation is readily accessible in the carotid triangle bounded by the sternocleidomastoid muscle, the posterior belly of the digastric muscle, and the anterior belly of the omohyoid muscle. The area between the carotid bifurcation and the base of the skull is a dense intertwining tangle of vessels, nerves, and muscles packed into a confined space behind the mandibular ramus. This is especially true of the anatomy surrounding the distal internal carotid artery. In order to ensure a safe surgical approach to this artery, a thorough grasp of its relationships is essential. The overall pattern of individual vessels and nerves in the neck will be considered first, followed by an in-depth look at the carotid triangle.

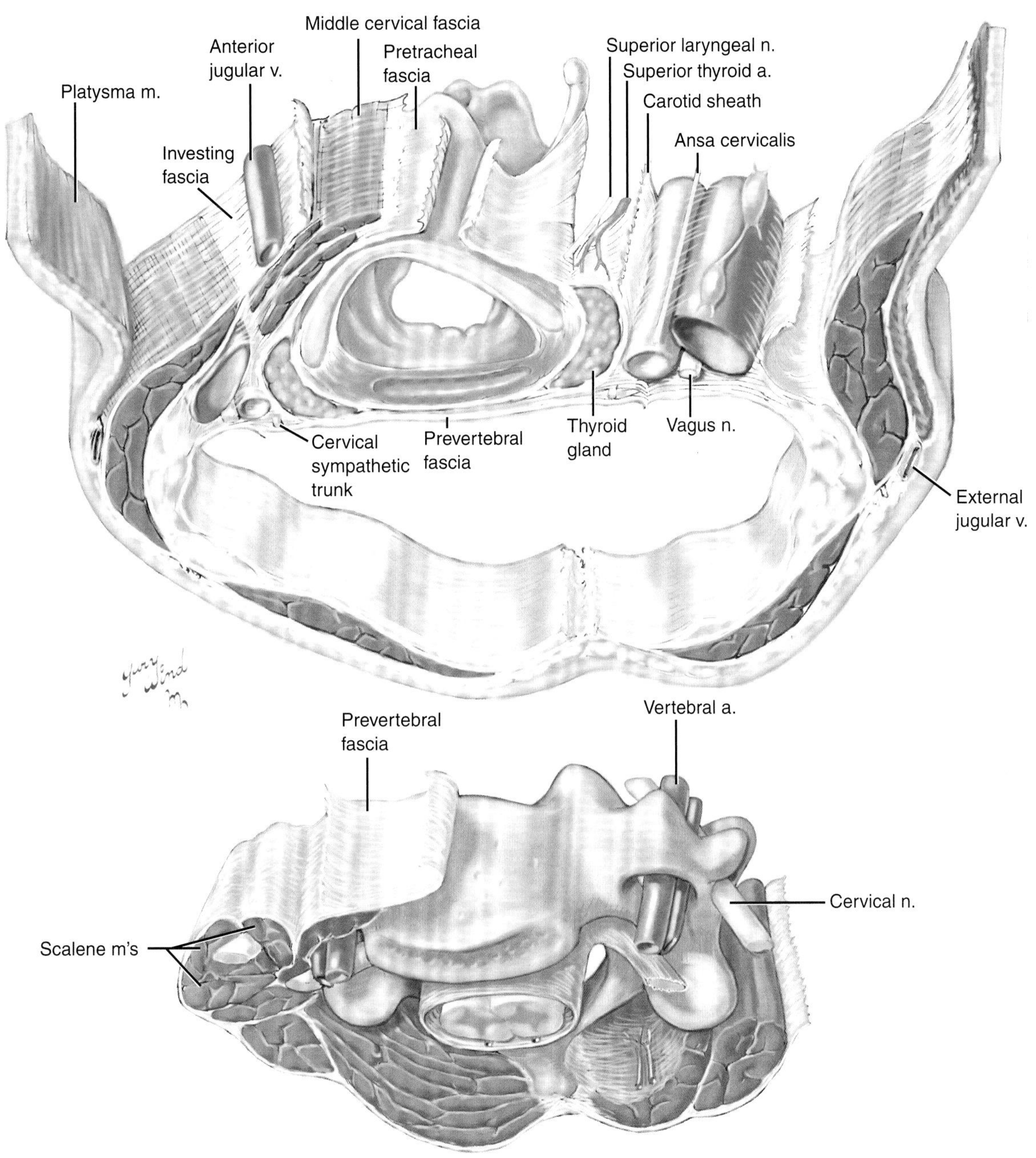

Fig. 1-7 A cross section of the neck shows the discrete boundary between the musculoskeletal element of the neck and the other components.

The Carotid Artery

The common carotid artery ascends in the neck medial to the internal jugular vein and normally has no branches (Fig. 1-8). Occasionally, the superior thyroid artery arises proximal to the bifurcation into internal and external carotid arteries. The bifurcation is usually located at the level of the superior border of the thyroid cartilage. Variations in the levels at which the carotid bifurcates are more often above this position than below. The external carotid artery, supplying the extracranial structures of the head, gives off several branches before its terminal bifurcation into the internal maxillary and superficial temporal arteries. These are the superior thyroid, ascending pharyngeal, lingual, facial, occipital, and posterior auricular arteries. The internal carotid artery proceeds posteromedially to enter the carotid canal at the base of the skull without giving off any branches. On the medial side of the bifurcation lie the small, oval carotid body, a chemoreceptor, and the carotid sinus, a pressure receptor intrinsic to the wall of the common and internal carotid arteries.

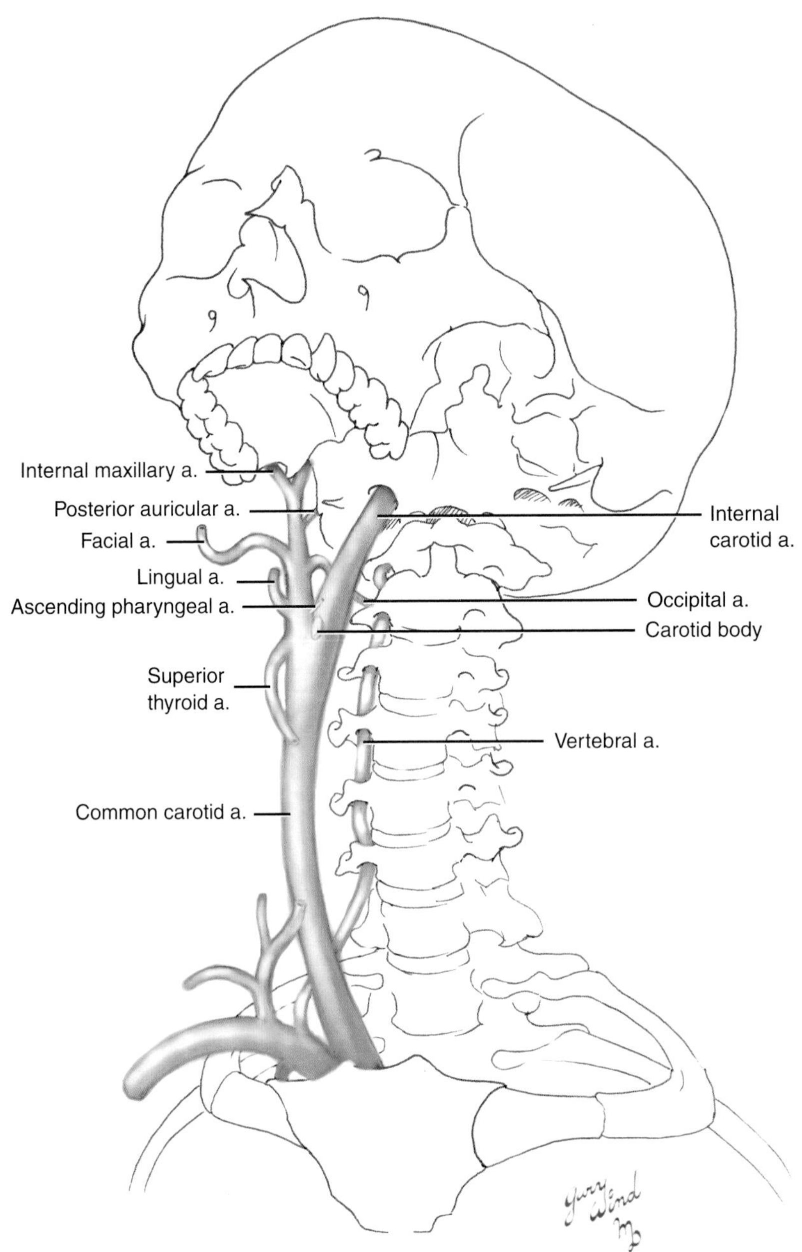

Fig. 1-8 The common carotid artery ascends two-thirds of the length of the neck without branches until it bifurcates. The external carotid has multiple extracranial ramifications while the internal carotid is branchless.

The Jugular Veins

The internal and external jugular veins sandwich the sternocleidomastoid muscle between them, following a somewhat diagonal course from the distal anterior margin to the proximal posterior margin of that muscle (Fig. 1-9). The two veins communicate distally through the retromandibular veins. The external jugular lies deep to the platysma for most of its course, and the internal jugular vein lies deep to the sternocleidomastoid muscle. The common facial vein usually enters the internal jugular vein at the level of the carotid bifurcation.

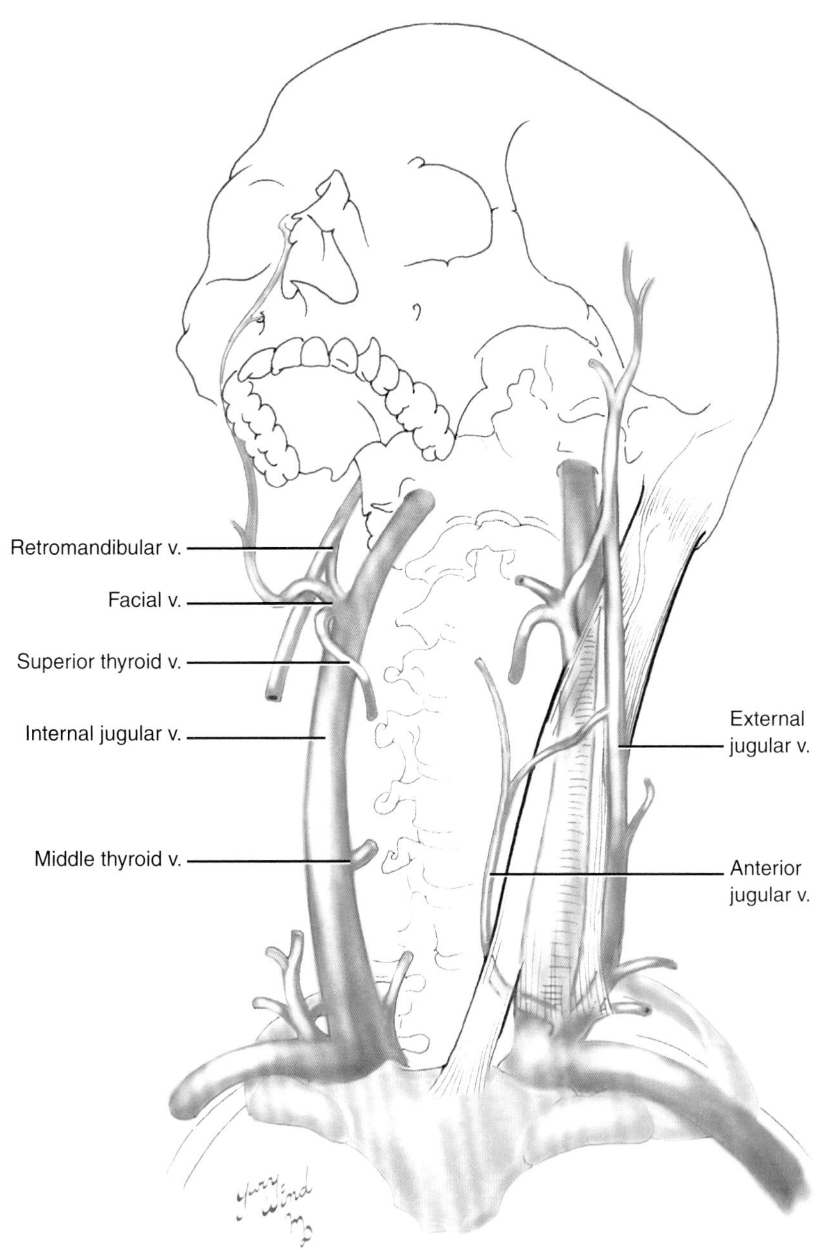

Fig. 1-9 The internal jugular vein lies immediately beneath the sternocleidomastoid muscle and is paralleled by the smaller external jugular vein crossing the superficial surface of that muscle. The pattern of the smaller venous branches is more variable than that of the corresponding arteries.

The Nerves of the Neck

There are three groups of nerves in the neck: the cranial nerves, the nerves of the cervical plexus, and the nerves of the brachial plexus (Fig. 1-10). Only the first group is of major concern when considering approaches to the distal carotid artery. Of the cranial nerves, the facial (VII), glossopharyngeal (IX), vagus (X), spinal accessory (XI), and hypoglossal (XII) are intimately related to the distal internal carotid artery and are discussed further below. In the midneck, the vagus, cervical sympathetic chain, and ansa cervicalis (also called ansa hypoglossi) share the carotid sheath. The cutaneous branches of the cervical plexus emerge from the prevertebral fascia deep to the sternocleidomastoid muscle and then pierce the investing fascia at the posterior border of that muscle.

The nerve roots of the brachial plexus emerge between the anterior and middle scalene muscles and lie lateral to the course of the common carotid arteries. This relationship is examined in more detail in Chapter 4.

The final key to understanding the approach to the carotid bifurcation and internal carotid artery is knowing the relationships of the pharynx, the cranial nerves mentioned above, the vessels, and the ramus of the mandible.

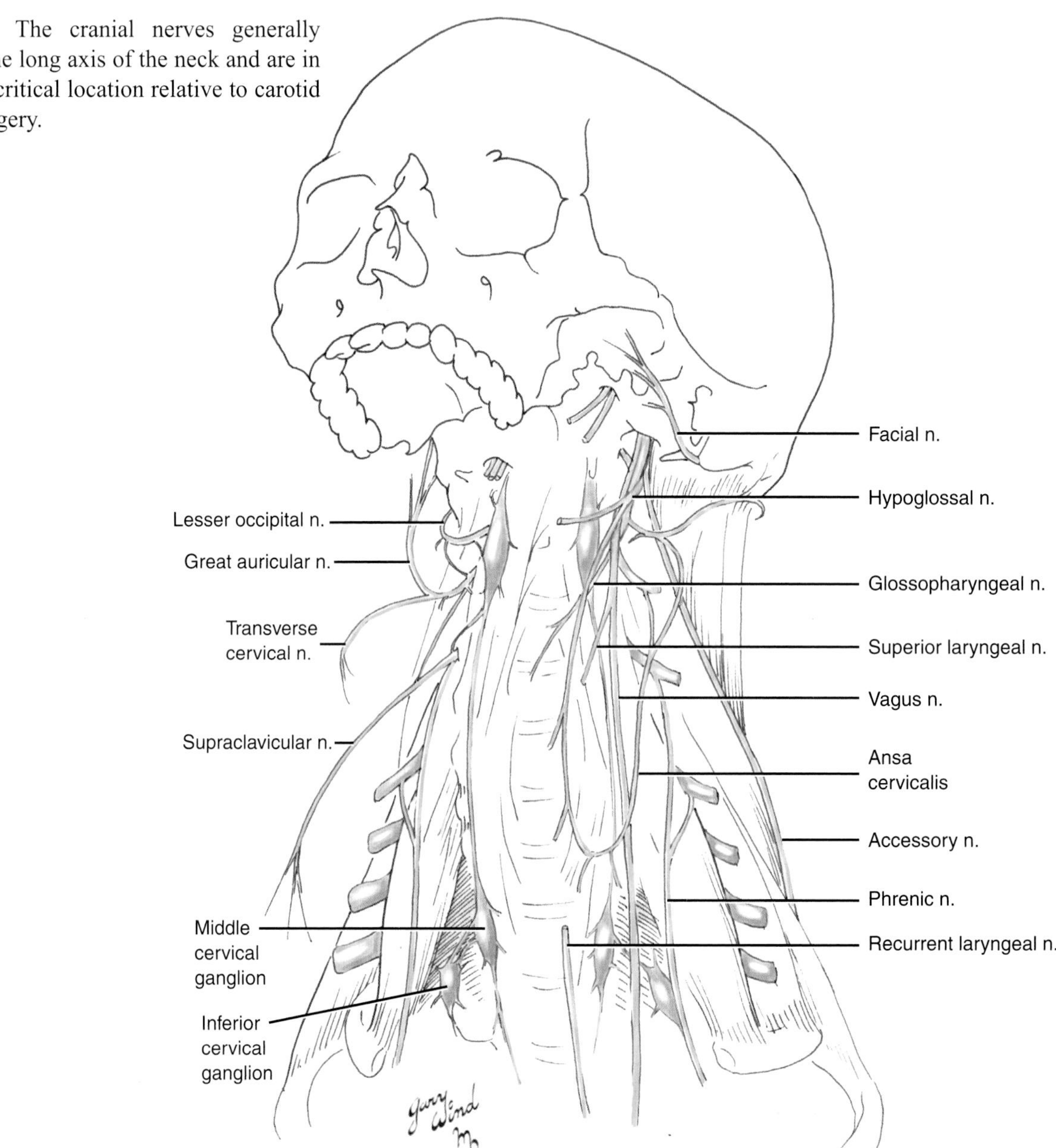

Fig. 1-10 The cranial nerves generally parallel the long axis of the neck and are in the most critical location relative to carotid artery surgery.

The Pharynx

The focal point of the posterior suspension of the pharynx from the base of the skull is the styloid process (Fig. 1-11). The stylohyoid ligament, styloglossus, stylopharyngeus, and stylohyoid muscles originate on this bony spine and attach in a fan-shaped pattern to the upper pharyngeal wall and hyoid bone. The digastric muscle provides additional support. Interleaved among these structures are the carotid and jugular arborizations and the cranial nerves.

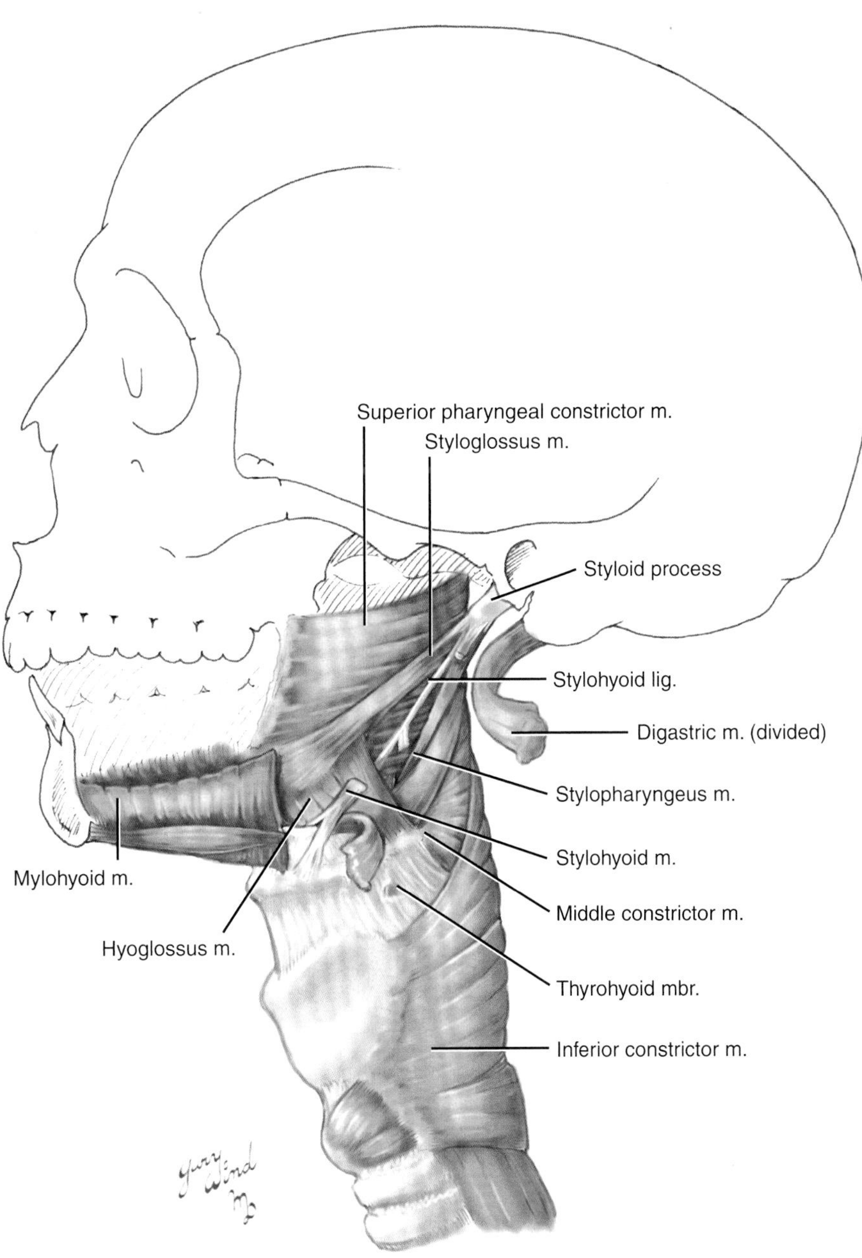

Fig. 1-11 The pharynx and its related muscles constitute the deep surface on which the carotid vessels lie.

The Internal and External Carotid Arteries

The internal carotid artery passes deep to the styloid process and all associated structures to reach the base of the skull (Fig. 1-12). The external carotid artery divides the posterior suspensory complex of the larynx by passing between the digastric and stylohyoid muscles laterally and the styloglossus and stylopharyngeus muscles medially. Beneath the posterior belly of the digastric muscle, the occipital artery crosses the distal internal carotid artery.

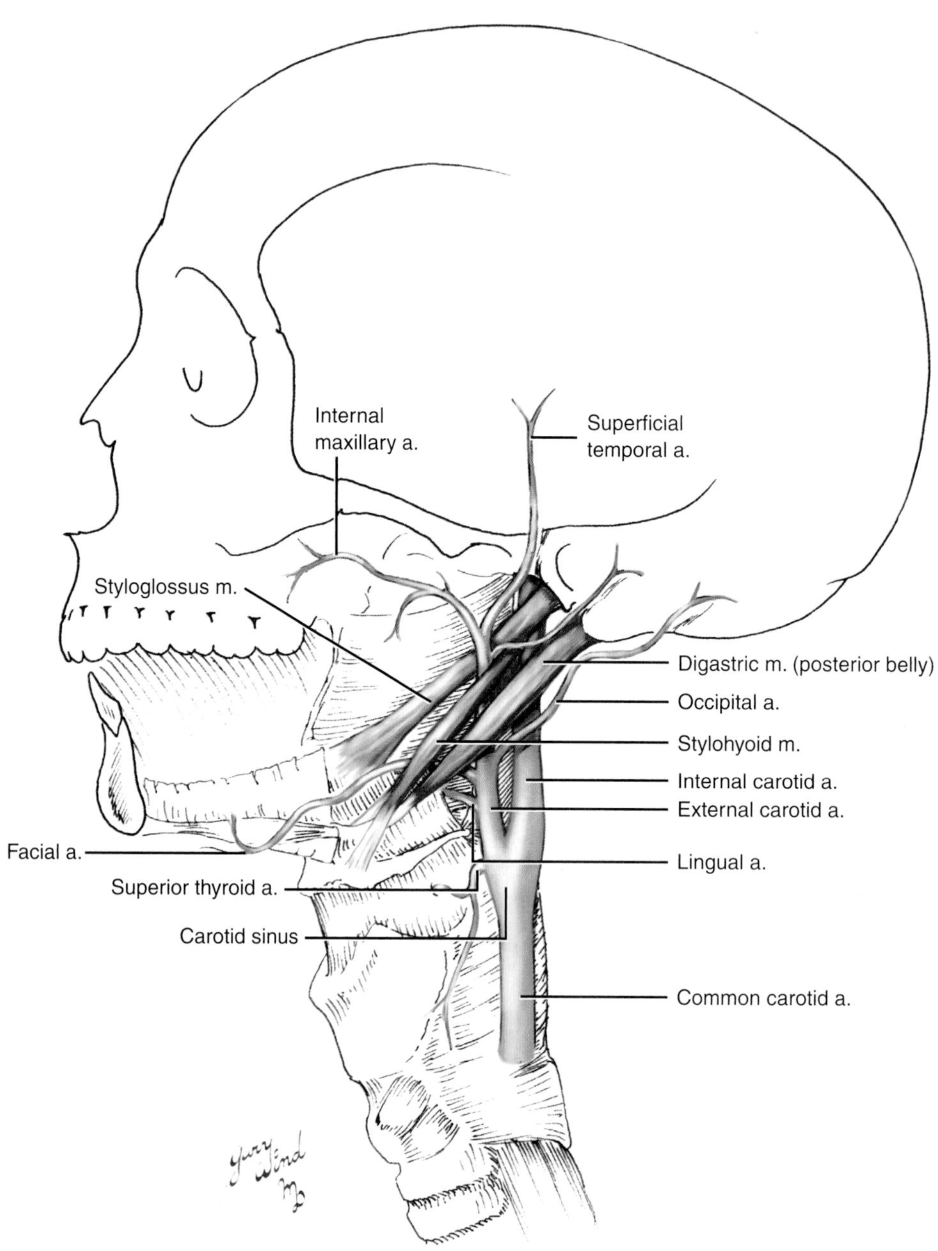

Fig. 1-12 The internal carotid artery passes deep to the posterior suspensory muscles of the pharynx to terminate medial to the styloid process, while the continuation of the external carotid passes between these muscles.

The Distal Jugular Vein

Just outside the jugular foramen, the internal jugular vein lies between the internal carotid artery and the root of the styloid process (Fig. 1-13). The retromandibular and facial branches of the common facial vein lie superficial to the digastric and stylohyoid muscles. However, cephalad to the stylohyoid muscle, the retromandibular vein and external carotid artery pass between the parotid gland and the ramus of the mandible, a relationship usually described as being within the substance of the parotid gland. Both vessels lie deep to the branches of the facial nerve fanning out through the parotid.

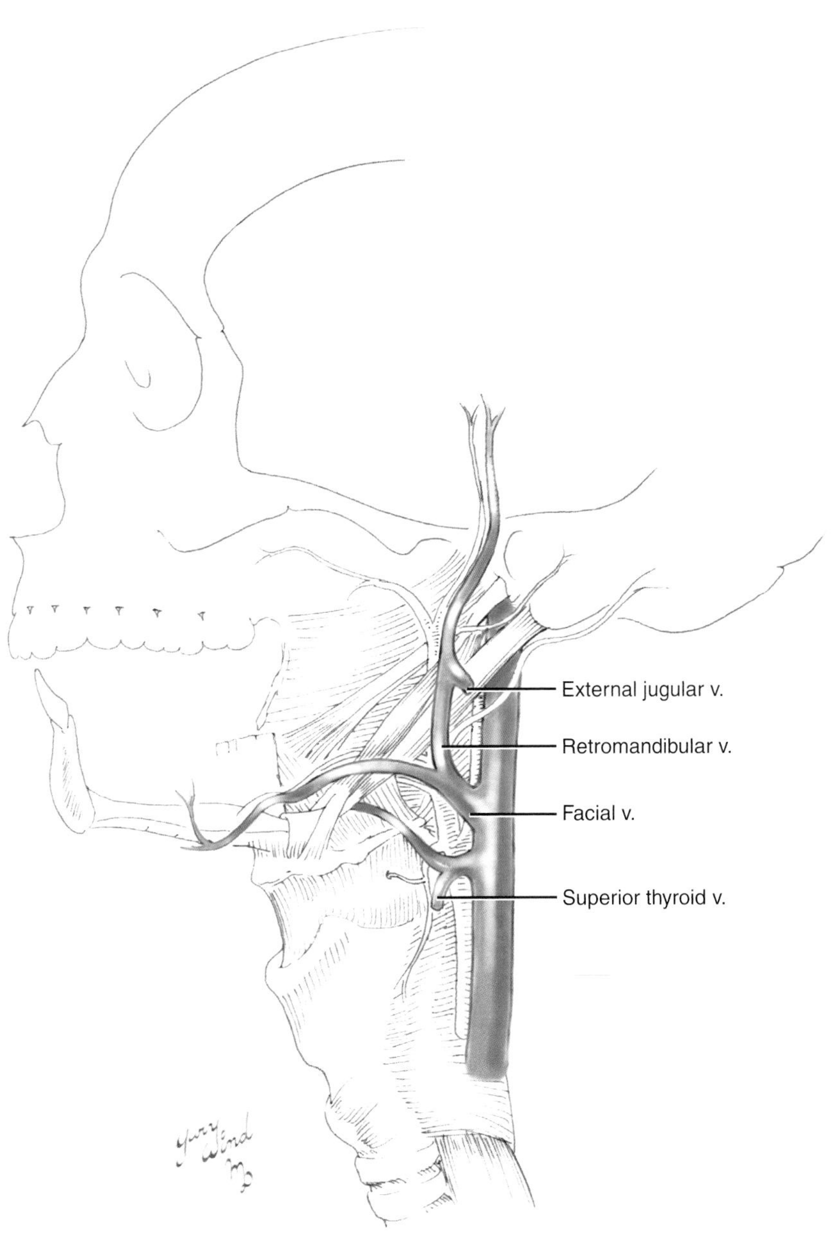

Fig. 1-13 The internal jugular vein runs posterolateral to the internal carotid artery and follows a similar course. The superficial veins of the face drain via the relatively constant facial vein, which crosses the carotid bifurcation to reach the internal jugular.

The Cranial Nerves

The immediate extracranial portions of the cranial nerves mentioned above intertwine with the muscular and vascular structures we have been discussing, putting them at risk for injury during carotid surgery (Fig. 1-14). Although most iatrogenic nerve injuries resulting from carotid surgery are temporary and subtle, careful examination will reveal such injuries in 5% to 21% of patients.[1-5] Detailed postoperative evaluations by neurologists documented cranial nerve injuries in 4.7% of the 1,240 patients randomized to the surgical arm of the Carotid Revascularization vs. Stenting Trial,[1] which was lower than the 8.6% of 1,415 patients randomized to surgery in the North American Carotid Endarterectomy Trial reported two decades prior.[3] The frequency of cranial nerve injury is higher in patients undergoing repeat carotid endartarectomy.[4] The frequency of individual nerve injuries remains controversial, but most authors report that either the hypoglossal nerve[2] or the recurrent laryngeal nerve[3,4] is most commonly injured. The glossopharyngeal nerve is among the least frequently injured, but permanent damage is associated with severe impairment due to swallowing difficulties.

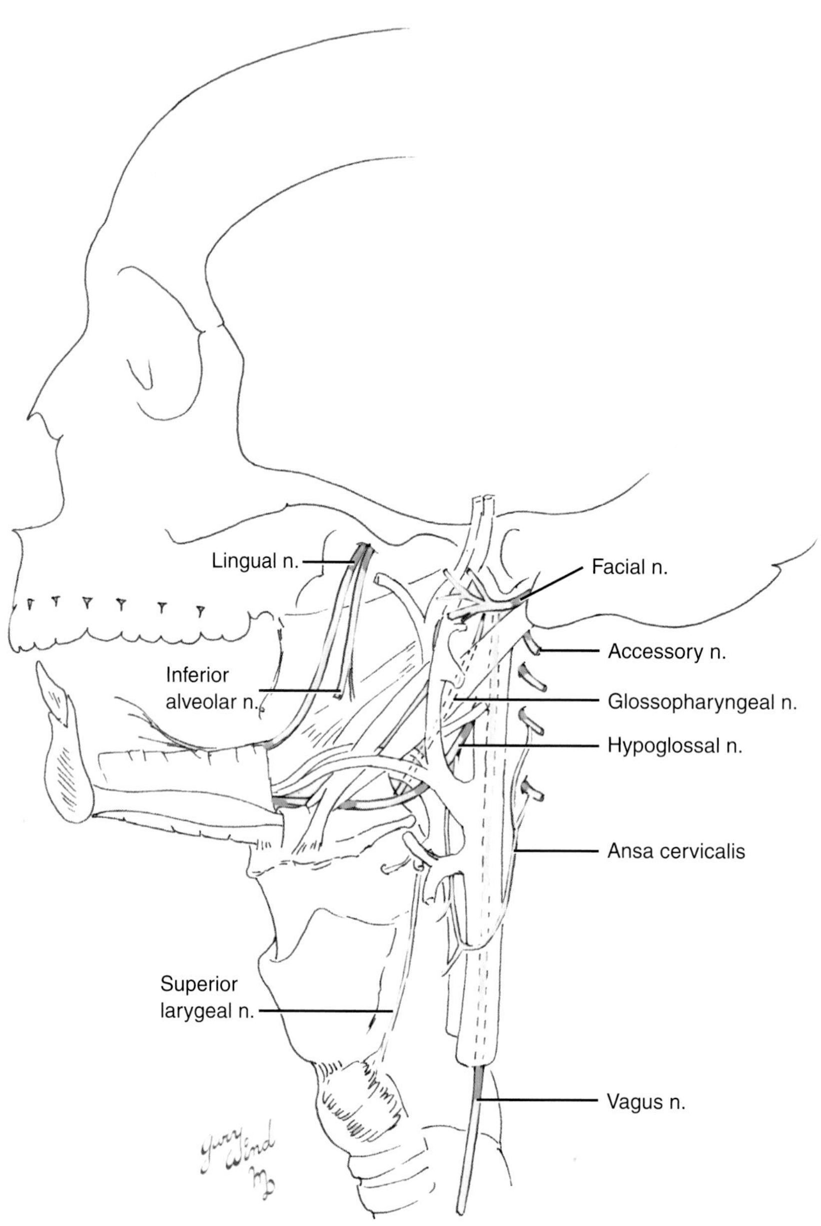

Fig. 1-14 The hypoglossal nerve swinging down superficial to the carotid vessels is often visualized during carotid surgery. The limb of the ansa cervicalis running with the hypoglossal nerve is often sacrificed with no ill effect during carotid surgery.

The emergence of the cranial nerves from the base of the skull provides orientation for describing their subsequent paths (Fig. 1-15). The facial nerve arises posterior to the base of the styloid process and immediately passes anterolaterally to enter the parotid gland. The accessory, vagus, and glossopharyngeal nerves exit from the jugular foramen. The hypoglossal nerve emerges from the hypoglossal canal just medial to the jugular foramen. The superior cervical sympathetic ganglion has a cephalic connection via the small carotid nerve arising at its cephalad pole.

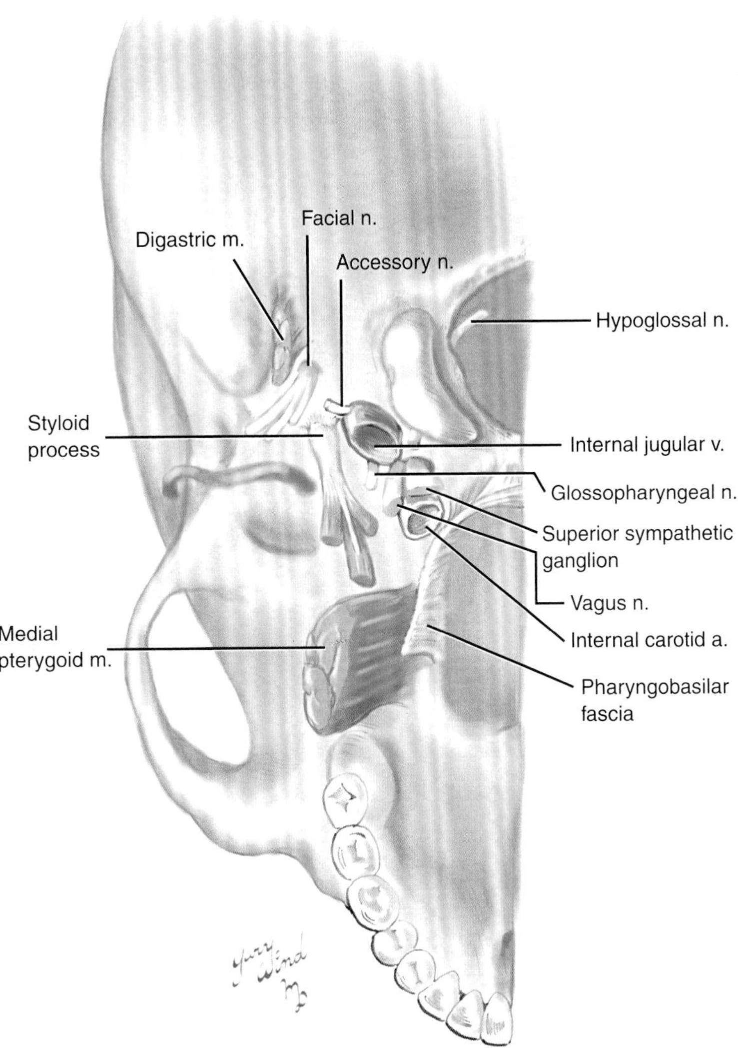

Fig. 1-15 An understanding of the emergence of the cranial nerves at the base of the skull helps prevent injury to these nerves during operations on the distal internal carotid artery.

The marginal mandibular branch of the facial nerve (ramus mandibularis) emerges from behind the parotid gland and runs below the angle of the mandible before turning upwards to run parallel with the mandibular ramus (Fig. 1-16). Although the nerve is usually within one finger's breadth of the inferior border of the mandible,[6] variants can course significantly below this level, making them prone to injury during carotid endarterectomy. The nerve innervates the muscles of the lower lip; injury results in the inability to draw the angle of the mouth downward, with compensatory drooping of the contralateral lip.[6,7] The ramus mandibularis is prone to injury from longitudinal incisions that are placed too far anteriorly and from retractors that are placed on the angle of the mandible.[5] Positioning retractors superficial to the platysma and curving the longitudinal incisions posteriorly toward the mastoid process may help to reduce injuries to the ramus mandibularis.

The vagus nerve and sympathetic chain lie posteriorly in the groove between the internal jugular vein and the internal and later common carotid artery (Fig. 1-17). Occasionally, the vagus nerve is located in a more anterior position in relation to the carotid artery at the base of the neck. The superior and inferior laryngeal branches of the vagus supply the muscles of the larynx, and varying degrees of dysphonia result when they are injured. The superior laryngeal nerve accompanies the artery of the same name from its origin high in the neck and is at direct risk from mobilization of the artery. The recurrent laryngeal nerve, arising low in the neck, is at indirect risk from injury to the main vagal trunk in the midneck. In rare cases, a nonrecurrent laryngeal nerve may branch directly from the vagus at the level of the carotid bifurcation and course medially behind the carotid bulb to reach the larynx. This anomaly is usually seen on the right side, associated with an aberrant right subclavian artery.

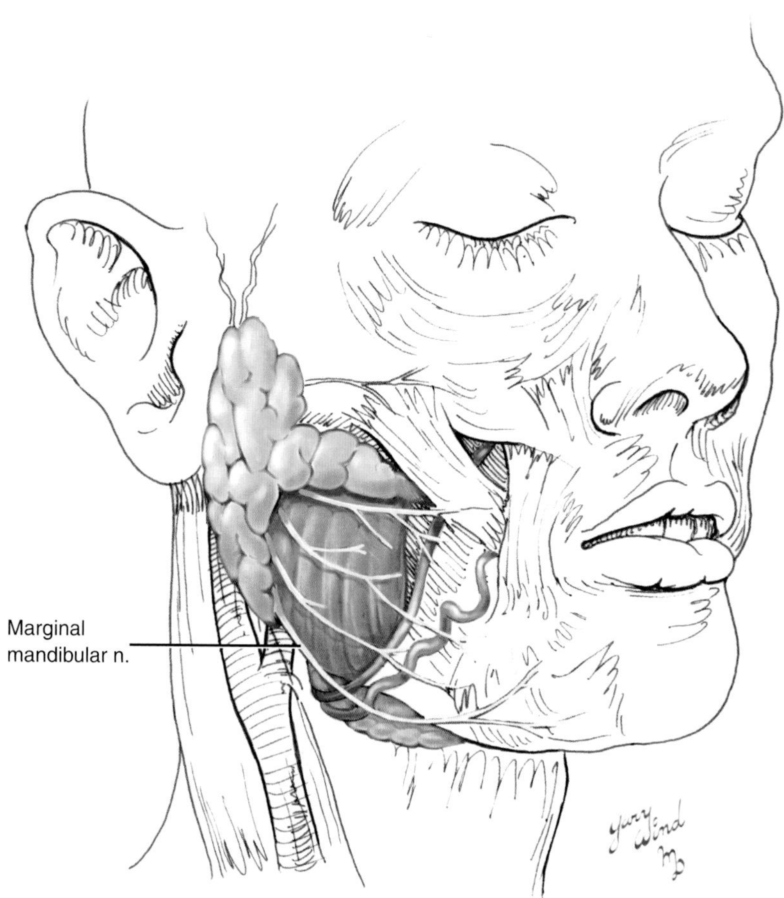

Fig. 1-16 The ramus mandibularis branch of the facial nerve runs below the edge of the mandible and is prone to injury during carotid endarterectomy.

The spinal accessory nerve penetrates and supplies the sternocleidomastoid muscle before passing across the posterior triangle of the neck to the trapezius. Its high location puts it at low risk for injury.

The hypoglossal nerve passes between the internal carotid artery and internal jugular vein. It turns anteriorly, spiraling around the internal carotid artery, and passes under the occipital artery along its course. It loops across the lateral surface of the external carotid artery and passes deep to the stylohyoid insertion and digastric sling before disappearing beneath the posterior edge of the mylohyoid muscle. Although usually found about 2 cm cephalad to the carotid bifurcation, its location may vary. The hypoglossal nerve is tethered by the descendens hypoglossi and by the sternomastoid artery and vein; the nerve can be mobilized during high carotid dissections by careful division of these structures. Nerve injury impairs motor function of the tongue and may cause dysarthria and dysphagia.

The glossopharyngeal nerve also passes superficial to the internal carotid artery to reach the posterior edge of the stylopharyngeus muscle. It spirals to the anterior surface of that muscle and disappears beneath the posterior edge of the hyoglossus muscle. Loss of its sensory and motor fibers to the tongue and pharynx may result in aspiration in the rare instances when it is injured.

At the carotid bifurcation, there is a fine network of nerves providing complex innervation to the carotid body and carotid sinus.[8] The carotid body is a discrete flat ovoid chemoreceptor located on the posterior aspect of the carotid bifurcation. It is one of several such receptors in the body, probably of neural crest origin, which are sensitive to hypoxia, hypercarbia, and acidosis and cause reflex respiratory stimulation. Nerve twigs to the carotid body from glossopharyngeal, vagus, and superior cervical sympathetic ganglion lie between the internal and external carotid arteries.

The carotid sinus nerve arises from the glossopharyngeal nerve and descends to the carotid sinus receptors in the dilated bulb and proximal internal carotid artery. In its course, it anastomoses with the vagus, superior cervical sympathetic ganglion, and carotid body. Its distal segment is entwined with the plexus of nerves associated with the carotid body. Besides the normal stimulus of elevated blood pressure, surgical manipulation of the carotids may also cause reflex bradycardia and hypotension.

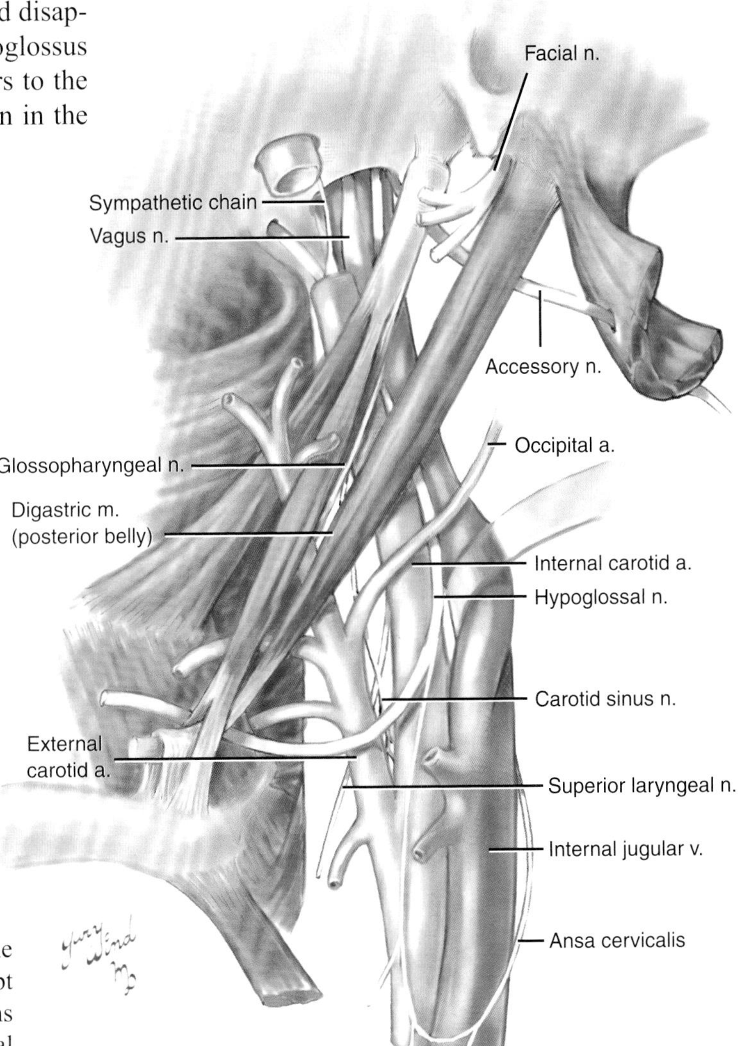

Fig. 1-17 All the major cranial nerves in the neck originate deep to the styloid process except the facial nerve. They reach their destinations through paths intimately related to the internal carotid artery.

Access to a highly placed bifurcation and to the distal common carotid is limited because of the proximity of the mandibular ramus and the mastoid process (Fig. 1-18). Strategies for dealing with this special situation are discussed in the second half of this chapter.

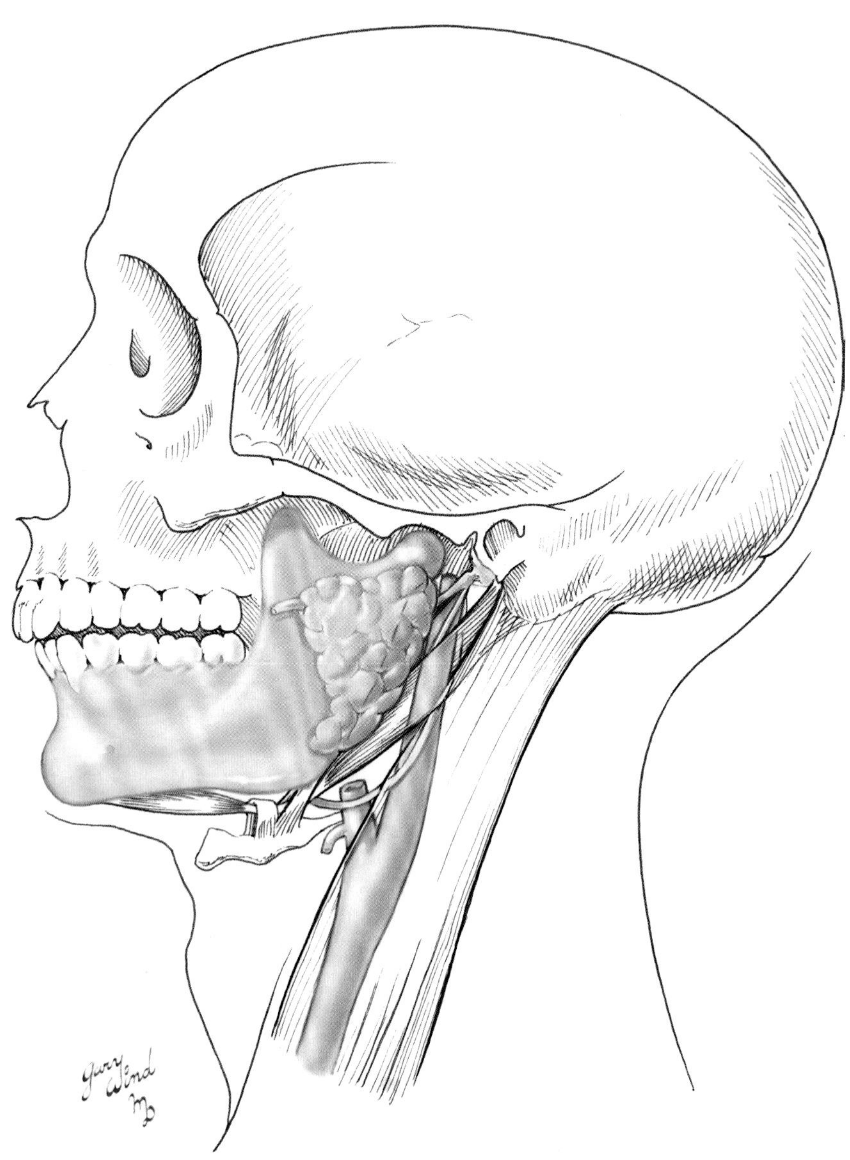

Fig. 1-18 The distal internal carotid artery is cramped in a narrow space behind and deep to the ramus of the mandible, making access difficult.

Exposure of the Carotid Artery and Its Branches

Optimal approaches to the extracranial carotid artery depend on the segments that are to be exposed. The major portion of the cervical carotid artery is relatively superficial and is approached through a single anterior cervical incision. However, exposure of the carotid segments located near the base of the skull and at the base of the neck may require specialized maneuvers[9] to achieve adequate circulatory control. In planning approaches for carotid surgery, we have found it useful to divide the neck into three anatomic regions as recommended by Monson et al.[10] (Fig. 1-19). Zone I extends from the base of the neck to 1 cm above the clavicle, zone II is the segment from 1 cm above the clavicle to the angle of the mandible, and zone III extends from the angle of the mandible to the base of the skull. For carotid exposure confined to zone II, a single anterior cervical incision is appropriate. Concomitant median sternotomy should be considered to ensure adequate proximal circulatory control in patients who may require carotid arterial exposure in zone I. Exposure of the carotid segment in zone III may require mandibular subluxation and periauricular extension of the cervical incision.

The following discussion considers exposure of the carotid artery in zones II and III. Performance of median sternotomy for exposure of the proximal carotid artery segment will be considered in Chapter 3.

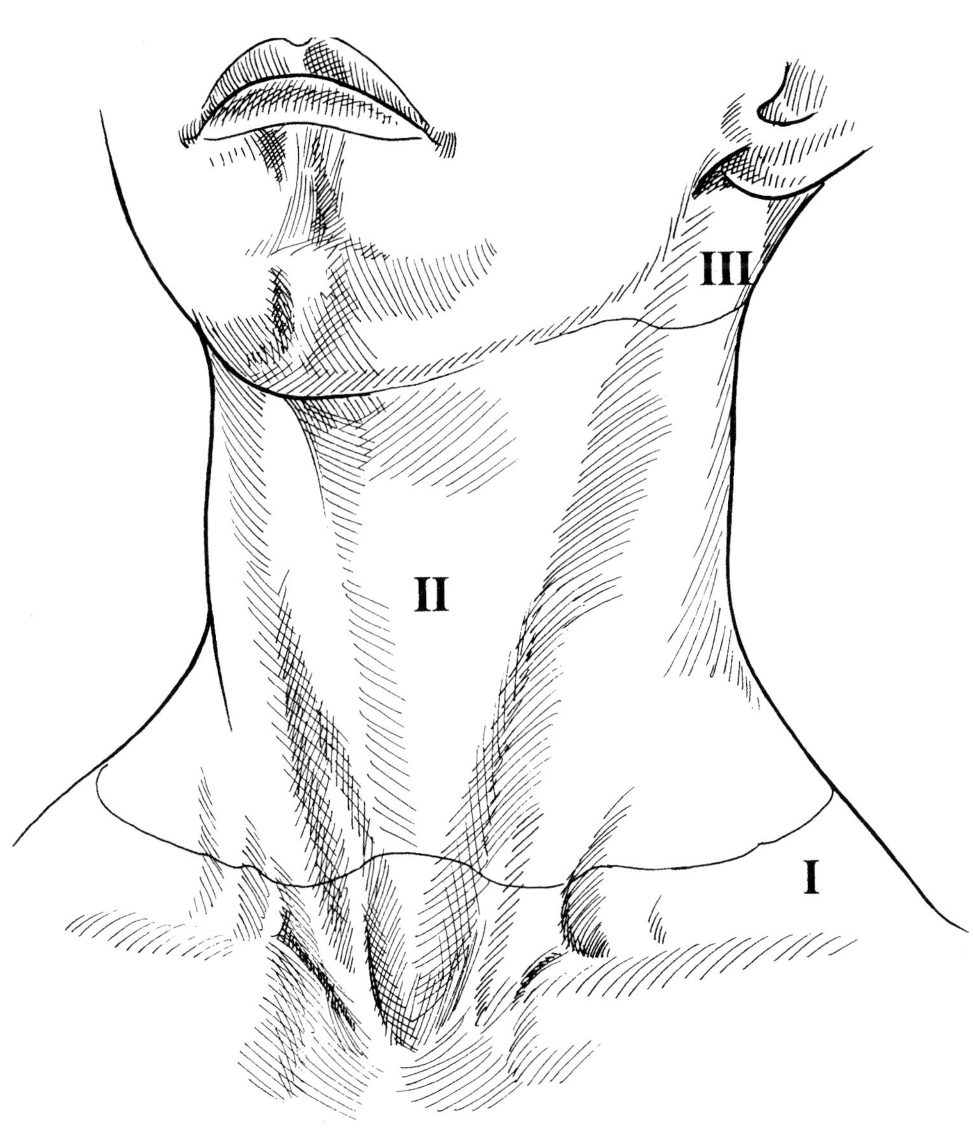

Fig. 1-19 A conceptual division of the neck into three zones helps to determine appropriate surgical approaches to different regions of the carotid arteries.

Exposure of the Carotid Bifurcation in the Neck (Zone II)

The neck is slightly extended, and the head is turned opposite the side of the intended incision and placed upon a gel ring. Elevation of the shoulders with a rolled sheet will enhance neck extension, especially in patients with short, broad necks. The upper chest, lower face, and lower ear are prepped and draped.

A longitudinal incision is made along the anterior border of the sternocleidomastoid muscle, extending from the clavicular head to the retromandibular area (Fig. 1-20). The incision should be curved slightly and extended just inferior to the lobe of the ear at its distal end. This posterior displacement of the incision helps avoid injury to the marginal mandibular branch of the facial nerve.[11] Alternatively, a transverse cervical incision may be used, but this oblique incision is associated with limited carotid exposure and a higher risk of injury to the marginal mandibular nerve.[11]

The incision is deepened through the platysma muscle, and the investing layer of the deep

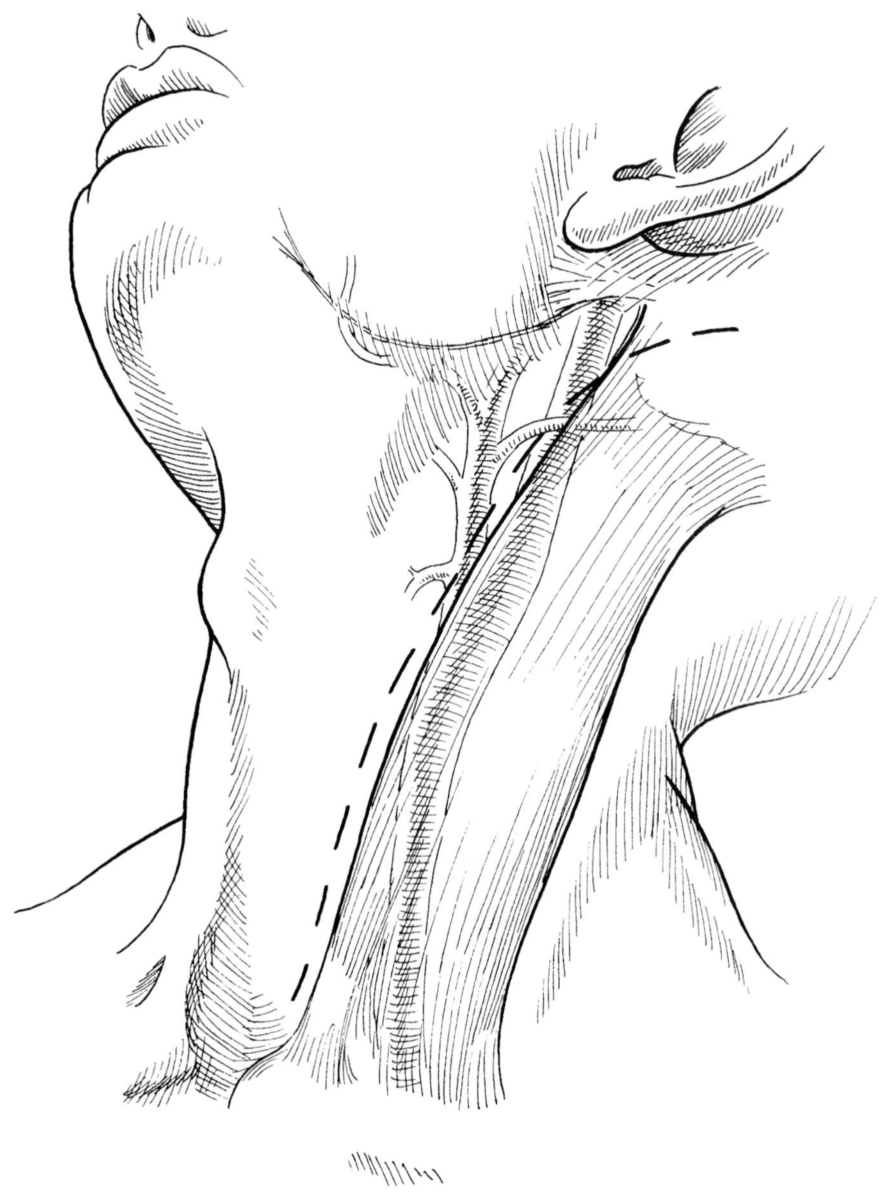

Fig. 1-20 Postauricular extension of the cephalad end of the longitudinal neck incision avoids injury to the ramus mandibularis of the facial nerve.

cervical fascia is opened on the anterior border of the sternocleidomastoid muscle. The sternocleidomastoid muscle is separated from the underlying vascular sheath by sharp dissection on its medial border (Fig. 1-21). The small sternomastoid branch of the superior thyroid artery will require ligation during this maneuver. More distal mobilization will require division of the sternocleidomastoid branch of the occipital artery near the superior part of the incision.[12] Care should be taken not to injure the accessory nerve, which crosses the superior aspect of the wound to pierce the sternocleidomastoid muscle.[13] By retracting the freed sternocleidomastoid posteriorly, the vascular sheath is identified. The sheath is opened superior to the omohyoid muscle; more proximal exposure necessitates division of the muscle. The internal jugular vein is dissected free along its anterior border in the central part of the wound and retracted posteriorly with the sternocleidomastoid muscle. This maneuver requires division

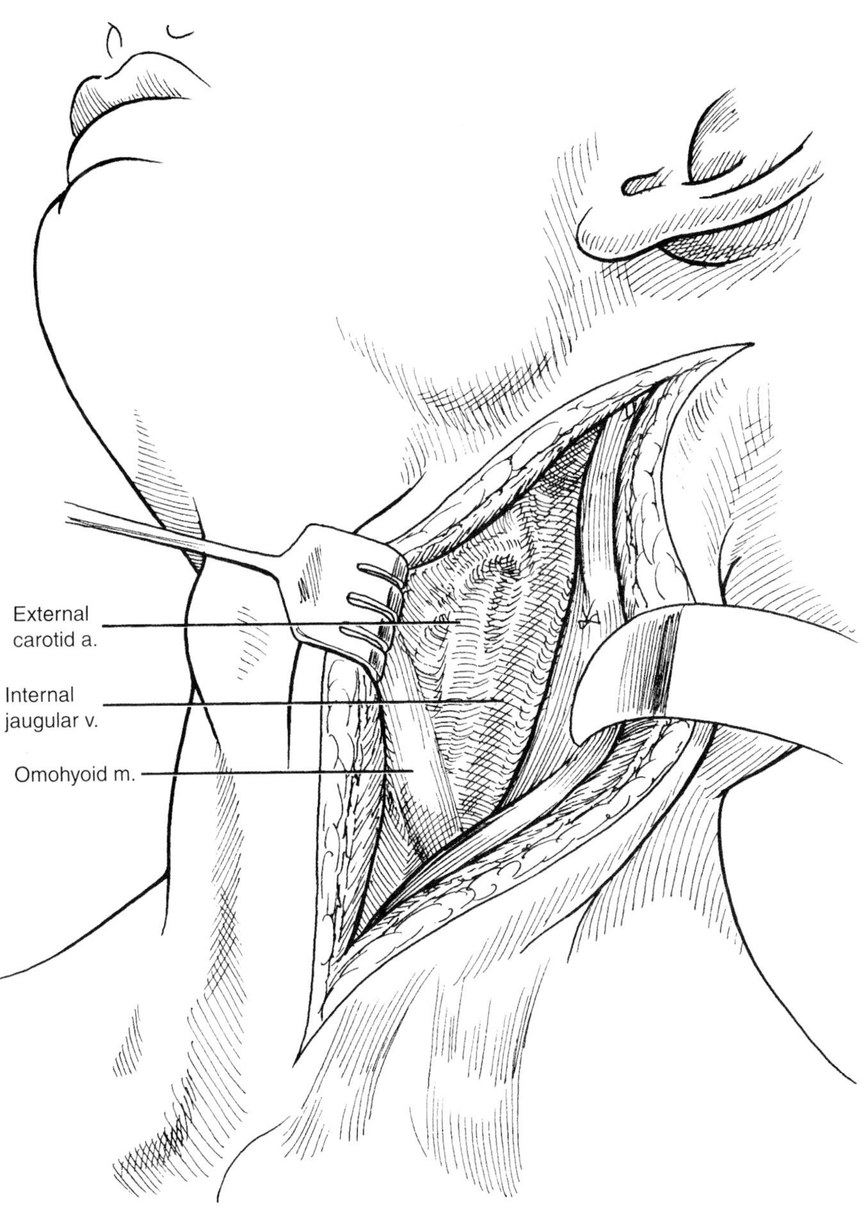

Fig. 1-21 Posterior retraction of the sternocleidomastoid muscle exposes the carotid sheath.

of the common facial vein (Fig. 1-22). The common facial vein is usually well-defined, and its division can be likened to the of a trap door, immediately exposing the carotid arteries.

Dissection of the common carotid artery and its branches is performed next. It is important to use exact and careful movements during arterial mobilization to prevent dislodgement of small emboli from irregular luminal surfaces. We favor the isolation of the common carotid and its branches away from the bifurcation, which is dissected last. This allows vessels with relatively normal surfaces to be dissected before manipulation of the atherosclerosis-prone bifurcation. The common carotid artery is isolated first, using sharp dissection. The vagus nerve usually lies posterior to the common carotid artery, but it is occasionally found anterior and lateral to the artery.[11] The recurrent laryngeal nerve is usually located in the tracheoesophageal groove, well removed from injury during carotid dissection. However, a nonrecurrent laryngeal nerve anomaly may be present that renders it more susceptible to injury. Although this anomaly is usually associated with aortic arch anomalies,

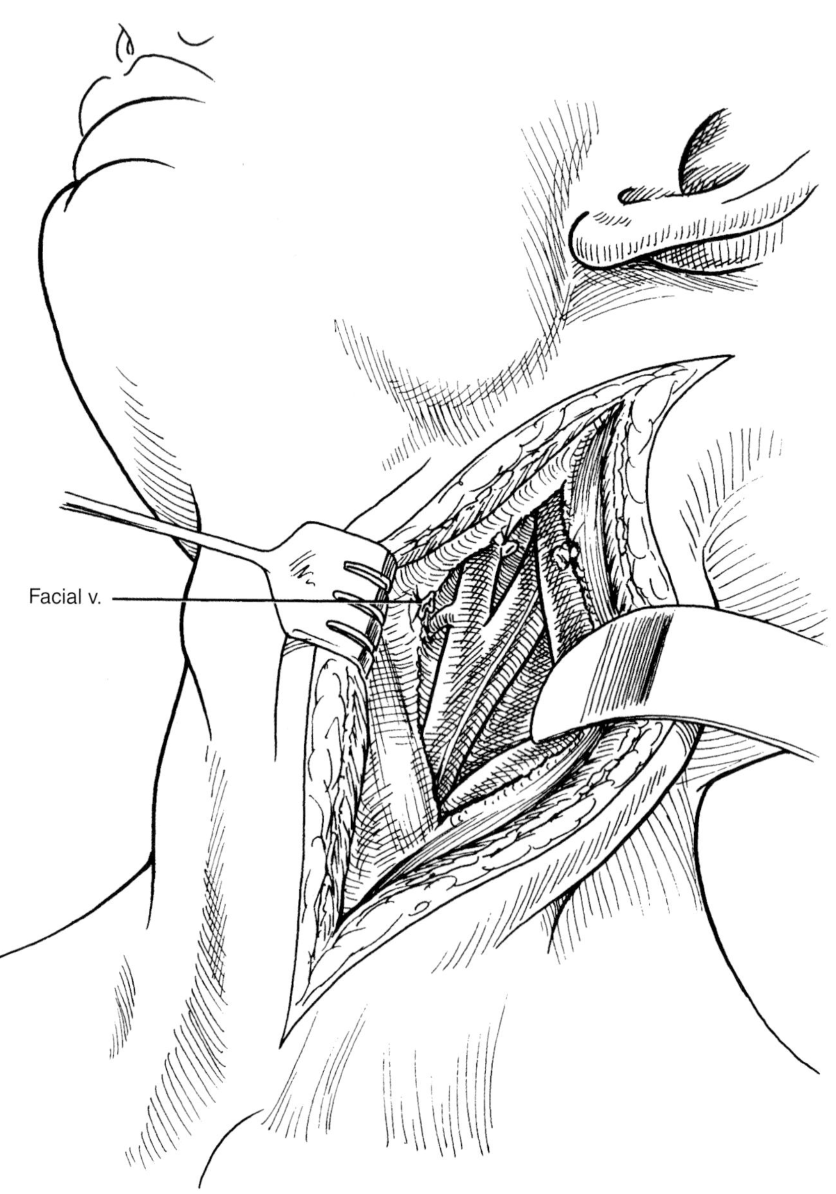

Fig. 1-22 After division of the facial vein, the jugular vein can be mobilized posteriorly to expose the carotid bifurcation cephalad to the anterior belly of the omohyoid muscle.

it has been reported in patients with normal arch anatomy.[14] A nonrecurrent laryngeal nerve occurs more frequently on the right side with an incidence of 0.3% to 0.8% and is usually associated with an aberrant right subclavian artery.[14] The nonrecurrent laryngeal nerve leaves the vagus at the level of the carotid bifurcation and is at risk of injury if the dissection is extended either medial to or posterior to the bulb area. Once the common carotid is completely freed from surrounding tissue, it is encircled with an elastic vascular loop away from the bifurcation area (Fig. 1-23). Clearance of tissues from the anterior surface of the common carotid may be facilitated by transection of the ansa hypoglossi nerve.

The internal carotid artery is isolated next. It is located posterior and medial to the external carotid artery and found deep to the internal jugular vein (Fig. 1-23). Dissection along the medial border of the internal jugular vein in the superior wound will allow exposure of the internal carotid away from the bifurcation. Lymphatic tissue overlying the vein requires division. Small venous branches draining into the anterior vein surface above the level of the facial vein should be identified and ligated to prevent troublesome bleeding.[12] Isolation of the artery requires careful sharp dissection. The hypoglossal nerve trunk crosses the internal carotid artery at a variable distance from the bifurcation and must be avoided during dissection. Identification of the hypoglossal nerve is facilitated by following the ansa hypoglossi nerve to its junction with the hypoglossal trunk.[15] The hypoglossal nerve is tethered by the sternocleidomastoid branch of the occipital artery.[11] If not already ligated during the initial dissection, this branch should be divided to mobilize the nerve at the time of distal internal carotid artery exposure. Once the internal carotid artery is freed, it is encircled with an elastic vascular loop.

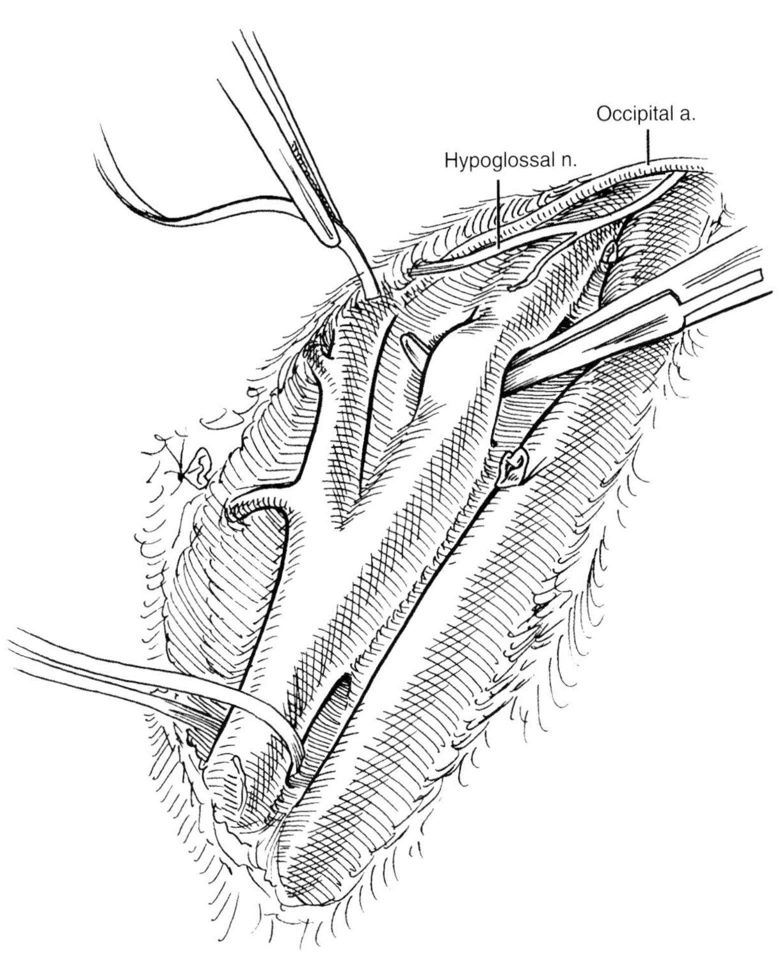

Fig. 1-23 Proximal and distal control is obtained before the carotid bifurcation is mobilized.

The external carotid artery is isolated at the bifurcation and encircled with an elastic vessel loop (Fig. 1-24). The superior thyroid artery requires isolation when it branches directly from the common carotid artery. The superior laryngeal nerve courses behind the external carotid artery[16] and is avoided by encircling the artery at its most proximal point. If not previously identified, the hypoglossal nerve can be avoided by dissection in the periadventitial tissues.

The carotid bifurcation area can now be dissected from surrounding tissues. A great deal of attention has been paid to the carotid sinus nerve (nerve of Herring). The carotid sinus is a collection of pressure receptors located at the junction of the common and internal carotid arteries. It has been suggested that changes in these baroreceptors induced by endarterectomy are associated with a reflex increase in vagal nerve function, resulting in hypotension and bradycardia.[17,18] In order to interrupt the reflex arc between the baroreceptors and the vagus nerve, some authors advocate inactivating the carotid sinus nerve by injecting local anesthesia at the carotid bifurcation or by dividing the nerve plexus containing the carotid sinus nerve posterior to the bifurcation area.[17,18] Citing a propensity toward development of hypertension after these maneuvers, other authors do not routinely inactivate the nerve but do so only after the development of vagal hyperactivity.[19] Once the decision to anesthetize the carotid sinus has been made, the carotid bifurcation should be mobilized completely to facilitate endarterectomy. Previous isolation of the common carotid artery and branches greatly facilitates dissection and minimizes injury to surrounding nerves and veins.

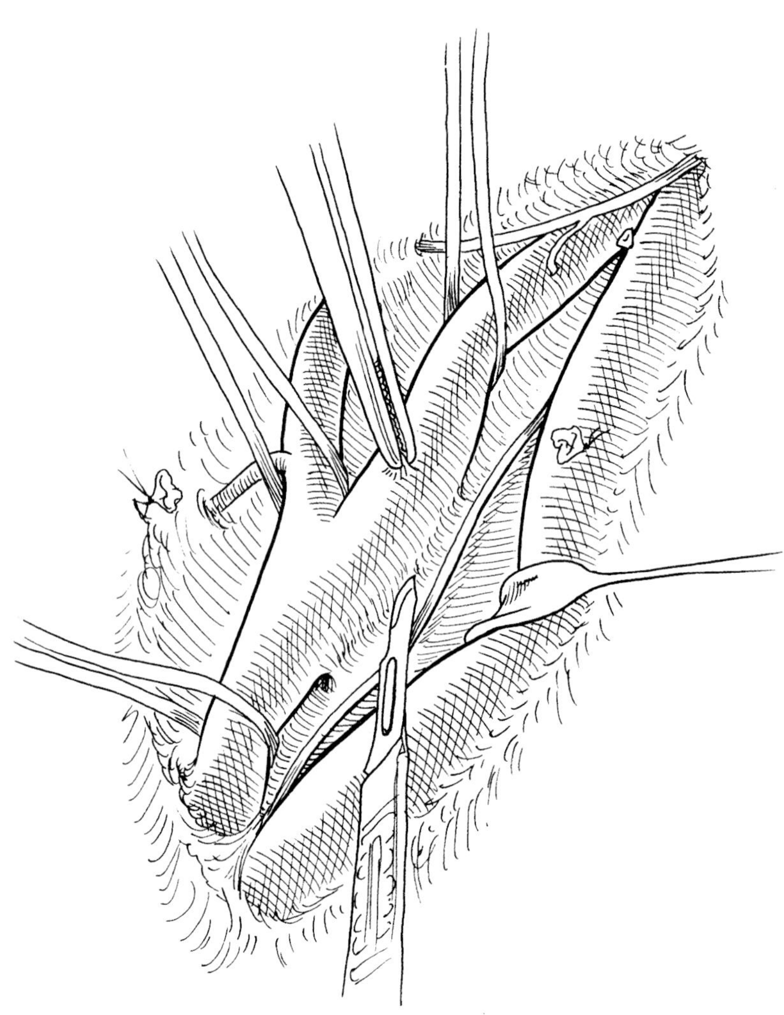

Fig. 1-24 Periadventitial dissection minimizes risk to adjacent cranial nerve branches.

Exposure of the Internal Carotid Artery in the Upper Neck (Zone III)

Arterial pathology may extend into the upper cervical segments of the internal carotid artery, an area considered to be relatively inaccessible. Common lesions in this segment include aneurysms from trauma, intimal dissection, or atherosclerosis, and luminal disease from atherosclerosis or fibromuscular hyperplasia. Exposure of the distal carotid artery near the skull may be required in the surgical repair of these lesions, as simple carotid ligation may have undesired consequences in noncomatose patients.[20] Many approaches have been described in the exposure of the distal internal carotid artery, including mandibular osteotomy,[21] creation of pre- and postauricular flaps,[22] removal of a portion of the mastoid bone,[23] and radical mastoidectomy with obliteration of the middle ear cavity.[24] We have come to rely on exposure through the standard vertical incision described above, using the technique of mandibular subluxation described by Fisher et al.[25]

General anesthesia with nasotracheal intubation is required for this approach. The mandibular condyle on the side to be operated is subluxed and transfixed with transnasal/oral wiring (Fig. 1-25).

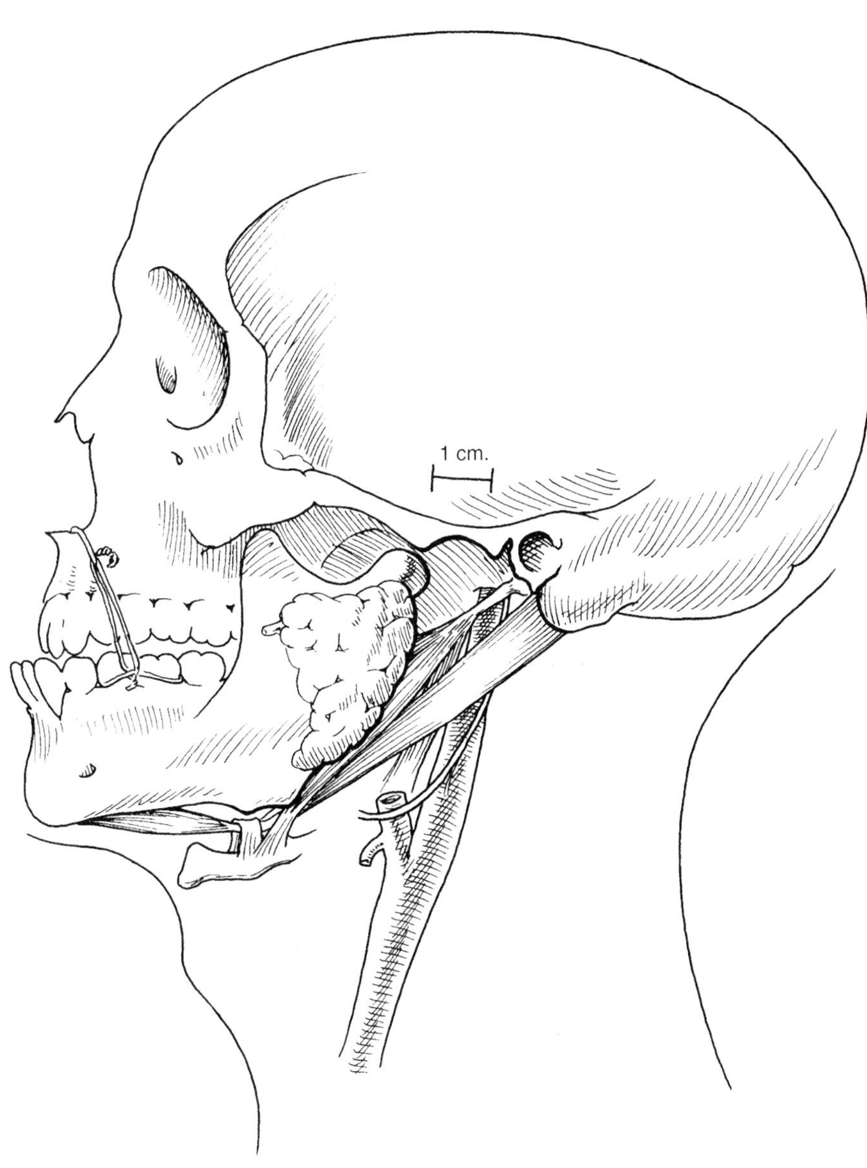

Fig. 1-25 Unilateral subluxation of the mandibular condyle provides an additional 1 cm of working space in the area of the distal internal carotid artery.

The optimal technique for temporary fixation depends on the presence of adequate dental stability, and a number of wiring options have been described by Simonian et al.[26] Yoshino et al. have recently described a less invasive method of subluxation using a mouthpiece made by a dentist to stabilize the mandible in the subluxated position.[27] The patient is positioned and surgically prepared as above, and the incision is made along the anterior border of the sternocleidomastoid muscle. The incision should be extended as high as possible and curved posteriorly just behind the lobe of the ear. Exposure of the common and internal carotid arteries proceeds as above. The hypoglossal nerve should be identified and protected, sometimes necessitating division of the occipital artery and ansa hypoglossi to allow optimal mobilization. In isolating the internal carotid artery, care should be taken to identify and ligate small crossing branches of the jugular vein. The lower edge of the parotid gland is retracted anteriorly during this maneuver.

Division of the posterior belly of the digastric muscle allows exposure of the internal carotid artery within 2 cm of the skull base (Fig. 1-26).

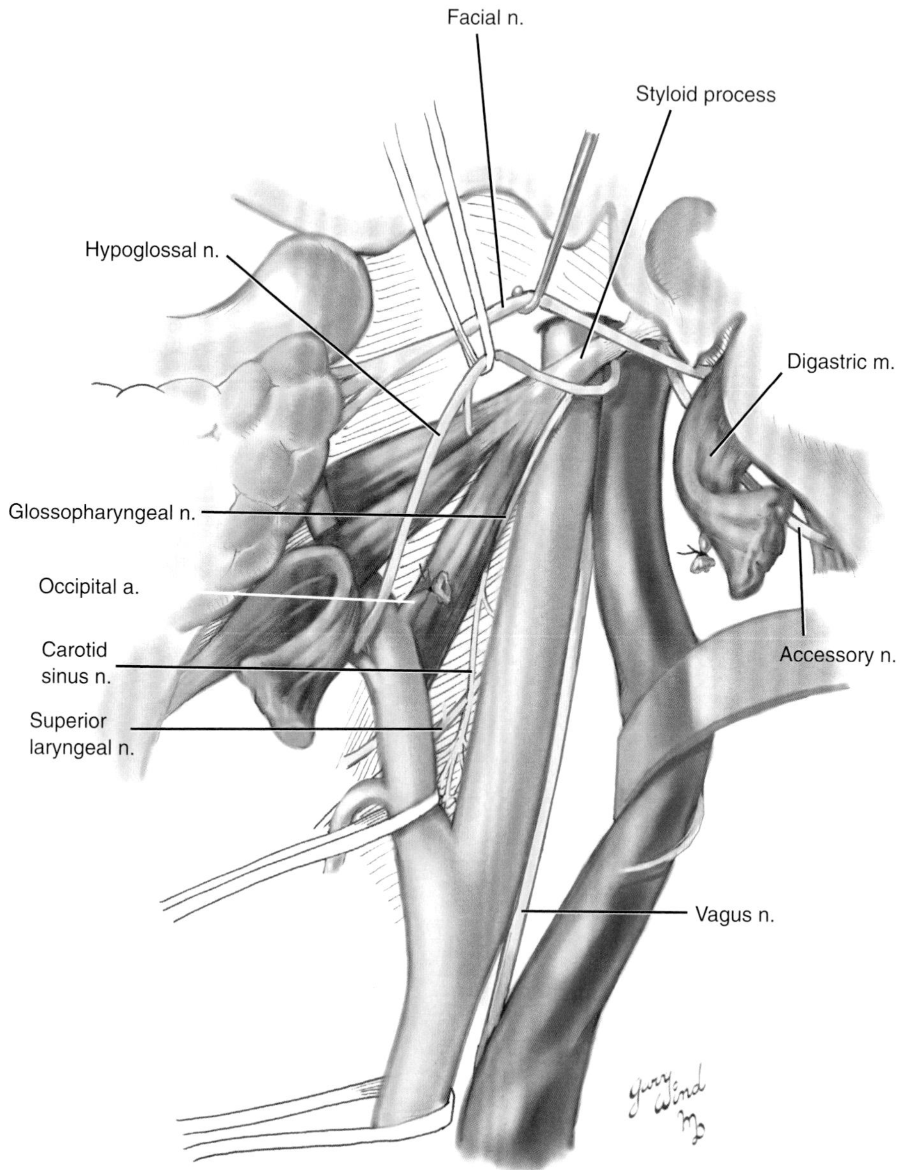

Fig. 1-26 Division of the posterior belly of the digastric muscle and of the occipital artery allows cephalad mobilization of the hypoglossal nerve. If the styloid process is divided, dissection must adhere closely to the bone to avoid injury to the immediately subjacent glossopharyngeal nerve.

The occipital artery and its accompanying vein course near the lower margin of the posterior belly of the digastric muscle and should be ligated at the time of muscle division. Higher exposure of the internal carotid artery is obtainable by dividing the stylohyoid ligament and stylohyoid, stylopharyngeus, and styloglossus muscles to permit removal of the styloid process.[28] The glossopharyngeal nerve is at risk for injury during these maneuvers. The nerve courses between the internal carotid artery and internal jugular vein, lying deep to the styloid process and attached muscles. Although the nerve may not be adequately exposed, the risk of injury can be lessened by confining dissection of the internal carotid to its periadventitial tissues.[29]

Should more superior isolation of the internal carotid artery be desired, exposure and gentle retraction of the facial nerve are required. Excision of the tail of the parotid will assist soft tissue exposure behind the mandible.[28] A preauricular extension of the cervical incision may be required to expose the facial nerve safely. The intrapetrosal internal carotid artery can be exposed using an anterior infratemporal approach described by Thomassin and Branchereau.[30]

References

1. Brott TG, Hobson RW II, Howard G, et al. Stenting versus endarterectomy for treatment of carotid-artery stenosis. *N Engl J Med.* 2010;363(1):11–23.
2. Cunningham EJ, Bond R, Matberg MR, et al. Risk of persistent cranial nerve injury after carotid endarterectomy. *J Neurosurg.* 2004;101:445–448.
3. Ferguson GG, Eliasziw M, Barr HWK, et al. The North American symptomatic carotid endarterectomy trial: surgical results in 1,415 patients. *Stroke.* 1999;30:1751–1758.
4. AbuRahma AF, Choueiri MA. Cranial and cervical nerve injuries after repeat carotid endarterectomy. *J Vasc Surg.* 2000;32(4):649–654.
5. Basile RM, Sadighi PJ. Carotid endarterectomy: importance of cranial nerve anatomy. *Clin Anat.* 1989;2(3):147–155.
6. Moffat DA, Ramsden RT. The deformity produced by a palsy of the marginal mandibular branch of the facial nerve. *J Laryngol Otol.* 1977;91:401–406.
7. Tulley P, Webb A, Chana JS, et al. Paralysis of the marginal mandibular branch of the facial nerve: treatment options. *Br J Plast Surg.* 2000;53(5):378–385.
8. Tchibukmacher NB. Surgical anatomy of carotid sinus nerve and intercarotid ganglion. *Surg Gynecol Obstet.* 1938;67:740–745.
9. Perry MO. Basic considerations in the diagnosis and management of carotid artery injuries. *J Vasc Surg.* 1988;8(2):193–194.
10. Monson DO, Saletta JD, Freeark RJ. Carotidñvertebral trauma. *J Trauma.* 1969;9(12):987–999.
11. Schauber MD, Fontanelle LJ, Soloman JW, et al. Cranial/cervical nerve dysfunction after carotid endarterectomy. *J Vasc Surg.* 1997;25:481–487.
12. Fróes LB, Castro de Tolosa EM, Camarga RD, et al. Blood supply of the human sternocleidomastoid muscle by the sternocleidomastoid branch of the occipital artery. *Clin Anat.* 1999;12(6):412–416.
13. Yagnik PM, Chang PS. Spinal accessory nerve injury: a complication of carotid endarterectomy. *Muscle & Nerve.* 1996;19:907–909.
14. Coady MA, Adler F, Davila JJ, et al. Nonrecurrent laryngeal nerve during carotid artery surgery: case report and literature review. *J Vasc Surg.* 2000;32:192–196.
15. Demos NJ. The ansa hypoglossi as a guide to the hypoglossi nerve during carotid endarterectomy and related anatomy. *Surg Rounds.* 1984;7(12):50–52.
16. Hertzer NR, Feldman BJ, Beven EG, et al. A prospective study of the incidence of injury to the cranial nerves during carotid endarterectomy. *Surg Gynecol Obstet.* 1980;151:781–784.
17. Bove EL, Fry WJ, Gross WS, et al. Hypotension and hypertension as consequence of baroreceptor dysfunction following carotid endarterectomy. *Surgery.* 1979;85:633–637.
18. Tarlov E, Schmidek H, Scott RM, et al. Reflex hypotension following carotid endarterectomy: mechanism and management. *J Neurosurg.* 1973;39:323–327.
19. Elliott BM, Collins GJ, Youkey JR, et al. Intraoperative local anesthetic injection of the carotid sinus nerve: a prospective, randomized study. *Am J Surg.* 1986;152(6):695–699.
20. Reva VA, Pronchenko AA, Samokhvalov IM. Operative management of penetrating carotid artery injuries. *Eur J Vasc Endovasc Surg.* 2011;42(1):16–20.
21. Nelson SR, Schow SR, Stein SM, et al. Enhanced surgical exposure for the high extracranial carotid artery. *Ann Vasc Surg.* 1992;6:467–472.
22. Perdue GF, Pellegrini RV, Arena S. Aneurysms of the high carotid artery: a new approach. *Surgery.* 1981;89(2):268–270.
23. Pellegrini RV, Manzetti GW, DiMarco RF, et al. The direct surgical management of lesions of the high internal carotid artery. *J Cardiovasc Surg.* 1984;25:29–35.
24. Fisch UP, Oldring DJ, Senning A. Surgical therapy of internal carotid artery lesions of the skull base and temporal bone. *Otolaryngol Head Neck Surg.* 1980;88(5):548–554.
25. Fisher DF, Clagett GP, Parker JI, et al. Mandibular subluxation for high carotid exposure. *J Vasc Surg.* 1984;1(6):727–733.

26. Simonian GT, Pappas PJ, Padberg FT Jr, et al. Mandibular subluxation for distal internal carotid exposure: technical considerations. *J Vasc Surg.* 1999;30:1116–1120.
27. Yoshino M, Fukumoto H, Mizutani T, et al. Mandibular subluxation stabilized by mouthpiece for distal internal carotid artery exposure in carotid endarterectomy. *J Vasc Surg.* 2010;52:1401–1404.
28. Shaha A, Phillips T, Scalea T, et al. Exposure of the internal carotid artery near the skull base: the posterolateral anatomic approach. *J Vasc Surg.* 1988;8(5):618–622.
29. Rosenbloom M, Friedman SG, Lamparello PJ, et al. Glossopharyngeal nerve injury complicating carotid endarterectomy. *J Vasc Surg.* 1987;5:469–471.
30. Thomassin JM, Branchereau A. Intrapetrosal internal carotid artery. In: Branchereau A, Berguer R, eds. *Vascular Surgical Approaches*. Armonk, NY: Futura; 1999:15–20.

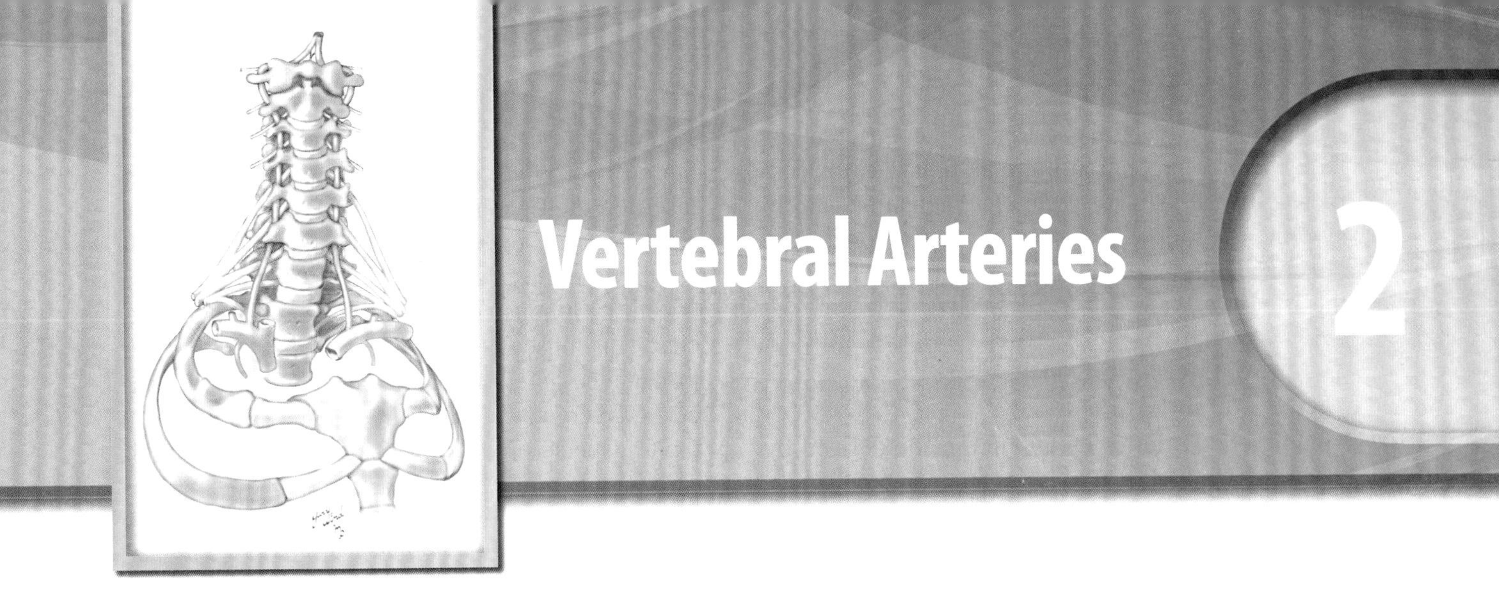

2 Vertebral Arteries

Surgical Anatomy of the Vertebral Arteries

Deep in the root of the neck, the vertebral arteries run the first third of their course from the proximal subclavian arteries to the transverse processes of the sixth cervical vertebrae (Fig. 2-1). For the remaining two-thirds of their course to the foramen magnum, the arteries are encased in a ladder-like bony lattice made up of the fenestrated transverse processes of the upper cervical vertebrae. The foramina for the artery occupy the anterior portion of the trough-like transverse processes, while the roots of the cervical nerves occupy the posterior position.

After passing through the transverse processes of the atlas, the arteries loop behind the articular processes and follow an anterior converging course upward through the foramen magnum. Within the cranium, the vertebral arteries unite at the lower border of the pons to form the basilar artery.

Vertebral a.
Carotid tubercle (C6 transverse process)
Thyrocervical trunk
Subclavian a.
Internal thoracic a.

Fig. 2-1 The proximal third of the vertebral artery lies in the deepest plane at the root of the neck. The remainder of the vessel lies within the bony lattice of the cervical transverse processes anterior to the cervical nerve trunks.

The deep central location of the vertebral arteries affords protection but makes surgical access more difficult than access to the companion carotid system. The following discussion focuses on the details of important relationships at different levels of the arteries.

Anterior Paravertebral Musculature

The vertebral arteries lie within a plane defined by a delta-shaped array of muscles attaching to the vertebral bodies and transverse processes (Fig. 2-2). The longus colli and longus capitis muscles provide anterior support to the cervical vertebrae and bracket the anterior longitudinal ligament of the spine between them. Laterally, the scalene muscles fan out from the cervical transverse processes and insert on the first and second ribs. The lower cervical nerve roots emerge between anterior and middle scalene muscles, while the upper roots appear between the longus capitis and levator scapulae muscles. This muscular delta is covered by prevertebral fascia. The anterior scalene and longus colli muscles converge at the prominent anterior tubercle of the transverse process of C6, sometimes called the carotid tubercle (of Chassaignac). In the inverted "V" formed by the muscles below this landmark, the first portion of the vertebral artery penetrates the prevertebral fascia to ascend through the C6 transverse foramen.

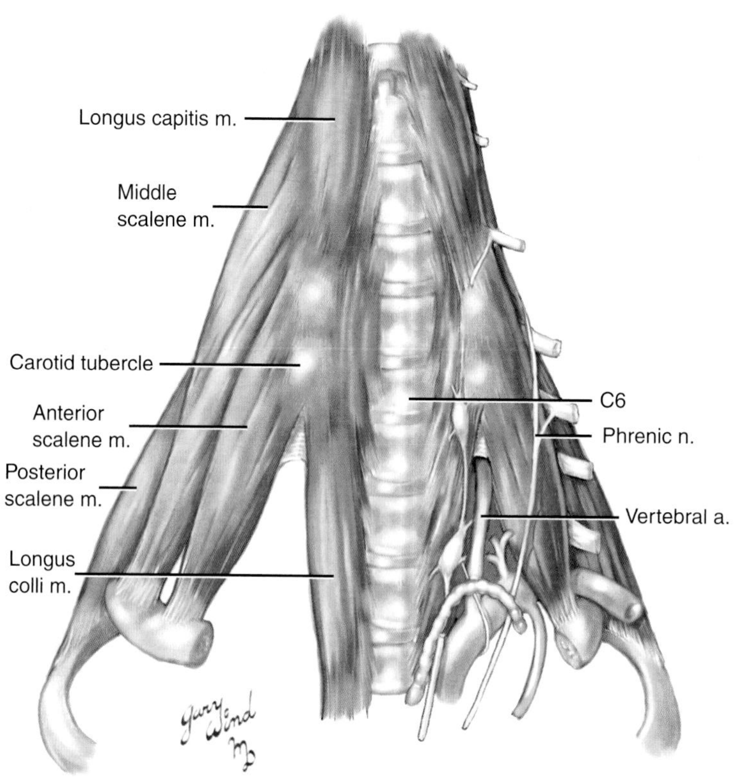

Fig. 2-2 The vertebral artery penetrates and lies buried beneath the delta of prevertebral and scalene muscles.

The Root of the Neck

The vertebral arteries originate from the first part of the subclavian arteries close to the origins of the internal thoracic (formerly internal mammary), thyrocervical, and costocervical vessels (Fig. 2-3). These origins are arrayed radially around the subclavian with the vertebral arising superiorly and posteriorly. The first portion of the vertebral arteries passes over the cupola of the lung to reach the scalenovertebral angle.

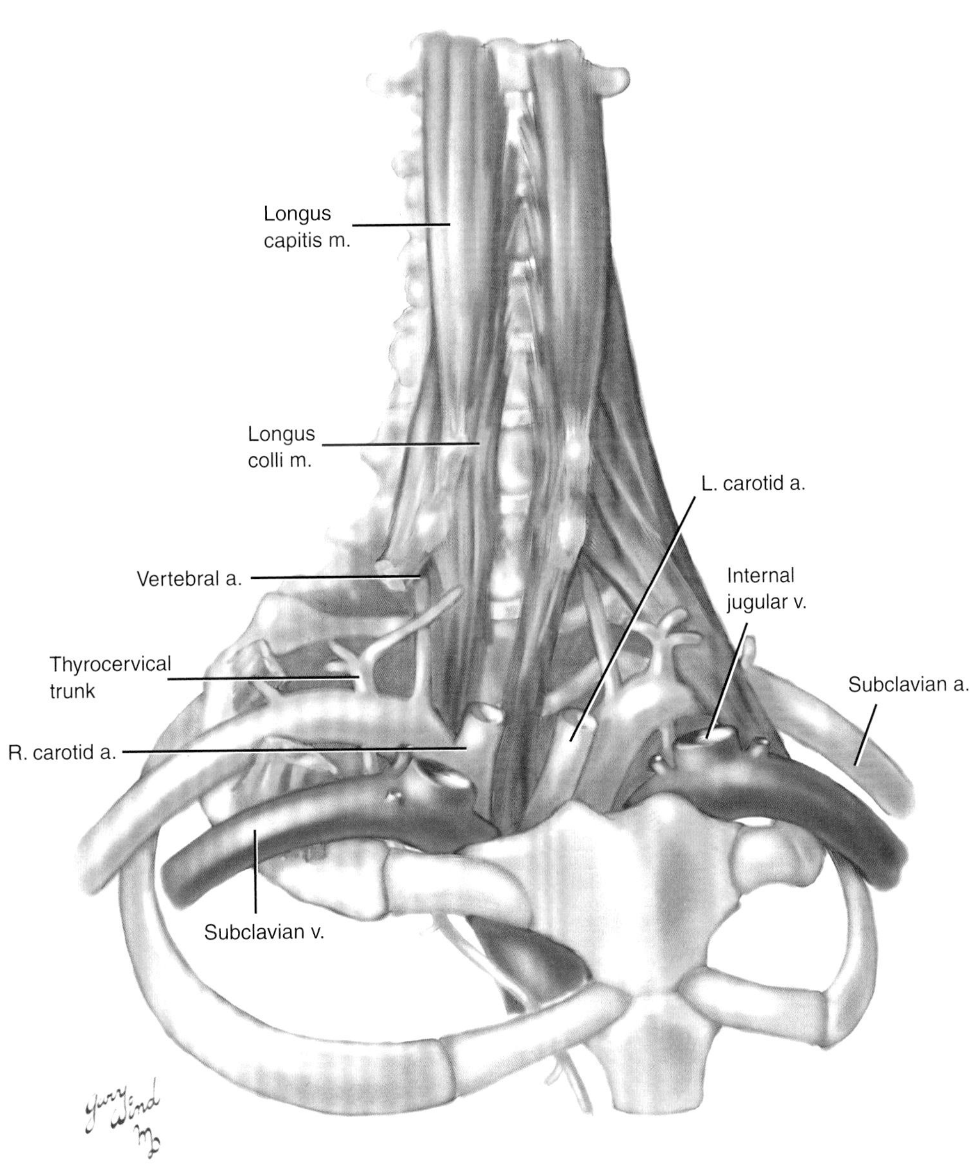

Fig. 2-3 The great vessels at the root of the neck overlie the vertebral arteries and must be mobilized during surgical approaches to the vertebral arteries.

The venous tributaries that accompany the distal vertebral artery converge to form a single vertebral vein on emerging from the sixth transverse process (Fig. 2-4). The vein enters the proximal subclavian vein just distal to the internal jugular vein. On the left side, the thoracic duct emerges from the posterior thorax, arches over the subclavian artery, and enters the subclavian vein between the internal jugular and vertebral veins.

The cervical sympathetic chain lies on the prevertebral fascia anterior to the longus colli and capitis muscles, which in turn lie anterior to the transverse processes housing the vertebral arteries. The middle cervical sympathetic ganglion lies at about the level of the carotid tubercle, and the inferior ganglion lies posteromedial to the origin of the vertebral artery. The inferior ganglion gives off fibers that wrap around and ascend with the vertebral artery.

The costocervical trunk arises posteriorly from the subclavian. Its cervical division ascends in the deep posterior cervical muscles and communicates with the vertebral along its course and with descending branches of the occipital artery.

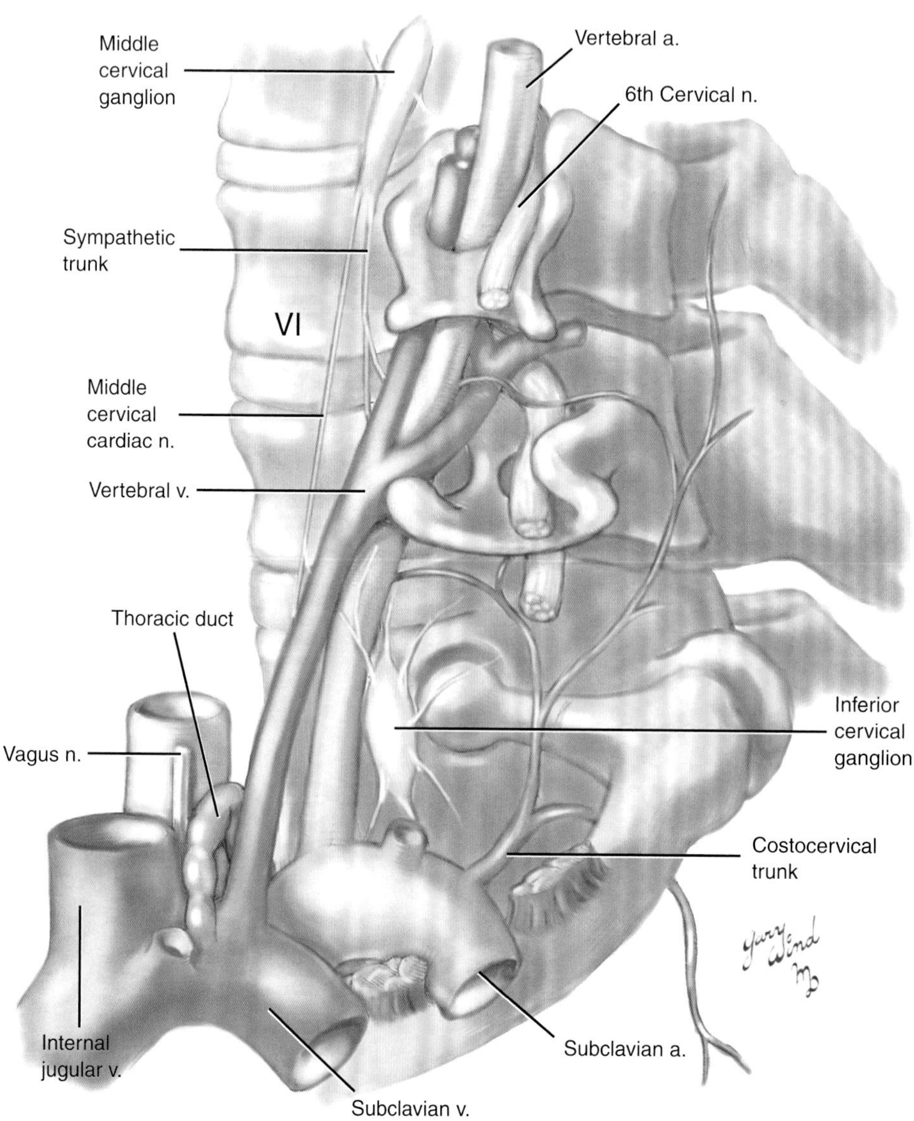

Fig. 2-4 In this lateral view of the proximal left vertebral artery, the scalene fat pad has been removed to show relationships to the thoracic duct, venous, and neural structures.

Anterior Relations of the Proximal and Midvertebral Artery

Beneath skin and platysma, the sternocleidomastoid muscle and investing fascia constitute the first layer to unroof on the way to the vertebral arteries (Fig. 2-5). The omohyoid muscle runs diagonally between the sternocleidomastoid and the underlying carotid sheath. The carotid sheath lies between the sternocleidomastoid muscle and prevertebral fascia medially, and lateral to the sheath, the scalene fat pad directly overlies the first portion of the vertebral artery.

In and around the fat pad are critical structures that must be respected when approaching the vertebral artery. Medially on the left side is the previously described thoracic duct. Deep to the fat pad laterally, the phrenic nerves descend diagonally across the anterior scalene muscles, pass lateral to the thyrocervical trunks, and dip between subclavian artery and vein to enter the chest. The inferior thyroid artery crosses anterior to the proximal vertebral artery.

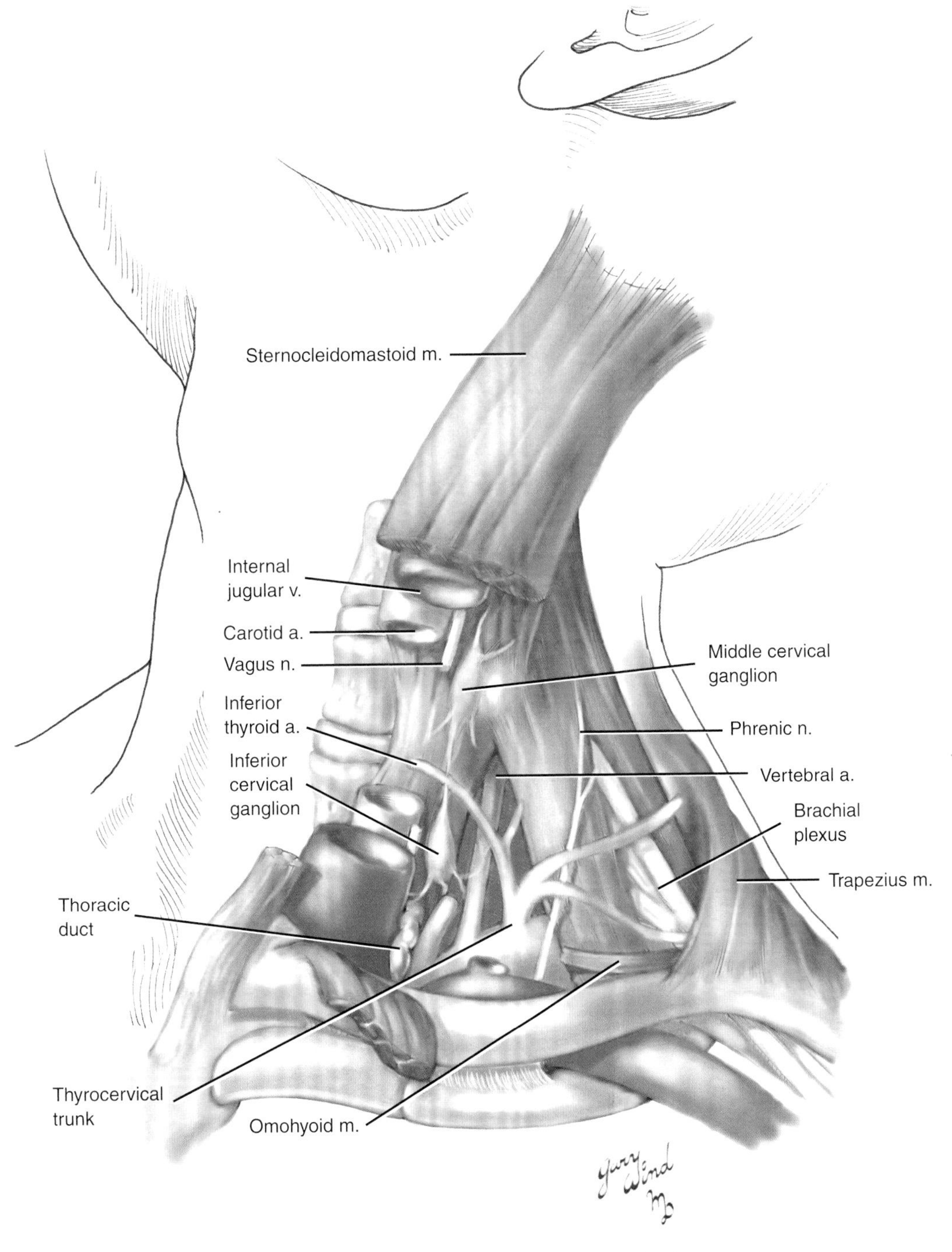

Fig. 2-5 This cut-away view shows the major anatomic landmarks that must be negotiated to reach the vertebral artery.

The Distal Vertebral Artery

Between the transverse processes of the atlas and axis vertebrae, there is more space for access to the vertebral arteries than in other interspaces due to the decreased bulk of the bony arches posteriorly (Fig. 2-6). After emerging through the foramina of the atlas, the arteries take a sharp bend backward and lie in grooves encircling the posterior rims of the bony articular plateaus. They then course anteriorly, medial to the atlantooccipital articulation, and pass through the foramen magnum.

At the level of the posterior groove, the arteries give off branches to the deep muscles of the neck that anastomose with ascending cervical, occipital, and deep cervical arteries. Medial to the articular facets, the arteries give off branches that descend within the vertebral canal, supplying vertebral bodies and meninges. Prior to converging at the level of the pons, small descending branches fuse to form a midline vessel along the ventral surface of the medulla.

The tortuous terminal extracranial vertebral arteries lie deep within the suboccipital muscular triangles and are difficult to expose (Fig. 2-7).

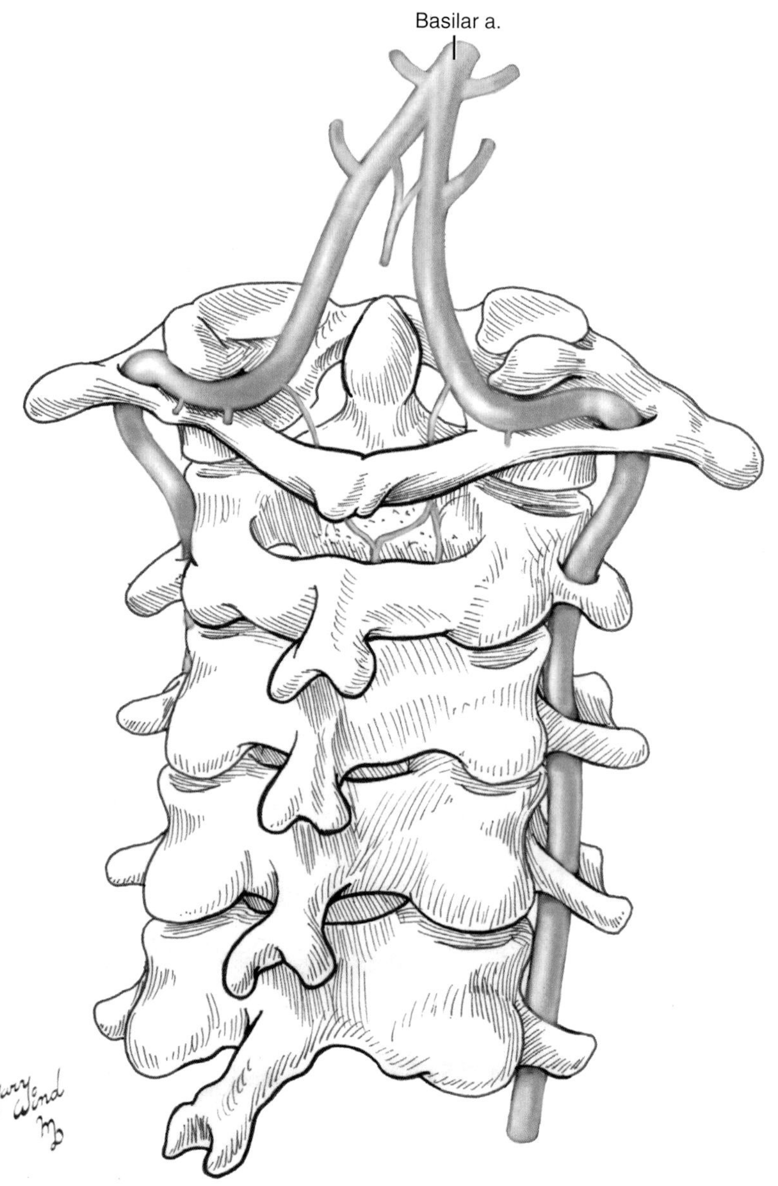

Fig. 2-6 The space between the transverse processes of the atlas and axis vertebrae affords the best exposure of the distal vertebral artery. The arterial segment above the atlas is the site of collateral arterial connections and is surrounded by a prohibitively dense venous plexus.

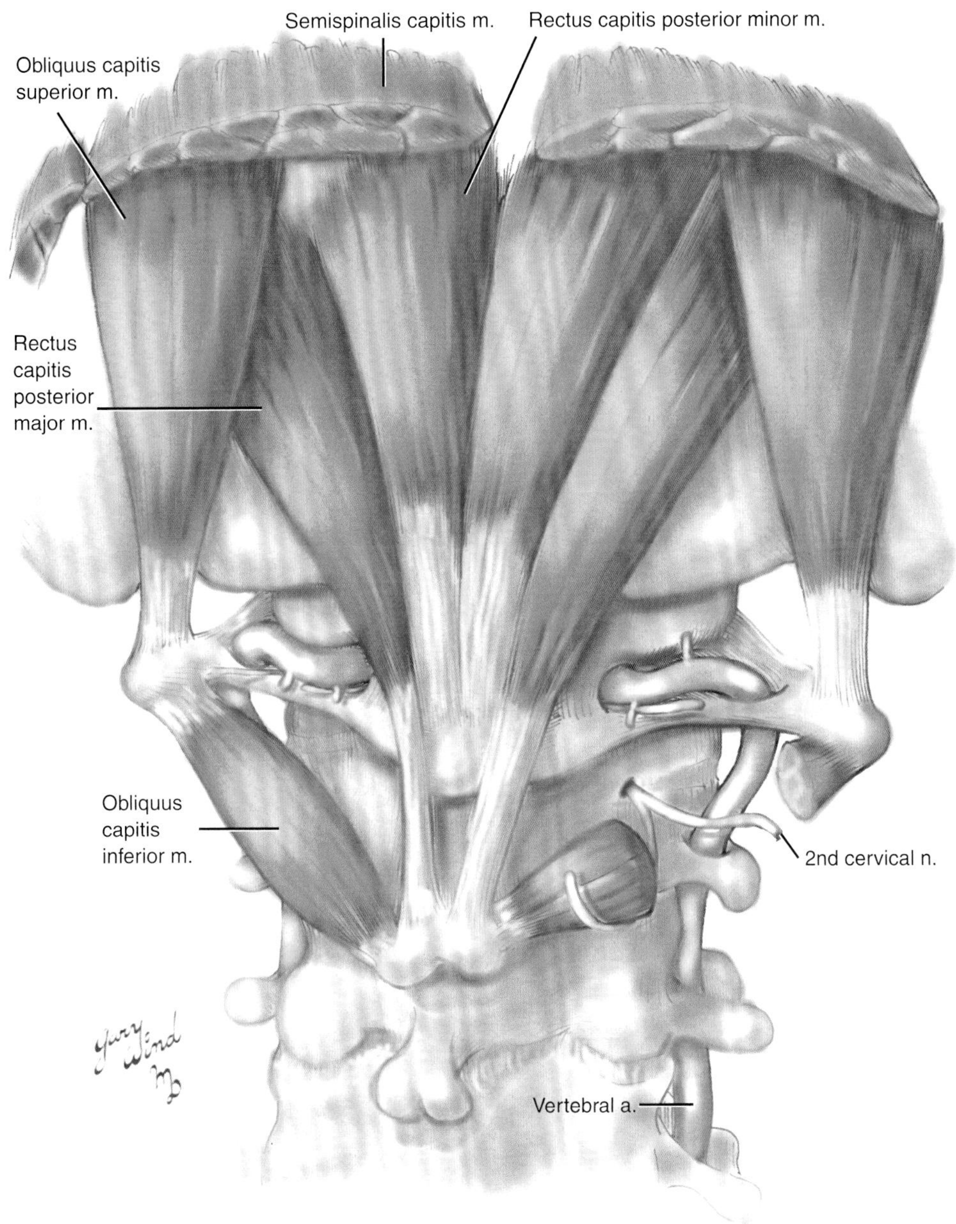

Fig. 2-7 The depth of the vessel in the posterior cervical triangle is shown in this view.

An anterolateral approach to the C1 to C2 segment is possible by detaching the levator scapulae origins from the tips of the transverse processes (Fig. 2-8).

After passing around the posterior part of the articular process, the vertebral artery penetrates first the atlantooccipital ligament and then the dura on its way to the foramen magnum (Fig. 2-9).

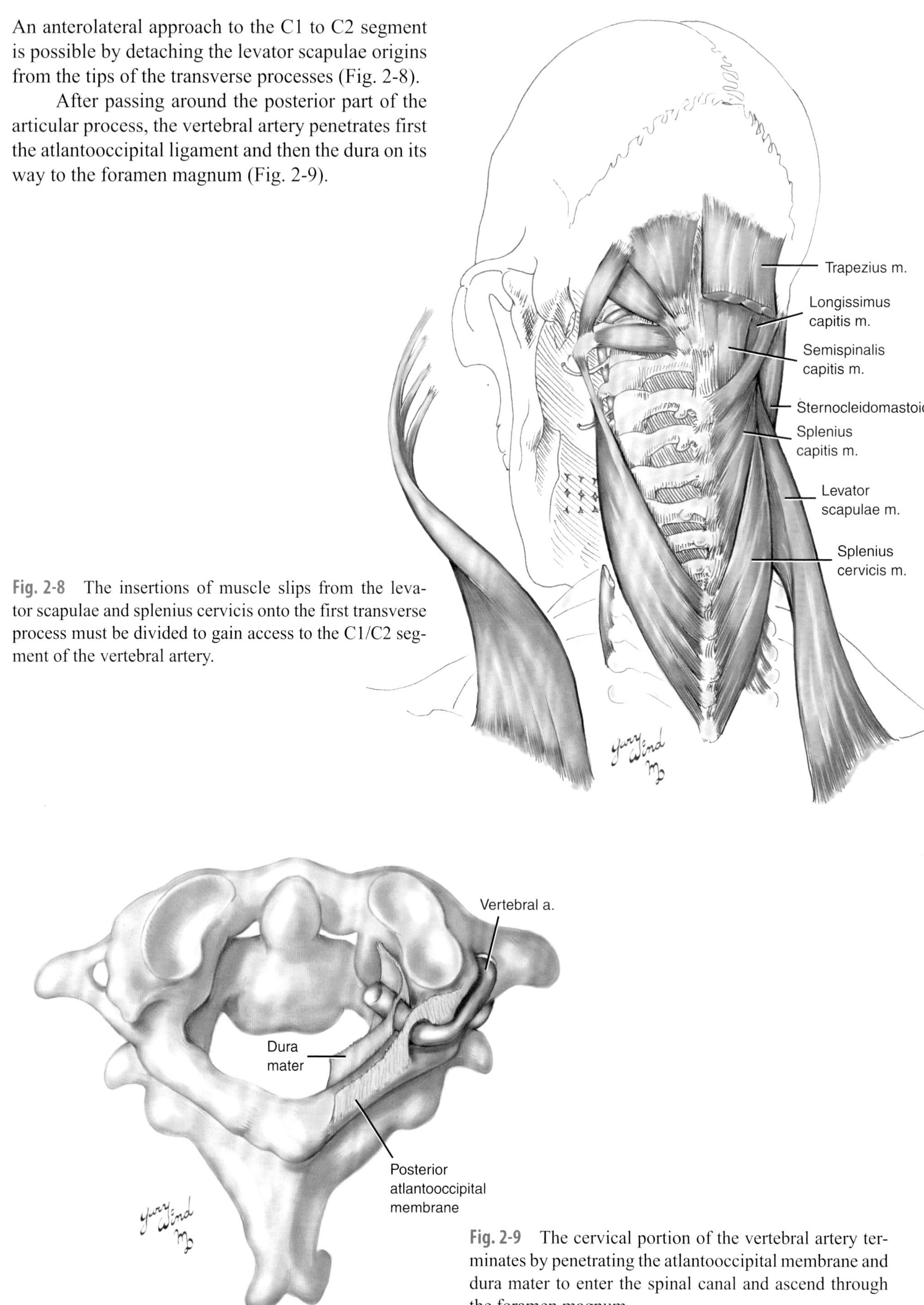

Fig. 2-8 The insertions of muscle slips from the levator scapulae and splenius cervicis onto the first transverse process must be divided to gain access to the C1/C2 segment of the vertebral artery.

Fig. 2-9 The cervical portion of the vertebral artery terminates by penetrating the atlantooccipital membrane and dura mater to enter the spinal canal and ascend through the foramen magnum.

Exposure of the Vertebral Artery in the Neck

A number of approaches are available to expose the extracranial vertebral artery, depending on the segment. A useful classification for describing the regional anatomy of the vertebral artery has been highlighted by Morasch[1] (Fig. 2-10). The most proximal segment (V1) extends from the subclavian origin of the vertebral artery to the level at which the artery enters the transverse process of C6. The interosseous segment (V2) courses within the transverse processes of the cervical vertebrae from C6 to C2. The third segment (V3) begins at the top of the C2 transverse process and terminates at the base of the skull. The intracranial portion (V4) begins at the atlantooccipital membrane and terminates at the basilar artery.

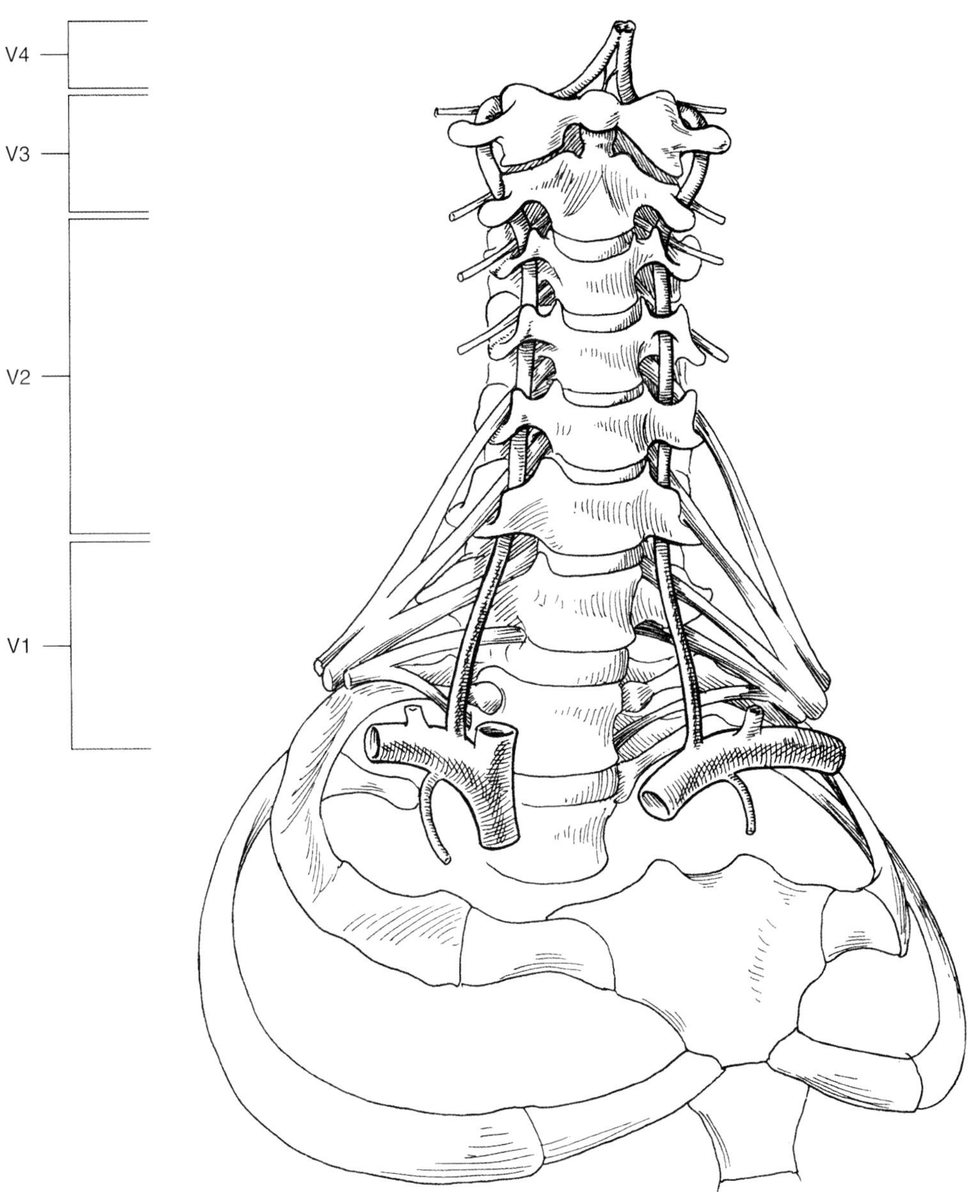

Fig. 2-10 The surgical segments of the vertebral arteries are shown.

Exposure of the Extraosseous Vertebral Artery (V1 Segment)

There are two main options for exposure of the most proximal portion of the vertebral artery: the transverse supraclavicular approach and the vertical anterior cervical approach. Although the supraclavicular approach affords excellent exposure of the vertebral artery at its origin, the exposure is relatively limited and requires transection of the sternocleidomastoid muscle. The anterior cervical approach does not require muscular transection, and it permits rapid extension of the incision for vascular control of more distal vertebral artery segments. However, exposure of the vertebral artery is more difficult through a cervical incision. In general, the supraclavicular approach is employed for elective operations involving vertebral artery reimplantation into the adjacent common carotid artery, and the anterior cervical approach is favored during emergency explorations for suspected vertebral artery injury.[1–4]

Supraclavicular Approach

The patient is supine, and the head is turned away from the side of surgery. The incision is made approximately 1 cm above the clavicle, beginning at the clavicular head and extending laterally for a distance of 7 or 8 cm (Fig. 2-11). The incision is

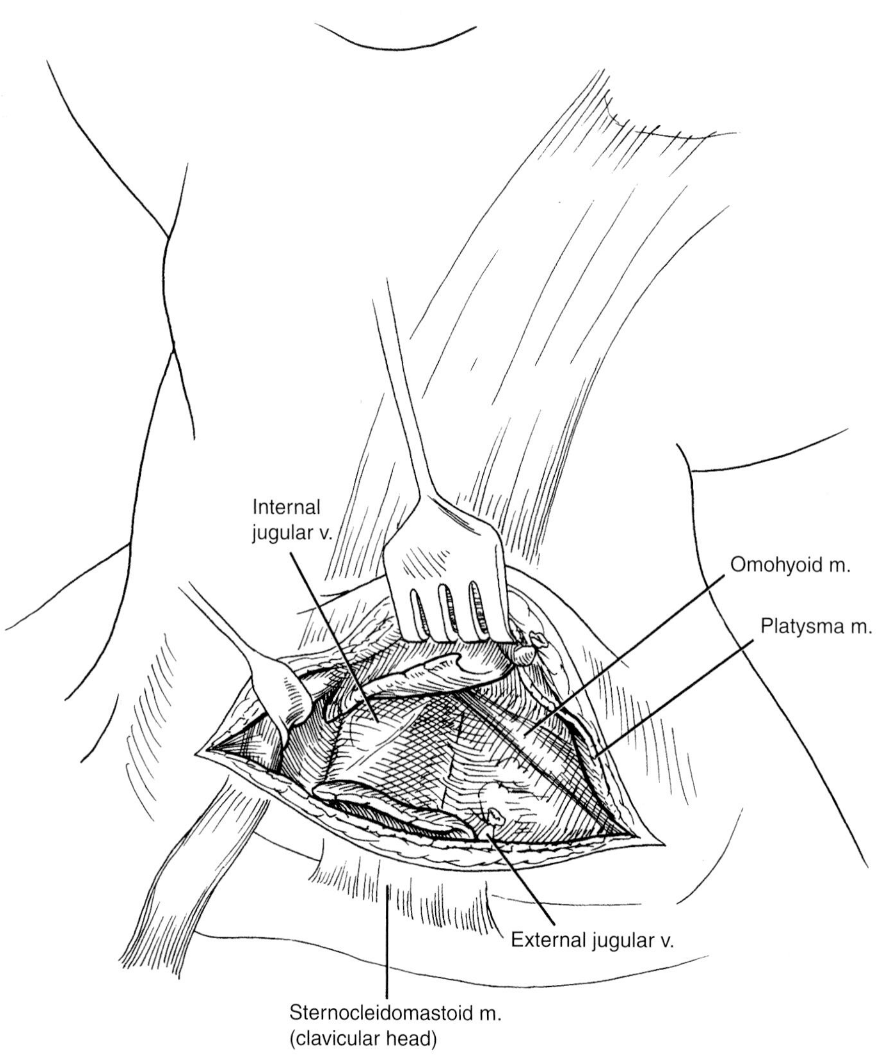

Fig. 2-11 The transverse supraclavicular incision is carried down through the clavicular head of the sternocleidomastoid muscle.

deepened through the platysma muscle and superficial fascia. The external jugular vein is divided at the lateral border of the sternocleidomastoid muscle.

Division of the clavicular head of the sternocleidomastoid muscle and retraction of the sternal head exposes the underlying carotid sheath. The sheath is mobilized by vertical dissection along the lateral border of the internal jugular vein, and the omohyoid muscle is divided (Fig. 2-12). When operating on the left side, the thoracic duct should be ligated and divided near its termination at the angle of the junction of the left internal jugular and subclavian veins. If the common carotid artery is needed for subsequent vertebral artery reimplantation,[1,2,5,6] it is carefully isolated at this time and encircled with a silastic loop. Caution should be exercised during these dissections to avoid injury to the vagus nerve and to the sympathetic chain, which usually course in the posterolateral aspect of the carotid sheath. After dissection is complete, the carotid sheath contents are gently retracted into the medial incision with the sternal head of the sternocleidomastoid muscle.

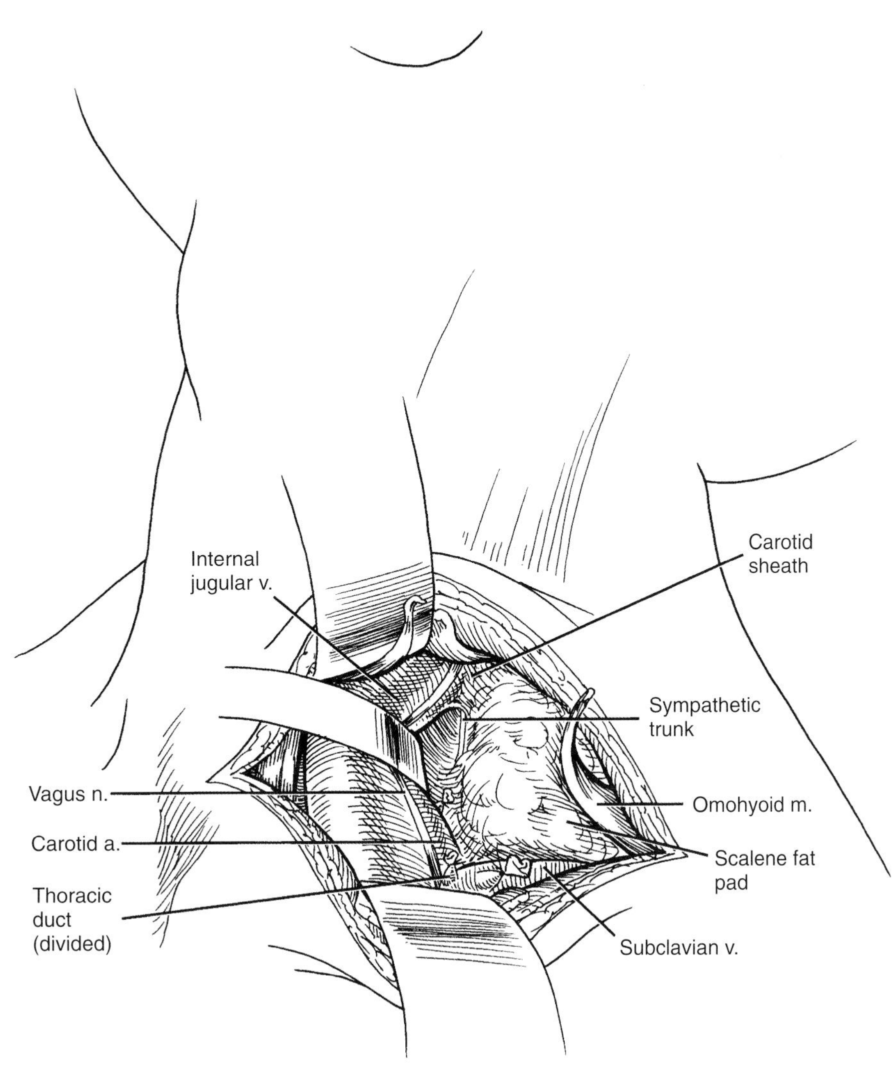

Fig. 2-12 Omohyoid muscle, external jugular vein, and thoracic duct (*on the left*) are divided, and the carotid sheath is mobilized medially.

The medial margin of the scalene fat pad is next mobilized, and the fat pad is retracted laterally. Careful sharp dissection is required in order to identify superficial vascular structures coursing within the fat pad, which must be individually ligated to ensure good hemostasis. Mobilization of the fat pad exposes the underlying anterior scalene muscle. The phrenic nerve is located on the ventral surface of the anterior scalene muscle and is usually found coursing near the muscle's medial border (Fig. 2-13). Edwards and Edwards[2] note that visualization of the phrenic nerve and anterior scalene muscle should alert the surgeon that the dissection has proceeded too far laterally. However, identification of these structures helps to insure that the phrenic nerve will not be inadvertently injured from a poorly positioned retractor.

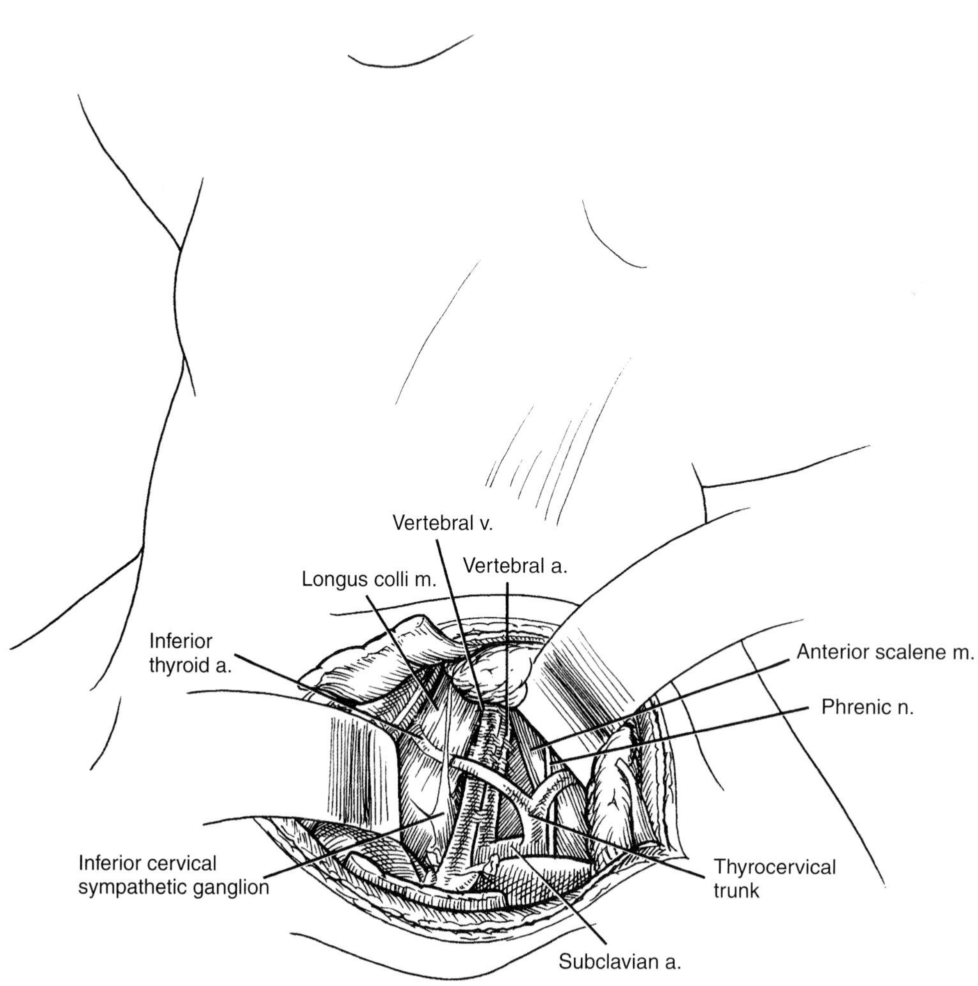

Fig. 2-13 Careful medial to lateral dissection of the scalene fat pad reveals the sympathetic chain, anterior scalene muscle, and phrenic nerve. The inferior thyroid artery and vertebral vein overlie the proximal vertebral artery.

The vertebral artery is located in the center of the angle formed by the anterior scalene and longus colli muscles. The artery is most easily identified and isolated by retracting the anterior scalene laterally (Fig. 2-14). Some authors advocate division of the anterior scalene muscle,[7] but this is rarely necessary. The vertebral artery should be exposed proximally to its origin at the subclavian artery. The nearby thyrocervical trunk can be differentiated from the vertebral artery by its multiple branches. The latter has no branches at this level. The inferior thyroid branch of the thyrocervical trunk crosses anterior to the vertebral artery and should be ligated. The accompanying vertebral vein should also be ligated. By continuing the dissection craniad, the entire extraosseous vertebral artery can be exposed to the level of the sixth cervical vertebrae, where the artery dips under the longus colli muscle to enter the transverse process of C6.

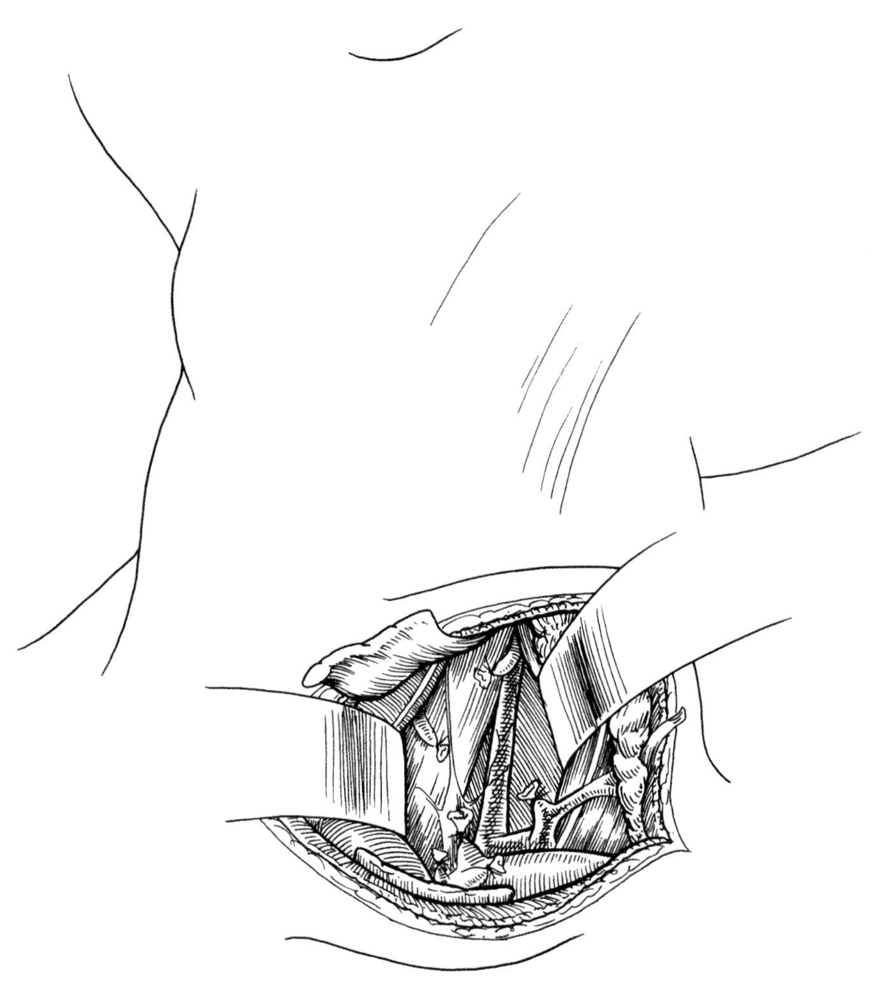

Fig. 2-14 Division of the inferior thyroid artery and vertebral vein exposes the artery.

Anterior Cervical Approach

The patient is placed in the supine position with the neck extended and head turned away from the side of the intended incision. A vertical incision is made along the anterior border of the sternocleidomastoid muscle, extending from the retromandibular area to the clavicular head. The incision is deepened through the platysma muscle and investing fascia to reach the anterior fibers of the sternocleidomastoid muscle. This muscle is dissected away from the underlying carotid sheath and retracted laterally (Fig. 2-15). The superior belly of the omohyoid muscle may be divided at this point to achieve adequate exposure in the inferior aspect of the wound. The carotid sheath and its contents are carefully freed by vertical dissection along the lateral border of the internal jugular vein. Great care

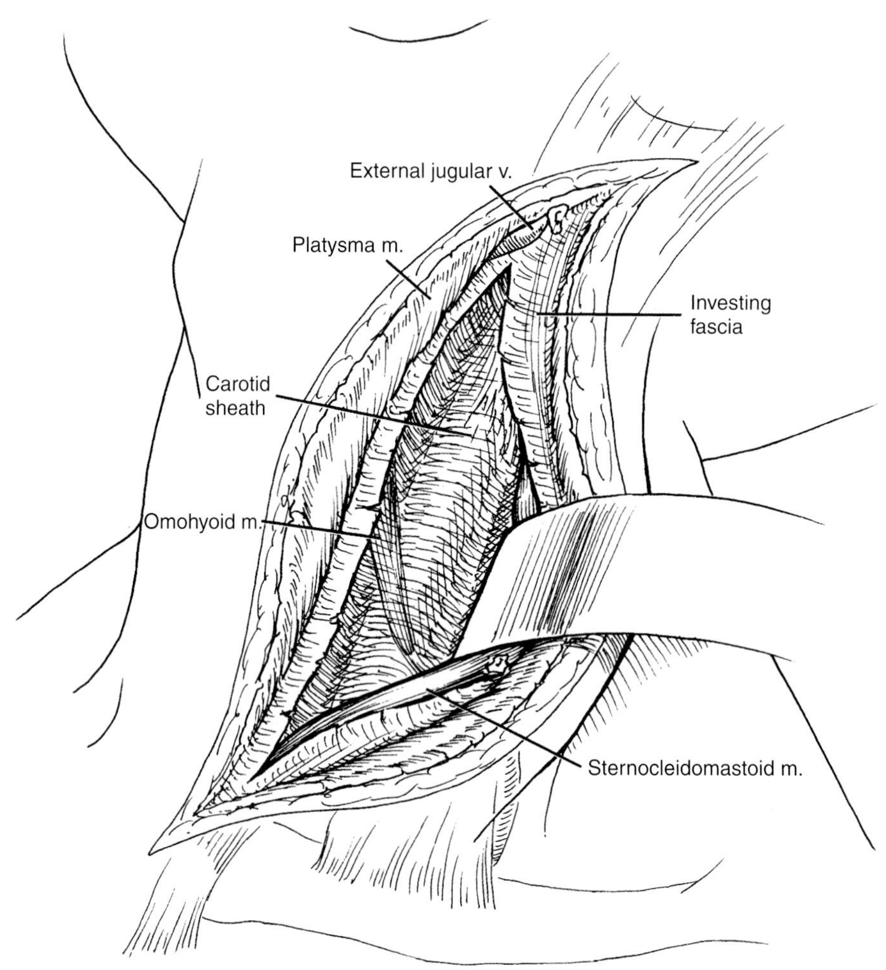

Fig. 2-15 An anterior longitudinal neck incision can be used to expose all three cervical segments of the vertebral artery.

should be taken to avoid injury to the vagus nerve and sympathetic chain, which course in the posterolateral aspect of the carotid sheath. Once freed from surrounding tissue, the carotid sheath and its contents are retracted medially[3] (Fig. 2-16). The scalene fat pad is mobilized along its medial border and retracted laterally, exposing the underlying anterior scalene muscle in the lateral wound. The phrenic nerve should be identified on the ventral border of the anterior scalene and protected from injury. The inferior thyroid artery should be ligated and divided as it crosses the medial border of the anterior scalene muscle. The vertebral artery is identified by retracting the anterior scalene muscle fibers laterally. The remainder of the dissection proceeds as above.

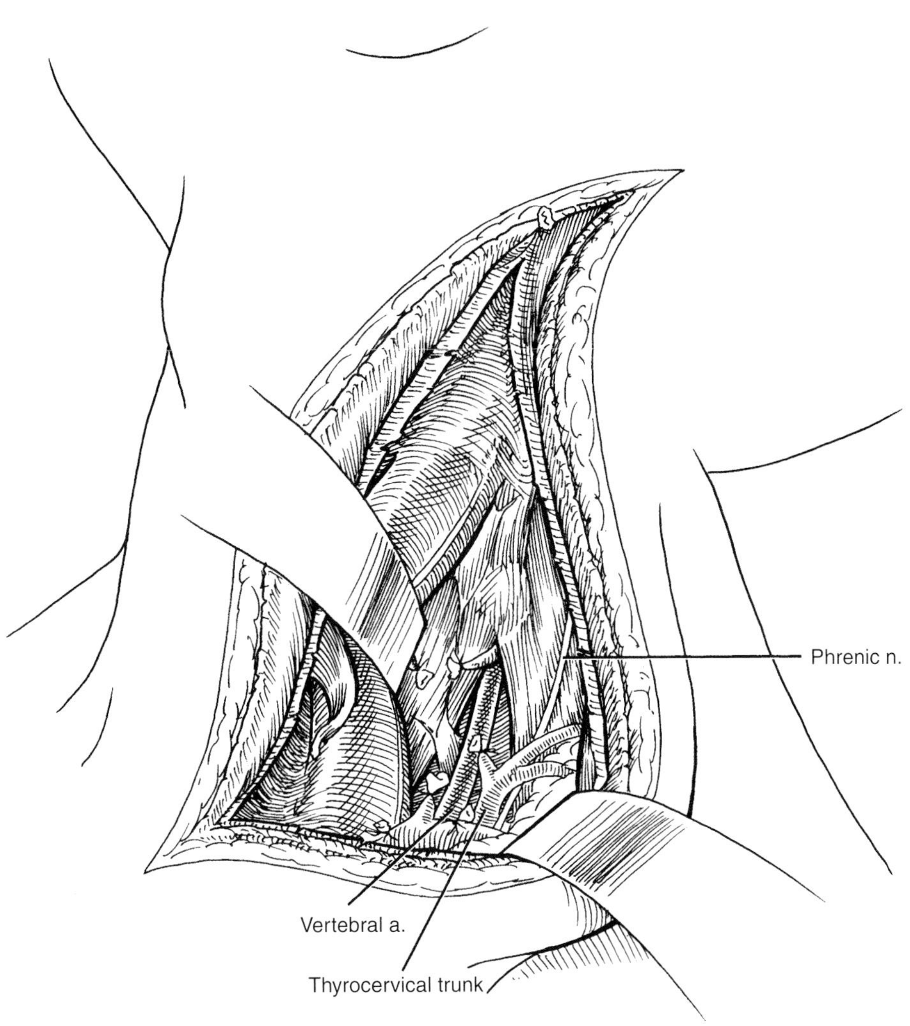

Fig. 2-16 Medial mobilization of the carotid sheath and proximal neck dissection as previously described exposes the proximal vertebral artery.

Exposure of the Interosseous Vertebral Artery (V2 Segment)

Control of hemorrhage is the most common indication for exposure of the vertebral artery segment lying within the foramina of the cervical transverse processes. Although the majority of vertebral injuries are now treated using endovascular means, there are still situations such as severe hemorrhage or endovascular failure when surgical control is necessary.[8] Ligation of vertebral arteries injured in this segment is appropriate and has not been associated with worsening neurologic sequellae.[3,9,10] Distal ligation is performed one transverse process above the injured interosseous vertebral artery, or higher if necessary. Direct exposure of the vertebral artery is best performed within the bony canal by unroofing the transverse process, as originally described by Shumacker.[11] Proximal ligation is performed in the extraosseous (V1) segment (see above).

The patient is placed in the supine position with the neck slightly extended and turned away from the side of operation. The same anterior cervical approach is used as shown in Figures 2-15 and 2-16. A vertical incision is made along the anterior border of the sternocleidomastoid muscle from the clavicular head to the mastoid process. The superior incision should be curved posteriorly at its uppermost margin, such that it passes just inferior to the lobe of the ear. The incision is deepened through the platysma muscle and investing fascia. The sternocleidomastoid muscle is freed from medial attachments and retracted laterally to expose the underlying carotid sheath. The carotid sheath, pharynx, and larynx are next freed from the prevertebral fascia by clearing attachments between the visceral and prevertebral fasciae in the retropharyngeal space. The carotid

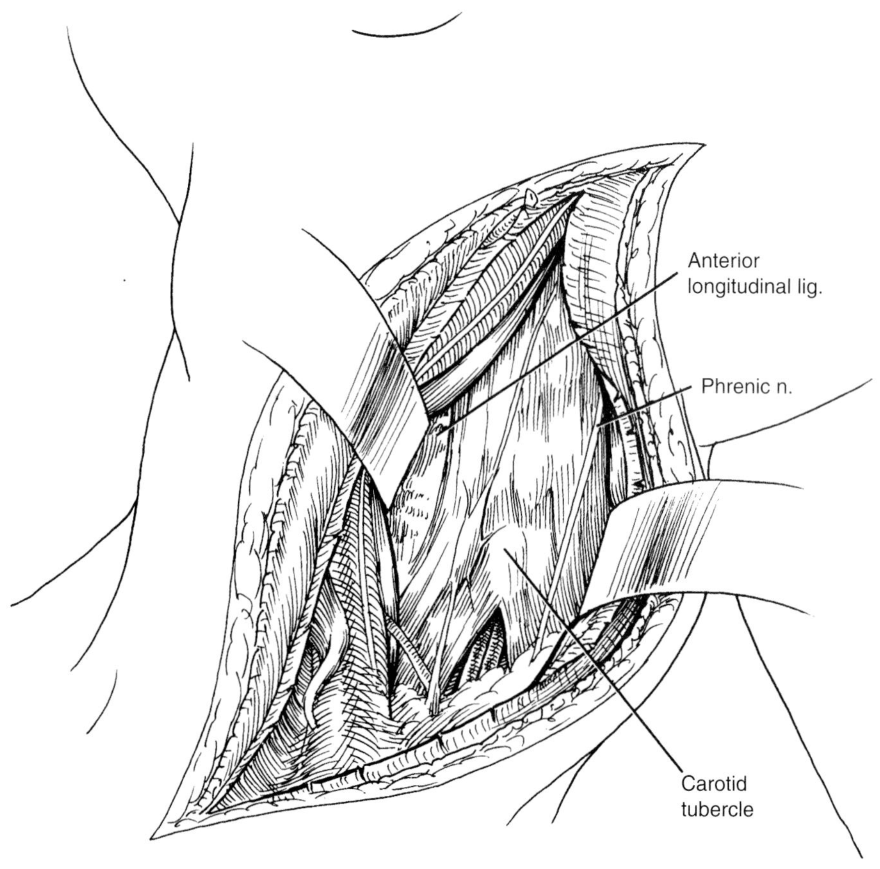

Fig. 2-17 Medial retraction of the carotid sheath and cervical viscera exposes the cervical vertebrae covered by the anterior longitudinal ligament.

sheath and visceral contents are retracted as far medially as possible, leaving the sympathetic ganglia lying on the prevertebral muscles just medial to the bulge of the transverse processes. The anterior longitudinal ligament is exposed deep in the medial wound (Fig. 2-17). It is incised vertically over the vertebral column for the length of the incision (Fig. 2-18). A periosteal elevator is used to separate the prevertebral fascia, longus colli, and longus capitis muscles away from the vertebral bodies and transverse processes.[3] It is extremely important to avoid extending the dissection beyond the lateral border of the transverse processes to prevent injury to the cervical nerve roots.[3]

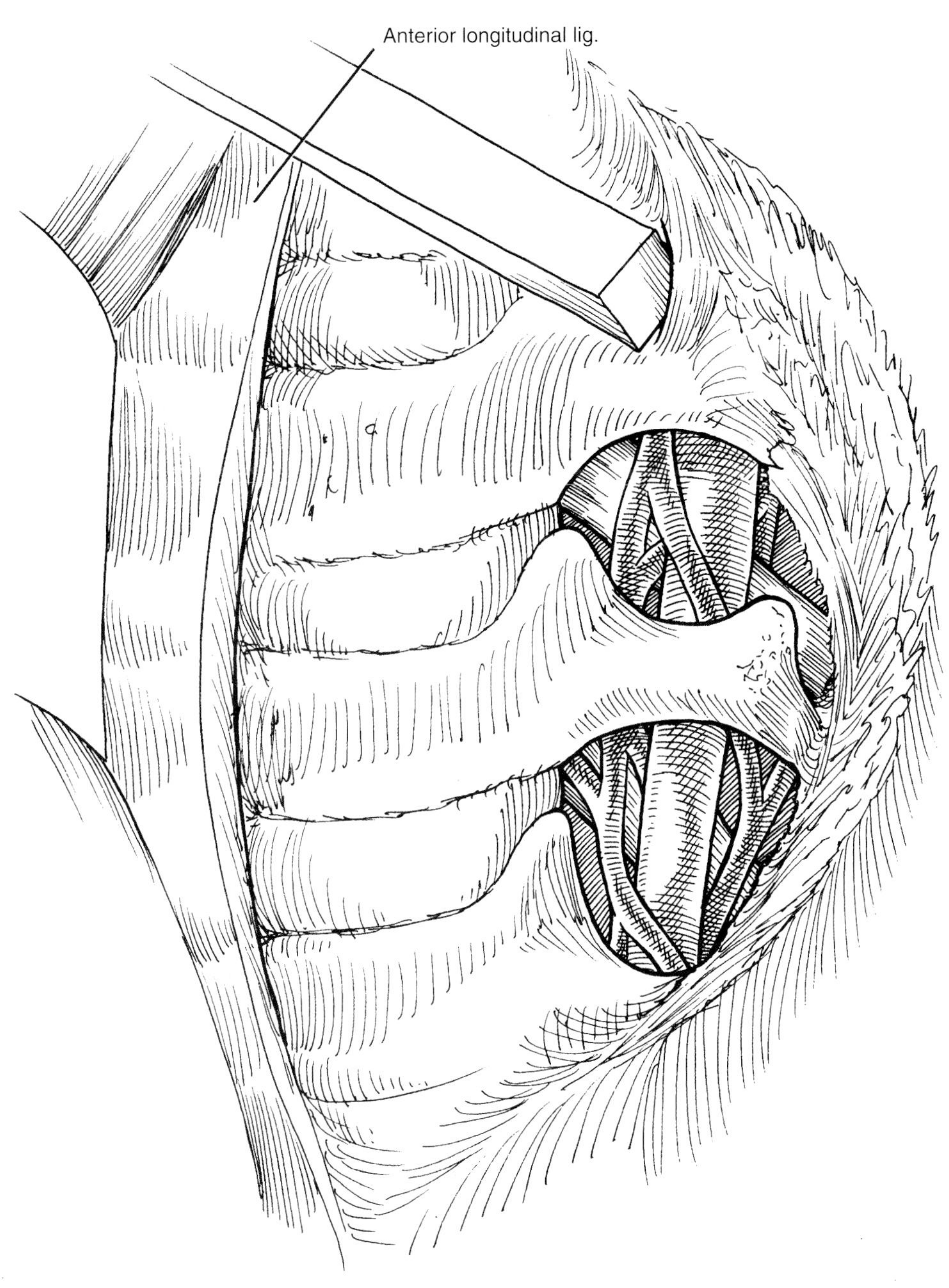

Fig. 2-18 Lateral retraction of anterior longitudinal ligament and anterior paraspinous muscles unroofs the transverse processes encasing the vertebral artery and veins.

The vertebral artery lies directly behind the bone forming the anterior border of the canal in the transverse process. The artery is most conveniently controlled within the bony canal rather than between the transverse processes because of the multiple venous tributaries that surround the artery in the latter segments.[3] The increased exposure afforded by entering the bony canal provides safer control of the artery. The bony canal is opened by removing the bone forming its anterior border. This can be accomplished with a small rongeur, working from cephalad to caudad[3] (Fig. 2-19).

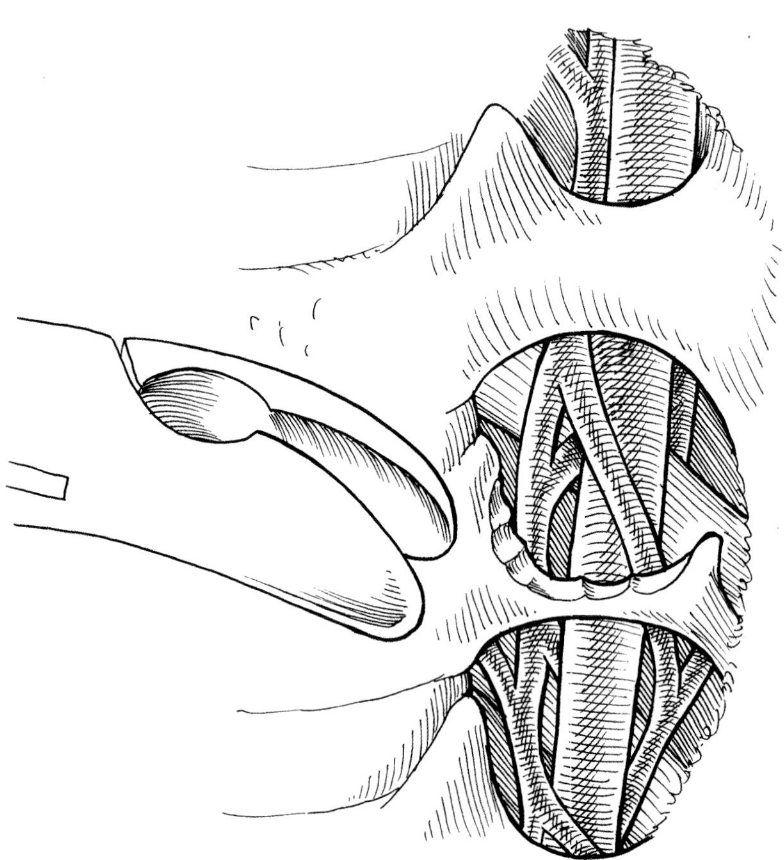

Fig. 2-19 Optimal access to the vertebral artery is obtained by removing the anterior arch of the transverse process.

Exposure of the Distal Extracranial Vertebral Artery (V3 Segment)

Berguer[12] has stated that the distal vertebral artery is surgically accessible within the space between the transverse processes of C1 and C2, the widest gap between the transverse processes of the cervical spine. Berguer's surgical approach was first described for use in constructing bypasses to the V3 artery segment.[12] In a 23-year experience with over 320 patients, Kieffer[13] has reported excellent long-term outcome after distal vertebral artery reconstruction. However, outside of specialized centers, the need to perform anastomoses in this area of the vertebral artery is very rare in clinical practice. The approach is more practical in the control of traumatic injuries to the distal vertebral artery. It may be a useful site for proximal control of the vertebral artery segment between C1 and the base of the skull, which is difficult to expose and has been associated with dangerous bleeding from the surrounding venous plexus.[3] Injuries to this arterial segment that require surgical control should be treated with proximal ligation of the artery in the space between the transverse processes of C1 and C2. As noted above, these injuries are more frequently treated with transcatheter techniques, which appear to be simpler, safer, and more rapid compared with operation. However, when endovascular techniques are not appropriate,[8] rapid proximal and distal ligation may be necessary. Proximal ligation is easily accomplished in the V1 segment, as described above. The following discussion concerns surgical exposure of the V3 segment at the space between the C1 and C2 transverse processes.

The patient is positioned as before. A vertical incision is made along the anterior border of the sternocleidomastoid muscle, extending from the level of the cricoid to the mastoid process (Fig. 2-20).

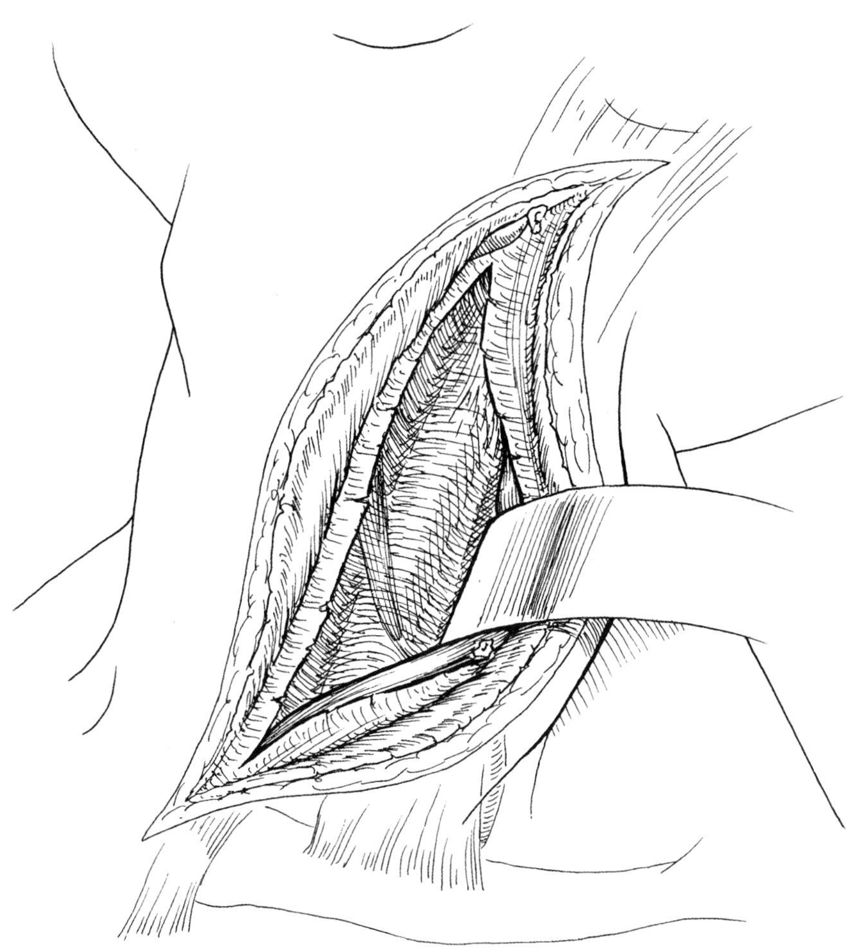

Fig. 2-20 The longitudinal incision is used for exposure of the distal vertebral artery.

The distal incision should be curved posteriorly just beneath the lobe of the ear to cross over the mastoid. The incision is deepened through the platysma muscle and investing fascia, and the sternocleidomastoid is dissected free and retracted laterally. The carotid sheath and contents are retracted medially as before. Some authors[3,14] prefer to detach the sternocleidomastoid and splenius capitis muscles from the mastoid process, but others[12] have found this to be unnecessary. Our dissections would strongly suggest that partial or complete detachment of the sternocleidomastoid origin greatly enhances exposure (Fig. 2-21). With either technique, it is important to identify the spinal accessory nerve, which usually enters the sternocleidomastoid 2 to 3 cm below the mastoid tip.[4,11] The nerve should be mobilized and gently retracted anteriorly.

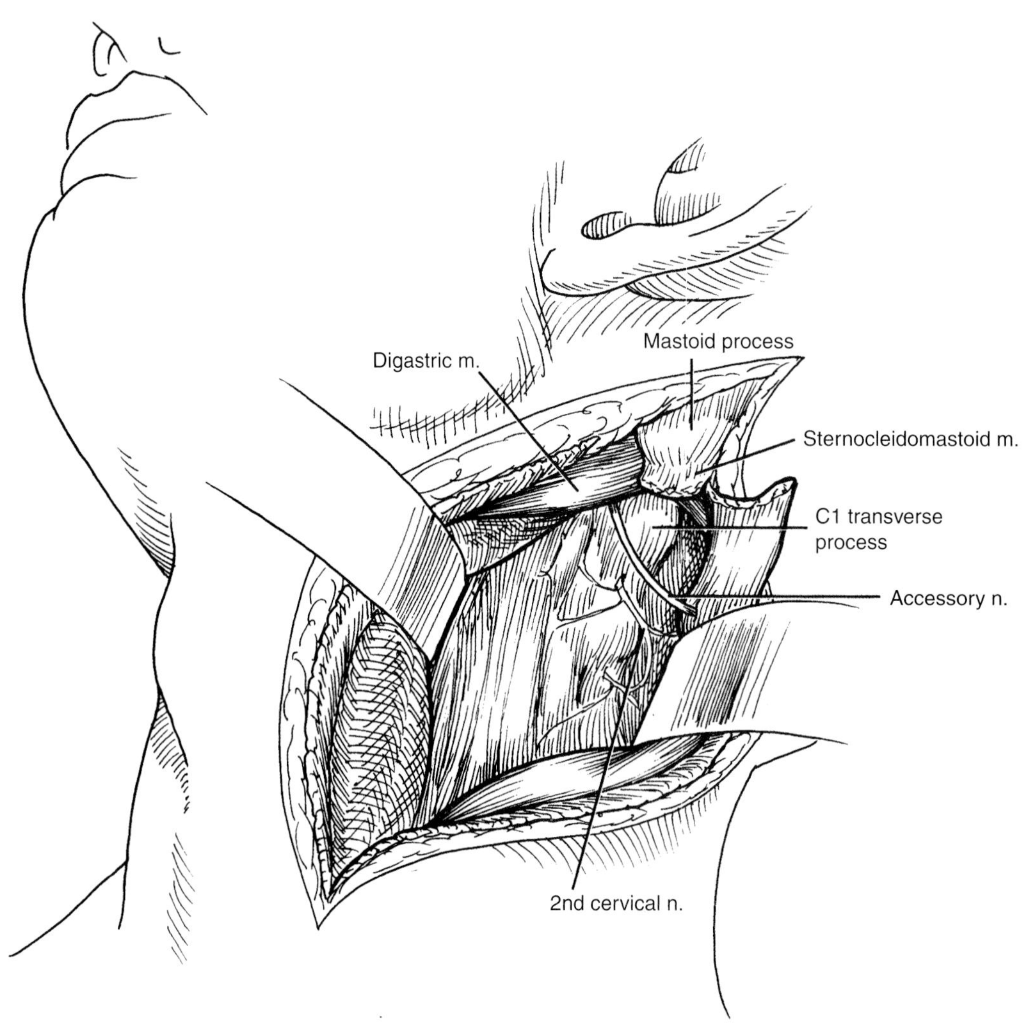

Fig. 2-21 Access to the upper two transverse processes is greatly facilitated by detaching the insertion of the sternocleidomastoid muscle, especially in a thick, short neck.

The tip of the transverse process of the atlas (C1) should be palpated in the superior wound deep to the digastric muscle. It should be noted that the tip of the transverse process of the atlas is anterior to the transverse process of the axis (C2) due to head rotation.[3] The prevertebral fascia is next incised posteriorly from the transverse process of C1 along a line parallel to the spinal accessory nerve. Once the spinal accessory nerve is retracted anteriorly, the levator scapulae and underlying splenius cervicis muscles are readily identified in the posterior wound (Fig. 2-22). These muscles cover the C1 and C2 interspace in which the vertebral artery is most accessible. The anterior ramus of the C2 nerve root emerges from under the anterior border of the levator scapulae and serves as an important landmark in the safe division of the covering muscles. A small retractor should be inserted between the C2 nerve ramus and the muscles.[12] The retractor serves as a guide as the levator scapulae and splenius cervicis muscles are divided as close to the transverse process of C1 as possible. Excision of these muscles over the C1 and C2 interspace will expose the vertebral artery. A 2-cm segment of vertebral artery is accessible in this interspace. The C2 nerve ramus will be noted to emerge behind the artery and will require protection during arterial manipulation. Many small venous tributaries enter the vertebral vein posterior to the artery. These tributaries are most dense near the transverse processes of C1 and C2; manipulation of the artery between these structures is least likely to cause troublesome bleeding.[12]

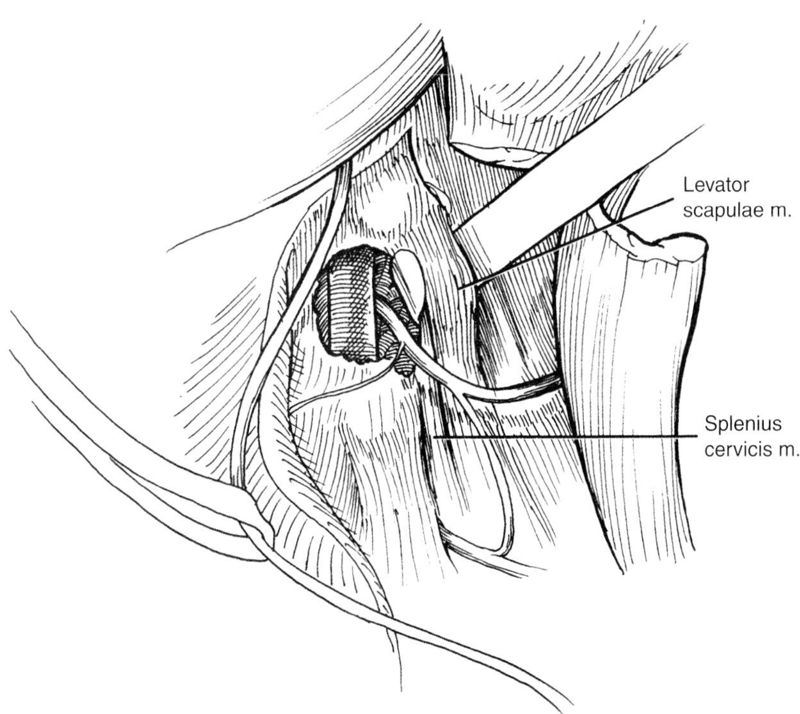

Fig: 2-22 With the accessory nerve retracted anteriorly, the highest slips of the levator scapulae and splenius cervicis are detached from the C1 transverse process to expose the vertebral artery between C1 and C2.

Posterior Exposure of the Suboccipital Vertebral Artery (V4) Segment

Berguer has described a now-classic approach to the portion of the V4 segment between the transverse process of C1 and the base of the skull.[15] This technique is applicable to treat rare pathologic lesions such as dissections or aneurysms involving the most distal portions of the extracranial vertebral artery. The posterior approach also allows exposure of the distal internal carotid artery, which can be used as a source of inflow in these cases.

The patient is placed in the prone position with the head turned toward the operative side. Berguer has recommended placing the patient in the "park bench" position, with the temple contralateral to the operative side resting on the forearm.[15] A curved transverse incision is made beginning at the occipital protuberance in the midline of the posterior neck and extended horizontally to the tip of the mastoid process. From there, it is curved downward and extended for 2 to 3 cm parallel to the posterior border of the sternocleidomastoid muscle (Fig. 2-23).

The incision is deepened by cutting the fibers of the trapezius, splenius capitis, semispinalis capitis, and longissimus capitis muscles. The greater occipital nerve (dorsal ramus of C2) courses upward over the semispinalis capitis muscle and may require division as it is encountered approximately 2 cm lateral to the posterior midline (Fig. 2-24). The sternocleidomastoid muscle should be divided at its mastoid insertion and reflected inferiorly. This will expose the internal jugular vein and the accessory nerve in the lateral wound. Palpation of the transverse process of C1 will aid in identifying the obliquus capitis superior muscle, which attaches to the superior margin of the bony prominence. The large condyloid emissary vein should be ligated and divided near the muscle's medial border (Fig. 2-25). Partial division of the rectus capitis posterior major muscle lying in the medial wound will expose the vertebral artery.

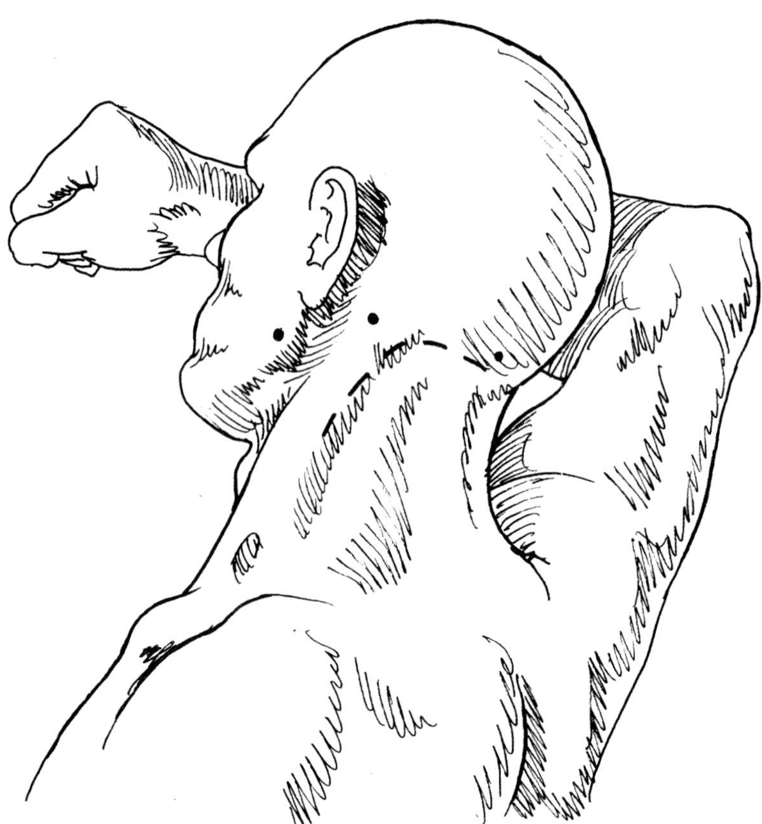

Fig. 2-23 The incision for posterior exposure of the suboccipital vertebral artery is shown.

Fig. 2-24 Deep exposure requires division of four muscle layers. The greater occipital nerve can be sacrificed to improve exposure in the lateral wound.

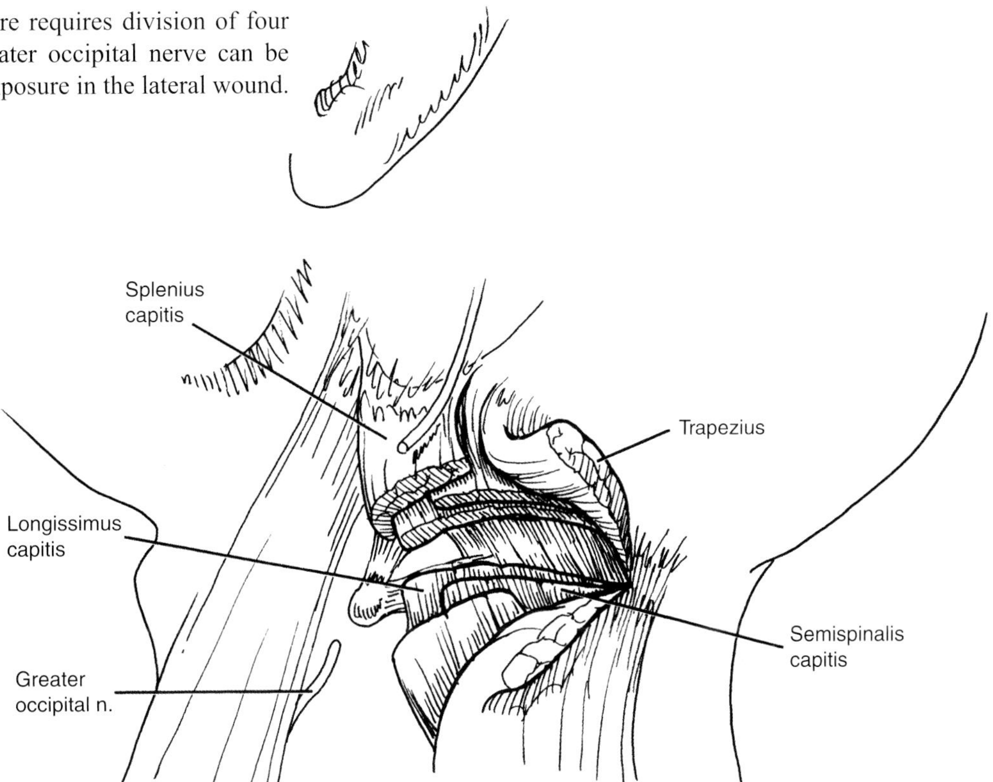

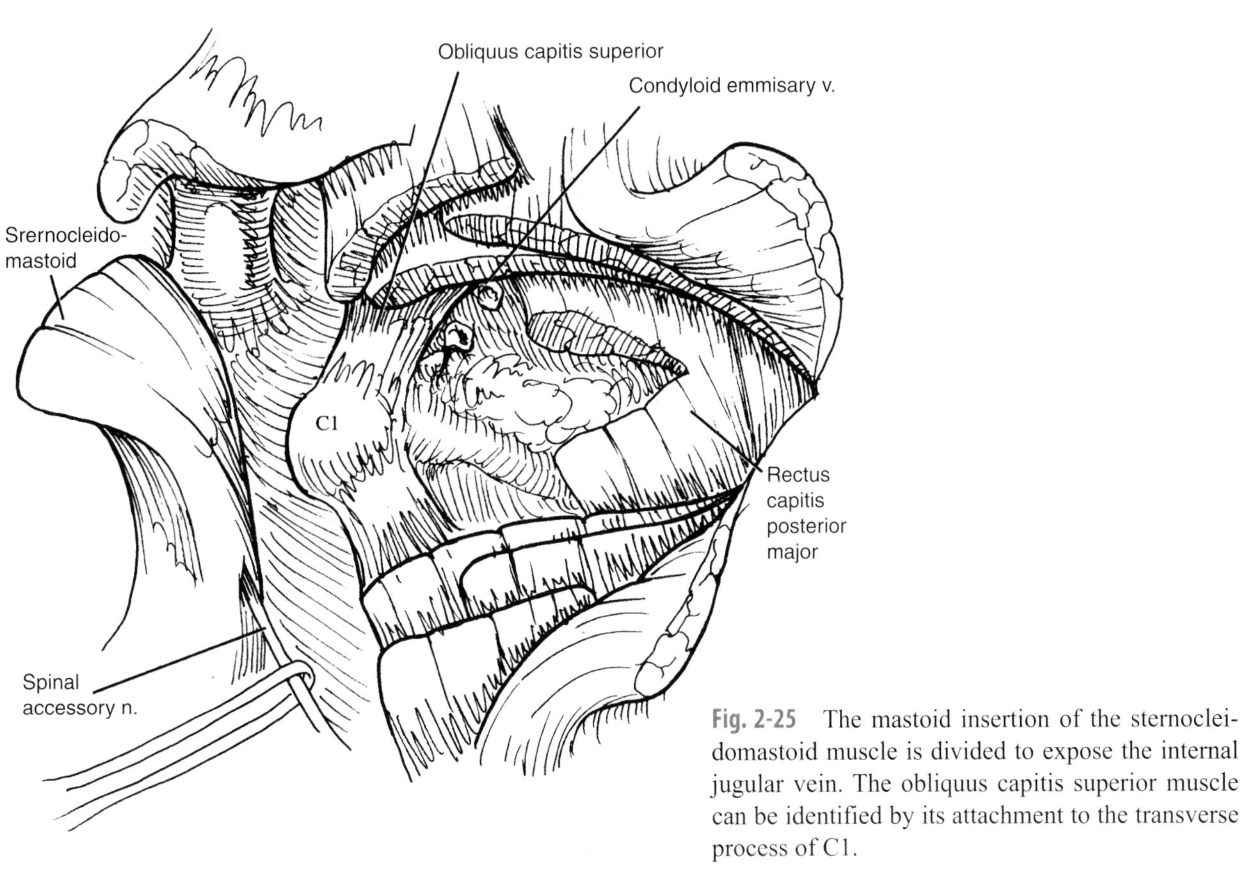

Fig. 2-25 The mastoid insertion of the sternocleidomastoid muscle is divided to expose the internal jugular vein. The obliquus capitis superior muscle can be identified by its attachment to the transverse process of C1.

A large venous plexus overlies the artery at this level (Fig. 2-26). Meticulous ligation and division of bridging vein segments will allow the plexus to be dissected away from the arterial adventitia. Branches of the suboccipital nerve should be divided as they cross the vessels at this level. The vertebral artery can then be mobilized to the level of the atlantooccipital membrane (Fig. 2-27). Care should be taken to avoid injury to the ventral ramus of the C1 root, which courses below the vertebral artery in this location. The distal internal carotid artery can be isolated in the lateral wound for use as inflow.[15] The artery can be exposed in the plane medial to the sternocleidomastoid muscle and isolated between the hypoglossal and vagus nerves (Fig. 2-28).

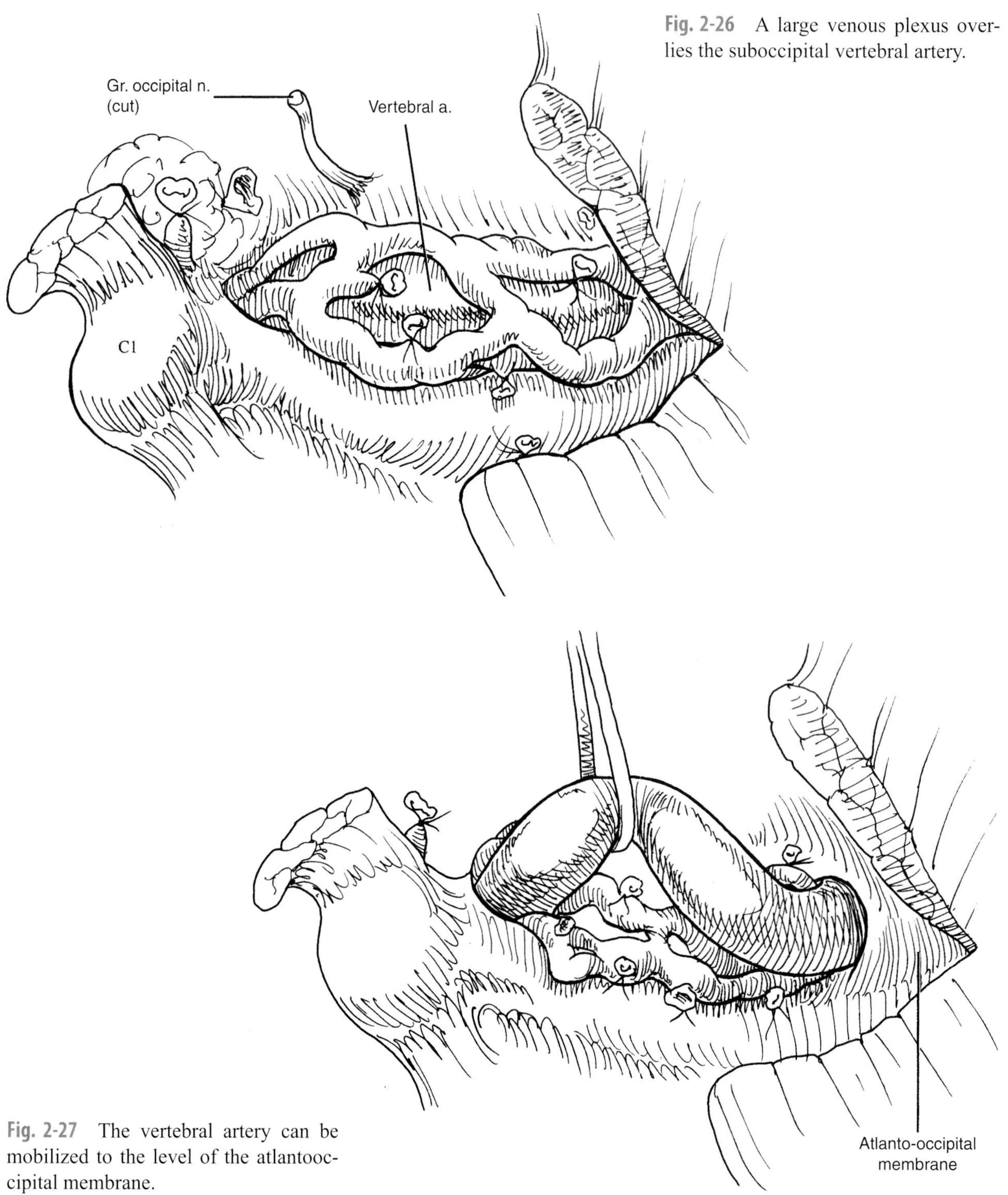

Fig. 2-26 A large venous plexus overlies the suboccipital vertebral artery.

Fig. 2-27 The vertebral artery can be mobilized to the level of the atlantooccipital membrane.

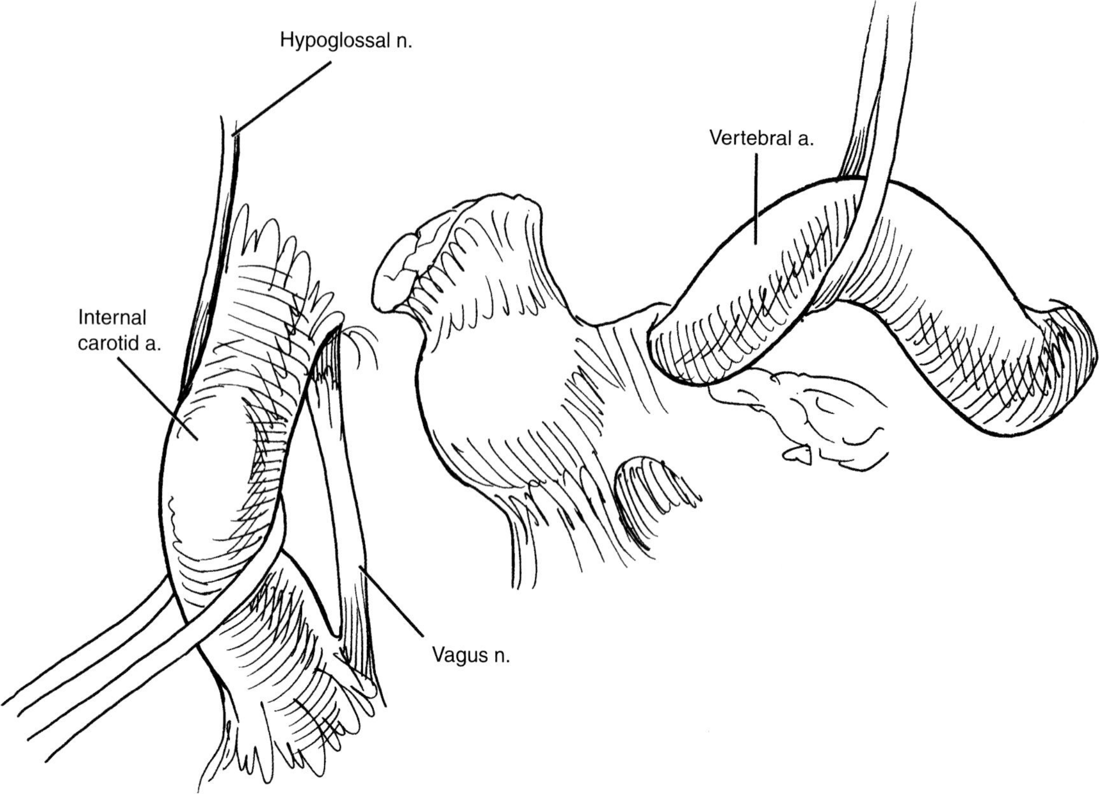

Fig. 2-28 The distal internal carotid artery can be isolated in the lateral wound and used as inflow for bypass to the suboccipital vertebral artery.

References

1. Morasch MD. Vertebral artery disease. In: Cronenwett JL, Johnston KW, eds. *Rutherford's Vascular Surgery.* 7th ed. Philadelphia, PA: Saunders Elsevier; 2010:1557–1574.
2. Edwards WH, Edwards WH Jr. Vertebral-carotid transpositions. *Semin Vasc Surg.* 2000;13(1):70–73.
3. Meier DE, Brink BE, Fry WJ. Vertebral artery trauma: acute recognition and treatment. *Arch Surg.* 1981;116(2):236–239.
4. Roberts LH, Demetriades D. Vertebral artery injuries. *Surg Clin North Am.* 2001;81:1345–1356.
5. Kline RA, Berguer R. Vertebral artery reconstruction. *Ann Vasc Surg.* 1993;7:497–501.
6. Berguer R, Flynn LM, Kline RA, et al. Surgical reconstruction of the extracranial vertebral artery: management and outcome. *J Vasc Surg.* 2000;31:9–18.
7. Imparato AM. Vertebral artery reconstruction: a nineteen-year experience. *J Vasc Surg.* 1985;2:626–634.
8. Kesser BW, Chance E, Kleiner D, et al. Contemporary management of penetrating neck injury. *Am Surg.* 2009;75:1–10.
9. Reid JDS, Weigelt JA. Forty-three cases of vertebral artery trauma. *J Trauma.* 1988;28:1007–1012.
10. Pearce WH, Whitehill TA. Carotid and vertebral injuries. *Surg Clin N Am.* 1988;68:705–723.
11. Shumacker HB. Arteriovenous fistulas of the cervical portion of the vertebral vessels. *Surg Gynecol Obstet.* 1946;83:625–630.
12. Berguer R. Distal vertebral artery bypass: technique, the "occipital connection," and potential uses. *J Vasc Surg.* 1985;2:621–626.
13. Kieffer E, Praquin B, Chickle L, et al. Distal vertebral artery reconstruction: long-term outcome. *J Vasc Surg.* 2002;36:549–554.
14. Henry AK. Sternomastoid eversion giving an exposure extensile to the vertebral artery. In: Henry AK, ed. *Extensile Exposure.* Edinburgh, England: Churchill Livingstone; 1973:58–74.
15. Berguer R. Suboccipital approach to the distal vertebral artery. *J Vasc Surg.* 1999;30:344–349.

VESSELS OF THE CHEST

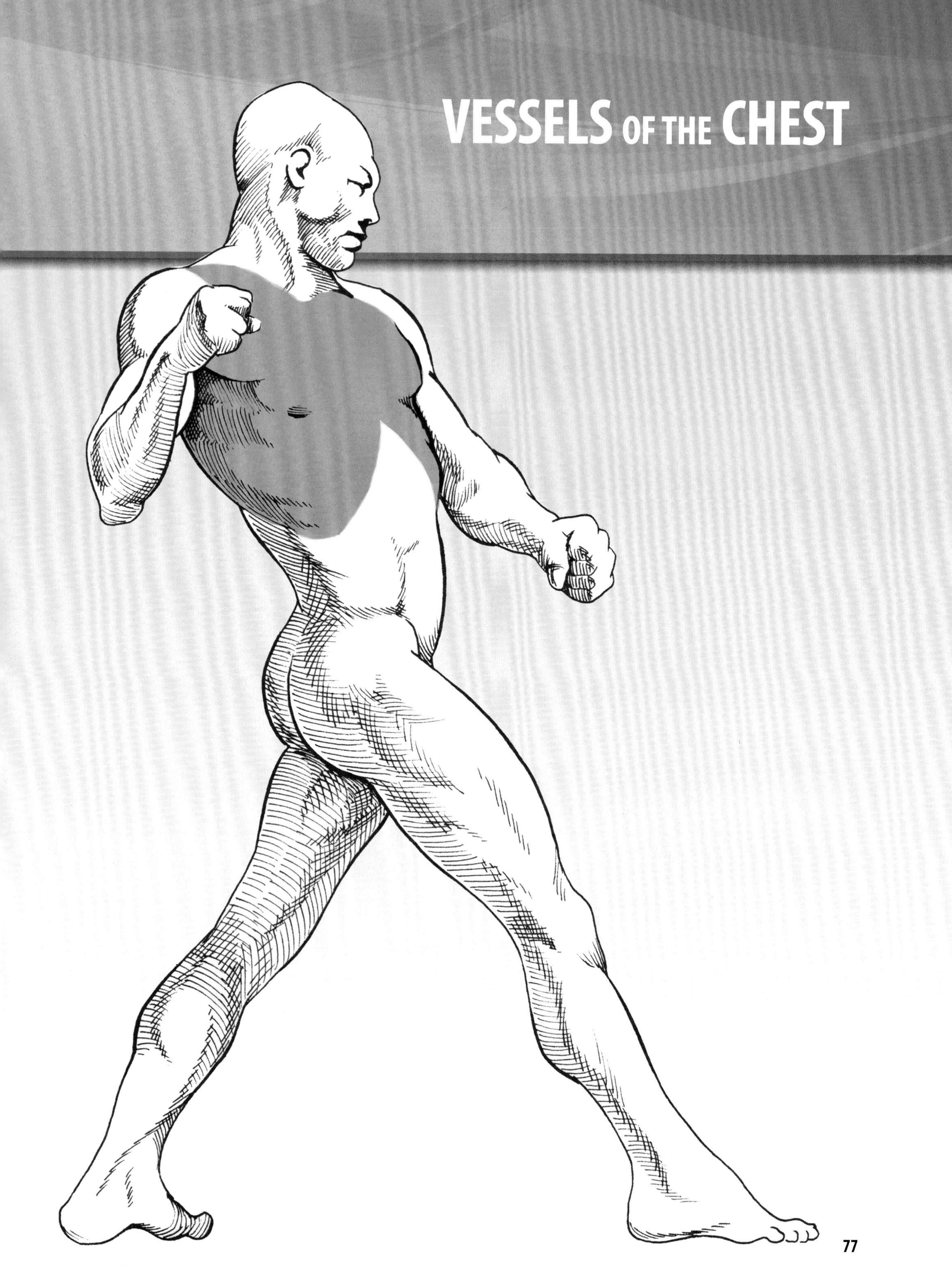

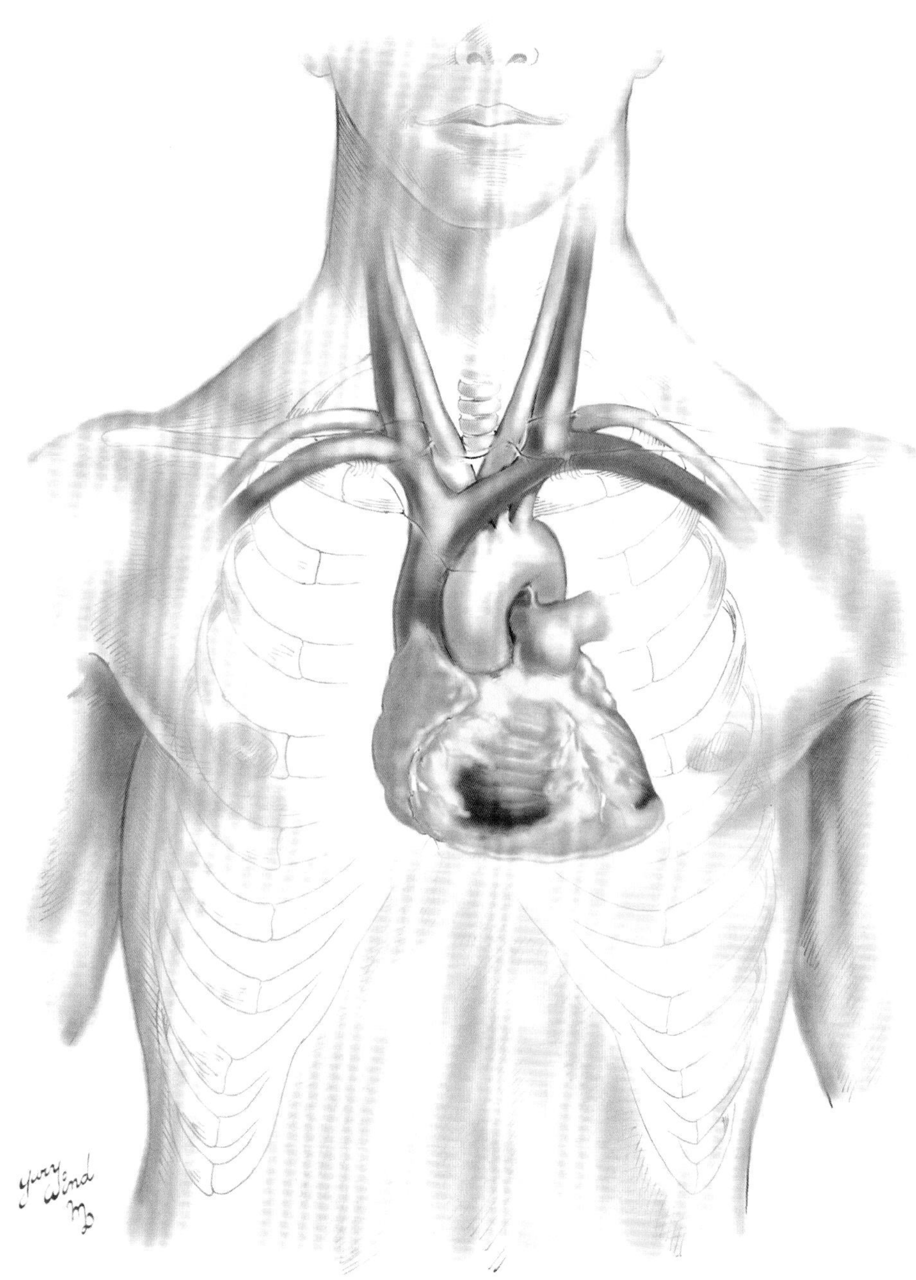

Fig. 3-1 The short span of the mediastinum is packed with vital structures connected via major conduits traversing the superior thoracic aperture.

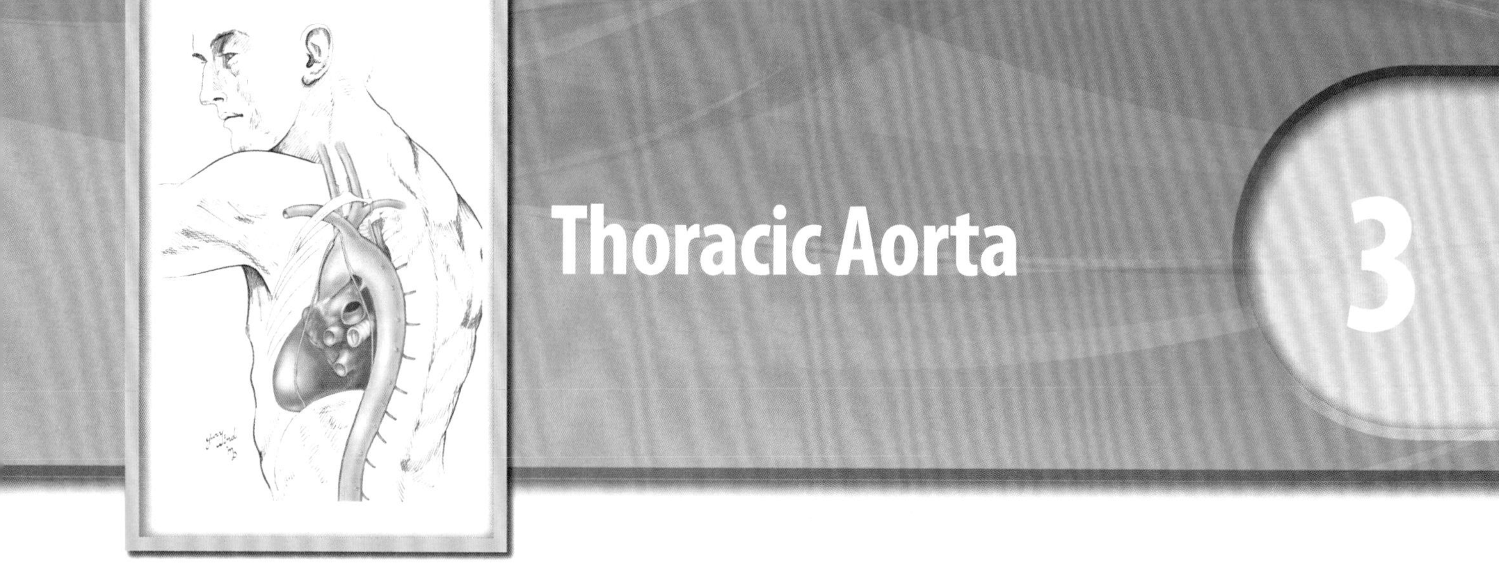

Thoracic Aorta

3

Surgical Anatomy of the Great Vessels of the Chest

Overview

To understand the anatomic disposition of the great vessels of the chest, one must view them in the context of the mediastinum and the superior thoracic aperture. The mediastinum is a short handspan in height from its base at the subcardiac portion of the diaphragm to the superior thoracic aperture (Fig. 3-1). The origin of the great vessels from the base of the heart lies at the midpoint of this length. The aortic arch, superior vena cava, and their branches lie closely packed with the trachea and esophagus in the superior mediastinum. At the superior thoracic aperture, the major branches blossom out to the arms and head. Understanding the relationships at these two key sites leads to an appreciation of the surgical approaches to these vessels.

The Mediastinum

At the level of the superior mediastinum, half the A-P diameter of the chest is occupied by the vertebrae (Fig. 3-2). In the small anterior component of this cross-section lie the great vessels, tracheobronchial tree, and esophagus. The lateral surfaces of this space are covered by closely applied parietal pleura, giving the underlying structures the appearance of having been shrink-wrapped.

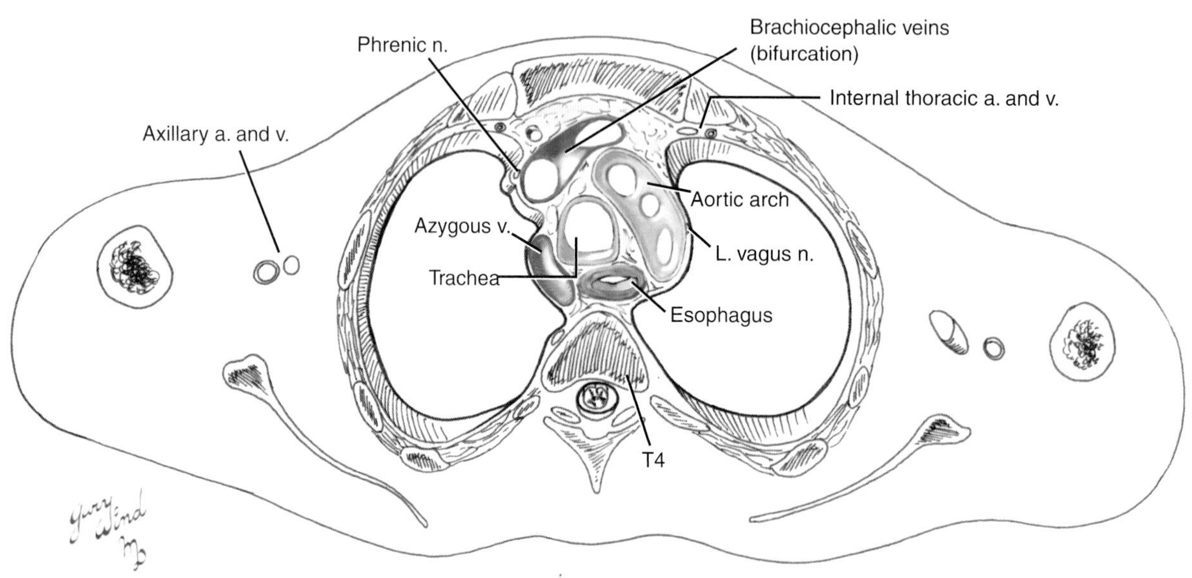

Fig. 3-2 At the level of the superior mediastinum, the anterior half of the A–P chest diameter is occupied by the great vessels, trachea, and esophagus.

The parietal pleura surrounds the pulmonary hilum, forming a short, broad-based bundle, and is reflected onto the medial lung surfaces (Fig. 3-3). The leaves of pleura surrounding the lung hila extend caudally between the lung and mediastinum to form the inferior pulmonary ligaments. The aorta frames the left lung root, and the ascending, transverse, and descending segments of the aorta are approached by reflecting the lung away in the appropriate direction. Between the pleura and pericardium, the phrenic nerves descend to the diaphragm accompanied by thin pericardiophrenic vessels (Fig. 3-4). The latter arise from the brachiocephalic vessels and/or from the internal thoracic (internal mammary) vessels.

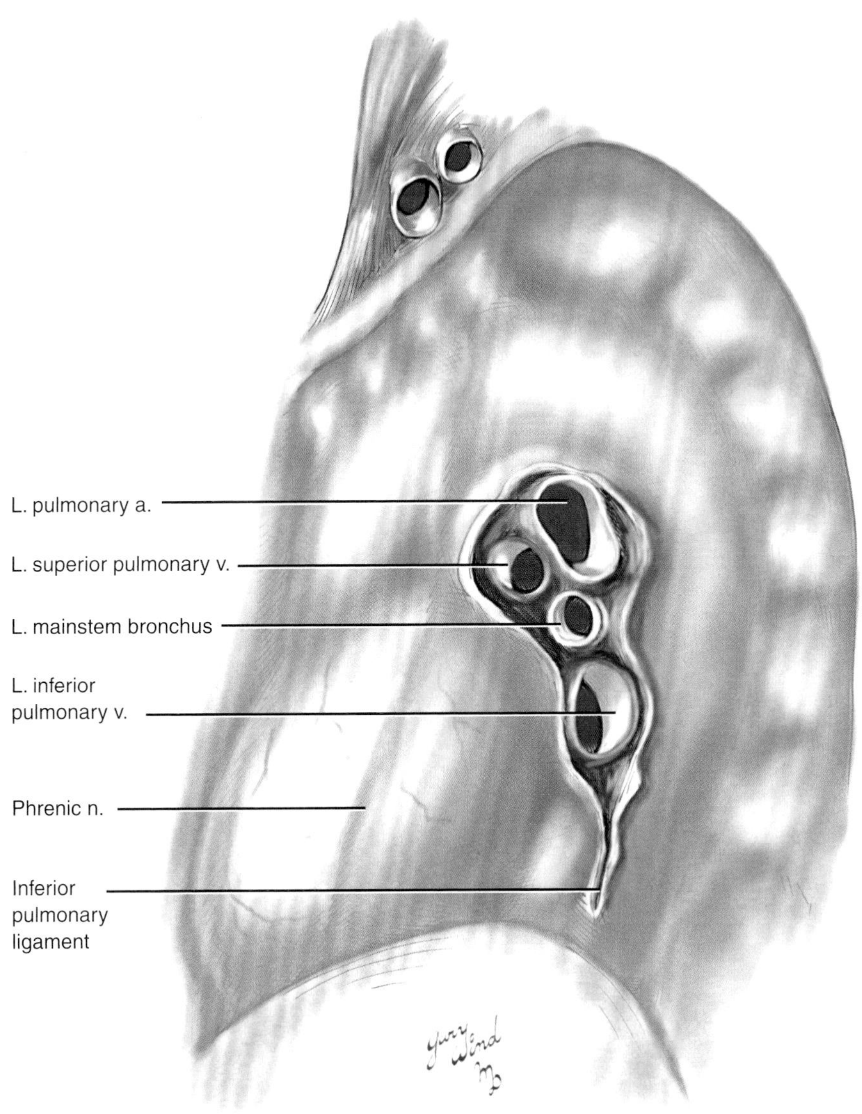

Fig. 3-3 The closely applied parietal pleura encloses the mediastinum laterally and surrounds the hilar stalks of the lungs.

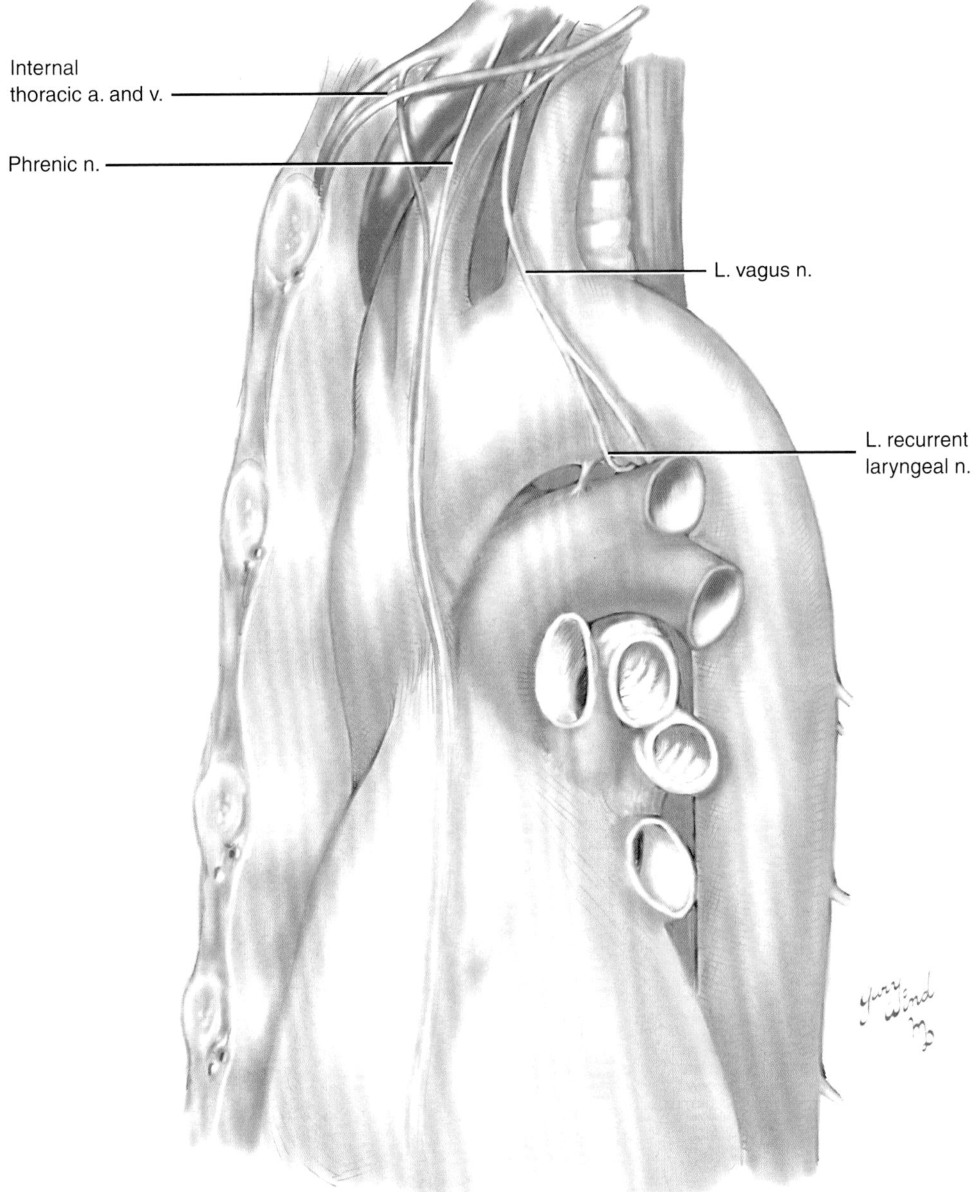

Fig. 3-4 The phrenic and vagus nerves lie beneath the parietal mediastinal pleura. The distal part of the phrenic nerve lies between pleura and pericardium.

The second set of major nerves traversing the mediastinum is the right and left vagus (Fig. 3-5). These are worth considering separately. The right vagus passes in front of the subclavian artery just lateral to its origin from the brachiocephalic artery. The right recurrent laryngeal nerve turns posteriorly beneath the subclavian artery and ascends in the tracheoesophageal groove, while the vagus descends behind the right main stem bronchus to reach the esophagus. The left vagus nerve passes between the left subclavian artery and left brachiocephalic vein to reach the lateral side of the aortic arch. Here the left recurrent laryngeal nerve diverges to pass beneath the aortic arch behind the ligamentum arteriosum. The vagus descends to reach the left side of the esophagus. At their junction with the esophagus, the vagi shift position, with the left moving anteriorly and the right moving posteriorly. Both trunks break up into multiple branches, which freely anastomose around the esophagus. This plexus coalesces into two major and several minor nerves at the distal esophagus. The major trunks lie anterior and posterior to the esophagus.

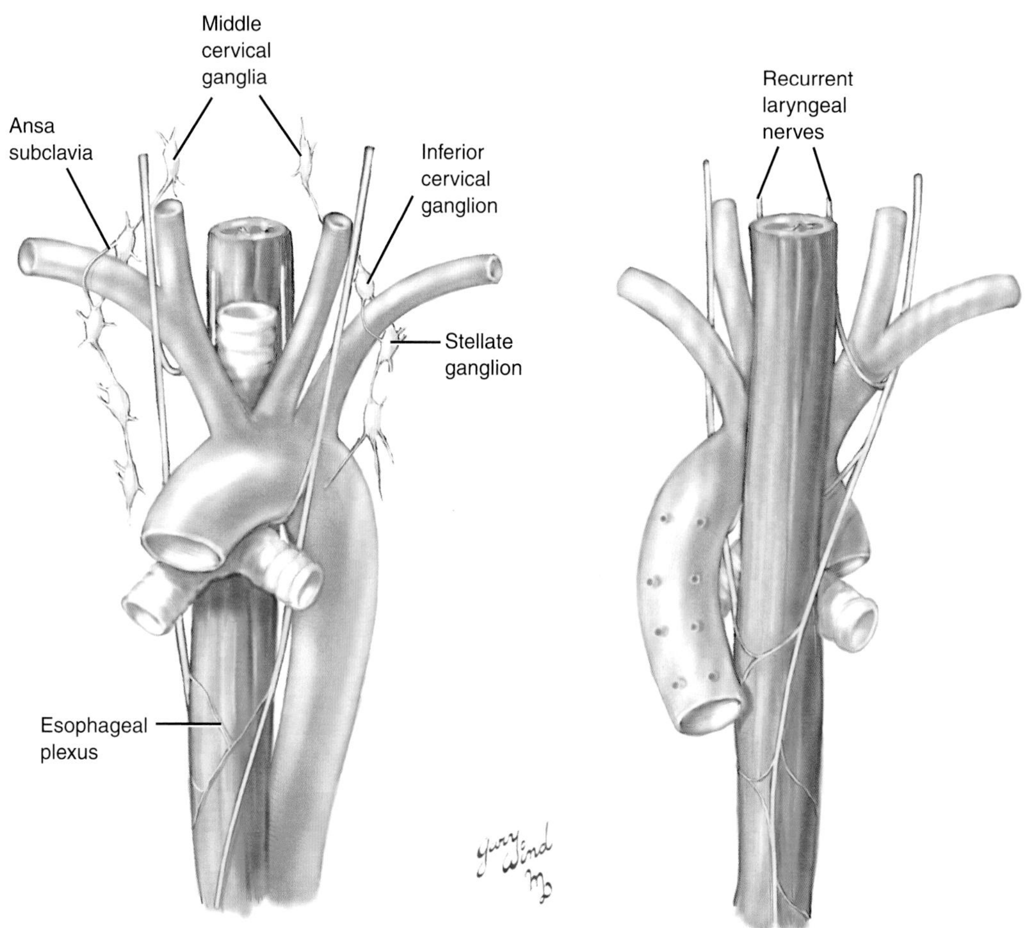

Fig. 3-5 The vagus nerves pass posterior to the lung roots to reach the midesophagus where they form an interconnecting plexus.

Two additional anatomic features should be noted for completeness. At the posterior limit of the mediastinum, the thoracic duct ascends between the esophagus and the vertebral bodies (Fig. 3-6). An extensive plexus of autonomic nerves surrounds the vascular and bronchial structures of the superior mediastinum.

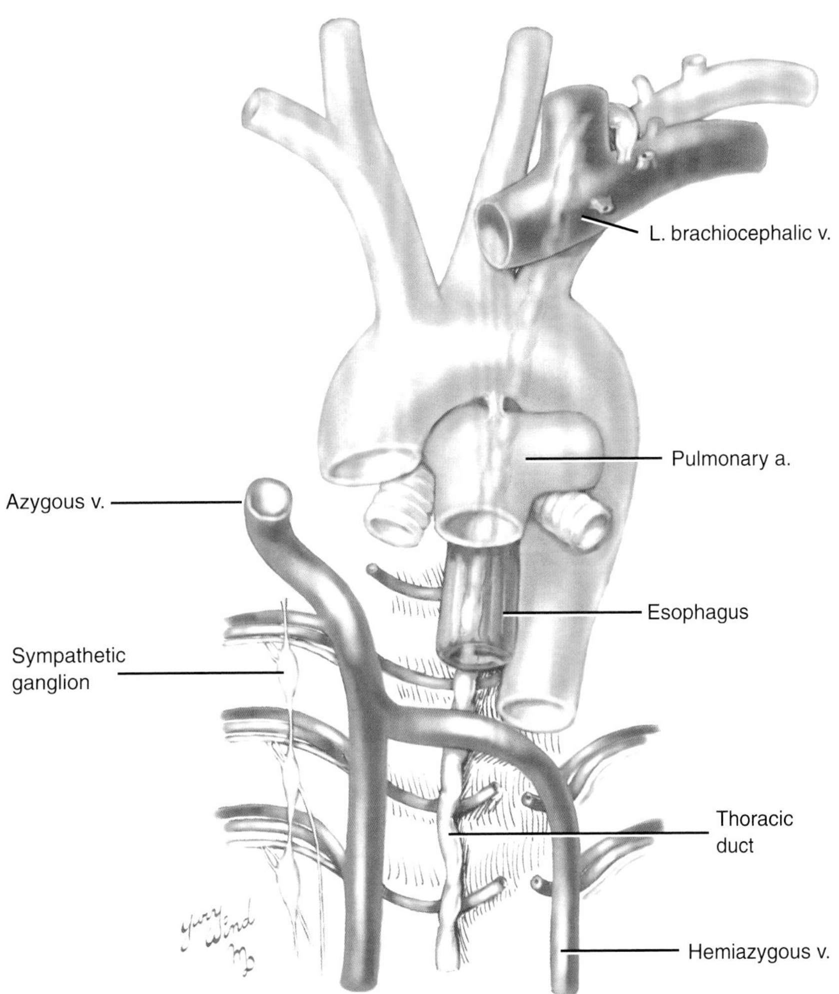

Fig. 3-6 The most posterior part of the mediastinum is occupied by the thoracic duct and the vessels supplying the chest wall.

The Aorta

The ascending aorta lies beneath the sternomanubrial joint and is accessible directly through the sternum (Fig. 3-7). The only intervening tissue is the remnant of the thymus gland. Flanking the sternum on either side are the internal thoracic vessels, which are tethered at their origins proximally. The medial pleural reflections closely approach the midline over the ascending aorta. The apex of the aortic arch lies

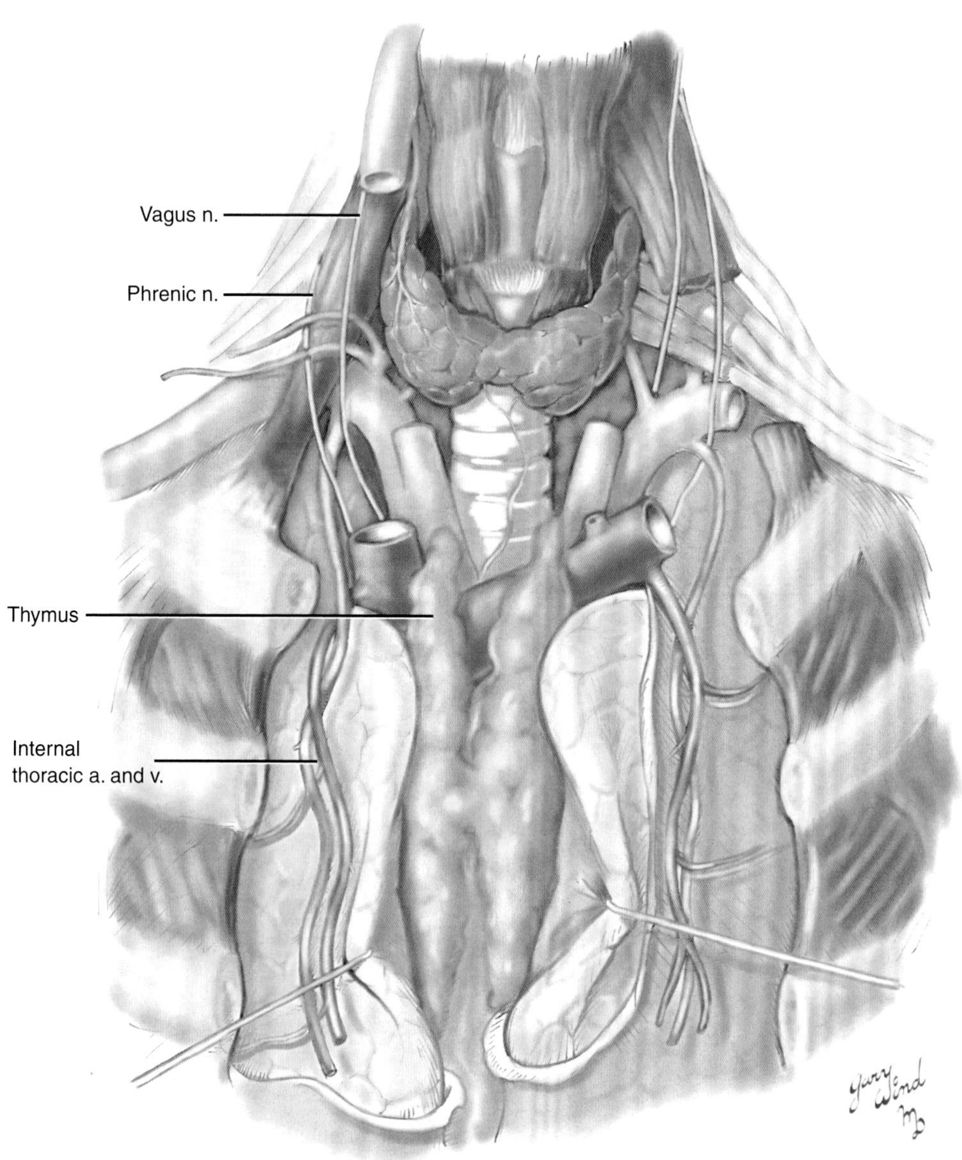

Fig. 3-7 The relationships of the vessels and lungs beneath the sternum are depicted.

in a diagonal direction relative to the sagittal plane of the chest (Fig. 3-8). As a result, the origins of the brachiocephalic and left common carotid arteries arise relatively anteriorly, while the left subclavian is more posteriorly placed. The confined space at the tapering lung apices restricts anterior access to the proximal left subclavian artery and mandates a left transthoracic approach for adequate exposure.

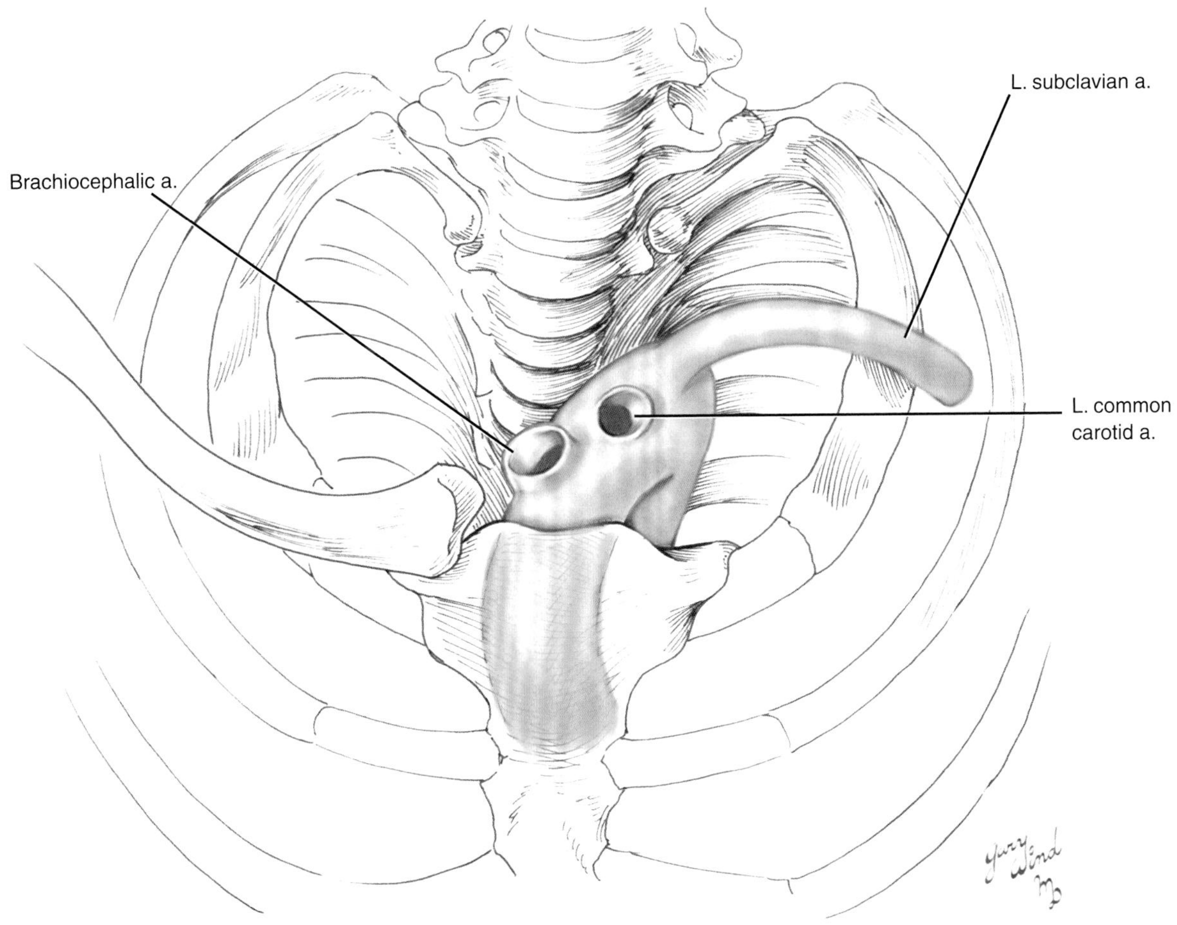

Fig. 3-8 The oblique axis of the aortic arch relative to the transverse plane of the chest places the origin of the left subclavian artery posteriorly.

As these vessels ascend and diverge, they surround the trachea and esophagus on three sides (Fig. 3-9). The arteries in turn are covered by an outer layer of major venous trunks. The superior vena cava lies lateral and parallel to the ascending aorta (Fig. 3-10). At the bifurcation of brachiocephalic veins, the right branch lies in the same coronal plane as the vena cava, inclined slightly to the right. The left brachiocephalic vein, on the other hand, arches anteriorly over the origins of the left common carotid and brachiocephalic arteries in its descent from left to right (Fig. 3-11). On the right side, the azygous vein drains into the superior vena cava just above the upper limit of the pericardium. On the left, the accessory hemiazygous vein drains into the brachiocephalic vein.

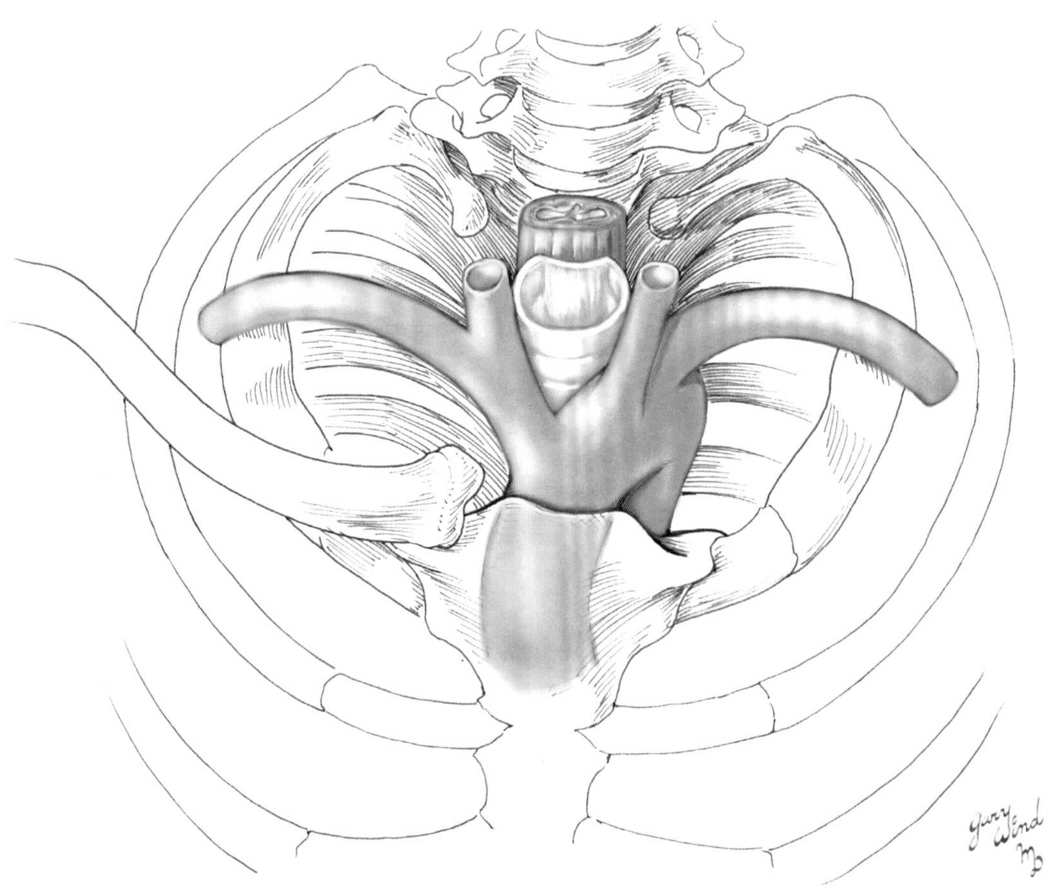

Fig. 3-9 The ascending and descending great vessels surround the trachea.

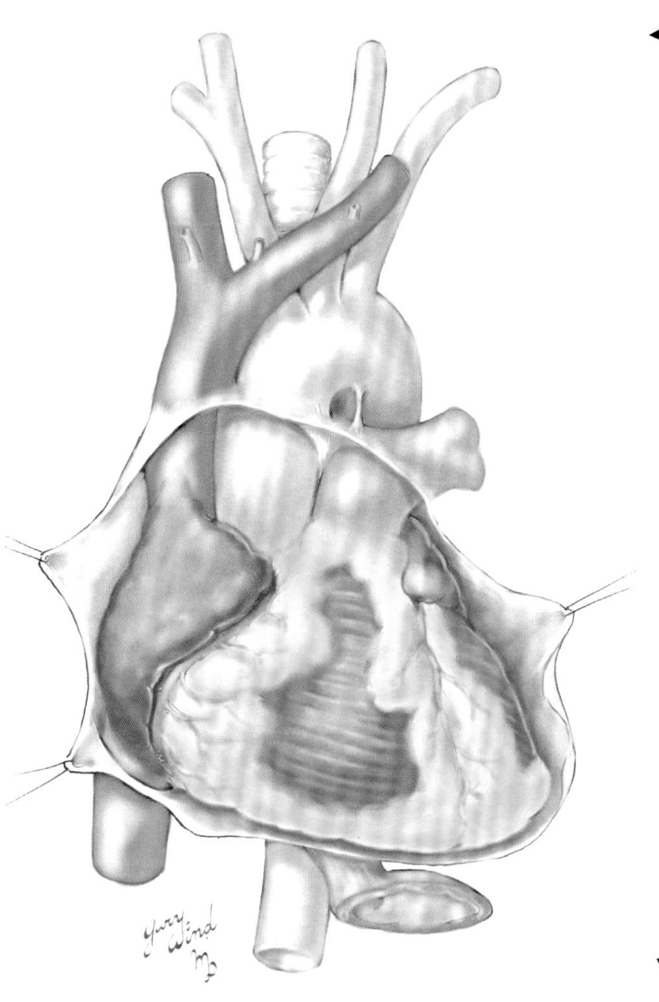

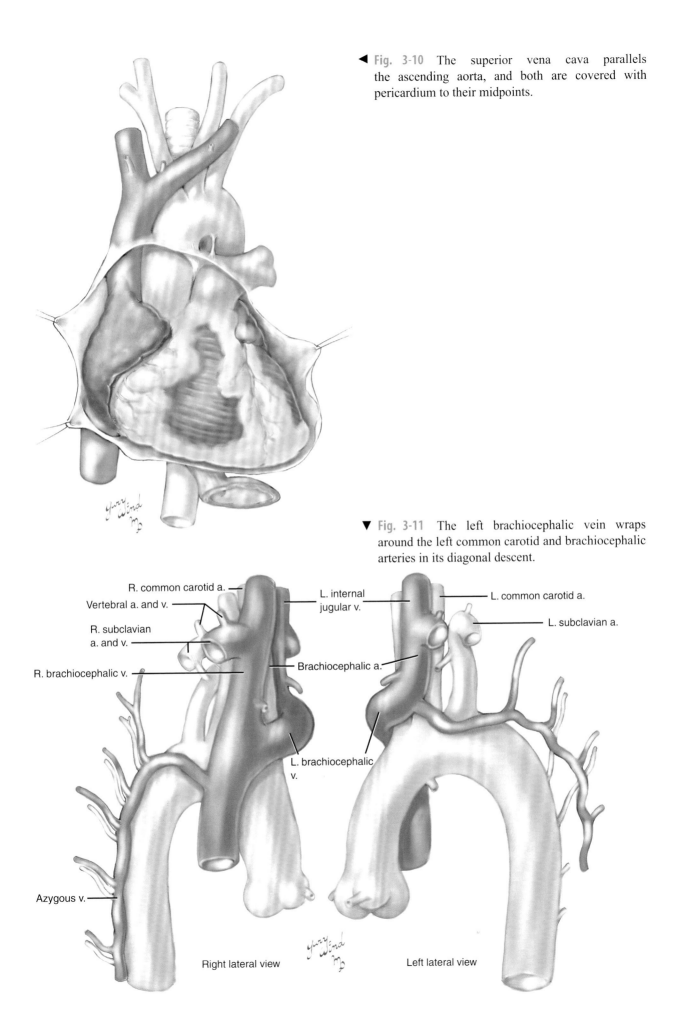

◀ Fig. 3-10 The superior vena cava parallels the ascending aorta, and both are covered with pericardium to their midpoints.

▼ Fig. 3-11 The left brachiocephalic vein wraps around the left common carotid and brachiocephalic arteries in its diagonal descent.

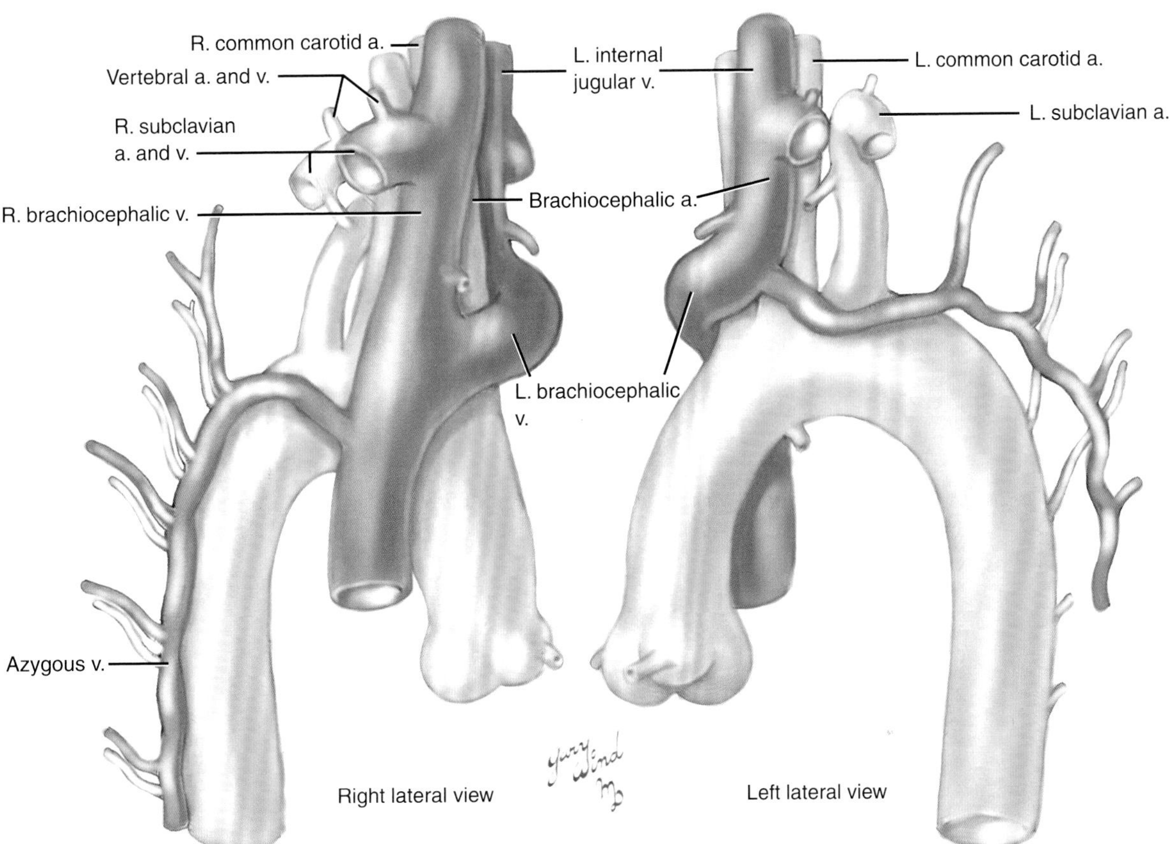

The central viscera at the thoracic aperture are confined anteriorly by the manubrium of the sternum and posteriorly by the vertebral column. A strong dome of fascia (Sibson's), continuous with the endothoracic fascia, covers the apex of each lung. The anterior halves of these domes support the arching subclavian vessels (Fig. 3-12). The cords of the brachial plexus descend over the posterior margin of the domes to converge with the subclavian arteries over the first ribs. Proximal branches of the subclavian vessels arise and ramify above these domes.

The clavicle articulates with the manubrium medially and acts as a protective barrier over the subclavian vessels. The costoclavicular ligament between the clavicle and the first rib forms the anterior

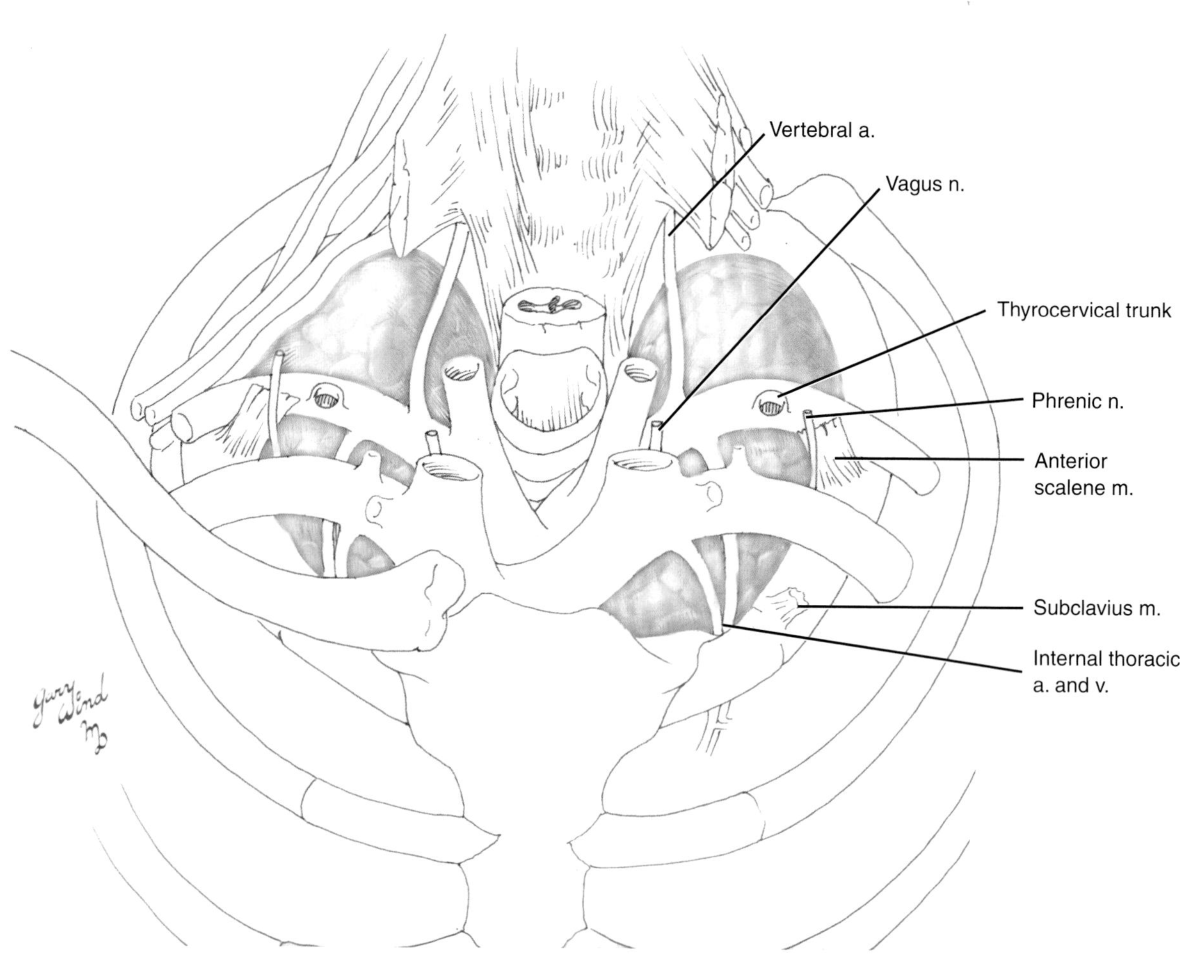

Fig. 3-12 The domes of the lung apices rise above the rim of the superior thoracic aperture and support the arching vessels and descending brachial plexus nerves. Sibson's fascia and pleura are removed in this illustration.

boundary of the aperture where the axillary vein passes over the first rib to become the subclavian. This structure marks the highest limit of an axillary dissection and is an important landmark for subclavian puncture.

An inverted cone of muscles attaches around the rim of the superior thoracic aperture (Fig. 3-13). The anterior and middle scalene muscles attach to the first rib, and the posterior scalene to the second rib, the strap muscles attach to the manubrium, and the sternocleidomastoid muscles attach to the medial part of the clavicle and to the manubrium. With all this protective architecture, it takes considerable force to fracture the first rib. When such a fracture occurs, associated major vessel injury must be suspected.

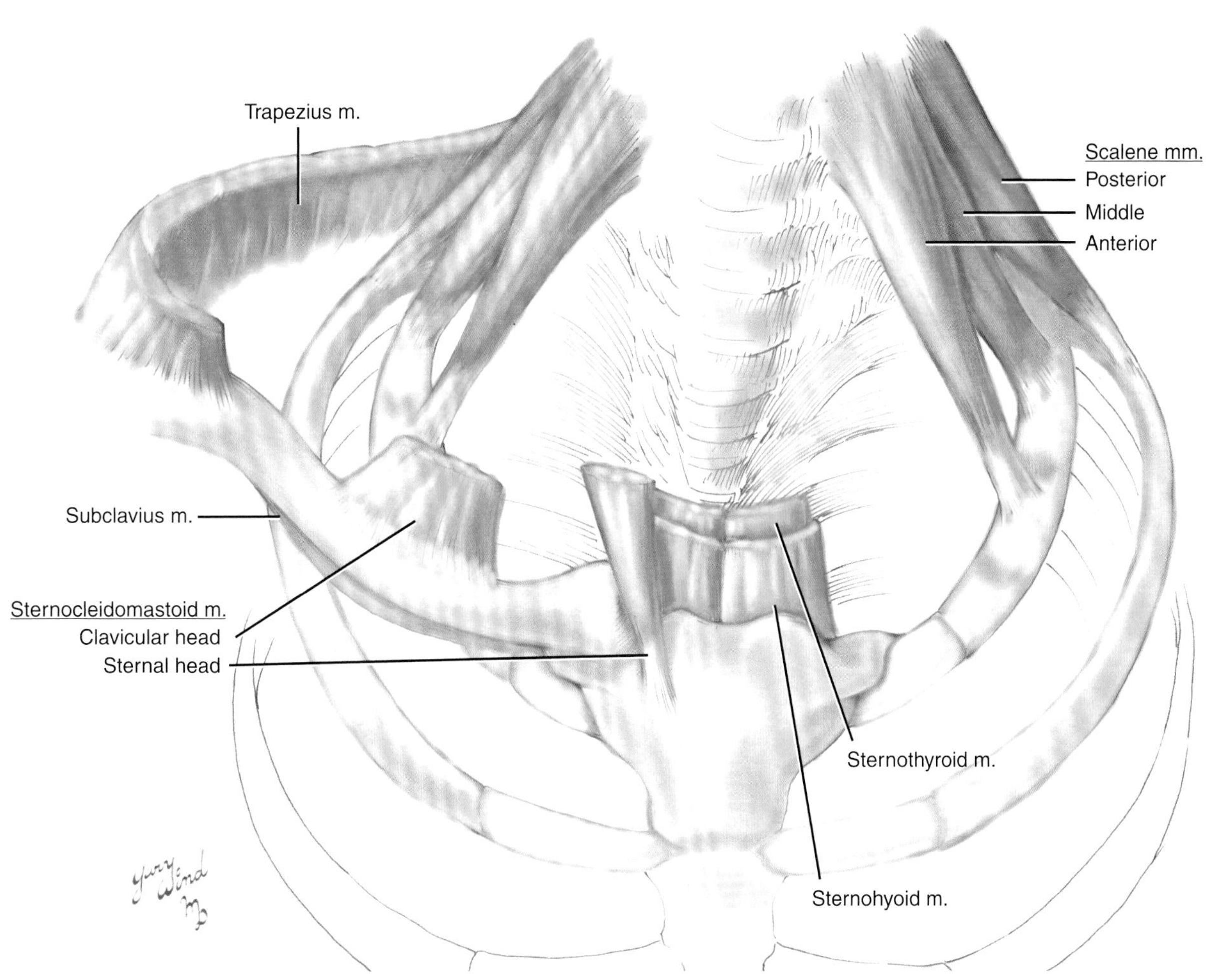

Fig. 3-13 The viscera of the superior thoracic aperture are covered by an inverted cone of muscles.

Beyond the arch, the proximal descending aorta lies to the left of the thoracic vertebral bodies (Fig. 3-14). It becomes progressively more midline as it approaches the aortic hiatus at the level of the twelfth thoracic vertebra. These relationships determine the optimal surgical approaches to the great vessels of the chest for control of hemorrhage in trauma and for elective surgical procedures.

Exposure of the Aortic Arch Branches

The importance of obtaining vascular control proximal and distal to an arterial injury is nowhere more evident than in the mediastinum. Rapid exsanguination, airway compromise, and cardiac tamponade threaten patients who have sustained injuries to the major branches of the aortic arch. Although endovascular management may have a place in the treatment of highly selected patients with contained hematomas, immediate open exploration is indicated in unstable patients.[1] Standard open surgical approaches remain the standard of care to treat blunt and penetrating injuries of the aortic arch branches because the long-term stent graft durability is unknown in the trauma population.[1,2]

The aortic arch branches include the left subclavian, left common carotid, and brachiocephalic arteries. Adequate exposure of these arteries without a thoracic incision is virtually impossible. Injuries to vascular structures at the base of the neck (zone I, see Chapter 1) are also difficult to manage without exposure of more proximal arteries in the chest. Early thoracotomy or sternotomy and rapid proximal arterial control in the chest can significantly reduce the mortality associated with injuries to the vessels of the mediastinum and base of the neck.[3–5] Although repair of aortic arch injuries almost always requires hypothermic cardiac arrest and or/cardiopulmonary bypass, arch vessels can usually be repaired without extracorporeal circulatory support or arterial shunts.[6]

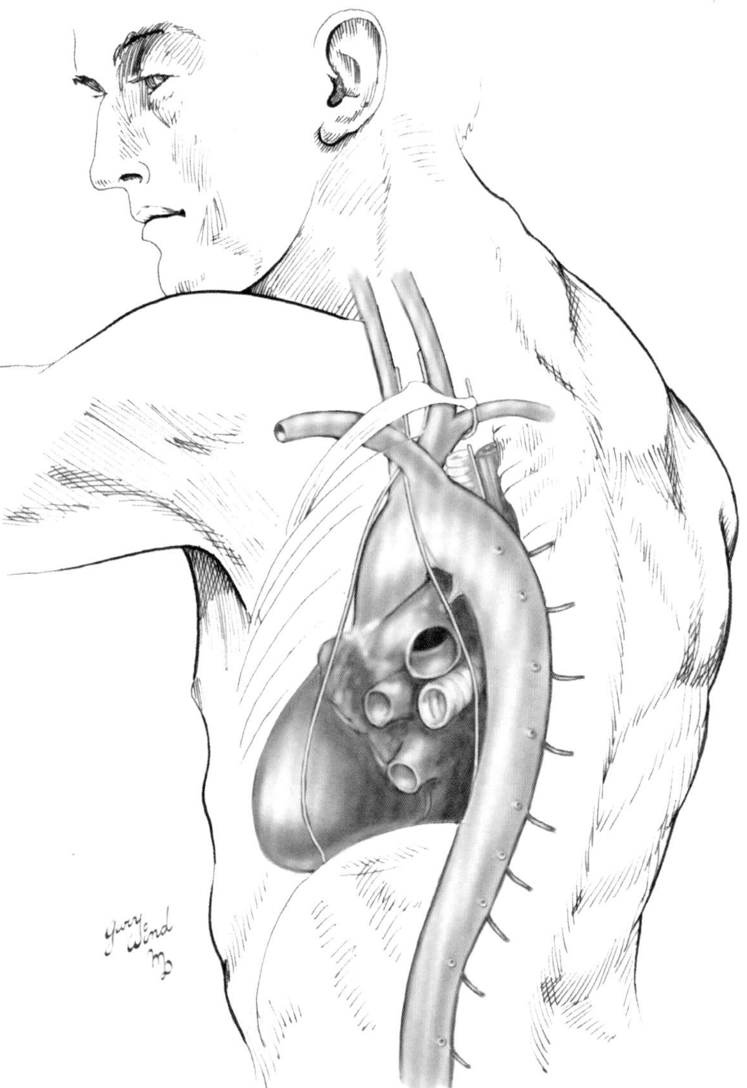

Fig. 3-14 The descending aorta initially lies anterolateral to the vertebral column and assumes a midline position at the aortic hiatus of the diaphragm in front of the twelfth thoracic vertebra.

Exposure of the brachiocephalic artery, proximal right subclavian and carotid arteries, and the proximal left common carotid artery requires median sternotomy.[4,5] Because of the relatively posterior location of the left subclavian artery in the mediastinum (see Fig. 3-9), a left thoracotomy is required for adequate proximal exposure of the proximal left subclavian artery, usually in combination with a separate supraclavicular incision or "trap door" extension.[4,7]

Patients with chronic occlusions of aortic arch branches rarely require thoracic incisions. Extrathoracic arterial revascularizations such as the carotid-subclavian bypass have been shown to be simple and durable approaches with low morbidity.[8] Likewise, preoperative revascularization of the left subclavian artery before thoracic endovascular aortic repair can be performed through an extrathoracic incision.[9] One notable exception is the repair of symptomatic brachiocephalic artery lesions, which are best treated with direct arterial repair or bypass through a median sternotomy.[10,11]

Exposure of the Anterior Branches: Brachiocephalic, Proximal Carotid (Zone I), and Proximal Right Subclavian Arteries

The most direct approach to the brachiocephalic and left carotid arteries at their respective origins is through a median sternotomy. This incision also provides rapid and complete access to the distal brachiocephalic artery and its branches in patients with right-sided zone I cervical injuries, particularly when combined with cervical or supraclavicular extensions.[4] The low morbidity of a median sternotomy has been well-established.[12]

Median Sternotomy

The patient is placed in the supine position with the arms drawn inward. The head should be turned toward the right in cases involving exposure of the left common carotid artery and toward the left for exposure of the brachiocephalic artery and its branches (Fig. 3-15). The anterior chest, abdomen, and neck are prepped and draped in the usual sterile fashion.

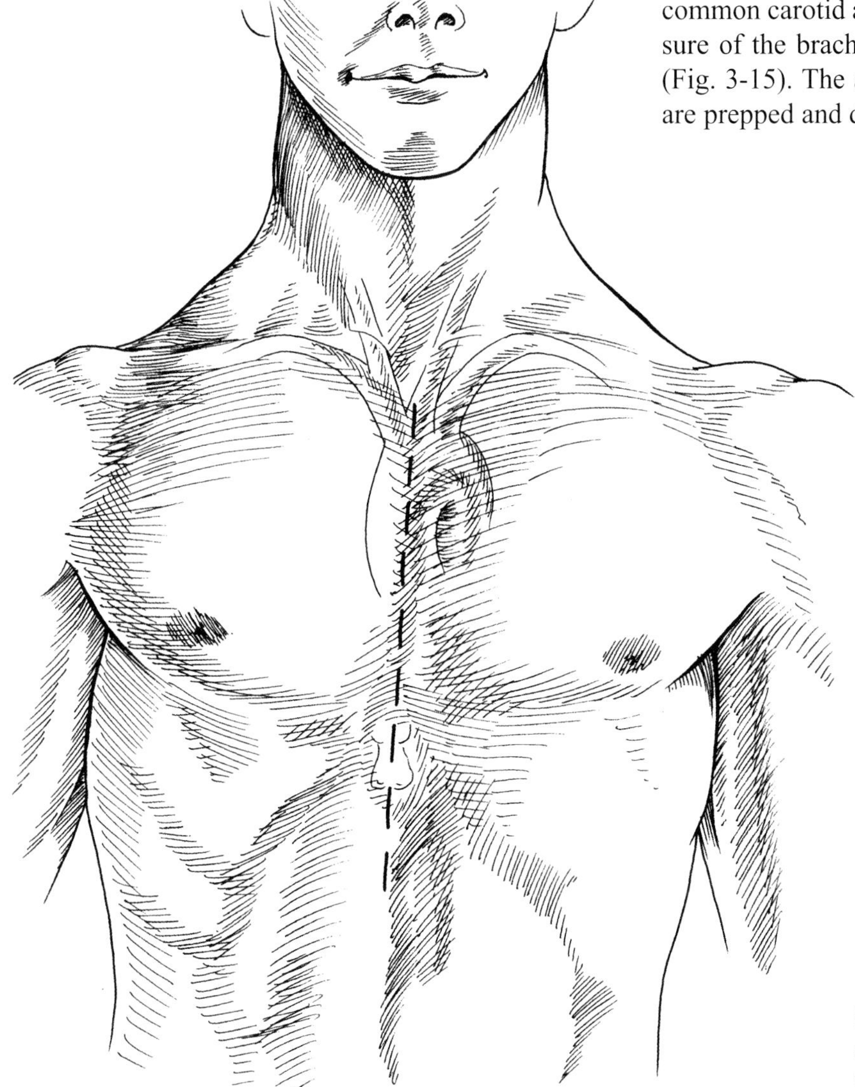

Fig. 3-15 The sternotomy incision extends from the suprasternal notch to the linea alba below the xiphoid process.

A vertical incision is made over the sternum from the suprasternal notch to a level 5 cm caudal to the xiphoid process. The incision is extended superiorly along the anterior border of the left sternocleidomastoid muscle when exposing the left carotid artery, or along the right sternocleidomastoid muscle when exposing the brachiocephalic artery and its branches. The cervical incision is deepened through the platysma, and the sternal incision is deepened through subcutaneous tissue to the periosteum of the sternum. The linea alba in the inferior wound is divided to the tip of the xiphoid process, allowing development of a plane between the peritoneum and the posterior rectus sheath. Using blunt finger dissection, this plane is extended behind the xiphoid and lower sternum (Fig. 3-16). A similar plane is developed behind the upper sternum at the suprasternal notch. It is not necessary to connect the two retrosternal planes.

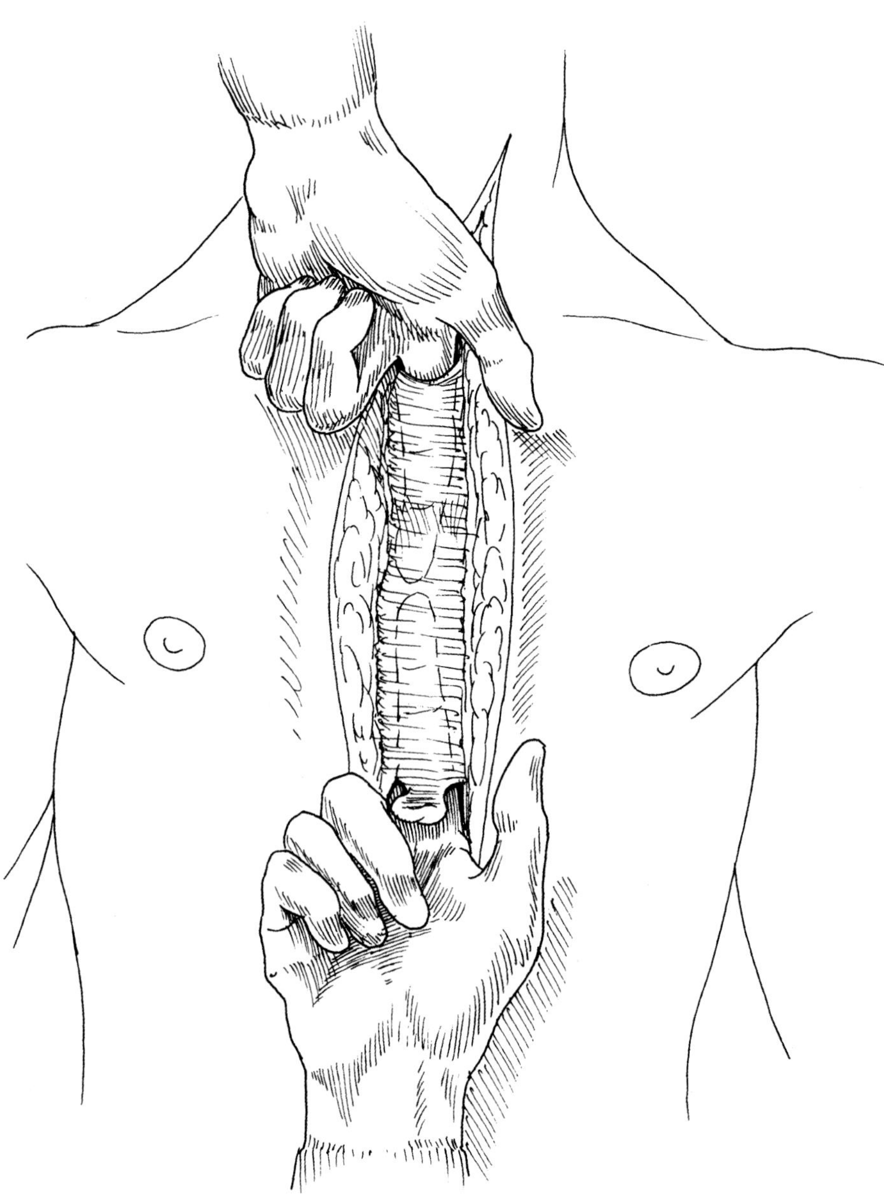

Fig. 3-16 The retrosternal plane is developed by blunt finger dissection.

In preparation for division of the sternum, the anesthesiologist should be directed to deflate the lungs temporarily. This may help avoid inadvertent entry into the pleural spaces. The sternum is next divided in the midline using either an electric sternal saw with a vertical oscillating blade or a Lebsche knife (Fig. 3-17). Maintaining the sternotomy in the midline is crucial to achieve an optimal closure and prevent dehiscence.[13] Bleeding from the edges of the sternal incision is best controlled with electrocautery. The use of bone wax on the sternal edges is contraindicated except in unusual circumstances because of the risks of impaired wound healing, increased infection, and embolization of wax to

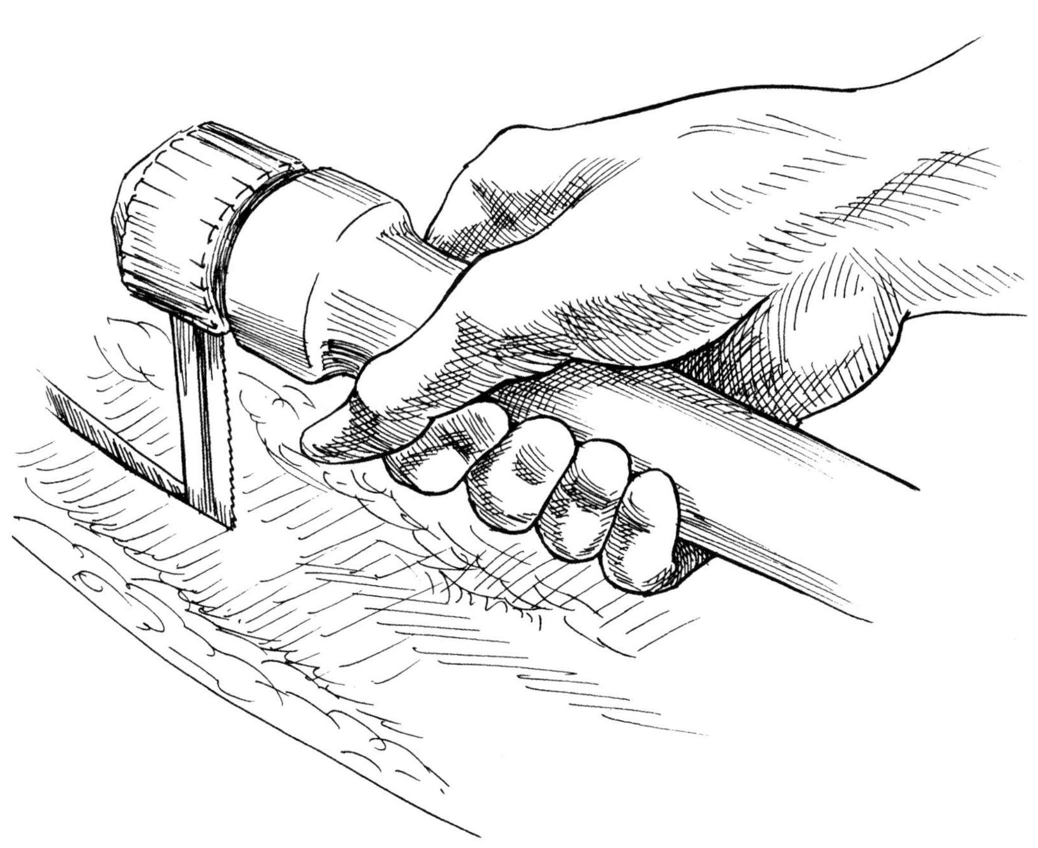

Fig. 3-17 The sternum is divided.

the lungs.[14] After hemostasis is obtained, a sternal retractor is carefully positioned and opened a few turns at a time to avoid sternal fractures (Fig. 3-18).

The carotid sheath is exposed through the cervical extension of the sternotomy (Fig. 3-19). The investing fascia is incised along the anterior border of the sternocleidomastoid muscle, which is freed on its medial surface. The underlying sternothyroid and sternohyoid muscles are divided. Lateral retraction of the sternocleidomastoid muscle will expose the internal jugular vein. After mobilizing the internal jugular vein and retracting it laterally, the common carotid artery can be identified and isolated (see Chapter 1).

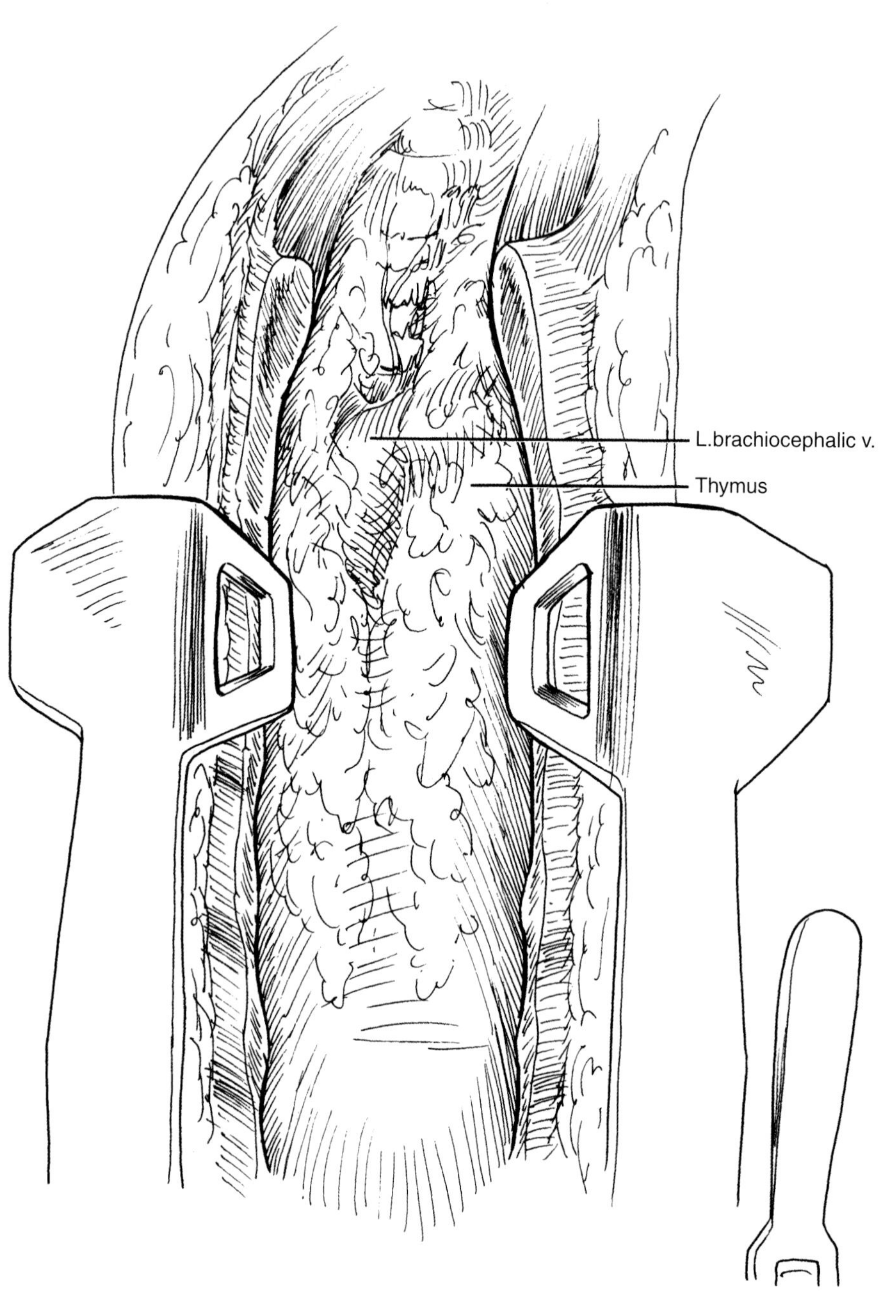

Fig. 3-18 The sternal retractor is opened slowly to allow strain to dissipate and avoid fracture. For clarity, all exposures are shown without laparotomy pads beneath retractors.

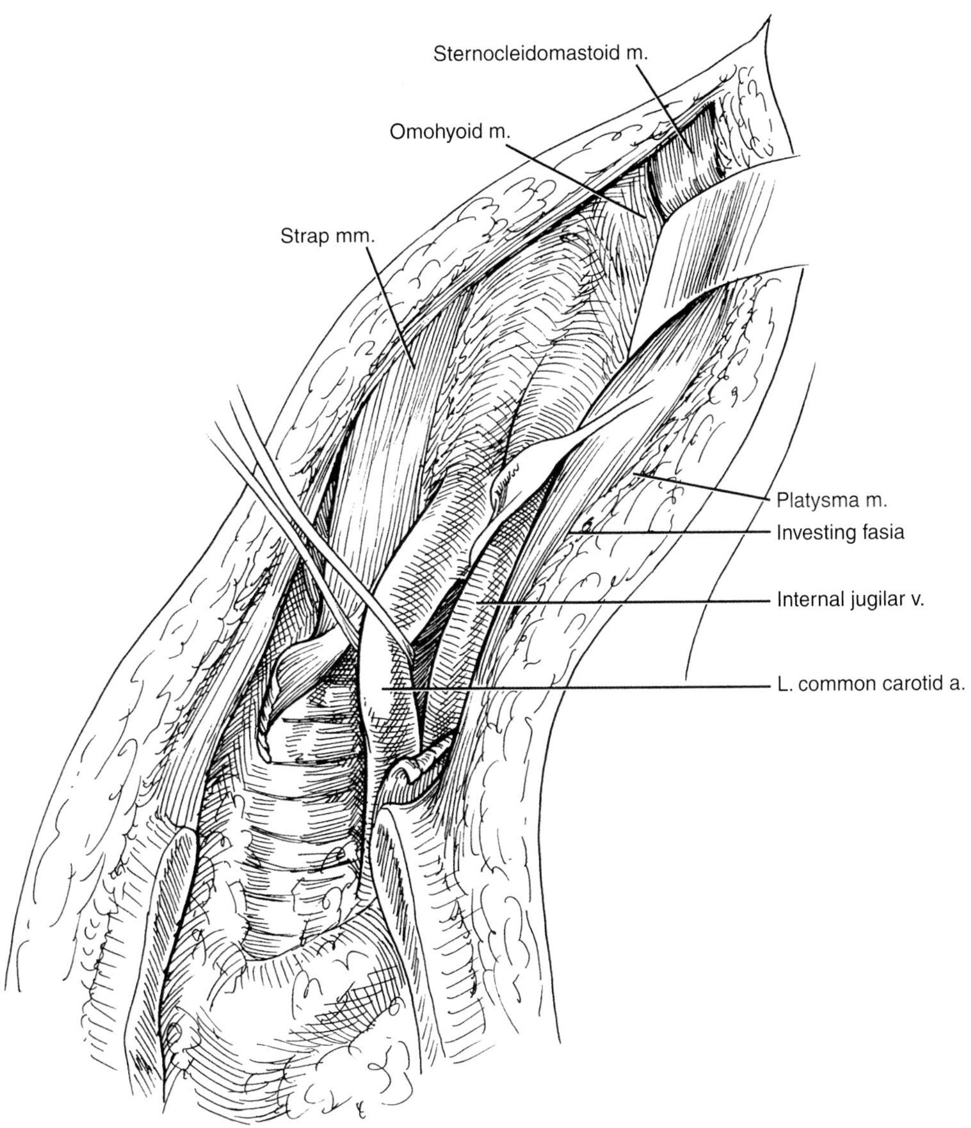

Fig. 3-19 A cervical extension of the sternotomy incision allows exposure of the carotid sheath.

Exposure of the aortic arch and its branches proceeds through the sternotomy incision (Fig. 3-20). The thymus gland is divided vertically in the midline and ligated. The left brachiocephalic vein is identified, mobilized, and encircled with a silastic loop. Although there are numerous venous tributaries that serve as collateral channels if the left brachiocephalic vein is occluded, intentional division of this vein is usually not required. Instead, the inferior thyroid vein and other tributaries of the left brachiocephalic vein should be divided to permit wide mobilization of the brachiocephalic vein. The brachiocephalic artery is identified superior to the left brachiocephalic vein; its origin at the aorta can be identified by retracting the left brachiocephalic vein superiorly. During mobilization of the brachiocephalic artery, care should be taken to identify the right vagus and recurrent laryngeal nerves. The right vagus nerve courses along the lateral aspect of the right carotid artery, crosses anterior to the right subclavian artery near its origin, and descends into the mediastinum posterior to the right brachiocephalic vein (Fig. 3-21). The recurrent laryngeal branch of the right vagus nerve loops around the inferior border of the proximal subclavian artery and courses medially to ascend in the neck between the trachea and esophagus. These nerves are best preserved in the periadventitial tissues. Lateral retraction of these

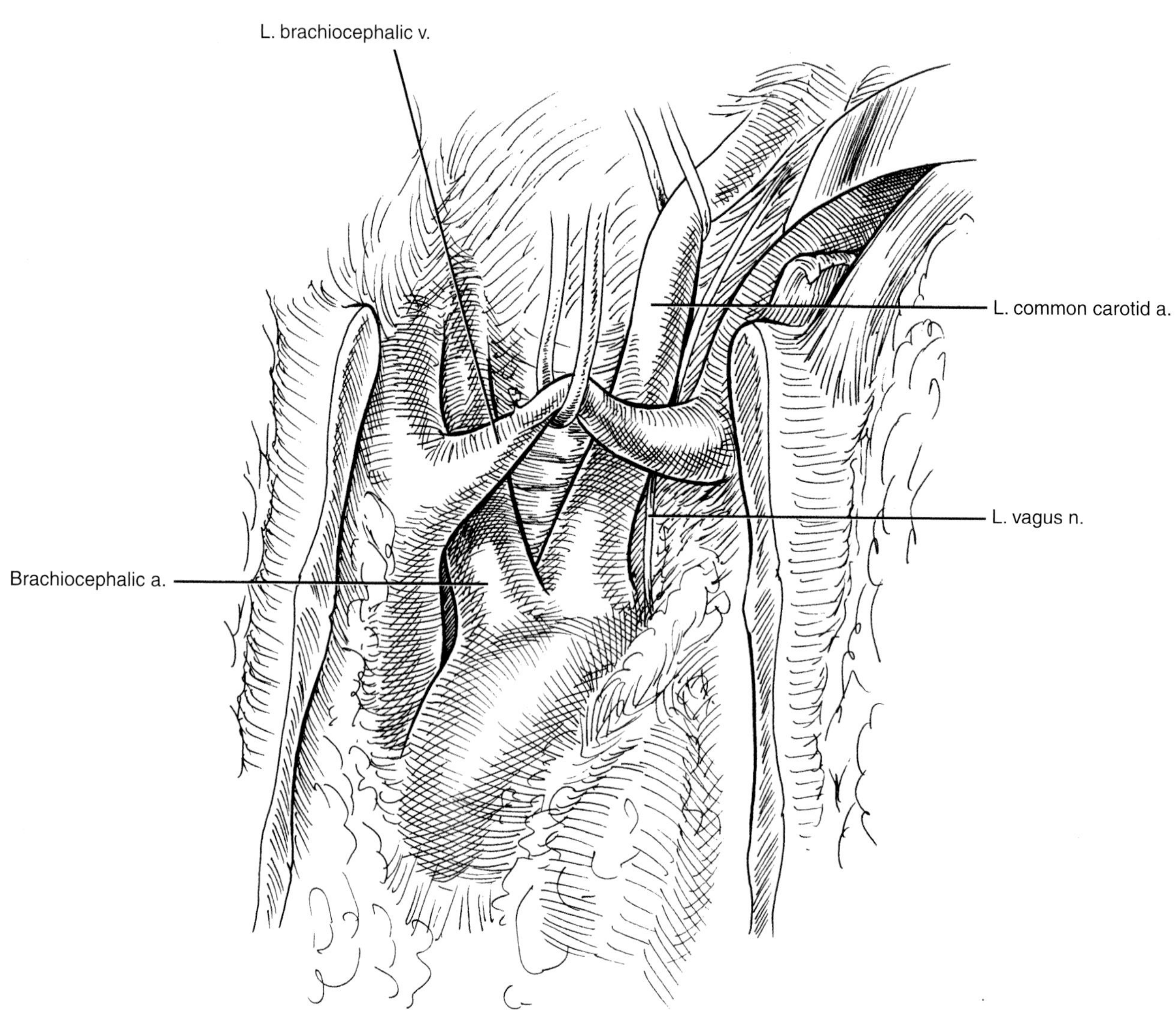

Fig. 3-20 Complete mobilization of the left brachiocephalic vein exposes the proximal brachiocephalic artery and left common carotid artery.

tissues during dissection of the distal brachiocephalic and proximal right subclavian arteries should prevent neural injury.

Isolation of the proximal right subclavian and common carotid arteries is performed just distal to the brachiocephalic bifurcation. Transection of the right-sided strap muscles is necessary to fully expose these vessels. More distal exposure of the right carotid artery may require superior extension of the cervical incision, with division of the omohyoid muscle (see Chapter 1). More distal exposure of the right subclavian artery may require a lateral extension of the midline wound across the right clavicle, with resection of the medial half of the clavicle or a separate right supraclavicular incision (see Chapter 5).

Identification of the proximal left common carotid artery proceeds in the left half of the sternotomy incision by retracting the brachiocephalic vein superiorly. Care should be taken to preserve the left vagus nerve, which descends into the mediastinum between the left common carotid and left subclavian arteries to cross the left side of the aortic arch. The left recurrent laryngeal branch passes under the aortic arch and ligamentum arteriosum, and then inclines medially to reach the tracheoesophageal groove.

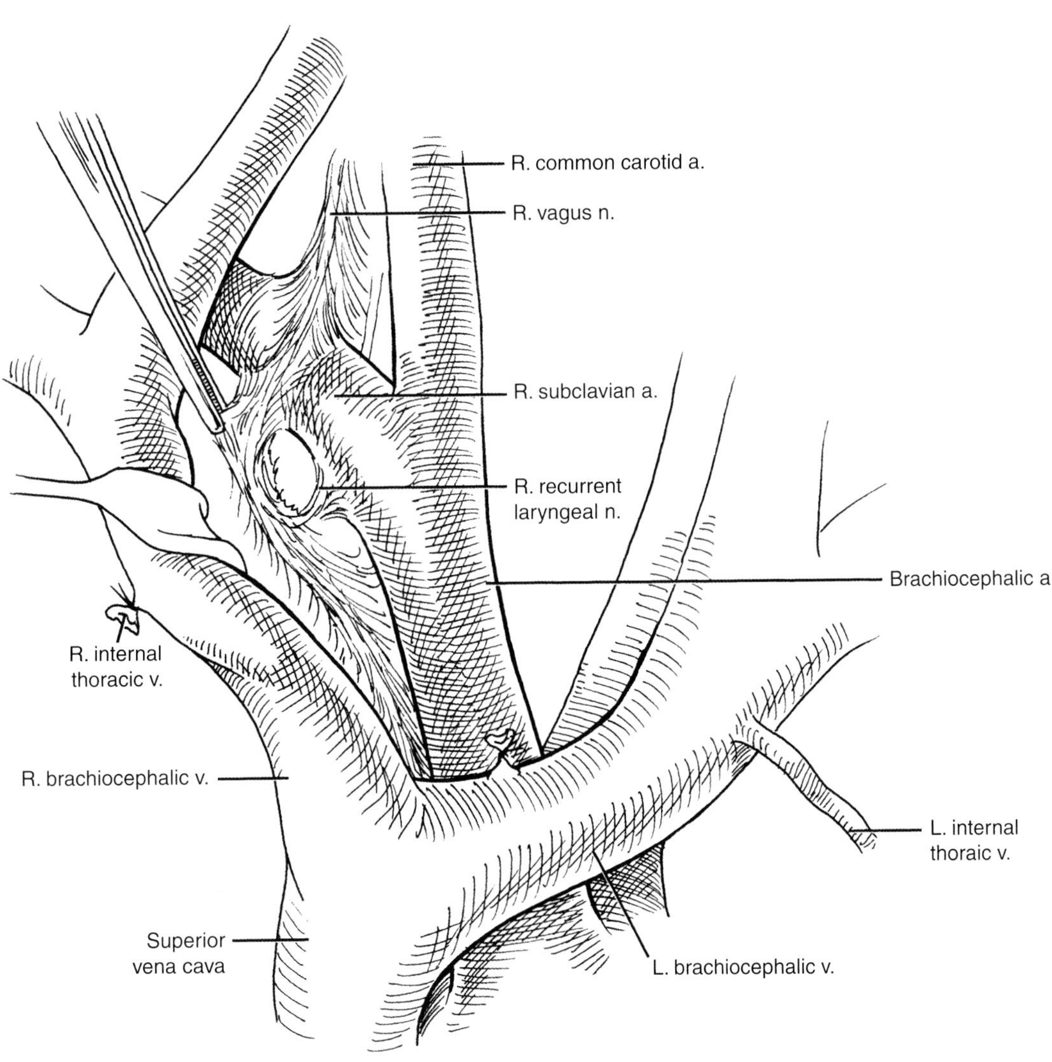

Fig. 3-21 On the right side, exposure of the bifurcation of the brachiocephalic artery and the proximal right subclavian and common carotid arteries requires mobilization of the vagus nerve.

Limited Upper Sternotomy

Full median sternotomy is recommended for most operations involving exposure of the aortic arch branches, especially in emergency situations when the exact location of injury has not been identified. In extremely limited circumstances, a complete sternotomy may not be necessary to expose the brachiocephalic and left common carotid arteries in the chest. Sakopoulos[15] has described a "ministernotomy" exposure for direct treatment of brachiocephalic and left common carotid lesions in elective circumstances. This less invasive approach is useful for amenable aortic arch branch lesions but should be avoided in patients with more extensive disease and in emergency circumstances.

The patient is placed supine with the arms drawn into the sides. The neck, chest, and upper abdomen are prepped and draped completely in the event a full sternotomy should become necessary. A vertical skin incision is made from the sternal notch to a level 2 cm below the angle of Louis. The sternum is divided in the midline from the manubrium to the third intercostal space using an oscillating saw (Fig. 3-22). The sternum is then transected horizontally in the third intercostal space to form an inverted "T" incision, taking care to avoid injury to the nearby internal mammary vessels. After hemostasis is obtained, the upper sternum is gently opened using a pediatric sternal retractor.[15] (Fig. 3-23) The underlying thymus is divided and ligated to expose the left brachiocephalic vein. Identification and exposure of the brachiocephalic and left common carotid arteries proceeds as above (Fig. 3-24). This approach is particularly suited for

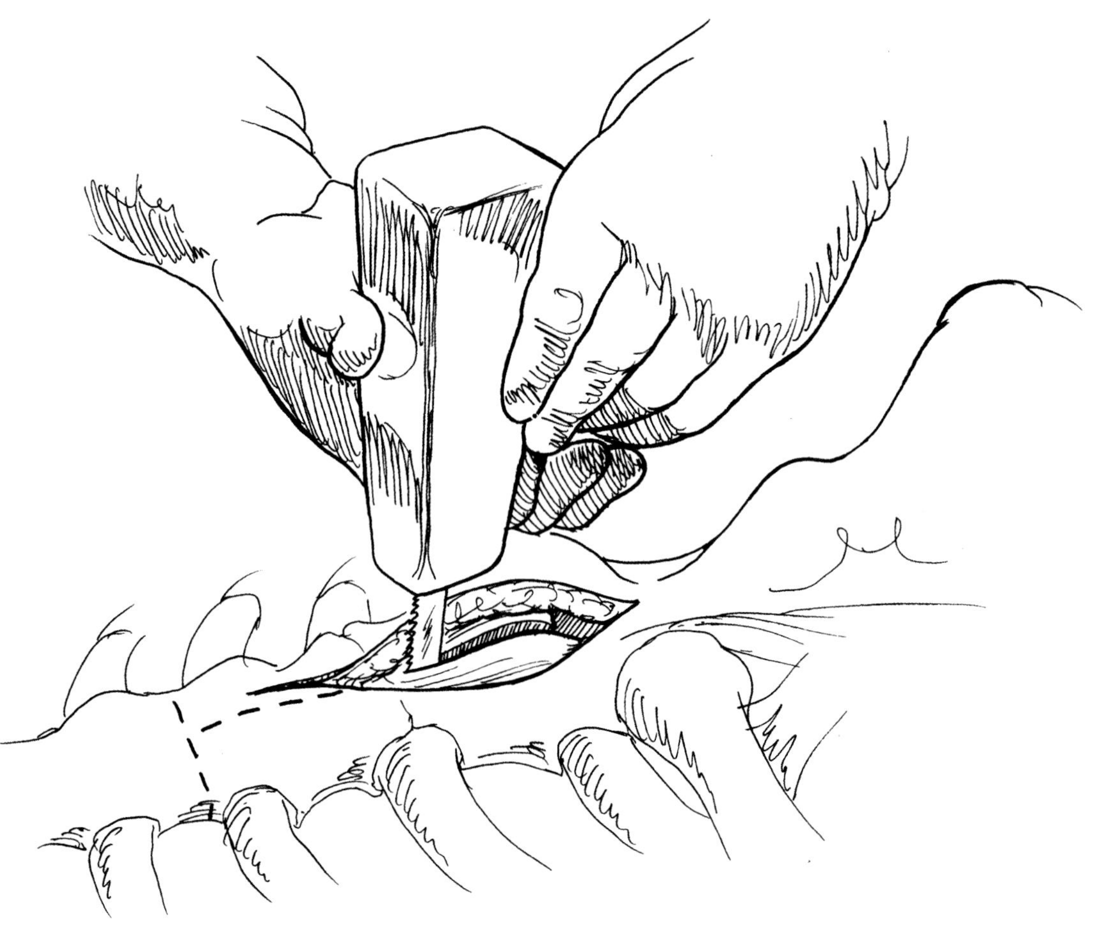

Fig. 3-22 The upper sternum is divided, then transected horizontally at the level of the third intercostal space to form an inverted "T."

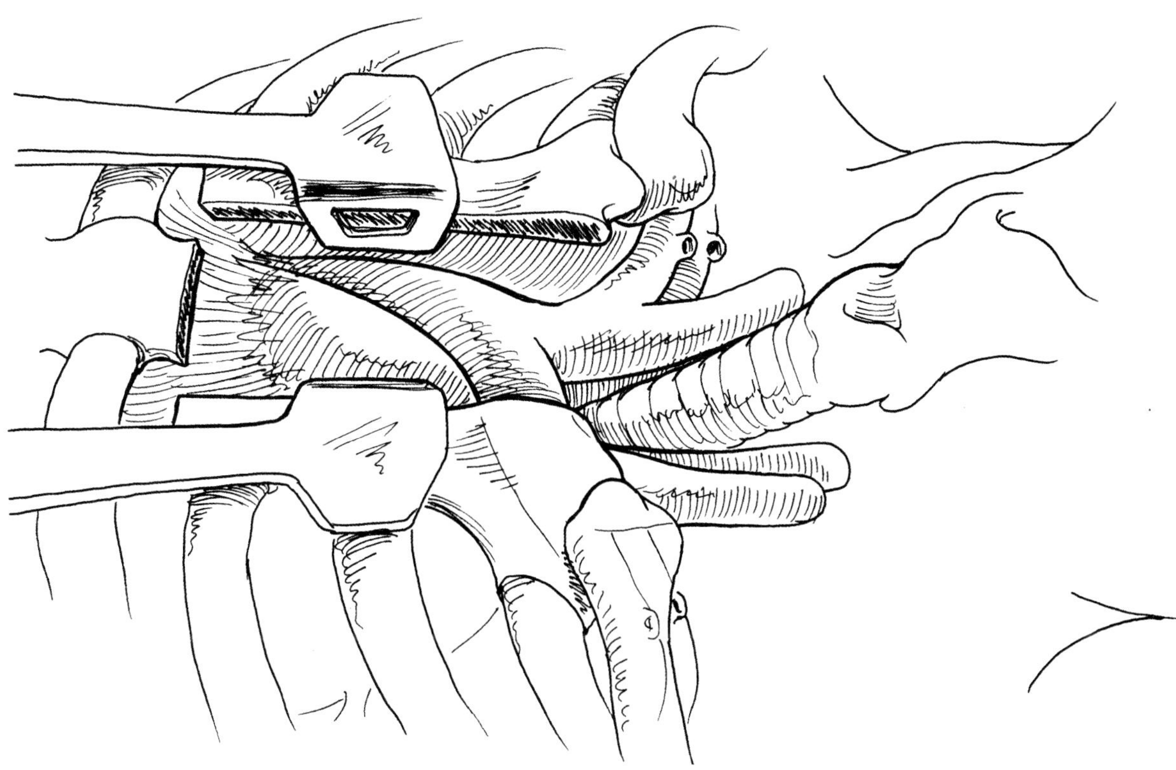

Fig. 3-23 The aortic arch and its proximal branches are readily exposed through the limited sternotomy.

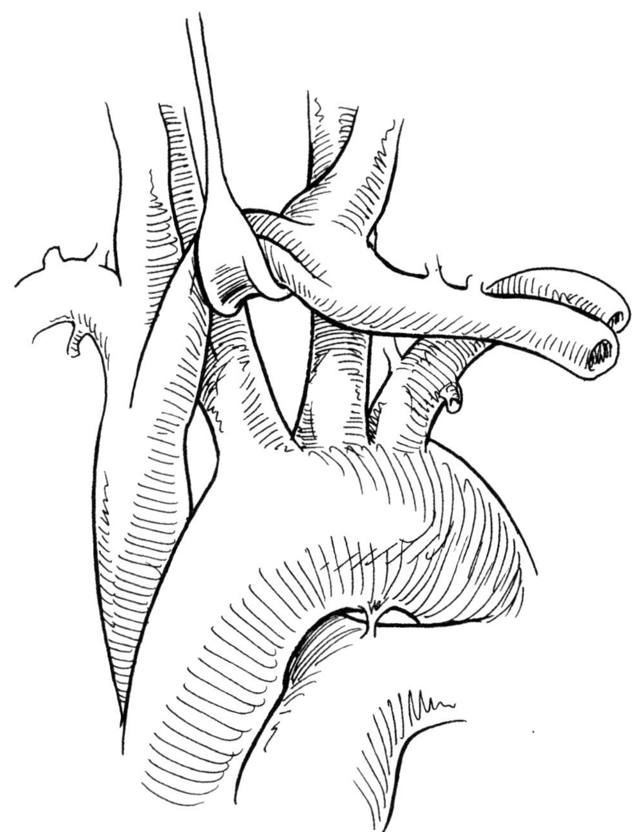

Fig. 3-24 Elevation of the left brachiocephalic vein exposes the origins of the brachiocephalic and left common carotid arteries.

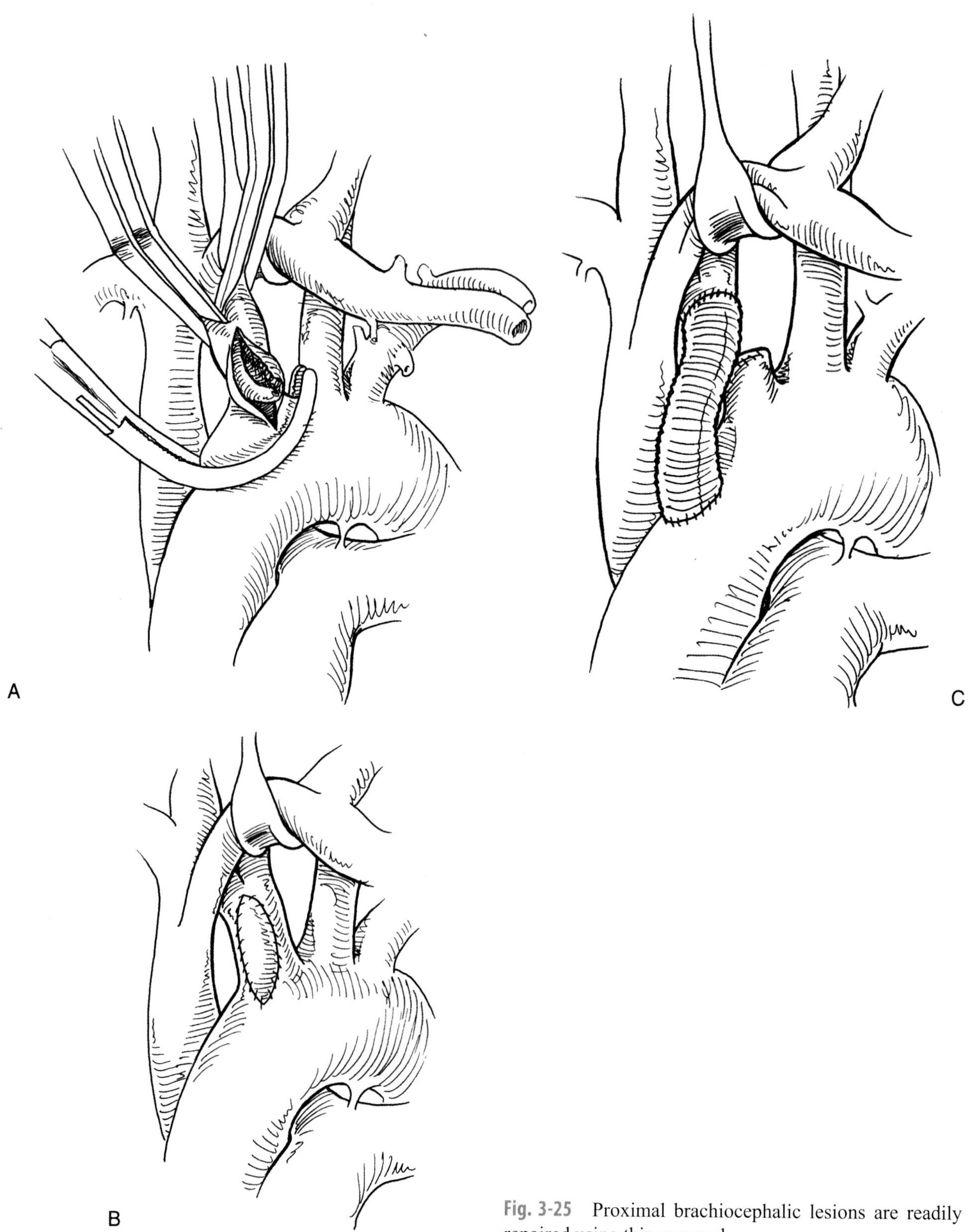

Fig. 3-25 Proximal brachiocephalic lesions are readily repaired using this approach.

direct repair of proximal brachiocephalic artery lesions (Fig. 3-25).

Exposure of the Proximal Left Subclavian Artery

Mediastinal exposure of the left subclavian artery is indicated in control of proximal injuries, which often result from penetrating trauma to the left mediastinum or base of the neck. Mediastinal control may also be urgently indicated in more distal subclavian artery injuries heralded by expanding supraclavicular hematomas. The need to expose this segment of the artery in cases of chronic occlusion has been superseded by the advent of extrathoracic bypass procedures, which are both durable and safe.[8]

The posterior location of the left subclavian artery relative to the other aortic arch branches renders it extremely difficult to expose through a median sternotomy (see Fig. 3-9). There are two surgical approaches that permit optimal exposure of the left subclavian artery at its origin: the anterolateral thoracotomy and the "trap door" thoracotomy. The former approach is optimal for emergency proximal control of the left subclavian artery and can be combined with a separate supraclavicular incision for definitive repair (see Chapter 5). The latter approach is a radical extension of the anterolateral thoracotomy and is ideal for control and repair of left subclavian artery injuries near the sternoclavicular joint. The "trap door" incision is limited in exposure, however, and should be reserved for injuries in the left side of the superior thoracic aperture.

Anterolateral Thoracotomy

The patient is placed in the supine position. A rolled sheet or pad should be placed behind the left scapula and hip to bring the left chest approximately 20° upward. The entire anterior and lateral chest, shoulder, axilla, and neck are prepped and draped.

A left transverse curvilinear incision is made over the fifth rib, just below the nipple. The incision may be made along the lower contour of the pectoralis major muscle to enhance cosmesis (Fig. 3-26).

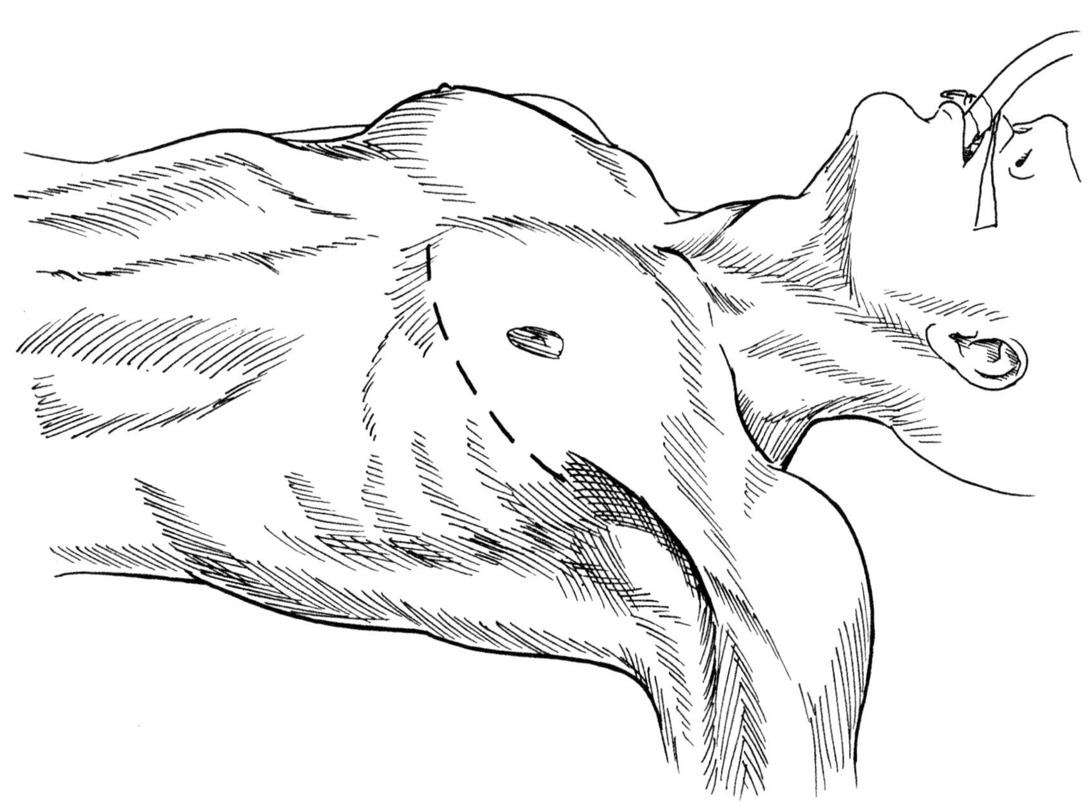

Fig. 3-26 Landmarks for a left anterolateral thoracotomy incision are demonstrated.

In females, it may be made just below the breast. Some authors advocate a third interspace incision above the nipple,[16–18] but we have found this to be somewhat limited by the bulk of the pectoralis major muscle and cosmetically inferior to the lower incision. The incision should extend from the lateral sternal border to the anterior axillary line. The fourth interspace is reached by dividing the tough pectoralis fascia and lower fibers of the pectoralis major muscle. The interspace is entered by dividing intercostal muscles along the top of the fifth rib (Fig. 3-27), which prevents injury to the neurovascular bundle lying just deep to the inferior border of the fourth rib. After incising the parietal pleura, the lung is allowed to collapse away from the chest wall, and the remainder of the wound is opened for the entire length of the skin incision. The internal thoracic artery and vein should be ligated and divided near the lateral sternal border. A rib spreader is placed in the wound and opened slowly to lessen the chance of rib fracture.

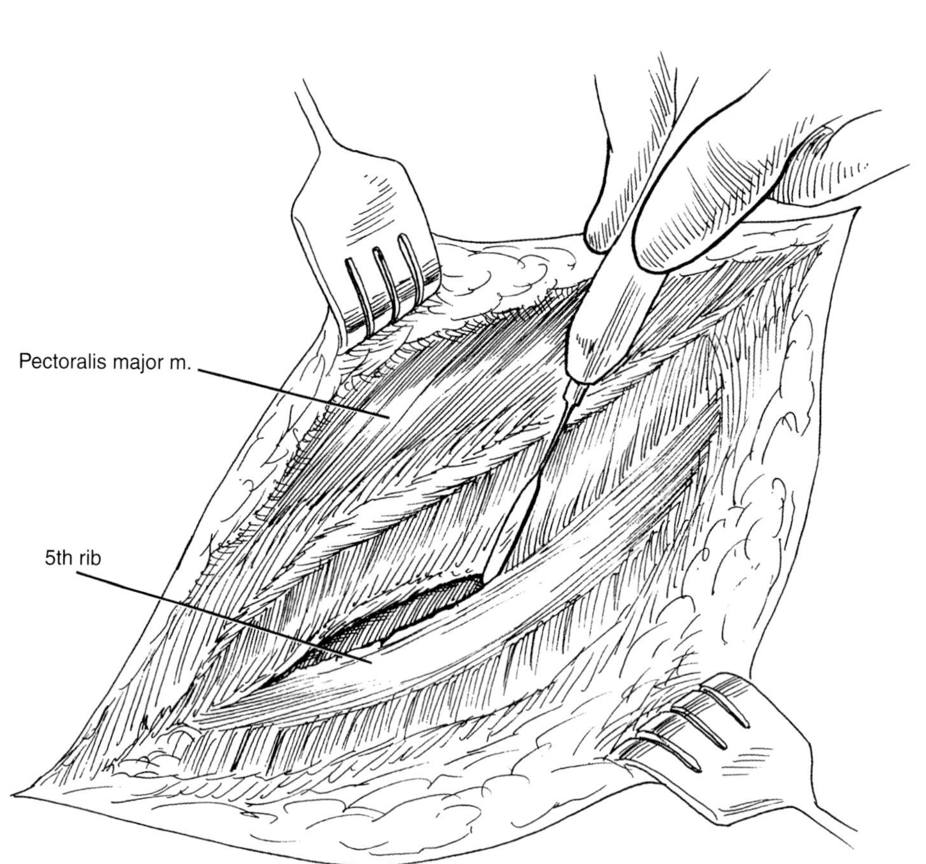

Fig. 3-27 The fourth interspace is entered over the top of the fifth rib.

By retracting the superior lobe of the left lung downward, the aortic arch can be readily seen under the glistening sheen of the mediastinal pleura (Fig. 3-28). The mediastinal pleura should be incised over the aortic arch at a point posterior to the left vagus nerve. The incision is then carried vertically

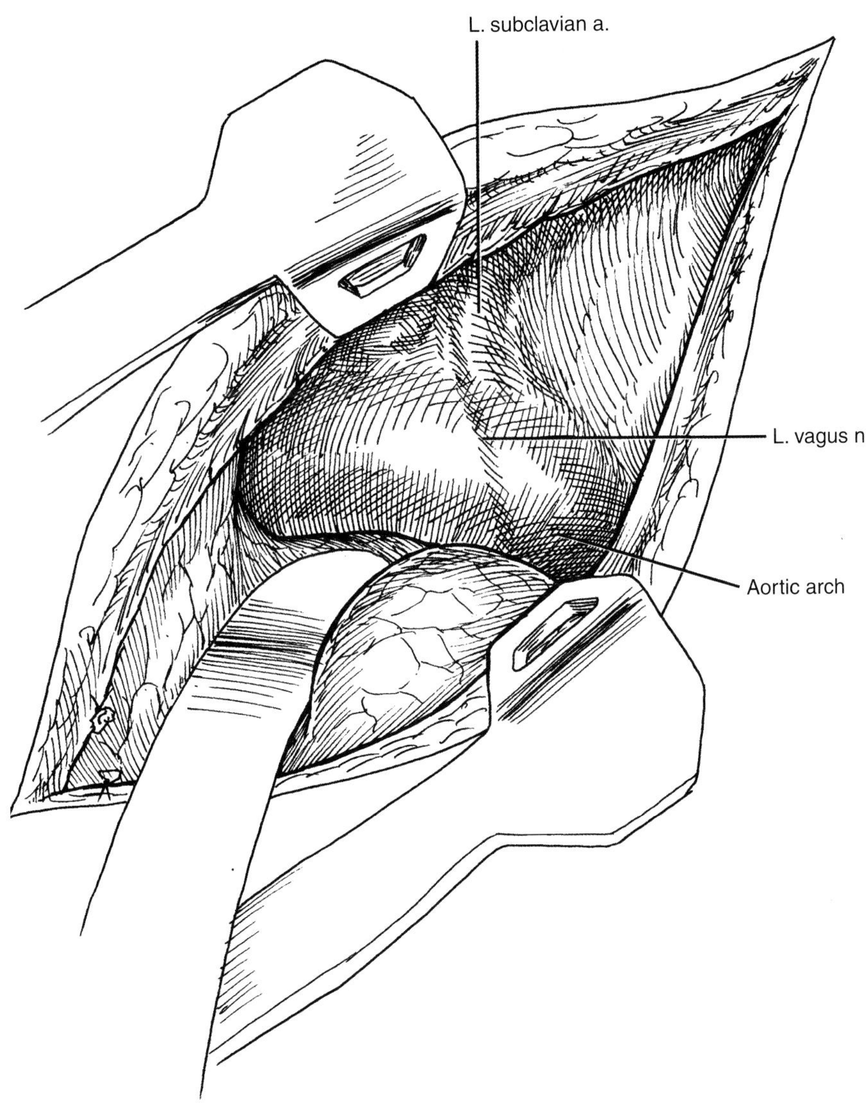

Fig. 3-28 The aortic arch is exposed by retracting the lung caudally.

over the left subclavian artery, which is most easily isolated just above its origin (Fig. 3-29). Care should be taken to avoid injuring the left vagus nerve and the thoracic duct during these maneuvers. The nerve should be recognizable under the mediastinal pleura as it courses anterolateral to the left subclavian artery and crosses the aortic arch. The thoracic duct is posteromedial to the left subclavian artery and is prone to injury during attempts at isolating the artery distal to its origin.

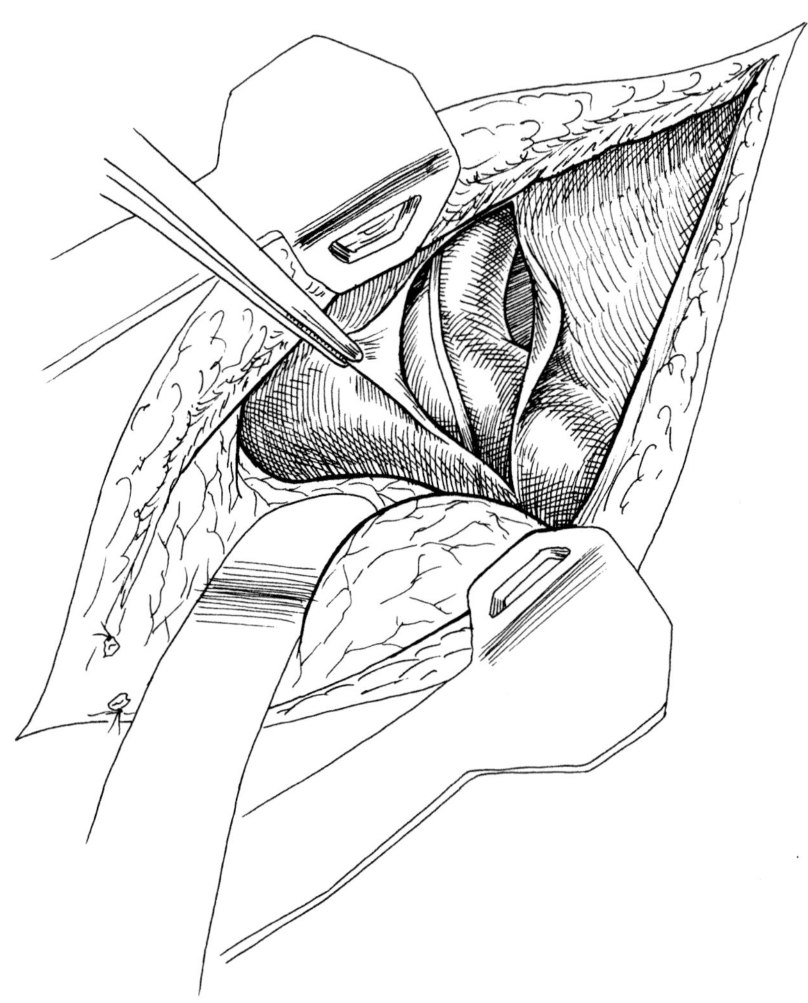

Fig. 3-29 The mediastinal pleura is opened over the arch and left subclavian artery posterior to the vagus nerve.

"Trap Door" Thoracotomy

This approach combines the left anterior thoracotomy with a left supraclavicular incision and an interconnecting upper median sternotomy (Fig. 3-30). The chest wall is not folded back as suggested by the nomenclature; rather, it is spread at the sternal division using a standard retractor.[18] Despite the criticisms[19,20] concerning the prolonged time involved in making the incision, pleural entry, excess bleeding, and a propensity for rib fractures, the "trap door" thoracotomy remains an important option for exposure of left-sided injuries at the superior thoracic aperture, particularly when the surgeon has already performed a left anterior thoracotomy in an unstable patient.

The patient is placed in the supine position. The entire chest, neck, and left shoulder are prepped and draped.

The anterolateral thoracotomy is performed first, as described above. We favor entry into the pleural space through the fourth interspace and perform an infra-areolar incision accordingly. Initial performance of this part of the incision permits early and rapid control of the left subclavian artery while

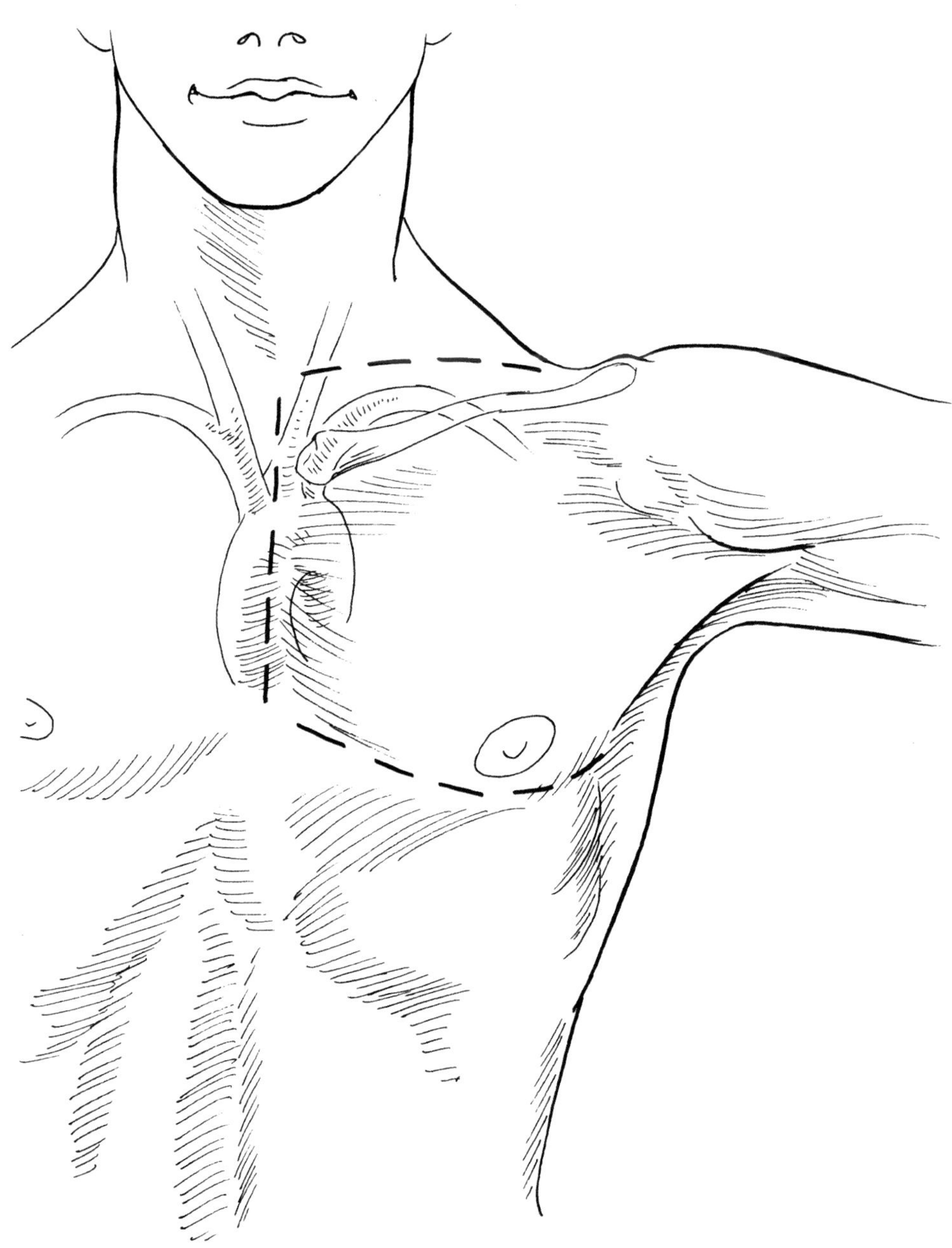

Fig. 3-30 The incisions for the "trap door" thoracotomy are outlined.

the incision is completed. The internal thoracic (mammary) vessels should be ligated and divided in the medial portion of the incision, near the sternum.

Exposure of the extrathoracic subclavian artery is performed next, allowing distal control of the arterial injury. The supraclavicular approach is preferred over resection of the medial half of the clavicle, since claviculectomy is time consuming and does not significantly improve exposure.[18,21] A transverse incision is made 2 cm above and parallel to the left clavicle, beginning at the sternal notch and extending laterally for 8 cm. The incision is deepened through subcutaneous tissues and the platysma muscle, exposing the sternocleidomastoid and omohyoid muscles. Both muscles are divided near their inferior attachments (Fig. 3-31). The external jugular vein is ligated and divided. The thin fascia overlying the supraclavicular fat pad is incised transversely, and the fat pad is swept laterally using sharp dissection. The thoracic duct should be ligated near the junction of the internal jugular and subclavian veins.

The carotid sheath is located on the medial edge of the fat pad. The lateral border of the internal jugular vein is freed, permitting medial retraction of the carotid sheath contents. This exposes the anterior scalene muscle in the medial wound (Fig. 3-32). The left phrenic nerve courses on the anterior surface of this muscle, and great care should be taken to isolate the nerve away from the anterior scalene muscle.

Once nerve protection is ensured, the anterior scalene muscle is divided near its attachment to the first rib. Division should be performed under direct vision, cutting a few fibers at a time to prevent injury to the left subclavian vein, which lies anterior to the muscle. The subclavian artery is isolated deep to the anterior scalene muscle (Fig. 3-33). The thyrocervical trunk and vertebral artery should be identified.

A vertical incision is made over the upper sternum to connect the medial borders of the

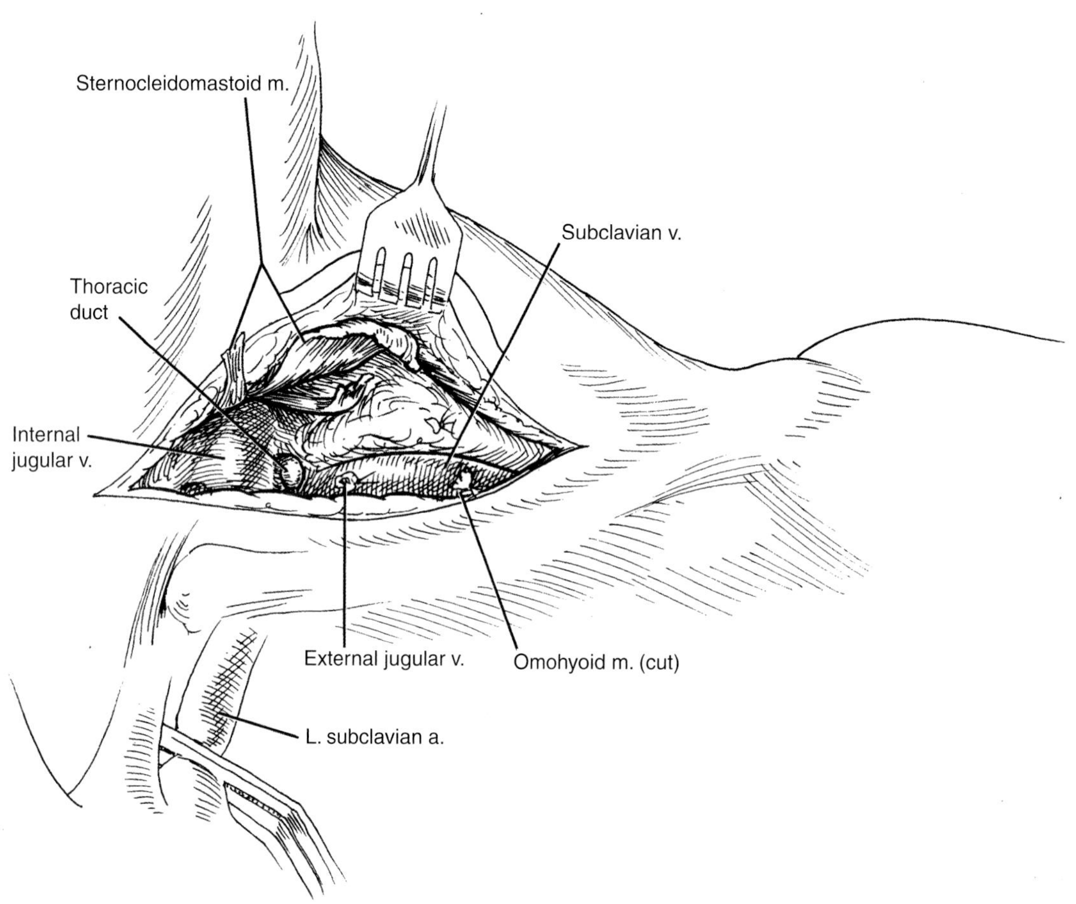

Fig. 3-31 The supraclavicular incision is developed after the anterolateral thoracotomy is complete.

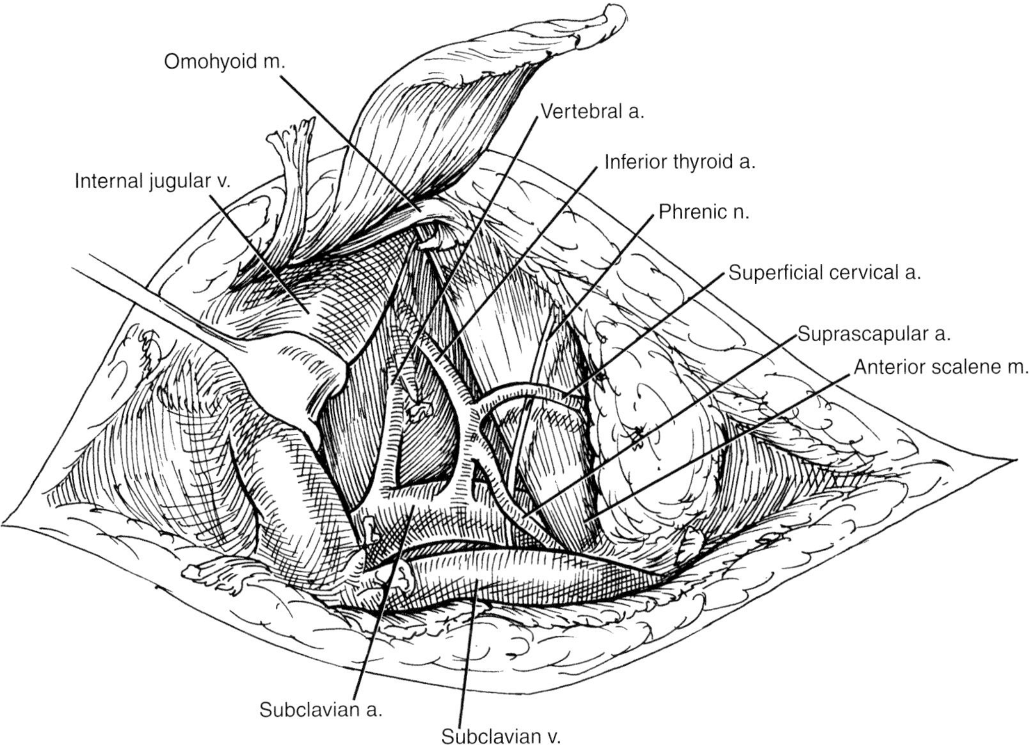

Fig. 3-32 Retraction of the carotid sheath and scalene fat pad exposes the subclavian vessels and anterior scalene muscle.

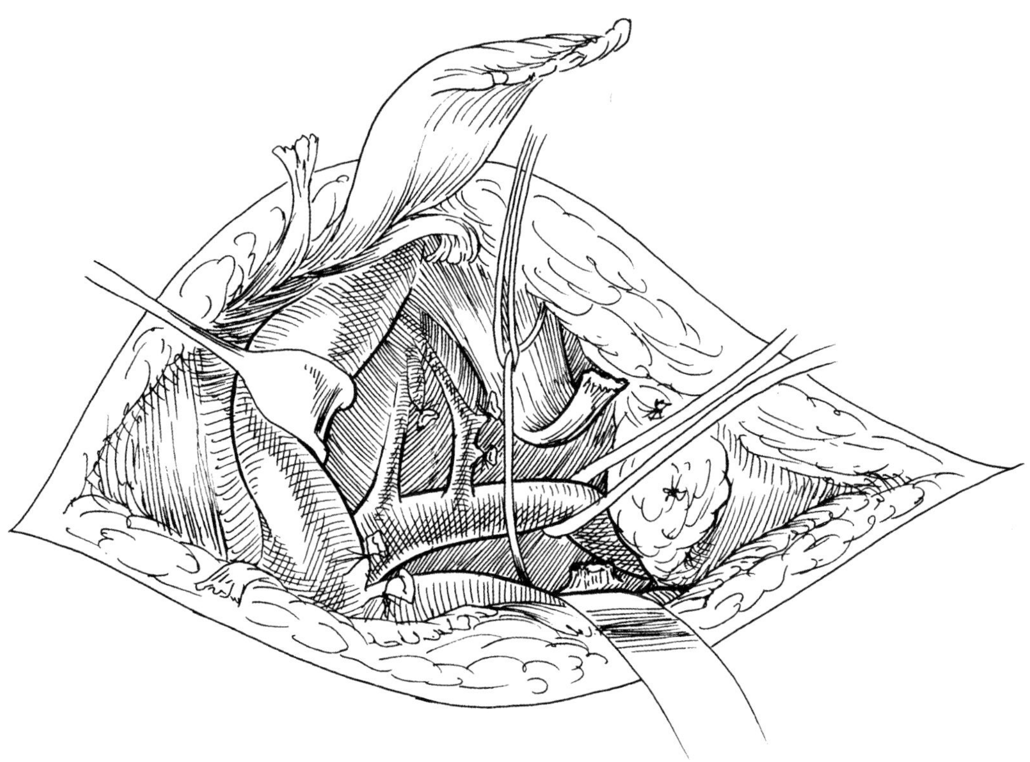

Fig. 3-33 The anterior scalene muscle is divided close to the scalene tubercle of the first rib.

supraclavicular and anterior thoracotomy incisions (Fig. 3-34). After deepening the sternal incision to the periosteum, a retrosternal plane is created at the suprasternal notch. The sternum is divided in the midline using a sternal saw or Lebsche knife (see above), beginning at the suprasternal notch and extending to the level of the fourth interspace. The sternotomy is extended laterally into the fourth interspace incision with the bone-cutting instrument.

The sternal retractor is placed in the sternotomy incision and opened slowly. The internal thoracic vessels should be ligated and divided as they are exposed during the sternal retraction. The entire length of the subclavian artery and vein are visible through this incision.

Exposure of the Descending Thoracic Aorta

The most common site of blunt injury to the thoracic aorta is just distal to the origin of the left subclavian artery, with the tear beginning at the ligamentum arteriosum.[22] Although a majority of victims who sustain such injuries are dead prior to arrival at treatment facilities, up to 20% may be alive.[23,24] Urgent diagnosis of this injury is crucial to survival, as the mortality rate rises with increasing time to definitive repair. Endovascular treatment has become a popular alternative to open repair, but the superiority of one technique over the other remains controversial. Although the endovascular approach appears to be

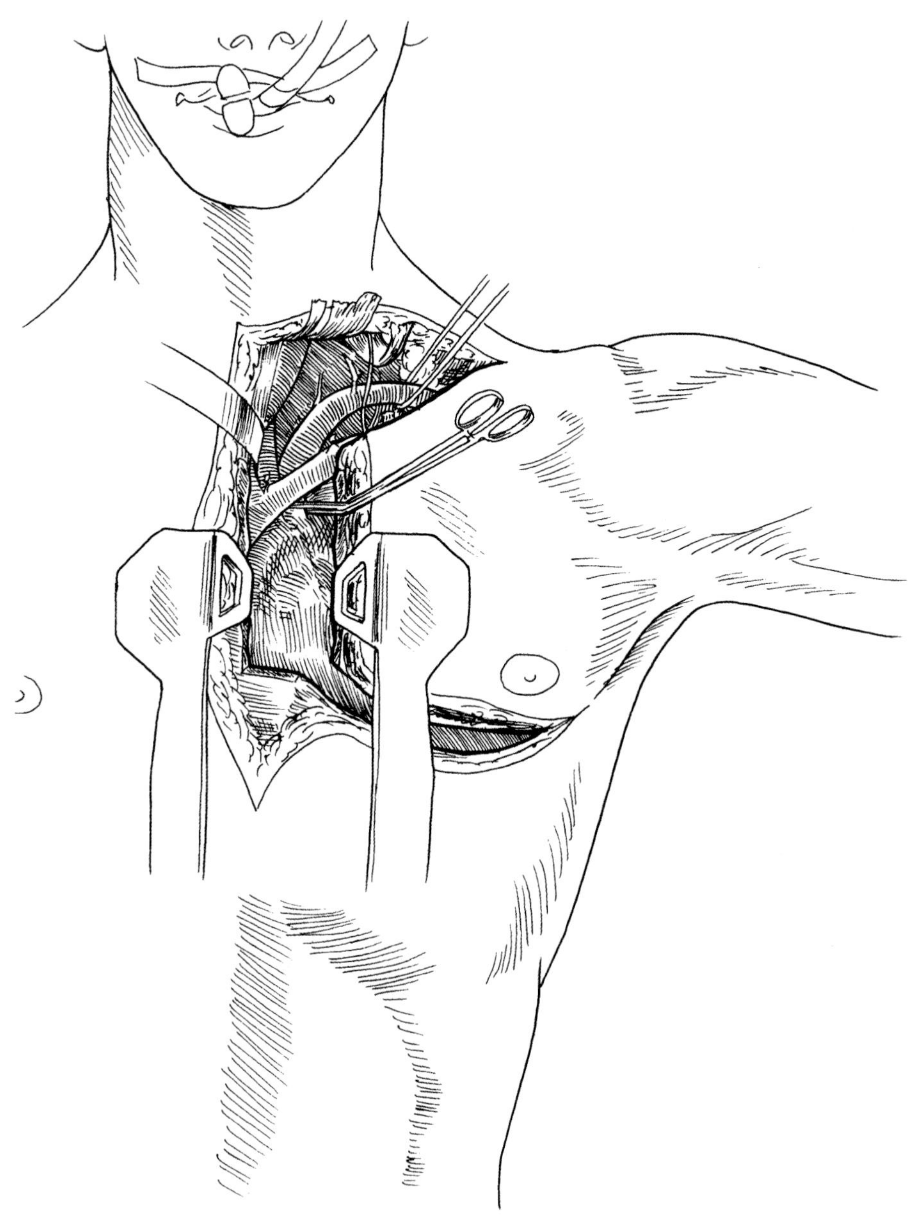

Fig. 3-34 A partial median sternotomy completes this incision.

associated with reduced morbidity and duration of hospitalization,[24,25] the durability of thoracic stent grafts in trauma patients who tend to be younger and resistant to follow-up remains unknown. Furthermore, a recent analysis suggests that survival in patients with blunt aortic injuries is determined by the extent of associated injuries and not influenced by the type or timing of surgical repair.[26] The following discussion describes exposure of the descending thoracic aorta for open repair, which is best obtained through a posterolateral thoracotomy.

Posterolateral Thoracotomy

The patient is placed in a true lateral position, with the right side down. A roll is placed beneath the right axilla. The right arm is placed on an armboard perpendicular to the patient, and the left arm is supported with pillows or on a Mayo stand. The right leg is flexed to 90°, and the left leg is extended and supported by pillows placed between the patient's knees (Fig. 3-35). Stabilization of the pelvis is ensured with wide tape that is brought from one side

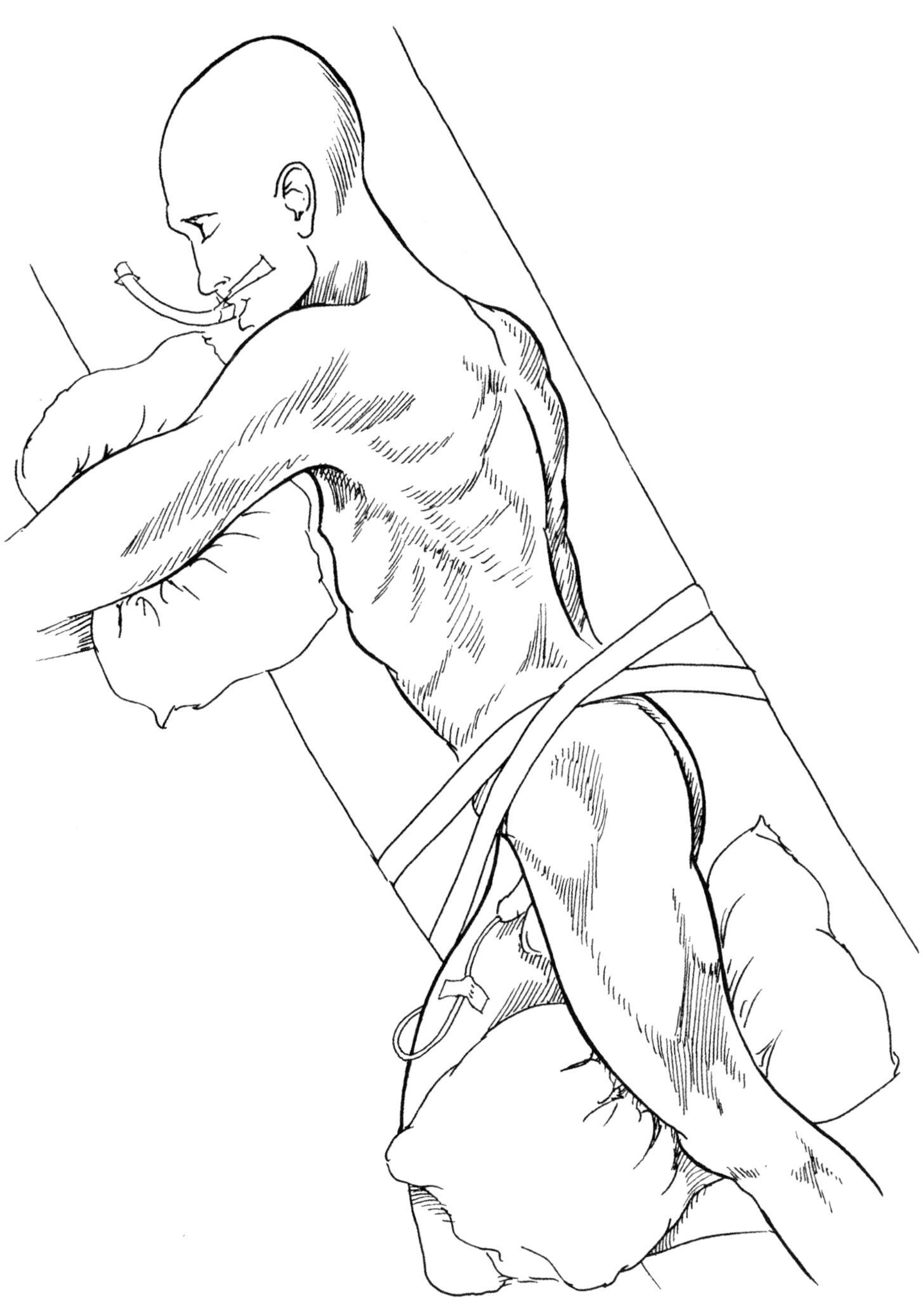

Fig. 3-35 Patient position for a left posterolateral thoracotomy incision is shown.

of the operating table to the other across the left hip. The exposed chest, flank, and left shoulder are prepped and draped.

The skin incision begins just below the left nipple and extends posteriorly to 1 inch below the tip of the scapula, then curves upward between the scapula and the spine (Fig. 3-36). The wound is deepened through the subcutaneous tissue and investing fascia. The latissimus dorsi, serratus anterior, and trapezius muscles are divided. Division of these muscles allows the shoulder girdle to move upward and the scapula to retract away from the incision. The optimal interspace through which the chest will be entered is determined by the level of aorta to be exposed. The proximal segment of the descending thoracic aorta is best exposed through the fourth interspace, and the distal segment is best exposed through the sixth interspace. The chosen interspace should be verified by counting the ribs from above downward. The surgeon's hand is placed beneath the scapula and pushed upward through loose areolar tissue toward the apex of the chest. The ribs are counted downward from the first. The fourth interspace is identified and entered by incising the intercostal muscles along the superior border of the fifth rib. After entering the pleural cavity, the left lung is

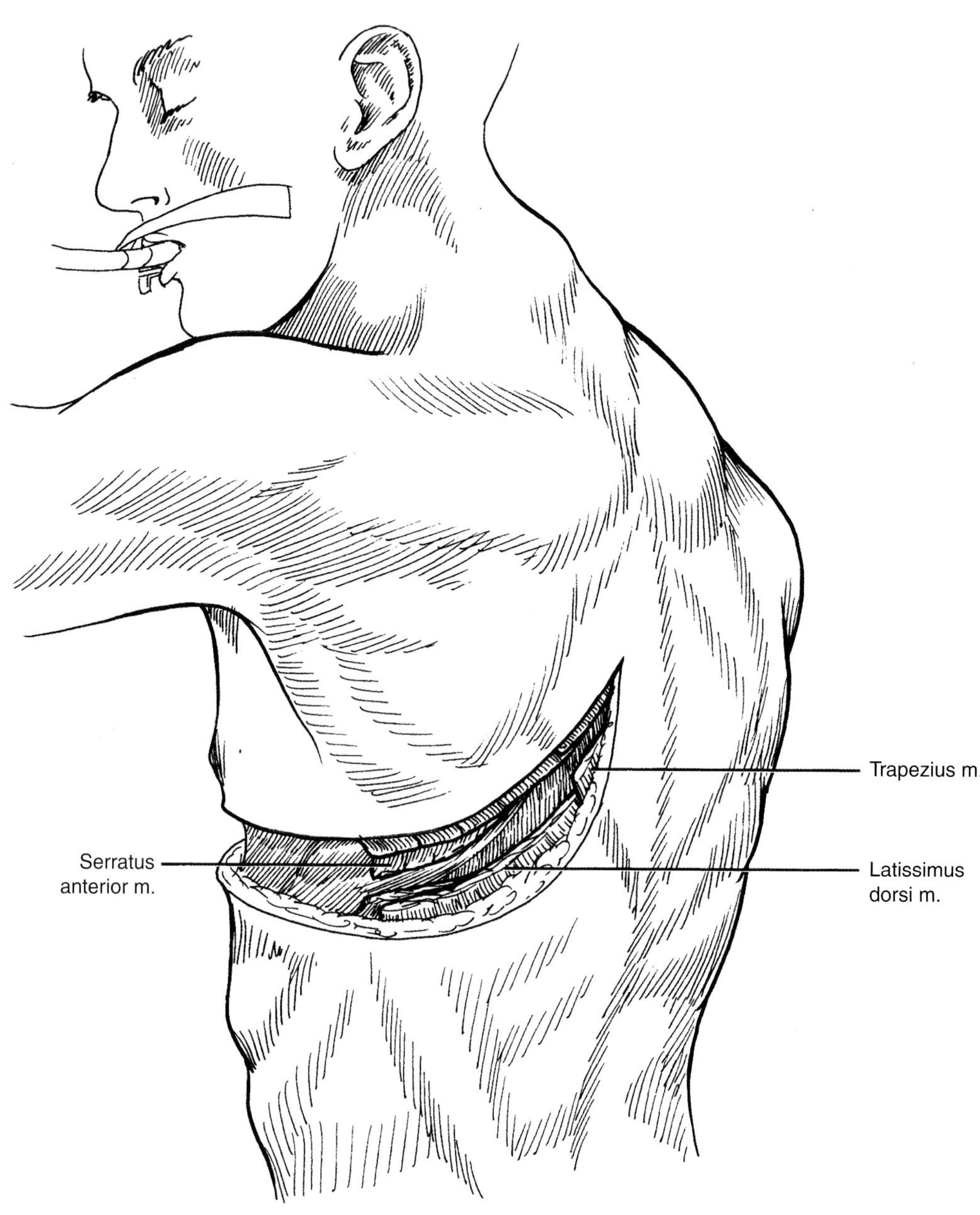

Fig. 3-36 Trapezius, latissimus, and serratus muscles are divided in turn.

allowed to collapse. Rib spreaders are placed in the wound and opened slowly to prevent rib fracture.

The descending thoracic aorta will be seen anterior to the vertebrae beneath the glistening surface of the mediastinal pleura. Control of the distal thoracic aorta is easily obtained by incising the mediastinal pleura directly over the vessel. The aorta is encircled with heavy tapes, taking care to preserve intercostal arteries.

Aortic tears at the level of the ligamentum arteriosum require control of the aorta between the left common carotid and left subclavian arteries, as well as control of the proximal left subclavian artery (Fig. 3-37). Control of the aorta at this level requires identification and protection of the vagus and phrenic nerves as they cross the aortic arch. This may be accomplished with vertical incision of the mediastinal pleura posterior to the vagus nerve. The left vagus nerve and surrounding periaortic tissues are bluntly swept forward until the aorta is sufficiently cleared to be clamped. The left phrenic nerve should be carefully dissected from the aortic arch and gently retracted away from the area of injury. The left subclavian artery can be controlled near its origin by extending the pleural incision superiorly (see above).

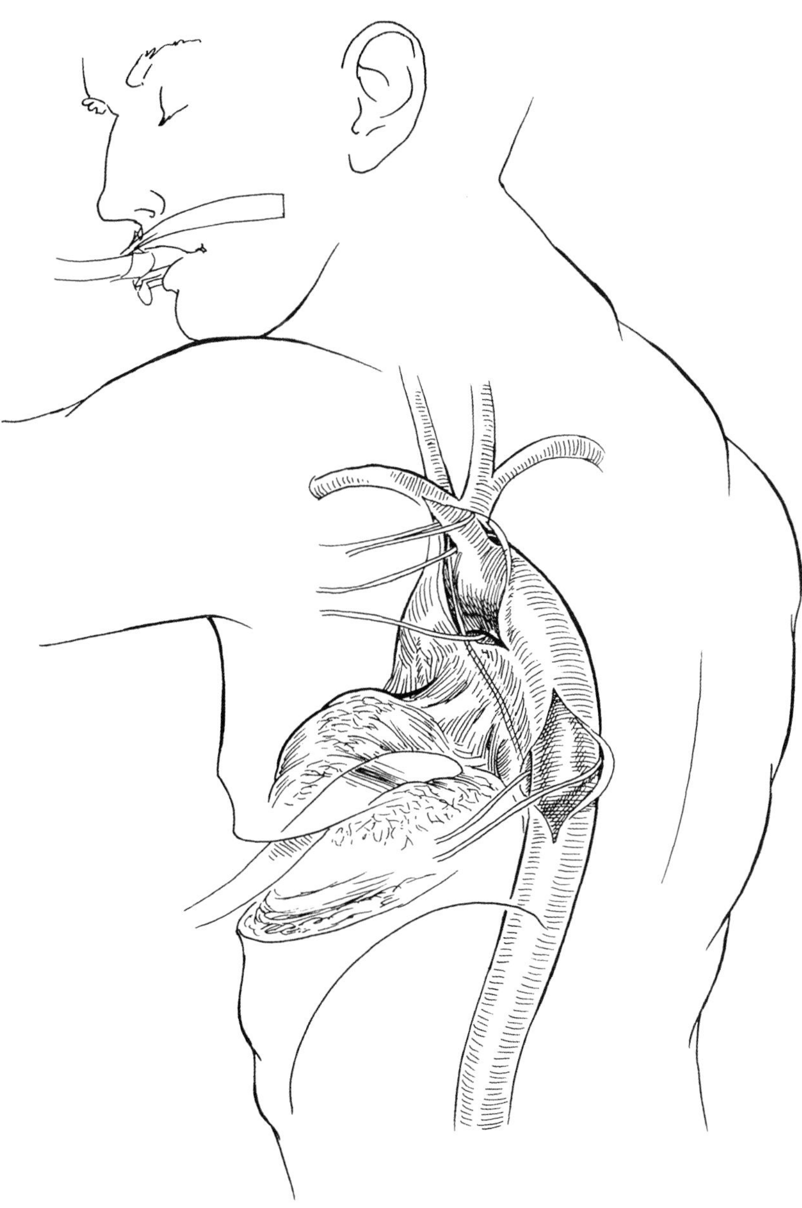

Fig. 3-37 Proximal and distal control is demonstrated for lesions of the proximal descending aorta.

References

1. Arthurs ZM, Sohn VY, Starnes BW. Vascular trauma: endovascular management and techniques. *Surg Clin North Am.* 2007;87:1179–1192.
2. Hershberger RC, Aulivola B, Murphy M, et al. Endovascular grafts for treatment of traumatic injury to the aortic arch and great vessels. *J Trauma.* 2009;67:660–671.
3. Cook CC, Gleason TG. Great vessel and cardiothoracic trauma. *Surg Clin North Am.* 2009;89:797–820.
4. Meredith JW, Hoth JJ. Thoracic trauma: when and how to intervene. *Surg Clin North Am.* 2007;87:95–118.
5. Hyre CE, Cikrit DF, Lalka SG, et al. Aggressive management of vascular injuries of the thoracic outlet. *J Vasc Surg.* 1998;27:880–885.
6. Pretre R, Chilcott M. Current concepts: Blunt trauma to the heart and great vessels. *N Engl J Med.* 1997;336:626–632.
7. McCoy DW, Weiman DS, Pate JW, et al. Subclavian artery injuries. *Am Surg.* 1997;63:761–764.
8. Berguer R, Morasch MD, Kline RA, et al. Cervical reconstruction of the supra-aortic trunks: a 16-year experience. *J Vasc Surg.* 1999;29:239–248.
9. Matsumura JS, Lee WA, Mitchell RS, et al. The Society for Vascular Surgery Practice guidelines: management of the left subclavian artery with thoracic endovascular aortic repair. *J Vasc Surg.* 2009;50:1155–1158.
10. Kieffer E, Sabatier J, Koskas F, et al. Atherosclerotic innominate artery occlusive disease: early and long-term results of surgical reconstruction. *J Vasc Surg.* 1995;21:26–337.
11. Ligush J Jr, Criado E, Keagy BA. Innominate artery occlusive disease: management with central reconstructive techniques. *Surgery.* 1997;121:556–562.
12. Cooper JD, Nelems JM, Pearson FG. Extended indications for median sternotomy in patients requiring pulmonary resection. *Ann Thorac Surg.* 1978;26:413–420.
13. Gopaldas RR, Chu D, Bakaeen FG. Acquired heart disease: coronary insufficiency. In: Townsend CM Jr, Beauchamp RD, Evars BM, Mattaox KL, eds. *Sabiston Textbook of Surgery.* 19th ed. Philadelphia, PA: Elsevier Saunders; 2012:1650–1678.
14. Robicsek F, Masters TN, Littman L, et al. The embolization of bone wax from sternotomy incisions. *Ann Thorac Surg.* 1981;31:357–359.
15. Sakopoulos AG, Ballard JL, Gundry SR. Minimally invasive approach for aortic arch branch vessel reconstruction. *J Vasc Surg.* 2000;31:200–202.
16. Schaff HV, Brawley RK. Operative management of penetrating injuries of the thoracic outlet. *Surgery.* 1977;82:182–191.
17. Kirschner RL. Management of penetrating injury to the vessels at the thoracic outlet. *Contemp Surg.* 1983;23:83–88.
18. Graham JM, Feliciano DV, Mattox KL, et al. Management of subclavian vascular injuries. *J Trauma.* 1980;20:537–544.
19. Symbas PN. Surgical anatomy of the great arteries of the thorax. *Surg Clin North Am.* 1974;54:1303–1312.
20. Robbs JV, Baker LW, Human RR, et al. Cervicomediastinal arterial injuries: a surgical challenge. *Arch Surg.* 1981;116:663–668.
21. Robbs JV, Reddy E. Management options for penetrating injuries to the great veins of the neck and superior mediastinum. *Surg Gynecol Obstet.* 1987;165:323–326.
22. Starnes BW, Lundgren RS, Gunn M, et al. A new classification scheme for treating blunt aortic injury. *J Vasc Surg.* 2012;55:47–54.
23. Morgan PB, Buechter KJ. Blunt thoracic aortic injuries: initial evaluation and management. *SMJ.* 2000;93:173–175.
24. Cindy M, Sabrina H, Kim D, et al. Traumatic aortic rupture: 30 years of experience. *Ann Vasc Surg.* 2011;25:474–480.
25. Patel HJ, Williams DM, Upchurch GR Jr, et al. A comparative analysis of open and endovascular repair for ruptured descending thoracic aorta. *J Vasc Surg.* 2009;50:1265–1270.
26. Lang JL, Minei JP, Modrall JG, et al. The limitations of thoracic endovascular aortic repair (TEVAR) in altering the natural history of blunt aortic injury. *J Vasc Surg.* 2010;52:290–297.

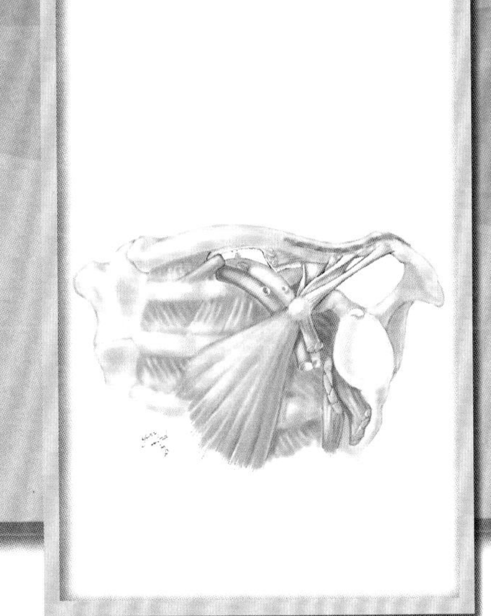

Superior Thoracic Aperture and Cervicothoracic Sympathetic Chain

4

Anatomy of the "Thoracic Outlet"

The superior opening of the bony thorax has come to be called the thoracic outlet. The anatomic term superior thoracic aperture and the term thoracic outlet will be used interchangeably in this chapter to designate the regional anatomy.

Compression of upper extremity neurovascular structures, collectively called the thoracic outlet syndrome, encompasses considerably more anatomy than the cephalad aperture of the bony thorax. The vessels exiting the chest and the nerves emerging from the spinal column pass between the scalene muscles above the rim of the superior thoracic aperture. They then pass through the triangle formed by the first rib, clavicle, and scapula and run beneath the coracoid process on their way to the brachium.

The following discussion considers all of the structures that can compress and compromise the nerves and blood vessels of the upper extremity. The basic surgical approaches to correcting such compression are addressed in the second part of the chapter.

The Cephalad Passages

The superior thoracic aperture is bounded by the first ribs, which connect the spinal column posteriorly with the sternum anteriorly (Fig. 4-1). The vertebral bodies indent the oval shape of this opening. The manubrium of the sternum rises above the plane of the first ribs to articulate with the heads of the clavicles. The mobile sternoclavicular joint is the only osseous connection between the axillary skeleton and the bones of the upper extremity. The mobility of the clavicle is important in determining the amount of space available for passage of the subclavian vessels and brachial plexus draped over the first rib. The costoclavicular ligament as well as the sternoclavicular joint attach the clavicle medially.

The transverse processes of the cervical vertebrae are trough-shaped and contain central apertures. The vertebral arteries normally enter the sixth transverse foramen and traverse the upper five foramina to reach the base of the skull. The transverse process of the seventh cervical vertebra is often quite large. Rarely, a cervical rib may be present, which attaches to this transverse process and lies in the path of the brachial plexus.

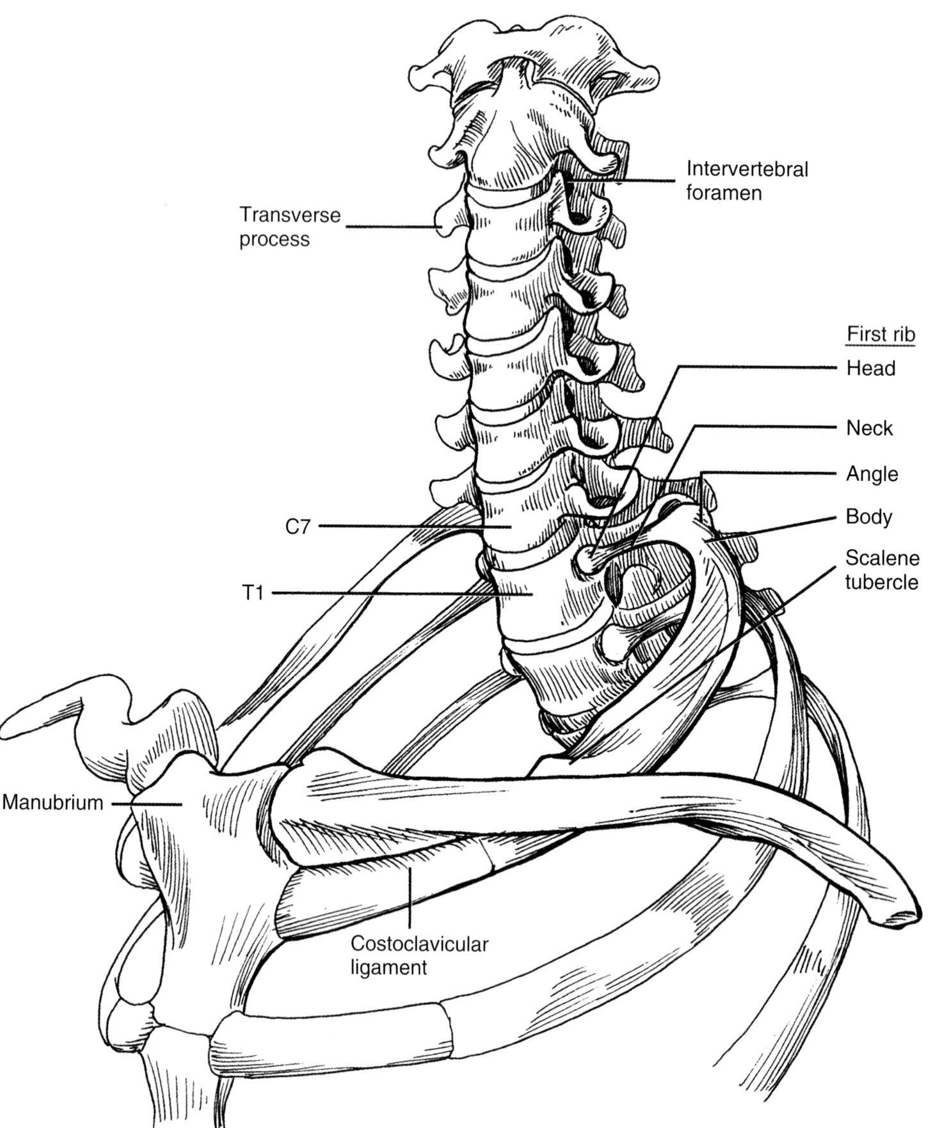

Fig. 4-1 The bony landmarks associated with the thoracic outlet include the obliquely angled face of the superior thoracic aperture between the spinal column posteriorly and the manubrium anteriorly. The clavicle and scapula constitute the pectoral girdle.

The fifth through the eighth cervical nerves and the first thoracic nerve give origin to the brachial plexus (Fig. 4-2). The nerves emerge through the intervertebral foramina and lie in the troughs of the transverse processes posterior to the vertebral vessels. The anterior and middle scalene muscles sandwich the roots of the brachial plexus. The anterior scalene muscles originate from the anterior tubercles of transverse processes three through six and insert on the scalene tubercle of the first rib between the subclavian artery and vein. The middle scalene muscles arise from the posterior tubercles of the lower six cervical transverse processes and attach more broadly to the posterior parts of the first ribs. The posterior scalene muscle rarely contributes to the thoracic outlet syndrome.

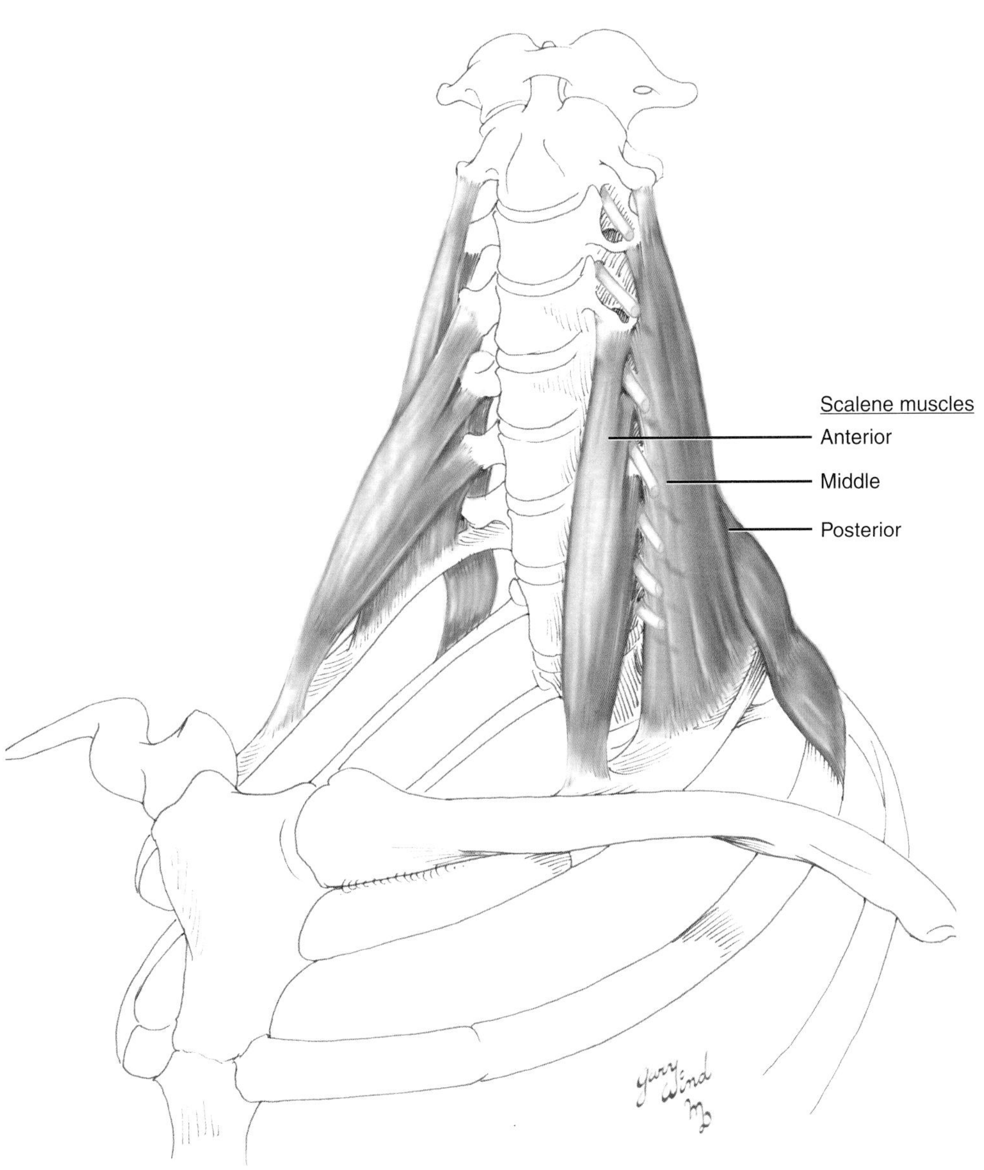

Fig. 4-2 The scalene muscles form struts between the cervical spine and the first ribs. The nerves to the upper extremity pass between the anterior and middle scalene muscles.

The Neurovascular Core

The *roots* of the brachial plexus are the ventral rami of the fifth through eighth cervical and first thoracic nerves, which lie between the anterior and middle scalene muscles (Fig. 4-3). Topographically these lie in the posterior triangle of the neck. As they emerge between the scalene muscles, the roots of the brachial plexus unite to form three *trunks*. At the level of the first rib, the trunks divide into anterior and posterior *divisions* which lie posterior to the first part of the axillary artery. The posterior divisions unite to form the posterior *cord* which continues behind the axillary artery to become the radial nerve. The anterior divisions form lateral and medial cords around the artery. The medial cord gives rise to the ulnar nerve. A branch of the medial cord unites with the lateral cord to form the median nerve anterior to the artery.

There are three important branches which deviate from the central location of the brachial plexus. Twigs from the roots of the fifth, sixth, and seventh nerves unite to form the long thoracic nerve and pass through the substance of the middle scalene muscle to reach the serratus anterior muscle on the chest wall. This relationship is important during the posterior dissection for first rib resection.

The phrenic nerve arises from the third, fourth, and fifth ventral nerve roots. It descends on the surface of the anterior scalene muscle, running from a lateral to a medial position. It enters the chest

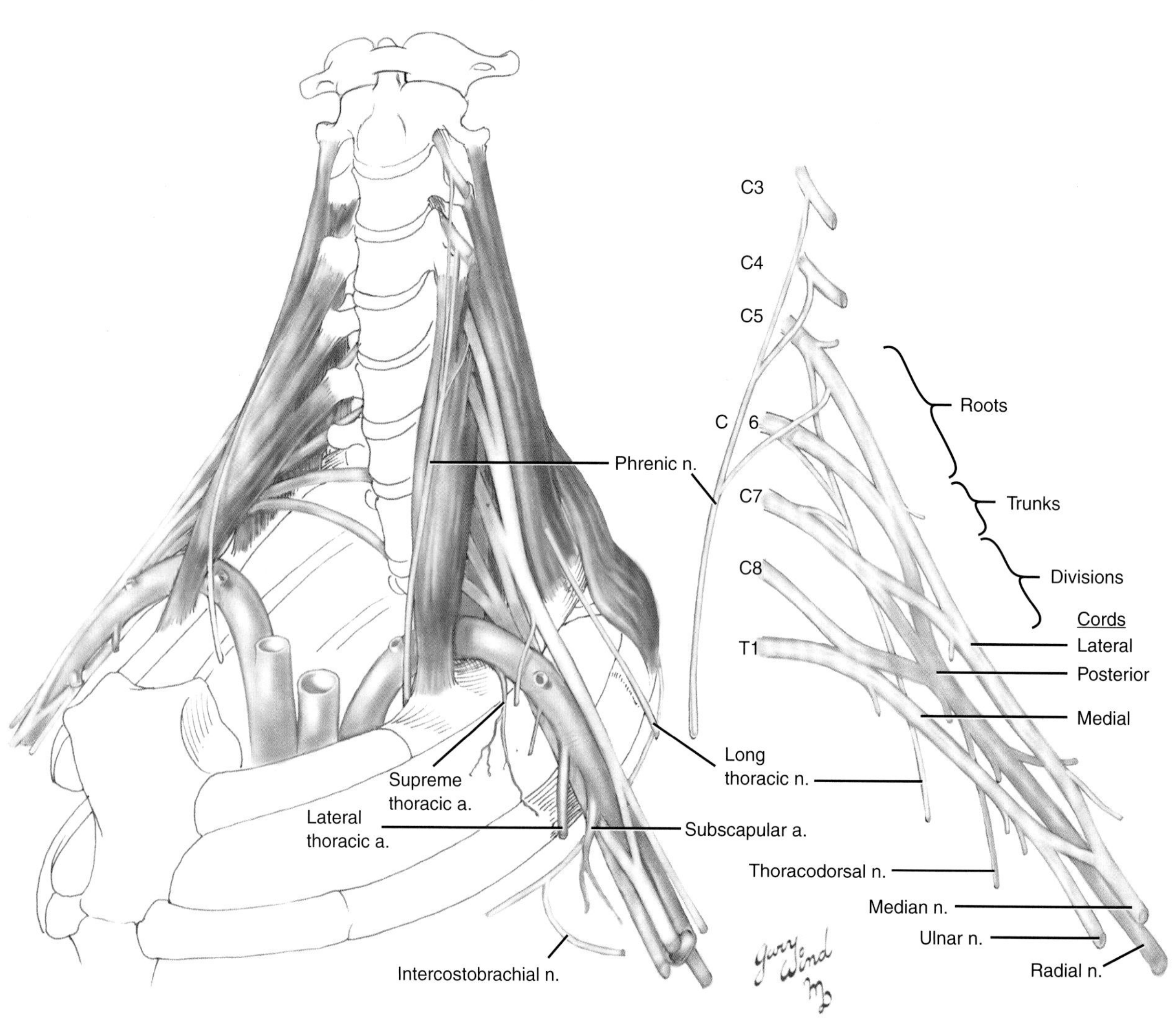

Fig. 4-3 The relationship between the brachial plexus and subclavian/axillary arteries is depicted in this illustration.

between the subclavian artery and vein at the inner margin of the first rib, just medial to the anterior scalene attachment to the scalene tubercle.

Another branch of the brachial plexus that is notable by its proximity during surgical correction of thoracic outlet compression syndromes is the thoracodorsal nerve. It arises from the posterior cord in the midaxilla and joins the thoracodorsal vessels to the latissimus dorsi muscle. Its lateral origin puts it at the periphery of the operative field when the arm is elevated.

The intercostobrachial nerve is a branch of the second intercostal nerve which crosses the center of the axillary space and usually joins the medial brachial cutaneous nerve. Some numbness on the inner aspect of the brachium may result from division of this nerve.

The axillary artery gives off the small supreme thoracic artery at the lateral margin of the first rib, the lateral thoracic artery in the midaxilla, and the subscapular artery in the distal axilla. The supreme and lateral thoracic vessels lie directly on the chest wall. The subscapular vessels arise more laterally and are not directly on the chest wall.

The Axillary Passages

The mobile pectoral girdle frames the upper border of the axilla (Fig. 4-4). The muscles attaching the clavicle and scapula to the chest wall form the boundaries of the axilla and create the neurovascular bundle's passageway to the upper extremity. Elevation of the pectoral girdle widens the passage, while depression and posterior displacement narrow the space.

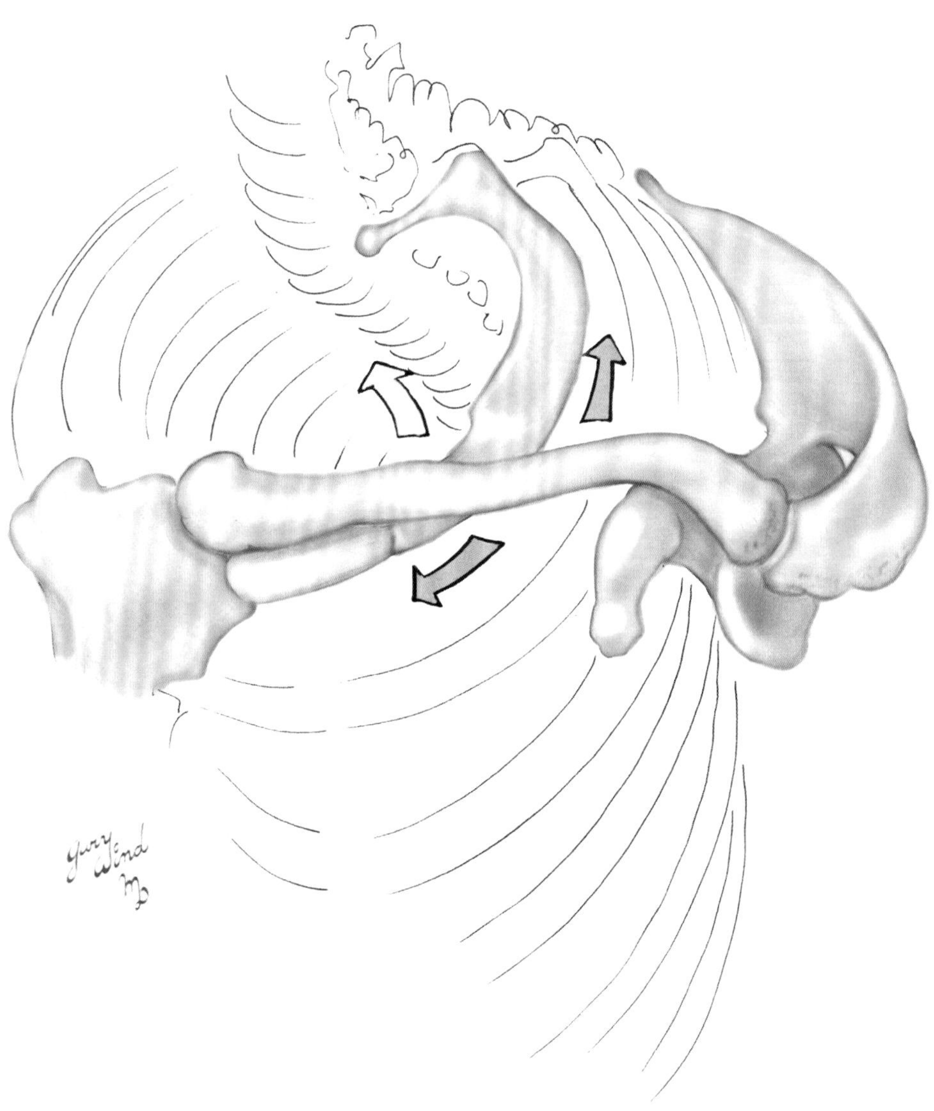

Fig. 4-4 The great mobility of the pectoral girdle affects the amount of space available for the nerve and vascular trunks to the upper extremity.

The serratus anterior muscle forms the majority of the medial axillary wall (Fig. 4-5). The subclavius muscle forms a bridge from the undersurface of the distal clavicle to the costochondral junction of the first rib. A second bridge is formed by the arching coracoid process and the origin of the pectoralis minor muscle. Subscapularis, teres major, and latissimus dorsi muscles form the posterolateral boundary of the axilla. The neurovascular bundle passes under these bridges to reach the axillary space.

The axillary space and neurovascular bundle are enclosed by several well-defined fascial layers. The prevertebral fascia surrounding the scalene muscles continues onto the surface of the vessels and nerves lying over the first rib, forming an axillary sheath. The clavipectoral fascia extends from the subclavius muscle across the pectoralis minor muscle, which it enfolds, and joins the axillary fascia. The latter spans from the lateral edge of the pectoralis major muscle to the anterior edge of the latissimus dorsi.

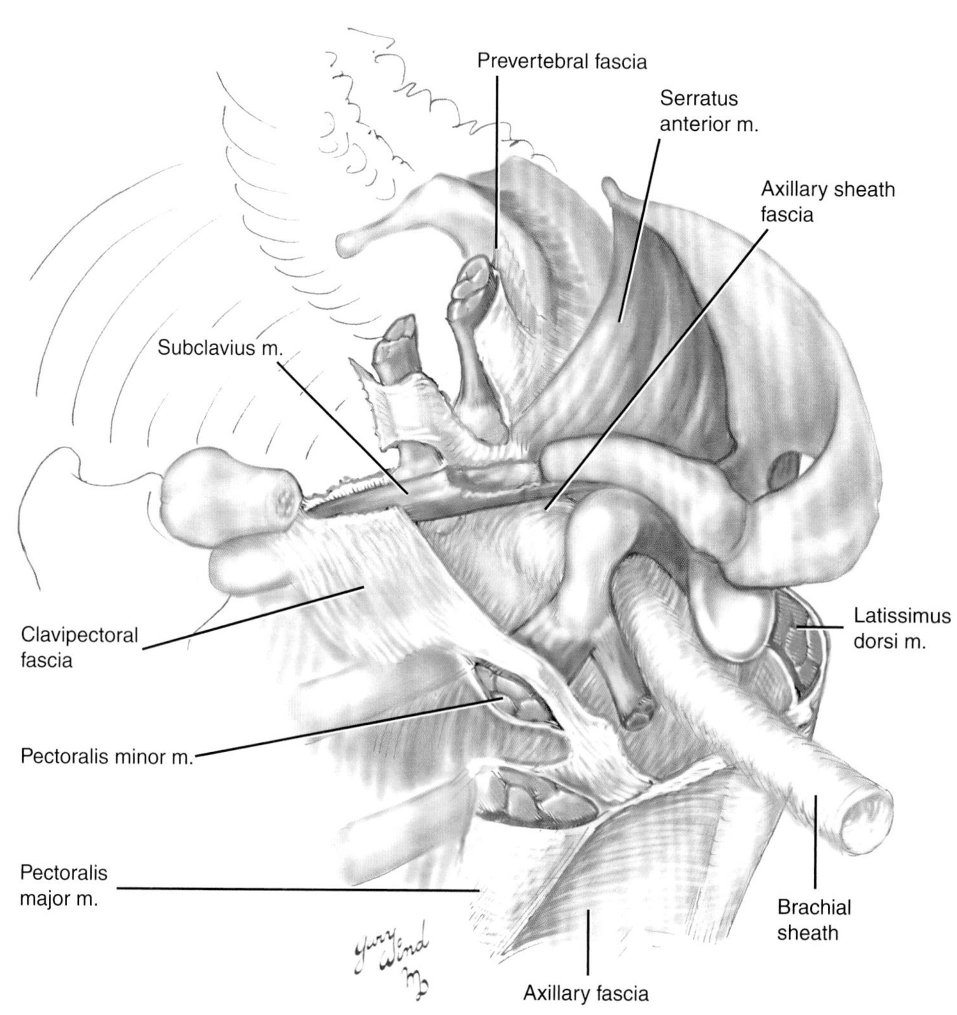

Fig. 4-5 The clavipectoral and axillary fasciae form anterior and lateral walls of the axillary space.

Looking from below the clavicle, one can see the geometry which causes compression of the costoclavicular passage with depression and posterior movement of the clavicle (Fig. 4-6). The angle between the clavicle and first rib is acute and subject to scissors-like closure, with the most pronounced effect being on the subclavian vein lying between them. The insertion of the subclavius muscle forms the medial margin of the foramen through which the subclavian vein enters the chest. It is an important landmark toward which the needle is directed when cannulating the subclavian vein, and it is the highest point of a complete axillary lymph node dissection.

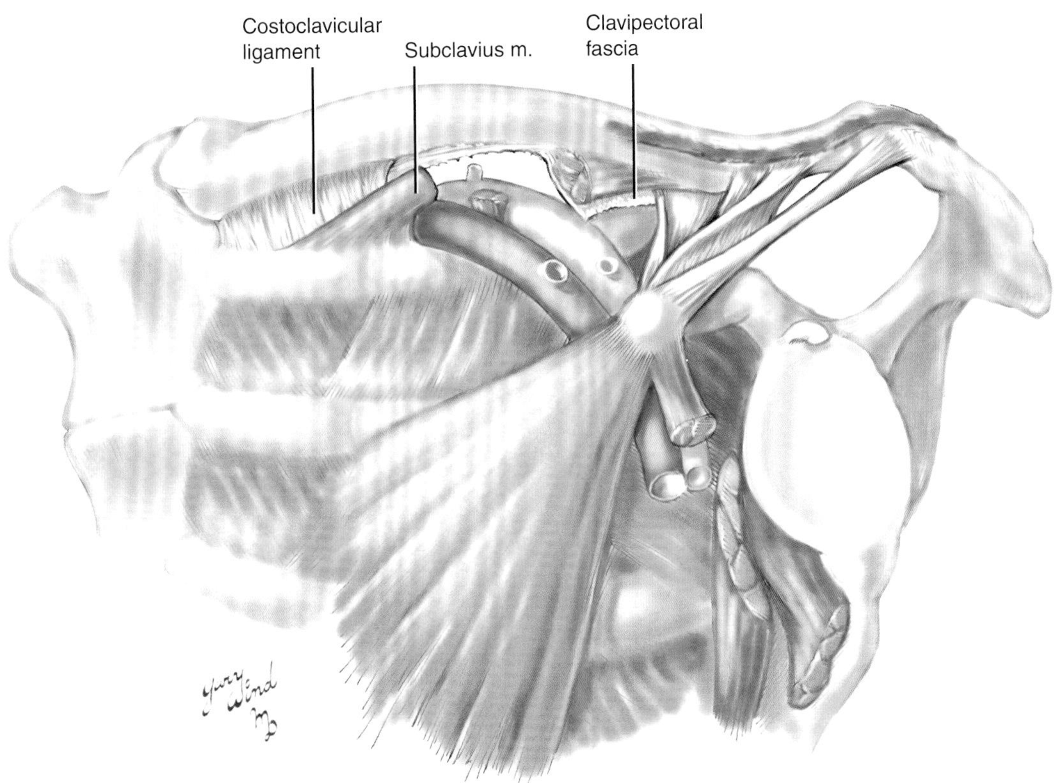

Fig. 4-6 Oblique fibers of the pectoralis minor and major and the latissimus dorsi make the distal clavicle a lever that closes the costoclavicular angle.

The surgical view of the axilla shows the relationships of the neurovascular bundle, its branches, and the surrounding structures (Fig. 4-7). The supreme thoracic and lateral thoracic vessels and thoracoepigastric vein cross the critical portion of the first rib and must be divided for access. The long thoracic and lateral thoracic nerves posterolaterally are important to preserve. The intercostobrachial nerve may be preserved or divided, depending on whether it interferes with exposure.

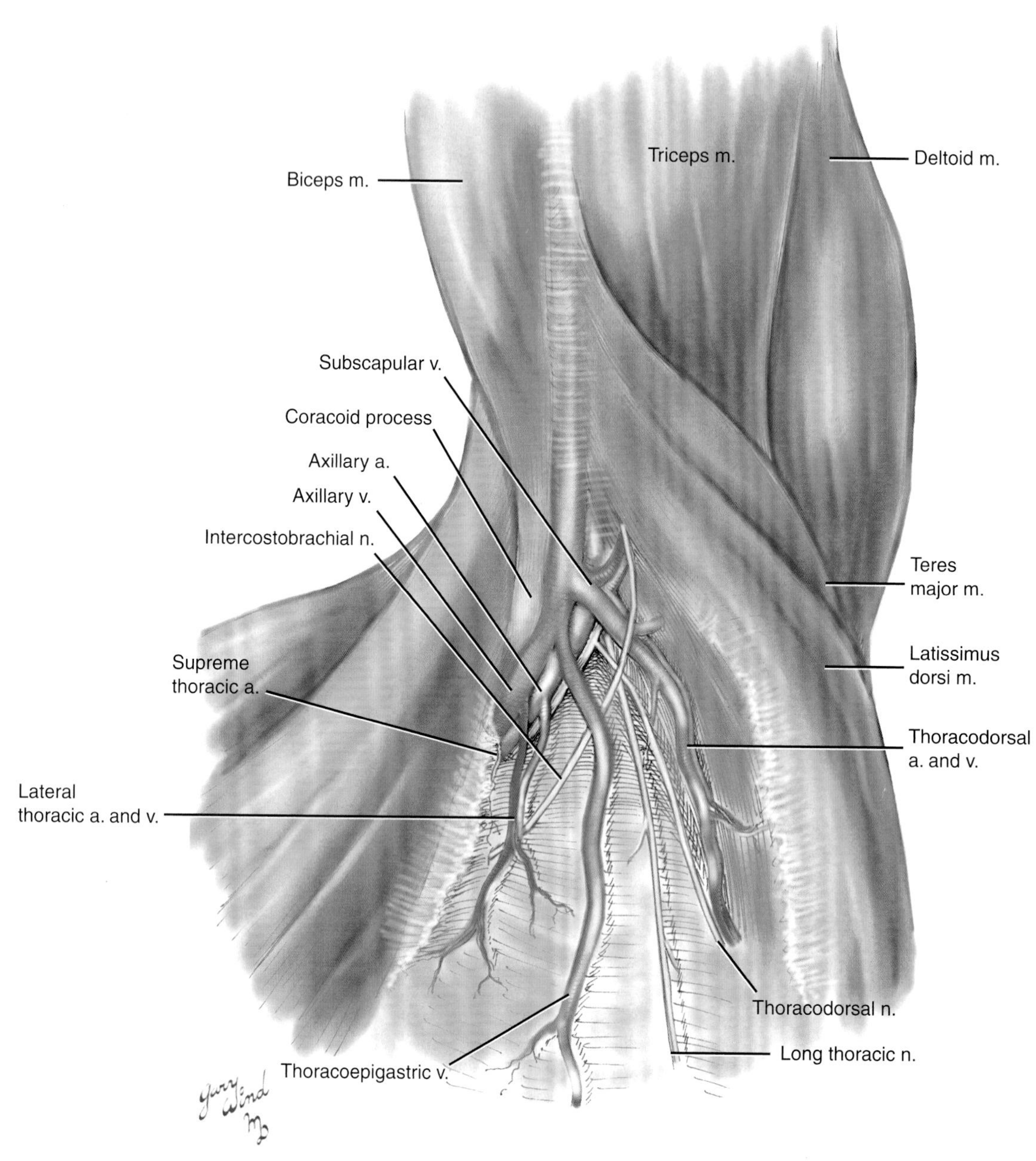

Fig. 4-7 Several nerves and vessels cross the axillary space and lie in the way of access to the first rib from below.

Vasomotor Sympathetics

Autonomic control of vascular tone in the upper extremity is regulated by sympathetic nerves whose preganglionic fibers originate in the lateral grey column of the second to eighth thoracic spinal cord segments. The axons pass from the cord through the ventral nerve root to the ventral rami where they exit via the white rami to the sympathetic trunk (Fig. 4-8). Within the sympathetic trunk, the preganglionic fibers synapse with multiple postganglionic neurons at various levels. Postganglionic axons from the middle cervical, stellate, and second thoracic ganglia join the roots of the brachial plexus or run directly in the adventitia of blood vessels. The majority of upper extremity vascular sympathetic nerves reach their destination through the lower trunk of the brachial plexus and the median and ulnar nerves.

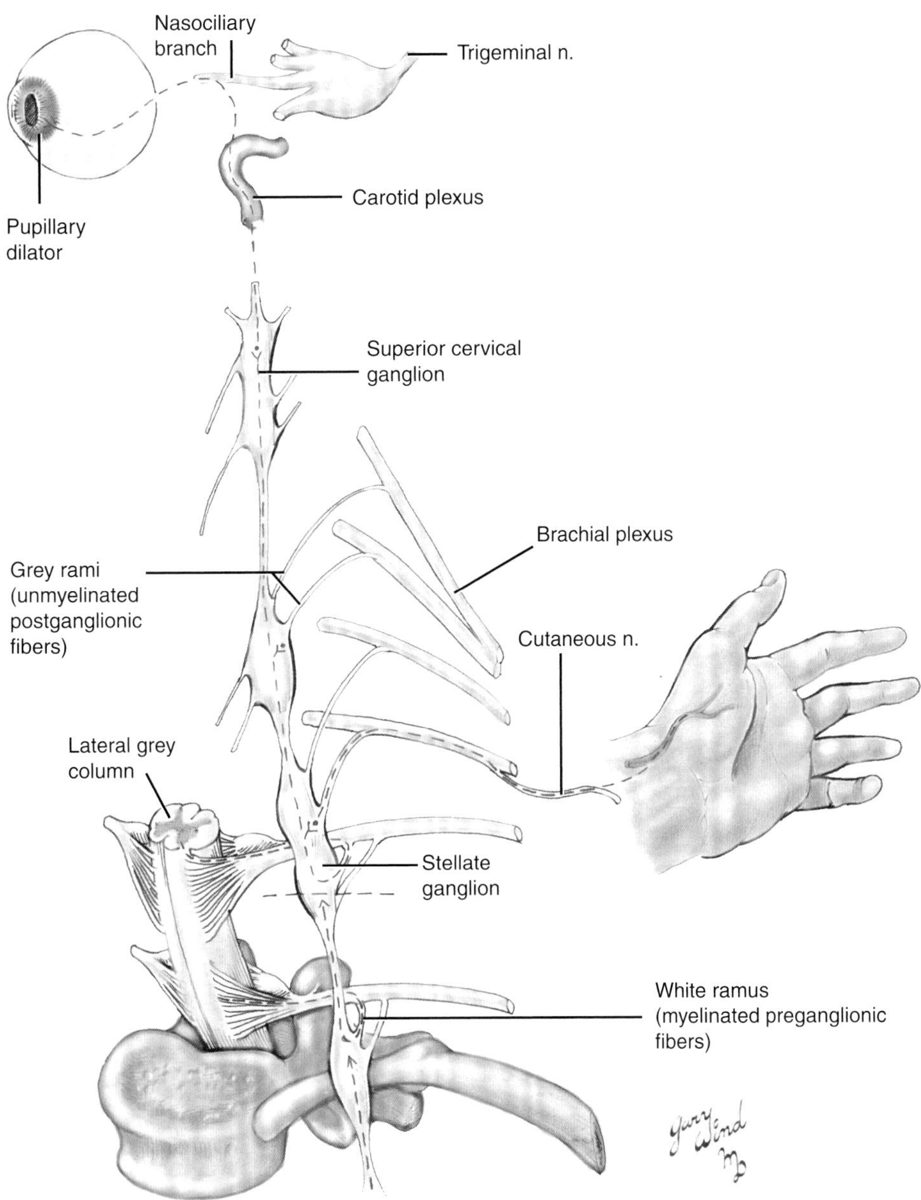

Fig. 4-8 Each sympathetic ganglion may have one to four communicating rami that connect to both contiguous spinal nerves and adjacent nerves. Interruption of the sympathetic trunk at the lower part of the stellate ganglion's thoracic component blocks the majority of sympathetic efferents to the upper extremity while preserving enough sympathetic innervation to prevent Horner's syndrome.

Anatomically, there are fewer thoracolumbar sympathetic ganglia than there are cord segments. The stellate ganglion found in most individuals represents the fusion of the inferior cervical and the first thoracic ganglia. The cervical sympathetic chain on each side lies between the carotid sheath and the prevertebral fascia anterior to the transverse processes of the cervical vertebrae (Fig. 4-9). The middle cervical ganglion lies at the level of the C6 transverse process (carotid tubercle) medial to the vertebral artery as it enters the vertebral foramen. The trunk then turns posterolateral to assume a paravertebral position. The thin ansa subclavia loops around the subclavian artery between the middle cervical ganglion and the stellate ganglion. In the chest, the sympathetic trunks and ganglia lie beneath the parietal pleura on the necks of the ribs.

Complete interruption of the sympathetic innervation of the upper extremity also interrupts the innervation of the pupillary dilator, local facial sweat glands, and blood vessels, resulting in Horner's syndrome. Section of the sympathetic chain at the lowermost part of the stellate ganglion preserves enough TI sympathetic outflow in most cases to avoid a Horner's syndrome. The amount of sympathetic innervation left in the upper extremity is not felt to be clinically significant by advocates of this procedure.

An older controversy involved the denervation hypersensitivity to circulating catecholamines, which results from interruption of postganglionic sympathetic fibers. Older procedures to selectively divide white rami only have been abandoned, since this syndrome is rarely observed clinically.

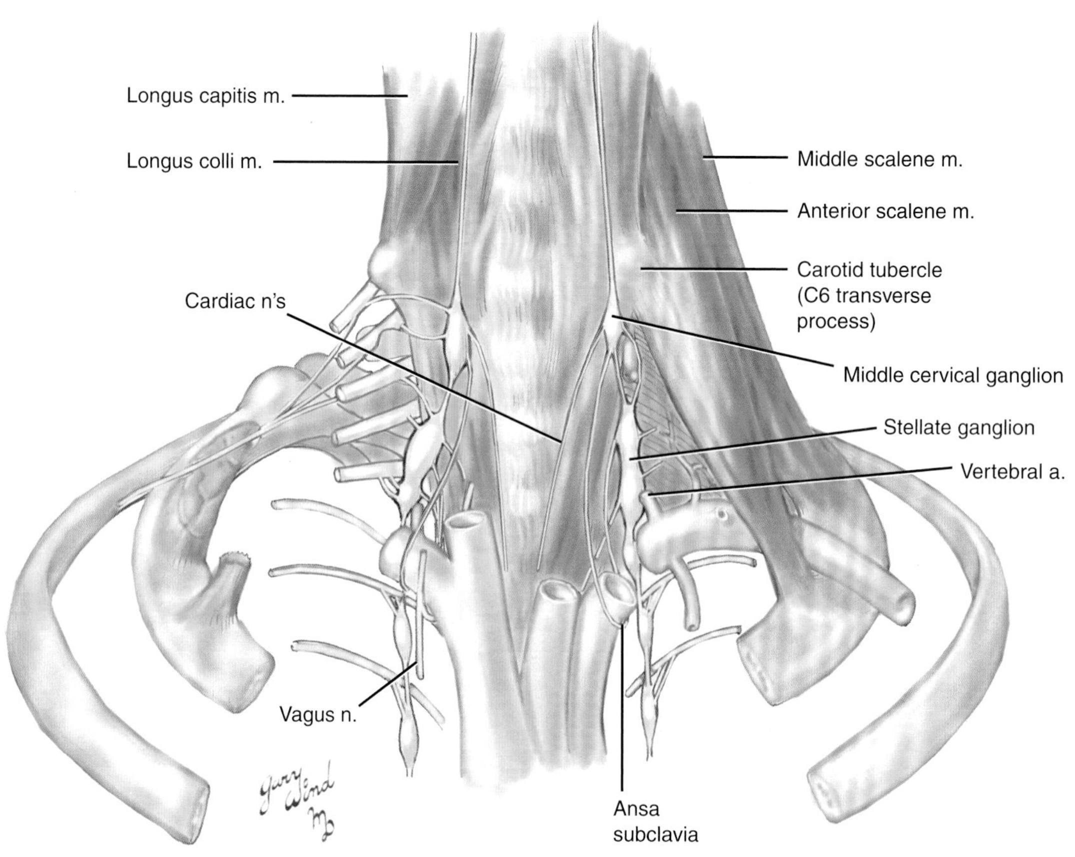

Fig. 4-9 The stellate ganglion lies dorsal to the vertebral artery.

Exposure of the Thoracic Outlet

Compression syndromes involving neurovascular structures in the thoracic outlet have been recognized for many years. The anatomic situation underlying compression in this area is the normal existence of four narrow spaces through which the neurovascular bundle must pass in coursing from the neck to the axilla: the superior thoracic aperture, interscalene triangle, costoclavicular passage, and subcoracoid space. Thyromegaly, thymic lesions, or adenopathy may reduce space availability within the superior thoracic aperture[1] (Fig. 4-10A). The interscalene triangle is a narrow confine bordered by the anterior scalene muscle anteriorly, the middle scalene muscle posteriorly, and the first rib inferiorly. The presence of first rib anomalies, fibromuscular bands, or abnormal muscular insertions can result in a fibromuscular vise that compresses the subclavian vessels and brachial plexus in this area.[2–4] The costoclavicular passage is a second triangle made up of the subclavius muscle and clavicle anteriorly, the first rib posteromedially, and the scapula and subscapularis muscle posterolaterally. This area is a common site of subclavian vein compression in patients with effort thrombosis.[5,6] A third anatomic triangle exists in the subcoracoid space, where the neurovascular bundle passes between the coracoid process and the pectoralis minor tendon. A tight band of superior clavipectoral fascia, the costocoracoid ligament, may narrow the subcoracoid space during shoulder abduction. Hypertrophy of the pectoralis minor muscle in athletes may also cause subcoracoid space narrowing.[7] More laterally, an accessory muscle that crosses the axilla from the latissimus dorsi to the pectoralis major muscle, Langer's axillary arch (Fig. 4-10B), has been reported to cause upper limb deep vein thrombosis from compression.[8]

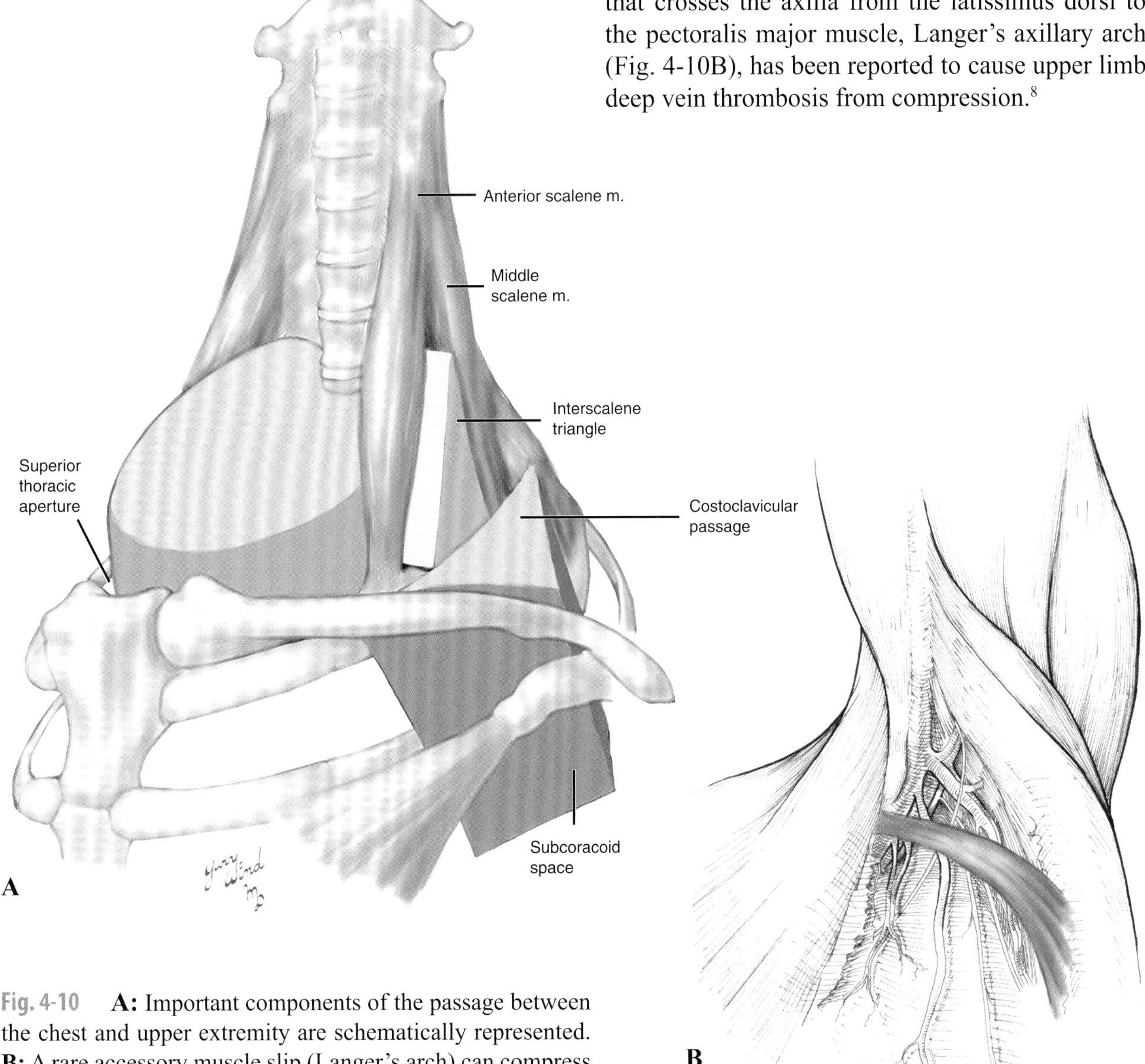

Fig. 4-10 **A:** Important components of the passage between the chest and upper extremity are schematically represented. **B:** A rare accessory muscle slip (Langer's arch) can compress the distal axillary structures.

Space availability within the confines of these narrow apertures may be further reduced by a combination of physiologic, anthropometric, and pathologic factors (Fig. 4-11). Hypertrophy of the anterior scalene or the pectoral muscles, scoliosis, abnormal shoulder posture, existence of cervical ribs, and clavicular fracture malunions, and other shoulder injuries have all been implicated in compression syndromes.[2,3,9] In addition, the existence of abnormal myofascial bands or anomalous scalene muscle insertions may underlie compression symptoms. Roos[11] feels that congenital fibrous bands or abnormal muscle insertions are the most common causes of this disorder. However, since these anomalies are common in the general population,[4,9,12] others have suggested that local trauma may be an important causative influence in patients who are predisposed to compression syndromes by congenital anomalies.[2,9]

There are three discrete types of thoracic outlet compression syndromes: brachial plexus compression, subclavian artery compression, and subclavian vein compression. Neural compression is by far the most common type, accounting for nearly 97% of thoracic outlet compression symptoms.[2,3,13] Diagnosis and evaluation of patients with all three types of suspected thoracic outlet compression are well-described elsewhere.[2,3,14] It should be stressed that a majority of patients will experience relief of

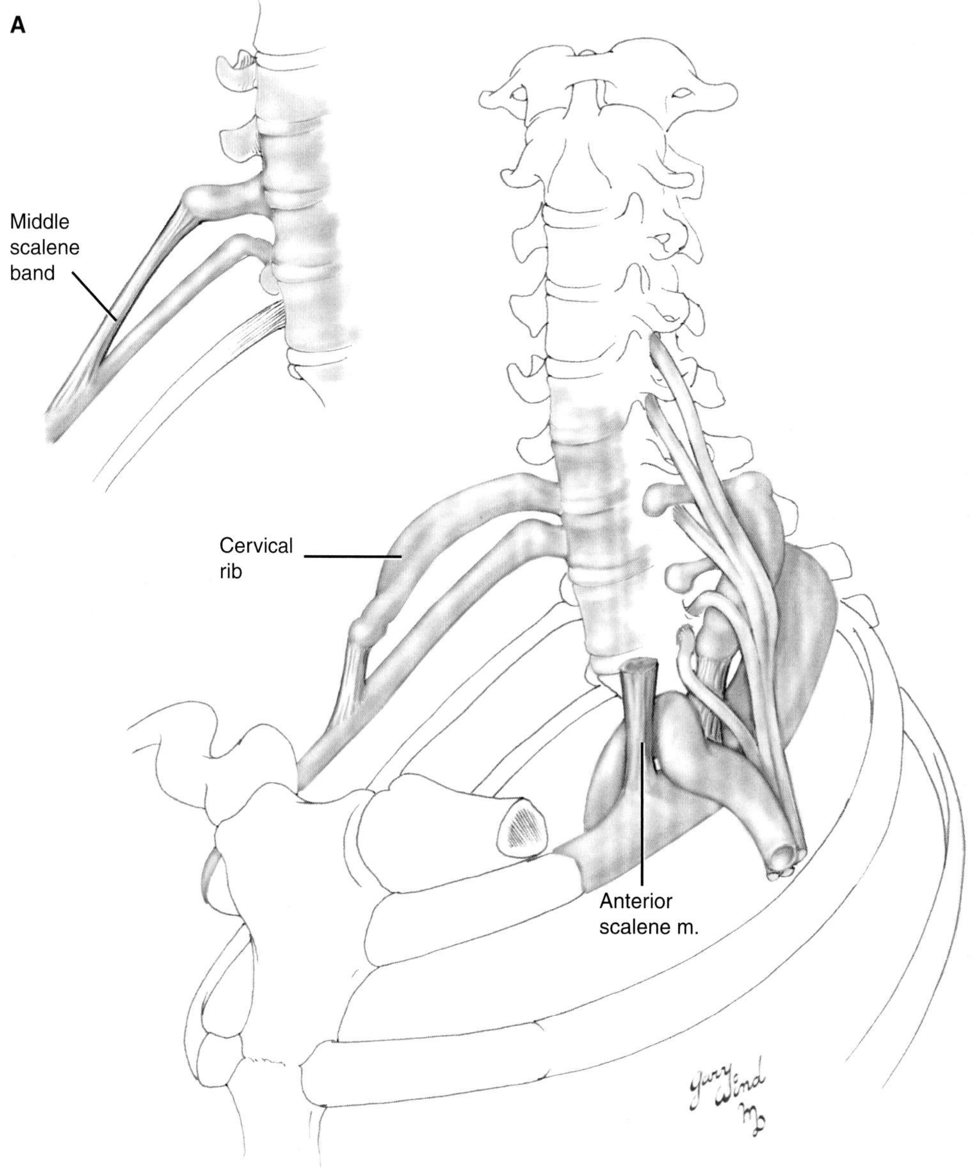

Fig. 4-11 Several different pathologic conditions are associated with the thoracic outlet syndrome. These include cervical ribs (usually embedded within the middle scalene muscle) and middle scalene bands (**A**); anomalous muscle insertions, fascial bands, and clavicular compression (**B**); and osseous anomalies and traumatic malformations (**C**).

Fig. 4-11 *(Continued)*

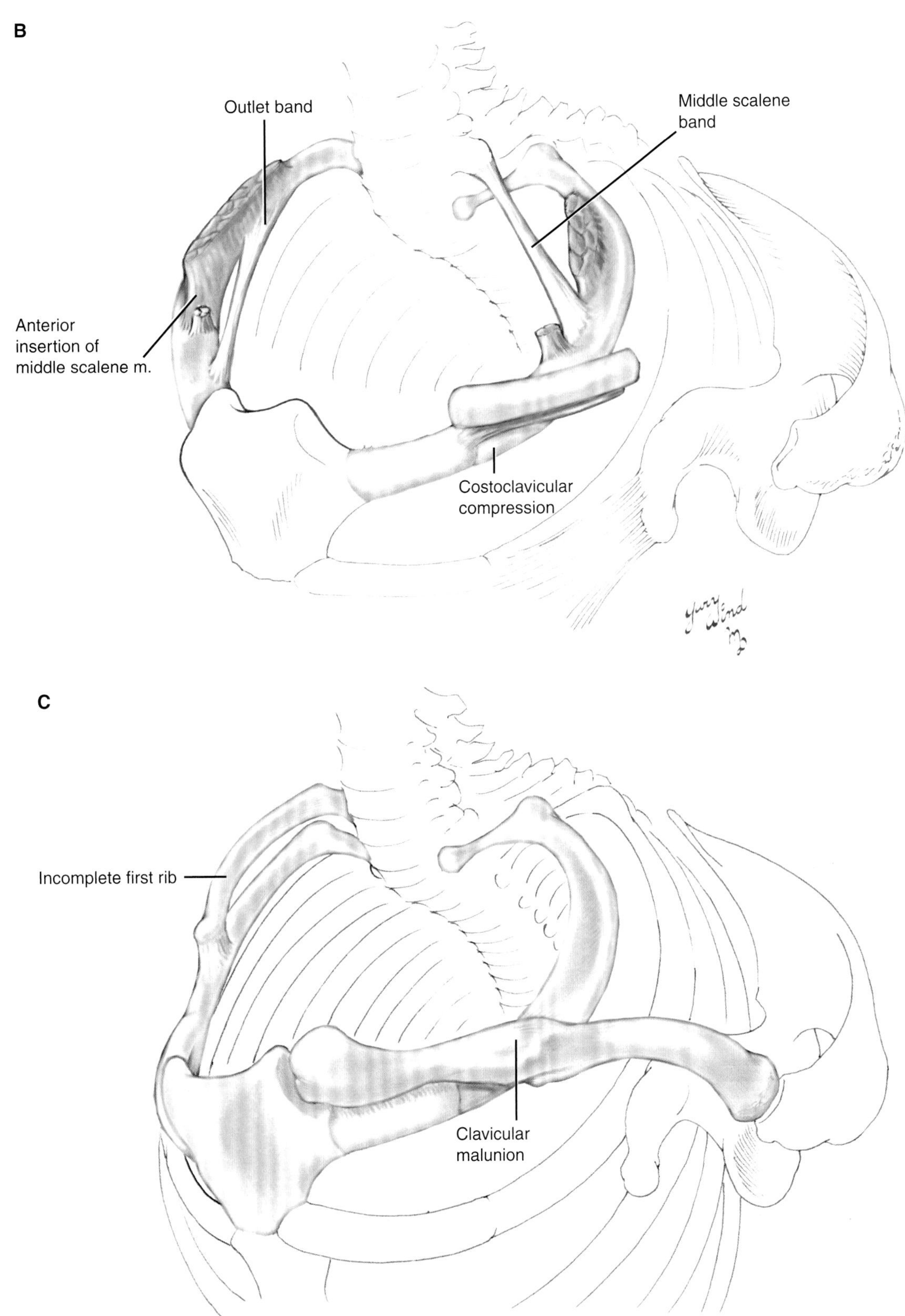

neurologic symptoms with nonoperative therapy.[2,3] In a recent review, Brooke and Freischlag[13] noted that injecting lidocaine or botulinum toxin A (botox) into the anterior scalene muscle at its insertion onto the first rib may provide durable symptom relief of neurogenic thoracic outlet syndrome for up to 3 months. Moreover, the degree of symptom relief appears to correlate with successful response to physical therapy and surgical intervention.

Several surgical procedures have been described for the treatment of thoracic outlet compression syndromes. Early reports suggested that simple scalenectomy was effective in alleviating symptoms.[15] Although some authors suggest that anterior scalene muscle excision may be appropriate in highly selected patients,[2,16] the consensus of opinion is that the first rib should be removed because it is the anatomic structure common to all three of the narrow thoracic apertures described above (Fig. 4-12). Clagett[17] was the first to recommend routine resection of the first rib as a way to alleviate symptoms regardless of the site of compression. Most modern surgeons have adopted this view and remove the first rib through one of two approaches, transaxillary and supraclavicular.

The transaxillary approach has been favored for many years. It is cosmetically superior but difficult to perform in muscular individuals. The anterior supraclavicular approach has undergone rejuvenation and is currently favored by some.[18–20] This approach should be used in cases involving agenesis of the first rib and when arterial reconstruction is planned. The posterior approach originally described by Clagett[17] has been abandoned because it

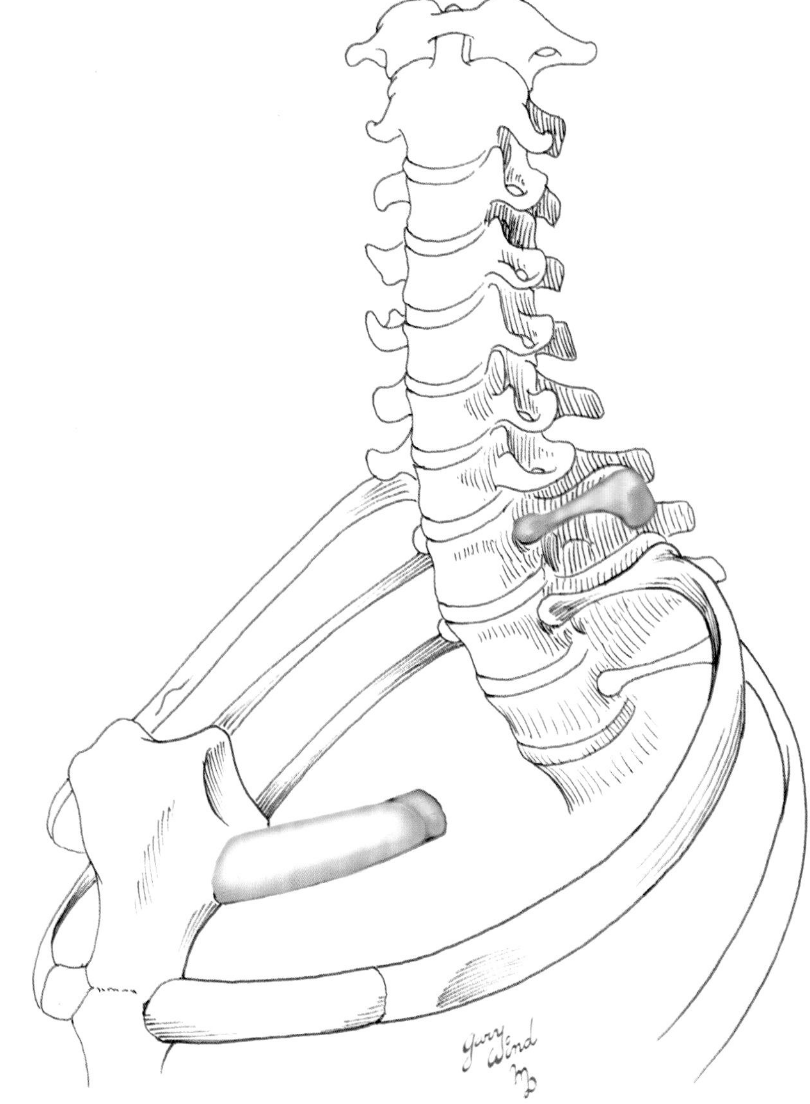

Fig. 4-12 The compression from a variety of causes responds to removal of the body of the first rib.

is technically demanding. The anterior infraclavicular approach[21] offers only limited first rib resection, and the view of the neurovascular structures is obstructed by the clavicle. It is most useful to ensure sternal disarticulation of the first rib and complete resection of the subclavius muscle in patients with venous thoracic outlet compression (see below). The transclavicular approach requires resection of the clavicle and is most useful in cases involving clavicular pathology. Because of the high reported risk of postoperative shoulder pain, claviculectomy is not recommended for thoracic outlet decompression in most cases.[22] The following discussion concerns the three currently popular approaches to thoracic outlet decompression.

Anterior Supraclavicular Approach

The principal advantage of this approach is that it provides wide exposure of all anatomic structures of the thoracic outlet. It can also be combined easily with other incisions to correct arterial pathology at the time of outlet decompression. Although the supraclavicular approach has been used since 1910, it has become a popular method of thoracic outlet decompression within the last three decades.[23] Long-term results attest to its efficacy in correcting neural compression symptoms.[19,20]

The patient is placed supine with the head turned away from the operative side (Fig. 4-13). The head of the table should be elevated slightly

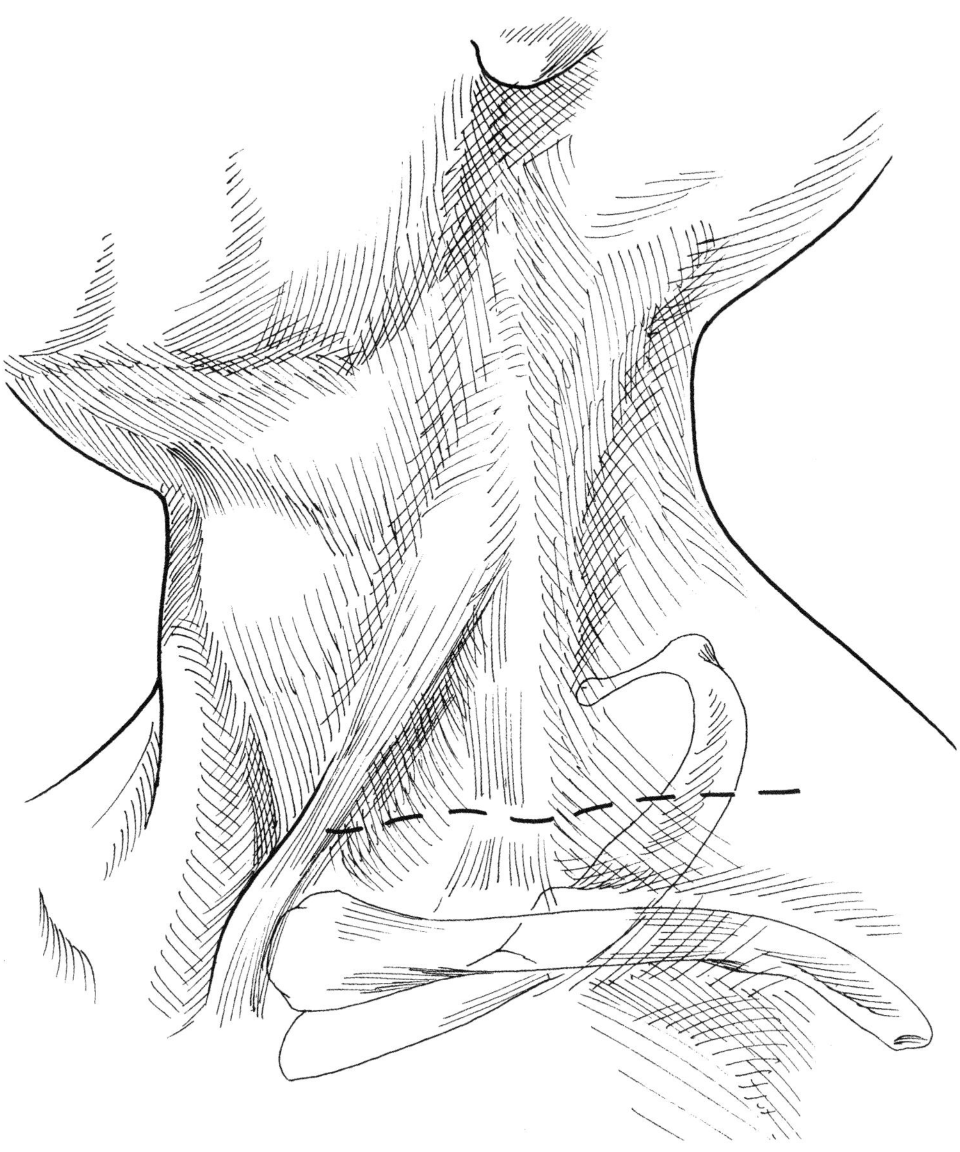

Fig. 4-13 The incision for the supraclavicular approach to the first rib is shown. The ideal exposures shown in the following illustrations for clarity are seldom achieved in reality due to the funnel-like depth of the operative field.

to reduce venous pressure in the operative field. A rolled towel placed vertically between the scapulae may help extend the shoulder and flatten the supraclavicular fossa. The neck, shoulder, and upper chest are prepped and draped in sterile fashion.

An incision is made 1 to 2 cm above and parallel to the clavicle, beginning at the clavicular head and extending approximately 8 cm laterally (Fig. 4-14). The incision is deepened through subcutaneous tissue and the platysma. Subplatysmal flaps are developed in the superior wound to the level of the cricoid cartilage and in the inferior wound to the clavicle.[23,24]

The external jugular vein and the omohyoid muscle are divided in the midwound. The clavicular head of the sternocleidomastoid muscle should be divided to enhance medial exposure at the time of first rib resection. Just deep to the divided sternocleidomastoid fibers is the internal jugular vein, which should be dissected on its lateral border and carefully retracted medially. The underlying scalene fat pad is mobilized along its medial, superior, and inferior borders and then reflected on a pedicle in the lateral wound.[24] On the left side, the thoracic duct should be identified and carefully ligated as it arches through the inferomedial corner of the scalene fat pad toward its termination near the junction of the left internal jugular and subclavian veins.

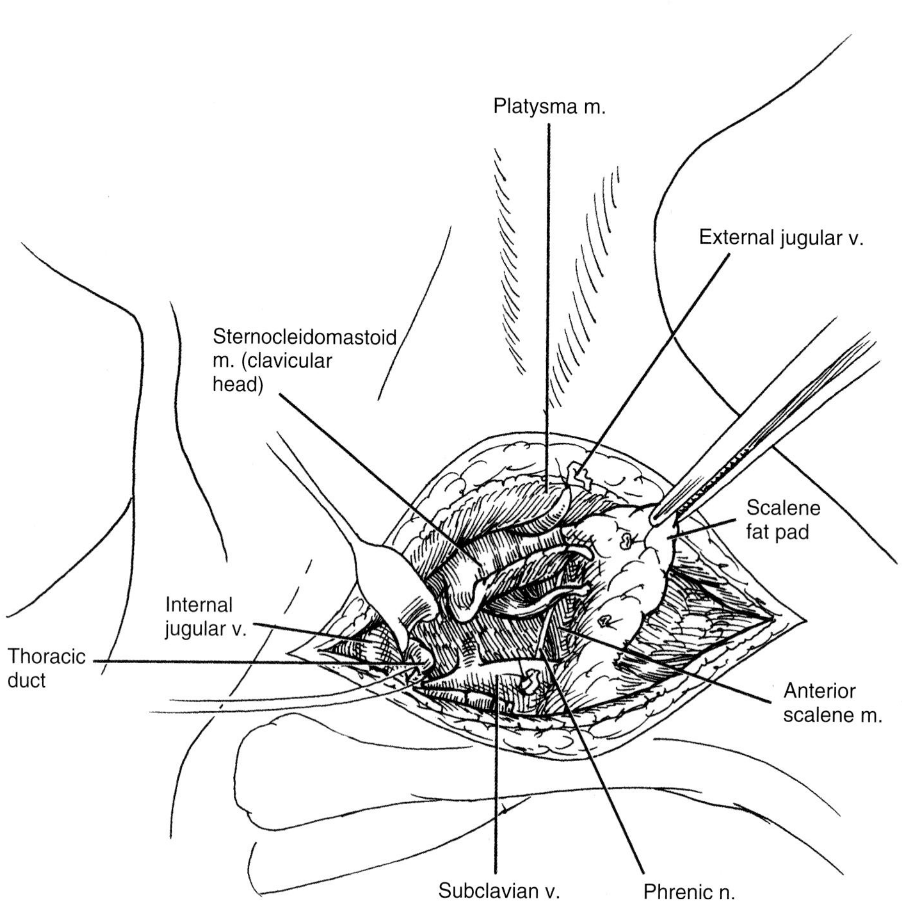

Fig. 4-14 The clavicular head of the sternocleidomastoid muscle and the omohyoid muscle are divided, and the scalene fat pad is separated from the internal jugular vein. The fat pad and vein are retracted in opposite directions, and the thoracic duct is ligated and divided on the left side.

The anterior scalene muscle lies directly beneath the fat pad. Coursing on the anterior surface of this muscle, usually near the medial border, is the phrenic nerve. The nerve should be freed from the adjacent fascia of the anterior scalene muscle and carefully protected during the ensuing dissection. The nerve should not be forcibly retracted because even minimal compression can result in a temporary diaphragmatic palsy.[23] The anterior scalene muscle is next divided at its insertion on the first rib (Fig. 4-15). The muscle should be divided a few millimeters at a time under direct vision to avoid injury to the overlying subclavian vein. The muscle can then be divided as close to its transverse process origins as possible to complete the resection. The subclavian artery lies in the inferior wound and is easily isolated should associated arterial pathology warrant surgical correction.

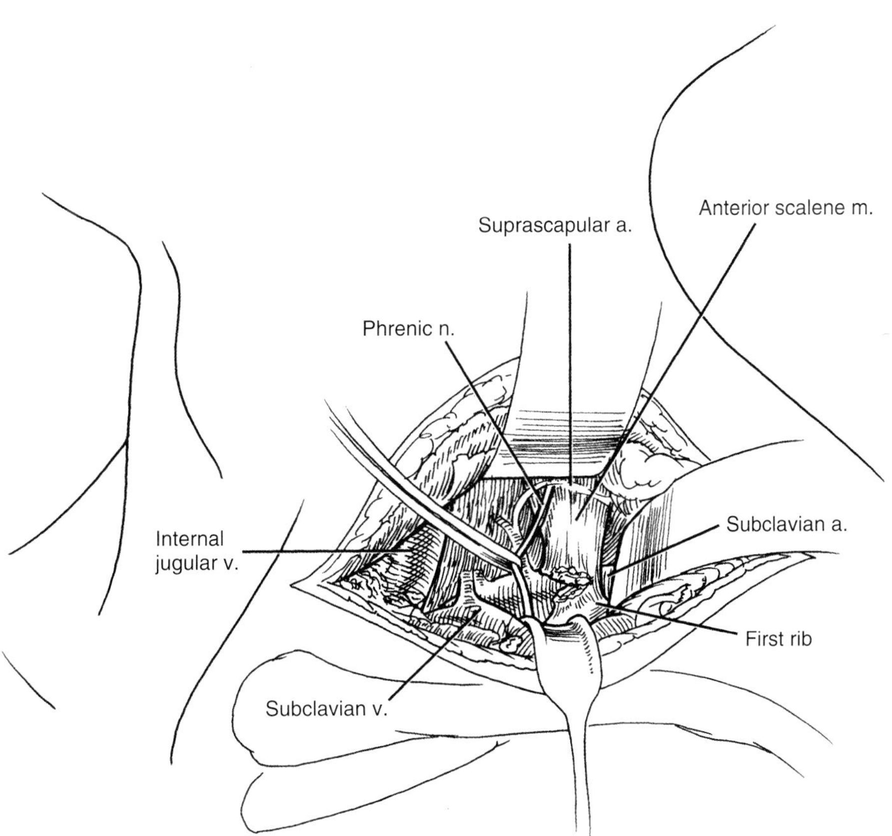

Fig. 4-15 The phrenic nerve is protected as the anterior scalene muscle insertion is divided.

Because of its possible contribution to compression problems at the thoracic outlet, the middle scalene muscle is resected next. It is located posterior and lateral to the roots of the brachial plexus. To facilitate exposure of the middle scalene, the C5 and C6 nerve trunk is mobilized along its lateral border and gently retracted downward. After the long thoracic nerve is identified and protected on the muscle's anterolateral surface, the middle scalene fibers are divided a few short segments at a time along the first rib attachments (Fig. 4-16). The long thoracic nerve marks the lateral boundary of muscle division. The most anterior portion of the middle scalene muscle may not be identified without undue traction on the brachial plexus. These fibers can be

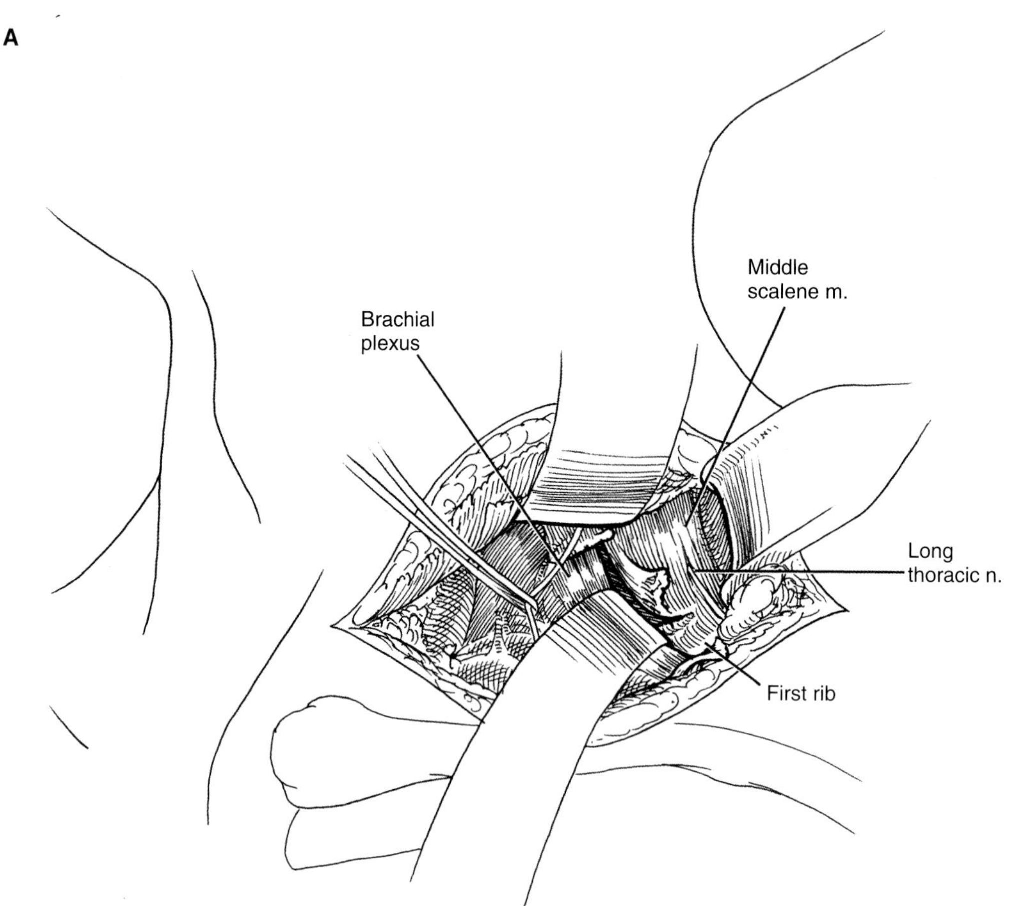

Fig. 4-16 The middle scalene muscle posterior to the brachial plexus is cautiously separated from the first rib (**A**), keeping in mind the location of the long thoracic nerve. The most anterior fibers of the middle scalene muscle may be approached between the subclavian artery and the lower nerve trunk as shown or may be approached between the seventh and eighth nerve roots to avoid undue traction on the brachial plexus (**B**).

divided in the space between the subclavian artery and the lower nerve trunk. Although most compressing bands will be removed with resection of the anterior and middle scalene muscles, the operative field should be palpated to detect the presence of any other fibrous constrictions. It is particularly important to remove any fibromuscular bands associated with the exposed areas of the brachial plexus, including those associated with C7 vertebrae and Sibson's fascia. Likewise, certain muscle anomalies, such as split middle scalene insertions and posterior scalene hypertrophy,[1] should be recognized. Cervical ribs are usually embedded within the fibers of the middle scalene muscle and are easily resected at the time of middle scalenectomy.[23]

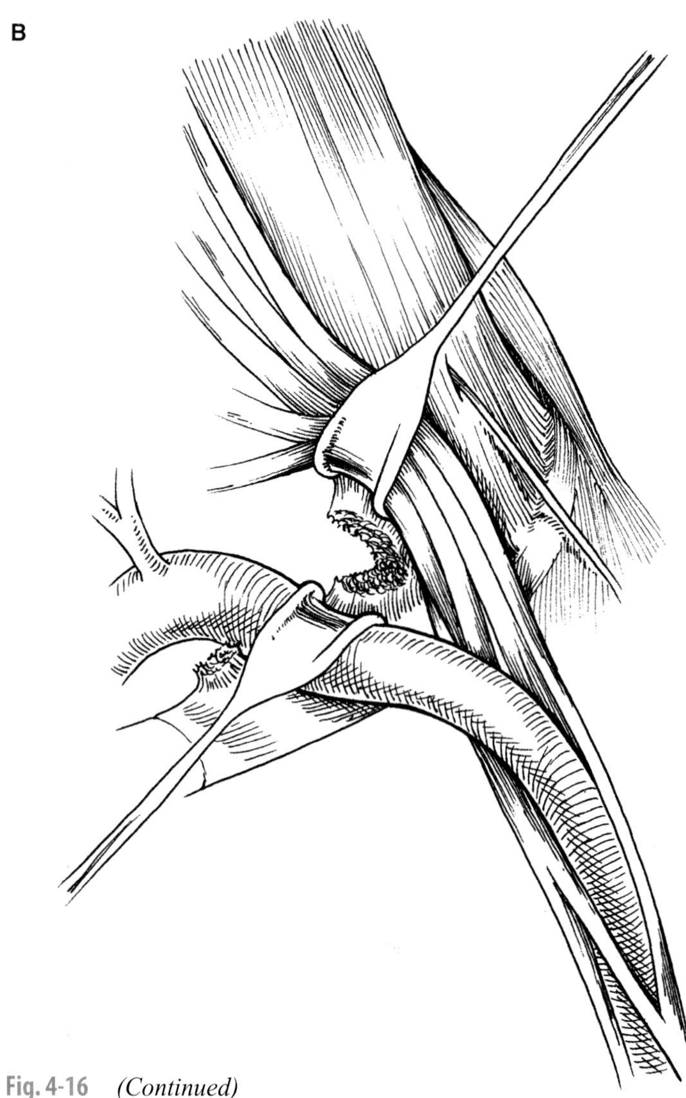

Fig. 4-16 *(Continued)*

The first rib is now ready for resection. Extraperiosteal resection is preferred over the subperiosteal approach because the former is simpler, and removal of the periosteum may prevent reossification of the periosteal bed and associated recurrent symptoms.[25] The rib is freed by blunt finger dissection along the inferior rib surface to detach intercostal muscle fibers. In the lateral wound, the brachial plexus is gently displaced anteromedially while the body of the first rib is divided cleanly just distal to the tubercle using a sagittal air-drive saw[24] or piecemeal with a narrow rongeur[23] (Fig. 4-17). The posterior rib remnant is removed as close to the transverse process as possible with a rongeur. This maneuver should be performed under direct vision to minimize the possibility of damage to the C8 and TI nerve roots, which pass near the neck of the first rib. If the jaws of the rongeur cannot

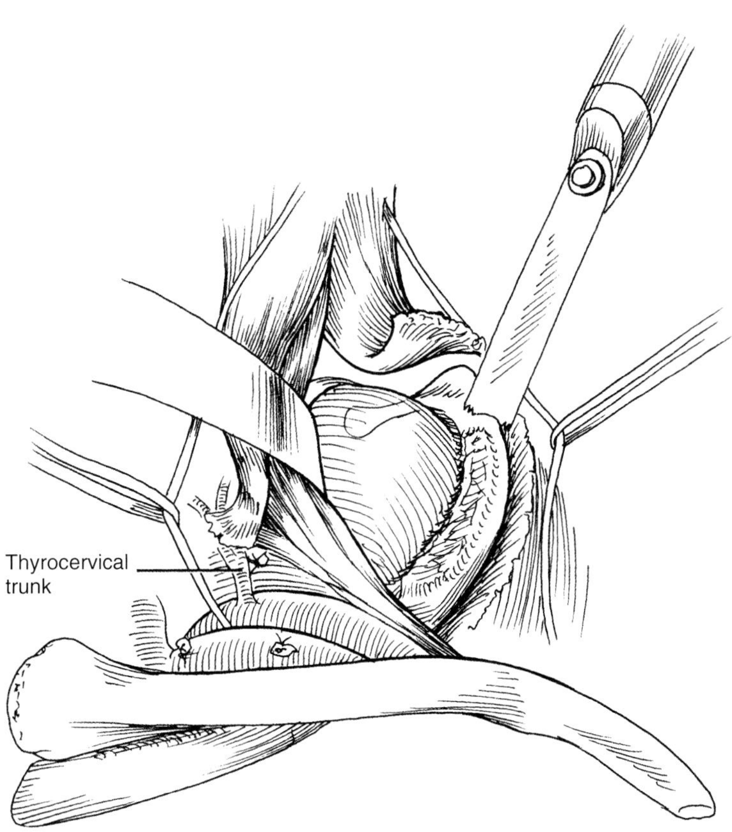

Fig. 4-17 In the extraperiosteal approach shown here, the intercostal and scalene muscles and endothoracic fascia are separated from the rib before it is divided anterior to the costal angle.

be seen, it is better to leave the posterior rib remnant in place.[24] The subclavian artery is carefully separated from flimsy periadventitial attachments to the top of the first rib, and the intercostal muscle and pleura are separated from the rib's underside using the extraperiosteal technique. The rib is now completely free of all attachments and ready for anterior division, which is performed in front of the anterior scalene tubercle. This portion of the rib is exposed by elevation and retraction of the clavicle and subclavian vein, with posterior retraction of the subclavian artery (Fig. 4-18). If exposure is too difficult or if the saw or rongeur cannot be visualized, an infraclavicular counterincision can be made to allow rib division at the costochondral junction (see below).

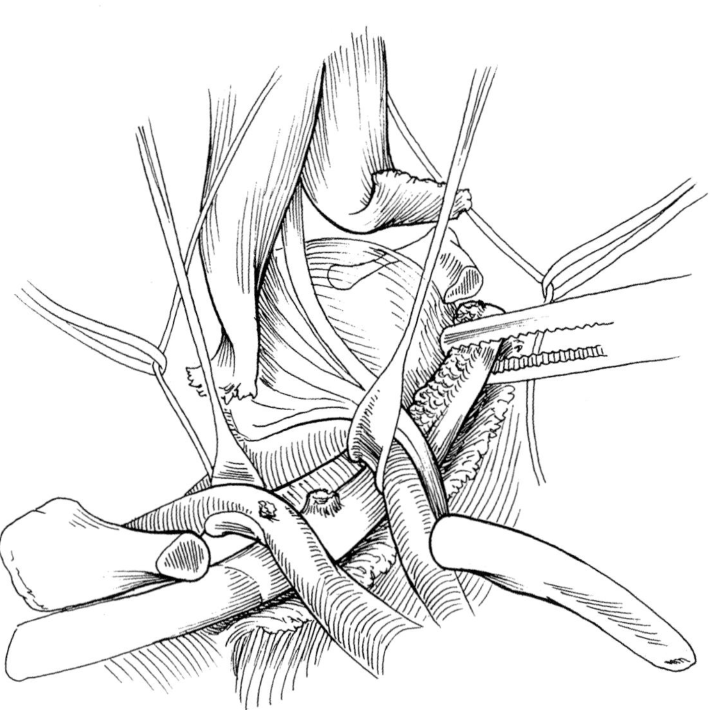

Fig. 4-18 The posterior rib is held as a lever while the subclavian artery and vein are separated for a clear view of the anterior division site.

Transaxillary Approach

Since its original description by Roos[26] in 1966, this approach has become a "gold standard" among surgeons performing thoracic outlet decompression. It offers a rapid approach to the first rib, and the incision is cosmetically appealing. However, several drawbacks of the transaxillary approach have been recognized. The most important is that visualization of the anatomic structures is limited within a relatively deep hole, making them prone to injury, especially the TI nerve root and the subclavian vein. In addition, the transaxillary approach affords incomplete exposure of the elements comprising the scalene triangle: most of the congenital fibromuscular bands are medial to the first rib and thus hidden by the neurovascular trunks in this approach. Complete excision of the anterior and middle scalene muscles is also difficult. Finally, correction of associated arterial pathology requires a second operation. Despite these shortcomings, a large amount of literature has been accumulated, attesting to the success of this approach.[2,27–29]

The patient is placed in a true lateral position with a soft pad placed under the opposite axilla to prevent neurovascular compression (Fig. 4-19).

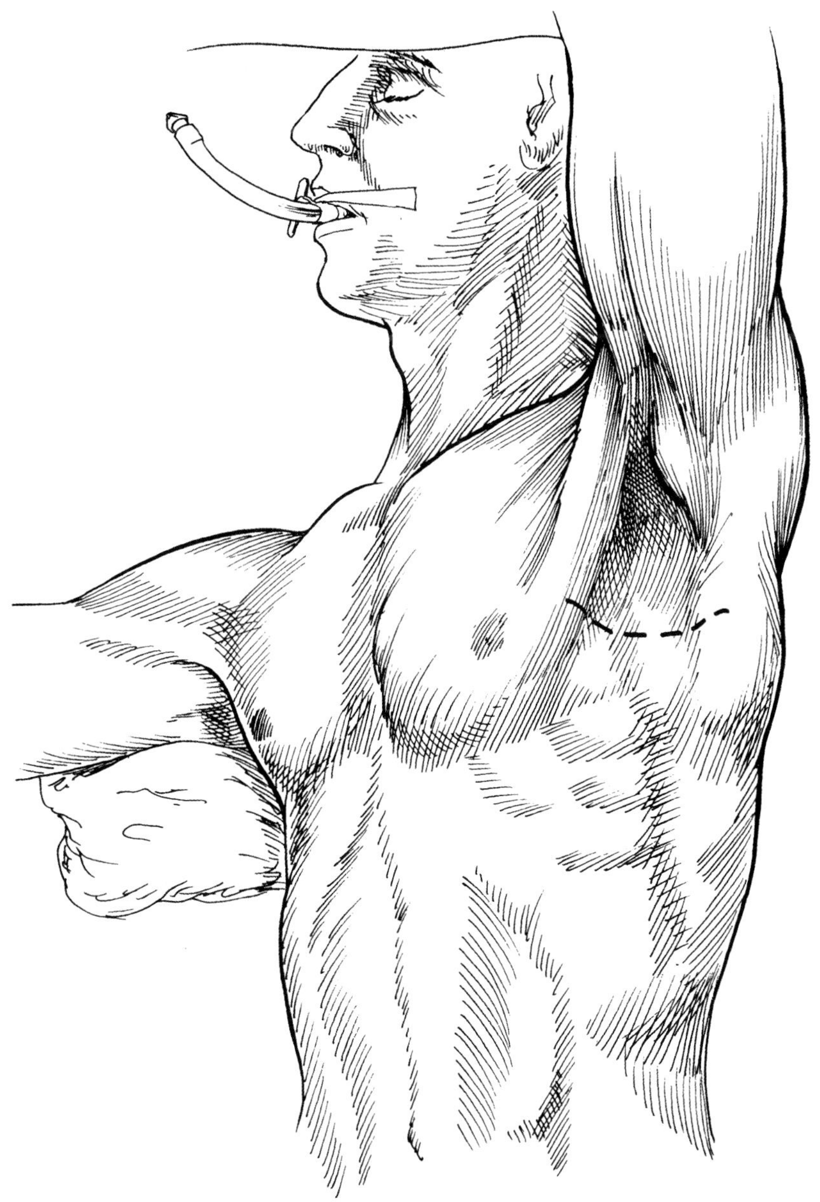

Fig. 4-19 A true lateral position with the affected extremity left free is used for the transaxillary approach to the first rib.

The ipsilateral arm remains free and is held and positioned by an assistant throughout the operation. The axilla, back, chest, shoulder, and arm are prepped and draped. A stockinette covers the distal arm.

The second assistant elevates the arm and shoulder using the double wristlock described by Roos[25] (Fig. 4-20). Arm retraction should be released on an intermittent basis during the operation to prevent arm ischemia and brachial plexus injury. As an alternative, Illig[30] has recently described a method of passive arm elevation using a shoulder suspension kit in which the arm is elevated by a weighted nylon cord suspended over a "shower curtain" assembly.

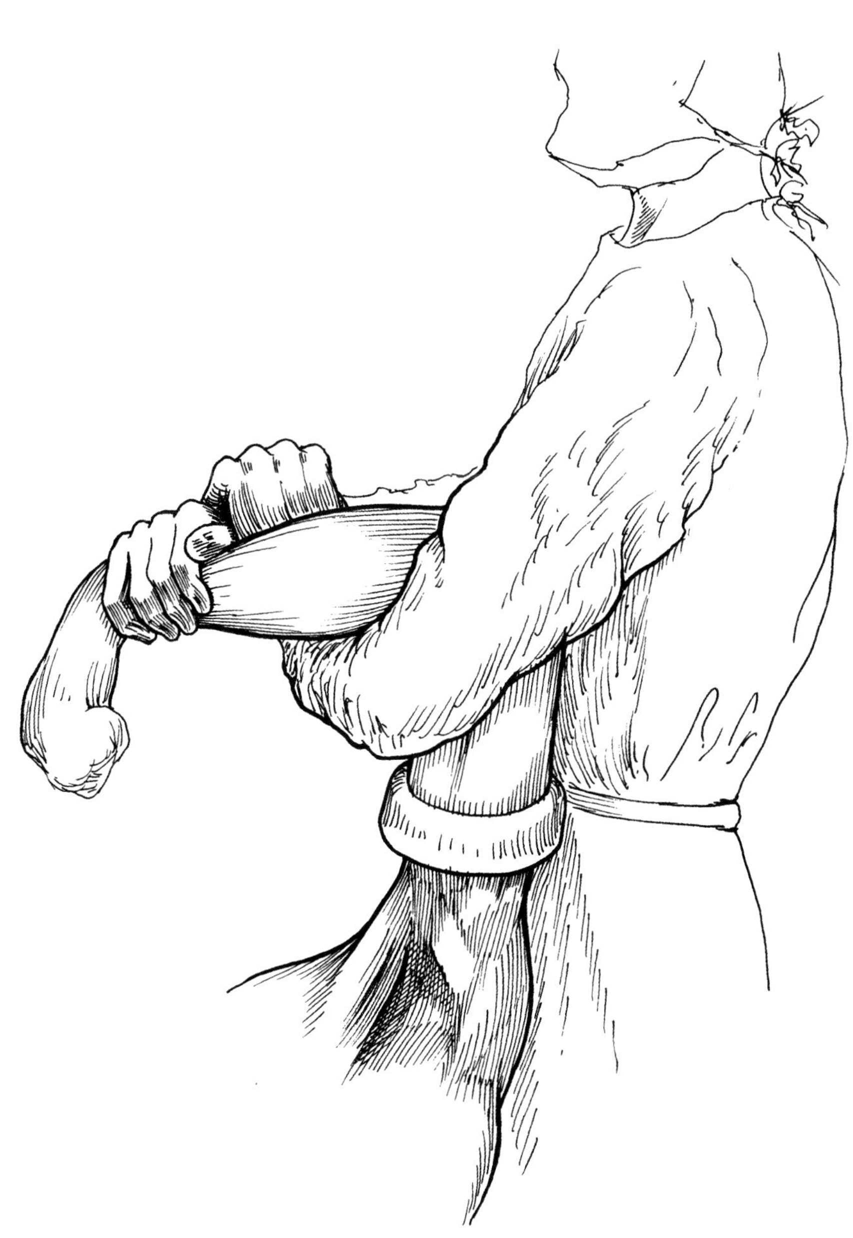

Fig. 4-20 The assistant holding the arm uses a wrist lock position for security and to minimize fatigue.

A transverse incision is made at the lower margin of the axillary hairline between the pectoralis major and latissimus dorsi muscles. The incision is deepened through subcutaneous tissue and the axillary fascia to reach the fascia of the serratus anterior at the level of the third rib (Fig. 4-21). The thoracoepigastric vein and lateral thoracic artery cross the incision just deep to the subcutaneous tissue; these vessels should be ligated and divided. A tissue plane is begun deep to the axillary fascia and developed superiorly in the loose areolar tissue on the surface of the serratus anterior. The intercostobrachial nerve will be encountered at the level of the second intercostal space in the middle of the operative field. Roos[26] has recommended preservation of the nerve to avoid axillary and medial arm anesthesia, but Dale[31] has recommended nerve division to prevent postoperative neuritic pain. The dissection plane is continued to the level of the first rib. The supreme thoracic artery and vein cross the first rib in the anterior wound and will also require division.[25]

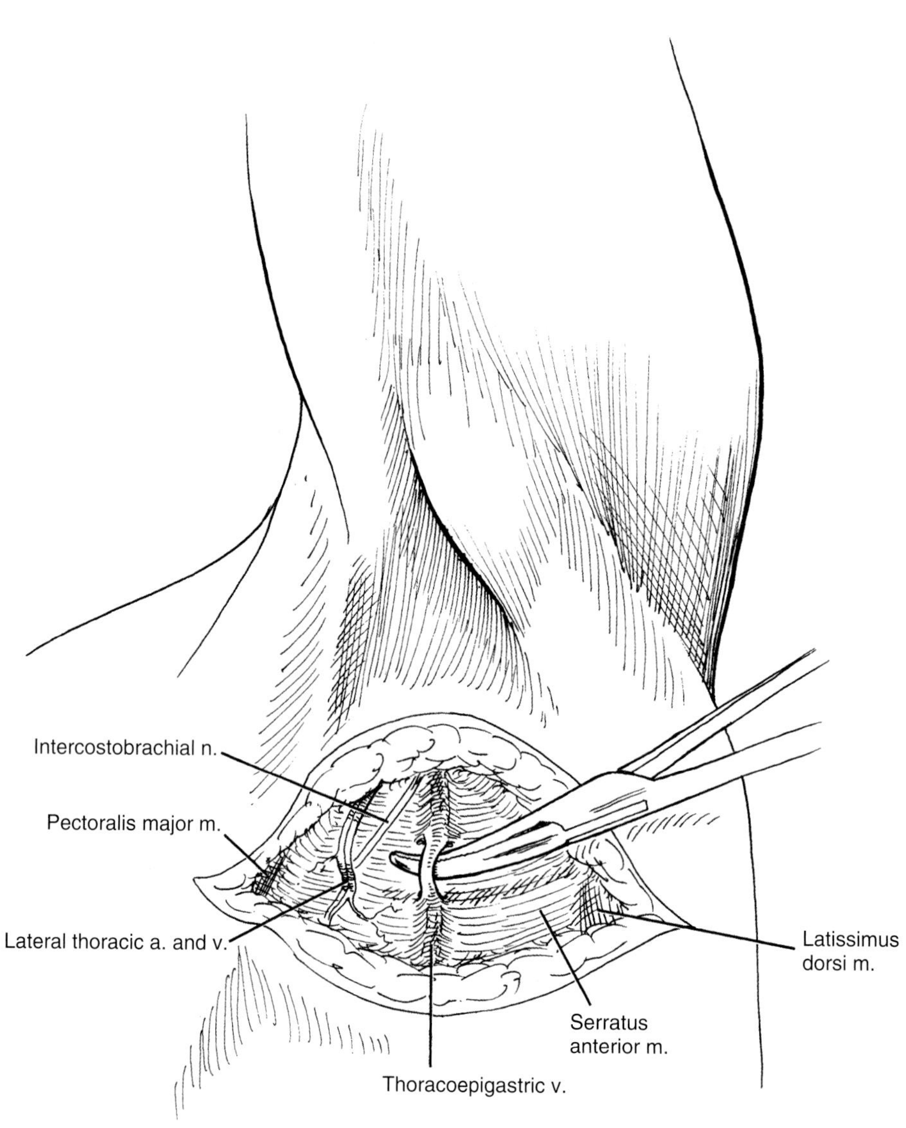

Fig. 4-21 Superficial axillary vessels are divided. The intercostobrachial nerve is mobilized or divided as necessary.

Roos[25] has noted that there is a cul-de-sac of fascia at the lateral border of the first rib that separates the axilla from the thoracic outlet. This tissue should be opened bluntly along the top of the first rib to expose the outlet structures (Fig. 4-22). Gentle elevation of the shoulder by the second assistant and retraction of the pectoralis major will greatly enhance exposure of the structures at the thoracic outlet. From anterior to posterior, one should identify the axillary vein, anterior scalene muscle, axillary artery, brachial plexus, and middle scalene muscle. The long thoracic nerve emerges dorsal to the brachial plexus and should be avoided as it passes along the lateral surface of the serratus anterior muscle in the posterior wound.

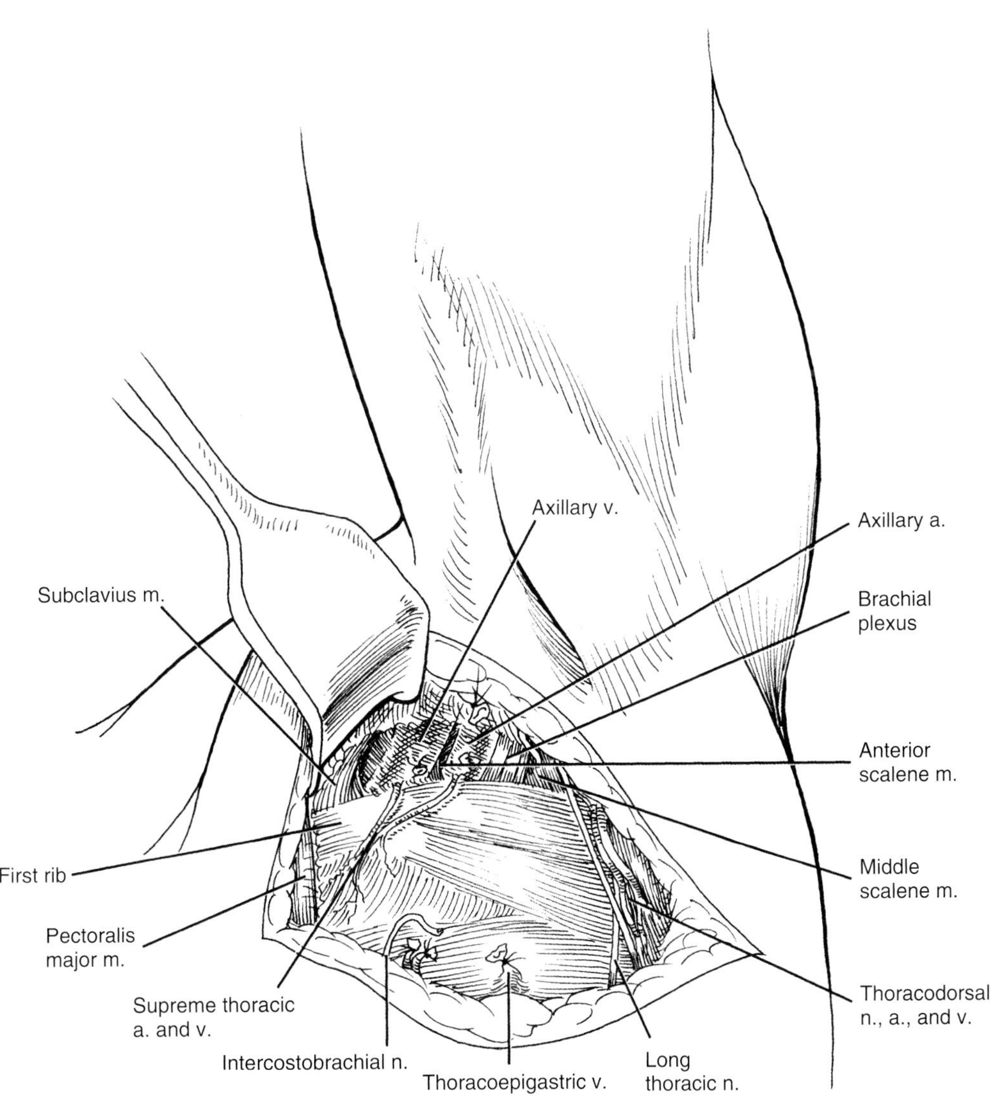

Fig. 4-22 The axillary fascia is opened, and the pectoralis major muscle is retracted to visualize the vessels and brachial plexus at the apex of the axilla.

In the anterior wound, the subclavius muscle is identified as a taut band under the clavicle. It is divided under direct vision and resected as medially as possible (Fig. 4-23). This provides increased exposure for rib resection and prevents subclavian vein compression by the subclavius muscle.[25] It cannot be overemphasized that to prevent vein injury, the subclavian vein requires careful and complete isolation from the subclavius before the muscle is divided. If the vein is adherent to the subclavius muscle, muscle resection should be abandoned to avoid tearing the thin-walled vessel.

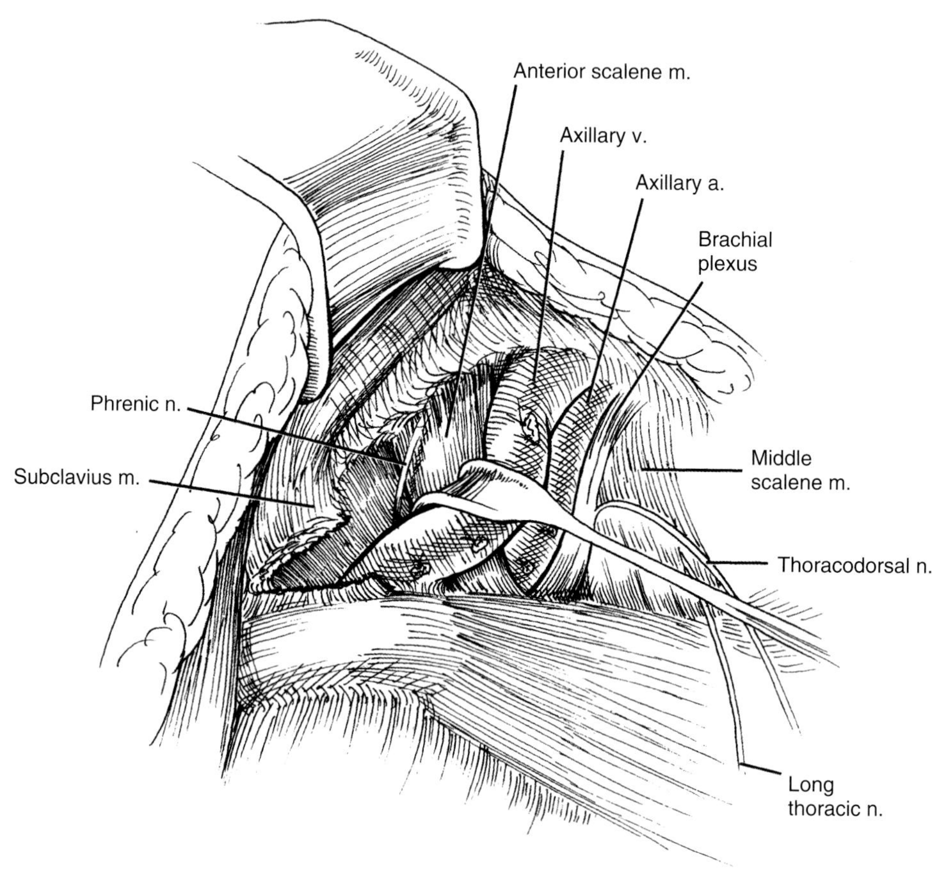

Fig. 4-23 Division of the subclavius muscle insertion allows elevation of the clavicle for improved visibility.

The anterior and middle scalene muscles are next separated from their attachments to the first rib. During division of the anterior scalene muscle, care should be taken to avoid injuring the subclavian artery that passes posterior and deep to the muscle at this level (Fig. 4-24). A right-angled hemostat can be used to retract the anterior scalene away from its surrounding vessels, and its division is best performed a few fibers at a time. The phrenic nerve passes medial to the muscle insertion. The middle scalene muscle is easily pushed off the first rib with a blunt-tipped elevator

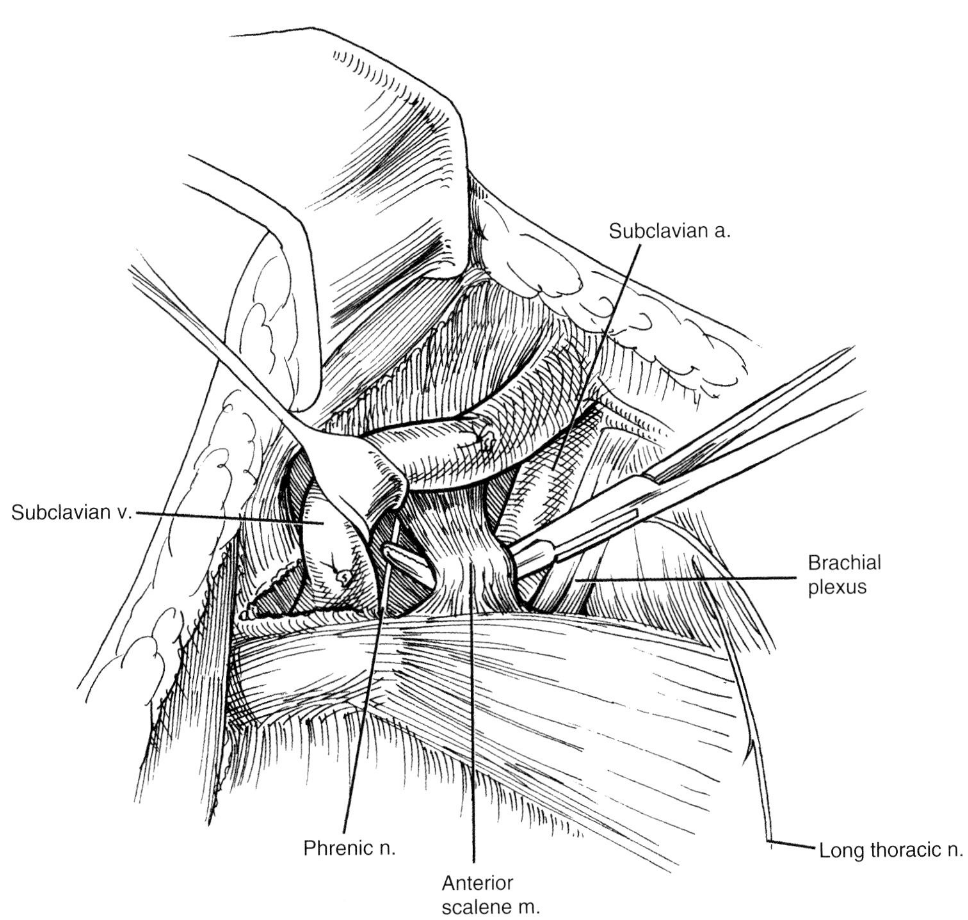

Fig. 4-24 When the anterior scalene insertion is isolated and divided, care must be taken not to injure the phrenic nerve.

(Fig. 4-25). After muscle separation is complete, the subclavian artery and brachial plexus should be freed by sharply dividing their delicate attachments to the first rib. In cases involving arterial compression, the artery may be adherent to the rib, and its wall may be thinned from poststenotic dilatation. Development of a subperiosteal plane underneath the artery may allow its safe dissection away from the rib in these cases.

The rib can now be resected. Although a subperiosteal resection may help avoid injuring the intercostal vessels and avoid entry into the nearby pleural space, most authors[23,24] prefer an extraperiosteal resection (see above). The intercostal muscles are stripped from the undersurface of the first rib with a blunt-tipped elevator, then an Overholt #1 raspatory is used to separate the inside curve of the first rib from Sibson's fascia.[25] Once the rib is completely freed circumferentially from the TI transverse process posteriorly to the costal cartilage anteriorly, it is ready for resection. The TI nerve is carefully retracted laterally to protect it during posterior rib division. Angled rib shears are placed as far posteriorly as possible without injuring the long thoracic nerve, and the rib is cleanly divided (Fig. 4-26). The anterior division takes place at the costochondral junction, with the subclavian vein carefully pushed away (Fig. 4-27). Sharp bony remnants are smoothed with rongeurs.

Cervical ribs are separated from the surrounding middle scalene muscle and resected with rongeurs as close to the spine as possible. Careful digital palpation of the wound is necessary to detect anomalous fibromuscular bands, especially in the area of the TI nerve.

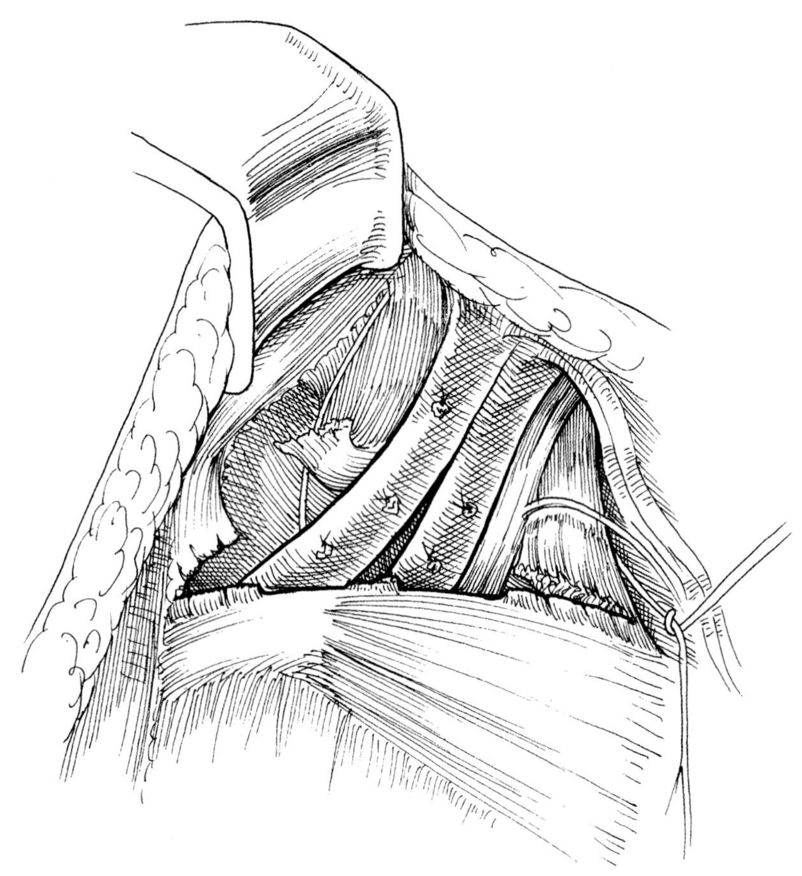

Fig. 4-25 Division of the middle scalene muscle insertion and separation of loose attachments between the first rib and the vessels completes the cephalad mobilization. The long thoracic nerve is again protected.

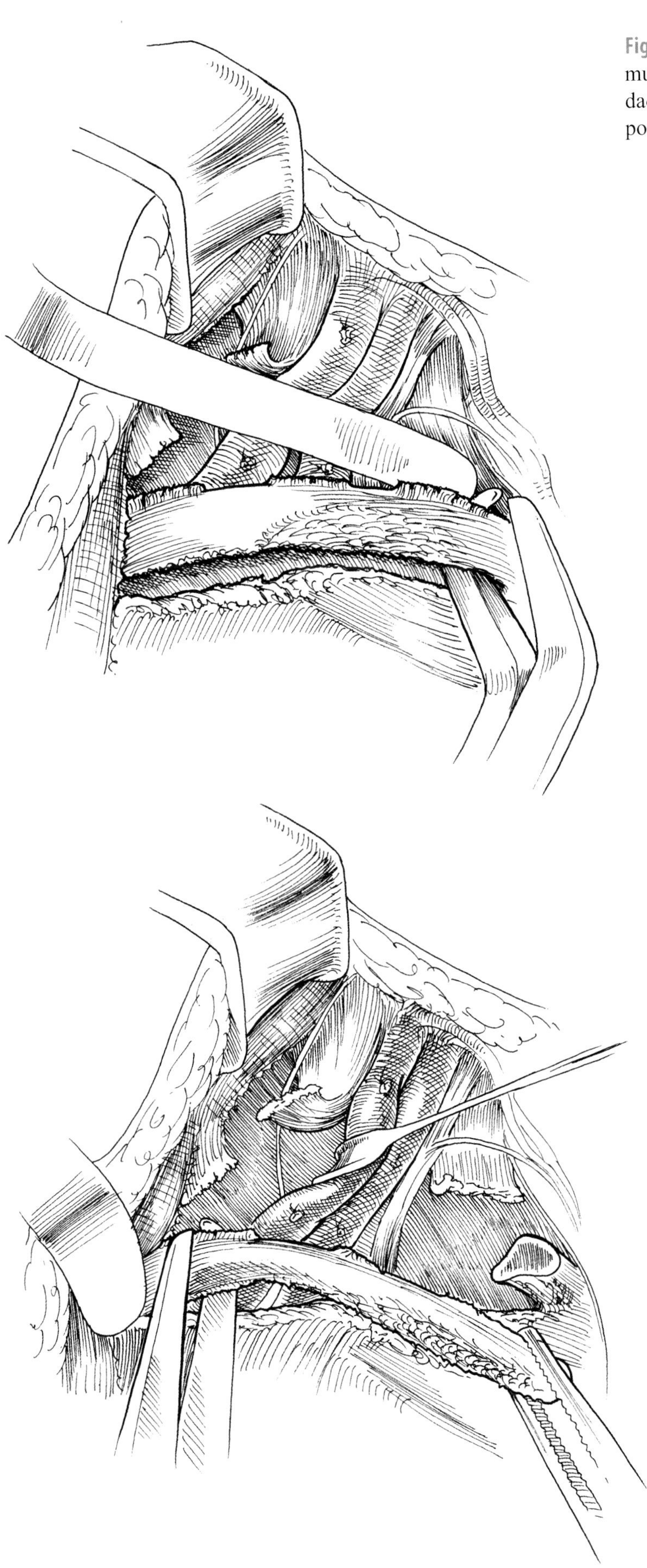

Fig. 4-26 After separation of the remaining muscular and fascial attachments to the caudad and deep rib surfaces, the rib is divided posteriorly.

Fig. 4-27 Anterior rib division completes the resection.

Infraclavicular Approach

Extrinsic compression of the subclavian vein at the level of the first rib can lead to spontaneous thrombosis in healthy patients. If recognized during the acute phase, this so-called effort thrombosis (Paget–Schroetter syndrome) can be treated using catheter-directed clot lysis followed by selective relief of thoracic outlet compression.[32–35] The most common site of compression occurs within the costoclavicular space, where excessive narrowing due to first rib anomalies or hypertrophy of the subclavius muscle can lead to compressive occlusion[3,6,35] (Fig. 4-28). Successful treatment usually requires removal of the first rib and complete venolysis.[33] In many cases, this can be successfully accomplished using a transaxillary or supraclavicular approach,[32–35] but complete resection to the costosternal junction is not always possible. In these circumstances, direct vision of the proximal first

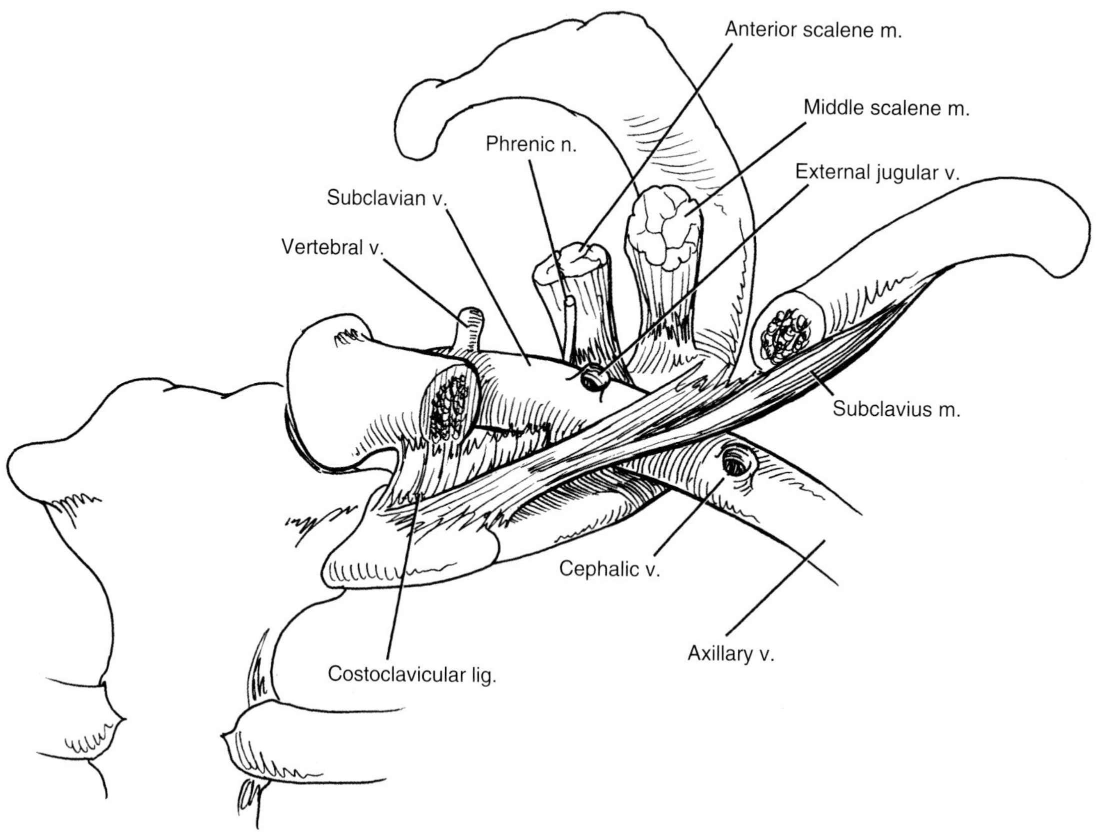

Fig. 4-28 The subclavian vein can be compressed within the costoclavicular space by bony or ligamentous abnormalities.

rib may be indicated; the infraclavicular approach affords direct exposure of this segment.[36] This approach may also be required for visualization of the proximal subclavian vein to allow complete venolysis, as recommended by Thompson et al.[37] Medial claviculectomy is another option that provides direct exposure of the subclavian vein, but clavicular resection has been associated with bothersome symptoms in up to half of patients.[22] The infraclavicular approach allows excellent exposure of the subclavian vein, preserves shoulder function, and is cosmetically superior to claviculectomy.

The patient is placed supine with the arms drawn inward. A transverse skin incision is made 2 cm below the clavicle, extending approximately 5 cm from the lateral border of the sternum (Fig. 4-29). The incision is deepened through the pectoral fascia, and the pectoralis major muscle is split in the direction of its fibers to expose the junction between the first rib and the sternum.[36]

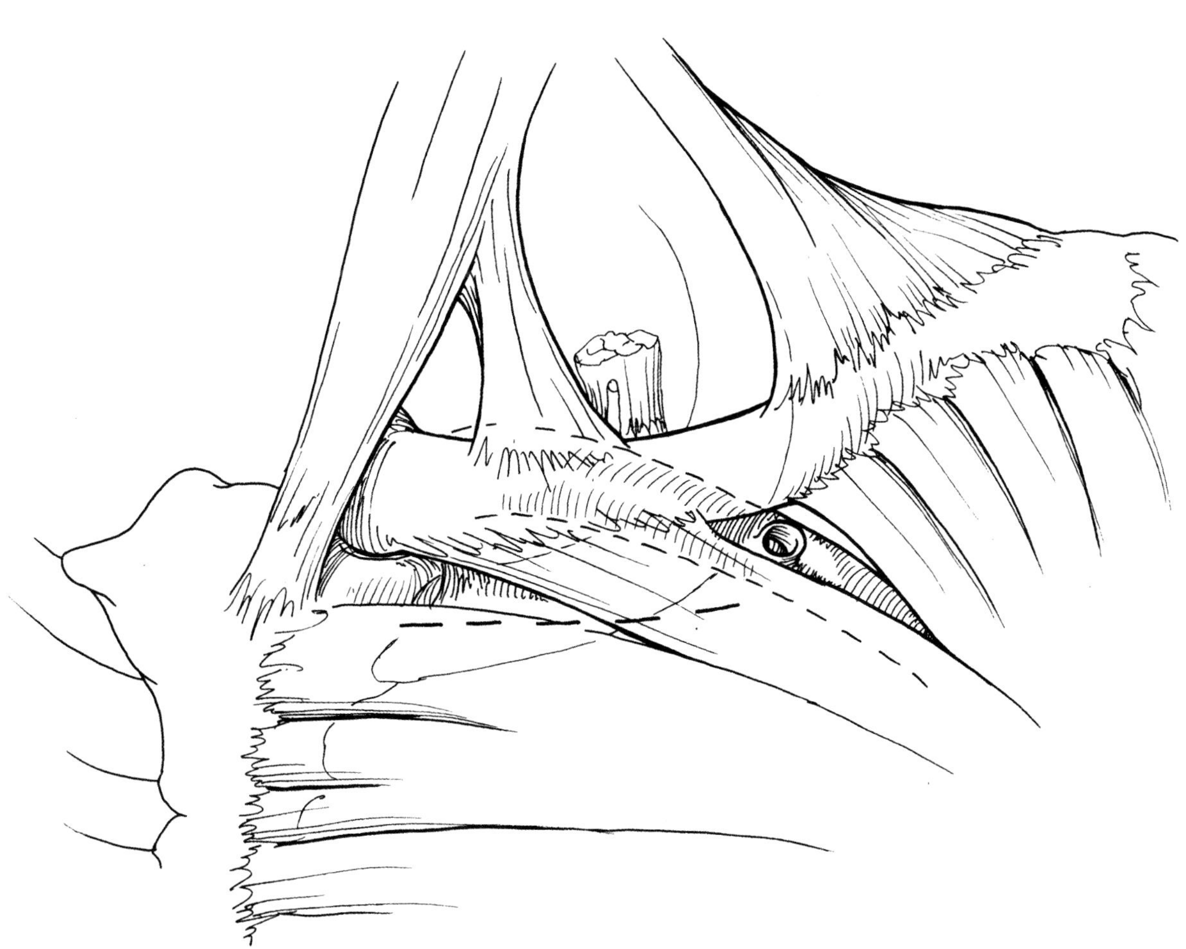

Fig. 4-29 The incision for infraclavicular approach to the first rib is made 2 cm below the clavicle.

The subclavius muscle tendon is divided at its insertion onto the superior surface of the first rib and excised (Fig. 4-30). The underlying subclavian vein can be freed using circumferential dissection. The costoclavicular (Halsted's) ligament lies just behind the insertion of the subclavius muscle. This ligament should be divided because its medial fibers may impinge on the subclavian vein along with the subclavius. Complete division will also simplify removal of the first rib at the sternoclavicular junction. Once all areas of extrinsic venous compression have been released, the subclavian vein will be soft and easily compressible[37] (Fig 4-31).

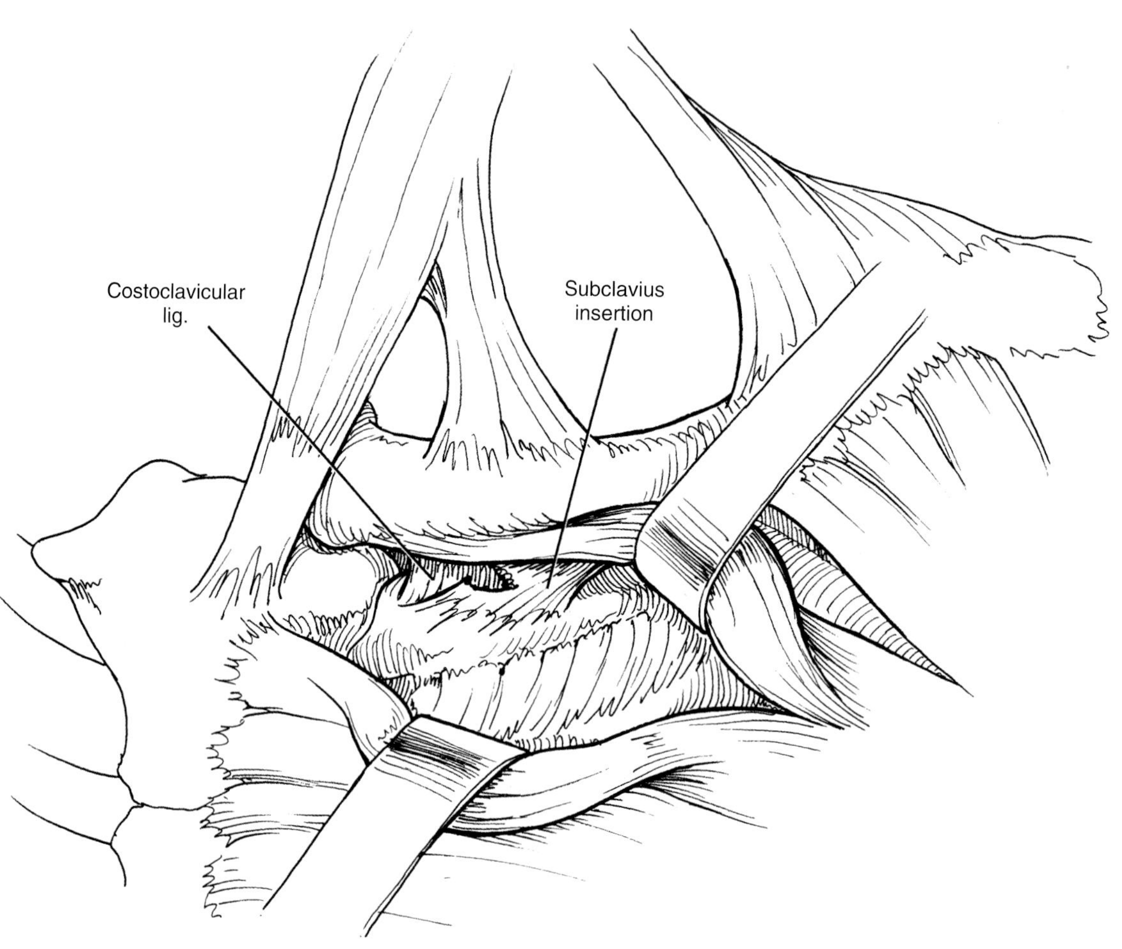

Fig. 4-30 The subclavius muscle is divided and excised. The nearby costoclavicular ligament should also be divided, since medial fibers may contribute to vein compression.

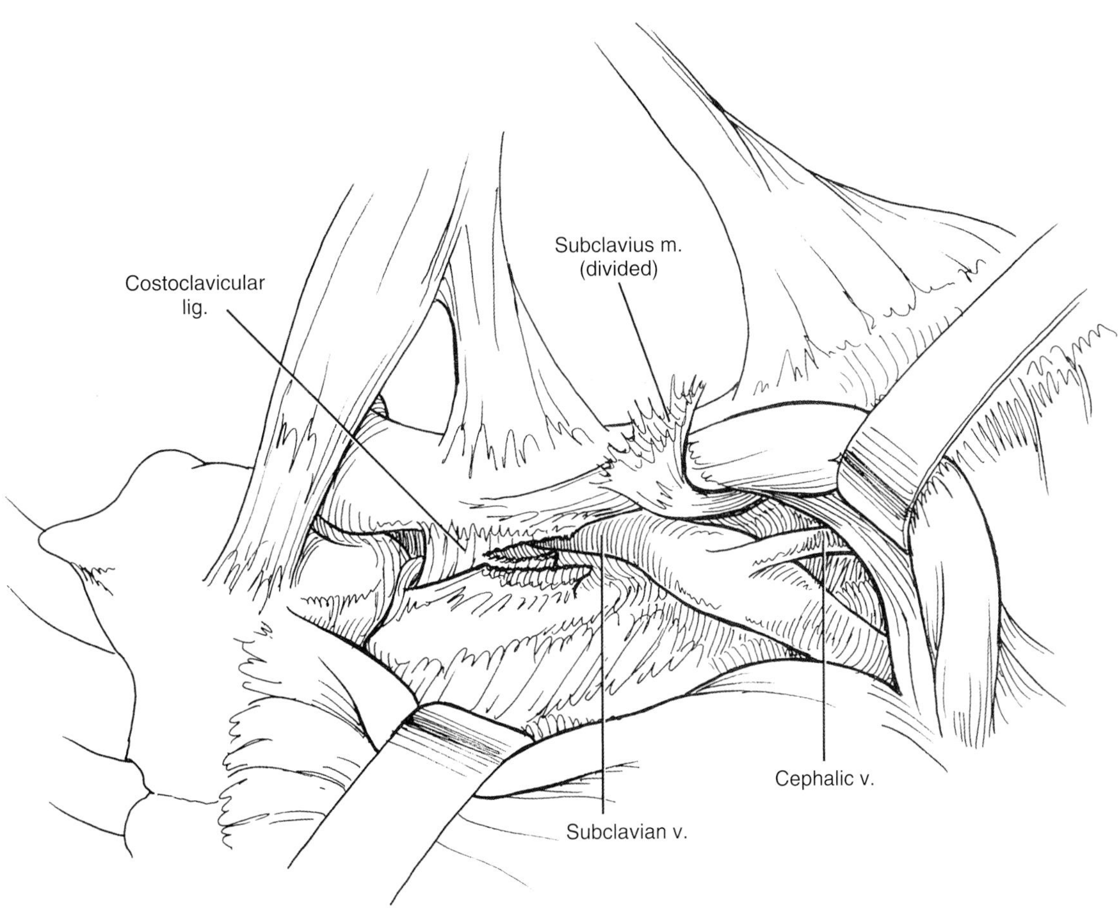

Fig. 4-31 The subclavian vein is freed using circumferential dissection.

In situations when most of the first rib has been resected using the supraclavicular or transaxillary approach (see above), the first rib remnant and its short costal cartilage are easily removed using downward tension and detachment at the costosternal junction. If the first rib is intact, the intercostal muscles along the rib's inferior border are divided. The pleura is carefully displaced from the inner border of the rib using blunt dissection, starting in the lateral wound and proceeding medially.[36] The anterior end of the first rib should be divided under direct vision, and any medial remnant can be removed as above (Fig. 4-32). Downward traction on the anterior end of the divided rib will help expose the anterior scalene muscle insertion. The subclavian vein should be retracted superiorly with a Langenbeck retractor as the anterior scalene is divided (Fig. 4-33). The phrenic nerve should be identified and carefully protected during this maneuver. The middle scalene muscle can be visualized by retracting the vein and artery together into the superior wound. Molina[36] has recommended that the rib be divided at least 1 cm behind the subclavian artery after the middle scalene has been transected (Fig. 4-34).

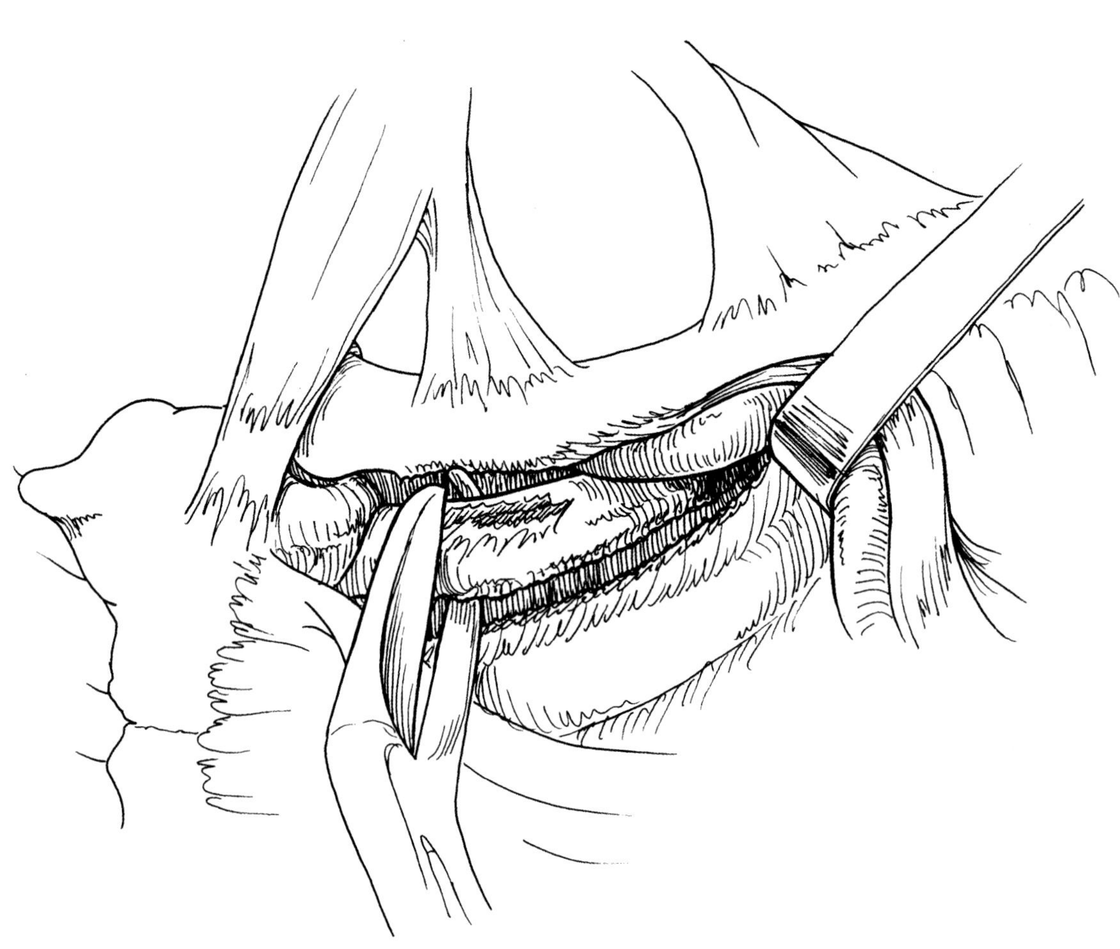

Fig. 4-32 The anterior end of the first rib is divided under direct vision.

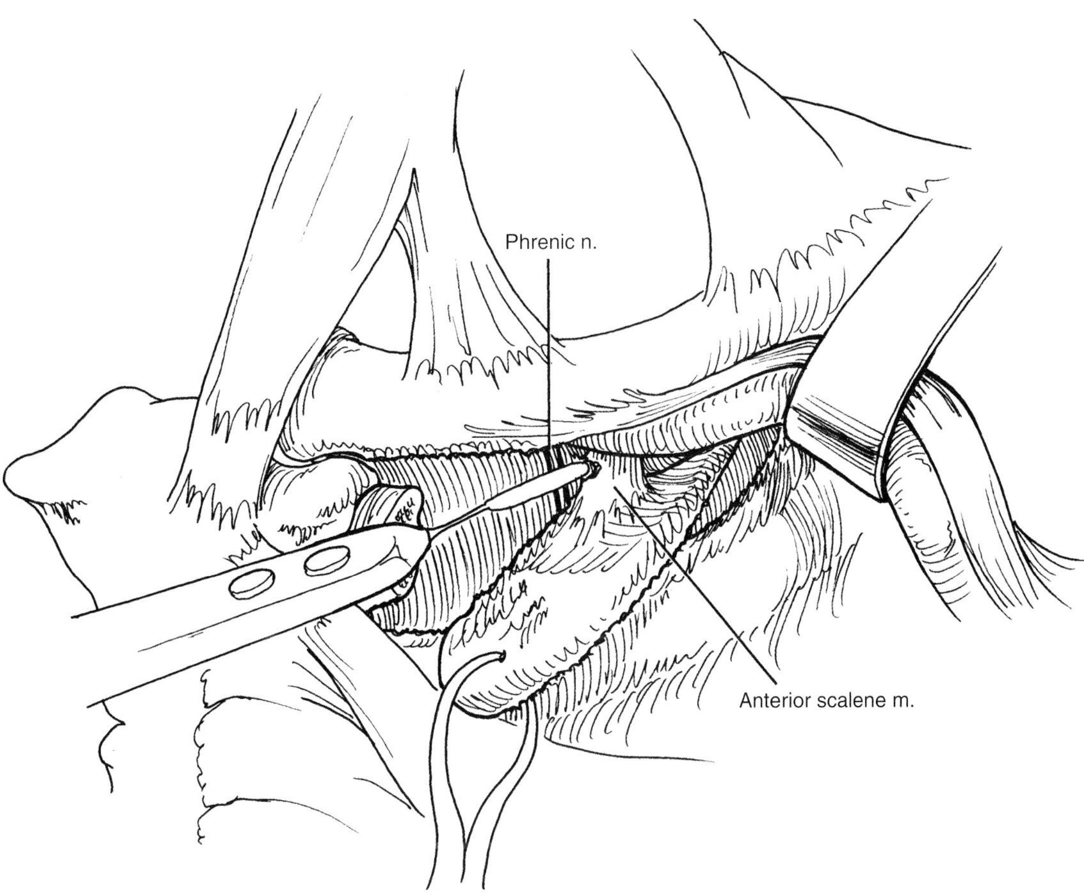

Fig. 4-33 Downward traction on the anterior end of first rib helps expose the anterior scalene muscle. The phrenic nerve should be identified and carefully protected during muscle division.

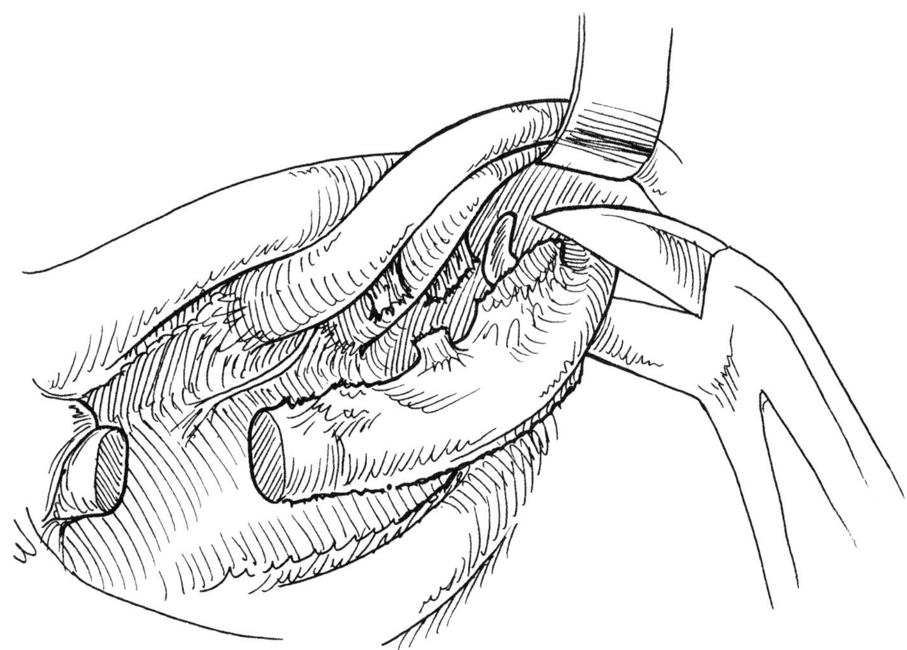

Fig. 4-34 The rib is divided at least 1 cm behind the subclavian artery.

Exposure of the Cervicothoracic Sympathetic Chain

The role of open cervicothoracic sympathectomy has become increasingly limited for two reasons. First, recent experience suggests that the procedure is best performed with endoscopic technology.[38–41] Second, few of the indications for the procedure have withstood the test of time. Most modern surgeons agree that cervicothoracic sympathectomy is indicated for treatment of upper extremity causalgia,[38,42] reflex sympathetic dystrophy,[38,43] and palmar hyperhidrosis.[38–41] The role of sympathectomy in the treatment of primary Raynaud's symptoms and thromboangiitis obliterans is somewhat more controversial. Sympathectomy is no longer indicated for treatment of disorders such as angina pectoris, epilepsy, thoracic outlet syndrome, migraine headaches, and systemic hypertension.

The proper extent of sympathectomy is also somewhat unsettled. To ensure a complete and permanent sympathetic denervation, some authors believe that the sympathetic chain should be resected from the inferior cervical ganglion to the third dorsal ganglion.[44] This will result in a permanent Horner's syndrome. To prevent this, most experienced surgeons prefer to spare at least the upper half of the stellate ganglion.[38–41,43] The second through third and possibly fourth dorsal thoracic ganglia and their interconnecting rami should be removed in all cases. Sympathectomies extending from T2 to T4 appear to be adequate for patients with palmar hyperhidrosis.[38–41]

There are four traditional approaches for exposing the cervicothoracic sympathetic chain: anterior transthoracic, posterior paravertebral, anterior supraclavicular, and transaxillary. The anterior transthoracic approach provides wide and direct exposure of the sympathetic chain,[45,46] but it has lost favor because of the large anterior thoracotomy that is required. The posterior paravertebral approach requires third rib resection and is limited in exposure, especially of the stellate ganglion.[45,47] The following discussion concerns the two remaining popular techniques for sympathetic chain exposure. Although modern endoscopic technology may have diminished the value of these exposures to little more than historical interest, they are included in this chapter for the sake of completeness.

Anterior Supraclavicular Approach to Dorsal Sympathectomy

This approach is direct, and it offers the advantage of reduced postoperative incisional pain.[45,48] A singular disadvantage is the limited exposure of the lower sympathetic chain, leading to potential problems of inadequate sympathectomy and uncontrolled hemorrhage in the deep wound. Despite this limitation, the procedure is considered simple and effective, with operative results similar to other techniques.[45,49]

The patient is placed in the supine position with the head turned toward the opposite side. The supraclavicular incision and deep dissection proceed as described in detail above. The fat pad is dissected away from underlying structures, and the sternocleidomastoid muscle and carotid sheath are mobilized and retracted medially. After the phrenic nerve is identified and protected, the anterior scalene muscle is divided near its first rib attachment, exposing the subclavian artery directly beneath (Fig. 4-35). The subclavian artery should be mobilized extensively and encircled with a vessel loop. The vertebral artery is similarly mobilized in the medial wound, beginning at its origin at the subclavian and extending as far cephalad as possible. This may require ligation of the vertebral vein. The stellate ganglion lies posterior to the vertebral artery, on the anteromedial surface of the brachial plexus. The ganglion is most easily exposed by retracting the subclavian artery downward and dissecting in the deep tissues behind the vertebral artery (Fig. 4-36). The thoracic sympathetic chain is exposed by freeing Sibson's fascia from the inferior border of the first rib and bluntly entering the retropleural space. The pleura is further dissected away from the chest wall until the first four ribs and associated ganglia are exposed.

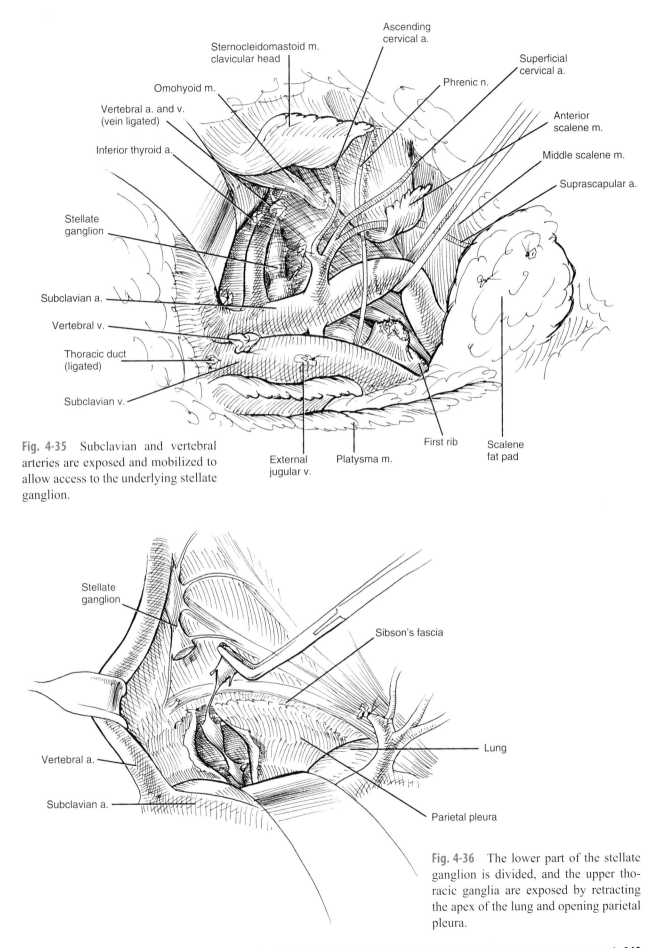

Fig. 4-35 Subclavian and vertebral arteries are exposed and mobilized to allow access to the underlying stellate ganglion.

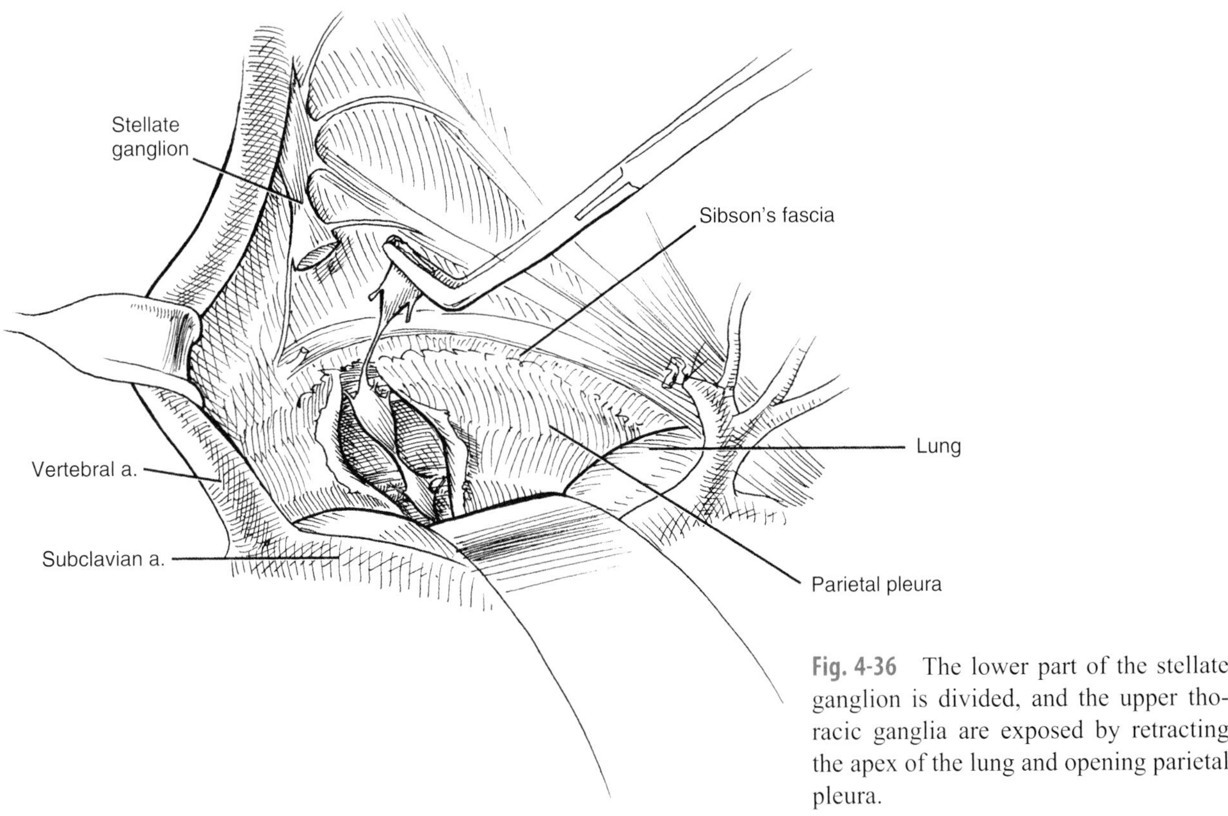

Fig. 4-36 The lower part of the stellate ganglion is divided, and the upper thoracic ganglia are exposed by retracting the apex of the lung and opening parietal pleura.

Transaxillary Approach to Dorsal Sympathectomy

This approach offers complete exposure of the sympathetic chain and a superior cosmetic result.[45,50,51] The principal disadvantage is the relatively narrow wound, through which dissection may be cumbersome in muscular individuals. Although the transpleural approach is preferred, an extrapleural approach may be used in individuals with pleural adhesions.[53]

The patient is placed in a lateral position, with the ipsilateral arm placed on an overhanging support (see Fig. 4-19). Although Haimovici[45] prefers entering the pleural space through the bed of the third rib, others have described entrance through the second intercostal space.[44,51,52] Accordingly, a transverse incision is made parallel to the second intercostal space, extending from the pectoralis major muscle anteriorly to the latissimus dorsi posteriorly. The wound is deepened through subcutaneous tissue and the axillary fascia to reach the lateral chest wall. The long thoracic and thoracodorsal nerves lie near the border of the latissimus dorsi in the posterior wound and should be carefully protected during muscle retraction. The wound is further deepened through the serratus anterior and intercostal muscle fibers, which should be divided on the superior border of the second rib. After the pleural space is entered, the second and third ribs are slowly spread apart with a small rib retractor (Fig. 4-37). The apex of the lung is retracted caudally, and the sympathetic chain is readily identified beneath the posterior parietal pleura. The pleura is opened directly over the sympathetic chain, which is lifted with a nerve hook. The sympathectomy is performed by dividing the branching rami of the fourth thoracic ganglion and progressing cephalad. The stellate ganglion is identified near the border of the first rib; at least half of this structure should be left intact to prevent a Horner's syndrome. On the left side, care should be taken to identify the thoracic duct, which courses near the stellate ganglion in the superior chest.

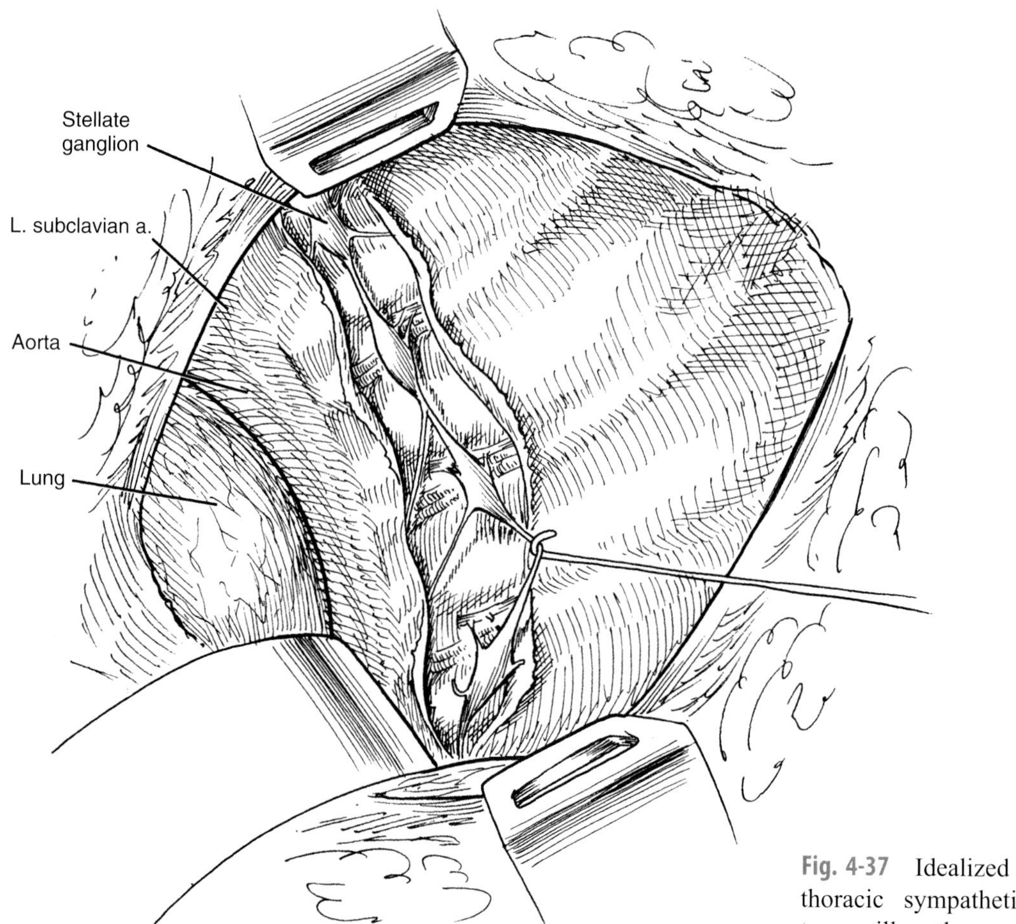

Fig. 4-37 Idealized exposure of the left thoracic sympathetic chain through a transaxillary thoracotomy is shown.

References

1. Pollak EW. Surgical anatomy of the thoracic outlet syndrome. *Surg Gynecol Obstet.* 1980;150:97–102.
2. Sanders RJ, Hammond SL, Rao NM. Thoracic outlet syndrome: a review. *Neurologist.* 2008;14:365–373.
3. Mackinnon SE, Novak CB. Thoracic outlet syndrome. *Curr Prob Surg.* 2002;39:1070–1145.
4. Fodor M, Fodor L, Ciuce C. Anomalies of the thoracic outlet in human fetuses: anatomical study. *Ann Vasc Surg.* 2011;25:961–968.
5. Doyle A, Wolford HY, Davies MG, et al. Management of effort thrombosis of the subclavian vein: today's treatment. *Ann Vasc Surg.* 2007;21:723–729.
6. Illig KA. Management of central vein stenosis and occlusions: the critical importance of the costoclavicular junction. *Semin Vasc Surg.* 2011;24:113–118.
7. McCarthy WJ, Yao JST, Schafer MF, et al. Upper extremity arterial injury in athletes. *J Vasc Surg.* 1989;9:317–327.
8. Magee C, Jones C, McIntosh S, et al. Upper limb deep vein thrombosis due to Langer's axillary arch. *J Vasc Surg.* 2012;55:234–236.
9. Brantigan CO, Roos DB. Etiology of neurogenic thoracic outlet syndrome. *Hand Clin.* 2004;20:17–22.
10. Sanders RJ, Hammond SL. Etiology and pathology. *Hand Clin.* 2004;20(1):23–26.
11. Roos DB. The place for scalenectomy and first-rib resection in thoracic outlet syndrome. *Surgery.* 1982;92:1077–1085.
12. Juvonen T, Satta J, Laitala P, et al. Anomalies at the thoracic outlet are frequent in the general population. *Am J Surg.* 1995;170:33–37.
13. Brooke BS, Freischlag JA. Contemporary management of thoracic outlet syndrome. *Curr Opin Card.* 2010;25:535–540.
14. Sanders RJ, Hammond SL, Rao NM. Diagnosis of thoracic outlet syndrome. *J Vasc Surg.* 2007;46:601–604.
15. Adson AW. Surgical treatment for symptoms produced by cervical ribs and the scalenus anticus muscle. *Surg Gynecol Obstet.* 1947;85:687–700.
16. Rochkind S, Shemesh M, Patish H, et al. Thoracic outlet syndrome: a multidisciplinary problem with a perspective for microsurgical management without rib resection. *Acta Neurochir Suppl.* 2007;100:145–147.
17. Clagett OT. Research and prosearch. *J Thorac Cardiovasc Surg.* 1962;44:153–166.
18. McCarthy MJ, Varty KV, London NJM, et al. Experience of supraclavicular exploration and decompression for treatment of thoracic outlet syndrome. *Ann Vasc Surg.* 1999;13:268–274.
19. Axelrod DA, Proctor MC, Geisser ME, et al. Outcomes after surgery for thoracic outlet syndrome. *J Vasc Surg.* 2001;33:1220–1225.
20. Maxwell-Armstrong CA, Noorpuri BSW, Haque SA, et al. Long-term results of surgical decompression of thoracic outlet compression syndrome. *J R Coll Surg Edinb.* 2001;46:35–38.
21. Gol A, Patrick DW, McNeel DE. Relief of costoclavicular syndrome by infraclavicular removal of first rib: technical note. *J Neurosurg.* 1968;28:81–84.
22. Green RM, Waldman D, Ouriel K, et al. Claviculectomy for subclavian venous repair: long-term functional results. *J Vasc Surg.* 2000;32:315–321.
23. Sanders RJ, Raymer S. The supraclavicular approach to scalenectomy and first rib resection: description of technique. *J Vasc Surg.* 1985;2:751–756.
24. Reilly LM, Stoney RJ. Supraclavicular approach for thoracic outlet decompression. *J Vasc Surg.* 1988;8:329–334.
25. Roos DB. Transaxillary first rib resection for thoracic outlet syndrome: indications and techniques. *Contemp Surg.* 1985;26:55–62.
26. Roos DB. Transaxillary approach for first rib resection to relieve thoracic outlet syndrome. *Ann Surg.* 1966;163:354–358.
27. Fulford PE, Baguneid MS, Ibrahim MR, et al. Outcome of transaxillary rib resection for thoracic outlet syndrome–a 10 year experience. *Cardiovasc Surg.* 2001;9:620–624.
28. Leffert RD, Perlmutter GS. Thoracic outlet syndrome: results of 282 transaxillary first rib resections. *Clin Orthop.* 1999;368:66–79.
29. Karamustafaoglu YA, Yoruk Y, Tarladacalisir T, et al. Transaxillary approach for thoracic outlet syndrome: results of surgery. *Thorac Cardiovasc Surg.* 2011;59:349–352.
30. Illig KA. An improved method of exposure for transaxillary first rib resection. *J Vasc Surg.* 2010;52:248–249.
31. Dale WA. Thoracic outlet compression syndrome: critique in 1982. *Arch Surg.* 1982;117:1437–1445.
32. Lokanathan R, Salvian AJ, Chen JC, et al. Outcome after thrombolysis and selective thoracic outlet decompression for primary axillary vein thrombosis. *J Vasc Surg.* 2001;33:783–788.
33. Angle N, Gelabert HA, Farooq MM, et al. Safety and efficacy of early surgical decompression of the thoracic outlet for Paget-Schroetter syndrome. *Ann Vasc Surg.* 2001;15:37–42.
34. Caparrelli DJ, Freischlag J. A unified approach to axillosubclavian venous thrombosis in a single hospital admission. *Semin Vasc Surg.* 2005;18:153–157.
35. Illig KA, Doyle AJ. A comprehensive review of Paget-Schroetter syndrome. *J Vasc Surg* 2010;51:1538–1547.
36. Molina JE. A new surgical approach to the innominate and subclavian vein. *J Vasc Surg.* 1998;27:576–581.
37. Thompson RW, Schneider PA, Nelken NA, et al. Circumferential venolysis and paraclavicular thoracic outlet decompression for "effort

thrombosis" of the subclavian vein. *J Vasc Surg.* 1992;16:723–732.
38. Ahn SS, Machleder HI, Concepcion B, et al. Thoracoscopic cervicodorsal sympathectomy: preliminary results. *J Vasc Surg.* 1994;20:511–519.
39. Alric P, Branchereau P, Berthet JP, et al. Video-assisted thoracoscopic sympathectomy for palmar hyperhidrosis: results in 102 cases. *Ann Vasc Surg.* 2002;16:708–713.
40. Krasna MJ. Thoracoscopic sympathectomy: a standardized approach to therapy for hyperhidrosis. *Ann Thorac Surg.* 2008;85:S764–S767.
41. Dumont P, Denoyer A, Robin P. Long-term results of thoracoscopic sympathectomy for hyperhidrosis. *Ann Thorac Surg.* 2004;78:1801–1807.
42. Hassantash SA, Maier RV. Sympathectomy for causalgia: experience with military injuries. *J Trauma.* 2000;49:266–271.
43. Schwartzman RJ, Liu JE, Smullens SN, et al. Long-term outcome following sympathectomy for complex regional pain syndrome type I (RSD). *J Neurol Sci.* 1997;150:149–152.
44. Goetz RH. Sympathectomy for the upper extremities. In: Dale WA, ed. *Management of Arterial Occlusive Disease.* Chicago, IL: Year Book Medical Publishers; 1971:431–447.
45. Haimovici H. Cervicothoracic and upper thoracic sympathectomy. In: Haimovici H, ed. *Vascular Surgery: Principles and Techniques.* Norwalk, CT: Appleton-Century-Crofts; 1984:911–924.
46. Palumbo LT Anterior transthoracic approach for upper thoracic sympathectomy. *Arch Surg.* 1956;72:659–666.
47. Golucke PJ, Garrett WV, Thompson JE, et al. Dorsal sympathectomy for hyperhidrosis: the posterior paravertebral approach. *Surgery.* 1988;103:568–572.
48. Khanna SK, Sahariah S, Mittal VK. Supraclavicular approach for upper dorsal sympathectomy. *Vasc Surg.* 1975;9:151–159.
49. Conlon KC, Keaveny TV. Upper dorsal sympathectomy for palmar hyperhidrosis. *Br J Surg.* 1987;74(7):651.
50. Ellis H. Transthoracic sympathectomy. *Br J Hosp Med.* 1986;35:50–51.
51. Jochimsen PR, Hartfall WG. Per axillary upper extremity sympathectomy: technique reviewed and clinical experience. *Surgery.* 1972;71:686–693.
52. Atkins HJB. Sympathectomy by the axillary approach. *Lancet.* 1954;263:538–539.

VESSELS OF THE UPPER EXTREMITY

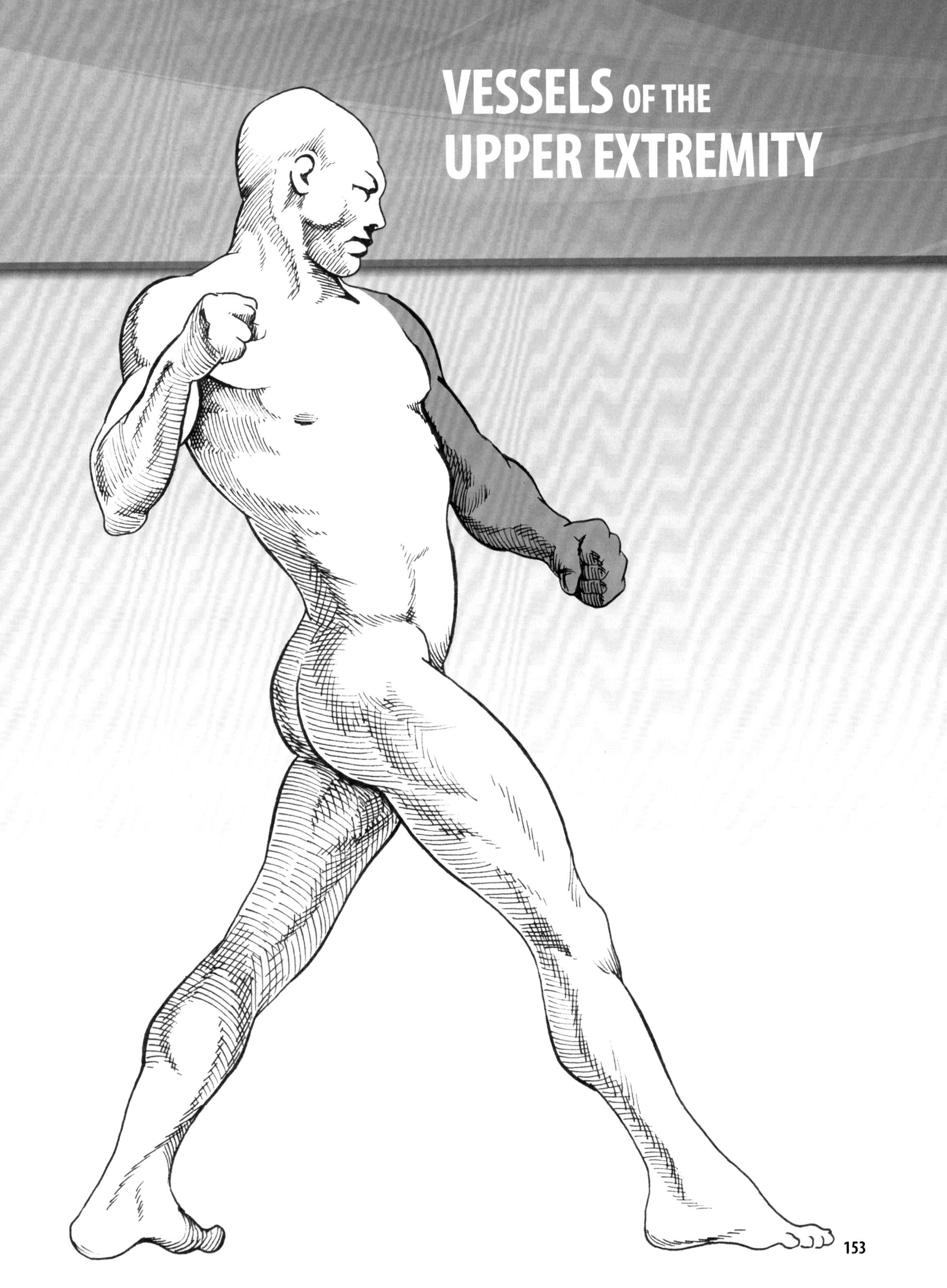

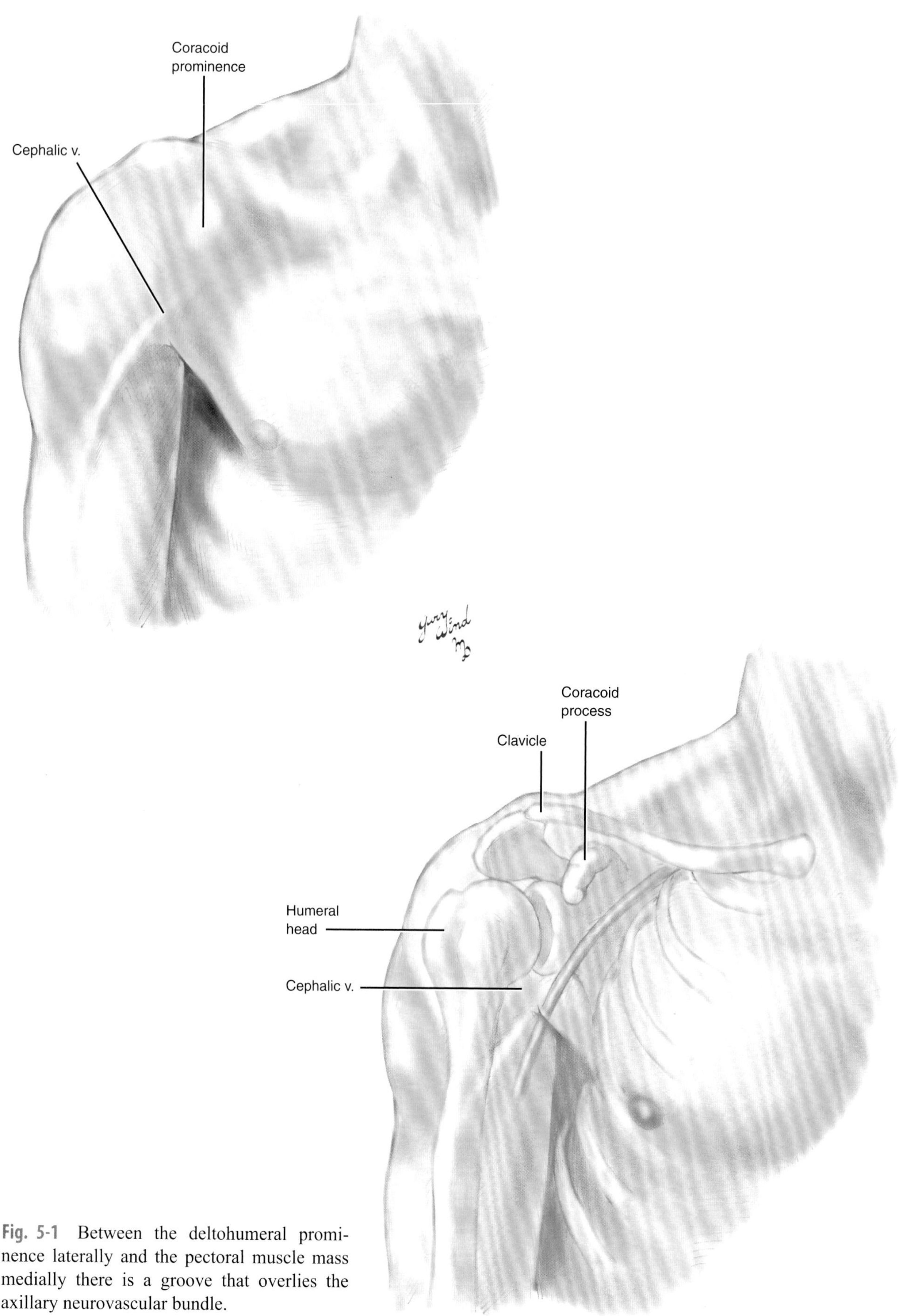

Fig. 5-1 Between the deltohumeral prominence laterally and the pectoral muscle mass medially there is a groove that overlies the axillary neurovascular bundle.

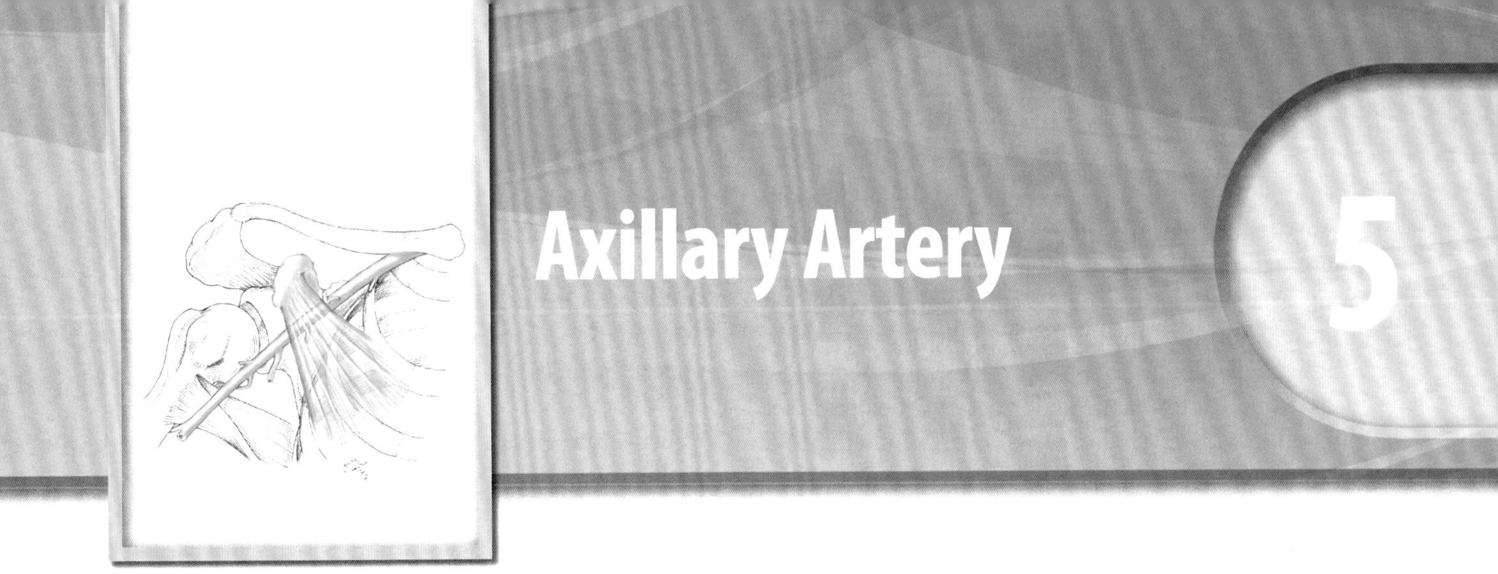

Axillary Artery

5

Anatomy of the Axillary Artery

When the arm is in its relaxed, adducted position, the axillary artery is enfolded on all sides by muscles of the chest wall, pectoral girdle, and proximal brachium. Surface landmarks help locate the position of the vessel in relation to the underlying musculoskeletal structures when the arm is at rest (Fig. 5-1). The recurved clavicle defines the upper frame of the axilla. The pectoral muscle mass follows the tapering contour of the upper chest wall beneath the clavicle medially. Laterally, the humeral head with its overlying deltoid and subscapular muscles forms a prominent bulge. The most medial component of this bulge is created by the coracoid process of the scapula pushing the medial part of the deltoid anteriorly. It is not generally appreciated that the corticoid is so clearly visible on surface inspection and requires no esoteric palpation to locate. The cephalic vein lies in the deltopectoral groove and may be visible in a thin or muscular individual. A depression is formed beneath the clavicle between the coracoid prominence of the shoulder and the lateral clavicular origin of the pectoralis major muscle. The axillary artery is most superficial within this depression and can be easily palpated. To follow the courses of the remainder of the vessel, it is necessary to unfold the muscular envelope and view the artery in its anatomic context.

The Muscular Boundaries

The axillary artery is anatomically defined by the lateral margin of the first rib proximally and the lateral edge of the teres major muscle distally. Along this span, the artery lies within a cleft formed by muscles originating on the scapula (Fig. 5-2). The broad subscapularis, converging toward the head of the humerus, forms the majority of the posterior bed on which the vessel lies. The lowest segment of the artery crosses the teres major and latissimus dorsi insertions.

The medial wall of the cleft consists of the serratus anterior, wrapping around the upper ribs from its origin on the medial border of the deep scapular surface. The coracoid process arches over the axillary neurovascular bundle and gives origin to muscles that lie anterior to the vessels. One of these, the pectoralis minor muscle, is used as a landmark to divide the axillary artery into three parts which are medial to, behind, and lateral to the muscle. The coracobrachialis, a small muscle analogous to the adductors of the thigh, and the short head of the biceps brachii also originate from the tip of the coracoid process. The neurovascular bundle parallels the course of these muscles. The pectoralis major adds the final anterior blanket of muscle over the axillary space.

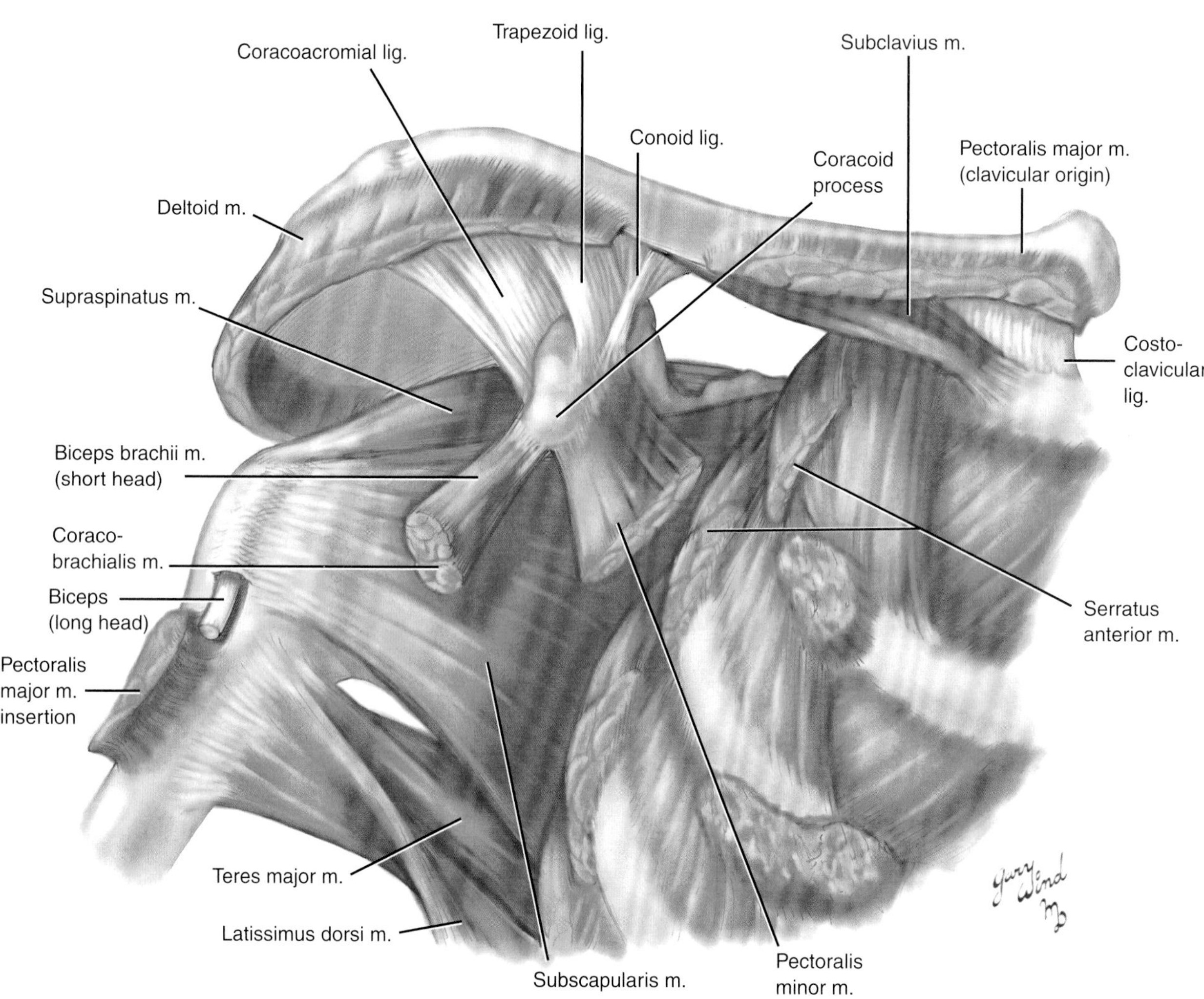

Fig. 5-2 The axillary contents are enclosed by pectoral girdle muscles.

Branches of the Axillary Artery

The first segment of the axillary artery has one branch, the second has two, and the third segment has three branches (Fig. 5-3). Immediately after passing over the outer rim of the first rib, the axillary artery gives origin to the small supreme thoracic artery.

Behind the medial margin of the pectoralis minor muscle, the second part of the axillary artery gives rise to the thoracoacromial artery from its anterior surface and the lateral thoracic artery from its inferior surface. After penetrating the clavipectoral fascia, the thoracoacromial artery divides into lateral acromial and deltoid branches, and medial clavicular and pectoral branches. The pectoral branch, with its accompanying vein and lateral pectoral nerve, forms the major neurovascular pedicle to the pectoralis major muscle. The lateral thoracic artery descends from the second part of the axillary artery to the lateral chest wall, pectoralis major muscle, and breast.

The largest branch of the axillary artery is the subscapular artery, which arises from the third part lateral to the pectoralis minor muscle. It is surrounded by the fat and lymph nodes of the central axilla. It divides into the circumflex scapular artery and thoracodorsal artery. The latter is joined by the thoracodorsal nerve to form the principal neurovascular pedicle of the latissimus dorsi muscle. The remaining two branches of the distal axillary artery are the medial and lateral humeral circumflex arteries. The medial branch runs between the subscapularis tendon and deltoid muscle. The lateral branch, accompanied by the axillary nerve, passes between the teres major, teres minor, long head of the triceps, and the humerus to reach the posterior aspect of the shoulder.

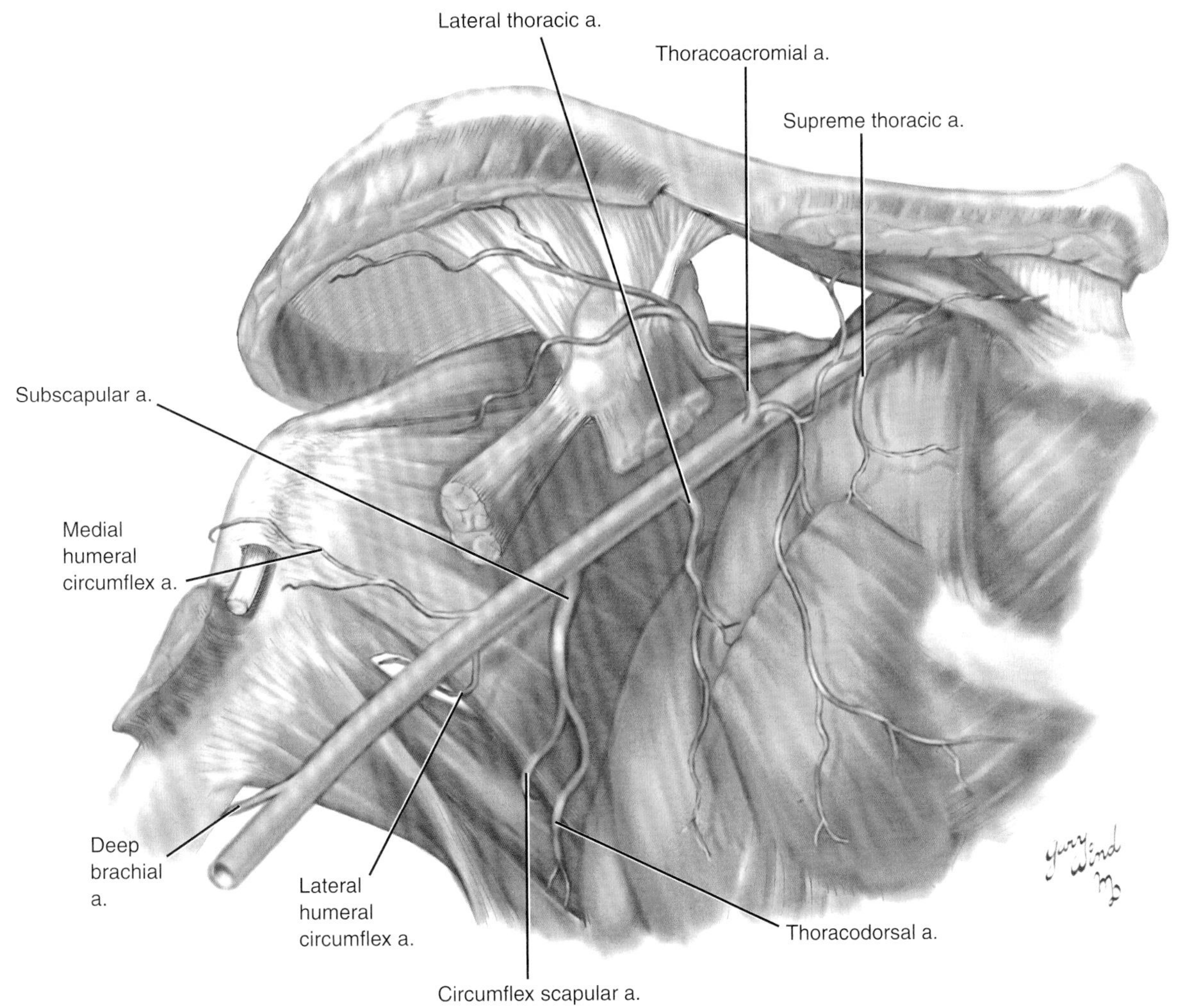

Fig. 5-3 The axillary artery branches are shown.

The Nerves of the Axilla

The divisions and cords of the brachial plexus interchange fibers in the proximal axilla and assume the final configuration of nerves to the arm around the third part of the axillary artery (Fig. 5-4). Several important branches arise from the roots, trunks, divisions, and cords of the brachial plexus and traverse the axillary space.

The nerve of the axilla with the most proximal origin is the long thoracic arising from the ventral primary rami of cervical nerves three, four, and five. The long thoracic nerve emerges through the body of the middle scalene muscle dorsal to the brachial plexus and lies on the serratus anterior muscle, which it innervates. It lies relatively far posterior in the serratus/subscapularis cleft described above.

The lateral and medial pectoral nerves are named for the cords of the brachial plexus from which they arise. Anatomically, they occupy relative positions opposite to what their names imply and have been described in clinical literature by positional designations.[1,2] The following discussion uses the descriptors based on origin. The pectoral nerves are important because they innervate the large pectoralis muscle. The lateral pectoral nerve usually divides into two to four branches and supplies the cephalad portion of the pectoralis major muscle. The branches that join the pectoral branch of the thoracoacromial artery form a neurovascular pedicle on which the pectoralis muscle can be transplanted. The medial pectoral nerve passes between the axillary artery and vein, penetrates and supplies the pectoralis minor muscle, and continues through that muscle as one or more branches to supply the caudal part of the pectoralis major muscle.

The musculocutaneous nerve arises from the lateral cord and supplies the coracobrachialis, biceps brachii, and the medial part of the brachialis muscles. The medial antebrachial and brachial cutaneous nerves arise from the medial cord in the midaxilla. The latter is usually joined by the intercostobrachial nerve spanning the distal axillary space from the second intercostal nerve. The thoracodorsal nerve arises from the posterior cord and joins the thoracodorsal artery to the latissimus dorsi muscle. The subscapular nerves to the subscapularis and teres major muscles also arise from the posterior cord. The last branch of the posterior cord is the axillary nerve to the teres minor and deltoid muscles and posterior shoulder.

The three major nerves to the upper extremity, the median, ulnar, and radial, surround the distal

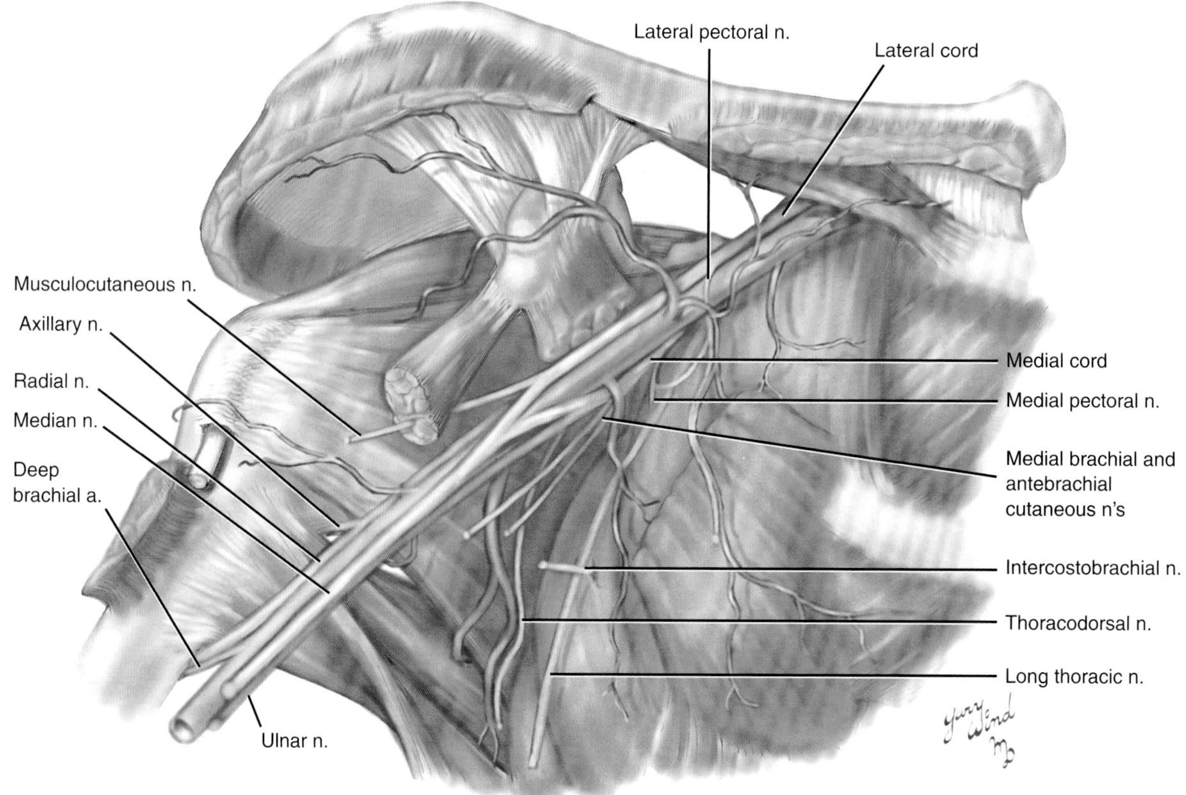

Fig. 5-4 The brachial plexus nerves surround the axillary artery within the axillary sheath.

axillary artery. The median and ulnar nerves accompany the brachial artery in the arm. The radial nerve deviates from the neurovascular bundle at the distal border of the latissimus tendon and passes posteriorly around the humerus with the deep brachial artery.

The Fasciae of the Axilla

The central compartment of the axilla is occupied by the neurovascular bundle and loose, fatty, areolar tissue containing lymphatics and lymph nodes (Fig. 5-5). The neurovascular bundle is surrounded by a fascial wrapping called the axillary sheath. Vascular and nerve branches exit the sheath and traverse the fatty axillary contents to reach their destinations. The bulk of the fatty axillary content is anterior, caudal, and posterior to the sheath. There is a clear plane between the sheath and fat along the anterior surface of the axillary vein. This plane is used to identify the neurovascular branches when beginning an axillary dissection. A second clear plane is found between the fat and the deep fascia over the serratus anterior muscle. The intercostobrachial nerve penetrates the axillary fat in the distal axilla and often must be divided to obtain a clean axillary dissection.

The next fascial layer anterior to the axillary contents is the clavipectoral fascia, which encloses the subclavius and pectoralis minor muscles. This layer is penetrated by the thoracoacromial vessels, pectoral nerves, and cephalic vein. Lateral to the pectoralis minor muscle, the clavipectoral fascia attaches to the axillary fascia and is thought to tether the latter, giving the axillary skin its concave shape. The outermost layer of fascia is the deep, investing pectoral fascia, which encloses the pectoralis major and deltoid muscles. The continuation of this fascia between the lateral edge of the pectoralis major and latissimus dorsi muscles is called the axillary fascia.

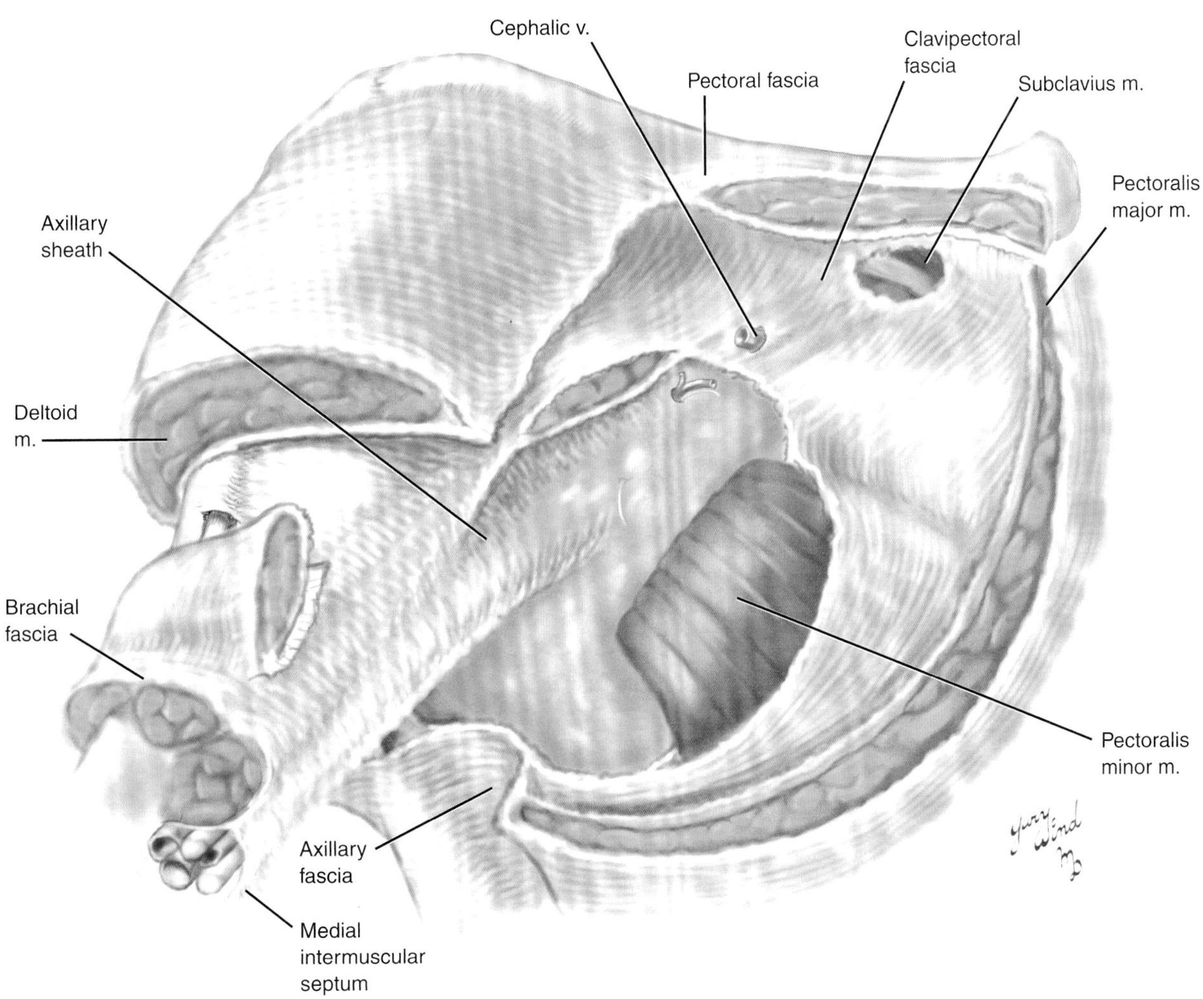

Fig. 5-5 The clavipectoral fascia is the outer envelope of the axillary contents.

Exposure of the Axillary Artery

The axillary artery is an ideal donor artery in extraanatomic bypasses to the opposite arm or to the lower extremities. It is a direct extension of major aortic arch branches and is usually free of flow-limiting arterial stenoses. Its location outside of the thorax and below the clavicle affords easy accessibility and allows construction of superficial bypasses. The physiologic advantage of these bypasses has been well-documented in elderly, poor-risk patients who would not tolerate more direct intraabdominal or intrathoracic bypasses.[3–5] Superficial bypasses are also indicated for lower extremity revascularization in cases of aortic sepsis.[6]

The superficial location of the axillary artery and its proximity to the brachial plexus also carry disadvantages, as the neurovascular bundle is prone to injury. The long-term consequences are determined by the degree of neurologic trauma.[7–9] Long-term functional deficits are rare after isolated axillary artery injuries, but patients with combined neurovascular trauma may experience severe disability and even require late arm amputation. In addition to injuries resulting from accidents or violence, the axillary artery is subject to iatrogenic trauma from invasive diagnostic tests, such as arteriograms. The tough axillary sheath prevents exsanguination from these injuries but permits rapid compression of its contents as blood accumulates. Symptoms of brachial plexus compression are reversible only with rapid evacuation of blood within the sheath.

Covered stents have become a popular alternative to open repair of axillary artery injuries in multiply injured patients and in selected patients with penetrating trauma.[10,11] However, the long-term results are not well established, due in large part to the notoriously poor follow-up of trauma patients. Limited data suggest that stent grafts may not be durable in large upper extremity arteries: one recent study of stented subclavian artery injuries reported that one-third of patients experienced stenosis or occlusion of the stent graft after a mean of 4 years.[12] Regardless of outcome, most surgeons agree that endovascular repair of an axillary artery injury is contraindicated in a hemodynamically unstable patient and in any injury resulting in vessel transection or an inadequate proximal fixation site.[13] Rapid open exposure of the axillary artery remains an important part of the modern vascular surgeon's armamentarium.

For purposes of exposure, the axillary artery can be considered in three anatomic sections (Fig. 5-6). The first part, extending from the edge

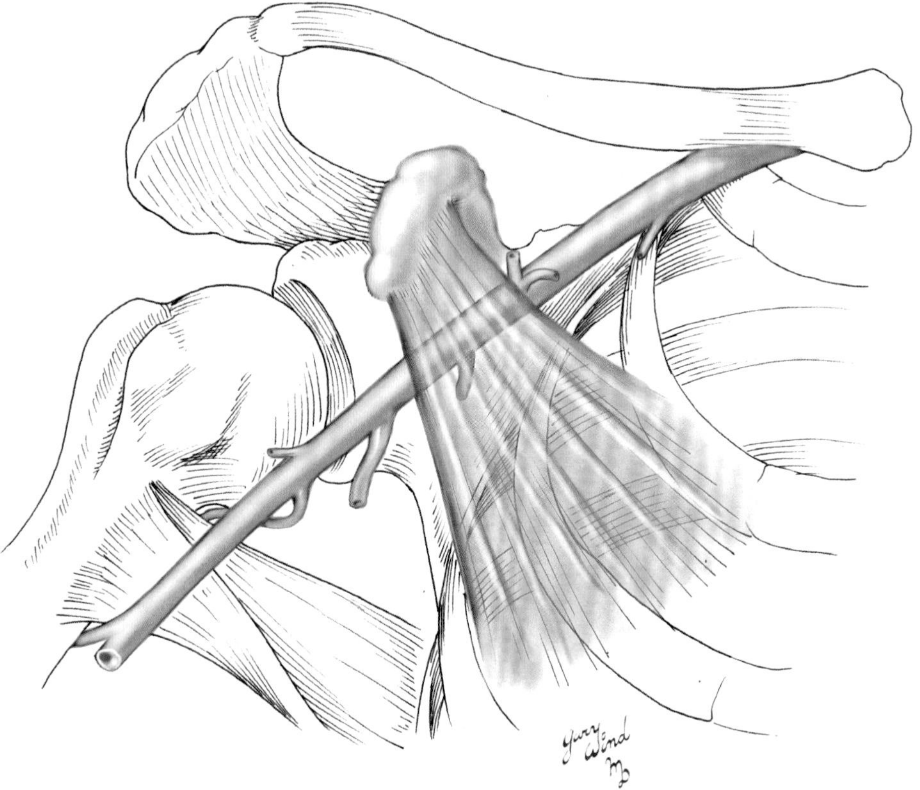

Fig. 5-6 The three parts of the axillary artery are marked by the borders of the pectoralis minor muscle.

of the first rib to the medial border of the pectoralis minor muscle, is relatively fixed and anterior to the brachial plexus. The second part courses beneath the pectoralis minor muscle and requires deep dissection for exposure. The third part extends from the lateral border of the pectoralis minor to the lateral border of the teres major; it is best approached through a lateral incision.

Infraclavicular Approach to the First Part of the Axillary Artery

The patient is placed supine with the ipsilateral arm abducted approximately 90° (Fig. 5-7). Arm abduction is important to ensure a proper amount of laxity in a graft that is anastomosed to the axillary artery,[14–16] but hyperabduction may be associated with traction

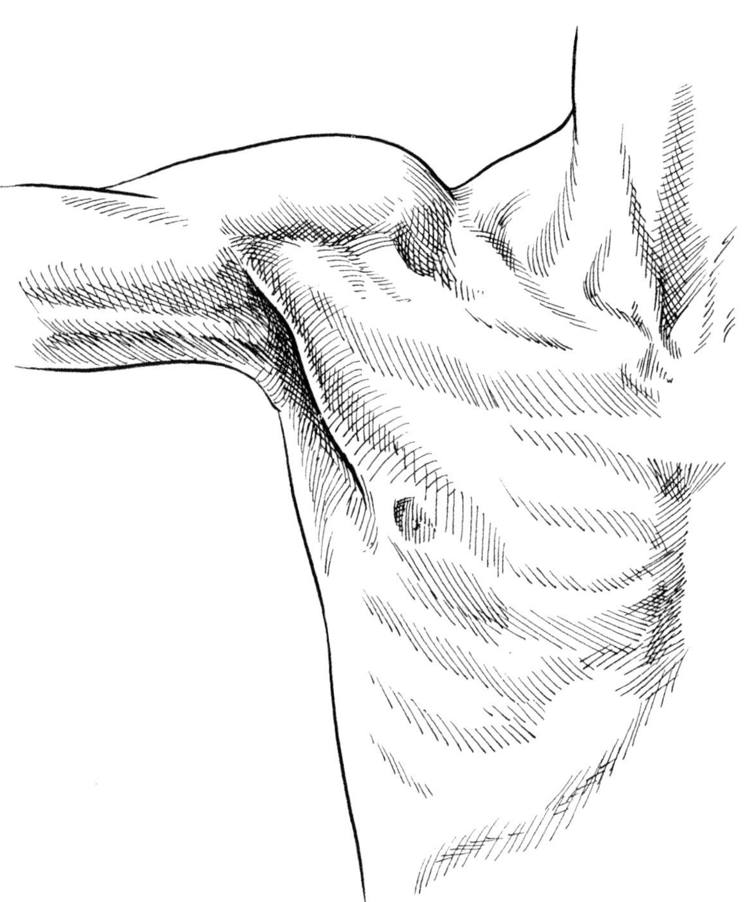

Fig. 5-7 The arm is abducted 90° for the infraclavicular approach to the axillary artery.

injury to the brachial plexus.[17] The shoulder, anterior chest, and axilla should be prepped and draped. In operations utilizing bypasses to groin arteries, the surgical prep should also include the anterior trunk and both legs, which are prepped and draped to the level of the midthigh.

A horizontal skin incision is made 2 cm below the middle third of the clavicle, extending for approximately 8 cm (Fig. 5-8). The incision is deepened through subcutaneous tissue and the pectoral fascia. The underlying pectoralis major muscle is split by bluntly separating its fibers for the length of the

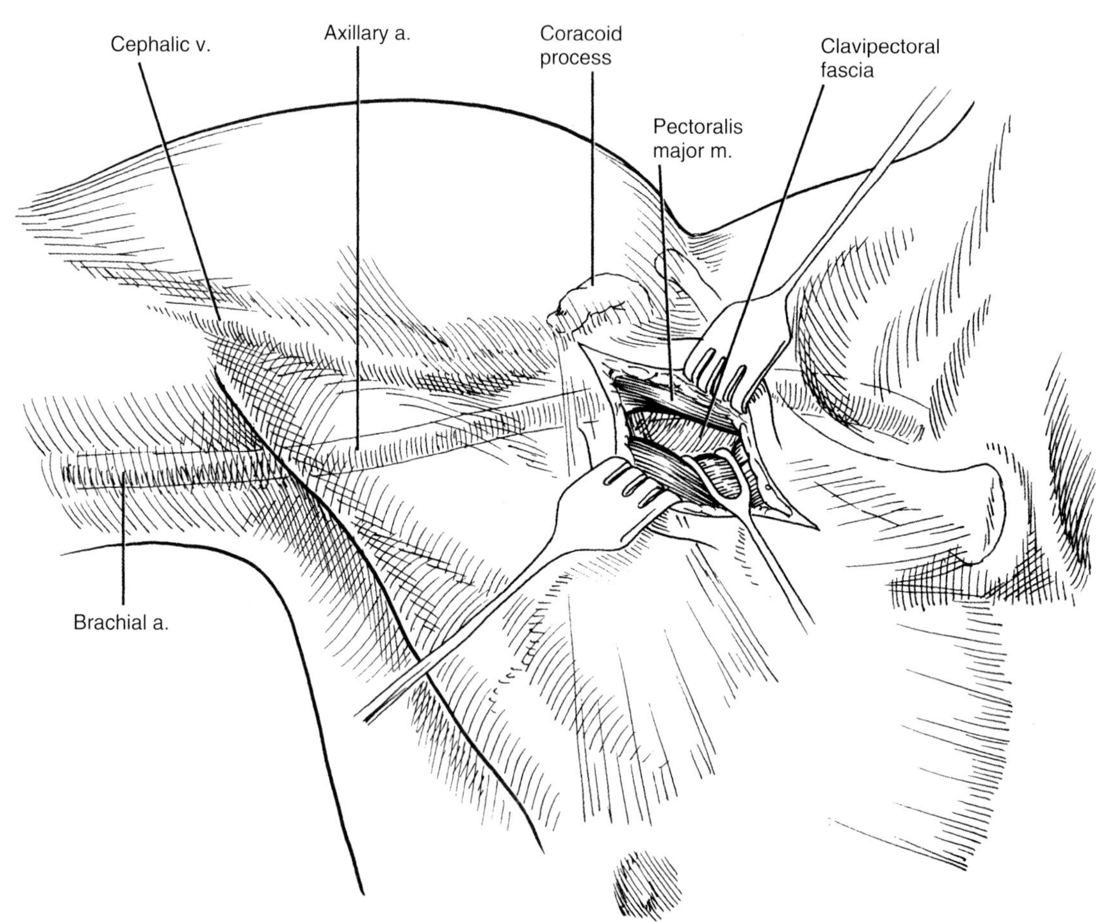

Fig. 5-8 The pectoralis fibers over the first portion of the axillary artery are separated.

wound, exposing the tough clavipectoral fascia. The neurovascular bundle and its enveloping axillary sheath are located in the adipose tissue deep to the clavipectoral fascia, which should be sharply incised. At the lateral wound margin, the pectoralis minor muscle can be freed and laterally retracted to enhance exposure of the first part of axillary artery (Fig. 5-9). Care should be taken to avoid injury to the lateral pectoral nerves during division of the pectoralis minor muscle.[1,2]

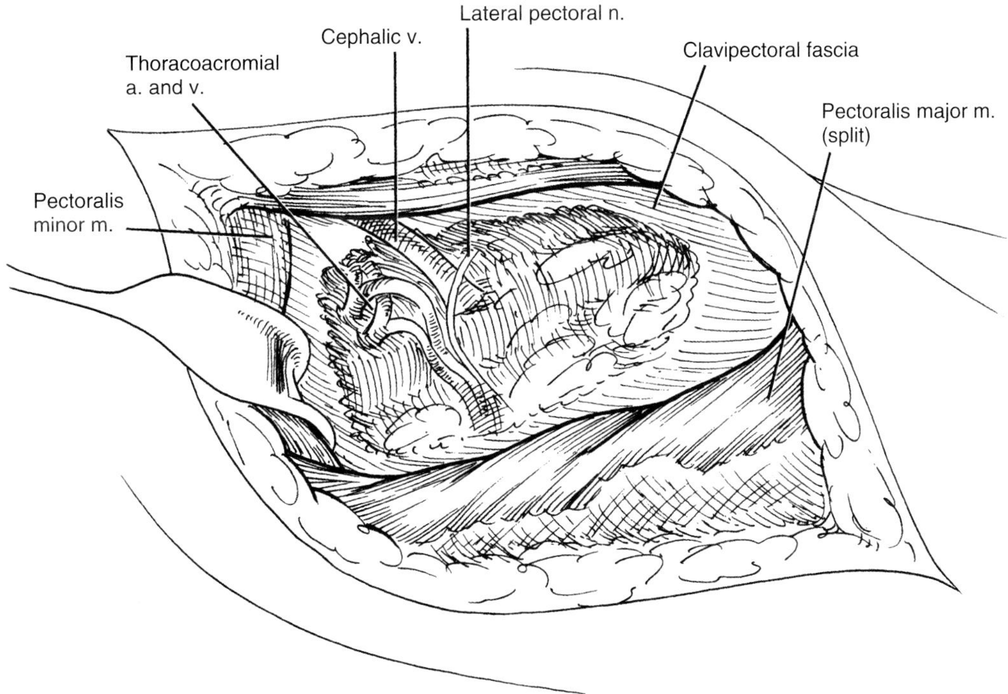

Fig. 5-9 Clavipectoral fascia is opened to expose the axillary sheath. Pectoral nerves and vessels as well as cephalic vein are seen in the operative field.

The axillary vein is the first structure to be encountered in the axillary sheath. The artery lies just superior and deep to the vein and is most conveniently exposed by mobilizing and retracting the vein caudally (Fig. 5-10). Several vein tributaries may require ligation during this maneuver. Most anastomoses will be created proximal to the thoracoacromial artery. This large branch is usually left intact but may be ligated at its origin to permit more adequate exposure of the axillary artery in small patients. The lateral pectoral nerve joining the pectoral branch of the thoracoacromial artery should be preserved when ligating the arterial trunk. The nerves of the brachial plexus lie deep to the first part of the axillary artery and are at risk for injury during blind placement of occluding arterial clamps. The artery should be mobilized as proximally as possible, taking care to identify the nearby pectoral nerves and their interconnecting loop[1] (Fig. 5-11). Once mobilized, the artery can be encircled with a vessel loop and elevated above the vein and brachial plexus to protect these structures prior to clamp placement.

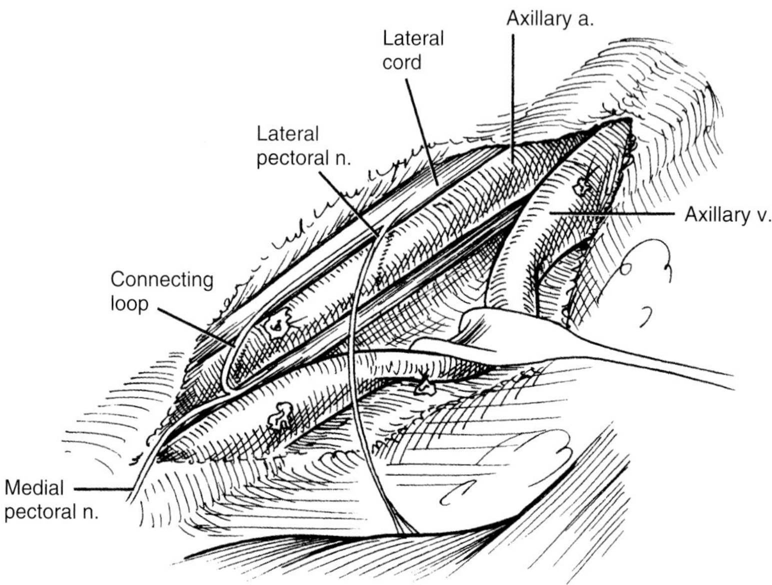

Fig. 5-10 The axillary vein is gently retracted to clearly expose the axillary artery.

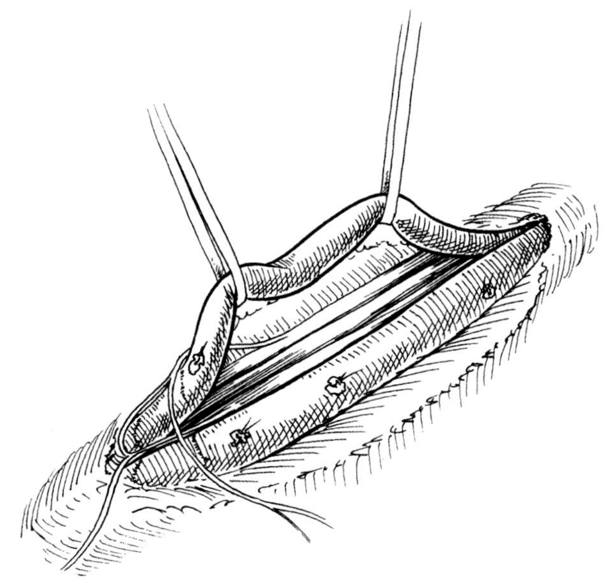

Fig. 5-11 The axillary artery is mobilized.

Proximal anastomoses of axillary artery bypasses should be constructed in the first portion, the area least likely to be stressed by shoulder motion. Proximal graft disruption has been reported in up to 5% of patients after axillofemoral bypass.[14] This catastrophe is usually associated with forceful arm abduction or shoulder trauma[14–16] (Fig. 5-12).

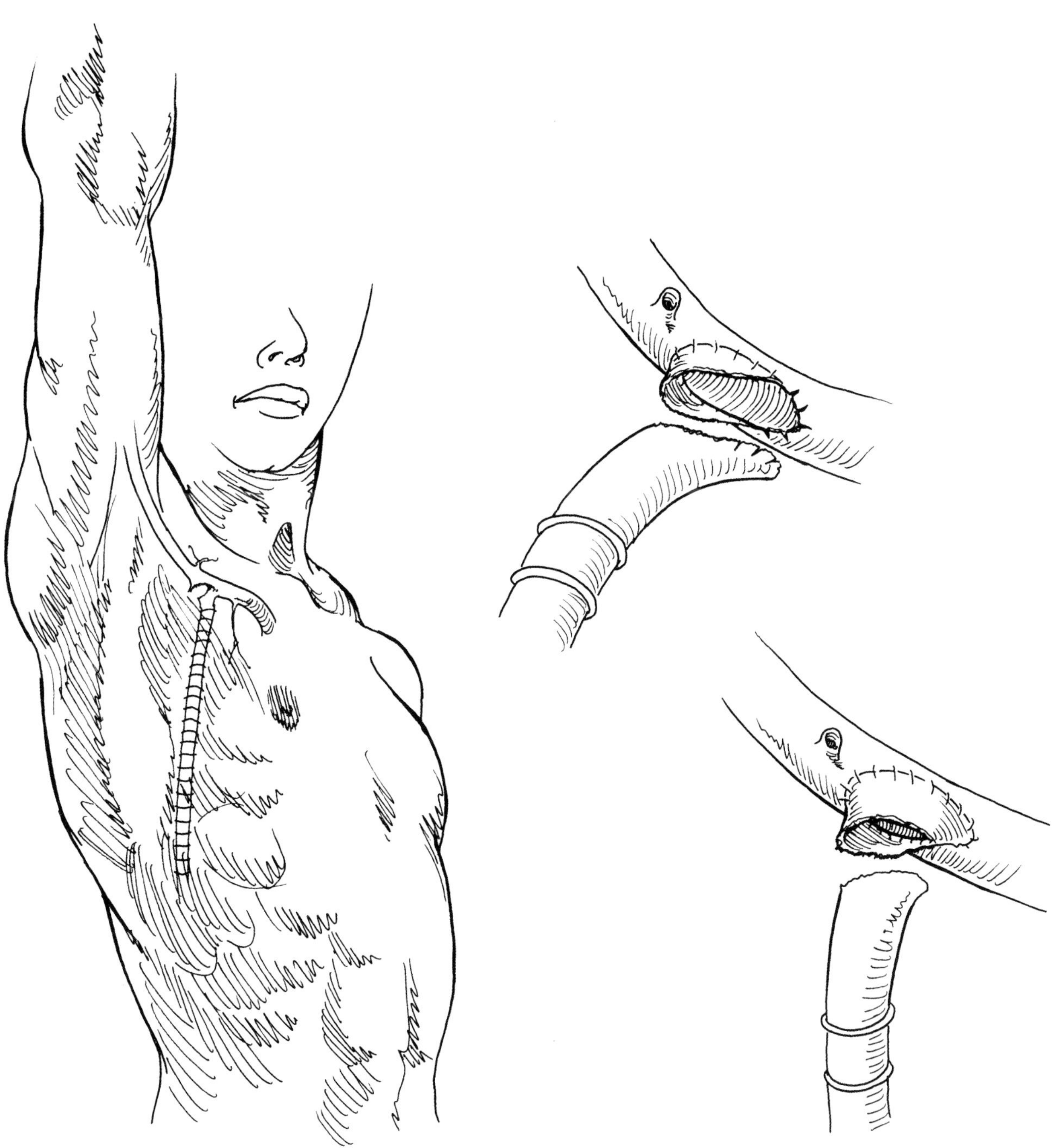

Fig. 5-12 Attention to the configuration of an axillofemoral bypass graft is important. Without sufficient laxity in the axillary portion, forceful arm abduction may lead to disruption of the anastomosis or fracture of the graft itself.

Deltopectoral Approach to All Parts of the Axillary Artery

This approach is somewhat difficult. The second and third parts of the axillary artery are located deep in a relatively narrow incision, and the precise determination of tissue planes necessary in this approach may be impeded by blood staining. Nevertheless, the deltopectoral incision is a very popular approach in cases of axillary vascular trauma, as it is a direct approach to all three parts of the axillary artery. It is particularly useful as an extension of the infraclavicular incision described above.

The patient is placed in the supine position with the arm abducted approximately 30° and externally rotated. An incision is made from the midpoint of the clavicle 5 to 7 cm along the anterior border of the deltoid muscle (Fig. 5-18). The incision is deepened through the subcutaneous tissue to reach the intermuscular groove between the pectoralis major and deltoid muscles, marked by the cephalic vein. The intermuscular groove is separated along the full extent of the wound, and the pectoralis major is retracted medially (Fig. 5-19). If increased lateral exposure is required, the pectoralis major tendon can be divided near its insertion. The cephalic vein, dissected along its medial border, is retracted laterally with the deltoid muscle. The underlying clavipectoral fascia and pectoralis minor muscle are now

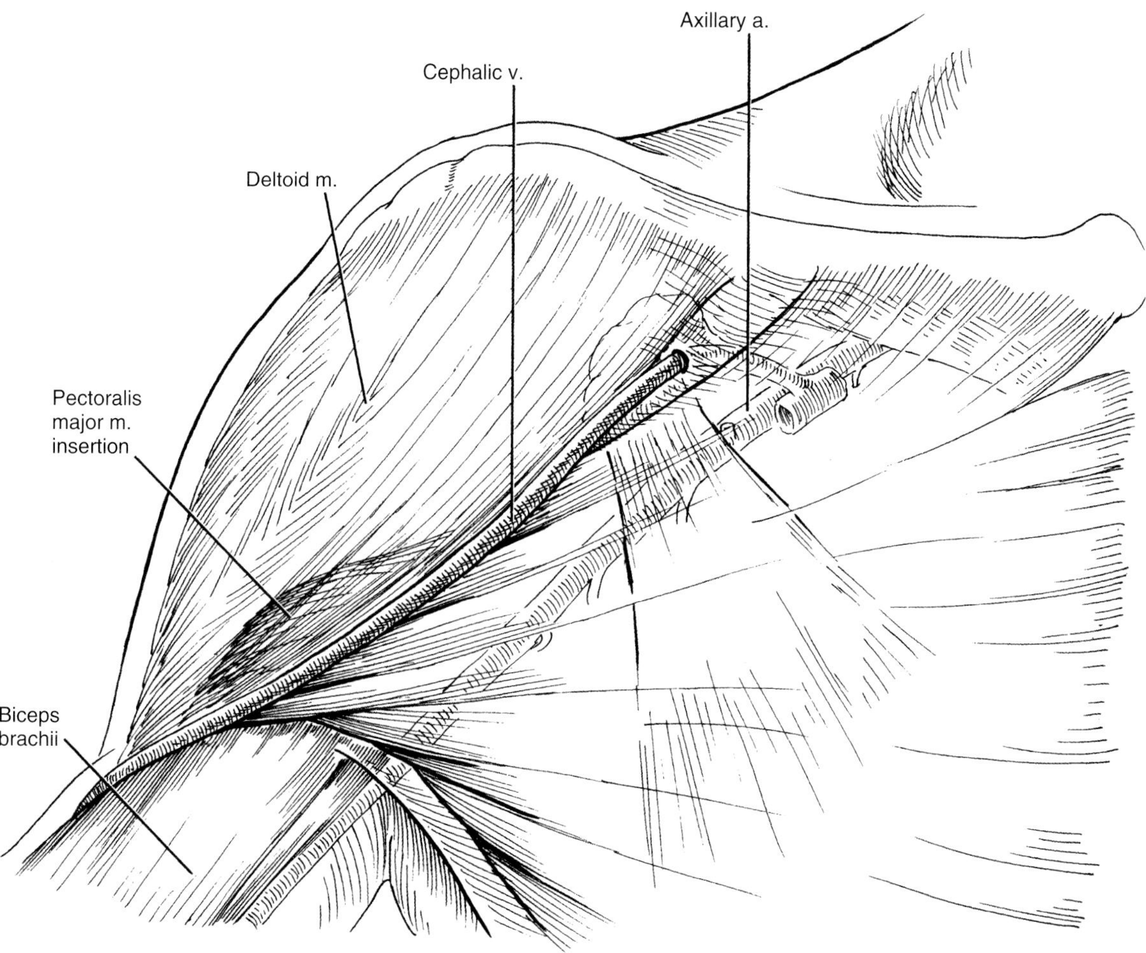

Fig. 5-18 The deltopectoral groove landmarks are shown.

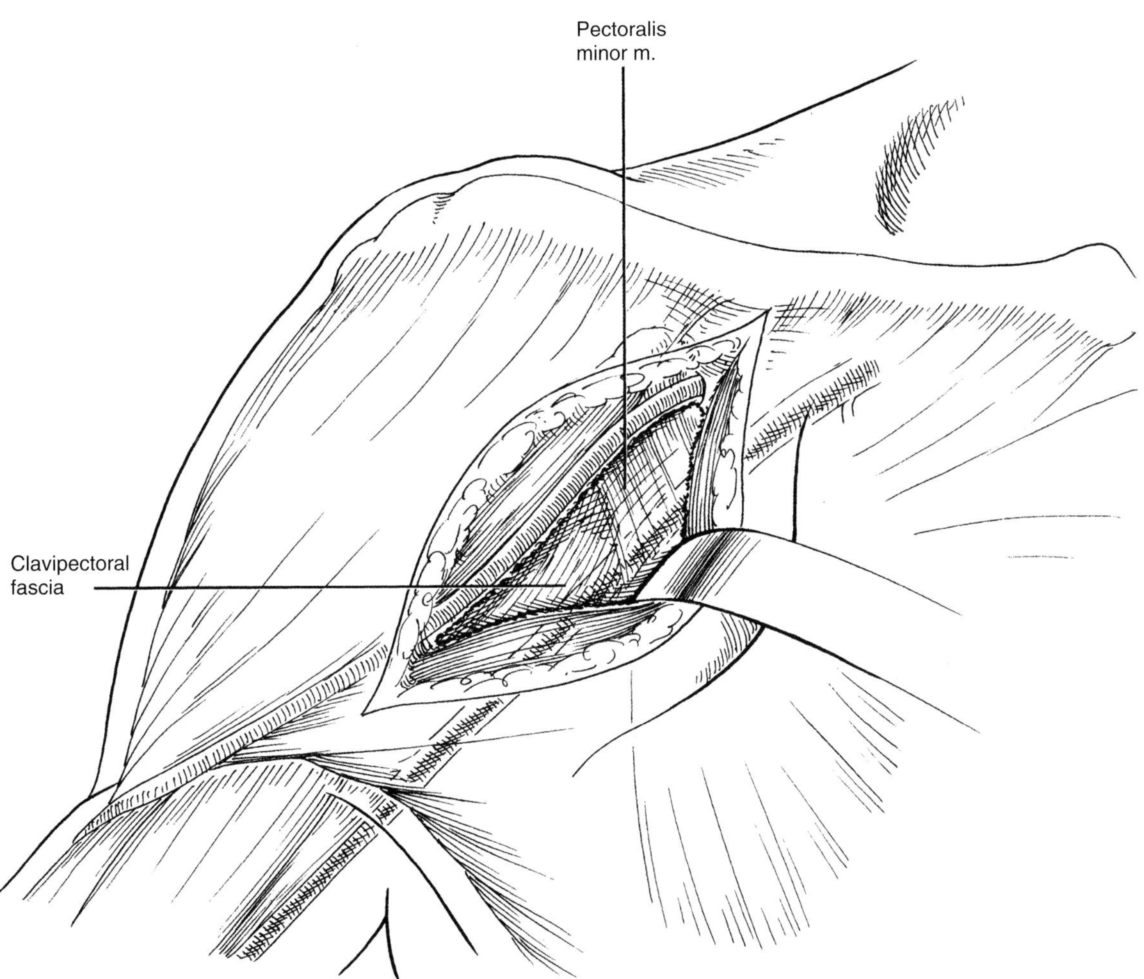

Fig. 5-19 Deep fascia is opened along the deltopectoral groove, and the pectoralis major muscle is retracted medially.

visible. The third part of the axillary artery is exposed by incising the clavipectoral fascia along the inferior border of the coracobrachialis muscle in the distal wound up to the coracoid process (Fig. 5-20). The neurovascular bundle is located in the areolar tissue beneath the clavipectoral fascia. The junction of the medial and lateral cords forming the median nerve is the most superficial structure within the axillary sheath. The third part of the axillary artery can be exposed by widely mobilizing the median nerve and retracting it cephalad. It is important not to mobilize more than a few centimeters of the cord junction to avoid undue nerve tension. The artery can be encircled with vascular tapes after careful isolation from the ulnar nerve and axillary vein near its medial border (Fig. 5-21).

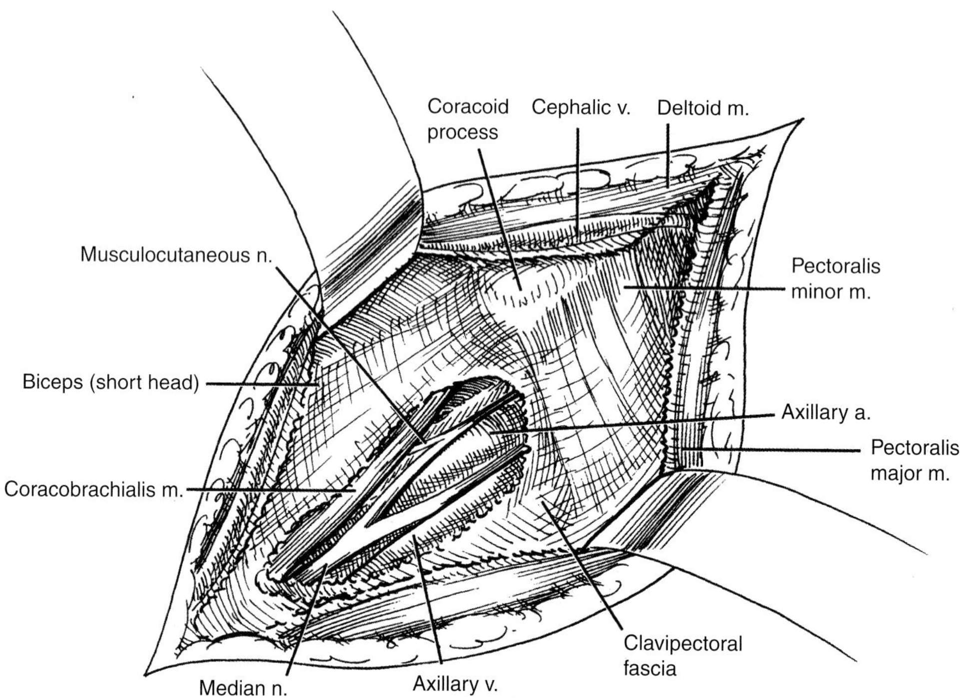

Fig. 5-20 To expose the third part of the axillary artery, the clavipectoral fascia is opened lateral to the pectoralis minor.

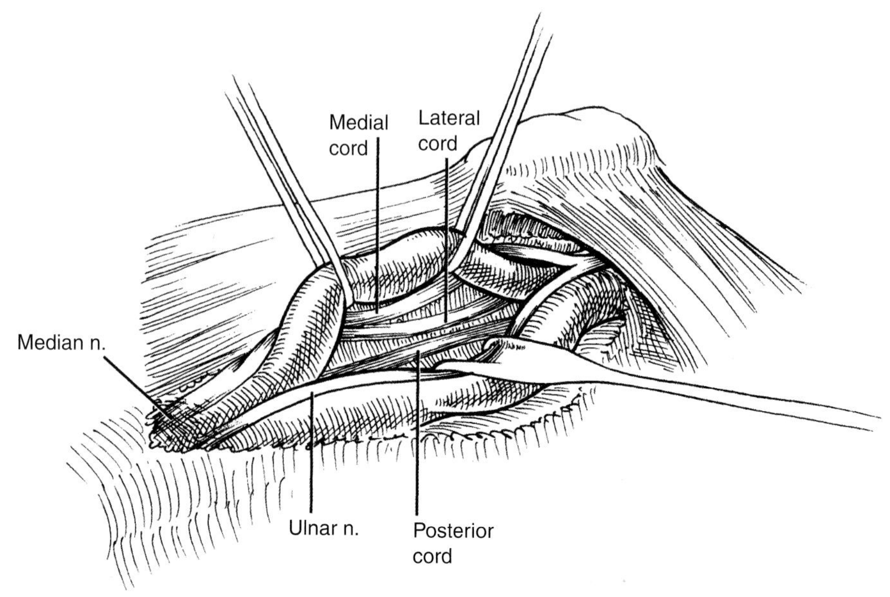

Fig. 5-21 The medial cord of the brachial plexus is reflected laterally, and the artery is mobilized.

The second part of the axillary artery is exposed by transecting the pectoralis minor muscle near the coracoid process (Fig. 5-22). Ligation and division of the thoracoacromial artery near its origin will help expose the boundaries of the pectoralis minor before muscle transection. The pectoral nerves should be identified and protected while the muscle is divided near the coracoid process.[1] The junction of the medial and lateral cords lies on the anterior surface of the axillary artery just distal to the lateral border of the pectoralis minor. The nerve loop connecting the pectoral nerves also crosses anterior to the axillary artery in this area and is prone to injury during dissection. The second part of the axillary artery is best isolated between the nerve loop and the cord junction. The lateral thoracic artery should be identified on the inferior surface of the axillary artery and ligated only if necessary to enhance exposure.

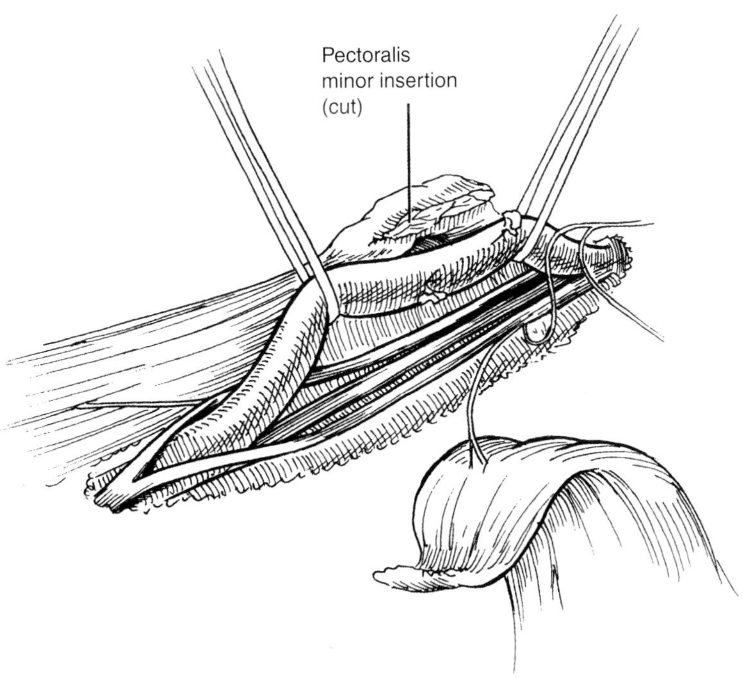

Fig. 5-22 The second part of the artery is exposed by dividing the pectoralis minor insertion.

The first part of the axillary artery is exposed in the wound proximal to the pectoralis minor muscle. Again, division of the thoracoacromial vessels allows increased exposure of the axillary artery in this segment. The clavipectoral fascia should be divided as proximally as possible, up to the level of the subclavius muscle (Fig. 5-23). The axillary sheath is found in the fatty areolar tissue beneath the clavipectoral fascia. The axillary artery lies just deep and slightly cephalad to the axillary vein. Mobilization and caudal retraction of the vein is required during dissection of the artery. As noted above, the artery is best encircled with vascular tapes and lifted into the wound above surrounding neurovascular structures before vascular clamps are applied.

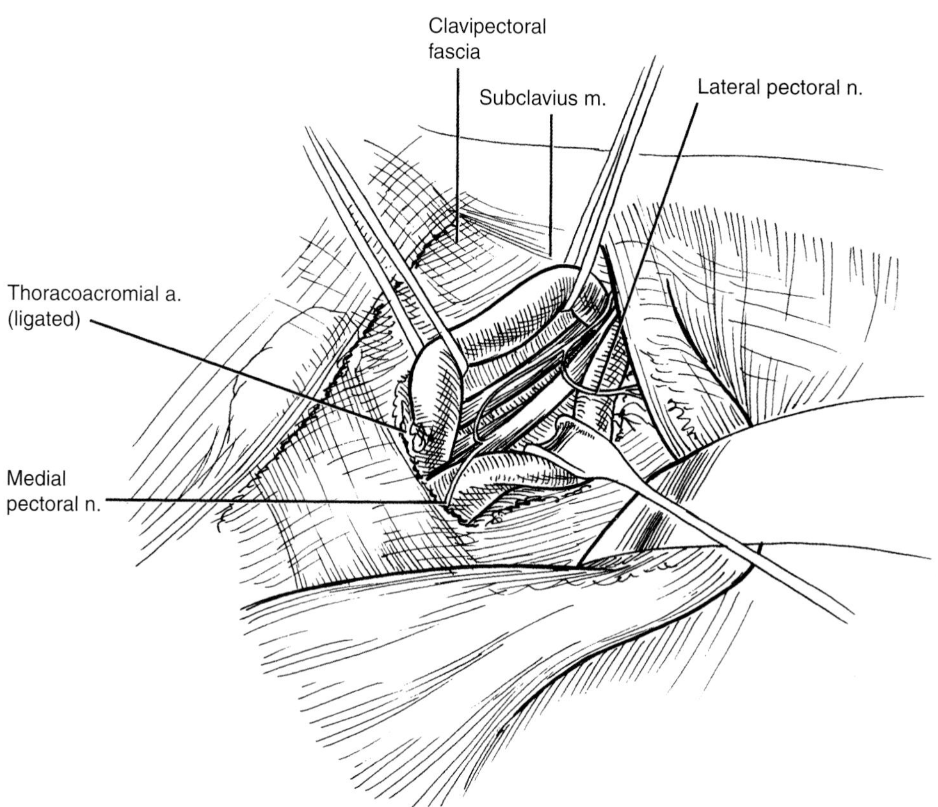

Fig. 5-23 The first part of the axillary artery is approached medial to the pectoralis minor.

References

1. Moosman DA. Anatomy of the pectoral nerves and their preservation in modified mastectomy. *Am J Surg.* 1980;139:883–886.
2. Porzionato A, Macchi V, Stecco C, et al. Surgical anatomy of the pectoral nerves and the pectoral musculature. *Clin Anat.* 2012; 25:559–575.
3. Martin D, Katz SG. Axillofemoral bypass for aortoiliac occlusive disease. *Am J Surg.* 2000;180:100–103.
4. Liedenbaum MH, Verdam FJ, Spelt D, et al. The outcome of the axillofemoral bypass: a retrospective analysis of 45 patients. *World J Surg.* 2009;33:2490–2496.
5. Passman MA, Taylor LM Jr, Moneta GL, et al. Comparison of axillofemoral and aortofemoral bypass for aortoiliac occlusive disease. *J Vasc Surg.* 1996;23:263–271.
6. Seeger JM, Pretus HA, Welborn MB, et al. Long-term outcome after treatment of aortic graft infection with staged extra-anatomic bypass grafting and aortic graft removal. *J Vasc Surg.* 2000;32:451–461.
7. Hyre CE, Cikrit DF, Lalka SG, et al. Aggressive management of thoracic injuries of the thoracic outlet. *J Vasc Surg.* 1998;27:880–884.
8. Weaver FA, Papanicolaou G, Yellin AE. Difficult peripheral vascular injuries. *Surg Clin North Am.* 1996;76:843–859.
9. Shaw AD, Milne AA, Christie J. Vascular trauma of the upper limb and associated nerve injuries. *Injury.* 1995;26:515–518.
10. Aksoy M, Tunca F, Yanar H, et al. Traumatic injuries to the subclavian and axillary arteries: a 13-year review. *Surg Today.* 2005;35:561–565.
11. Shalhub S, Starnes BW, Hatsukami TS, et al. Repair of blunt thoracic outlet arterial injuries: an evolution from open to endovascular approach. *J Trauma.* 2011;71:E114–E121.
12. Du Toit DF, Lambrechts AV, Stark H, et al. Long-term results of stent graft treatment of subclavian artery injuries: management of choice for stable patients? *J Vasc Surg.* 2008;47:739–743.
13. Danetz JS, Cassano AD, Stoner MC, et al. Feasibility of endovascular repair in penetrating axillosubclavian injuries: a retrospective review. *J Vasc Surg.* 2005;41:246–254.
14. Taylor LM Jr, Park TC, Edwards JM, et al. Acute disruption of polytetrafluoroethylene grafts adjacent to axillary artery anastomoses: a complication of axillofemoral grafting. *J Vasc Surg.* 1994;20:520–528.
15. Landry GJ, Moneta GL, Taylor LM Jr, et al. Axillofemoral bypass. *Ann Vasc Surg.* 2000;14:296–305.
16. Kitowski NJ, Gundersen SB. Traumatic fracture of polytetrafluoroethylene axillofemoral bypass graft. *Vasc Endovasc Surg.* 2010;44:131–133.
17. Kempczinski R, Penn I. Upper extremity complications of axillofemoral grafts. *Am J Surg.* 1978;136:209–211.
18. McKinley AG, Carrim AT, Robbs JV. Management of proximal axillary and subclavian artery injuries. *Br J Surg.* 2000;87:79–85.

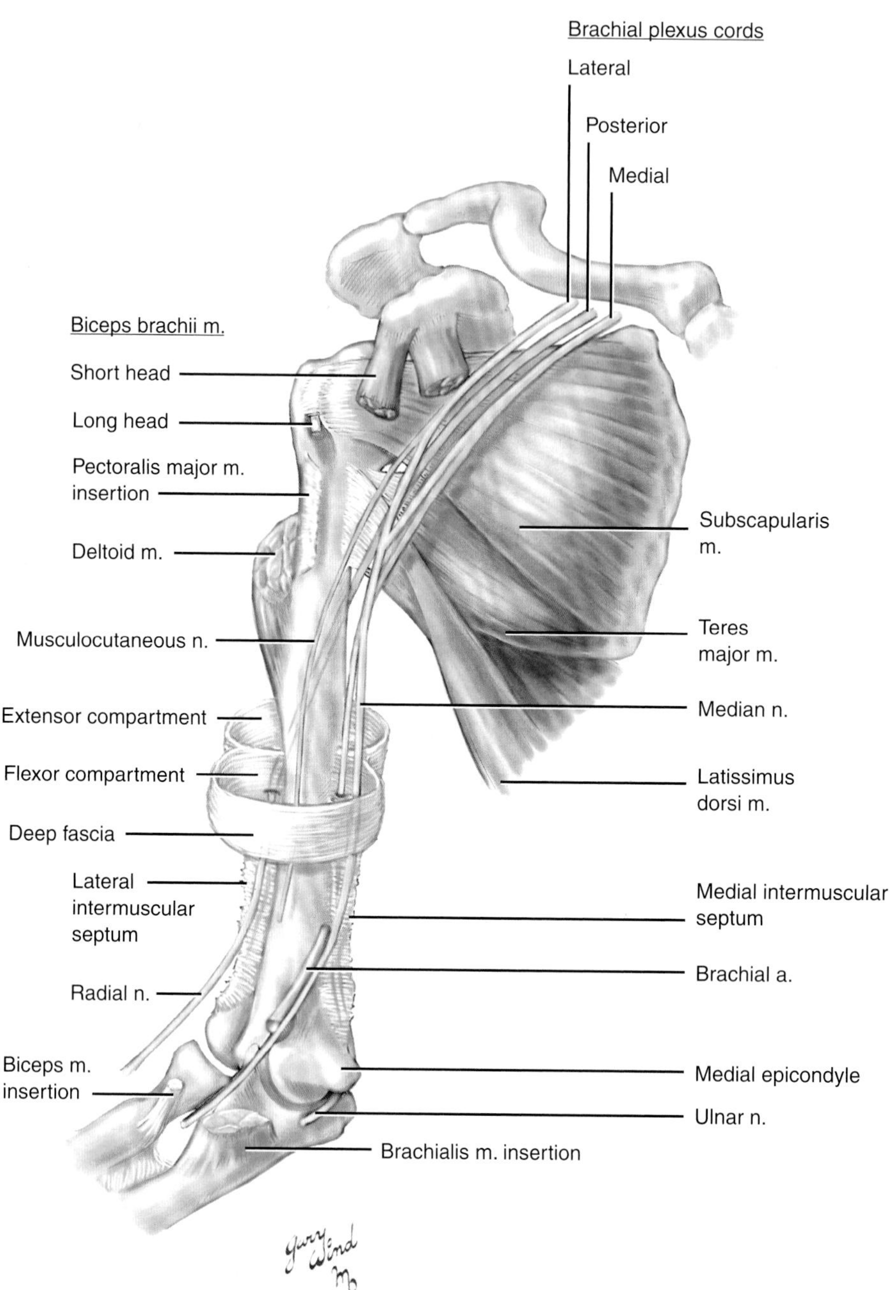

Fig. 6-1 The deep fascia and supracondylar septa of the arm contain the flexor muscles anteriorly and the triceps complex posteriorly. The brachial artery and median nerve are ensheathed in the anterior compartment, while the radial and ulnar nerves switch compartments through the intermuscular septa in the distal arm.

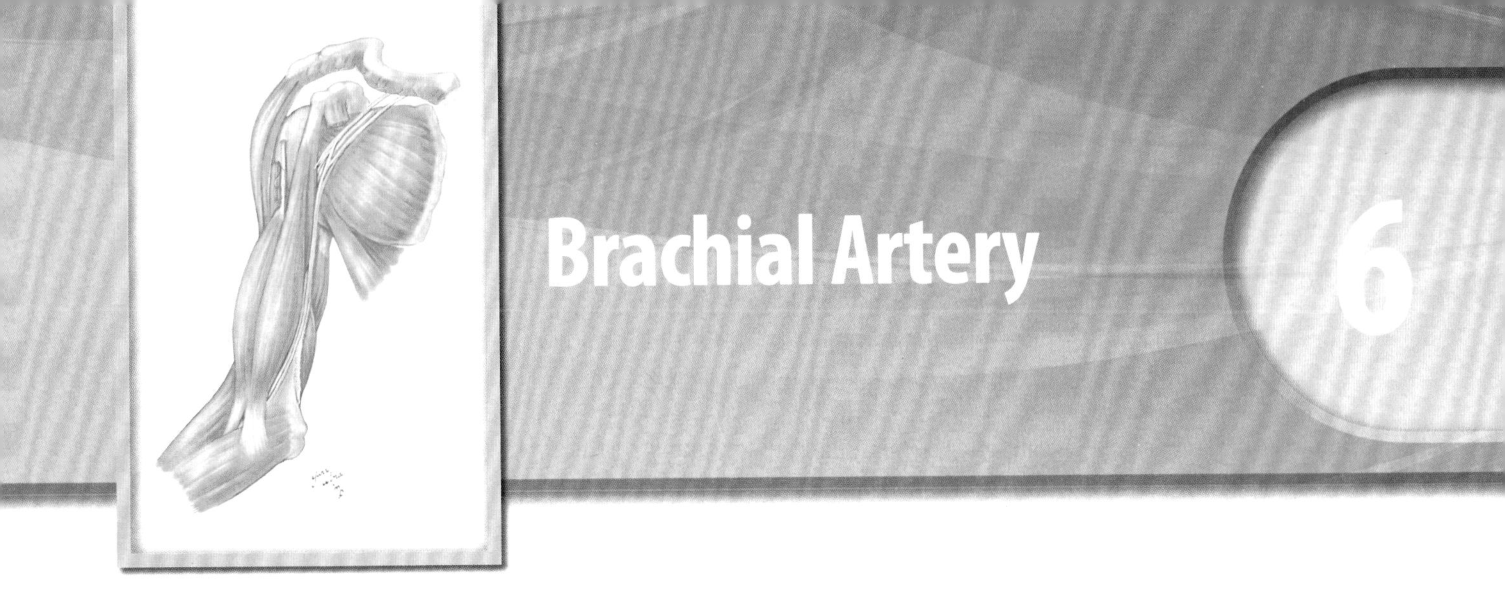

Brachial Artery

6

Surgical Anatomy of the Brachium

Unlike the leg, the brachium receives its major nerve and vessel trunks in a dominant single bundle. The muscles of the brachium are grouped into clearly defined flexor and extensor groups like the homologous structures of the leg, but the septae and fascial coverings are less robust. The neurovascular trunks should be considered in the context of the surrounding muscles and fasciae.

Brachial Fascia

The anterior flexor compartment and posterior extensor compartment of the arm are enclosed by a thin, firm sheath of deep fascia (Fig. 6-1). The compartments are separated by medial and lateral intermuscular septae originating from the supracondylar ridges of the distal humerus. The encircling fascia attaches to these partitions and to the olecranon and humeral epicondyles distally. The neurovascular bundle contained within the axillary sheath continues into the arm deep to the brachial fascia. The radial nerve and profunda brachii artery diverge posteriorly at the distal border of the latissimus tendon while the median, ulnar, and two medial cutaneous nerves accompany the brachial artery into the confined space of the well-defined neurovascular sheath of the brachium. This brachial sheath is subcutaneous in the midbrachium and is easily entered just anterior to the medial intermuscular septum.

Nerves of the Arm

At the lateral edge of the latissimus tendon, three major nerve trunks surround the brachial artery. The median nerve lies anterior, the ulnar nerve medial, and the radial nerve posterior to the vessel. The musculocutaneous nerve branches from the lateral cord of the brachial plexus in the midaxilla and follows an independent course through the coracobrachialis to the other brachial flexors.

The median nerve continues with the brachial artery through the length of the brachium and crosses the artery diagonally from a relatively lateral to a medial position. The ulnar nerve penetrates the medial intermuscular septum in midbrachium and continues posterior to that septum to reach the groove behind the medial epicondyle of the humerus. The radial nerve turns posteriorly at the caudal border of the latissimus tendon and follows a spiral course behind the humerus between the origins of the lateral and medial heads of the triceps muscle. In the midbrachium, the radial nerve penetrates the lateral intermuscular septum to reach the forearm extensor compartment. The cutaneous branches emanating from these major trunks will not be described here but should be reviewed in terms of incision placement and the potential for confusion with major nerves.

Brachial Vessels

Each major nerve of the arm is accompanied by an artery. As noted above, the brachial artery runs with the median nerve through the medial side of the anterior compartment (Fig. 6-2). Proximally, the profunda branch of the brachial artery joins the radial nerve and follows it through the lateral intermuscular septum, at which point it is called the radial collateral artery. The superior ulnar collateral artery arises from the midpoint of the brachial artery and accompanies the ulnar nerve through the medial intermuscular septum. A second ulnar collateral branch penetrates the septum more distally. In addition to muscular branches, the brachial artery sends a major nutrient vessel to the middle of the humeral shaft.

The brachial artery is usually accompanied by two veins. The basilic vein runs in a subcutaneous position from the antecubital fossa to the medial aspect of the midbrachium where it penetrates the deep fascia to join one of the brachial veins. The brachial veins make numerous deep and superficial anastomoses before uniting at the level of the teres major to form the axillary vein. The cephalic vein is superficial along its entire course to the deltopectoral groove. The vein accompanying the deep brachial artery empties into the transition between brachial veins and the axillary vein.

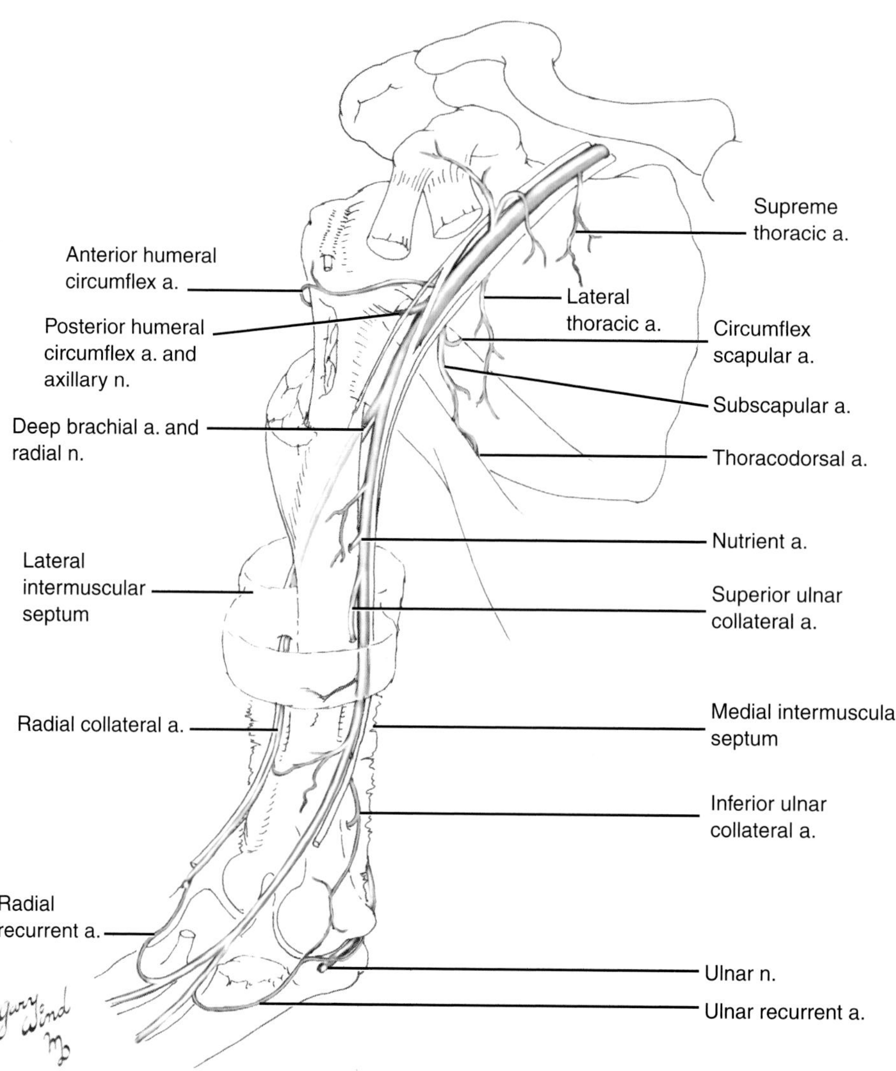

Fig. 6-2 The branches of the brachial artery accompany the nerve trunks and make collateral connections around the shoulder and elbow.

Anterior Brachial Muscles

Proximally, the humerus is attached to the pectoral girdle and chest wall by several powerful muscles that act around the shoulder joint (Fig. 6-3). Distally, the broad brachialis is the dominant anterior brachial muscle attached to the humerus. The small coracobrachialis muscle originates in common with the short head of the biceps brachii and is penetrated by the musculocutaneous nerve. The nerve then lies between the brachialis and biceps, supplying both.

The proximal brachial artery and its associated nerves first lie posterior to the coracobrachialis muscle close to the humeral shaft and then diagonally cross the medial part of the brachialis belly. The radial nerve emerges lateral to the distal belly of the brachialis.

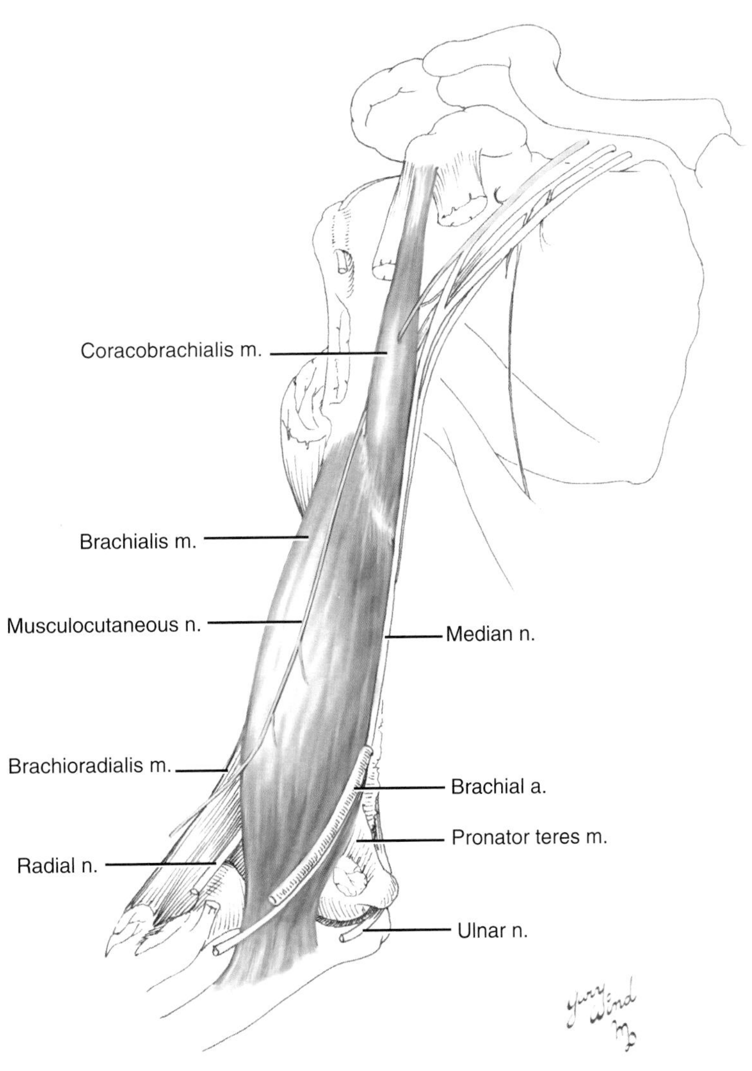

Fig. 6-3 The coracobrachialis and brachialis muscles, the deep muscles of the brachium, are supplied by the musculocutaneous nerve, which penetrates the former and then runs between the brachialis and biceps.

The biceps brachii muscle covers the length of the humerus anteriorly (Fig. 6-4). Proximally, the heads of the biceps are restrained by the tendon of the pectoralis major muscle crossing to insert into the lateral lip of the bicipital groove of the humerus. Distally, the biceps tapers to a strong tendon inserting on the bicipital tuberosity of the radius. From the distal muscle, a broad secondary tendinous expansion runs medially to attach to the deep fascia of the forearm flexors. This band bridges over the brachial artery and median nerve.

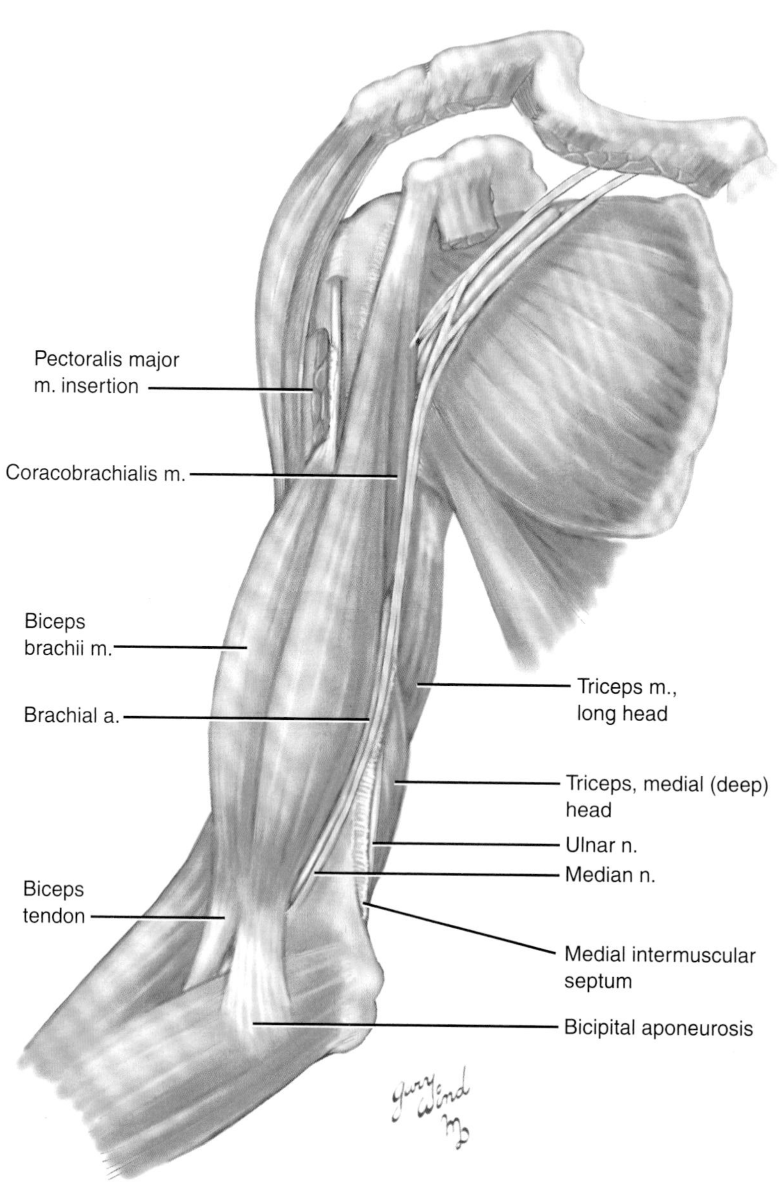

Fig. 6-4 The biceps brachii crosses both the shoulder and elbow joints and is bordered medially by the brachial artery and median nerve.

Posterior Brachium

The back of the arm is dominated by the mass of the triceps muscle (Fig. 6-5). The long head originates from the infraglenoid tuberosity of the scapula. The lateral and medial heads originate broadly from the posterior humerus. Running diagonally between these two heads in the spiral groove of the humerus are the deep brachial artery and the radial nerve. The deep brachial artery anastomoses with the posterior humeral circumflex artery. Before the artery and nerve penetrate the lateral intermuscular septum at the distal end of the spiral groove, the artery gives off a posterior descending branch that anastomoses with ascending collateral vessels at the elbow.

After penetrating the medial intermuscular septum, the ulnar nerve runs medial to the medial

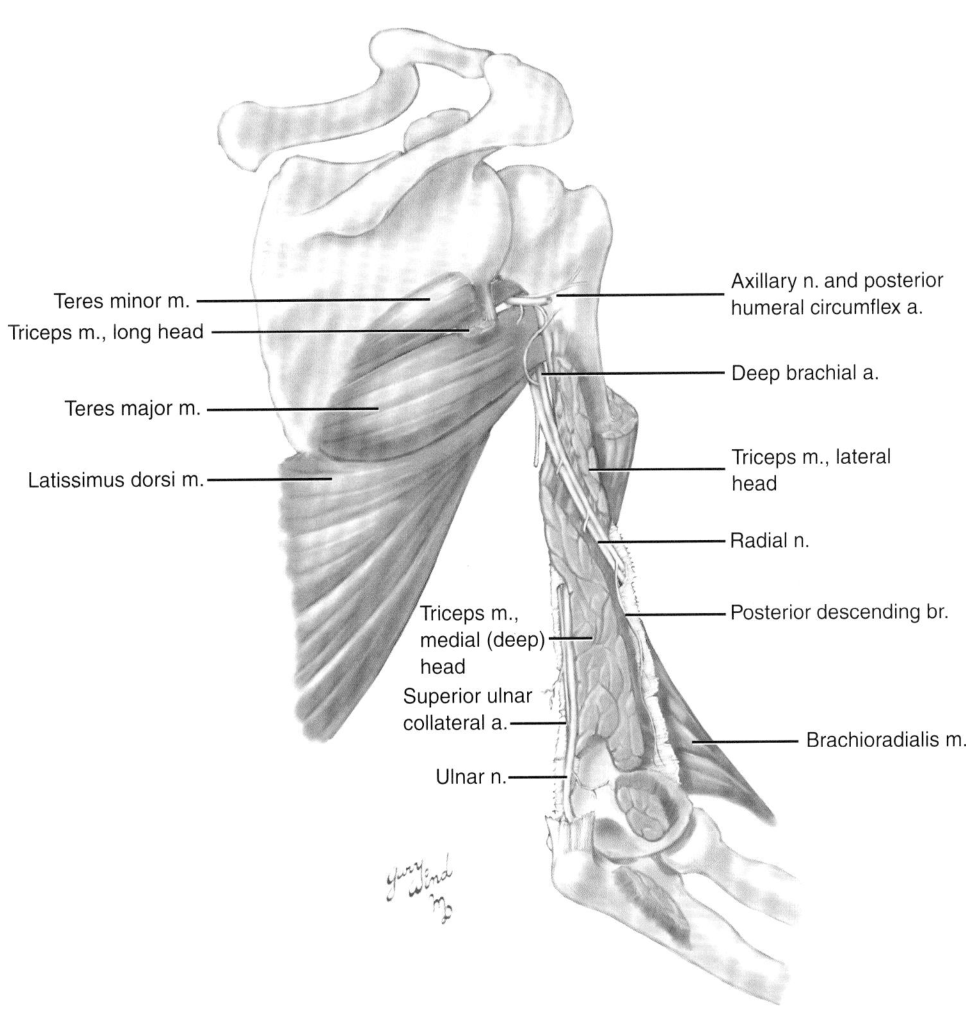

Fig. 6-5 The lateral and medial (or deep) heads of the triceps muscle originate from the humerus, leaving a spiral cleft between them which accommodates the deep brachial artery and radial nerve.

head of the triceps accompanied by the superior and inferior ulnar collateral branches of the brachial artery.

The three heads of the triceps muscle merge over the distal humerus and insert on the olecranon of the ulna by a broad, strong tendon (Fig. 6-6).

Topography

When the arm is abducted and extended, the neurovascular bundle is visible as a cord-like structure between the flexor and extensor compartments (Fig. 6-7). Note the mass of muscles forming a hood over the proximal humerus.

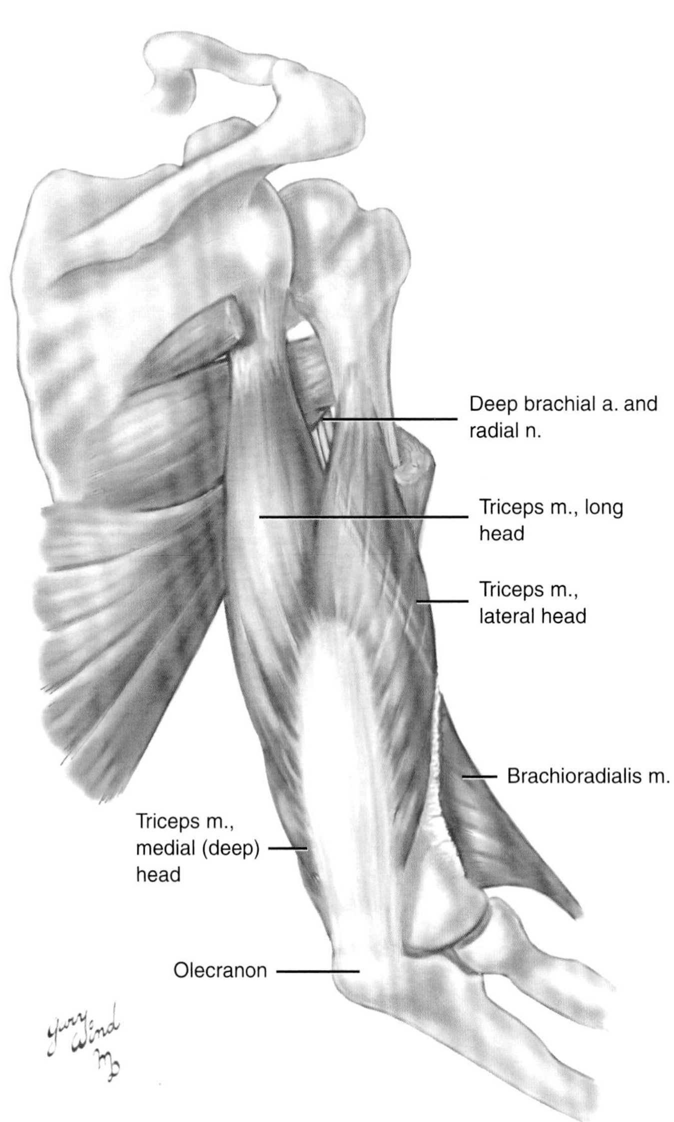

Fig. 6-6 The triceps muscle covers the posterior brachium.

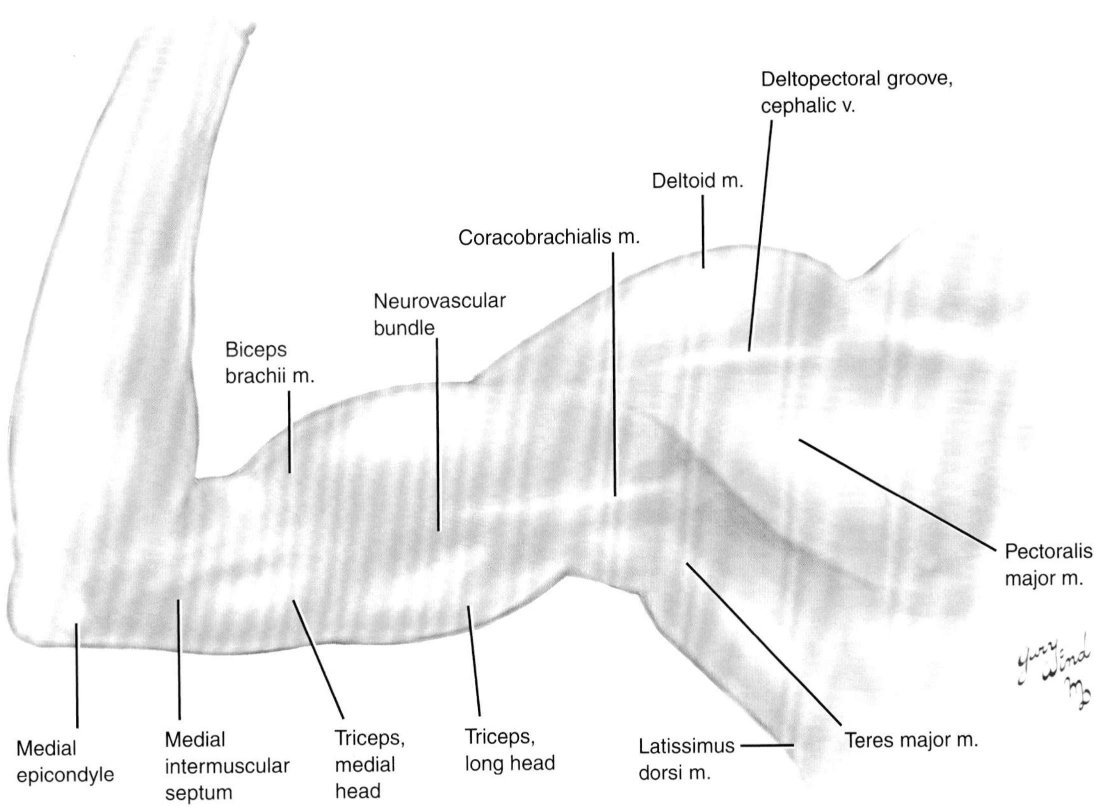

Fig. 6-7 The coracobrachialis muscle and adjacent neurovascular bundle form a cord-like ridge between biceps and triceps. The cephalic vein marks the deltopectoral groove.

Laterally, the course of the radial nerve is covered by the lateral head of the triceps (Fig. 6-8). The lateral intermuscular septum is evidenced by a ridge running proximally from the lateral epicondyle. The depression between the deltoid and the long head of triceps marks the beginning of the course of the radial nerve and deep brachial artery. The distal insertion of the deltoid and the proximal origin of the brachioradialis divide the humeral shaft into thirds. The penetration of the radial nerve through the lateral intermuscular septum occurs just distal to the start of the brachioradialis.

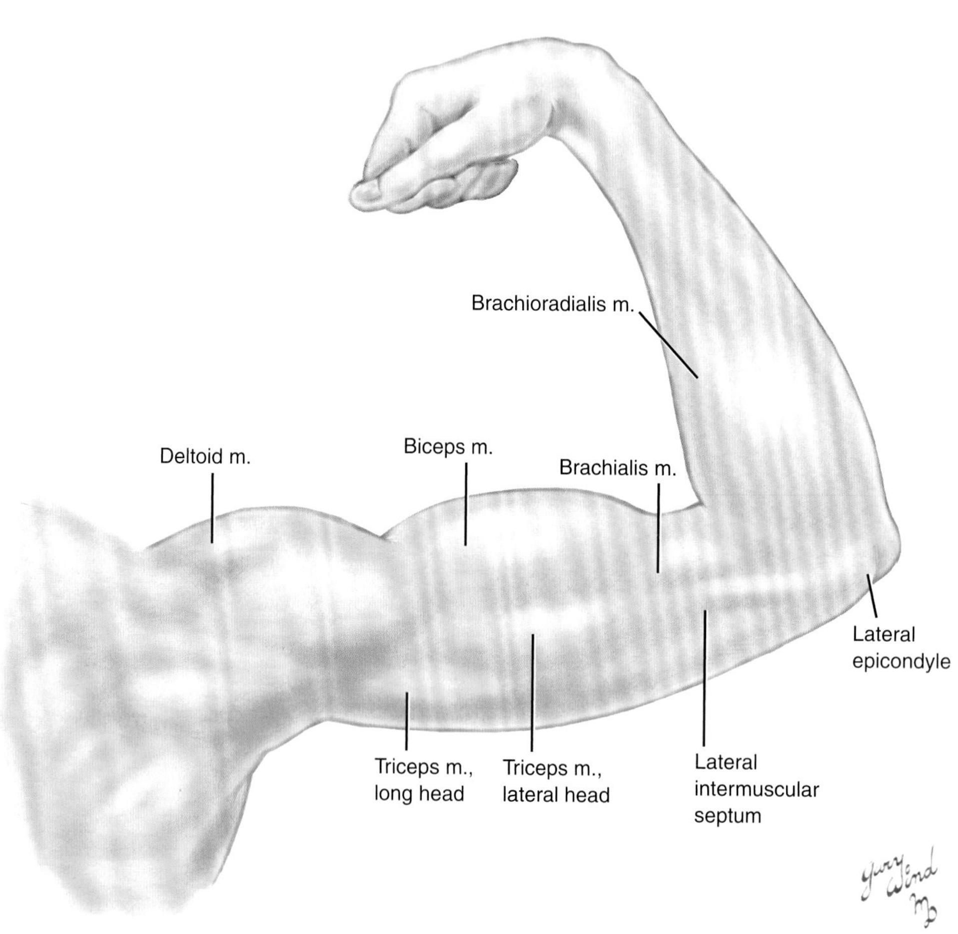

Fig. 6-8 The dimple between the deltoid and long head of the triceps marks the location of the deep brachial artery and radial nerve proximally.

Exposure of the Brachial Artery

The superficial location of the brachial artery and its proximity to the humerus makes it vulnerable to injury. Brachial artery trauma accounts for most vascular injuries of the upper extremity.[1–3] The vast majority of brachial injuries are associated with penetrating trauma,[1] but blunt injuries have been reported after posterior elbow dislocation and supracondylar fractures in children.[4,5] In supracondylar fractures, the direction of displacement determines the structures at risk: medial displacement of the distal fragment can result in injury to the radial nerve, while lateral displacement risks injury to the median nerve and brachial artery[4] (Fig. 6-2). Regardless of the mechanism of injury, the close proximity of major nerve structures commonly leads to permanent dysfunction due to associated trauma.[2,3]

The brachial artery is quite simple to expose. The following discussion concerns isolation of the brachial artery proximal to the antecubital fossa; exposure of the brachial artery at its bifurcation will be discussed in Chapter 7.

The patient is placed supine near the edge of the operating table with the arm abducted 90° and supported on an armboard. Shoulder hyperextension should be avoided to prevent stretch injury to the brachial plexus. The axilla, brachium, and hand are prepped and draped. The hand and forearm are covered with a stockinette to allow repositioning during the operation and to allow palpation of the radial pulse (Fig. 6-9).

A 5- to 8-cm longitudinal incision is made in the groove between the biceps and triceps muscles on the medial aspect of the arm. The incision can be extended as needed to increase proximal or distal exposure. In the lower half of the arm, care should be taken to prevent injury to the basilic vein as the incision is deepened through subcutaneous tissue. The vein perforates the deep fascia just distal to the middle of the arm and courses near the brachial vessels in the deep tissues proximal to this point. It is most convenient to retract the basilic vein into the posterior wound, ligating crossing vein branches as needed.

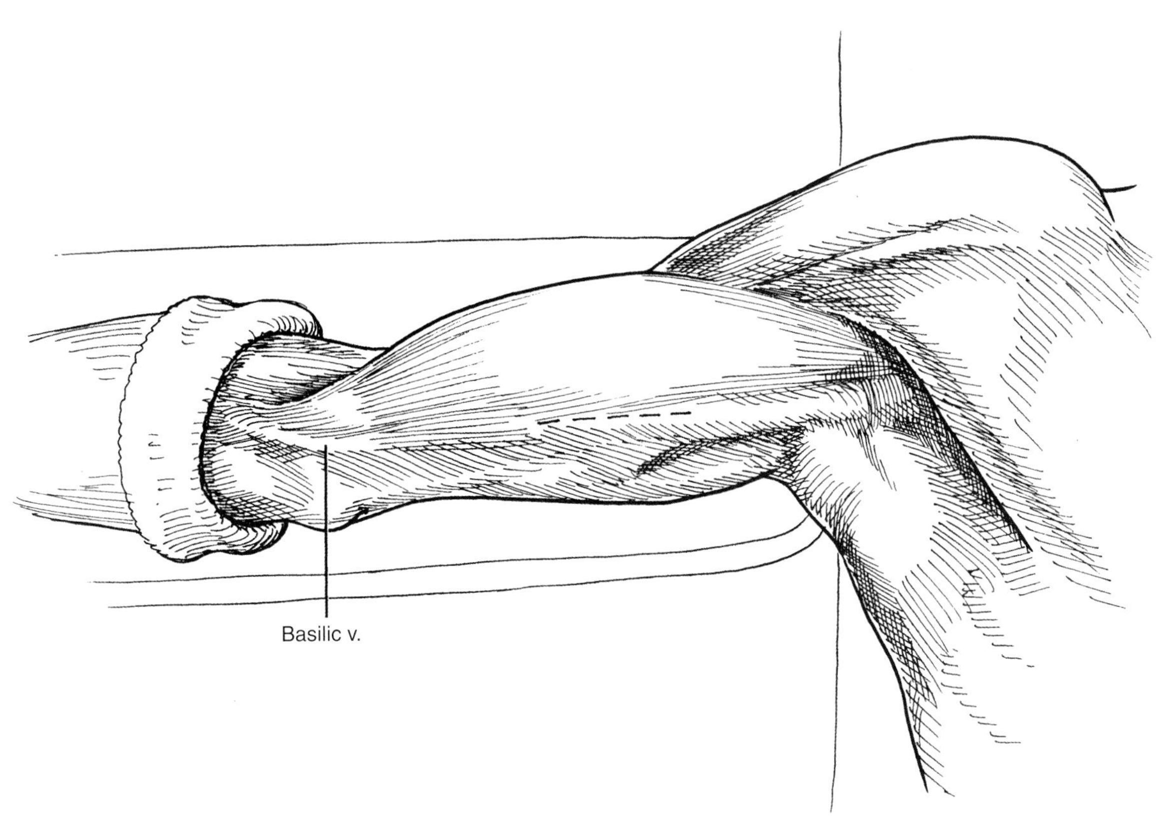

Fig. 6-9 To approach the brachial artery, the arm is abducted 90°.

The neurovascular bundle is exposed by incising the deep fascia at the medial border of the biceps muscle, which is retracted anteriorly (Fig. 6-10). The basilic vein should be identified coursing medial to the brachial sheath. After carefully retracting the vein into the posterior wound, the brachial sheath is opened. The median nerve is the most superficial structure encountered upon entering the brachial sheath. The nerve should be widely mobilized and gently retracted into the anterior

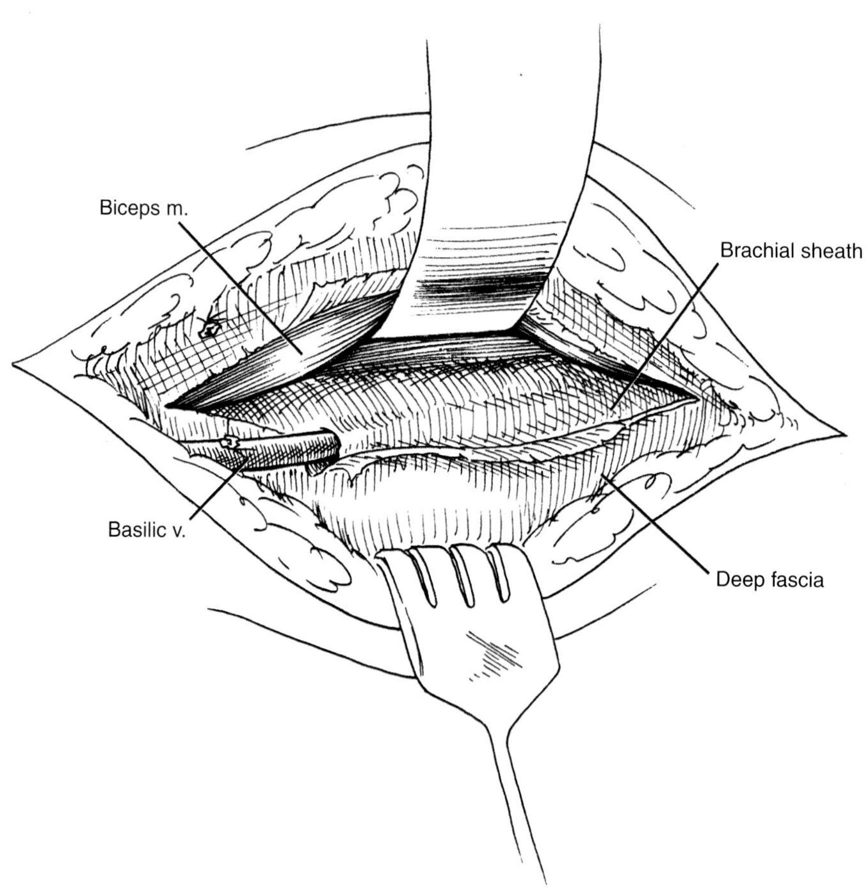

Fig. 6-10 The deep fascia at the medial border of the biceps muscle is incised, exposing the neurovascular bundle enclosed in its fascial sheath. The basilic vein penetrating the deep fascia is preserved.

wound (Fig. 6-11). The artery lies just deep to the median nerve, surrounded by two brachial veins and flanked posteriorly by the ulnar nerve. Isolation of the artery requires ligation of interconnecting vein branches that cross the artery's medial surface. In the proximal arm, the deep brachial artery should be identified and protected on the posteromedial surface of the brachial artery just distal to the lateral border of the teres major muscle. Two other branches, the superior and inferior ulnar collateral arteries, may require control during brachial artery isolation in the mid- and distal arm, respectively.

In some patients, two arteries may be seen running in parallel from the upper arm to the antecubital space. This variation is due to high bifurcation of the brachial artery, which occurs most commonly in the upper third of the arm.[6] The two arteries occupy the usual position of the brachial artery within the neurovascular bundle and continue in the forearm as the radial and ulnar arteries (see Fig. 19-7).

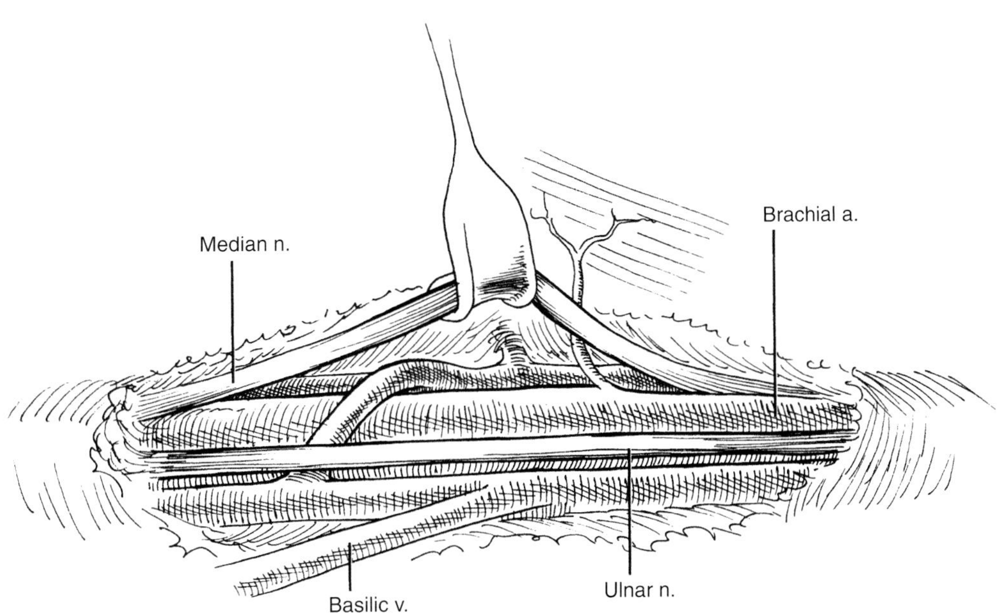

Fig. 6-11 The vessels and nerves are exposed, the median nerve is retracted gently, and vein branches are divided, allowing the artery to be mobilized.

References

1. Franz RW, Goodwin RB, Hartman JF, et al. Management of upper extremity arterial injuries at an urban level I trauma center. *Ann Vasc Surg.* 2009;23:8–16.
2. Stone WM, Fowl RJ, Money SR. Upper extremity trauma: current trends in management. *J Cardiovasc Surg.* 2007;48:551–555.
3. Topel I, Pfister K, Moser A, et al. Clinical outcome and quality of life after upper extremity arterial trauma. *Ann Vasc Surg.* 2009;23:317–323.
4. Brahmamdam P, Plummer M, Modrall JG, et al. Hand ischemia associated with elbow trauma in children. *J Vasc Surg.* 2011;54:773–778.
5. Korompilias AV, Lykissas MG, Mitsionis GI, et al. Treatment of pink pulseless hand following supracondylar fracture of the humerus in children. *Int Orthop.* 2009;33:237–241.
6. Bergman RA, Thompson SA, Afifi AK. *Catalogue of Human Variation.* Baltimore, MD: Urban & Schwarzenberg;1984:108–114.

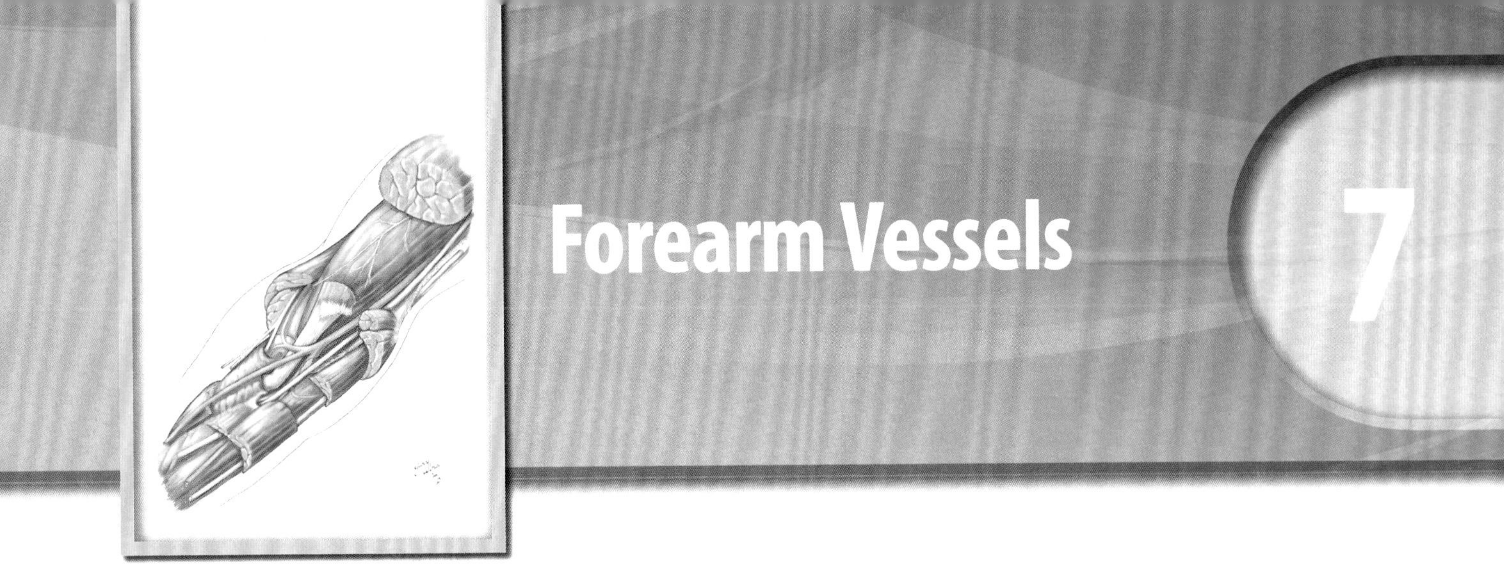

Forearm Vessels

Surgical Anatomy of the Forearm

The major nerves and arteries of the forearm run parallel with the two major muscle groups and lie between their layers as they converge toward the wrist. The axial rotation that uniquely characterizes the forearm is associated with a spiral disposition of the flexor/pronator muscle group and extensor/supinator muscle group from medial to volar and from lateral to dorsal, respectively. Safe surgical approaches to the arteries require a good three-dimensional appreciation of the relationships between vessels, nerves, and muscles, particularly in the area of the cubital fossa.

Superficial Veins and Nerves

The superficial veins of the distal forearm are highly variable, but as they converge toward the antecubital space they assume a more predictable pattern (Fig. 7-1). The most constant vein in the distal forearm is the cephalic, which starts along the lateral prominence of the radius. Before continuing up the arm along the lateral side of the biceps, it divides in front of the biceps tendon. There it sends a major tributary, the median cubital vein, diagonally across the biceps tendon to join the basilic vein. The basilic vein is formed from the veins draining the medial forearm and penetrates the deep fascia on the medial side of the brachium. The basilic vein is separated from the underlying brachial artery and median nerve by the biceps tendon in the antecubital fossa and by the deep fascia in the distal brachium.

Two superficial nerves run the length of the volar forearm and provide cutaneous sensation for two-thirds of its circumference. The medial antebrachial cutaneous nerve originates from the medial cord of the brachial plexus and accompanies the brachial artery to the midbrachium. There it exits the deep fascia through the same opening

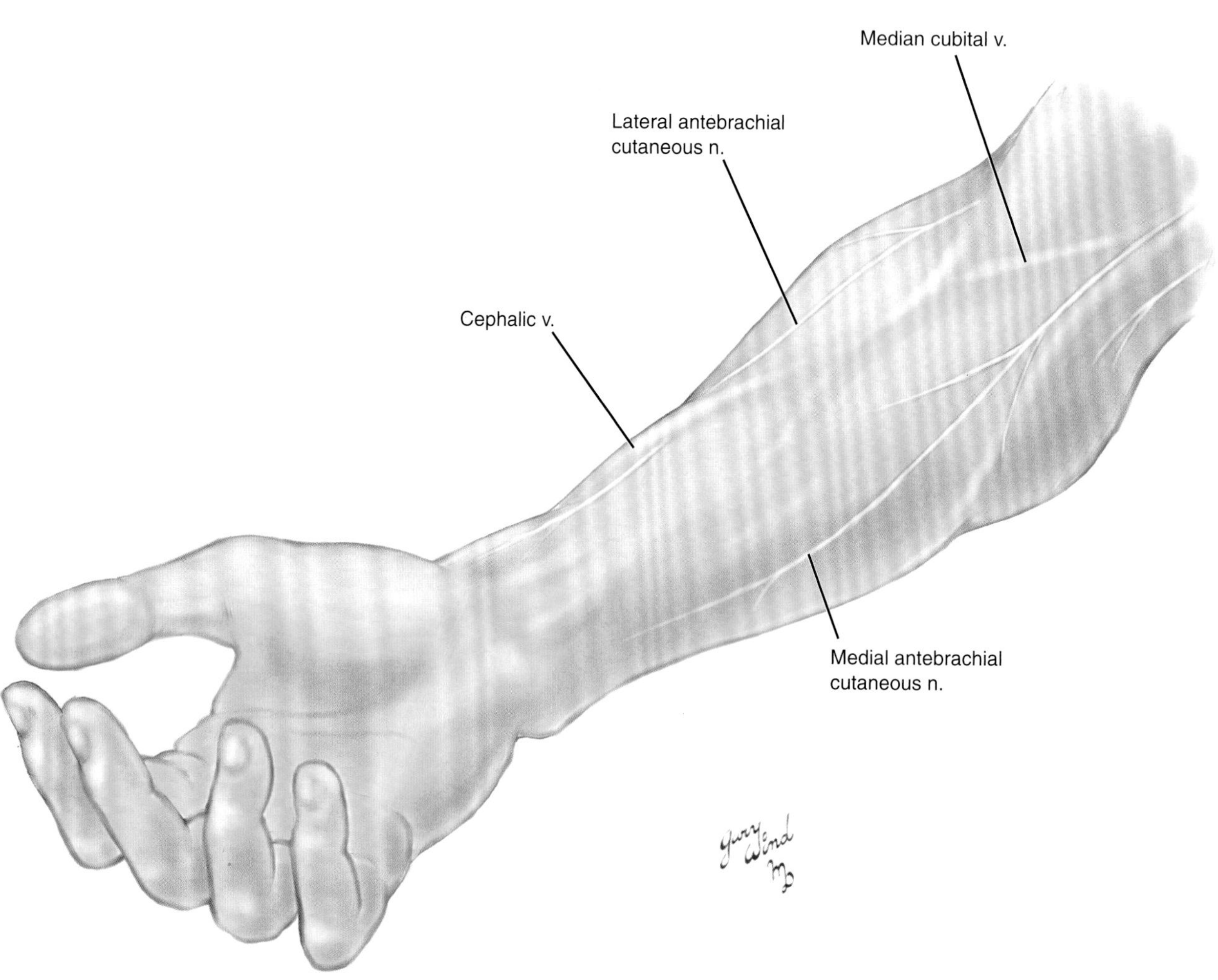

Fig. 7-1 The superficial veins and nerves of the volar forearm are depicted. The axially oriented medial and lateral antebrachial cutaneous nerves provide sensation for two-thirds of the forearm circumference.

traversed by the basilic vein and travels down the forearm toward the ulnar side. The lateral antebrachial cutaneous nerve is a continuation of the musculocutaneous nerve which innervated the biceps. This nerve emerges lateral to the biceps tendon, divides into two branches, and runs over the brachioradialis down the radial side of the forearm in the subcutaneous plane. Both of these nerves are subject to injury during venipuncture of the antecubital veins.

The remaining strip of extensor forearm is innervated by the posterior antebrachial cutaneous nerve (Fig. 7-2). This nerve arises from the radial nerve in the spiral groove and becomes subcutaneous at the lateral border of the triceps tendon. It passes behind the lateral epicondyle to reach the dorsal forearm.

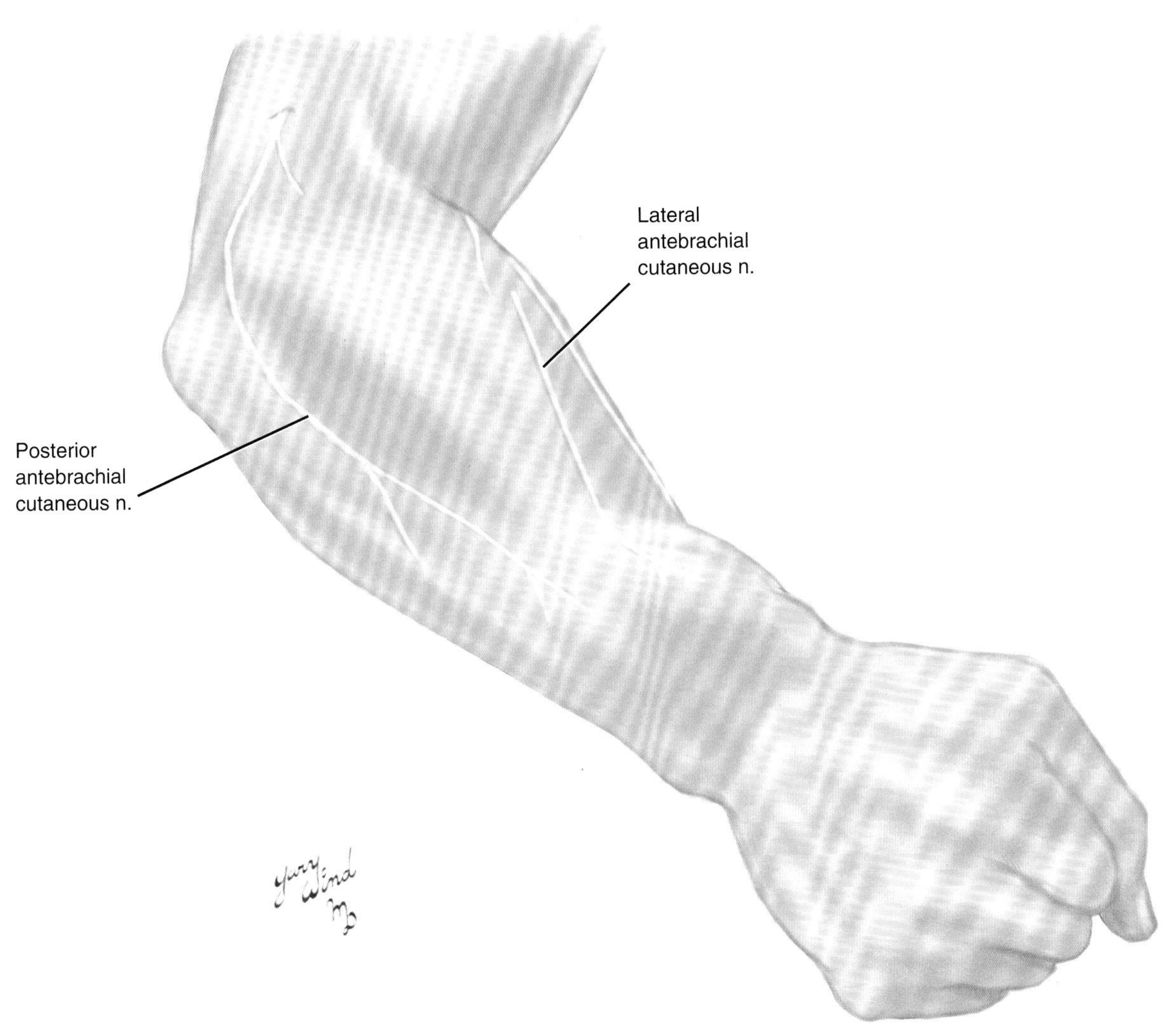

Fig. 7-2 The posterior antebrachial cutaneous branch of the radial nerve supplies the remaining extensor surface of the forearm.

Bony Anatomy and Muscle Overview

By virtue of its proximal and distal articulations, the radius is capable of virtually 180° rotation at its distal end (Fig. 7-3). Both the intrinsic supinator and pronators between radius and ulna and the major muscle groups effect this dramatic motion. The two-headed pronator teres acts proximally, and the flat pronator quadratus acts distally between the radius and ulna. The supinator wraps around the proximal radius from its origin on the posterior ulna.

Two large muscle groups, each arising from an epicondyle-based common tendon, dominate the forearm. The flexor/pronator group arises from the medial epicondyle of the humerus and fans out across the volar forearm. Beneath this group, a deep layer of flexor muscles arises from the radius, ulna, and interosseous membrane. The extensor/supinator muscle complex arises from the lateral epicondyle of the humerus and extends toward the dorsum of the wrist. It, too, overlies a deeper layer. Two additional muscles, the brachioradialis and extensor carpi radialis longus, are anatomically transitional between these two groups but are properly associated with the extensor group by virtue of their radial nerve innervation. Between the

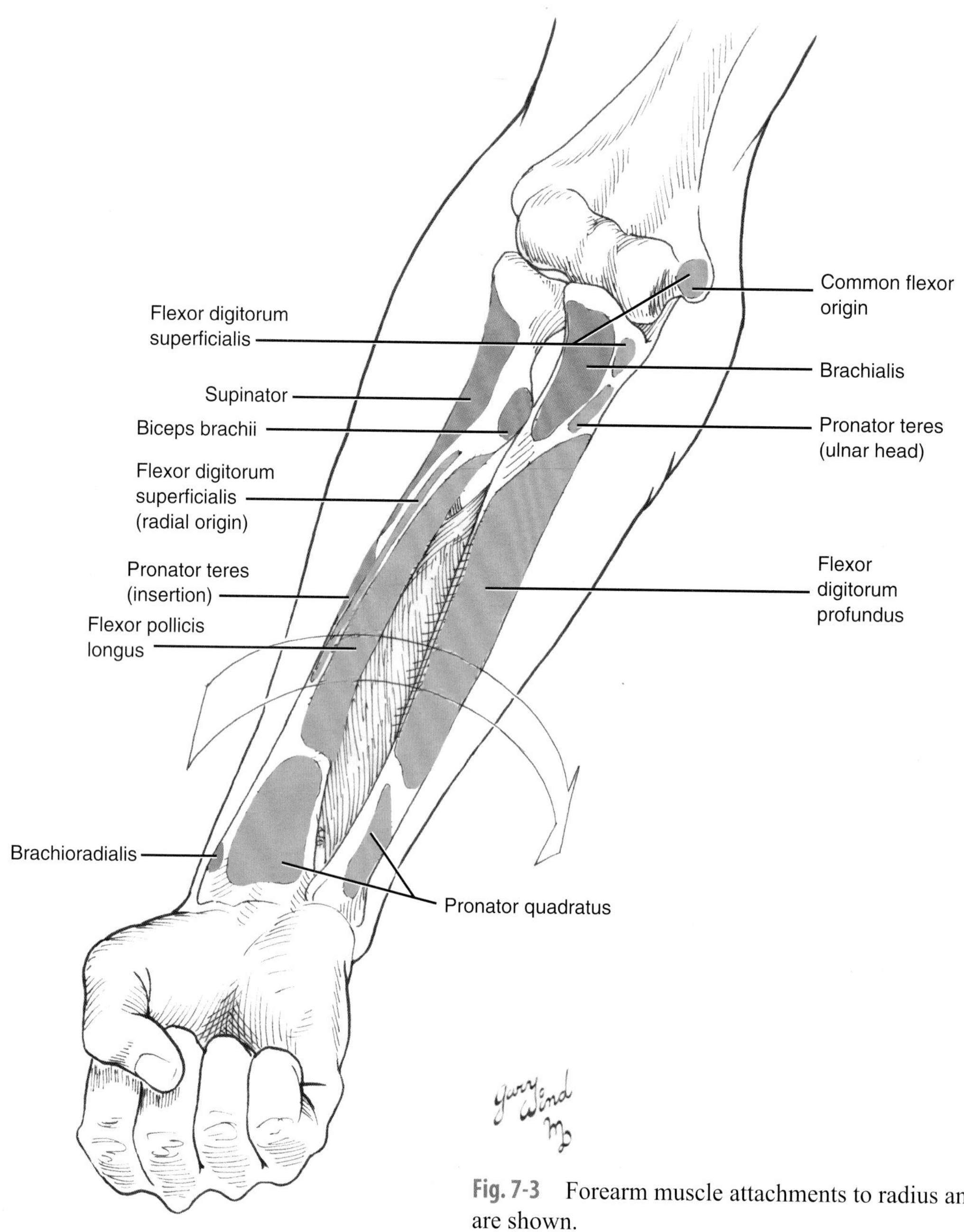

Fig. 7-3 Forearm muscle attachments to radius and ulna are shown.

brachioradialis and flexor muscles proximally is the deep cubital fossa.

The forearm is wrapped in a firm layer of deep fascia continuous with the fascia of the brachium. This is thickened around the biceps tendon, at the epicondyles, and at the wrist where it forms the dorsal and volar retinacula. In addition, there are septa from the deep fascia to the radius and ulna. This compartmentalization is completed by the dense interosseous membrane.

The Flexors

In the floor of the cubital fossa, the broad brachialis muscle converges to insert onto the proximal ulna (Fig. 7-4). The biceps tendon passes over the brachialis to reach the radial tuberosity which is virtually in the midline. A fascial expansion of the biceps tendon, the bicipital aponeurosis, extends down the medial forearm to spread over the proximal flexor muscles.

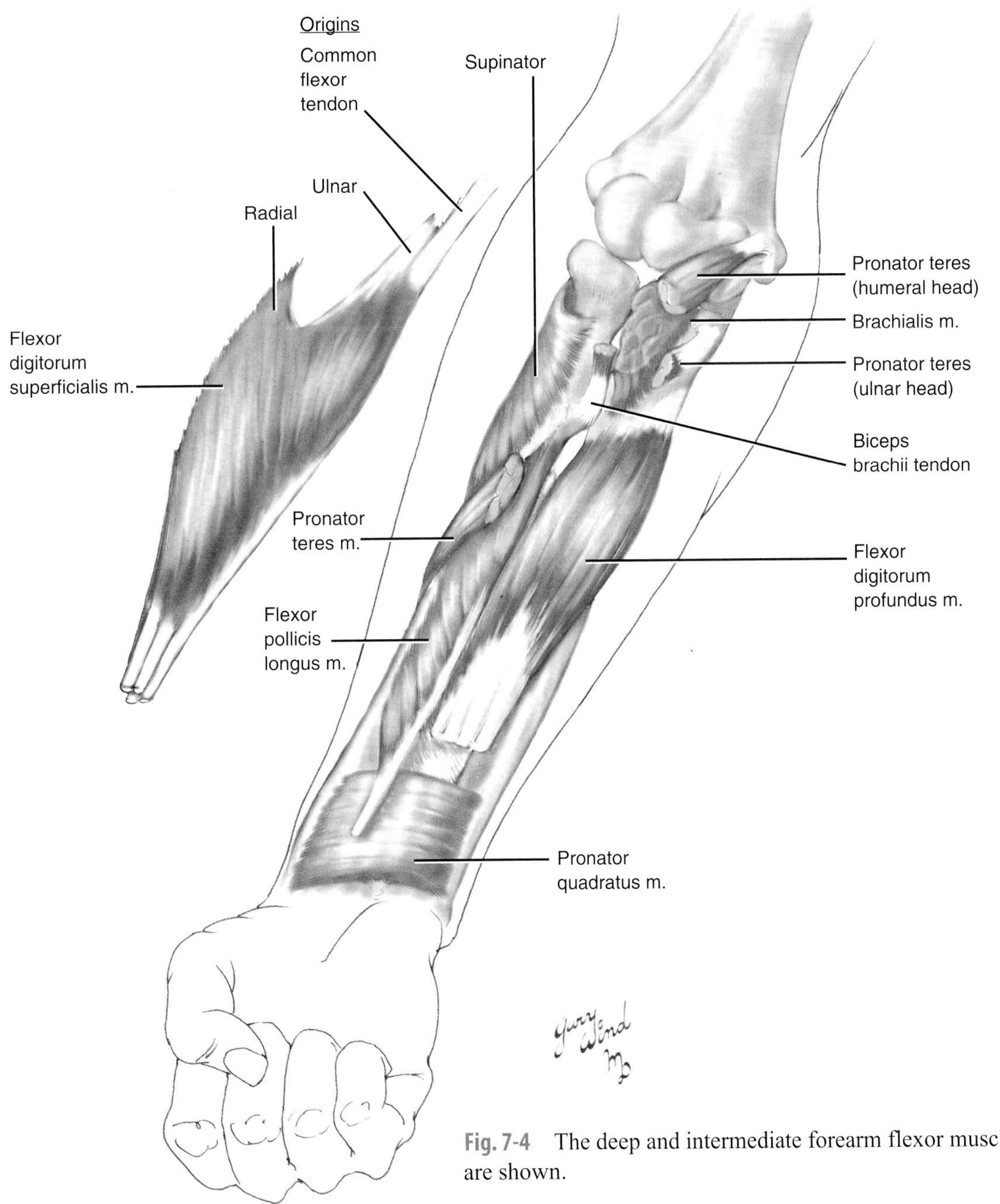

Fig. 7-4 The deep and intermediate forearm flexor muscles are shown.

The proximal flexor muscles lie on the medial side of the brachialis and biceps insertions. The deepest layer consists of flexor digitorum profundus and flexor pollicis longus. The flexor digitorum superficialis (FDS) which has humeral, ulnar, and radial origins is interposed as an intermediate layer. The most superficial layer consists of the muscles with a common origin at the medial epicondyle, including the pronator teres (Fig. 7-5).

All the flexors except the flexor carpi ulnaris (FCU) and the ulnar half of the flexor profundus are innervated by the median nerve. The exceptions are innervated by the ulnar nerve.

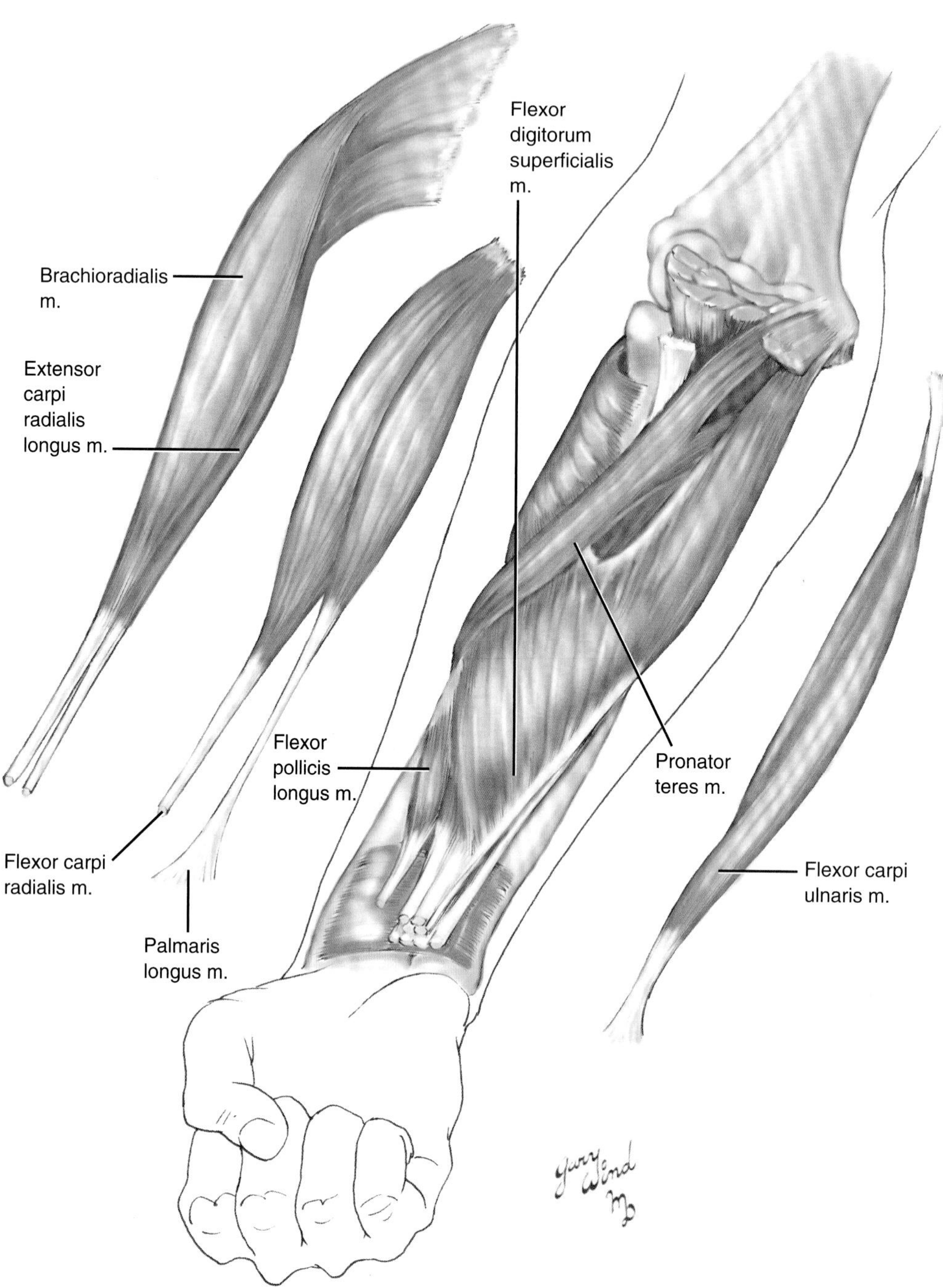

Fig. 7-5 The superficial forearm flexors fan out from a common tendon of origin at the medial epicondyle of the humerus.

Intermediate and Extensor Groups

The brachioradialis and extensor carpi radialis longus originate from the lateral supracondylar line of the humerus and the lateral intermuscular septum. They run in a direct line down the lateral side of the arm and are innervated at their proximal end by the radial nerve.

The dorsum of the forearm is also covered by a superficial group with a common epicondylar origin and a deep layer beneath (Fig. 7-6). An interesting feature of the dorsal forearm muscles is the interdigitation of the specialized thumb muscles with the other muscles of the extensor group.

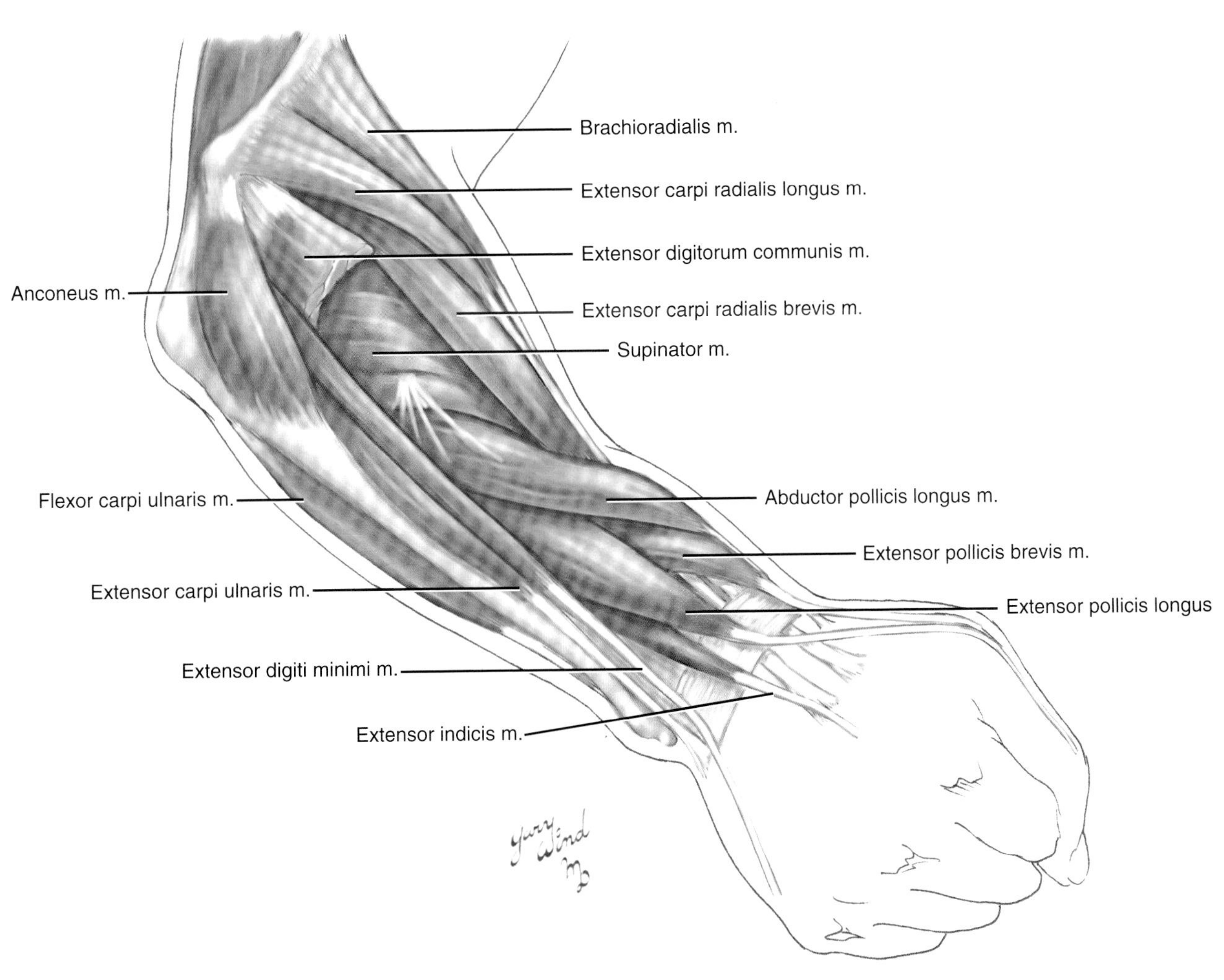

Fig. 7-6 The extensor muscle complex also consists of superficial and deep layers.

Like the popliteal artery at the knee, the brachial artery is the single major trunk supplying the distal extremity (Fig. 7-7). The artery bifurcates at the level of the radial tuberosity into radial and ulnar branches. The radial branch is the more direct continuation of the brachial artery, while the larger ulnar artery takes off at almost a right angle to the parent vessel. Immediately after its origin the ulnar artery gives off a short common interosseous branch which bifurcates at the hiatus in the proximal interosseous membrane. The dorsal and volar interosseous branches run on either side of the membrane to supply the deep muscles of each compartment.

The proximal radial and ulnar arteries give rise to recurrent collateral branches which anastomose with brachial tributaries around the elbow. The radial recurrent artery joins the radial collateral branch of the profunda brachii along the course of the radial nerve. The anterior and posterior ulnar recurrent vessels join the inferior and superior ulnar collateral branches of the brachial artery anterior and posterior to the medial epicondyle. An additional collateral artery, the interosseous recurrent, arises from the common interosseous artery and passes dorsal to the radius to join the

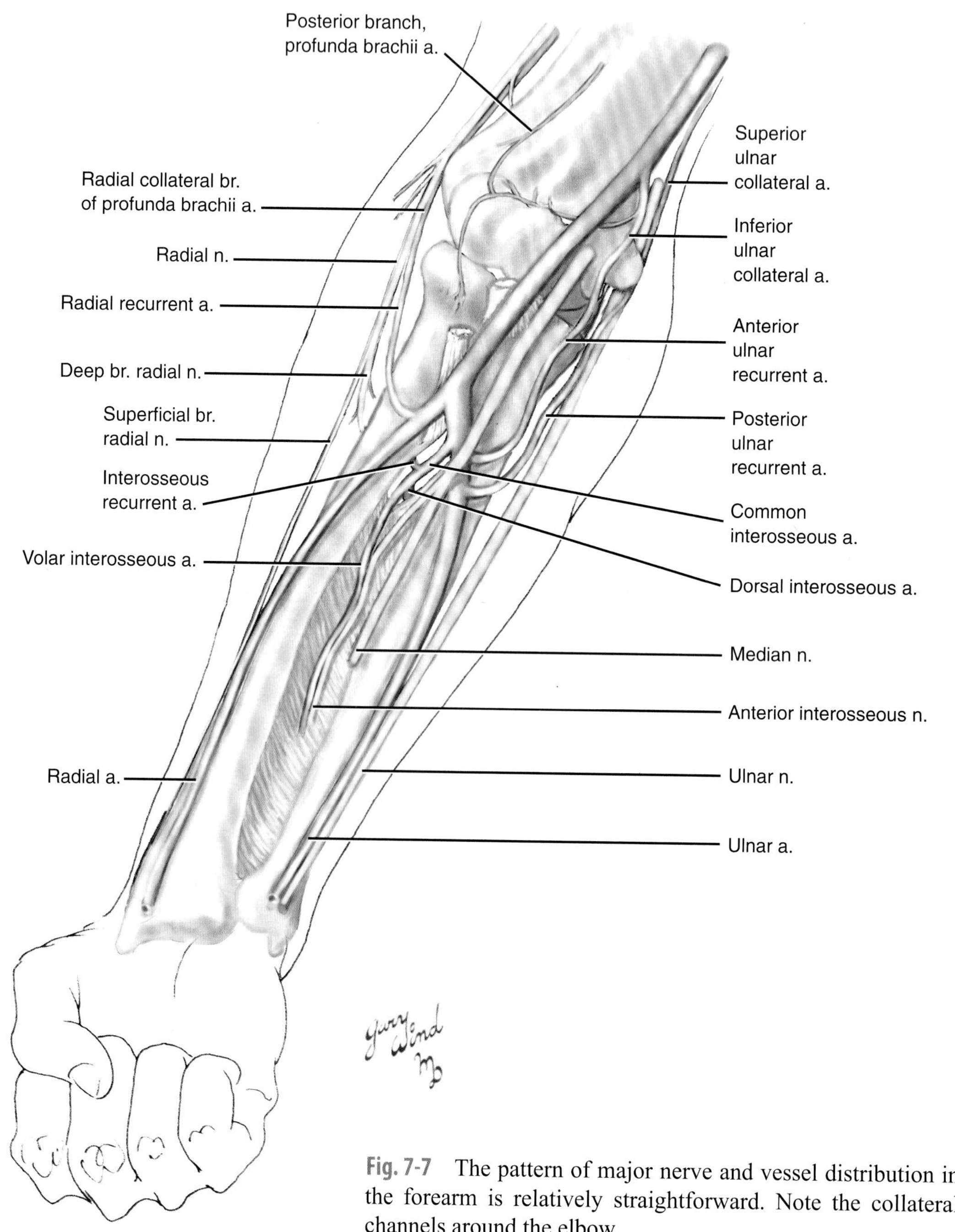

Fig. 7-7 The pattern of major nerve and vessel distribution in the forearm is relatively straightforward. Note the collateral channels around the elbow.

posterior branch of the profunda brachii as well as a branch of the inferior ulnar collateral artery.

The distal radial artery lies close to the superficial branch of the radial nerve, and the distal ulnar artery is joined by the ulnar nerve. The median nerve follows a central route down the forearm. A deep branch of the median nerve accompanies the anterior interosseous artery (AIA), and the posterior interosseous branch of the radial nerve passes through the supinator around the neck of the radius to reach the posterior interosseous artery and extensor muscles.

The Cubital Fossa

The relationship of the arteries to the surrounding muscles and nerves becomes somewhat complex in the depths of the cubital fossa (Fig. 7-8). Two elements of the regional anatomy are the keys to understanding the disposition of the forearm vessels. One is the structure of the pronator teres muscle, and the other is the structure of the FDS.

The pronator teres muscle arises from two heads. The humeral head is the most cephalad of the muscles originating from the common flexor tendon at the medial epicondyle. The ulnar head originates from the ulna lateral to the insertion of the brachialis muscle. This deep head rises between the median nerve and the ulnar artery to join the humeral head and separates the two structures. At the same time, it creates an isolated cleft through which the median nerve passes. The muscle is thus united as it passes over the ulnar artery. It then passes *under* the radial artery on its way to inserting on the lateral border of the midradius.

The FDS forms an intermediate muscle layer in the forearm. It has two origins medially, one from

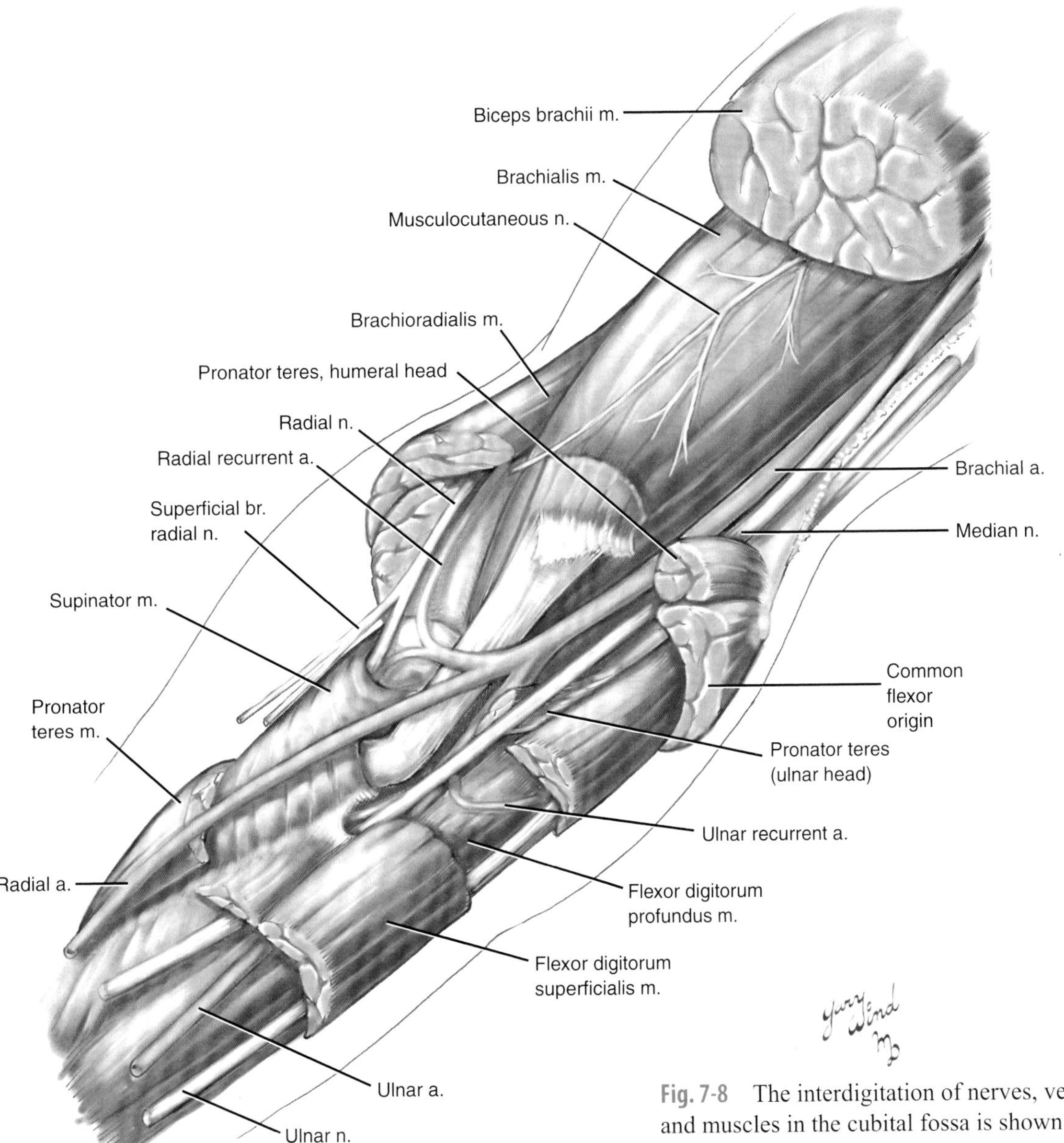

Fig. 7-8 The interdigitation of nerves, vessels, and muscles in the cubital fossa is shown.

the common tendon at the medial humeral epicondyle and the second from the ulna lateral to the brachialis insertion just cephalad to the origin of the deep pronator head. The broad lateral origin runs along the anterior radius between the insertion of the supinator and the origin of the flexor pollicis longus. The inverted arc formed by the junction of the heads is the gateway through which the ulnar artery and median nerve pass to reach the plane between the flexors digitorum superficialis and profundus. Near this arch, the artery and nerve reverse positions from medial to lateral. Also beneath this arch, the interosseous vessels and anterior interosseous nerve pass toward the interosseous membrane.

The courses of the superficial radial nerve, radial artery, and ulnar nerve are relatively straightforward as the following description demonstrates.

The Distal Forearm

The radial artery in the midforearm lies beneath the medial border of the brachioradialis muscle (Fig. 7-9). The ulnar artery becomes superficial in

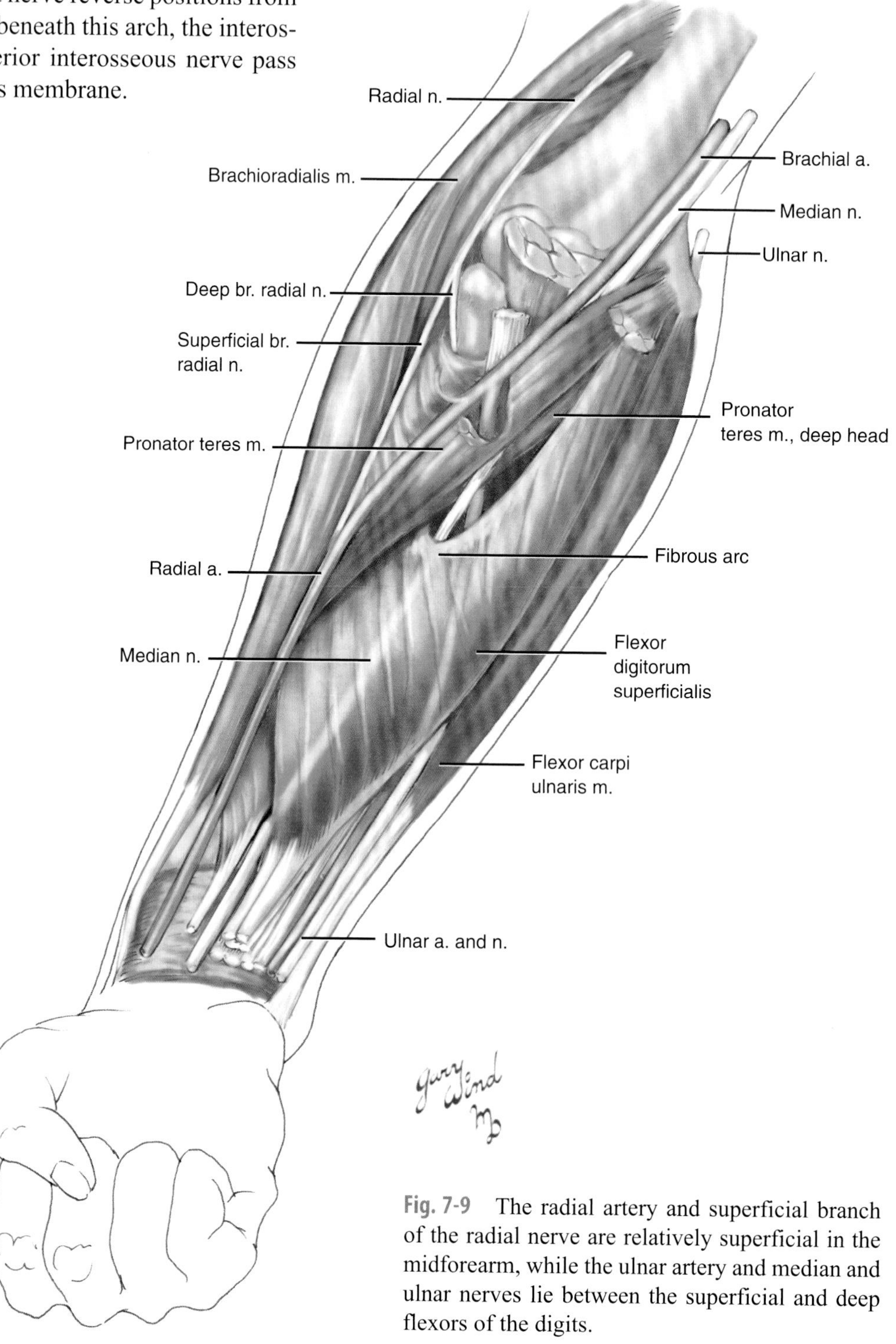

Fig. 7-9 The radial artery and superficial branch of the radial nerve are relatively superficial in the midforearm, while the ulnar artery and median and ulnar nerves lie between the superficial and deep flexors of the digits.

the distal forearm at the lateral border of the FDS. The ulnar nerve is covered along most of its course by the FCU. The median nerve traverses the forearm between the FDS and flexor digitorum profundus.

Near the wrist the radial artery becomes superficial, lying anterior to the radius and pronator quadratus, between the tendons of brachioradialis and flexor carpi radialis (Fig. 7-10). The ulnar artery and nerve are accessible on the radial side of the tendon of the FCU. The median nerve is found ulnar to the tendon of flexor carpi radialis between the tendons of the flexor pollicis longus and flexor digitorum profundus.

Exposure of Arteries in the Forearm

The superficial location of the radial and brachial arteries makes them ideal sites for arterial catheterization and for establishment of hemodialysis access. The radial artery is a common site of catheterization for indwelling arterial lines and for insertion of catheters during interventional radiologic procedures.[1–3] Radial artery occlusion occurs in 5% to 25% of patients undergoing these procedures,[4,5] but radial artery thrombosis does not usually lead to hand gangrene. Radial artery catheterization has a reported incidence of permanent hand ischemia of 0.09%;[1] in most cases, digital gangrene is thought to occur as a result of embolization from the site of initial arterial thrombosis.[6]

The arterial circulation of the hand is variable. In the vast majority of cases, the forearm arteries terminate in the superficial and deep palmar arches that interconnect the radial and ulnar circulations. Incomplete superficial and deep palmar arches are common, but one of the arches will be patent in most individuals (see Fig. 18-8). Because the ulnar artery is usually the dominant artery to the hand, many

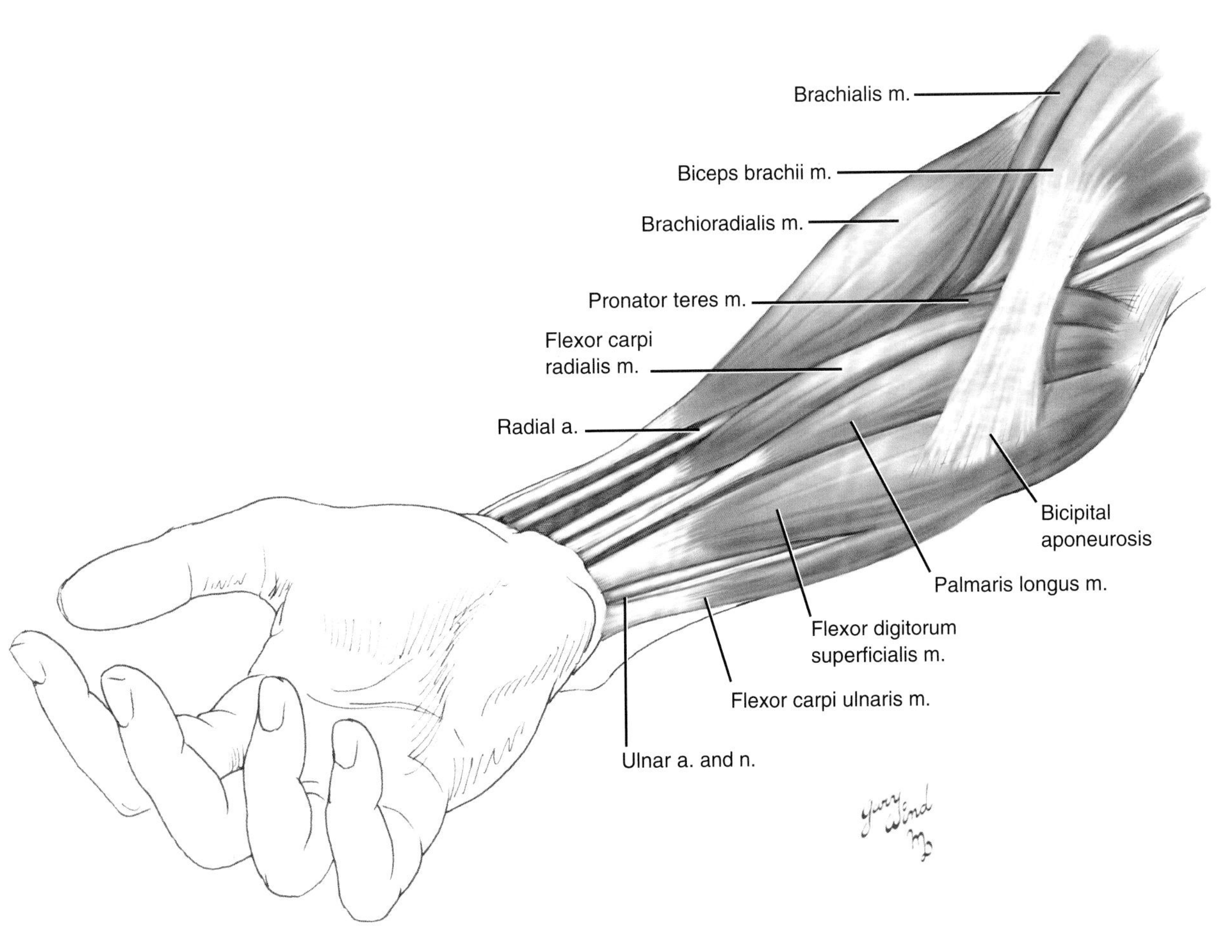

Fig. 7-10 The radial and ulnar arteries become superficial between the tendons of the wrist.

cardiovascular surgeons routinely harvest the radial artery for use as a coronary artery bypass conduit with minimal hand sequela.[7,8] However, it is important to keep in mind that some patients have disconnected ulnar and radial circulations. Radial artery harvest may result in mild to moderate hand ischemia in up to 10% of individuals;[8] it is critically important to identify patients with radial artery-dependent hand circulations prior to performing radial artery harvest. Physical examination using the Allen test has been favored by many as a simple and inexpensive method of assessing the collateral circulation of the hand, but there is a high rate of false-positive and false-negative results.[8] Complementary noninvasive tests such as the Allen test with Doppler insonation of the palmar arch,[9] finger pressure determinations,[10] or full-length scanning of the ulnar artery with ultrasonography[8] have been recommended for screening.

The brachial and radial arteries are commonly used to establish high-flow arteriovenous conduits for hemodialysis access. The size of the vessels appears to be ideal for balancing long-term conduit patency with avoidance of high-output congestive heart failure.[11] The most favorable patency rates are obtained with autogenous arteriovenous fistulas,[12] and published guidelines from the National Kidney Foundation indicate a strong preference for autogenous fistulas over prosthetic graft.[13] The first choice of arteriovenous fistula is the radiocephalic fistula originally described by Brescia,[14] followed by brachiocephalic and brachiobasilic fistulas.[12,13] Whereas synthetic conduits have inferior patency rates, favorable results have been obtained with prosthetic grafts in a variety of configurations, as long as the venous anastomosis is kept below the elbow.[12,15,16]

Exposure of the Distal Brachial Artery and Its Bifurcation

The patient is placed in the supine position with the arm abducted 90° and supported on a board attached to the operating table. The hand, forearm, and arm should be prepped circumferentially and draped away from the trunk.

To expose the brachial artery in the antecubital fossa, a transverse skin incision is made 1 cm distal to the midpoint of the antecubital crease and extended medially for a distance of 3 to 4 cm (Fig. 7-11). Longitudinal incisions across the antecubital crease should be avoided to prevent flexion

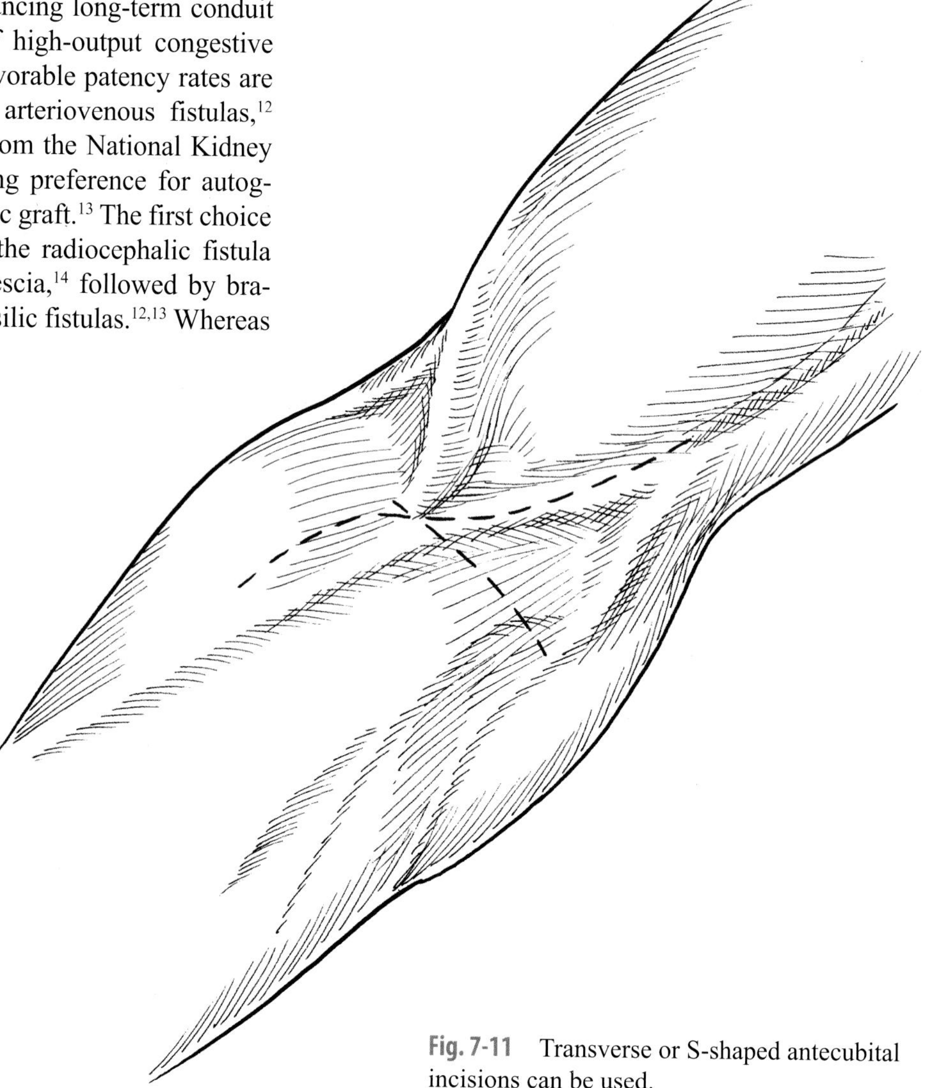

Fig. 7-11 Transverse or S-shaped antecubital incisions can be used.

contractures from hypertrophic scarring. Wider proximal exposure of the brachial artery and distal exposure of its branches can be gained by creating an S-shaped incision. The superior longitudinal portion is made along the medial border of the biceps muscle, and the horizontal portion is brought across the flexion crease. The inferior portion is made lateral to the midpoint of the volar forearm for a distance of 4 to 6 cm.

On deepening the incision, one should take care to avoid injuring subcutaneous veins, which may be used as outflow vessels in arteriovenous shunt procedures (Fig. 7-12). It is often necessary to mobilize the basilic vein and retract it medially. The medial antebrachial cutaneous nerve should be protected as well. When creating an S-shaped incision, it may be necessary to divide the median cubital vein if its course interferes with exposure.

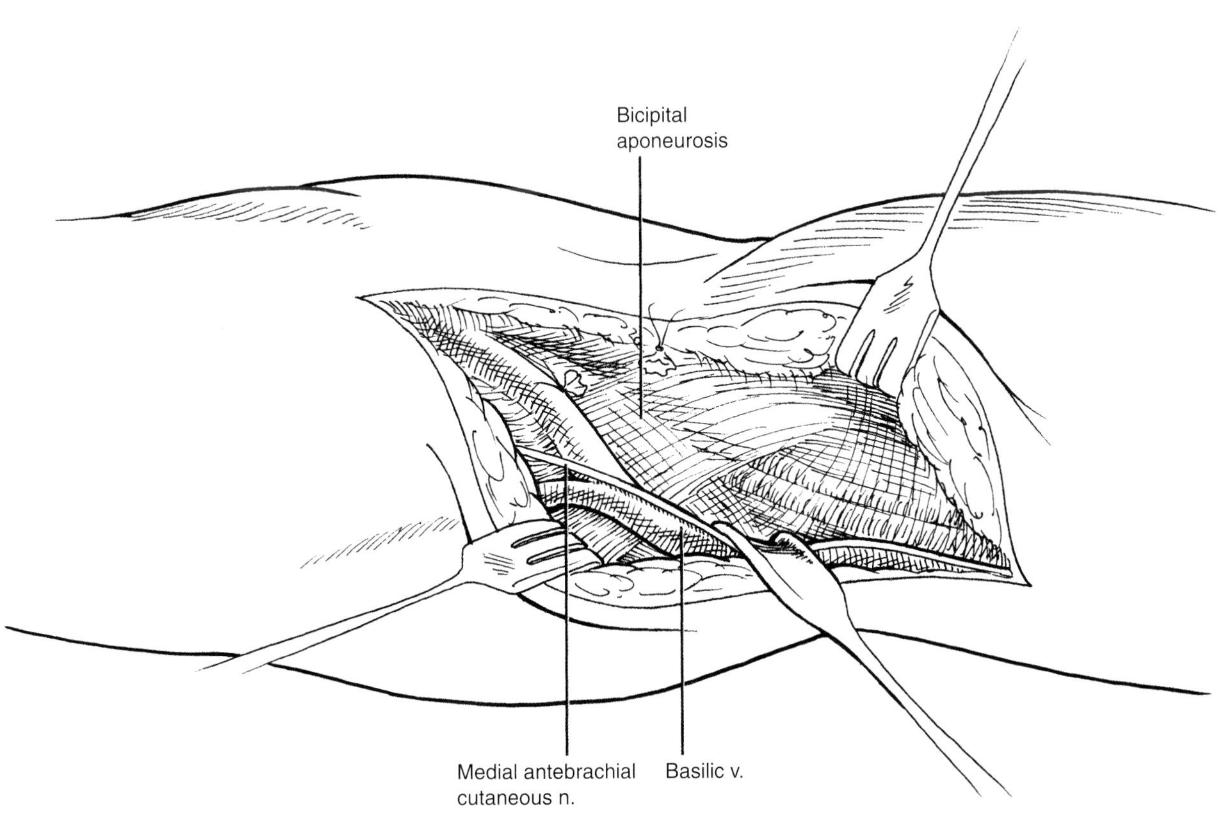

Fig. 7-12 The basilic vein and medial antebrachial cutaneous nerve are retracted, exposing the deep fascia and bicipital aponeurosis over the brachial artery and median nerve. An S-shaped incision has been depicted for clarity.

The bicipital aponeurosis is recognized in the center of the wound at the fascial level. Division of this aponeurosis exposes the brachial artery, which is flanked by two deep veins and crossed by their communicating branches (Fig. 7-13). Isolation of the brachial artery requires ligation and division of these crossing vein branches.

The radial and ulnar arteries are exposed by retracting the distal skin edge of the transverse skin incision or by deepening the distal portion of the S-shaped

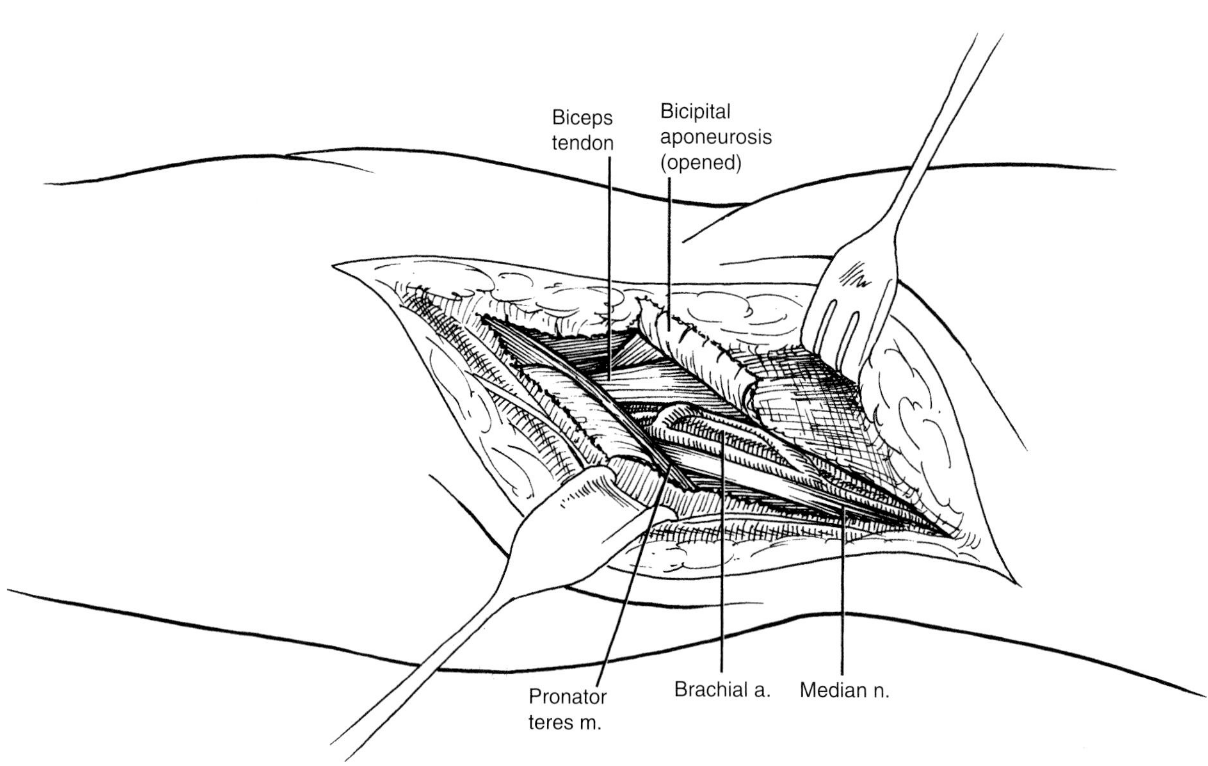

Fig. 7-13 The fascia is opened, revealing the artery and nerve medial to the biceps tendon. The artery is accompanied by two veins that intercommunicate.

incision. The brachial bifurcation is usually located in the antecubital fossa near the intersection of the brachioradialis and pronator teres muscles (Fig. 7-14). It is most easily identified by tracing the brachial artery distally. The radial branch courses in the same direction as the brachial artery toward the radial side of the forearm. It can be isolated at the brachial bifurcation or at any point along the medial border of the brachioradialis muscle. The ulnar branch dives beneath the pronator teres a short distance from its origin. Isolation of the ulnar artery distal to this small segment will require separate incisions (see below).

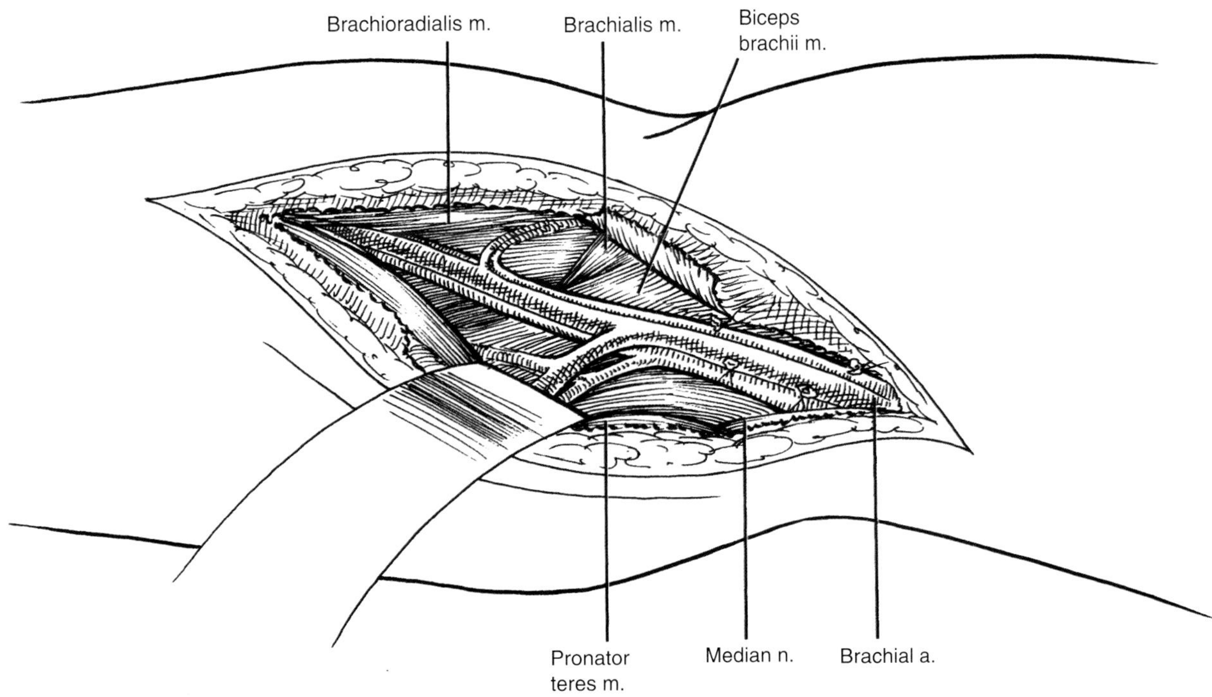

Fig. 7-14 The bifurcation of the brachial artery can be exposed by retracting the pronator teres and flexor muscle mass. The radial artery can be followed the length of the incision, but the larger ulnar artery dives between the heads of the FDS.

Exposure of the Radial Artery in the Midforearm

The patient is placed supine with the arm abducted at 90° on a supporting board. A 5-cm longitudinal incision is made over the portion of the artery to be exposed. Alternatively, a long incision across the volar forearm should be used when the entire radial artery is to be harvested for use in coronary bypass procedures.[17] The landmark for the incision follows a line from the midpoint of the antecubital crease to the styloid process of the radius, corresponding to the groove on the medial edge of the brachioradialis muscle (Fig. 7-15). Subcutaneous veins are ligated and divided as the wound is deepened, and the antebrachial fascia is incised along the medial border of the brachioradialis muscle. In the proximal and middle thirds of the forearm, the radial artery lies beneath the medial fibers of the brachioradialis muscle and can be exposed by retracting the brachioradialis and pronator teres muscles apart. In the distal forearm, the artery lies just beneath the antebrachial fascia between the tendons of the brachioradialis and flexor carpi radialis muscles. In the middle third of the forearm, the superficial radial nerve is closely associated with the lateral aspect of the radial artery and must be carefully preserved. The radial artery is accompanied by paired veins throughout its course, and care should be taken to separate these during arterial isolation.

Exposure of the Radial Artery at the Wrist

The patient is placed as described above, with the entire forearm and hand circumferentially prepped and draped. Proper placement of the incision will be determined by the indication for radial artery

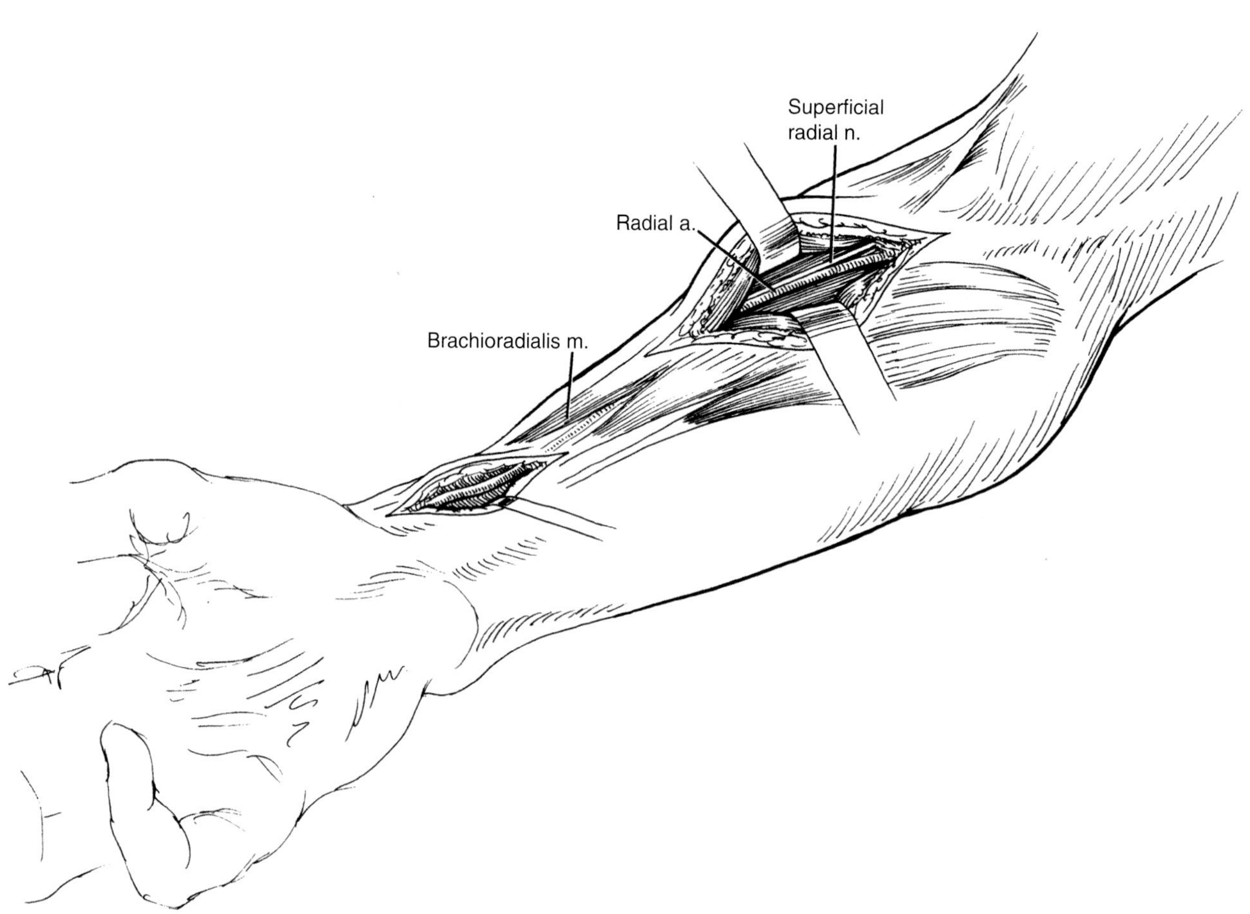

Fig. 7-15 The radial artery in the midforearm can be easily exposed beneath the brachioradialis.

exposure. In cases involving open arterial line placement or simple arterial ligation, a longitudinal incision should be made directly over the radial pulse, beginning just proximal to the level of the styloid process (Fig. 7-16). For creation of radiocephalic arteriovenous fistulas, a 2- to 3-cm longitudinal incision should be made approximately halfway between the radial artery and the cephalic vein, near the lateral border of the radius. Longitudinal incisions permit increased mobilization of the vein and artery; some authors prefer transverse, oblique, or sigmoid modifications.

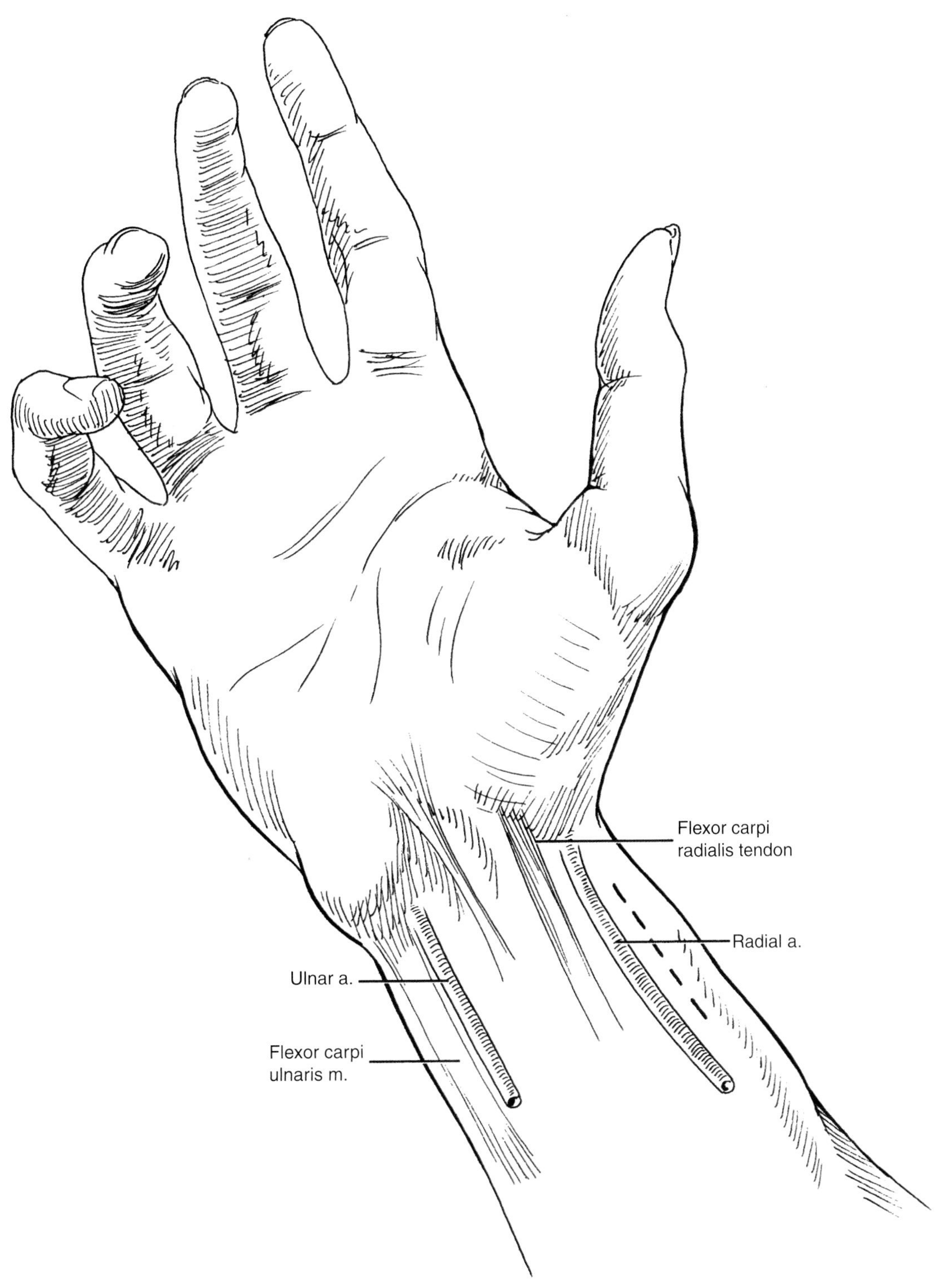

Fig. 7-16 The incision for exposing the radial artery is shown. A more lateral incision also gives access to the cephalic vein for creation of arteriovenous fistulas.

The cephalic vein is exposed in the subcutaneous tissues of the lateral skin flap (Fig. 7-17). The radial artery is exposed by incising the antebrachial fascia just medial to the radius. Two deep veins accompany the artery at this level and should be carefully dissected away during arterial isolation. The superficial radial nerve and its medial and lateral branches course between the cephalic vein and radial artery in this area. These nerves lie superficial to the antebrachial fascia and should be carefully preserved during creation of arteriovenous fistulas.

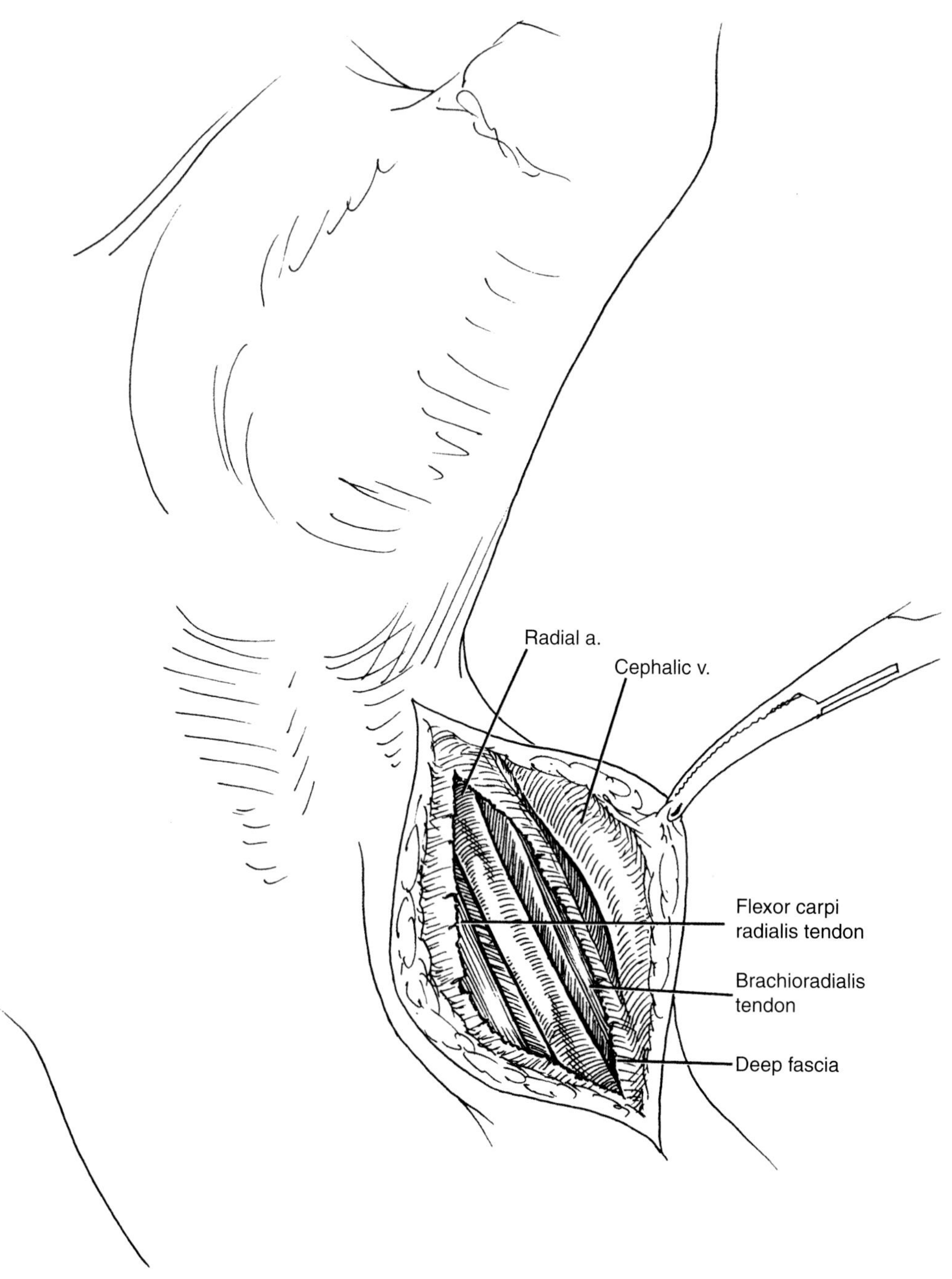

Fig. 7-17 The radial artery at the wrist lies just deep to the deep fascia between the flexor carpi radialis tendon and the insertion of the brachioradialis.

Exposure of the Ulnar Artery in the Forearm

The ulnar artery courses beneath the superficial flexor muscles in the proximal forearm, emerging near the ulnar border at a point midway between the elbow and the wrist. Because of its deep placement in the proximal third of the forearm, exposure is somewhat difficult.

The patient is placed in the supine position, with the arm supinated and the hand slightly flexed to relax the flexor muscles. In the proximal forearm, the ulnar artery is exposed between muscles of the superficial flexor group. An 8- to 10-cm incision is begun approximately four fingerbreadths below the medial epicondyle of the humerus, extending along a line from the medial epicondyle to the pisiform (Fig. 7-18). Superficial veins are ligated as necessary, and the antebrachial fascia is incised for the length of the incision. The ulnar artery is located by developing a plane between the FCU and FDS muscles. In the proximal third of the forearm, the artery and its accompanying veins can be identified by laterally retracting the FDS muscle. In the middle third of the forearm, the vessels lie just deep to the FCU, which should be retracted medially. The ulnar nerve joins the artery near the border of the upper and middle thirds of the forearm; the nerve should be identified on the artery's medial border in the distal wound and protected during arterial isolation.

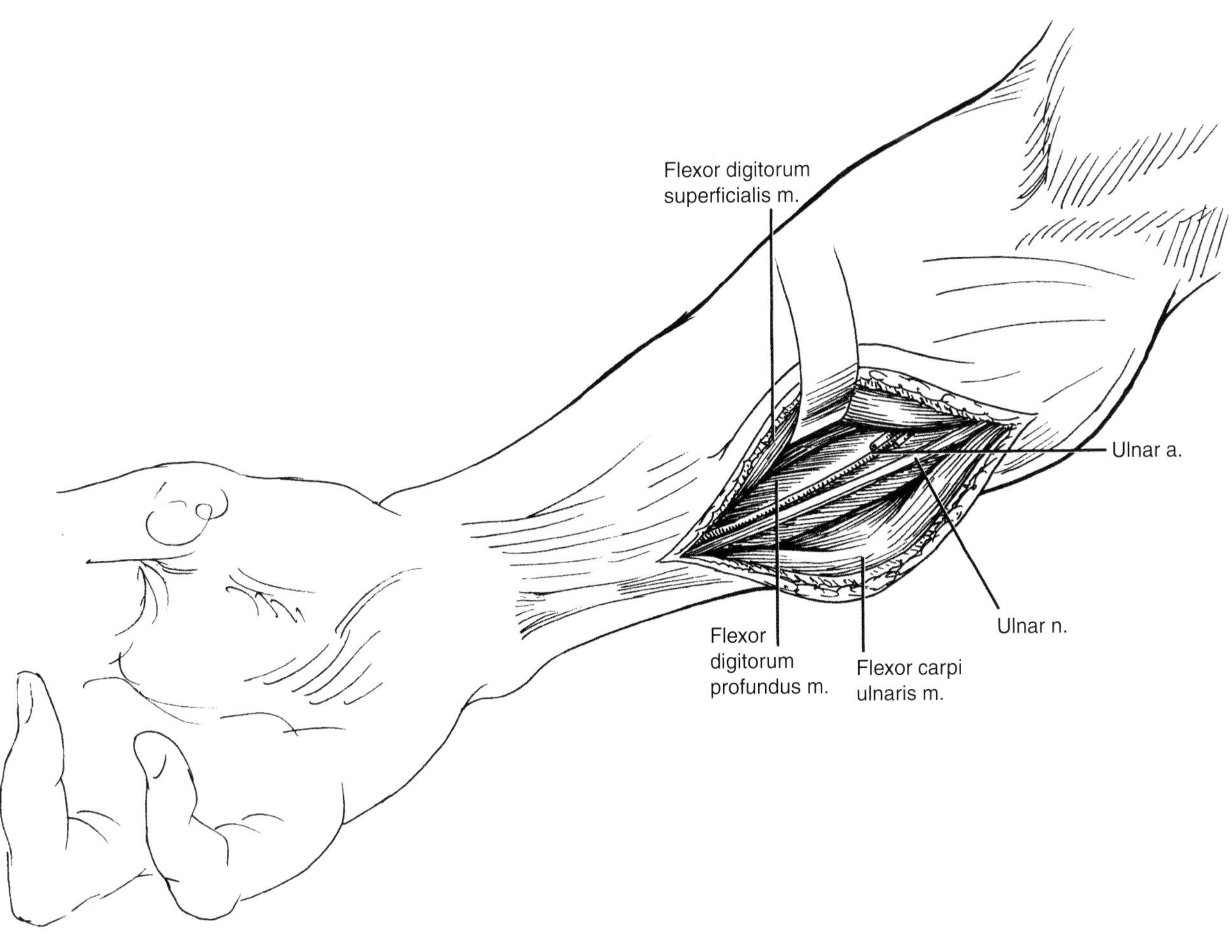

Fig. 7-18 The ulnar artery in the midforearm is reached between the FCU and FDS.

In the distal forearm, the ulnar artery courses just beneath the antebrachial fascia and is easily exposed through a longitudinal incision placed radial to the FCU (Fig. 7-19). The palmar branch of the ulnar nerve courses superficial to the antebrachial fascia and should be preserved during arterial exposure.

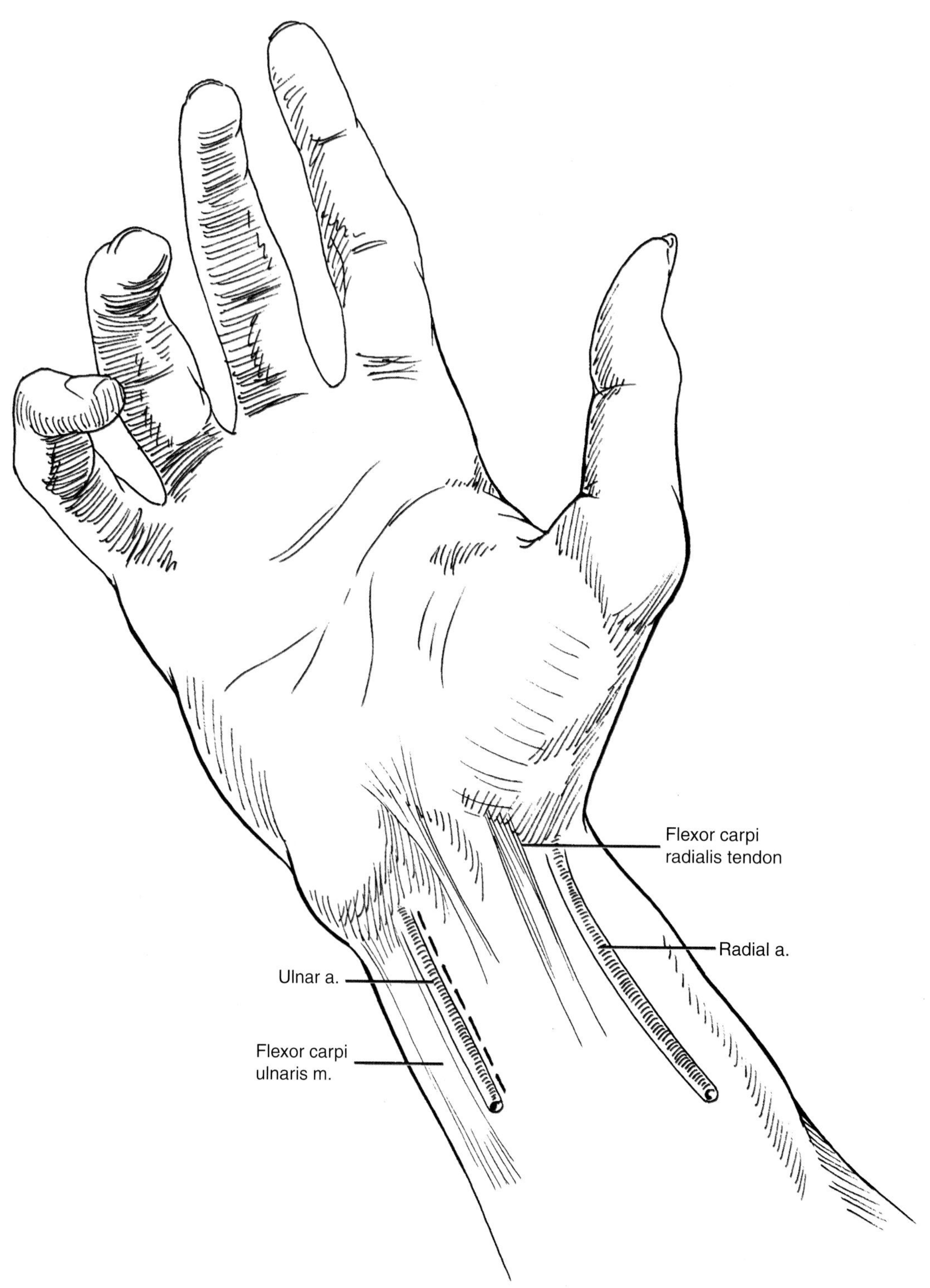

Fig. 7-19 The incision over the ulnar artery at the wrist is shown.

Forearm Fasciotomy

Compartment syndrome occurs whenever the interstitial tissue pressure within an enclosed anatomic rises sufficiently to impair tissue perfusion, ultimately resulting in ischemia and cell death (myonecrosis). The deep fascia of the forearm, like that of the leg, firmly encloses the underlying muscles (Fig. 7-20A, B). The diagnosis of acute compartment syndrome is based on history and physical

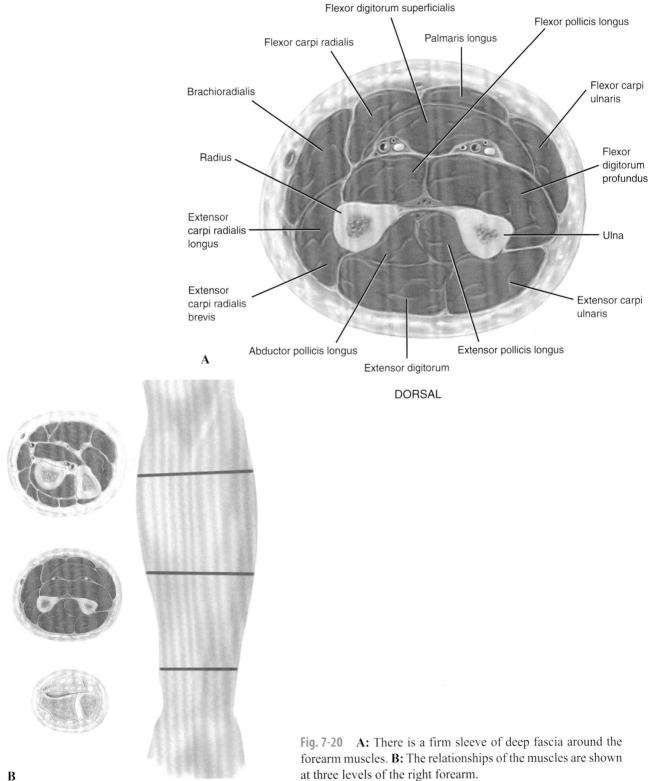

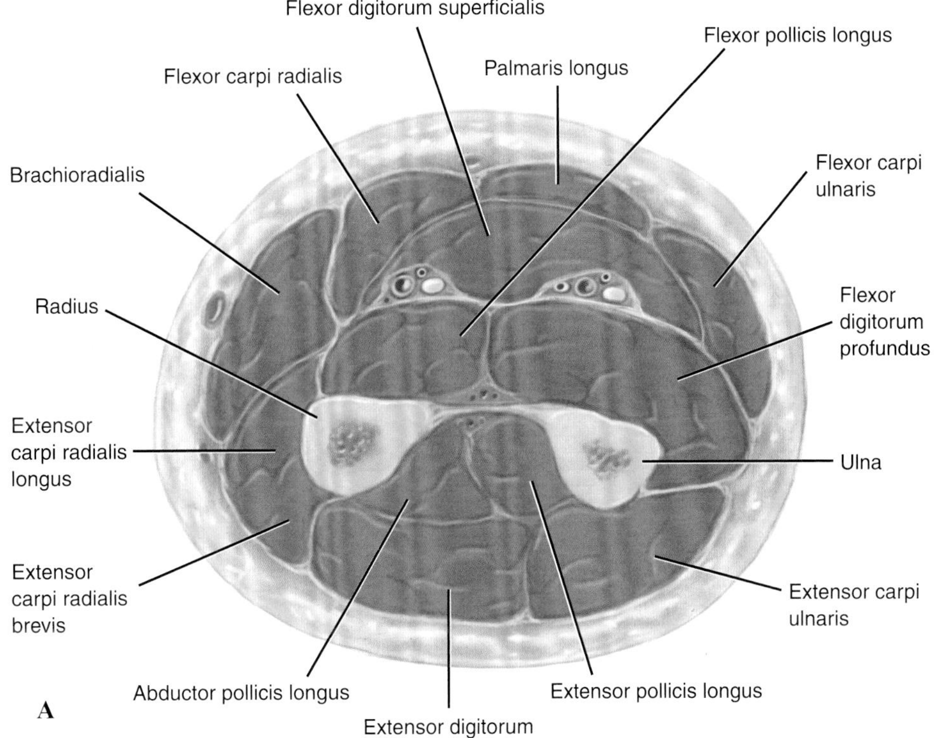

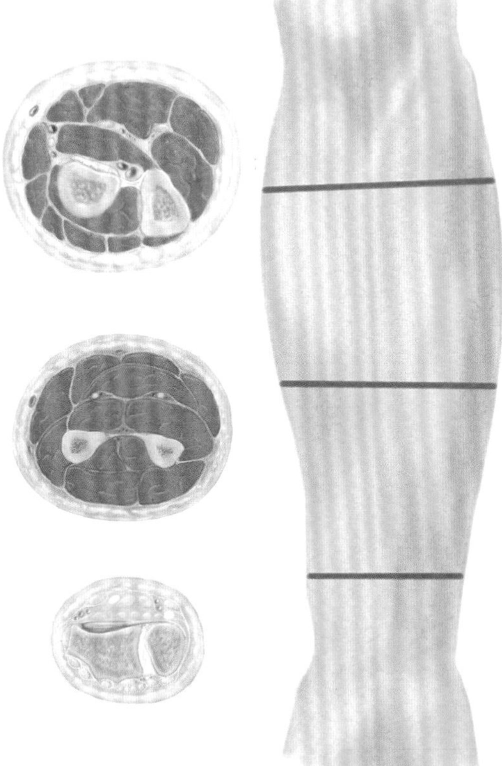

Fig. 7-20 **A:** There is a firm sleeve of deep fascia around the forearm muscles. **B:** The relationships of the muscles are shown at three levels of the right forearm.

examination and confirmed with interstitial pressure measurements.[18] In particular, the combination of certain types of injury (i.e., crush, fracture, electrical burn) and physical findings (i.e., pain with passive motion of the fingers, tense forearm, and neurologic findings referable to the compartment) should alert the surgeon that an acute compartment syndrome is developing.

The threshold interstitial pressure at which fasciotomy is warranted remains controversial. The most commonly quoted criteria for compartment syndrome is based on interstitial pressure related to either the mean arterial pressure or the diastolic pressure. Based on data from the classic paper of Whitesides et al.,[19] fasciotomy is indicated when the dynamic interstitial pressure rises to within 30 mm Hg of the mean arterial pressure or 20 mm Hg of the diastolic blood pressure. Regardless of the specific criteria used, prompt fasciotomy is indicated to relieve compartment ischemia and limit cell death. A properly executed forearm fasciotomy is crucial to minimize the morbidity of this procedure. A retrospective review of 84 forearm compartment syndromes found an overall complication rate of 42%, with neurologic deficits in 21%.[20] Particular attention should be given to the skin incision and to ensuring complete release of the deep muscles of the volar compartment.

The forearm consists of three primary compartments (Fig. 7-21): volar, dorsal, and lateral or mobile wad (brachioradialis, extensor carpi radialis longus, and brevis). The volar compartment includes three deep muscles supplied by the AIA: flexor digitorum profundus, flexor pollicis longus, and pronator quadratus. The long, small diameter AIA is especially prone to occlusion from compartment hypertension,[21] and the three deeper volar compartment muscles are subsequently the most commonly affected in forearm compartment syndromes. Hence, complete release of the "deep volar" compartment is paramount.

The use of a tourniquet is advocated by some. It is the author's preference to have one in place, but not elevated, to avoid further ischemic insult to the tissue. Multiple incisions have been described for volar forearm fasciotomy. Regardless of the specific configuration, the goal is to adequately decompress all compartments, minimize injury to the major nerves, and at the completion of the fasciotomy, be

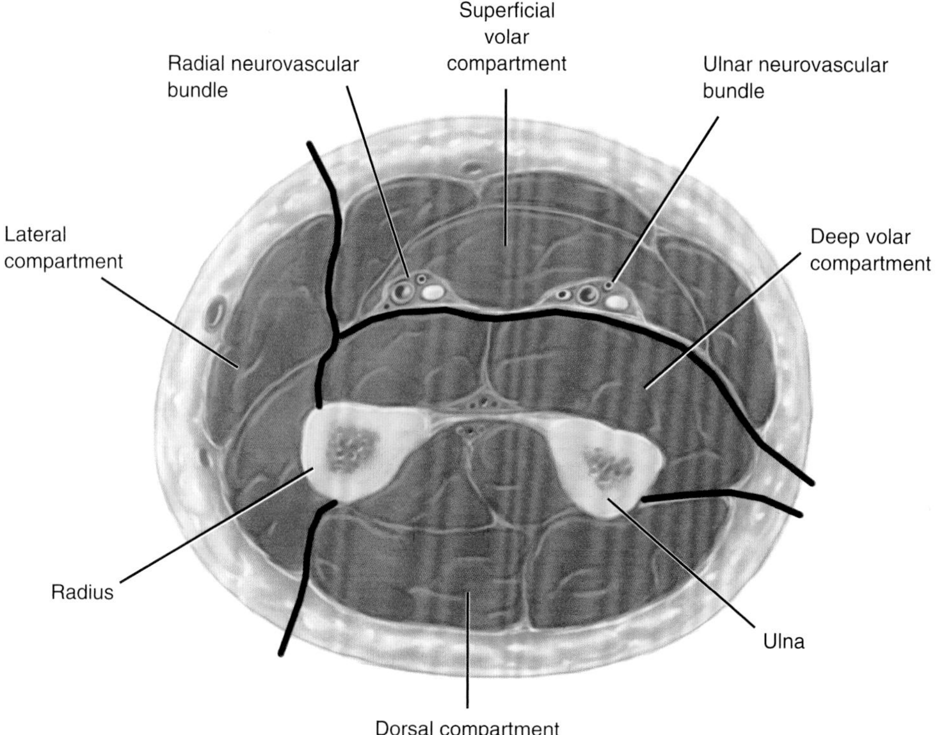

Fig. 7-21 The three main compartments of the right forearm are shown at midforearm level.

able to safely cover the distal 3 to 4 cm of the median nerve which becomes superficial and only partially covered by the palmaris longus tendon. Figure 7-22 shows our preferred incision.[22]

The incision begins on the palm with a classic carpal tunnel incision lying in line with the radial border of the ringer finger and extending 2 to 3mm ulnar to the thenar crease (Fig. 7-23). An incision from Kaplan's cardinal line to the wrist flexor crease will allow adequate access to the median nerve through the palmar fascia and transverse carpal ligament. The surgeon must not be unnecessarily rushed by the emergency of the situation when releasing the median nerve. Iatrogenic injury to this structure is the most debilitating complication related to the procedure.

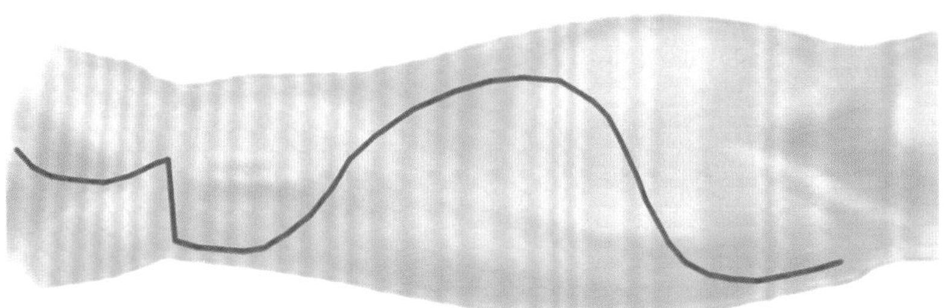

Fig. 7-22 The recommended incision is shown.

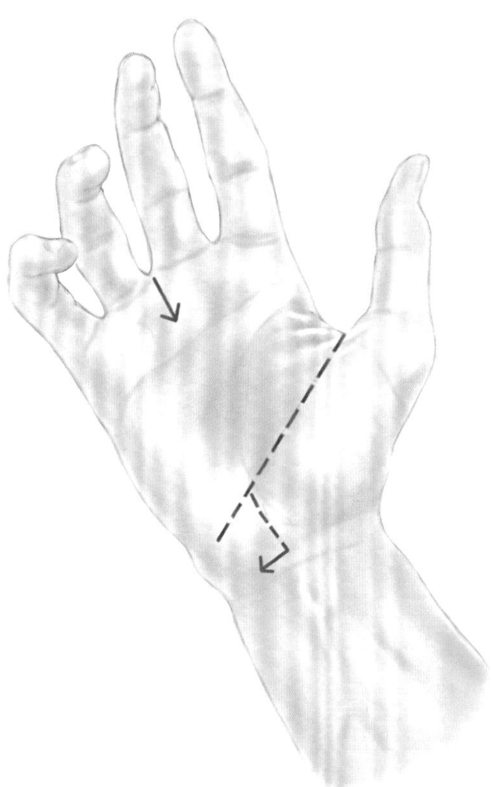

Fig. 7-23 The initial palmar portion of the incision is shown. Kaplan's cardinal line is shown in red.

The carpal tunnel incision is then carried ulnarly along the distal wrist flexor crease to the FCU tendon. At the ulnar side of the FCU tendon, the incision is brought proximally 4 to 5 cm before gently curving to the midline. This incision protects the ulnar nerve and artery, located radial to the tendon, and forms an adequate flap to cover the distal median nerve.

The skin incision is extended proximally and toward the midline for simultaneous decompression of the mobile wad muscles. The large veins crossing the incision path often require suture ligation. Superficial nerves crossing the forearm will be sacrificed and the patient should be counseled preoperatively if possible. Sharp and blunt dissection will allow elevation of the fascia with the ulnarly based full thickness skin flap. Once the plane between fascia and muscle is defined, the flap is elevated along its entire length (Fig. 7-24). The flap is raised off of the FCU tendon with the paratenon left intact, thereby protecting the deeper ulnar nerve and vessels.

The ulnar neurovascular bundle is commonly adherent to the deep and ulnar aspect of the FDS muscle belly before becoming relatively superficial between the FCU and FDS tendons (see Fig. 7-9). Branches from the ulnar artery to the deep muscles can be sacrificed and the FDS elevated from the FCU to gain access to the flexor pollicis longus and

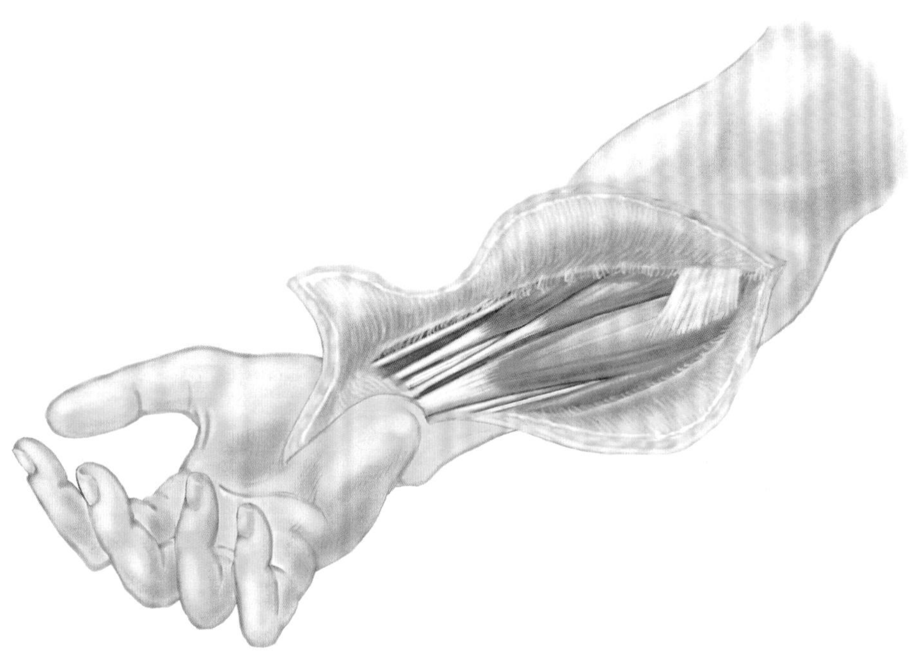

Fig. 7-24 The elevation of the fasciocutaneous flap is shown.

flexor digitorum profundus (Fig. 7-25). The muscle fascia overlying the deep compartment muscles will not be as thick as that overlying the FDS.

Upon completion of the release of the deep volar compartment, the midforearm portion of the incision lies adjacent to the mobile wad muscles (Fig. 7-26). Blunt subfascial dissection in a radial fashion (*arrow*) will allow entry into the lateral compartment. Proximal dissection will place radial nerve and artery at risk and is not necessary.

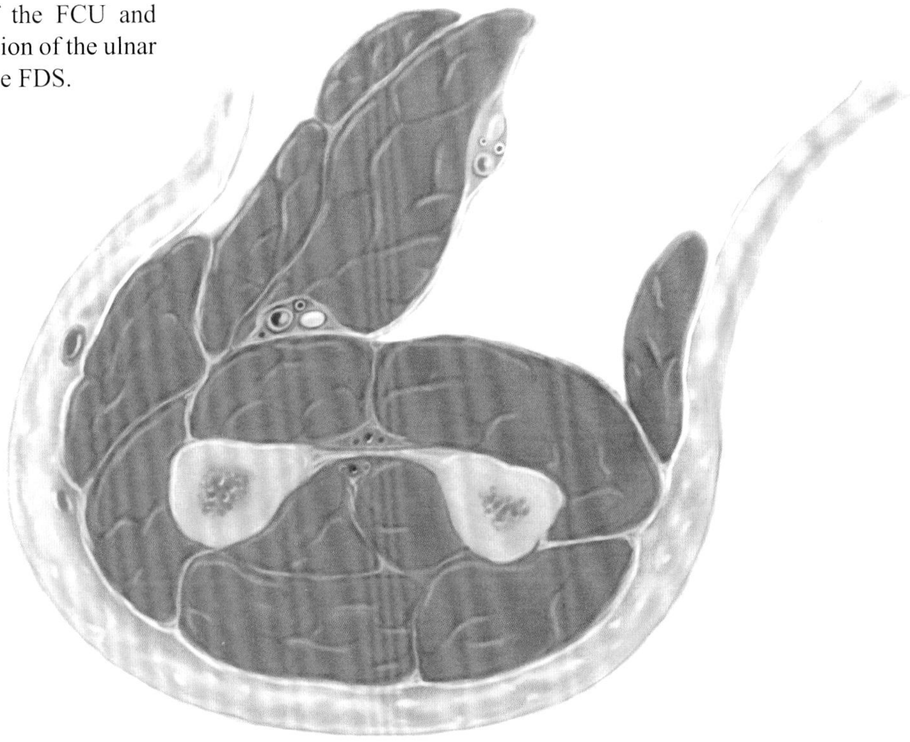

Fig. 7-25 The separation of the FCU and FDS is shown. Note the inclusion of the ulnar neuromuscular bundle with the FDS.

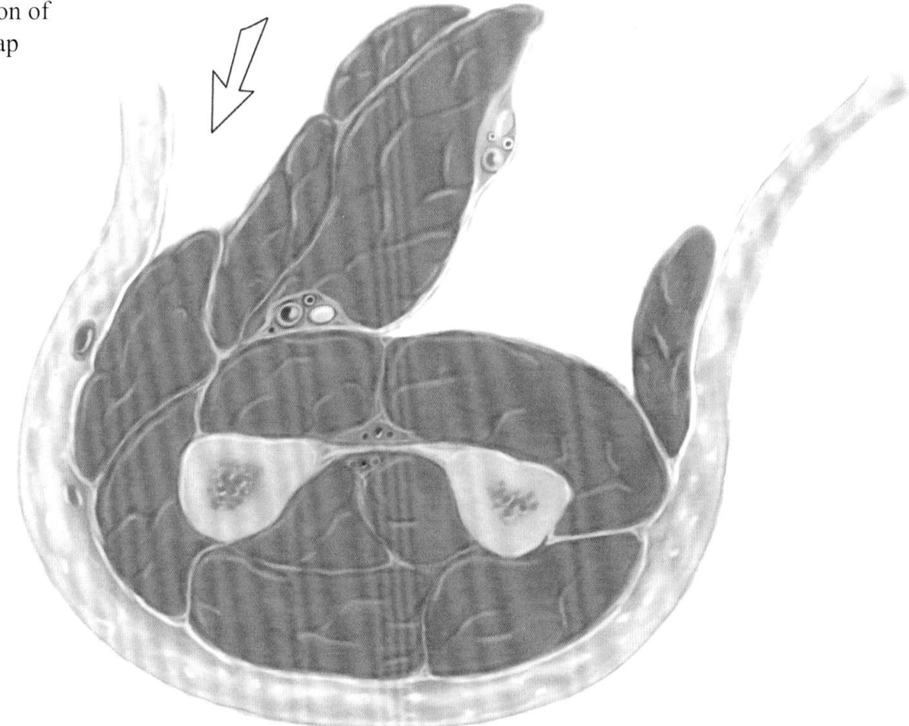

Fig. 7-26 Subfascial extension of the lateral fasciocutaneous flap decompresses the lateral compartment.

In most situations, the dorsal compartment muscles will be adequately decompressed by the full length volar decompression. However, some injuries, such as prolonged crush or electrical burn, will require dorsal compartment fasciotomy. A dorsal 6 to 8 cm incision in line from the lateral epicondyle to the radial styloid, ulnar to the mobile wad (Fig. 7-27), will allow release of the compartment fascia.

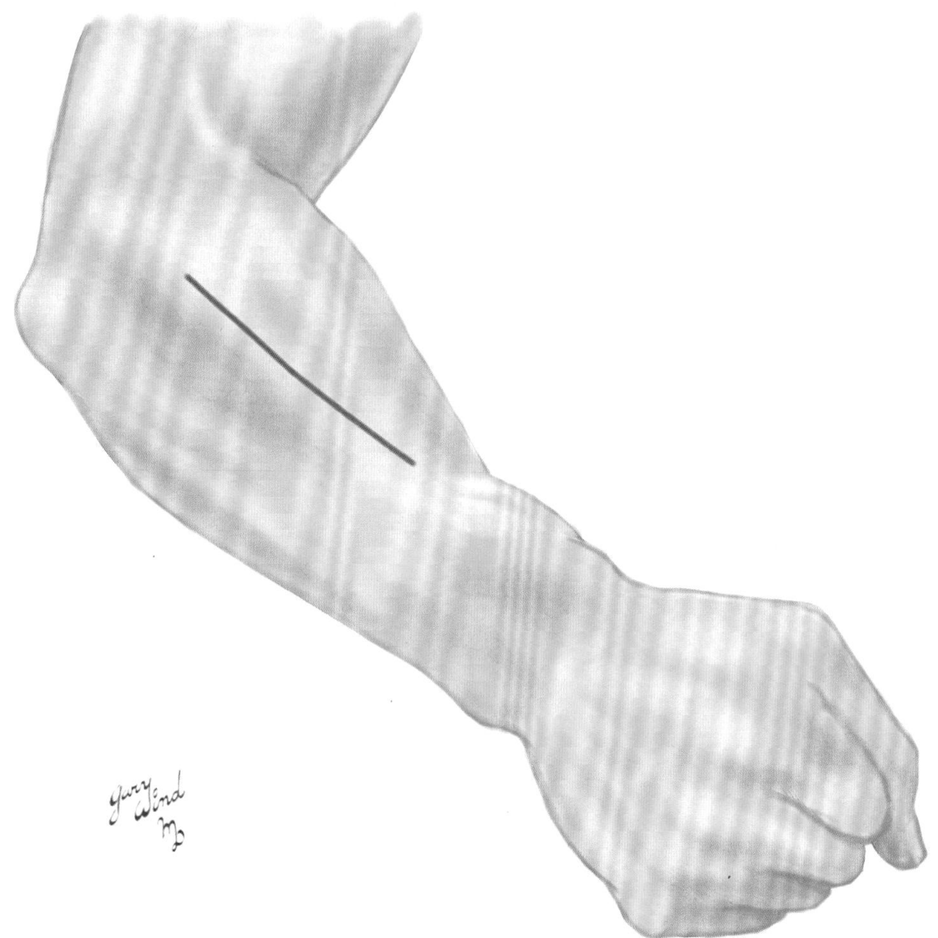

Fig. 7-27 Rarely, a dorsal counterincision will be necessary.

References

1. Brzezinski M, Luisetti T, London MJ. Radial artery cannulation: a comprehensive review of recent anatomic and physiologic investigations. *Anesth Analg.* 2009;109:1763–1781.
2. Nohara AM, Kallmes DF. Transradial cerebral angiography: technique and outcomes. *Am J Neuroradiol.* 2003;24:1247–1250.
3. Brueck M, Bandorski D, Kramer W, et al. A randomized comparison of transradial versus transfemoral approach for coronary angiography and angioplasty. *JACC Cardiovasc Interv.* 2009;2:1047–1054.
4. Stella PR, Kiemeneij F, Laarman GJ, et al. Incidence and outcome of radial artery occlusion following transradial artery coronary angioplasty. *Cathet Cardiovasc Diagn.* 1997;40:156–158.
5. Sfeir R, Khoury S, Khoury G, et al. Ischemia of the hand after radial artery monitoring. *Cardiovasc Surg.* 1996;4:456–458.
6. Valentine RJ, Modrall JG, Clagett GP. Hand ischemia after radial artery cannulation. *J Am Coll Surg.* 2005;201:18–22.
7. Sajja LR, Mannam G, Pantula NR, et al. Role of radial artery graft in coronary artery bypass grafting. *Ann Thorac Surg.* 2005;79:2180–2188.
8. Manabe S, Tabuchi N, Tanaka H, et al. Hand circulation after radial artery harvest for coronary artery bypass grafting. *J Med Dent Sci.* 2005;52:101–107.
9. Ruengsakulrach P, Brooks M, Hare DL, et al. Preoperative assessment of hand circulation by means of Doppler ultrasonography and the modified Allen test. *J Thorac Cardiovasc Surg.* 2001;121:526–531.
10. Starnes SL, Wolk SW, Lampman RM, et al. Noninvasive evaluation of hand circulation before radial artery harvest for coronary artery bypass grafting. *J Thorac Cardiovasc Surg.* 1999;117:261–266.
11. Youg PR Jr, Rohr MS, Marterre WF Jr. High-output cardiac failure secondary to a brachiocephalic arteriovenous hemodialysis fistula: two cases. *Am Surg.* 1998;64:239–241.
12. Sidawy AN, Spergel LM, Besarab A, et al. The society of vascular surgery: clinical practice guidelines for the surgical placement and maintenance of arteriovenous hemodialysis access. *J Vasc Surg.* 2008:48:2S–25S.
13. The Vascular Access Work Group. NKF-DOQI clinical practice guidelines for vascular access. Update 2000. *Am J Kidney Dis.* 2001;37:S137–S181.
14. Brescia MJ, Cimino JE, Appel K, et al. Chronic hemodialysis using venipuncture and a surgically created arteriovenous fistula. *N Engl J Med.* 1966; 275:1089–1092.
15. Hodges TC, Fillinger MF, Zwolak RM, et al. Longitudinal comparison of dialysis access methods: risk factors for failure. *J Vasc Surg.* 1997;26:1009–1019.
16. Kalman PG, Pope M, Bhola C, et al. A practical approach to vascular access for hemodialysis and predictors of success. *J Vasc Surg.* 1999;30:727–733.
17. Voucharas C, Bisbos A, Moustakidis P, et al. Open versus tunneling radial artery harvest for coronary artery grafting. *J Card Surg.* 2010;25:504–507.
18. Leversedge FJ, Moore TJ, Peterson BC, et al. Compartment syndrome of the upper extremity. *J Hand Surg.* 2011;36A:544–560.
19. Whitesides TE, Haney TC, Harada H, et al. A simple method for tissue pressure determination. *Arch Surg.* 1975;110:1311–1315.
20. Kalyani BS, Fisher BE, Roberts CS, et al. Compartment syndrome of the forearm: a systematic review. *J Hand Surg.* 2011;36A:535–543.
21. Ronel DN, Mtui E, Nolan WB. Forearm compartment syndrome: anatomical analysis of surgical approaches to the deep space. *Plast Reconstr Surg.* 2004;114:697–705.
22. Jones MD, Santamarina R, Warhold LG. Surgical decompression of the forearm, hand and digits for compartment syndrome. In: Wiesel SW, ed. *Operative Techniques in Orthopaedic Surgery.* Philadelphia, PA: Lippincott Williams & Wilkins; 2011:2875–2881.

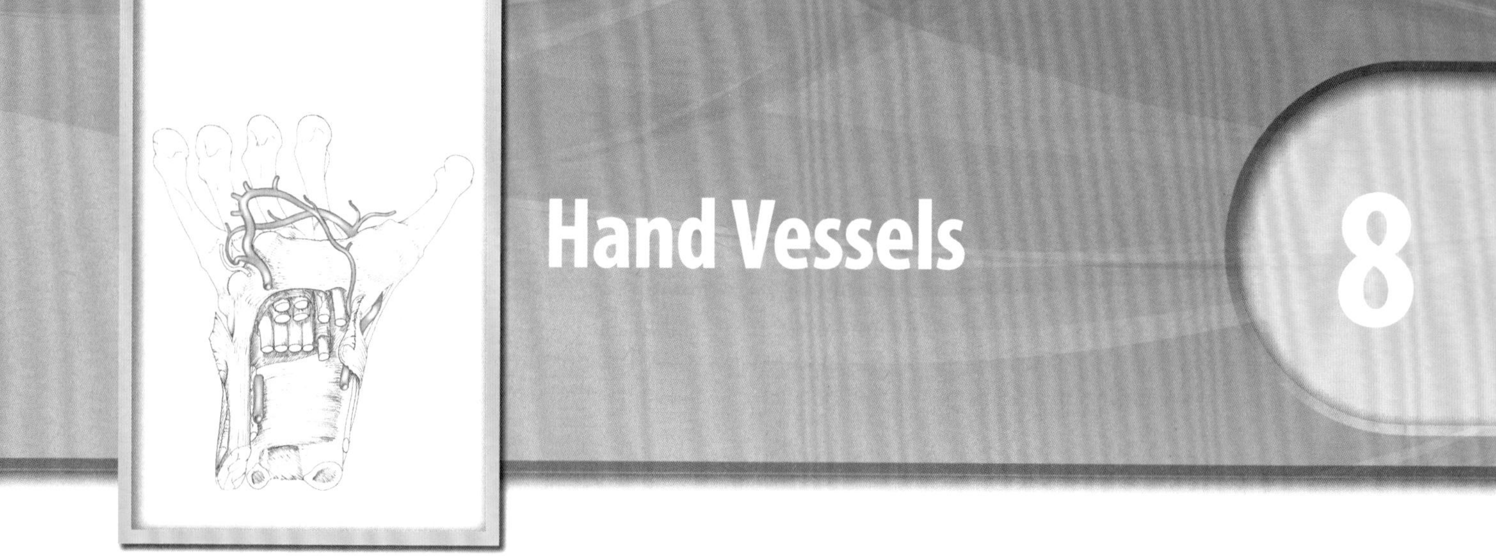

Hand Vessels

Vascular Anatomy of the Hand

The anatomy of the hand is complex, and the ramification of the blood vessels within the tightly packed musculoskeletal structures is difficult to visualize. The following discussion presents hand anatomy as a framework for understanding the paths of the blood vessels.

Cutaneous Nerves of the Hand

The superficial innervation of the hand is relevant to the vascular surgeon in choosing an approach to the underlying vessels. Sensation is more critical to the function of the hand than to any other area of the body. All three major nerves of the arm provide sensation to areas of the hand, and the nerve branches in adjacent territories interconnect.

On the volar surface of the hand (Fig. 8-1), two major areas are supplied by the median and ulnar nerves. The division lies along the middle of the ring finger. A palmar cutaneous branch arises from the median nerve in the midforearm. This branch penetrates the deep fascia at the wrist and supplies the skin over the thenar eminence. The remainder of the palm and the volar surface of the fingers are innervated by the common and proper digital nerves branching from the main trunks of the median and ulnar nerves beneath the palmar fascia. The superficial palmaris brevis muscle at the base of the hypothenar eminence is innervated by the ulnar nerve. The radial side of the thenar eminence and dorsal thumb is served by the lateral branch of the superficial radial nerve.

The dorsum of the hand is supplied by the ulnar and radial nerves. The dorsal branch of the ulnar

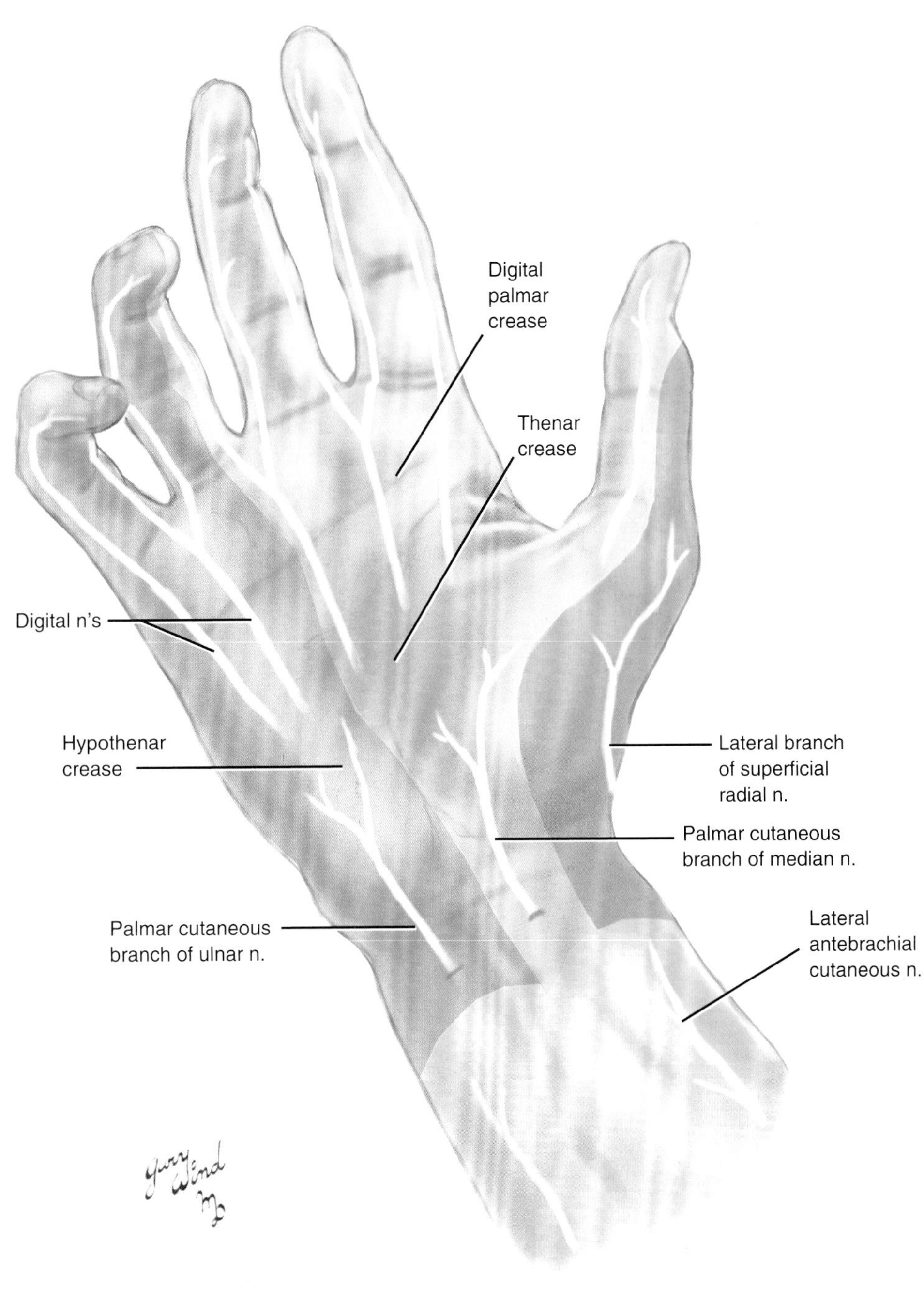

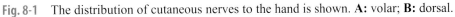

Fig. 8-1 The distribution of cutaneous nerves to the hand is shown. **A:** volar; **B:** dorsal.

nerve arises in the distal forearm 5 cm from the wrist flexion crease and passes between the flexor carpi ulnaris and the distal ulna to reach the ulnar side of the dorsum of the hand. Its territory is again marked by the midline of the ring finger. The superficial branch of the radial nerve passes under the tendon of the brachioradialis muscle and crosses the anatomic snuffbox. It divides over the first extensor compartment into the lateral branch described previously and a larger medial division that supplies the remainder of the dorsum. A peculiarity of this distribution is that the distal phalanges of the index and middle fingers and the radial half of the ring finger are supplied by the median nerve. The superficial radial nerve is at risk of injury when surgically approaching the radial artery in the anatomic snuffbox.

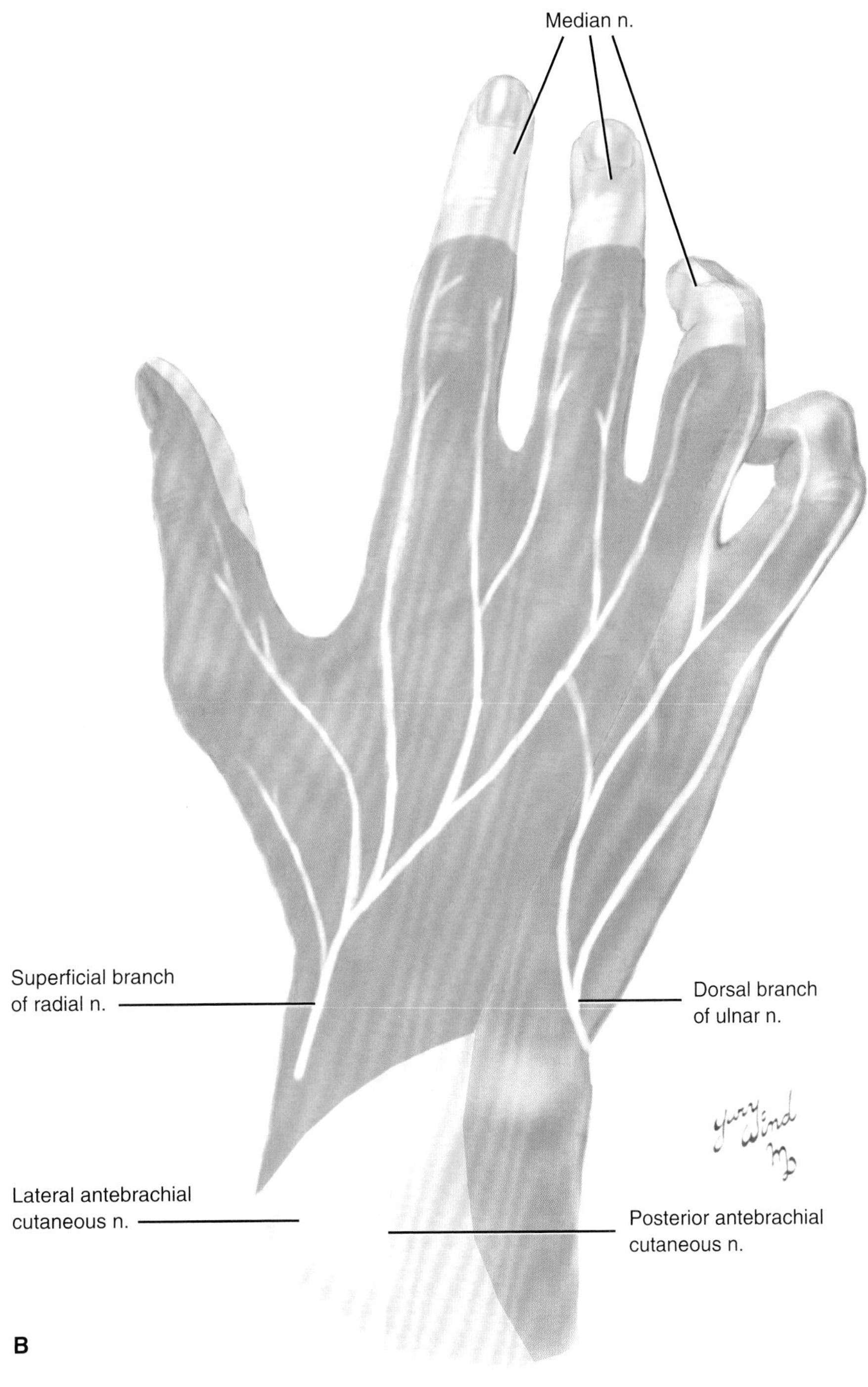

Fig. 8-1 *(continued)*

Bones of the Hand

The key to understanding the bony framework of the hand is the carpal arch (Fig. 8-2). The deep volar concavity of the carpal bones forms the channel through which the major tendons pass from forearm to hand and establishes the foundation for opposition between the thumb and little finger. The tunnel for the flexor tendons is closed by a dense transverse ligament extending from the trapezium and scaphoid tubercle radially to the pisiform bone and hook of the hamate bone on the ulnar end of the arch. Note that the pisiform bone and hook of the hamate bone are not aligned axially relative to the ulna but angle toward the base of the third metacarpal.

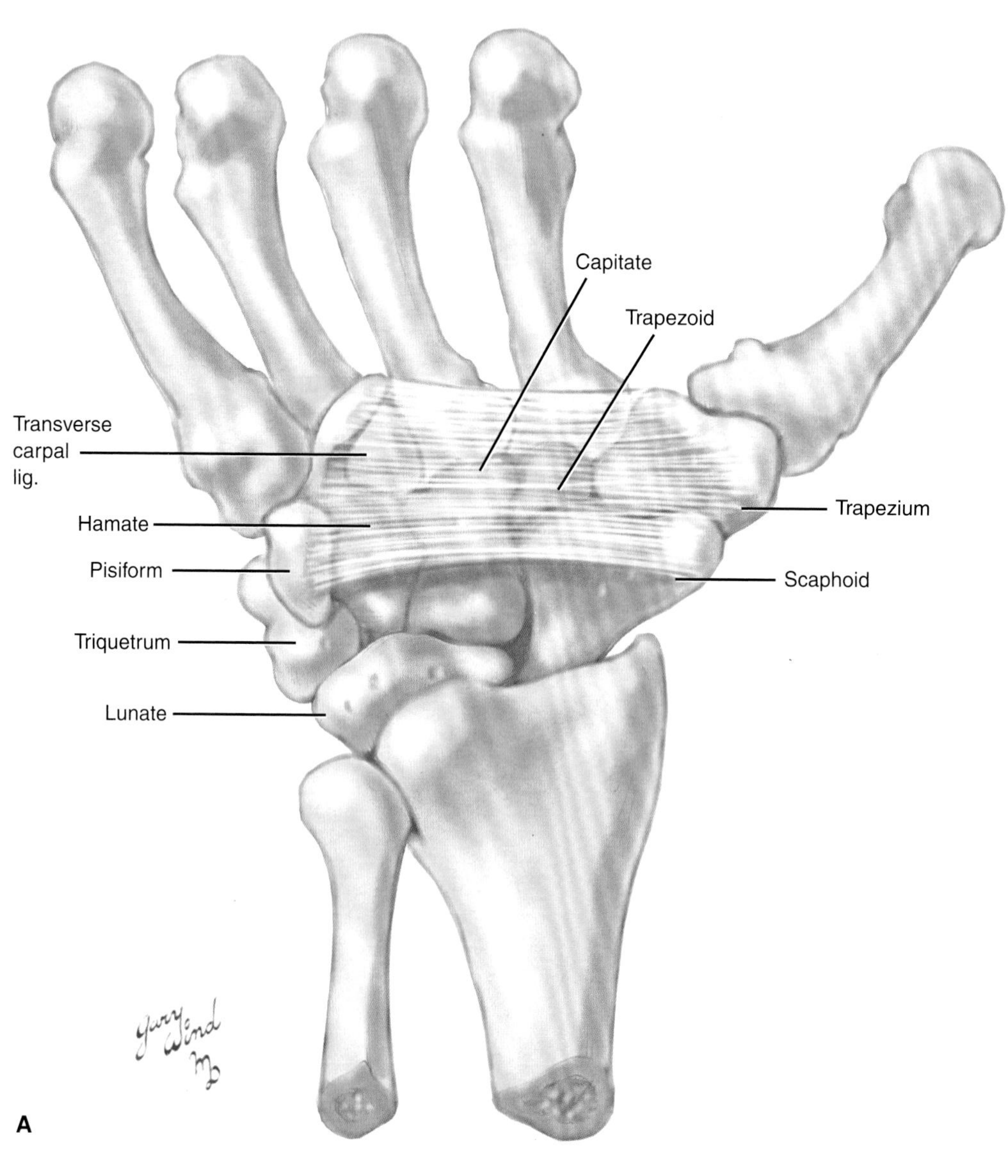

Fig. 8-2 The carpal bones form a deep arch that cradles the long flexor tendons. **A:** volar; **B:** proximal view.

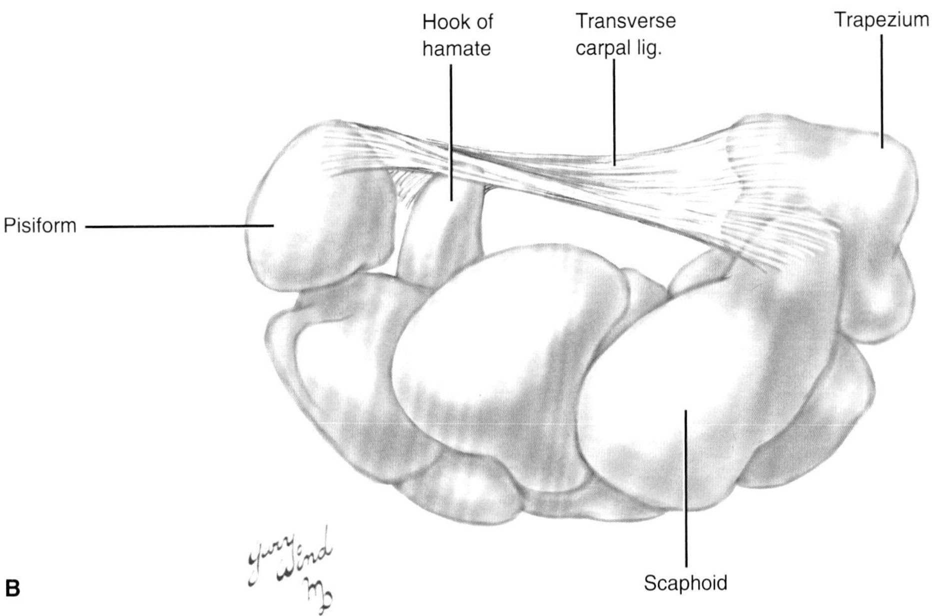

Fig. 8-2 *(continued)*

Fascia

The deep fascia of the forearm is thickened around the wrist, forming the extensor retinaculum on the dorsum and the volar carpal ligament on the volar side (Fig. 8-3). The palmaris longus tendon fuses with the volar carpal ligament at the wrist and fans out over the central palm, reinforcing the deep fascia there and forming the palmar aponeurosis. This layer of investing fascia is distinct from the underlying transverse carpal ligament, which bridges the carpal arch from end to end and forms the restraining retinaculum for the flexor tendons. The transverse carpal ligament is derived from carpal ligaments with a contribution from the tendon of flexor carpi ulnaris muscle, whereas the volar carpal ligament is a thickened band of deep fascia. The only complexity in this relationship is the midline adherence between the palmar aponeurosis and the transverse carpal ligament. This adherence creates a canal on the ulnar side of the wrist, with the ulnar artery and nerve sandwiched between the two fascial layers (the canal of Guyon). The radial attachment of the transverse carpal ligament divides to accommodate the passage of the flexor carpi radialis tendon through a separate tunnel.

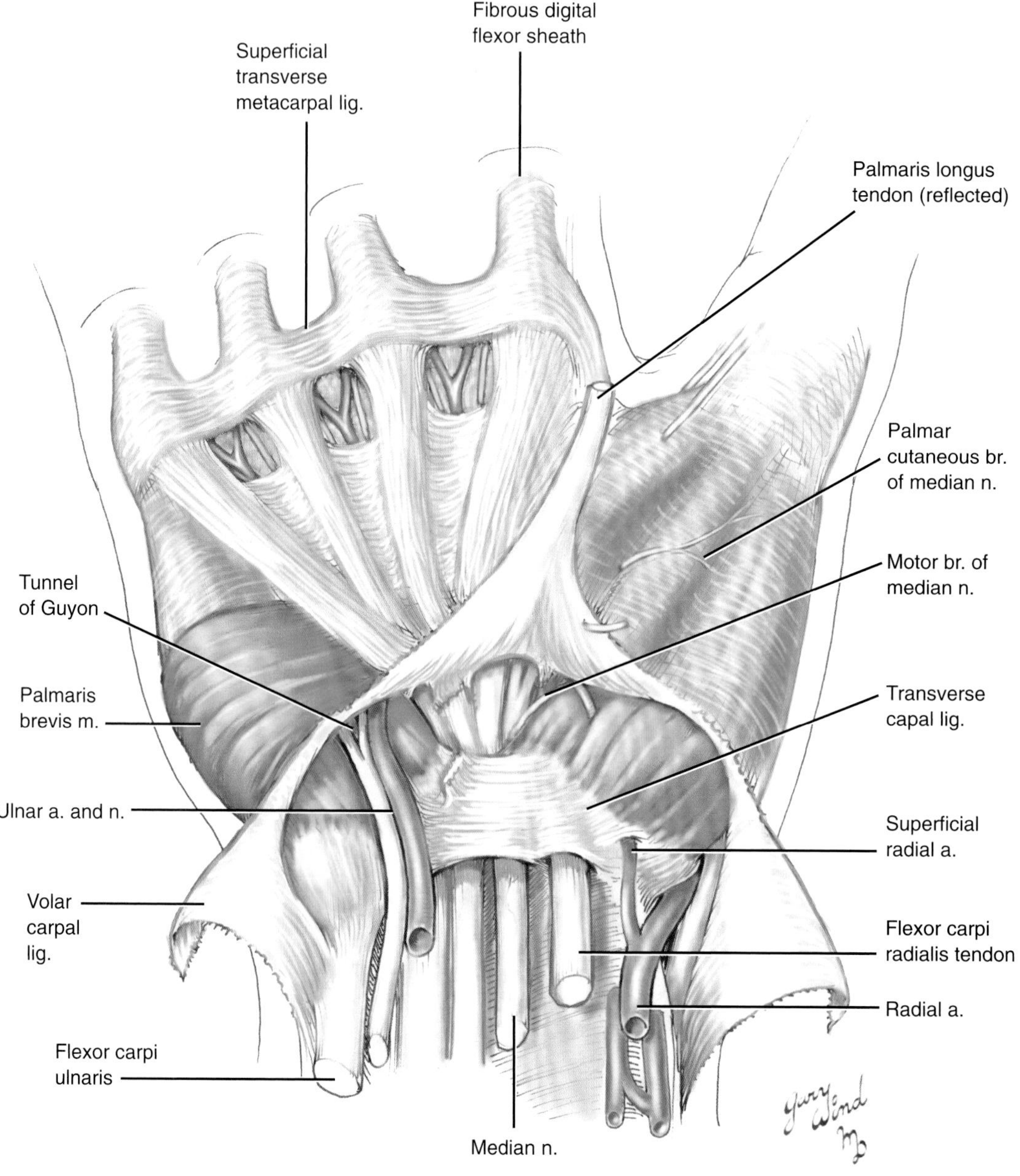

Fig. 8-3 The volar carpal ligament is a thickening of the deep fascia and is superficial to the transverse carpal ligament, which closes the carpal arch.

Beyond the wrist, the palm is divided into three compartments by two fascial septa that span between the palmar aponeurosis and the first and fifth metacarpals, respectively (Fig. 8-4). These septa separate the thenar and hypothenar spaces from the central palmar compartment. The eight digital flexors are enclosed in a common bursa and fill the central compartment. The lumbrical muscles, digital nerves, and vessels also occupy this space.

A deep oblique connective tissue septum runs between the undersurface of the common bursa and the shaft of the middle metacarpal. This septum divides the plane between flexor tendons and the metacarpal/interossei layer into the midpalmar space on the ulnar side and the thenar space on the radial side. These potential spaces are the sites of deep hand infections.

The palmar aponeurosis coalesces into four bands in the distal palm. These overlie and contribute to the fibrous flexor tendon sheaths at the distal end of the metacarpals. The interdigital space between the bands encloses the underlying digital nerves, arteries, and lumbrical muscles. Between the flexor sheaths, superficial and deep transverse metacarpal ligaments create three closed passages for these structures. The lumbrical muscles pass above the deep transverse metacarpal ligaments, and the tendons of the interosseous muscles pass below.

The radial bursa, the second palmar bursa, encloses the single tendon of the flexor pollicis

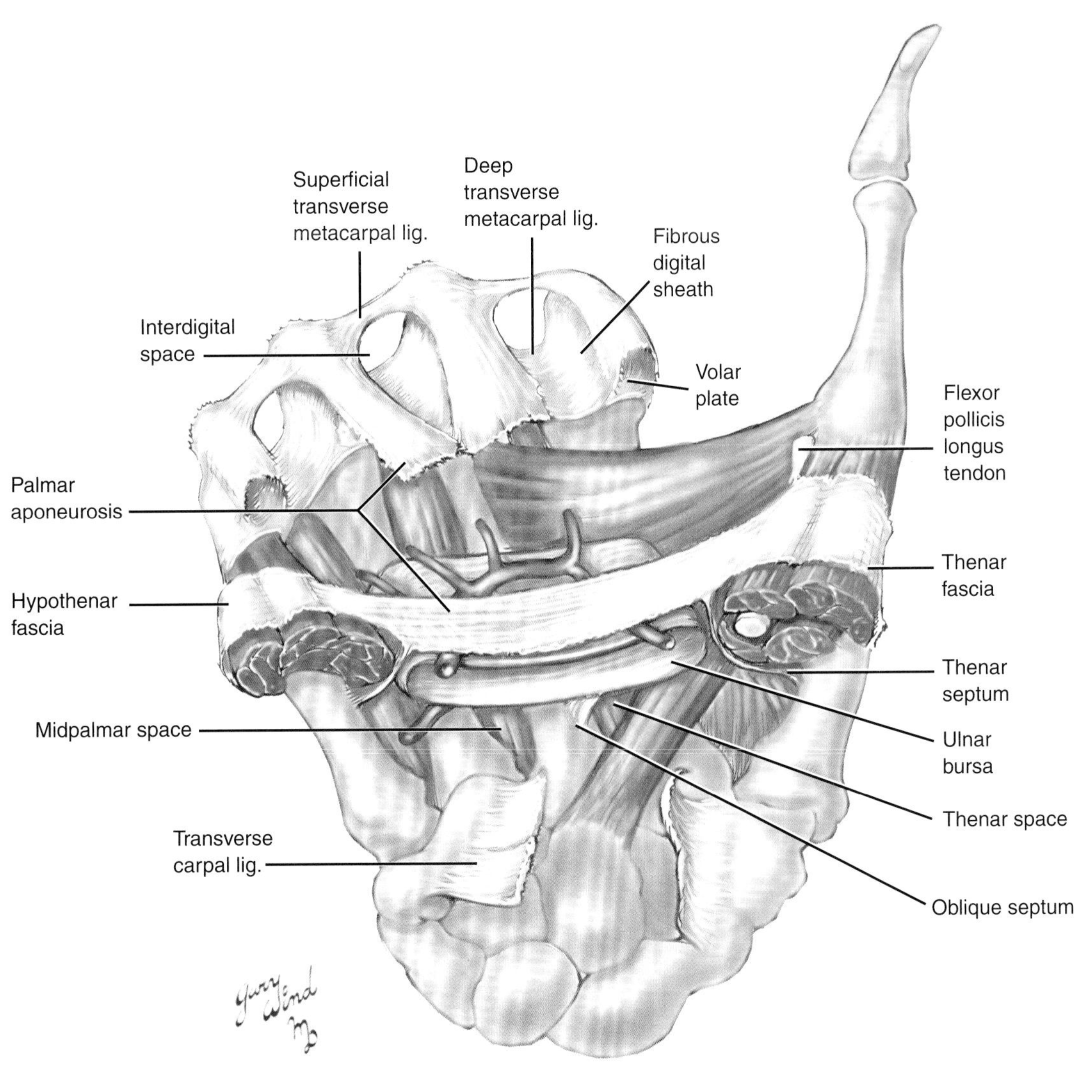

Fig. 8-4 The fascial compartments of the palm are shown.

longus muscle and passes between the heads of the flexor pollicis brevis muscle. This bursa and tendon are thus contained within the thenar compartment.

Intrinsic Hand Muscles

Three muscles, an abductor, flexor, and opponens, constitute both the thenar and hypothenar groups (Fig. 8-5). These muscles arise from both the end bones of the carpal arch and from the transverse carpal ligament. The hypothenar muscles are pierced at their base by the deep branches of the ulnar artery and nerve. The artery forms one side of the deep palmar arch, which lies in the potential space between the ulnar bursa and the metacarpal plane.

The recurrent motor branch of the median nerve arises just beyond the distal edge of the transverse carpal ligament and supplies the thenar muscles. The most volar of the thenar muscles, the abductor pollicis brevis muscle, is usually penetrated by the superficial thenar branch of the radial artery on its way to complete the superficial palmar arch. The thumb is moved by one additional intrinsic muscle,

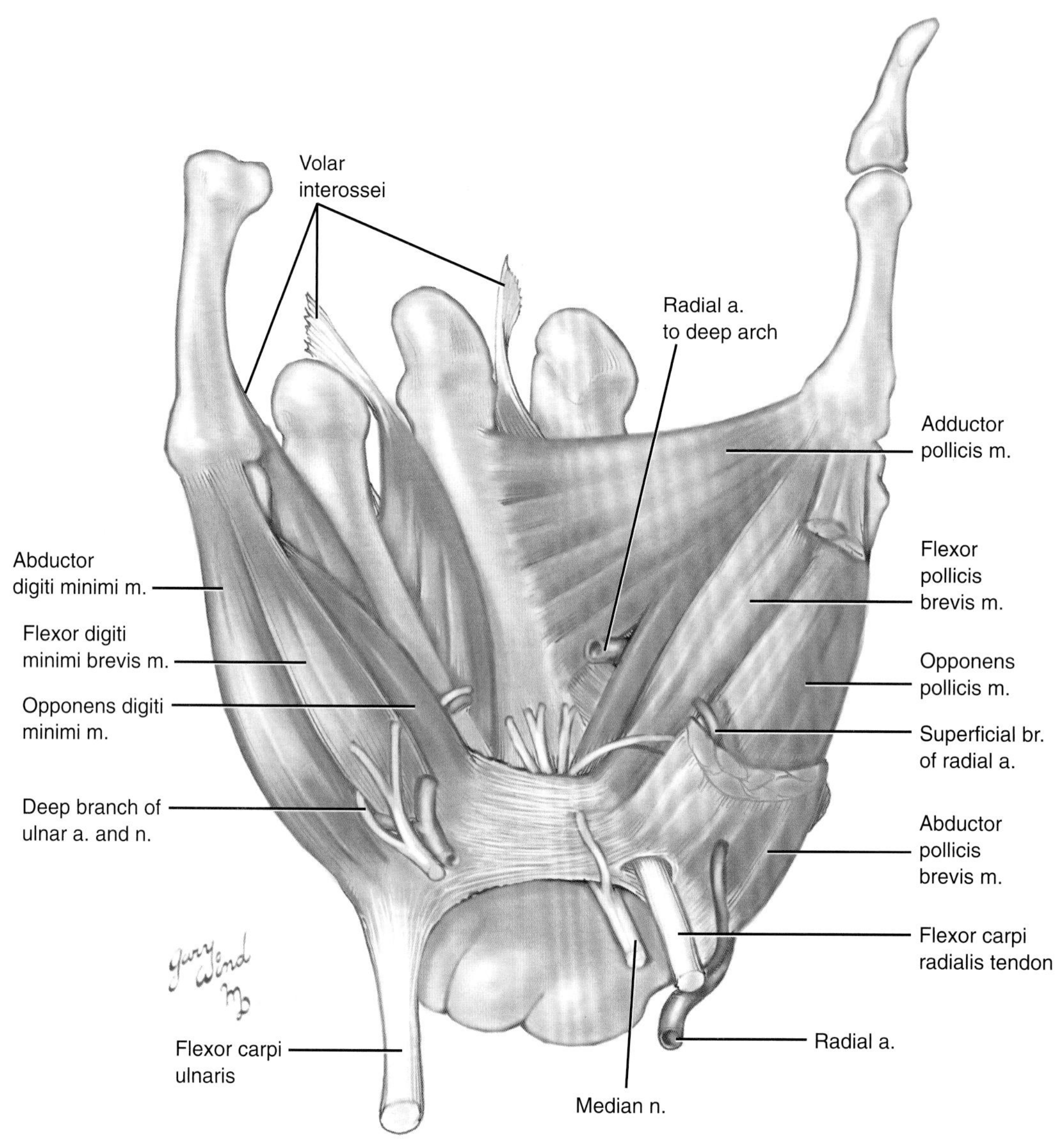

Fig. 8-5 The intrinsic muscles of the hand form a cup to contain the central tendons, nerves, and vessels.

the adductor pollicis. The radial artery reaches the deep palm between the transverse and oblique heads of the adductor. The ulnar nerve supplies the hypothenar muscles, all the interossei, the adductor pollicis muscle, the deep head of the flexor pollicis brevis muscle, and the two ulnar lumbrical muscles. The radial lumbrical muscles are supplied by the median nerve.

Path of the Radial Artery

The radial artery passes around the radial side of the carpal bones under the tendons of abductor pollicis longus and extensor pollicis brevis muscles (Fig. 8-6). The vessel then lies over the scaphoid in the depression between the extensor pollicis brevis and extensor pollicis longus tendons known as the

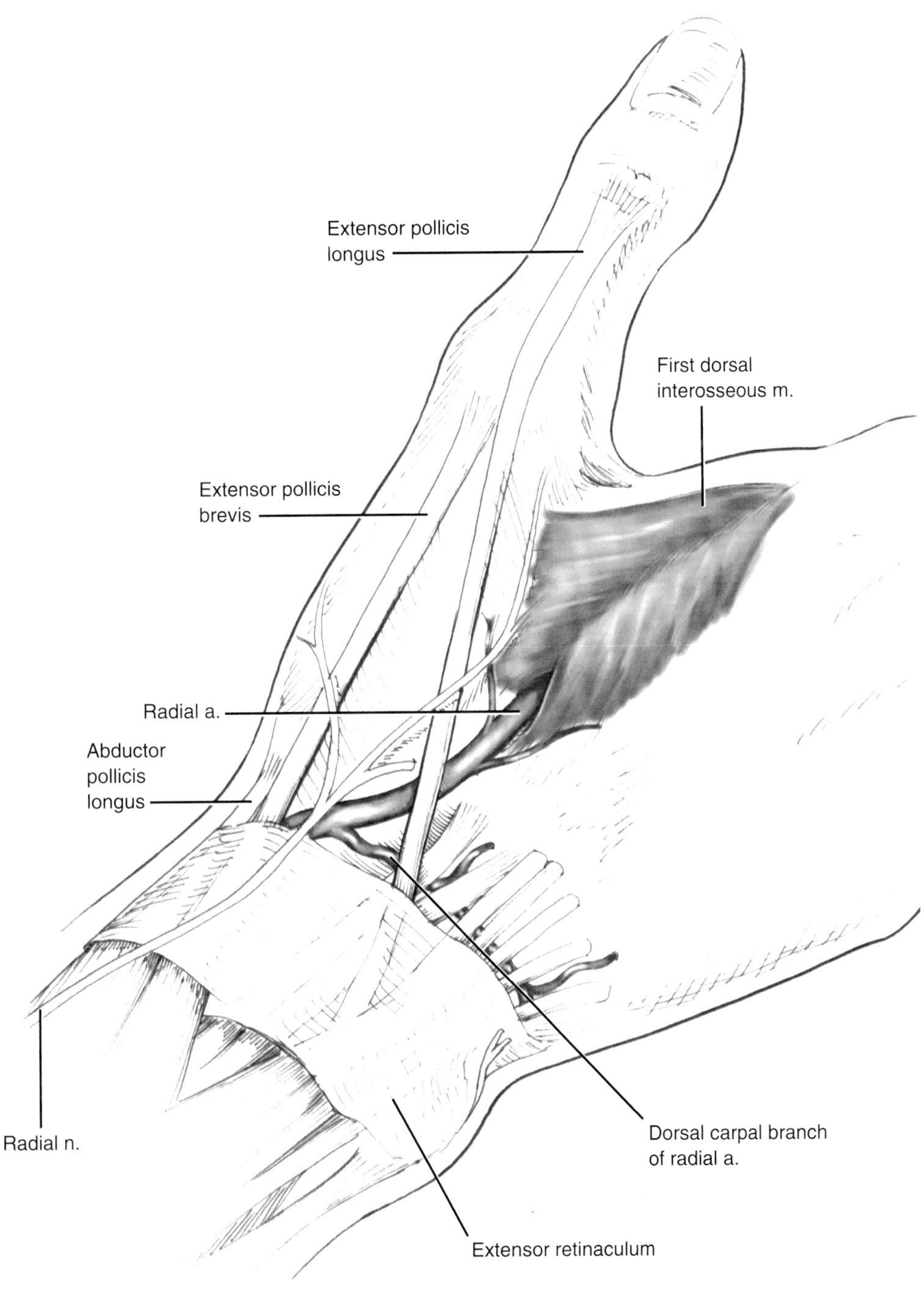

Fig. 8-6 The radial artery turns around the lateral border of the carpal bones and passes between the first two metacarpals to reach the palm.

anatomic snuffbox. There it gives off a dorsal carpal branch that runs beneath the extensor tendons. The superficial branch of the radial nerve overlies the artery outside the deep fascia. The artery then crosses beneath the tendon of extensor pollicis longus muscle and dives between the two heads of the first dorsal interosseous muscle and through the first two metacarpals toward the deep palmar space.

After passing between the metacarpals, the radial artery gives off two branches deep to the adductor pollicis muscle, the princeps pollicis and radialis indicis arteries. These branches may have a common origin (Fig. 8-7). The continuation of the radial artery passes between the heads of the adductor muscle to become one end of the deep palmar arch.

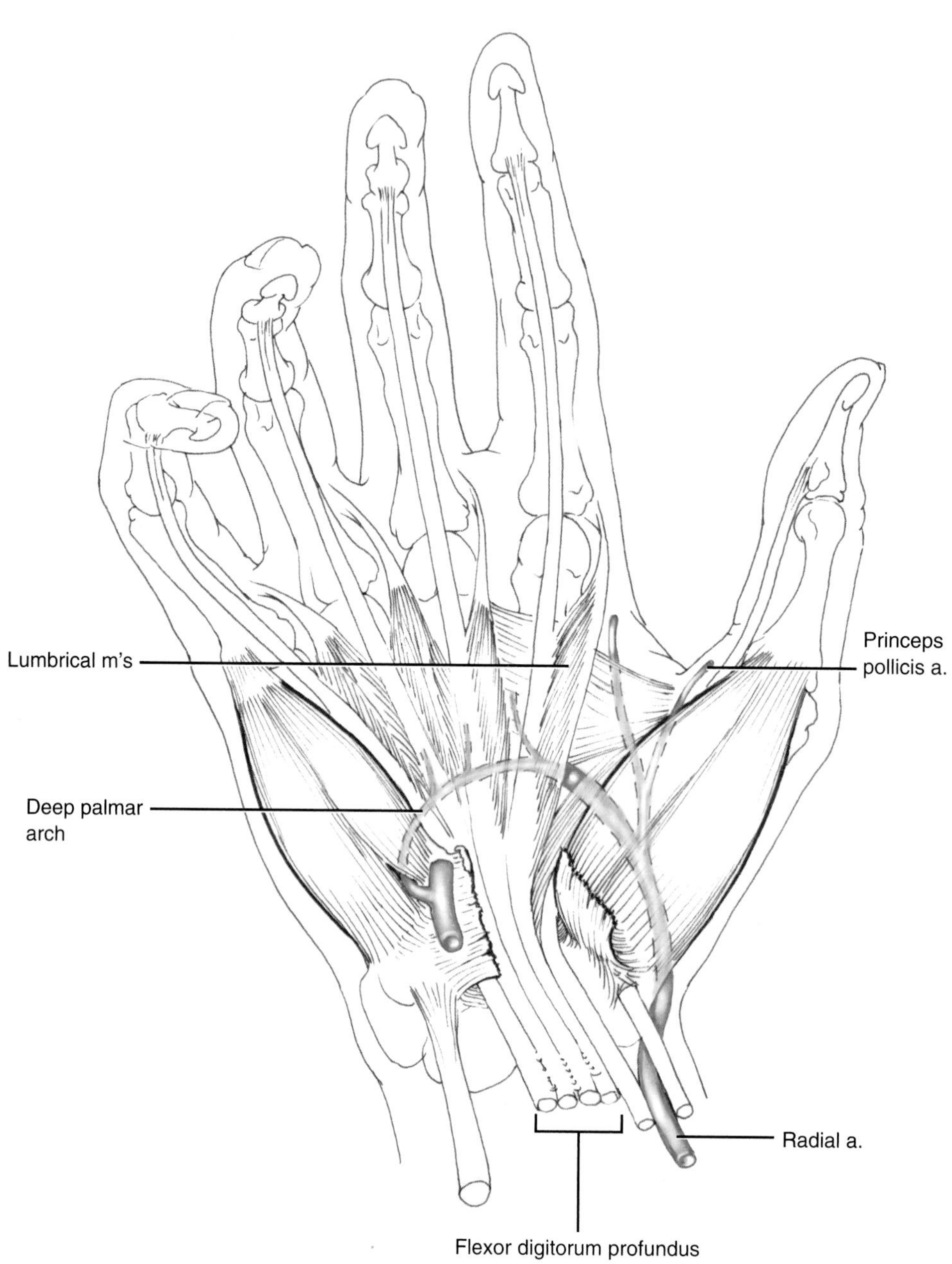

Fig. 8-7 The radial artery gives off two digital branches (shown with a common trunk) deep to the adductor pollicis muscle.

Palmar Arches

The superficial palmar arch has a dominant ulnar supply and a small radial end that may be absent in some cases[1] (Fig. 8-8). The apex of the superficial arch is at the level of the proximal palmar crease.

The deep arch has a dominant radial supply and is slightly more proximal, lying just beyond the bases of the metacarpals. The eight digital flexor tendons and the median nerve branches pass between the two arches.

Unroofing the palmar fascia reveals the superficial palmar arch lying on the digital nerves

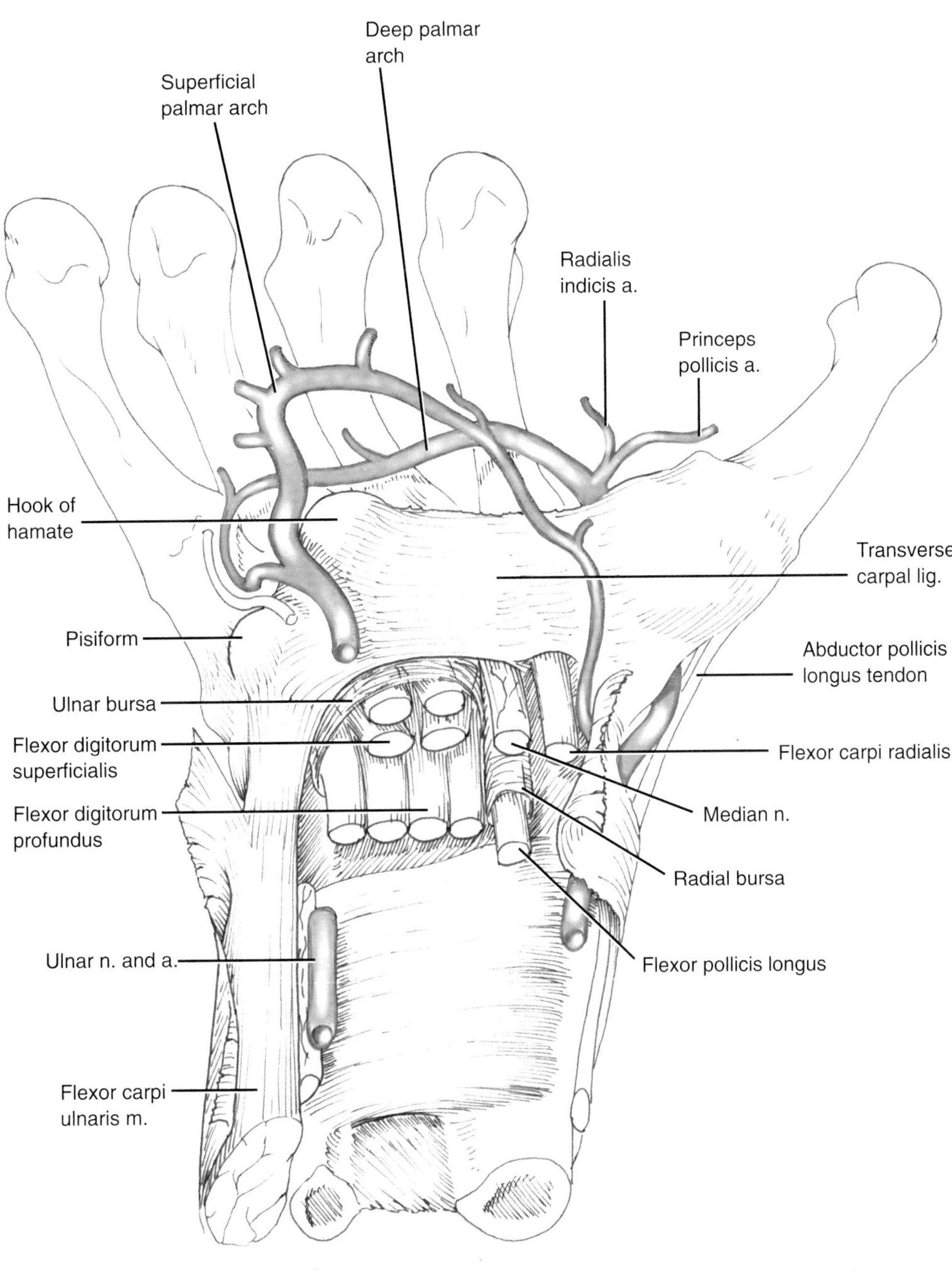

Fig. 8-8 The long digital flexors, lumbrical muscles, and digital nerves lie between the two palmar arches.

and flexor tendons (Fig. 8-9). The ulnar end of the arch starts in the cleft between the volar carpal ligament and transverse carpal ligament, crosses the base of the hypothenar muscles, and turns across the central palmar structures to meet the superficial branch of the radial artery. Remember that the arch is penetrating both the hypothenar and thenar septa connecting the palmar fascia to the first and fifth metacarpals in its course across the palm. The digital vessels lie superficial to the nerves near the arch

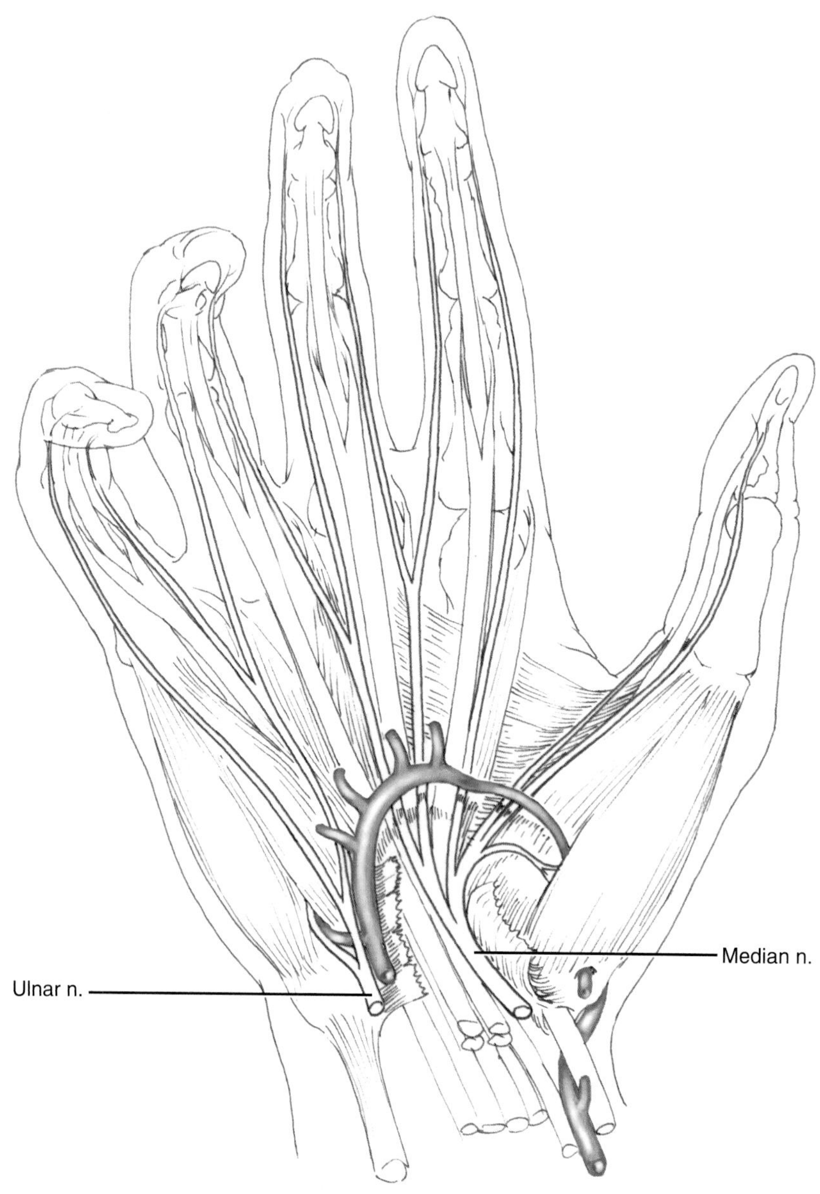

Fig. 8-9 The superficial arch lies just beneath the palmar aponeurosis.

but assume a dorsal position relative to the digital nerves in the fingers.

There is a rich communication at the base of the metacarpophalangeal joints between the branches of the deep and superficial arches in the palm (Fig. 8-10). In addition, there are anastomoses between the metacarpals from the deep arch branches to the dorsal arterial network.

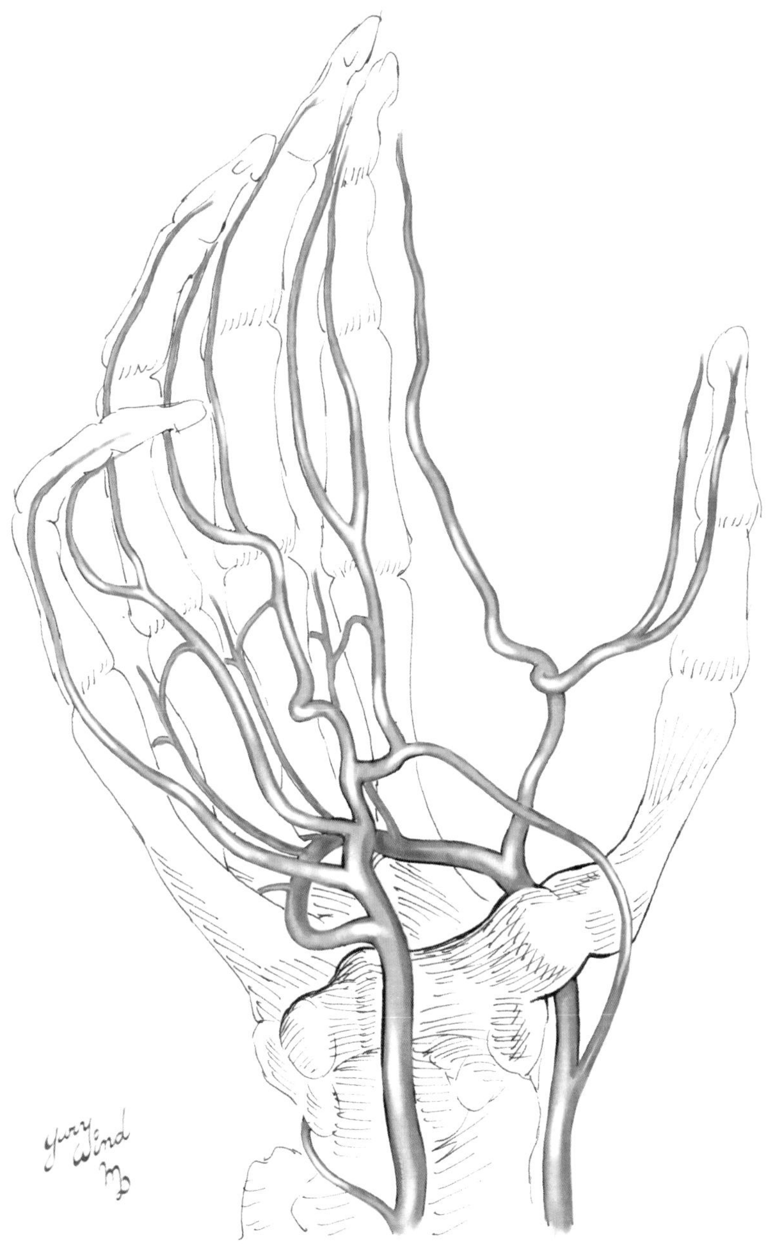

Fig. 8-10 There is a rich intercommunication among the vessels of the hand.

Exposure of Hand Arteries

There are two situations in which the vascular surgeon may become involved with exposure of arteries in the hand: creation of arteriovenous fistulae and resection of aneurysms or irregular arterial segments associated with finger embolization. Creation of a radiocephalic arteriovenous fistula within the anatomic snuffbox has been recommended because it results in a long segment of arterialized vein for access and because it spares more proximal vessels for secondary operations.[2] Repetitive blunt trauma on the ulnar aspect of the hand can result in formation of aneurysms or intimal irregularities in the ulnar artery at the level of the hamate bone.[3] The lesions associated with this so-called hypothenar hammer syndrome may thrombose or cause digital embolization, leading to finger gangrene.[4] Although this syndrome has been attributed to repetitive occupational trauma in patients with underlying arterial abnormalities,[4] some cases can arise from recreational activities or after a single traumatic episode.[5]

Exposure of the Radial Artery in the Anatomic Snuffbox

The patient is placed in the supine position with the arm abducted and placed on a supporting board. The arm should be pronated to allow the hand to rest on its ulnar surface, and the entire hand and forearm are prepped and draped.

A 3-cm longitudinal incision is made over the anatomic snuffbox, extending from the radial styloid to the base of the first metacarpal (Fig. 8-11).

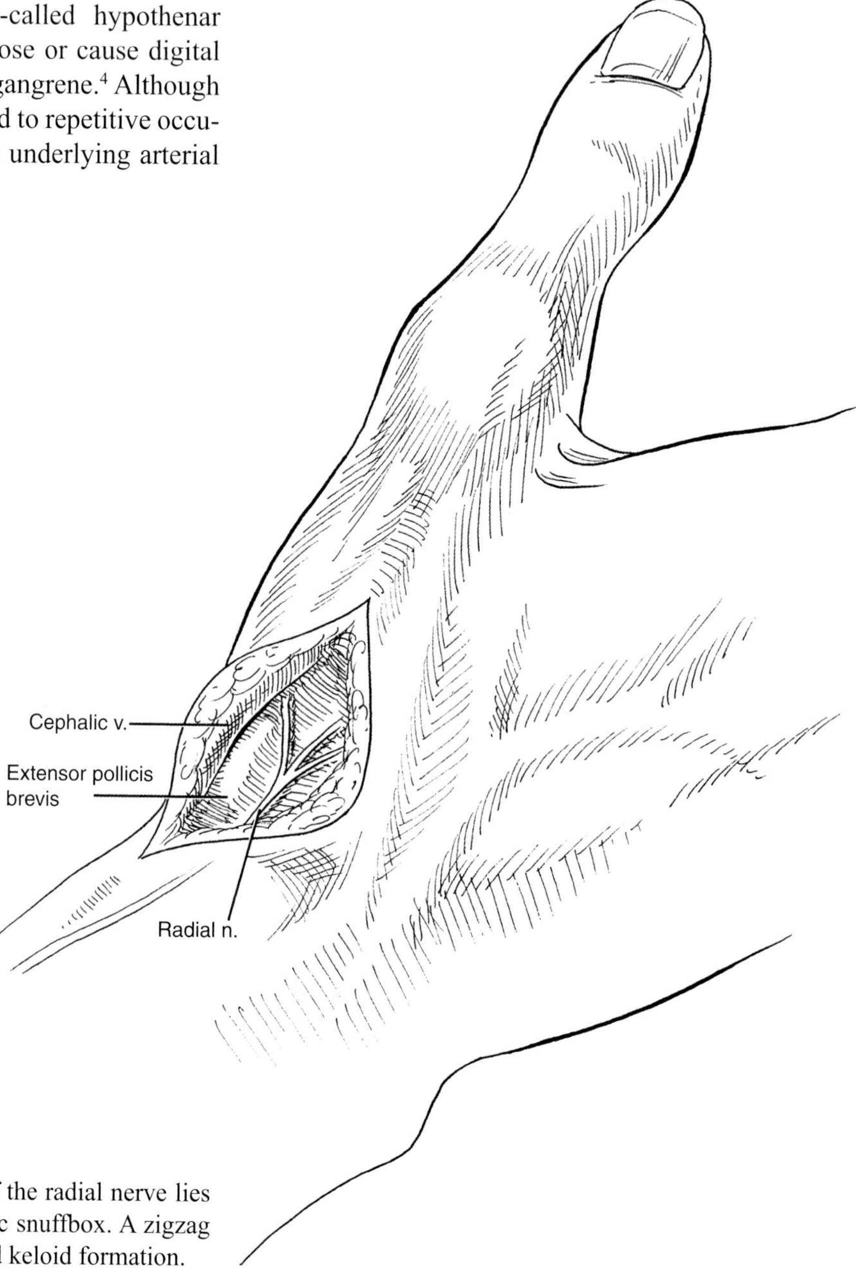

Fig. 8-11 The superficial branch of the radial nerve lies on the deep fascia over the anatomic snuffbox. A zigzag incision over this area helps to avoid keloid formation.

The cephalic vein of the thumb is located in the subcutaneous tissues and fully mobilized in cases involving arteriovenous fistula creation. Digital branches of the superficial radial nerve are identified on the surface of the deep fascia and protected. The nerves may require mobilization and gentle retraction toward the palmar or dorsal surface, depending on their location. The deep fascia is incised between the extensor pollicis longus and extensor pollicis brevis muscles to expose the radial artery (Fig. 8-12). Mobilization of the radial artery requires ligation of the dorsal carpal branch.

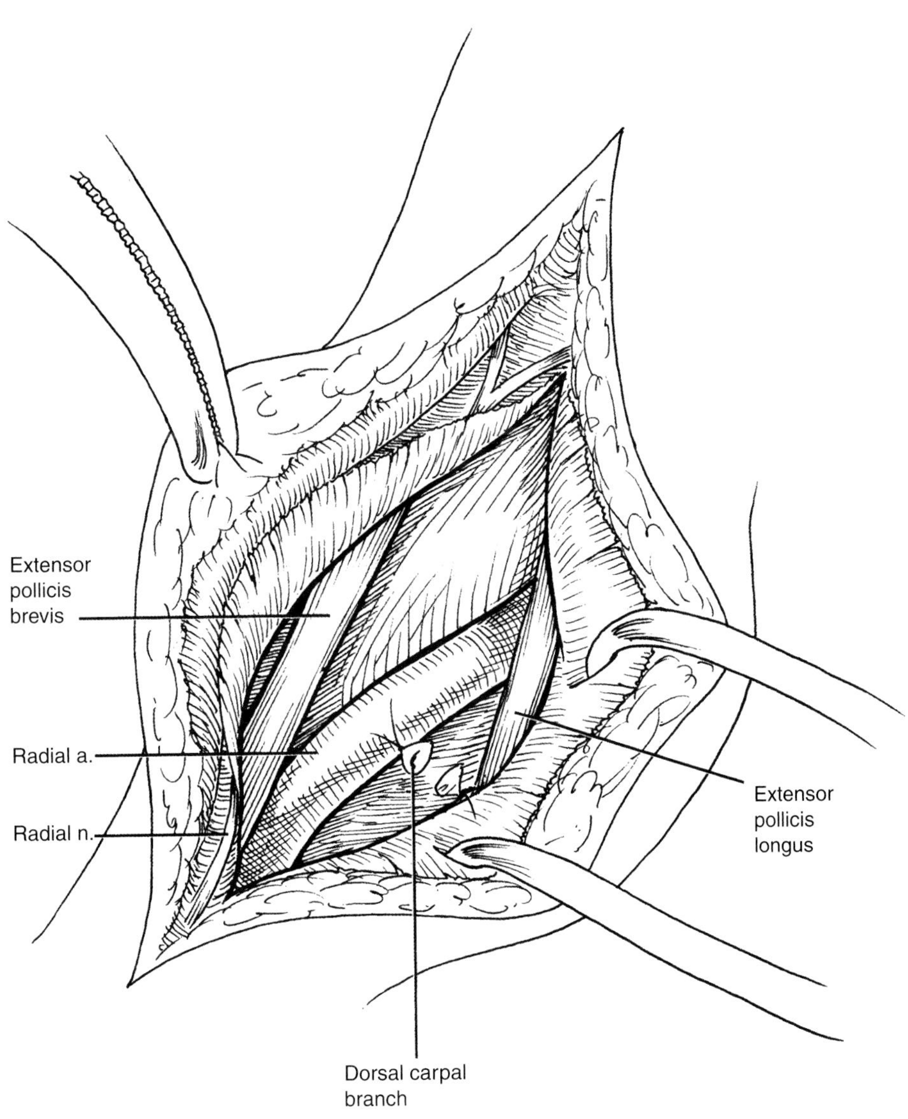

Fig. 8-12 The fascia is opened to expose the radial artery, and the dorsal carpal branch is divided.

Exposure of the Radial Artery in the Distal Hand

The patient is positioned and prepped as previously described. A longitudinal incision is made parallel to the second metacarpal on the dorsal surface of the first interosseous space (Fig. 8-13). The incision should begin at the level of the extensor pollicis longus muscle and extend approximately 3 cm. Superficial veins should be preserved and retracted in the subcutaneous tissue to expose the deep fascia. The fascia is incised between the two heads of the first dorsal interosseous muscle, which are carefully separated and retracted to expose the radial artery.

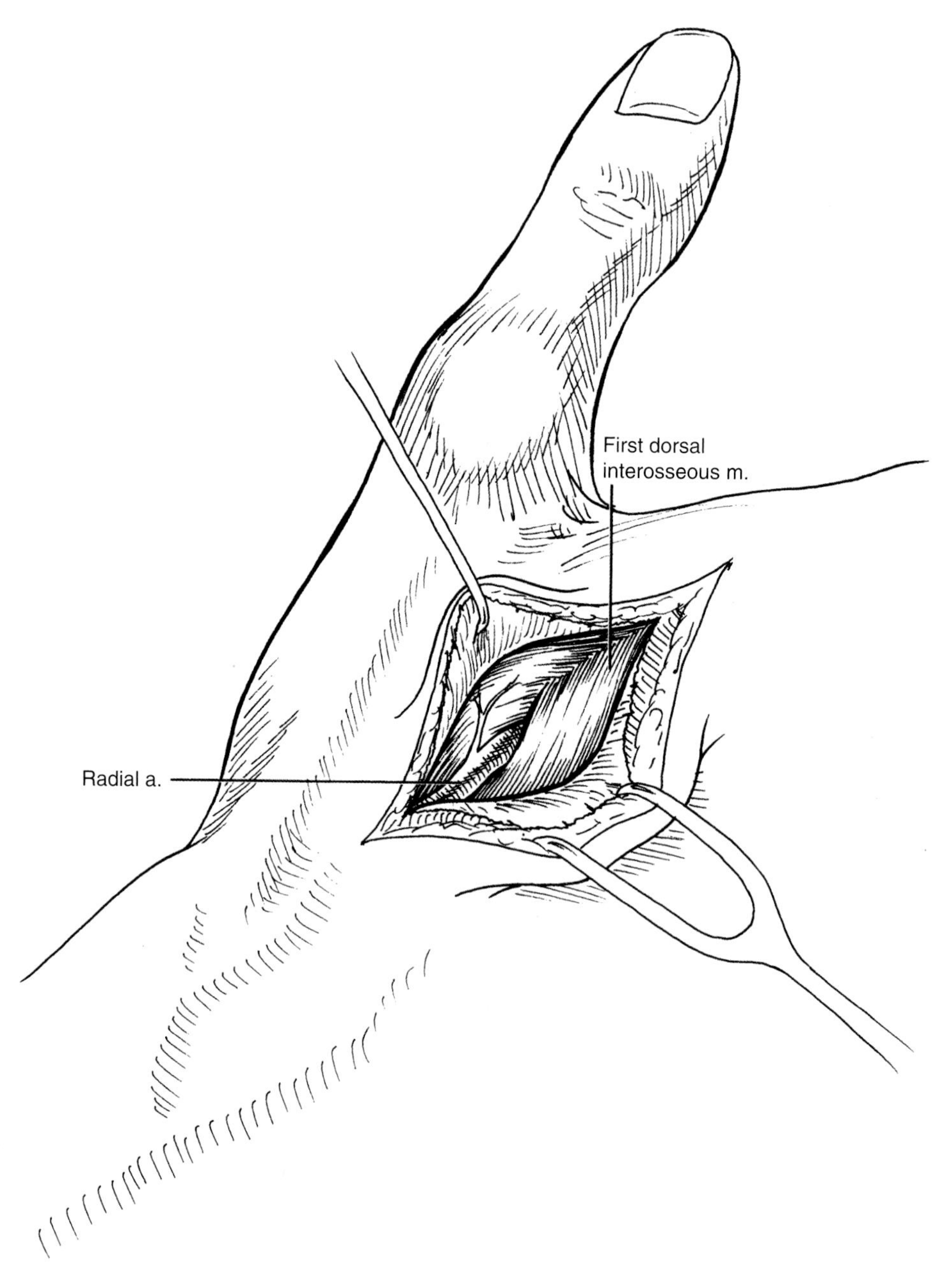

Fig. 8-13 The segment of radial artery beyond the extensor pollicis longus tendon is exposed.

Exposure of the Ulnar Artery and Superficial Palmar Arch

After the hand and forearm are prepped and draped, the hand is placed with the palmar surface up. An oblique incision is made in the hypothenar crease, extending from the radial border of the pisiform bone to the distal transverse palmar crease, crossing the proximal transverse crease obliquely to avoid scar contracture complications (Fig. 8-14). The incision is deepened to the level of the palmaris brevis muscle. The ulnar artery can be identified at the proximal edge of the muscle and traced distally as the muscle is incised. It is important to confine the dissection close to the palmar surface of the ulnar artery to avoid injuring its several branches. Palmar digital nerves of the superficial ulnar nerve course on the ulnar side of the ulnar artery and should be carefully preserved. By dividing

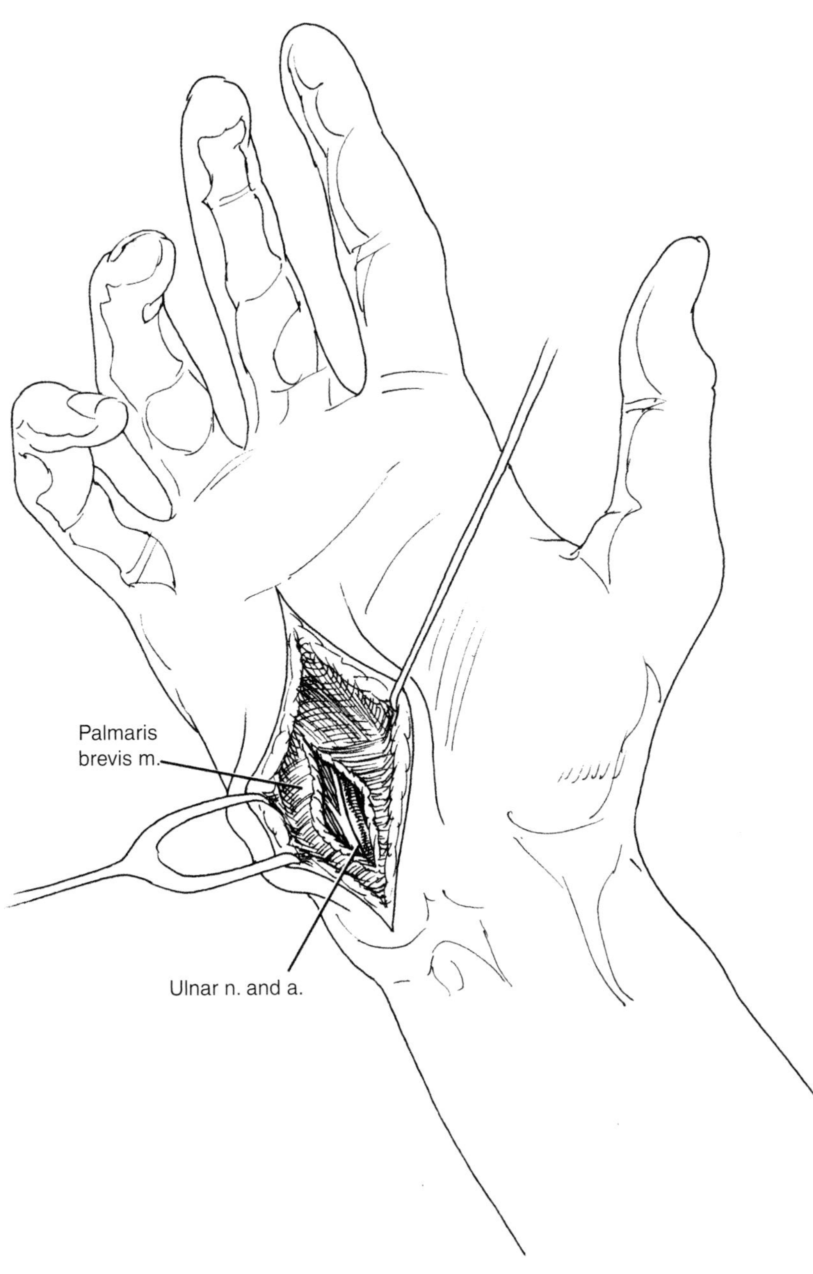

Fig. 8-14 The ulnar artery and nerve beyond the canal of Guyon are exposed beneath the palmaris brevis muscle and hypothenar fascia.

fibers of the palmar aponeurosis, the artery can be traced beyond the fifth digital artery branch, where it becomes the superficial palmar arch (Fig. 8-15). Digital branches of the median nerve course beneath the superficial palmar arch in this area and should be preserved.

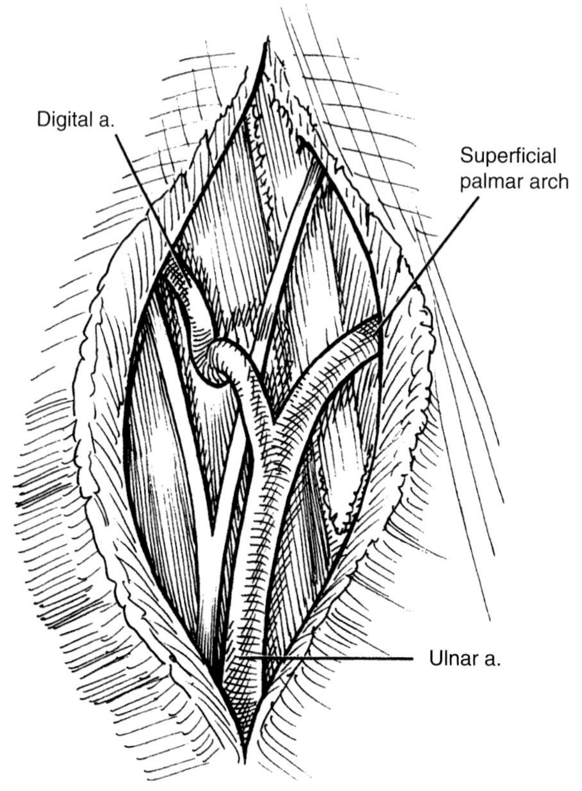

Fig. 8-15 The continuation of the ulnar artery toward the superficial palmar arch is exposed by opening through the hypothenar compartment septum into the palmar aponeurosis.

References

1. Gellman H, Botte MJ, Shankwiler J, et al. Arterial patterns of the deep and superficial palmar arches. *Clin Orthop.* 2001;383:41–46.
2. Wolowczyk L, Williams AJ, Donovan KL, et al. The snuffbox arteriovenous fistula for vascular access. *Eur J Endovasc Surg.* 2000;19:70–76.
3. Cooke RA. Hypothenar hammer syndrome: a discrete syndrome to be distinguished from hand-arm vibration syndrome. *Occup Med.* 2003;53:320–324.
4. Marie I, Herve F, Primard E, et al. Long-term follow-up of hypothenar hammer syndrome: a series of 47 patients. *Medicine.* 2007; 86:334–343.
5. Custer T, Channer LT, Hartranft T. Hypothenar hammer syndrome. Case report and literature review. *Vasc Surg.* 1999;33:567–577.

VESSELS OF THE ABDOMEN

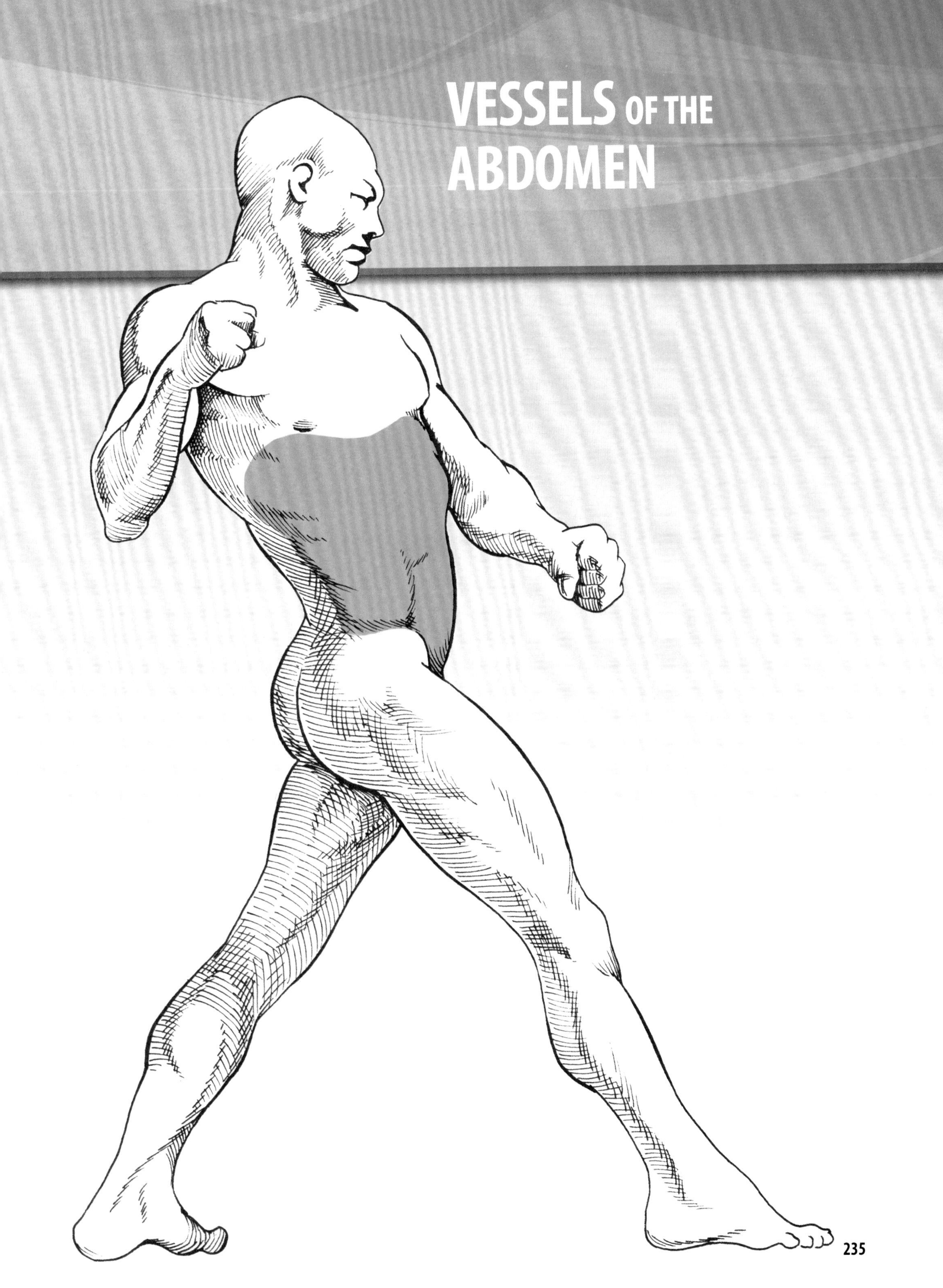

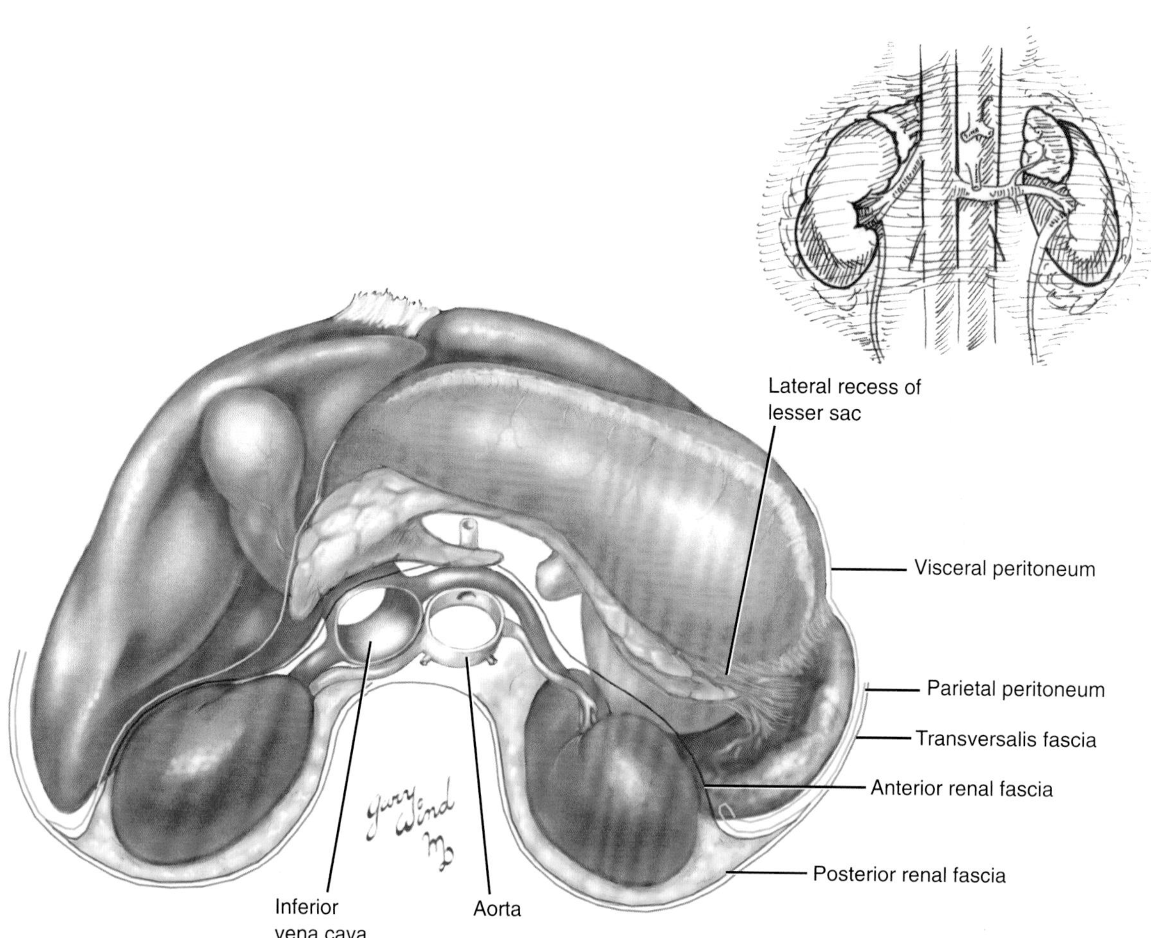

Fig. 9-1 The upper abdominal organs are arrayed around the central core of the great vessels. Note the relationship of the anterior renal fascia to the vessels in the retroperitoneum.

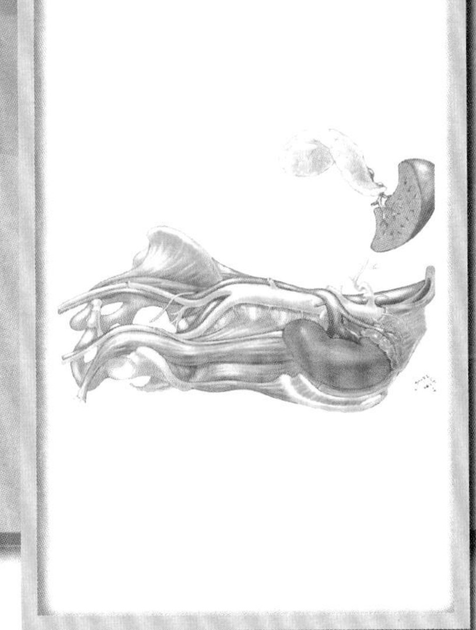

9 Upper Abdominal Aorta, Including the Visceral and Supraceliac Segments

Surgical Anatomy of the Abdominal Aorta

In its short span, the abdominal aorta is the center of some of the most complex anatomic relationships in the body. The unique problems of access to the various segments are dealt with separately in the following chapters. Before focusing on regional details, it is useful to review the disposition of the abdominal aorta in the context of the whole abdomen.

Overview

The aorta occupies a central position in the abdominal cavity. In the upper abdomen, the major organs are arranged in a semicircle around the great vessels and fill the domes of the diaphragm beneath the rib cage (Fig. 9-1). The vessels lie within the continuations of anterior and posterior renal fascia (Gerota's fascia) across the midline.[1] The viscera on the left side can be mobilized in the plane between the pancreas and anterior renal fascia. To mobilize the kidney along with the other viscera, the anterior renal fascia must be opened.

The profile of the midabdomen is flattened and relatively shallow from front to back (Fig. 9-2). The prominent vertebral bodies of the lumbar spine further impinge on the anterior-posterior diameter. Thus, the abdominal aorta, which caps the ridge of the lumbar spine, lies remarkably close to the anterior abdominal wall in thin individuals. From its central location overlying the first to fourth lumbar vertebrae, the aorta sends branches to the whole abdomen.

The abdomen consists of bony and muscular walls capped by diaphragms at each end and lined by transversalis fascia. Contained within the abdominal cavity is the envelope of parietal peritoneum surrounding most of the abdominal organs (Fig. 9-3).

The posterior wall of parietal peritoneum is invaginated in a complex pattern by the roots of the small bowel and the transverse and sigmoid colon

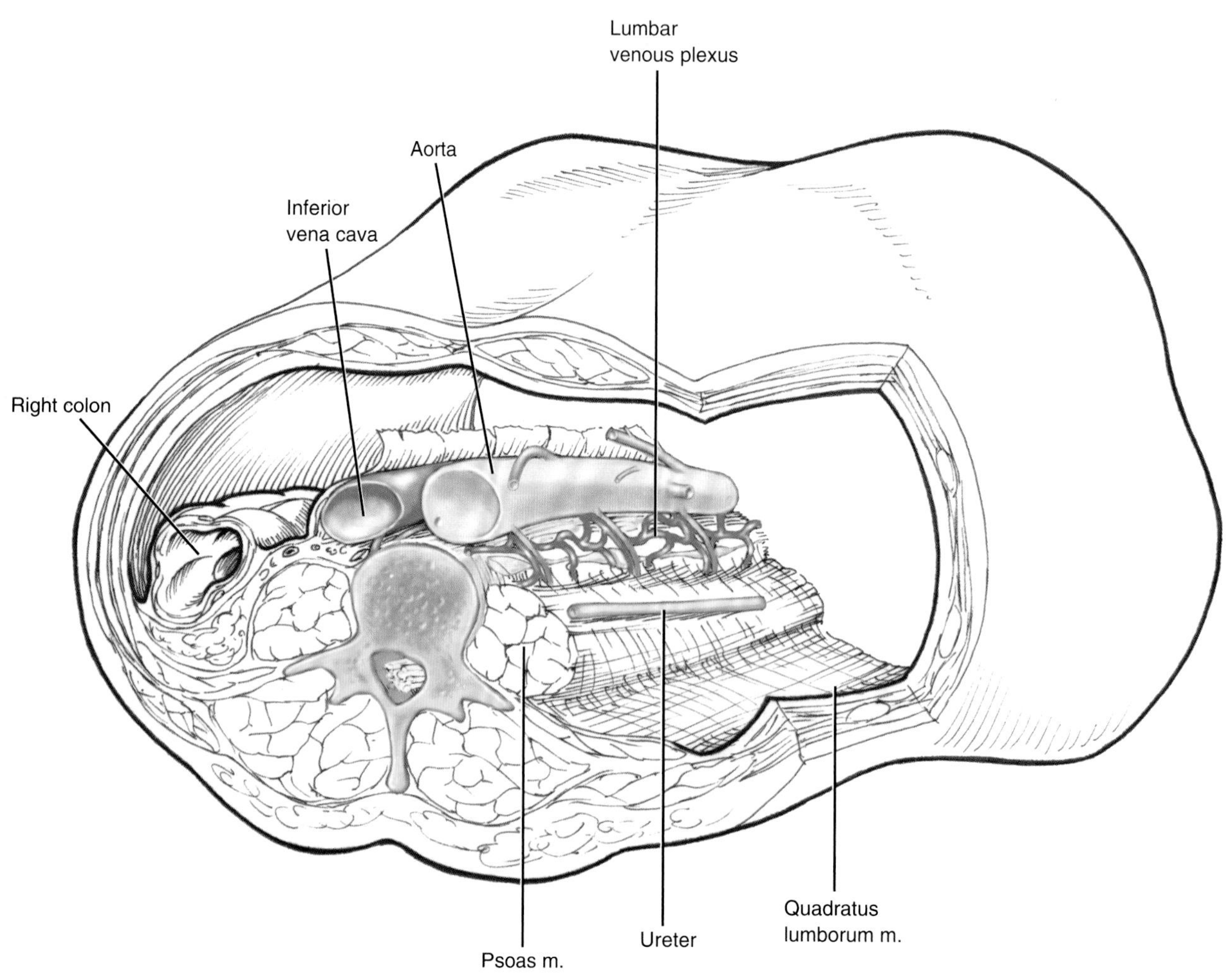

Fig. 9-2 The vessels cap the crest of the lumbar spine in the central abdomen.

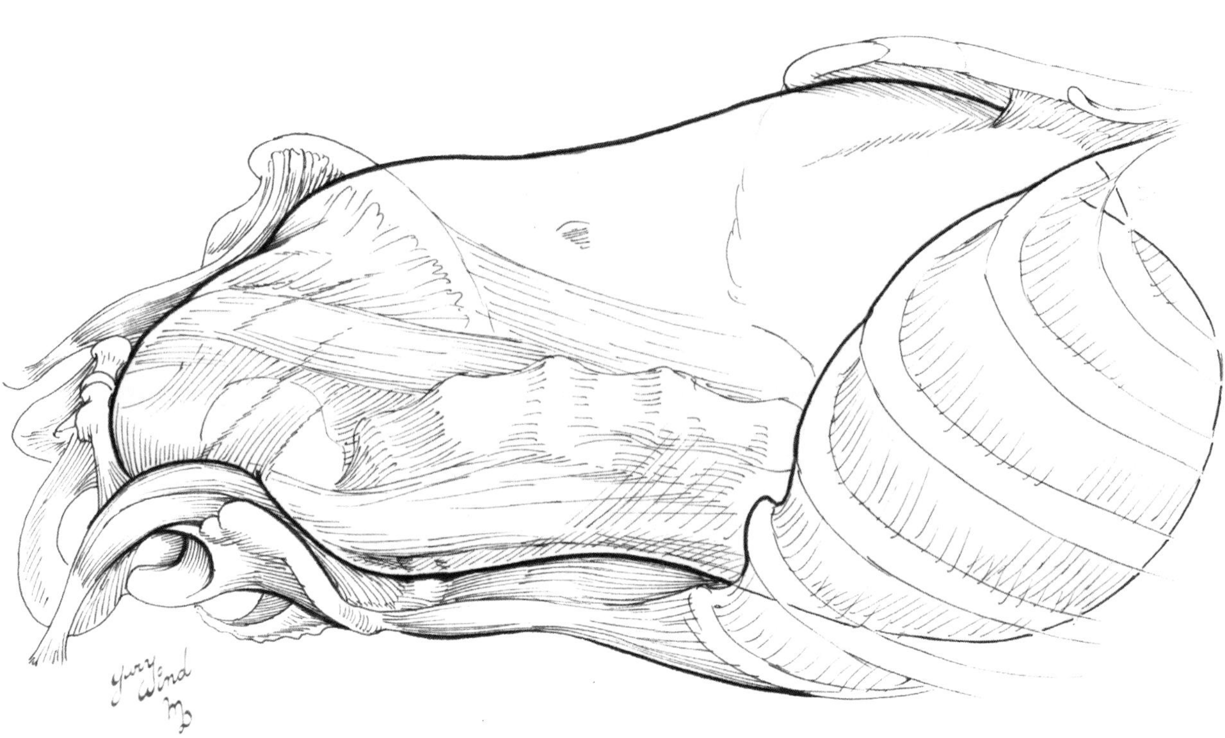

Fig. 9-3 The anterolateral surfaces of the parietal peritoneal envelope are smoothly continuous.

mesenteries as well as the broad attachments of the liver, spleen, and ascending and descending colon (Fig. 9-4). The great vessels and the urologic and pancreaticoduodenal complexes lie between the posterior peritoneal envelope and the posterior abdominal wall (Fig. 9-5). The stomach, colon, and small bowel fill the parietal peritoneum and blanket the great vessels (Fig. 9-6).

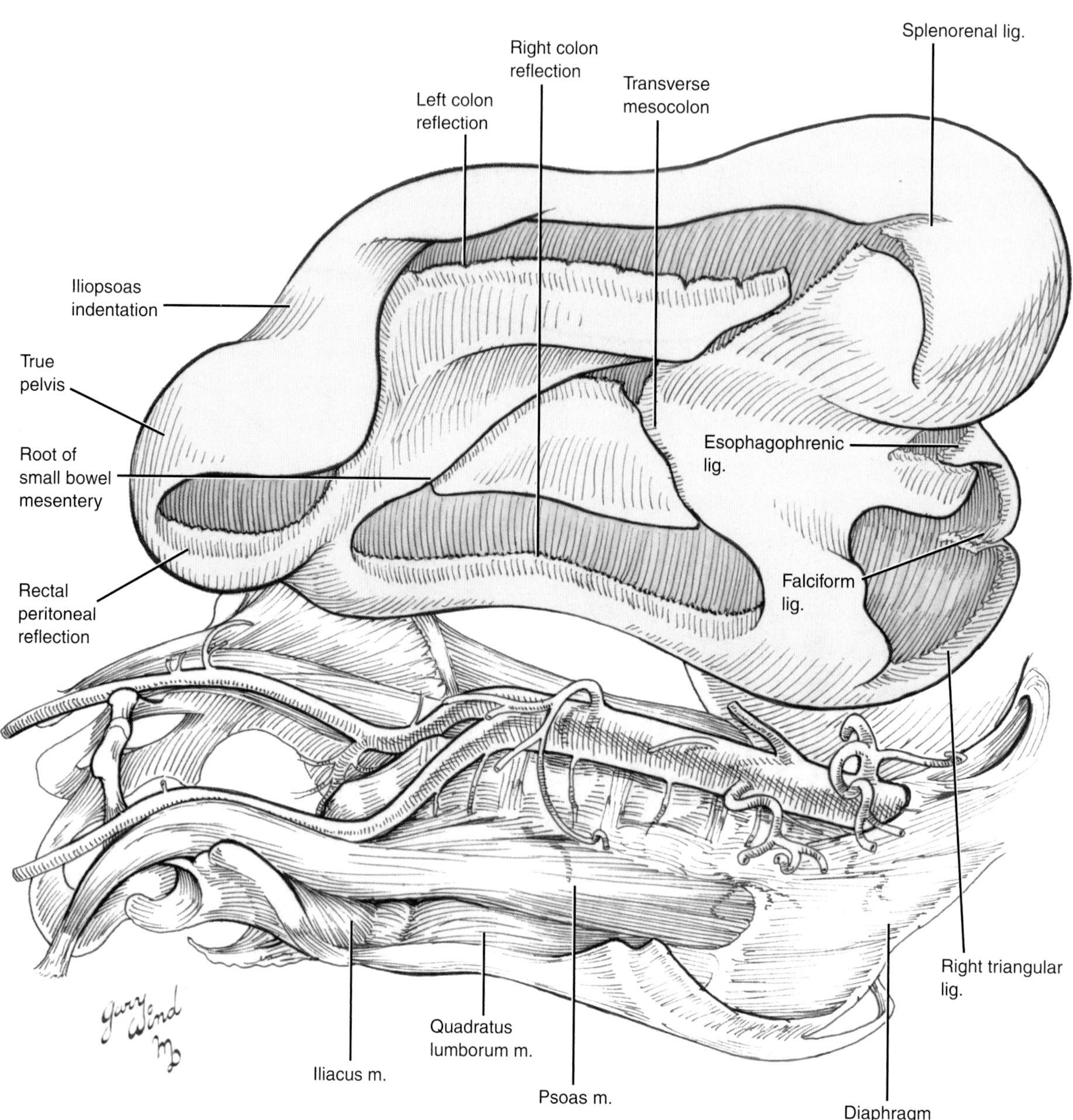

Fig. 9-4 The posterior parietal peritoneum is interrupted by numerous invaginations for colonic and mesenteric attachments.

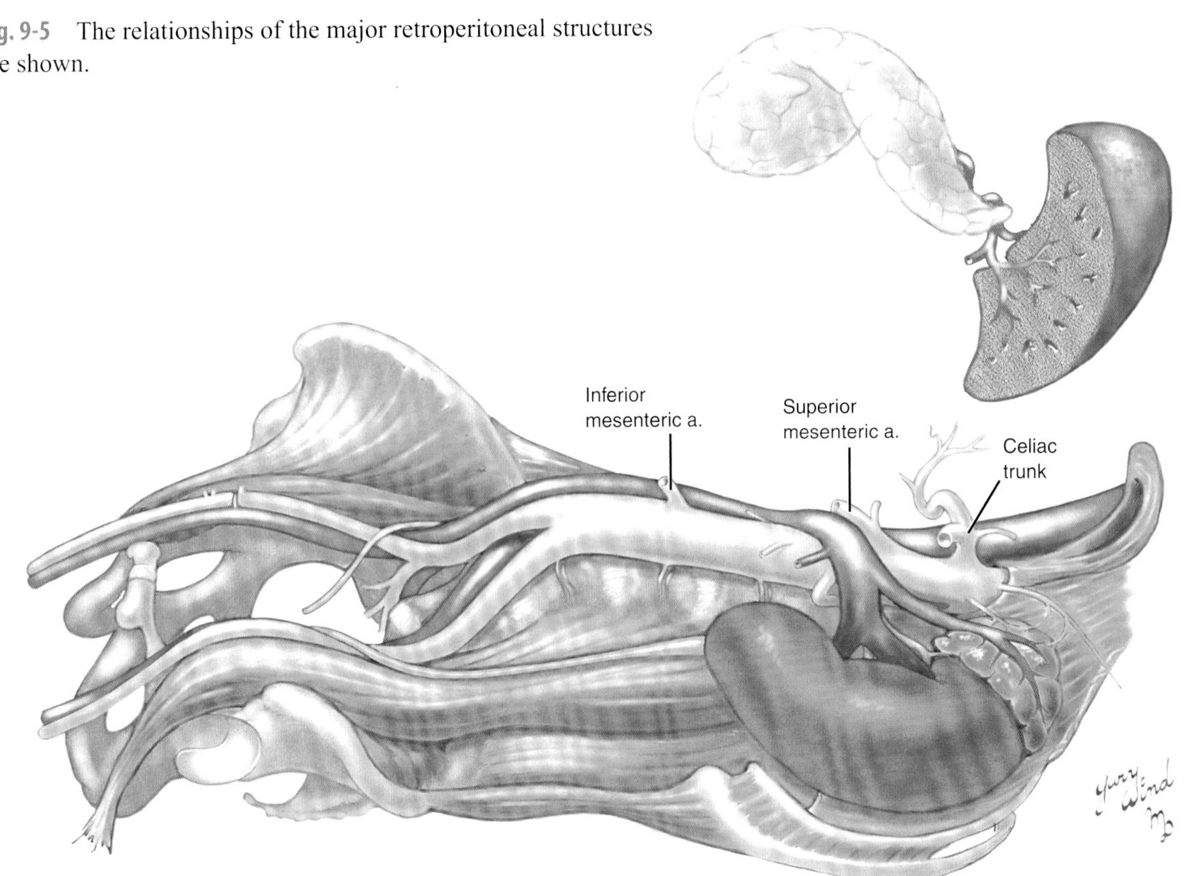

Fig. 9-5 The relationships of the major retroperitoneal structures are shown.

Fig. 9-6 The hollow viscera blanket the great vessels.

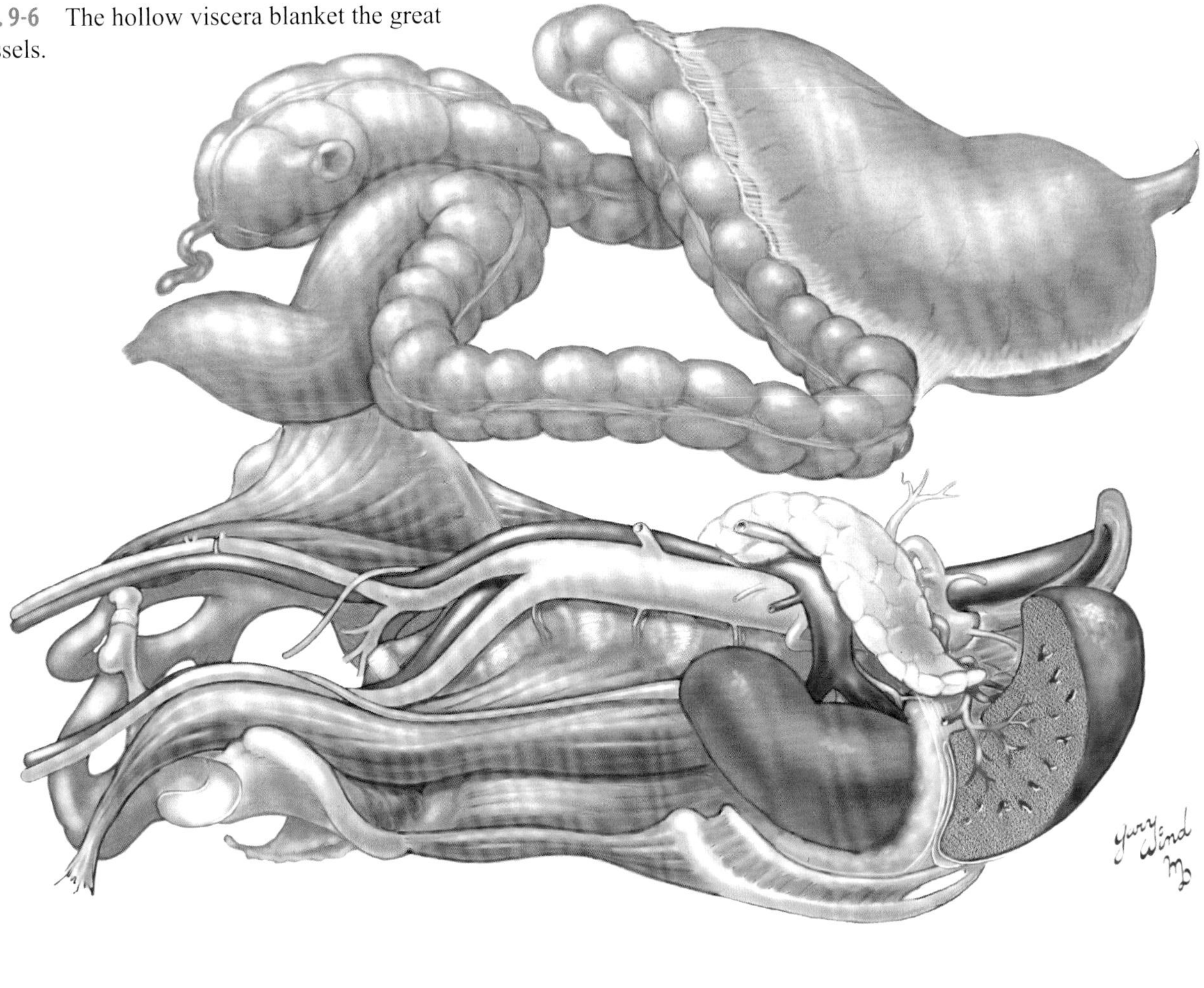

Diaphragm and the Supraceliac Abdominal Aorta

To understand the relationships and approaches to the proximal abdominal aorta, one must understand the anatomy of the diaphragm. The diaphragm consists of a crown of axial muscle fibers originating from the rim of the inferior thoracic aperture and inserting into a strong, aponeurotic, three-lobe central tendon (Fig. 9-7). The anterior two-thirds of the circumferential origin attach to the free margin of the costal cartilages and lower ribs. These slips of origin interdigitate perpendicularly with the origins of the transversus abdominis muscles. In the deepest angle of the anterior sulcus thus formed, the musculophrenic branches of the internal thoracic arteries course along the costal margin on

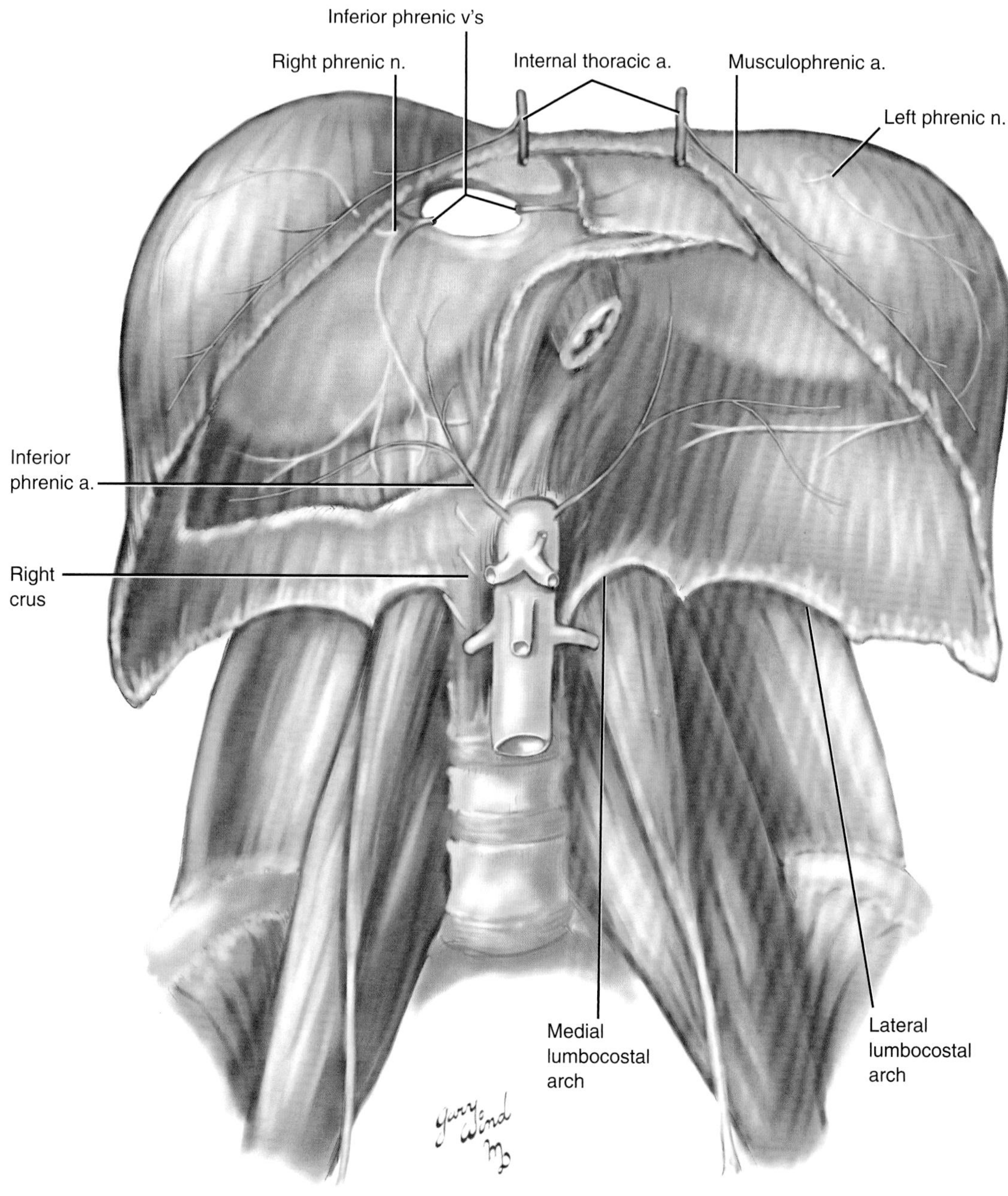

Fig. 9-7 The origins and neurovascular supply of the diaphragm are shown.

each side. These vessels are transected when the costal margin is divided. The internal thoracic arteries penetrate the diaphragm between the sternal and costal slips.

Posteriorly, the diaphragm originates from the lateral and medial lumbocostal arches spanning the quadratus lumborum and psoas muscles, respectively. The final components of the origins are the crura, which originate from the anterior surfaces and anterior longitudinal ligament of the first three lumbar vertebrae on the right and the first two on the left.

The main blood supply on the undersurface of the diaphragm consists of paired inferior phrenic arteries that have a variable origin from the aorta or its first major branches. These vessels have anterior and posterior divisions on each side. The veins follow the arterial pattern and drain into the vena cava.

The esophageal hiatus is muscular and consists primarily of fibers from the right crus. Note the ascending arrangement of aortic, esophageal, and inferior vena cava openings.

The topography of the diaphragm is best appreciated when viewed from above (Fig. 9-8). The rim of the diaphragm reflects the inverted V of the costal margin anteriorly, runs transversely around the posterior flanks, and appears to sprout from the roots of the crura. The domes present a bilobed mammillation depressed centrally at the seat of the heart and indented posteriorly by the vertebral column and aorta. In this view, the application of the crura to several centimeters of terminal thoracic aorta above the aortic hiatus can be appreciated.

The inferior vena caval aperture is the most cephalad and lies at the junction of the middle and

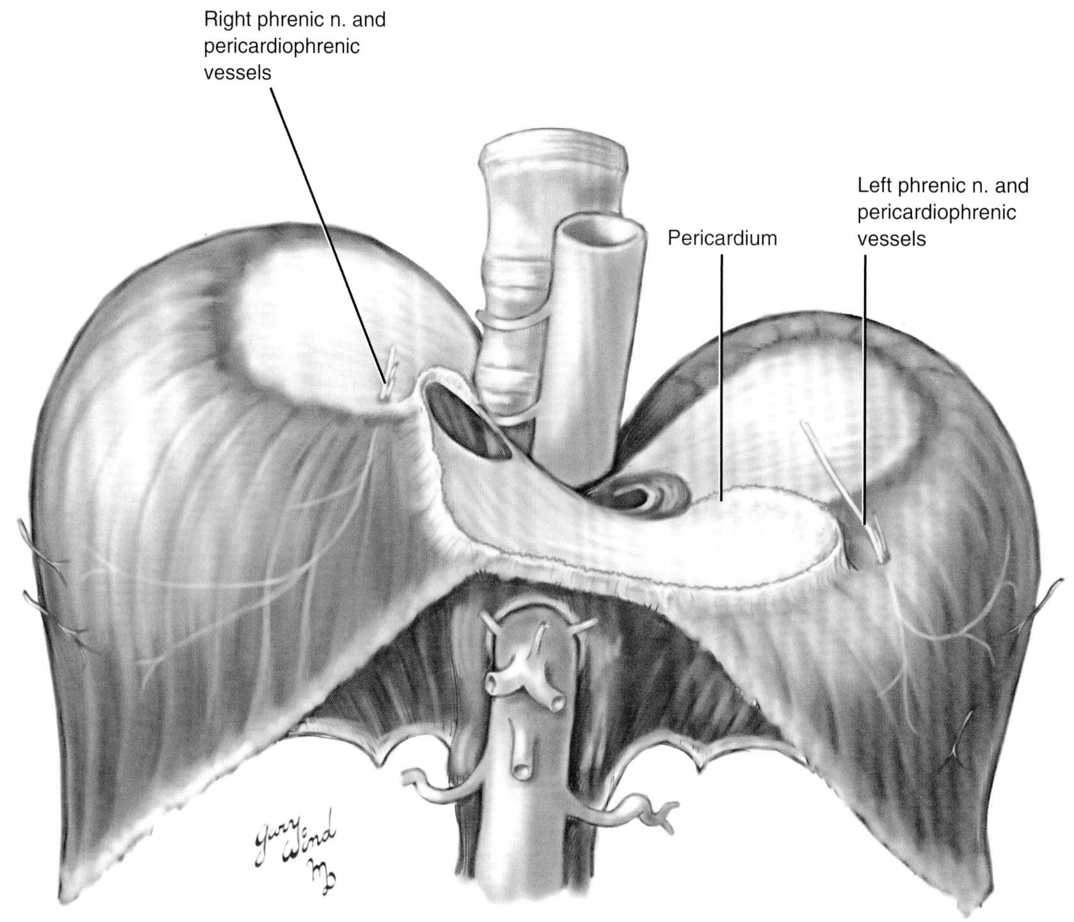

Fig. 9-8 The undulating diaphragmatic contours wrap around the aorta and vertebral bodies.

right lobes of the central tendon, directly beneath the right atrium. The esophageal hiatus lies at an intermediate level between the vena caval orifice and the aortic hiatus, slightly to the left of midline. It is surrounded by muscular fibers of the right diaphragmatic crus.

The motor innervation to the diaphragm is via the phrenic nerves, which also carry sensory fibers. Additional sensory fibers from the lower intercostal nerves serve the periphery. The right phrenic nerve sends a branch to the cephalad surface of the diaphragm and then penetrates the right leaf of the central tendon just lateral to the vena caval orifice. It divides into anterior and posterior branches on the undersurface. The left phrenic follows a similar pattern at the apex of the heart on the left.

Viewed from behind, the enfolding of the aorta by the diaphragmatic crura is evident, as is its anterior-posterior proximity to the lower esophagus (Fig. 9-9). The surest way to identify the esophageal hiatus on abdominal exploration is to locate the pulsations of the aorta transmitted through the esophageal walls. The aortic passage posterior to the diaphragm lies between the median arcuate ligament connecting the crura anteriorly and the body of the T12 vertebra posteriorly.

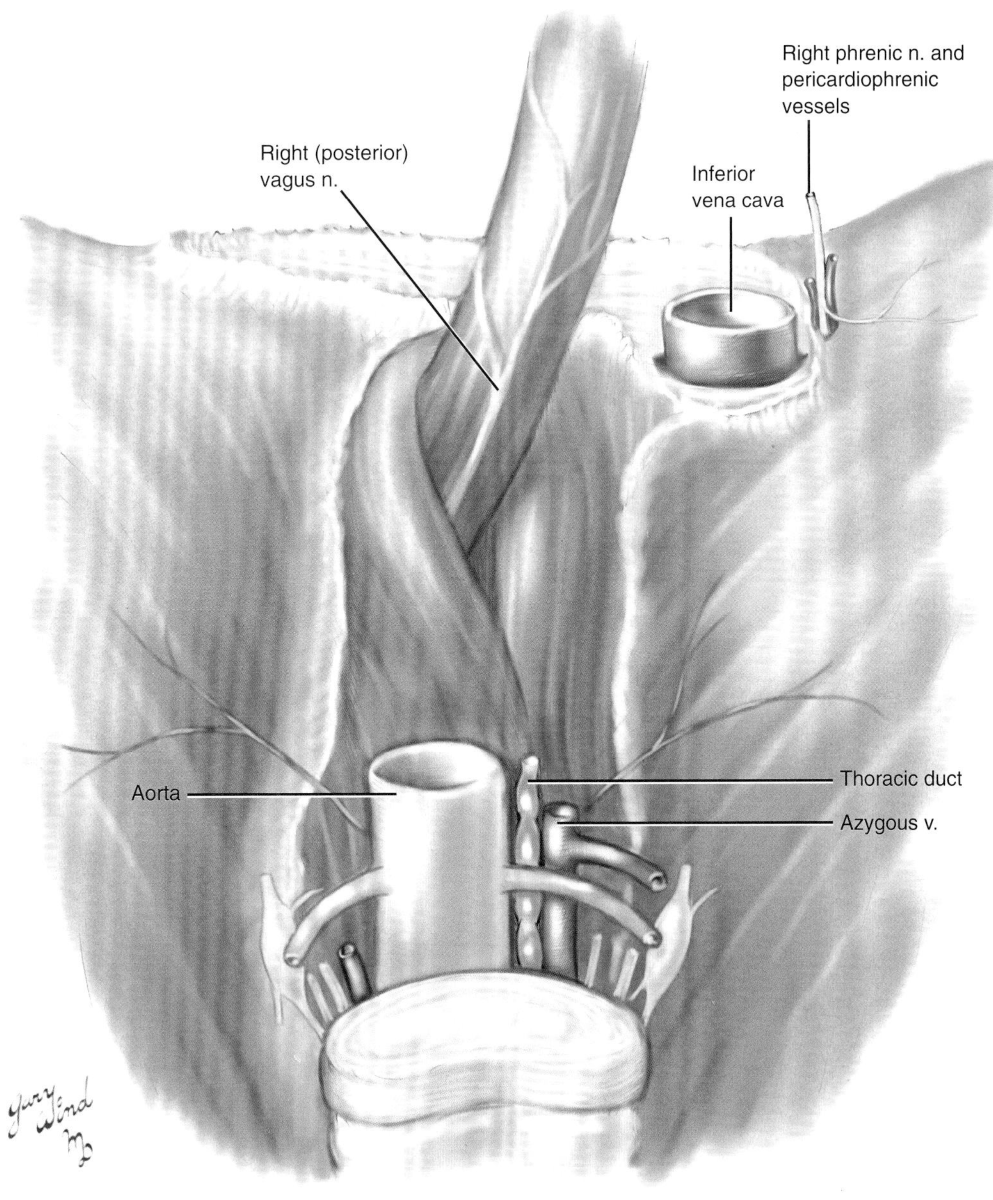

Fig. 9-9 The diaphragmatic crura separate the intraabdominal esophagus from the lower thoracic aorta.

Note the paraaortic structures and keep them in mind when considering the anterior approach to this segment of aorta.

The supraceliac abdominal aorta is only 1 to 2 cm in length (Fig. 9-10). Only the variable inferior phrenic and T12 lumbar vessels arise from this short segment. The origin of the thoracic duct from the cisterna chyli lies to the right of the aorta and passes beneath the right crus.

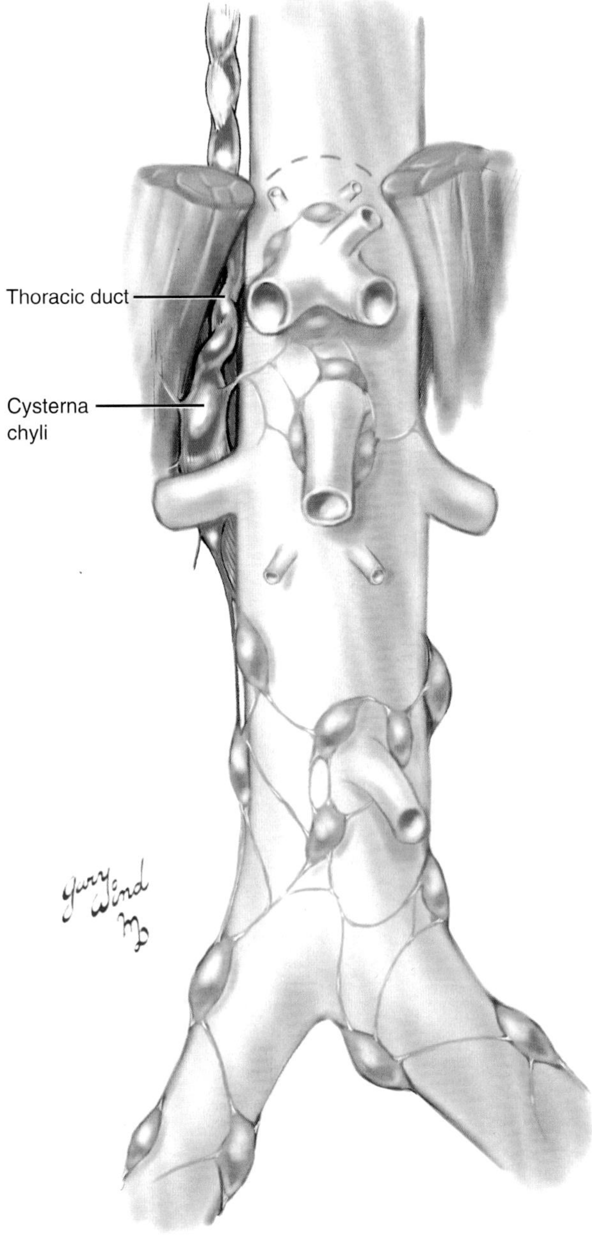

Fig. 9-10 The celiac trunk arises from the abdominal aorta within centimeters of the aortic hiatus.

Exposure of the Upper Abdominal Aorta

For purposes of discussion, the upper abdominal aorta can be anatomically divided into three segments by the large visceral and renal branches that originate in this area. The supraceliac aorta includes the portion between the celiac artery and the mediastinum. The visceral segment spans between the renal arteries and the celiac axis and includes the origin of the superior mesenteric artery. The juxtarenal area is the portion within 1 cm above and below the renal arteries that frequently overlaps with the visceral segment.

Exposure of the supraceliac aorta may be accomplished using transabdominal or retroperitoneal approaches. Because the transabdominal approach provides relatively limited exposure of the aorta above the celiac axis, its use should be restricted to situations in which more extensive exposure of the upper abdominal aorta is not required. The transabdominal approach is ideal for vascular control of the aorta above the celiac artery when control below the level of the renal arteries is technically difficult, such as pararenal aneurysms, inflammatory aneurysms, ruptured aneurysms with disruption of local tissue planes, and aneurysms with hostile infrarenal aortic necks or prior endovascular repair.[2–5] Clamp occlusion of the aorta above the celiac artery has been associated with fewer complications compared with occlusion between the renal and superior mesenteric arteries in these circumstances.[6,7] Limited exposure of the supraceliac aorta may also be indicated in the construction of prograde bypasses to the mesenteric and renal arteries.[8] The segment of aorta proximal to the celiac artery is often devoid of plaque and may be an ideal site for placement of a partial occlusion clamp during bypass construction.

The retroperitoneal approach allows more extensive exposure of the juxtarenal and visceral aorta. This approach has been used in the elective treatment of aortic diseases of all types and appears to confer important physiologic benefits compared with transperitoneal exposures.[9,10] We have found it especially useful to treat juxtarenal aneurysms, inflammatory aneurysms, and embolizing lesions of the visceral aorta ("coral reef" syndrome). However, because access to the right renal and right iliac arteries is limited, it should be avoided in patients with extensive atherosclerosis in these locations.[11]

Operations that require full exposure of the visceral, supraceliac, and lower thoracic segments of the aorta cannot safely be performed through a

simple abdominal incision.[12,13] Such exposure is most commonly gained by simultaneously entering the abdominal and left thoracic cavities, the so-called left thoracoabdominal approach. The unique characteristics of vascular disease in this area and the detrimental physiologic effects of thoracoabdominal incisions have been chronicled elsewhere.[14–16]

The following discussions concern the limited transabdominal exposure of the supraceliac aorta, the more extensive retroperitoneal exposure of the visceral aorta, and the complete thoracoabdominal approach to the lower thoracic and visceral aortic segments. Exposure of the infrarenal aorta is discussed in Chapter 12.

Transabdominal Exposure of the Supraceliac Aorta

The patient is placed in the supine position, and the chest, abdomen, groin, and thighs are prepped and draped. A longitudinal incision is made in the abdominal midline from the xiphoid process to the umbilicus. The peritoneal cavity is entered through the linea alba, and the abdominal viscera is packed into the lower half of the abdomen. The left lobe of the liver is retracted superiorly and to the patient's right. Increased exposure may be gained by dividing the left triangular ligament of the liver (Fig. 9-11) and folding the left lobe of the liver under a large Deaver retractor.

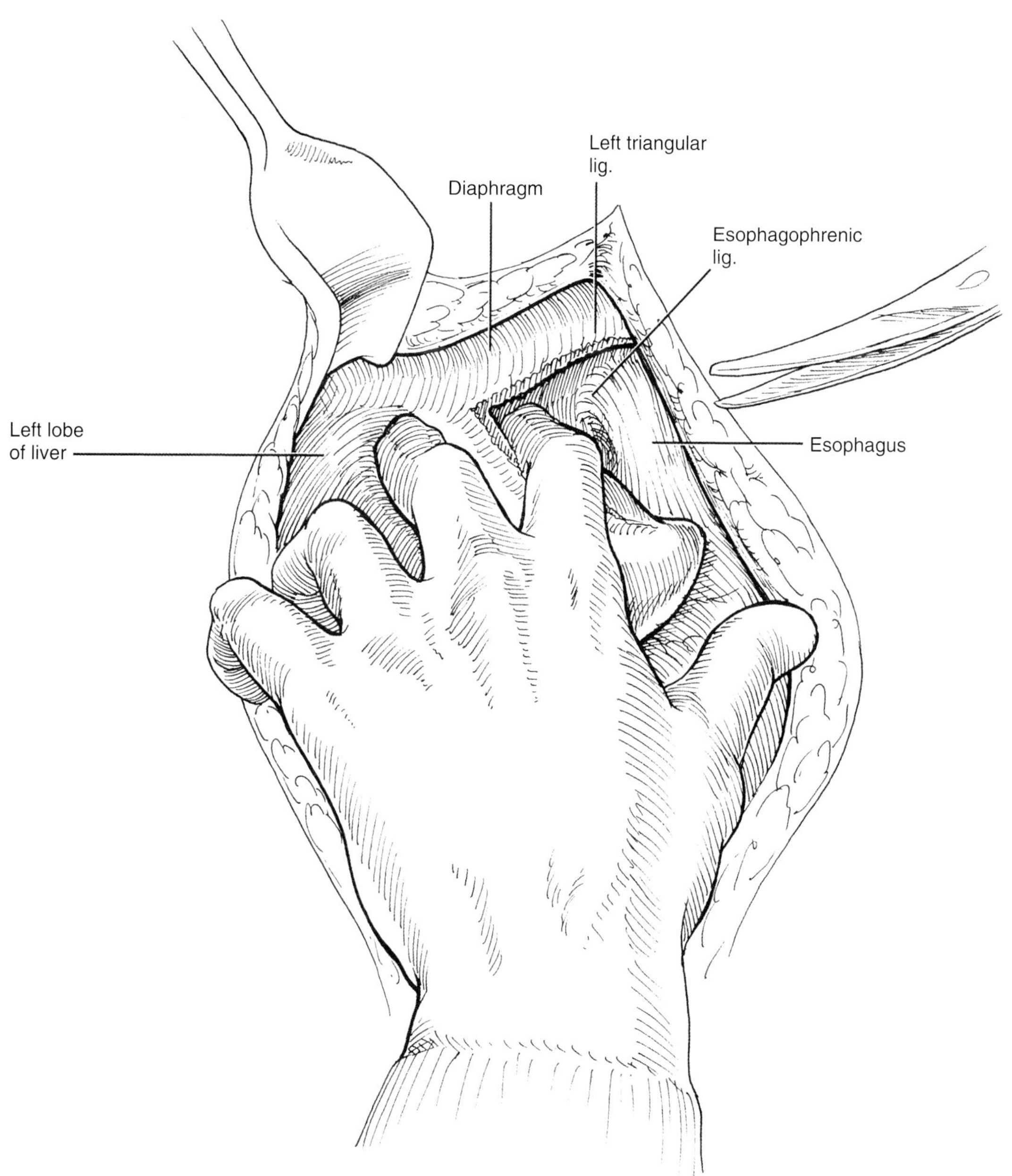

Fig. 9-11 When dividing the left triangular ligament to mobilize the lateral segment of the left lobe, keep in mind the proximity of the hepatic veins and vena cava at the dome of the liver.

The lesser sac is entered through a longitudinal incision in the gastrohepatic ligament made approximately 1 cm to the right of the esophagus and extended along the upper margin of the lesser curvature of the stomach (Fig. 9-12). Care should be taken to avoid injuring a replaced or accessory (50:50) left hepatic artery, arising from the left gastric in 10% to 15% of individuals. When present,

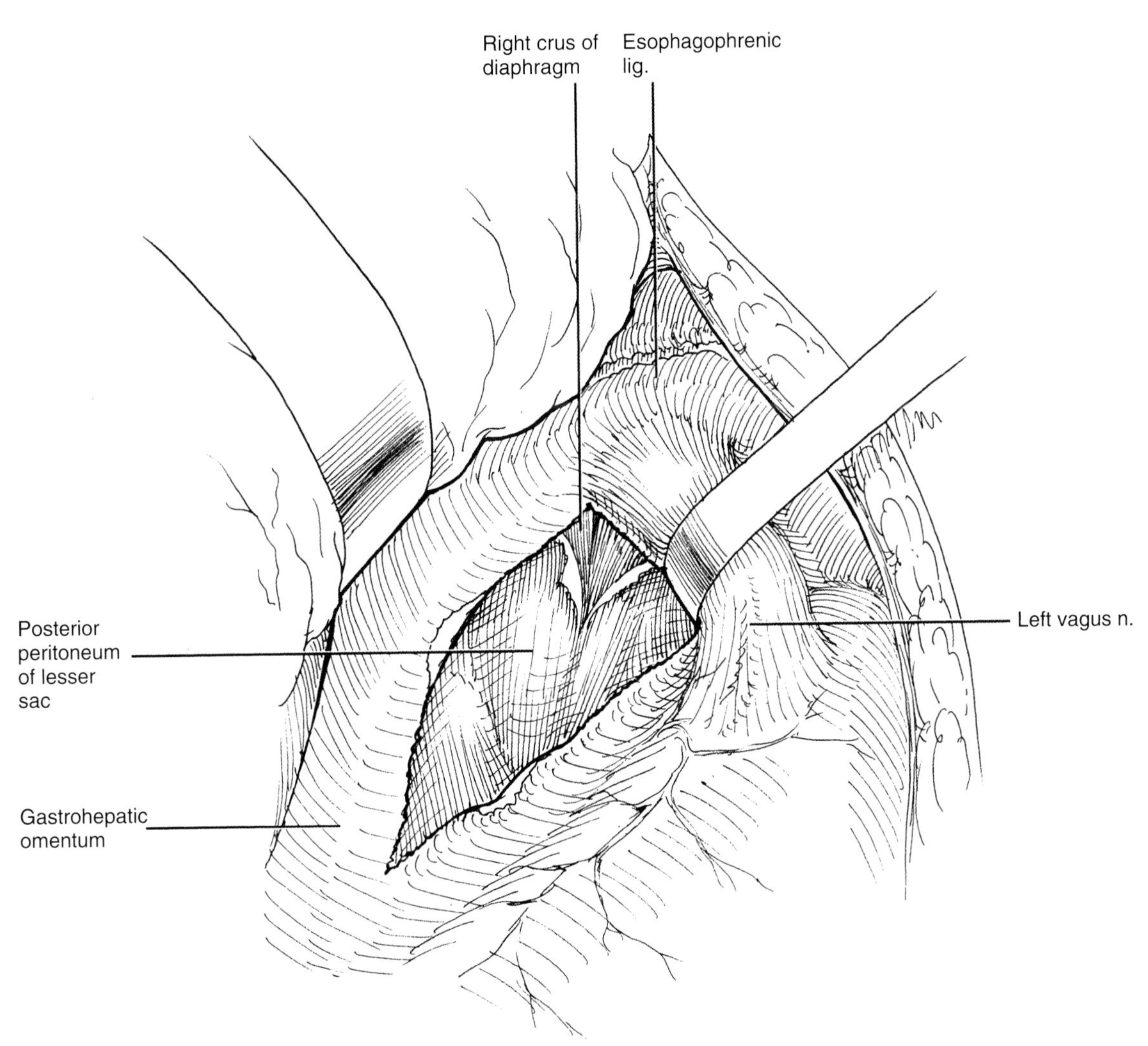

Fig. 9-12 Opening the gastrohepatic omentum exposes the right crus of the diaphragm.

this vessel runs in the cephalad portion of the gastrohepatic ligament (Fig. 9-13). Retraction of the esophagus and stomach to the left exposes the right crus of the diaphragm, which lies beneath the posterior peritoneum of the lesser sac. The aorta is exposed by incising the posterior peritoneum and separating the two limbs of the right crus to create a 5-cm opening over the anterior aortic wall

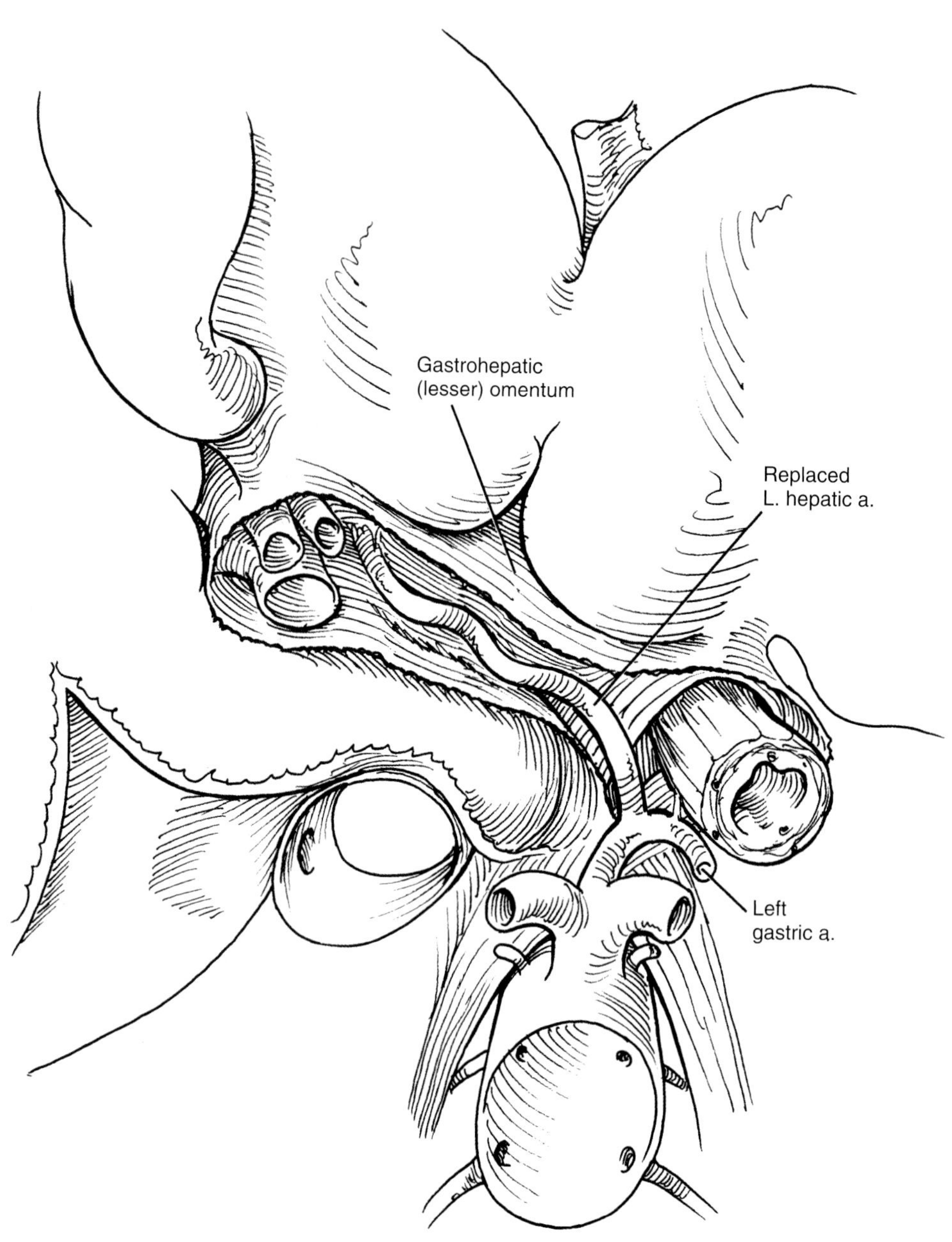

Fig. 9-13 In 10% to 15% of individuals, a replaced or accessory left hepatic artery arises from the left gastric artery and runs in the cephalad portion of the gastrohepatic ligament.

(Fig. 9-14). The medial and lateral walls of the aorta are cleared for a distance of 2 to 3 cm using blind finger dissection, which is not difficult because the aorta is devoid of periadventitial attachments in this area. The aorta should not be isolated circumferentially because of the limited exposure and access with this approach. The index and middle fingers of the left hand are placed astride the cleared aorta as a guide for placement of an occluding clamp. A large, slightly curved clamp can be

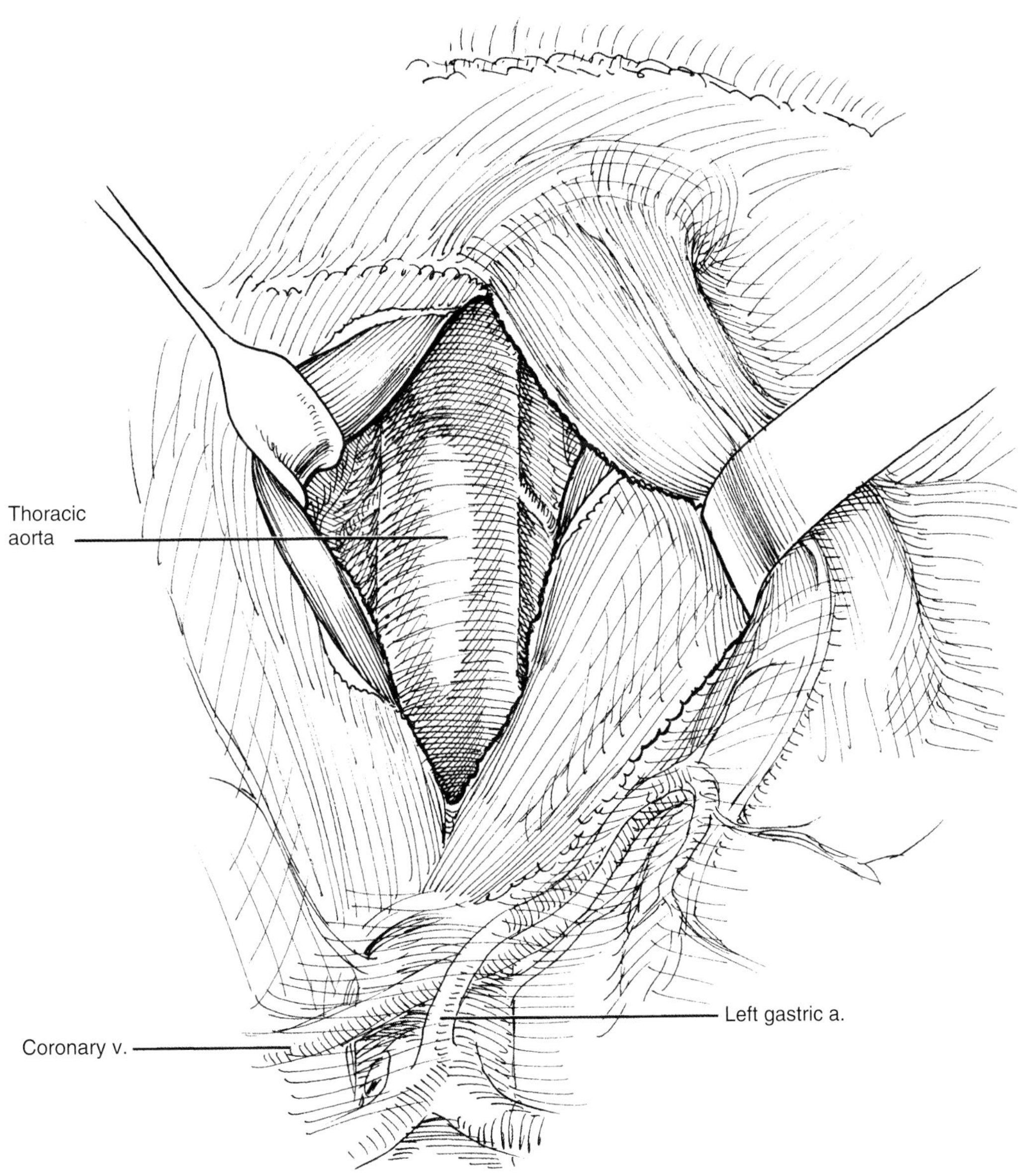

Fig. 9-14 The lower thoracic aorta can be exposed between the limbs of the right crus.

placed above and parallel to the fingers and pushed posteriorly toward the vertebral column for aortic occlusion (Fig. 9-15).

Complete exposure of the supraceliac aorta is performed by vertically incising the median arcuate ligament and the right crus over the anterior aorta (Fig. 9-16). The incision is continued superiorly into the posterior mediastinum until the entire crus has been divided. It is often necessary to divide venous and arterial branches that cross this area, but care should be taken to avoid transecting a replaced left hepatic artery (see above).[7] Once divided, the muscle tissue is dissected laterally to expose a 5- to 7-cm segment of aorta. The segment above the median arcuate ligament is actually the descending thoracic aorta in the posterior mediastinum. The inferior phrenic arteries arise from the aorta at variable levels in this area and should be identified to prevent injury.

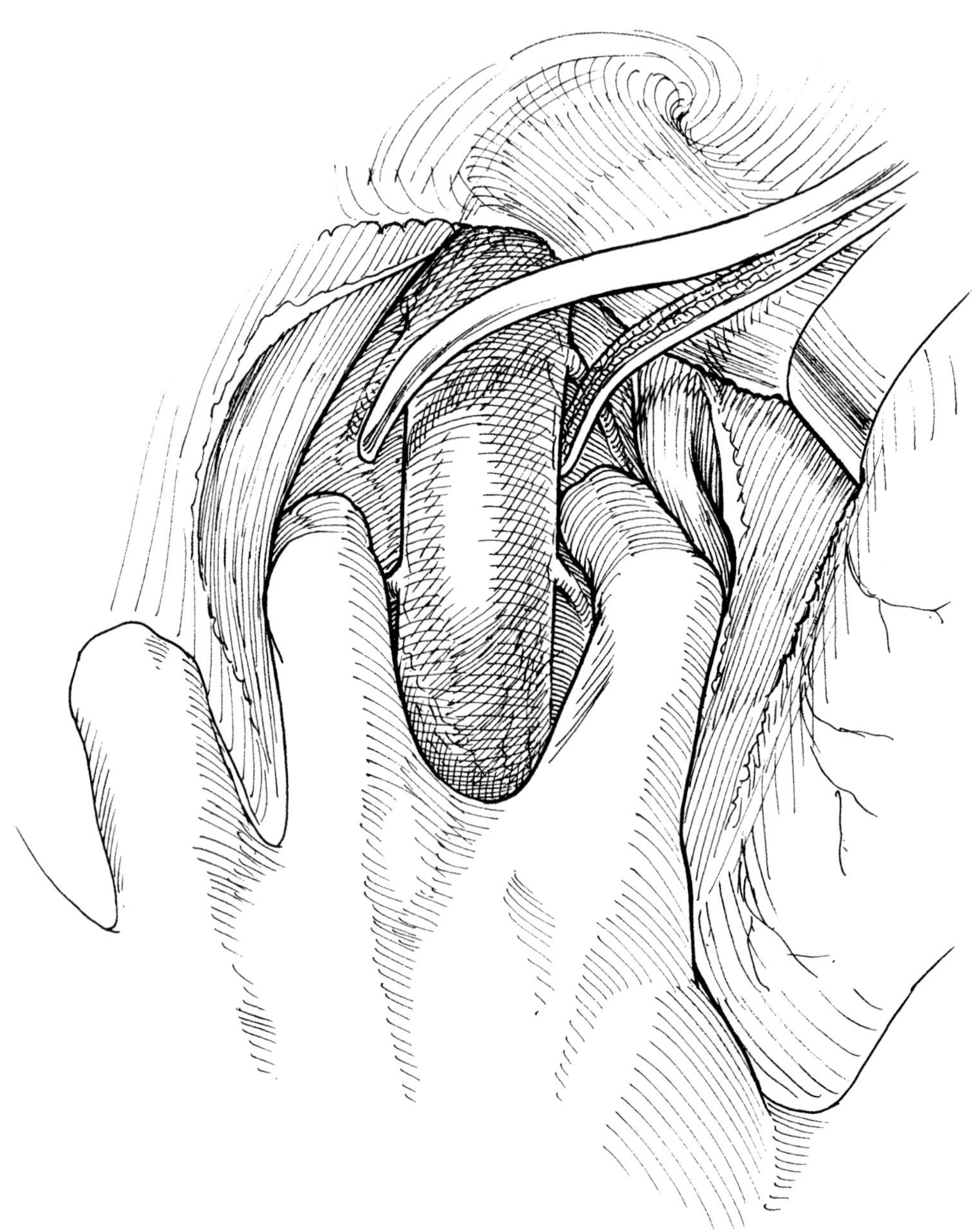

Fig. 9-15 Proximal control for operations on the supraceliac abdominal aorta is obtained by clamping the exposed thoracic aorta.

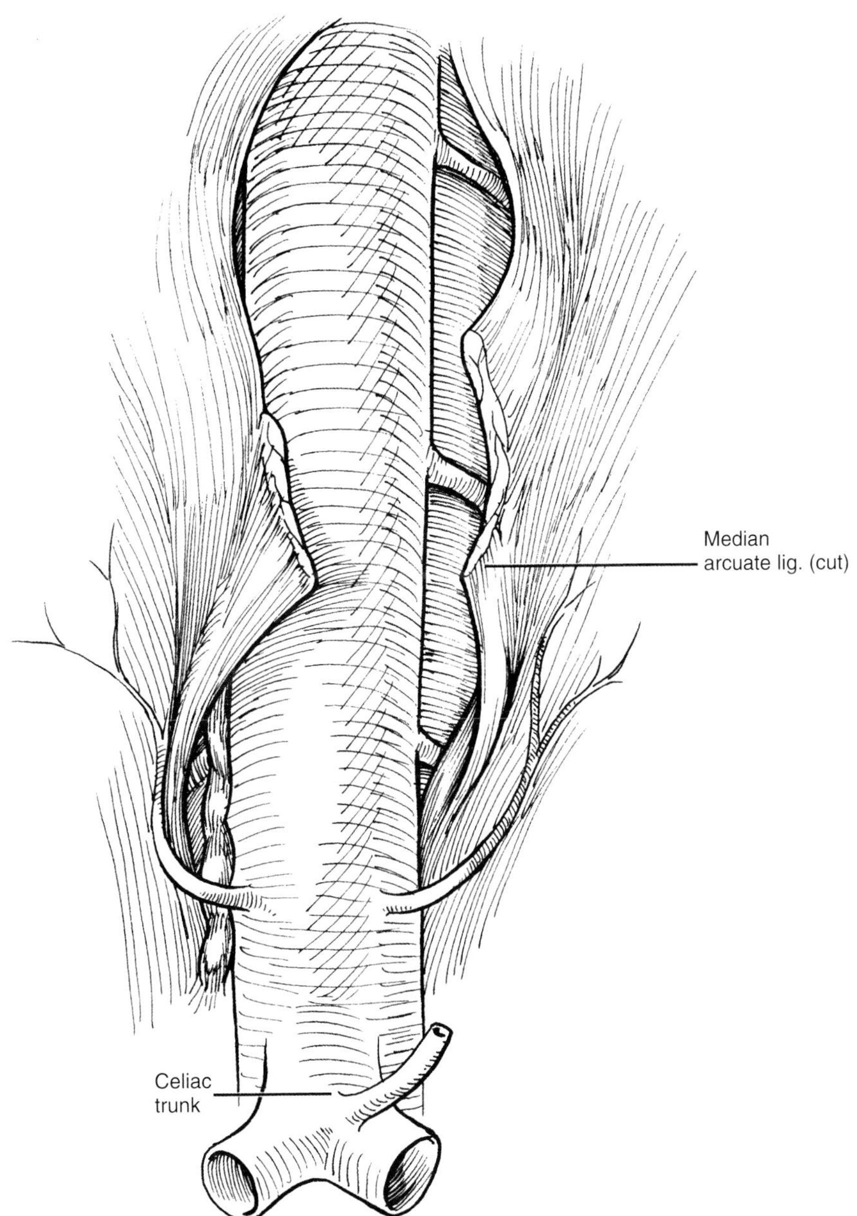

Fig. 9-16 Division of the aortic hiatus through the crura provides wider exposure of the aorta.

Retroperitoneal Exposure of the Visceral Abdominal Aorta

The patient is placed on a beanbag apparatus and the left chest is rolled upward so that the scapula is elevated approximately 90° from the table. The pelvis is twisted posteriorly to lie as flat as possible, and the left arm is placed on an overhanging support. The patient should be positioned so that the midpoint between the left costal margin and the left iliac crest is centered over the break in the table, then the table is jackknifed to widen the space between the costal margin and pelvic brim[17] (Fig. 9-17). After air is evacuated from the beanbag to make it firm, the left chest and pelvis should be further secured with wide adhesive tape.

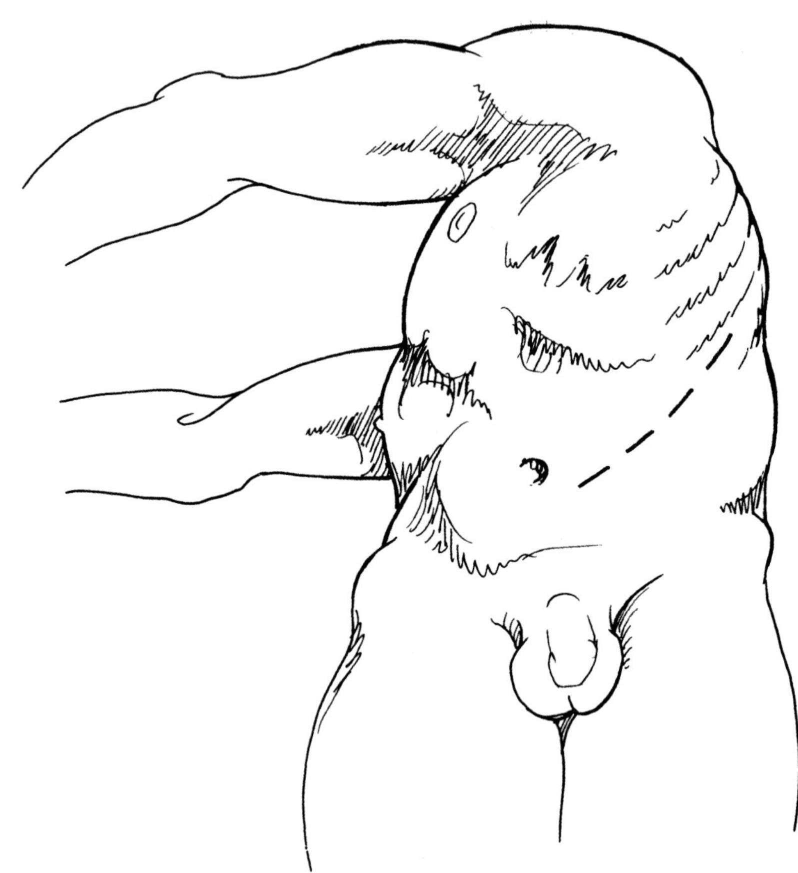

Fig. 9-17 Patient positioning for retroperitoneal exposure of the visceral aorta. **A:** The torso is twisted such that the pelvis lies horizontally and the left shoulder is rotated 90° from the operating table. **B:** The table is jackknifed to widen the space between the costal margin and pelvic brim.

To expose the most proximal portion of the abdominal aorta below the diaphragm, the incision should begin in the 10th interspace, extending from the posterior axillary line to the abdominal midline approximately 1 cm below the umbilicus. Lower aortic exposure can be accomplished through the 11th interspace.[17] The incision is deepened through subcutaneous tissues, the external abdominal oblique aponeurosis, and the anterior rectus sheath. The external abdominal oblique muscle is split in the direction of its fibers, and the internal oblique and the left rectus muscles are divided using electrocautery

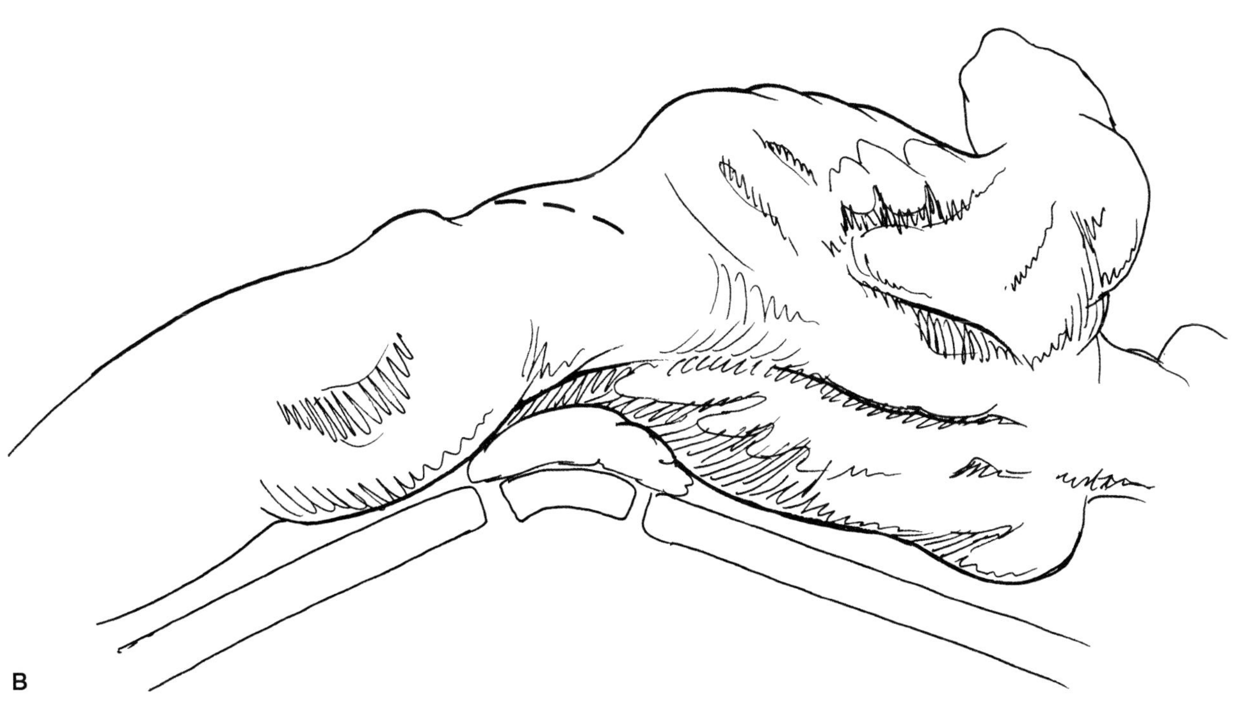

Fig. 9-17 *(continued)*

(Fig. 9-18). Branches of the epigastric vessels coursing posterior to the rectus abdominis should be carefully ligated.

The transversalis fascia is incised next, but the medial portion of the incision should stop 2 to 3 cm lateral to the midline because the underlying peritoneal surface may be adherent to the posterior rectus sheath in this area. To facilitate exposure in the lateral wound, we have found it advantageous to remove the 11th (or 12th) rib as far posteriorly as possible. The rib should be divided cleanly with a rib cutter, taking care to avoid injuring the neurovascular bundle that courses just underneath the inferior rib margin.

The retroperitoneal plane is most easily entered in the lateral wound by stripping the peritoneum away from the abdominal wall using blunt finger dissection. To enhance exposure, the peritoneum should be dissected from the abdominal wall as far superiorly and inferiorly as possible. Several small veins will be seen crossing the extraperitoneal space in the lateral wound and should be cauterized during this maneuver. Dissection of the peritoneum proceeds posteriorly, over the psoas muscle. To expose the visceral aorta on its anterolateral surface, the kidney should be mobilized anteriorly, allowing the ureter to be swept into the medial wound along with the

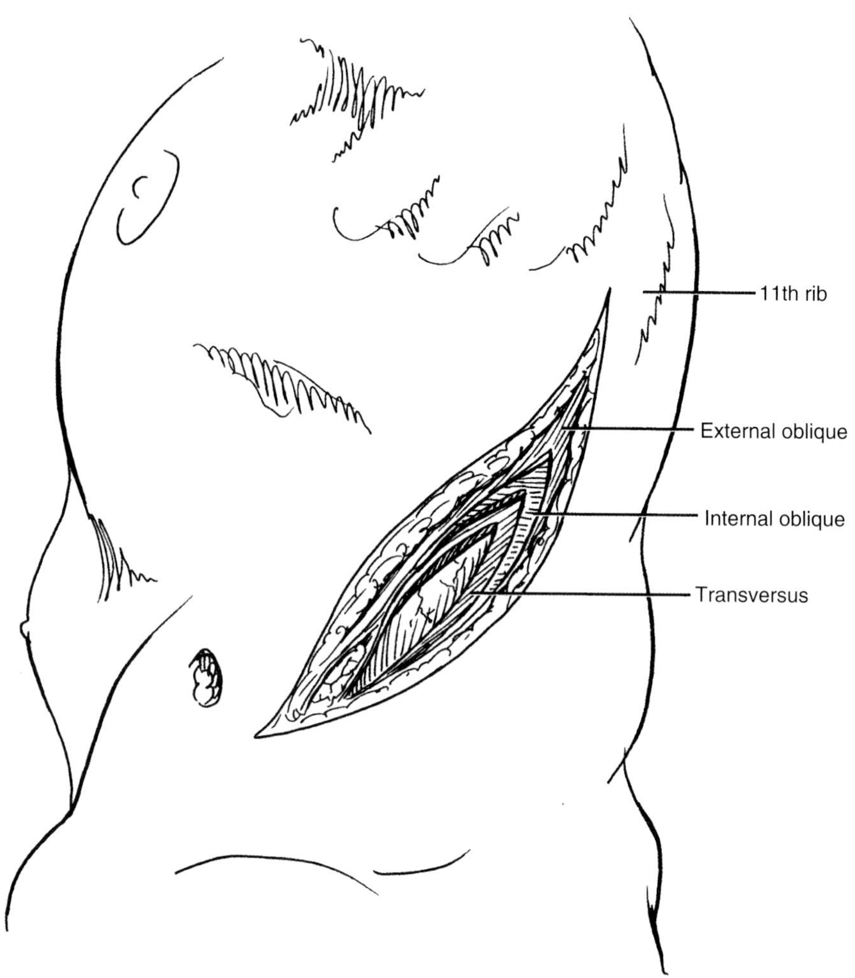

Fig. 9-18 The incision is begun in the 10th interspace and curved inferomedially to the abdominal midline below the umbilicus.

peritoneal contents (Fig. 9-19). This is accomplished by opening the anterior renal fascia and developing a plane posterior to the kidney. A large lumbar branch tethering the left renal vein on the lateral surface of the aorta should be carefully ligated and divided during this maneuver. Exposure is improved by inserting deep blades of a self-retaining retractor to hold the kidney and peritoneum anteriorly.

The left renal artery should be carefully identified in the areolar tissues overlying the left anterior surface of the aorta; Williams[18] noted this to be the first important step in aortic exposure because it is the only major structure that can be injured. After the left renal artery has been carefully exposed at its origin, dissection of the visceral aorta proceeds by incising tissue surrounding the anterior,

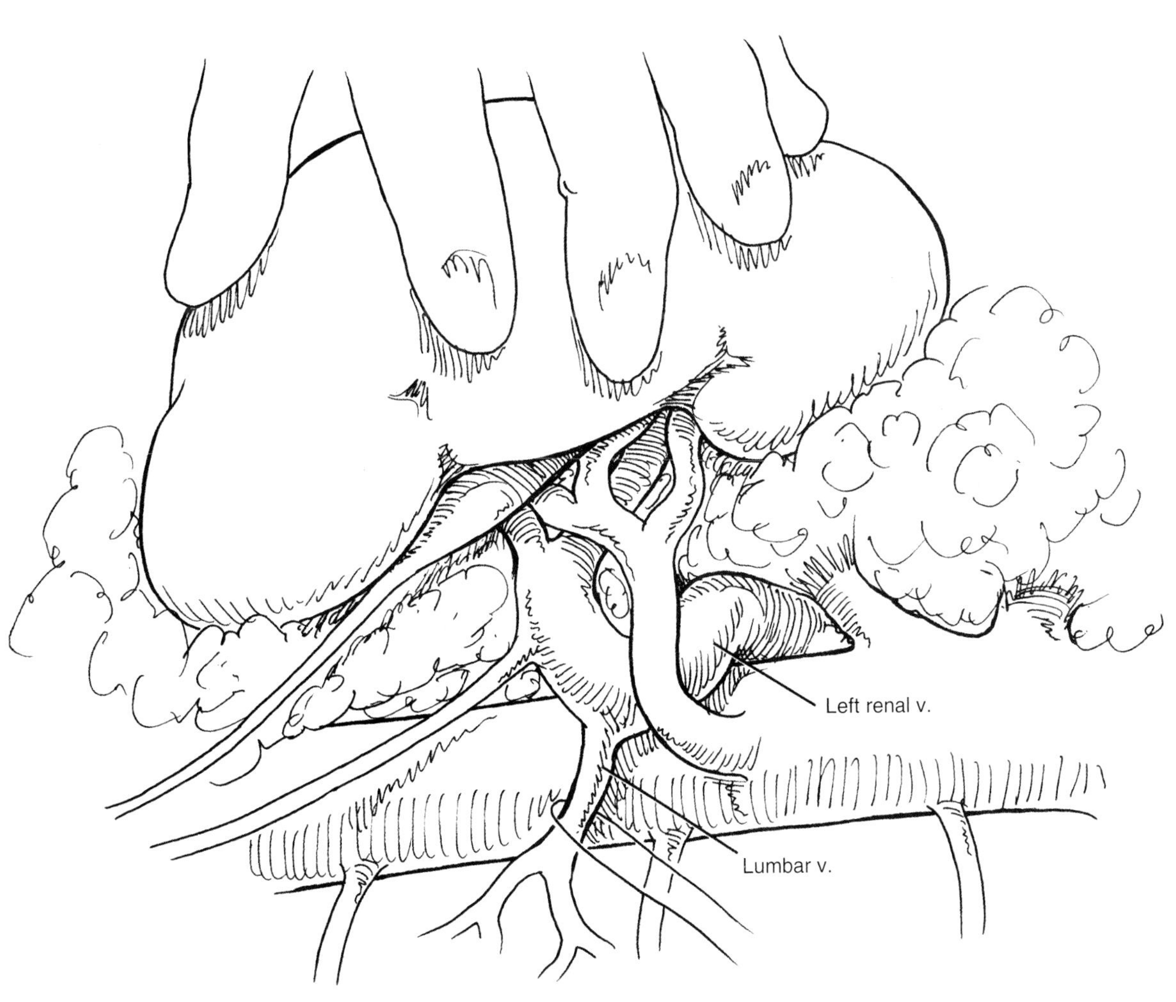

Fig. 9-19 Anterior mobilization of the left kidney requires careful ligation of a large lumbar vein.

left lateral, and posterior surfaces. Proximal exposure to the level of the supraceliac segment is readily obtained by dividing the diaphragmatic crus (Fig. 9-20). Vascular control of the aorta should be accomplished by confining dissection to the anterior and posterior surfaces; circumferential control risks injury to the vena cava or other large venous structures.[18]

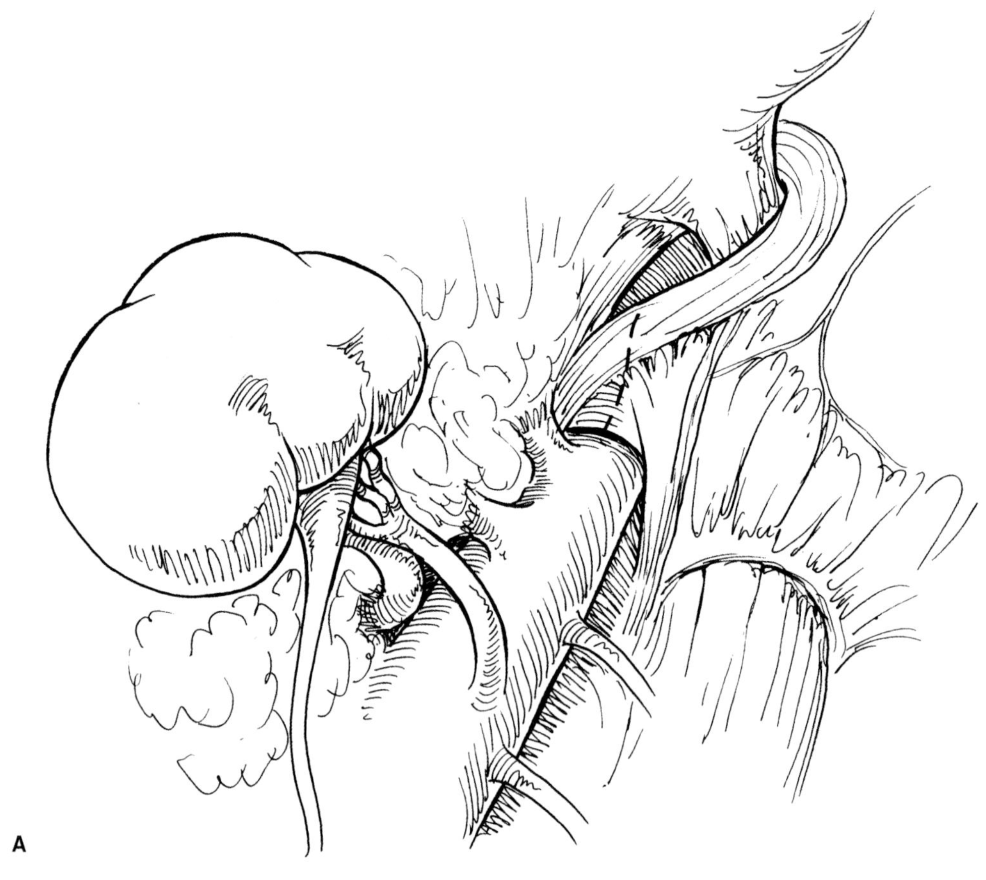

Fig. 9-20 By incising the crus anterior to the supraceliac aorta **(A)**, direct exposure can be obtained to the level of the lowest thoracic segment **(B)**.

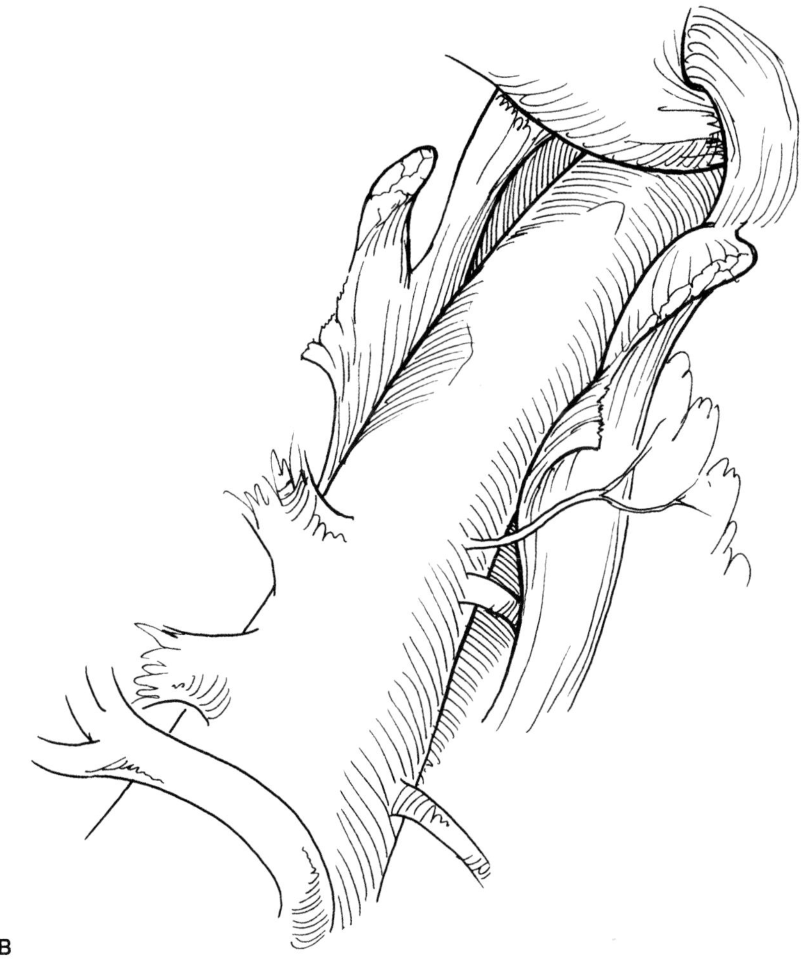

Fig. 9-20 *(continued)*

Thoracoabdominal Incision for Extensive Exposure of the Aorta, Including the Upper Abdominal and Lower Thoracic Portions

Preoperative planning is extremely important to minimize the morbidity of this approach. In addition to restoration of intravascular volume, all patients should undergo optimization of cardiac and pulmonary parameters. A central venous catheter should be placed to monitor cardiovascular dynamics; depending on the experience of the anesthesiologist, monitoring with a pulmonary artery catheter or transesophageal echocardiography may be desirable. Use of a double-lumen endotracheal tube enhances exposure of the thoracic aorta during the procedure by allowing the left lung to collapse while maintaining adequate right lung ventilation. To lessen the risk of spinal cord ischemia, many surgeons and anesthesiologists routinely advocate cerebrospinal fluid drainage,[16,19,20] epidural cooling,[21,22] distal aortic perfusion,[23] or a combination of techniques. Unfortunately, none of these adjunctive procedures is universally protective against paraplegia.[24]

After intubation, the patient is placed in the supine position on a beanbag apparatus. The left scapula is elevated approximately 60° away from the operating table so that the trunk is twisted. The left arm is placed on an overhanging support, and the beanbag is deflated. The left chest is further secured with wide adhesive tape (Fig. 9-21). This unusual position has two advantages over the more traditional lateral thoracic position: it allows access to the femoral arteries should exposure at this level become necessary, and the trunk torsion tends to widen the incision and lessen retraction requirements.

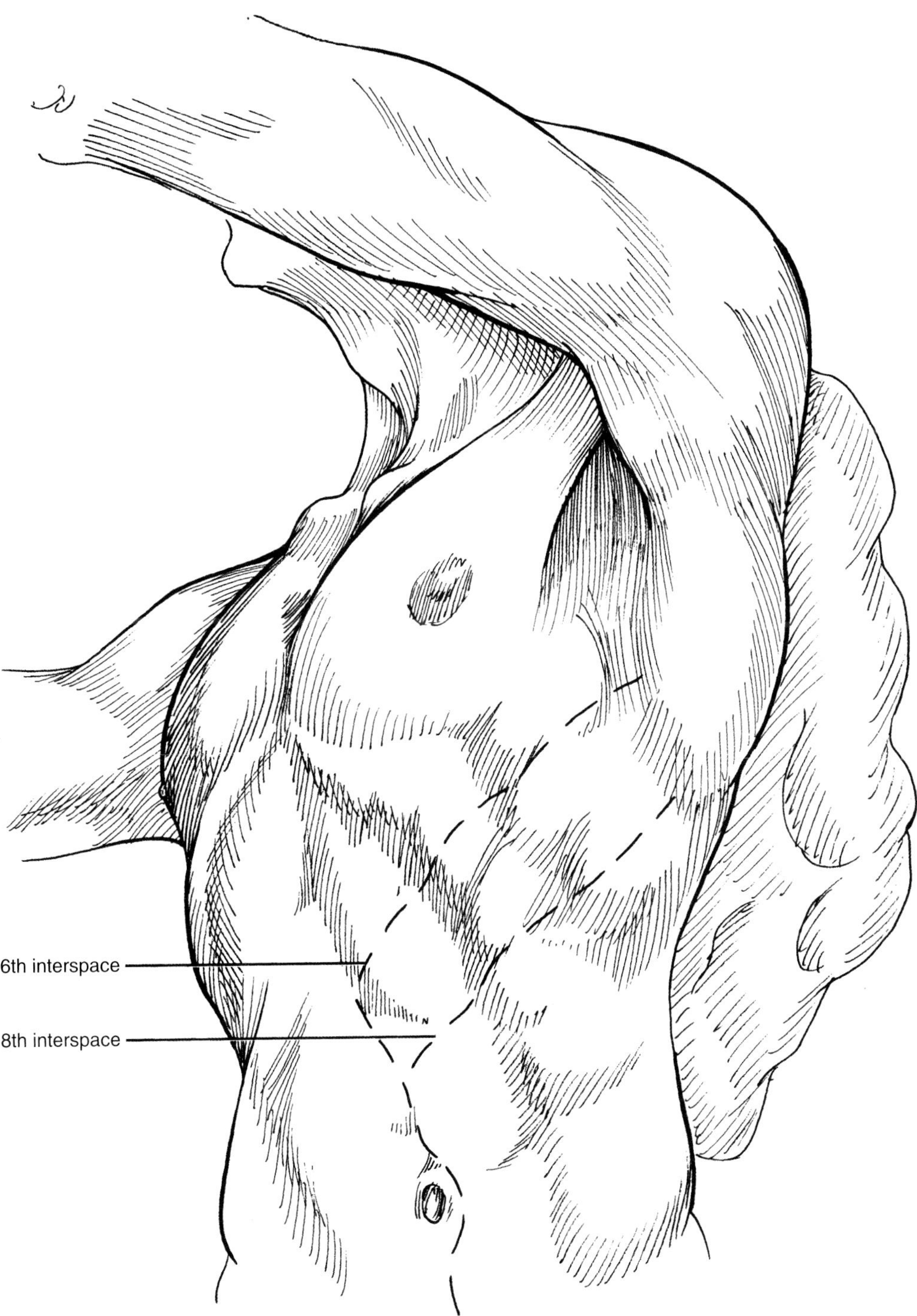

Fig. 9-21 Thoracoabdominal incisions in the sixth or eighth interspace can be extended down the midline of the abdomen.

The precise location and extent of the thoracoabdominal incision should be dictated by the specific area of aorta to be exposed. In most cases, this is determined by the extent of aneurysmal disease. The most widely used classification of thoracoabdominal aneurysms was originally proposed by Crawford et al.[25] (Fig. 9-22). A Crawford type I aneurysm begins just distal to the left subclavian artery and extends to the visceral aorta above the renal arteries. A type II aneurysm, the most extensive, descends from the left subclavian artery to the infrarenal aorta. A type III aneurysm extends from the middescending thoracic aorta to below the renal arteries, and a type IV aneurysm extends from the diaphragmatic aorta to the iliac bifurcation. In the modified classification proposed by Safi et al.,[26] a type V aneurysm extends from the middescending thoracic aorta to above the renal arteries.

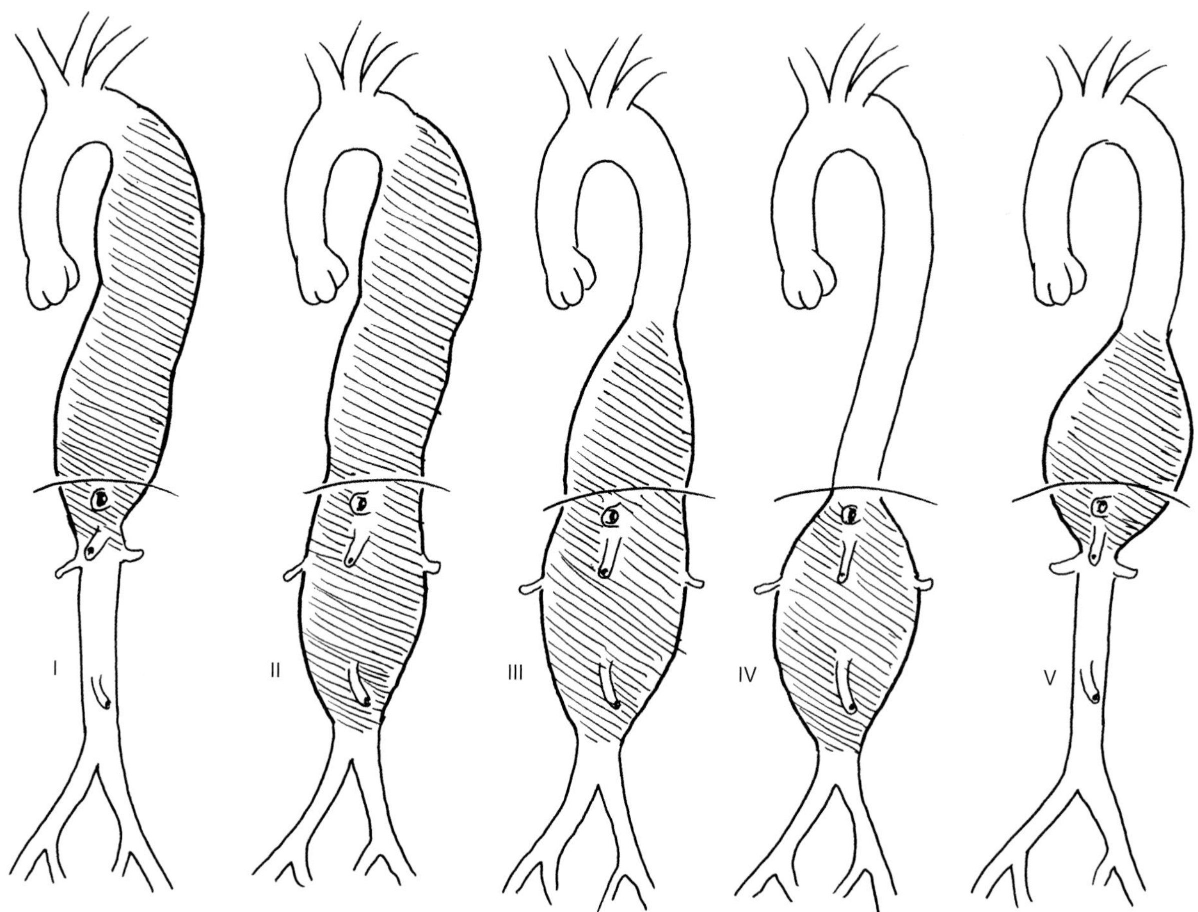

Fig. 9-22 Classification of thoracoabdominal aneurysms.

The appropriate interspace level for the thoracic portion of the incision is determined by the proximal extent of the aneurysm. Optimal exposure of the aorta at the level of the distal arch or subclavian artery (aneurysm types I and II) is through the fifth interspace. The descending thoracic aorta (aneurysm types III and V) is best exposed through the sixth interspace, whereas the eighth interspace is the optimal level for exposure of the aorta at the level of the diaphragm (type IV aneurysm)[26] (Fig. 9-23).

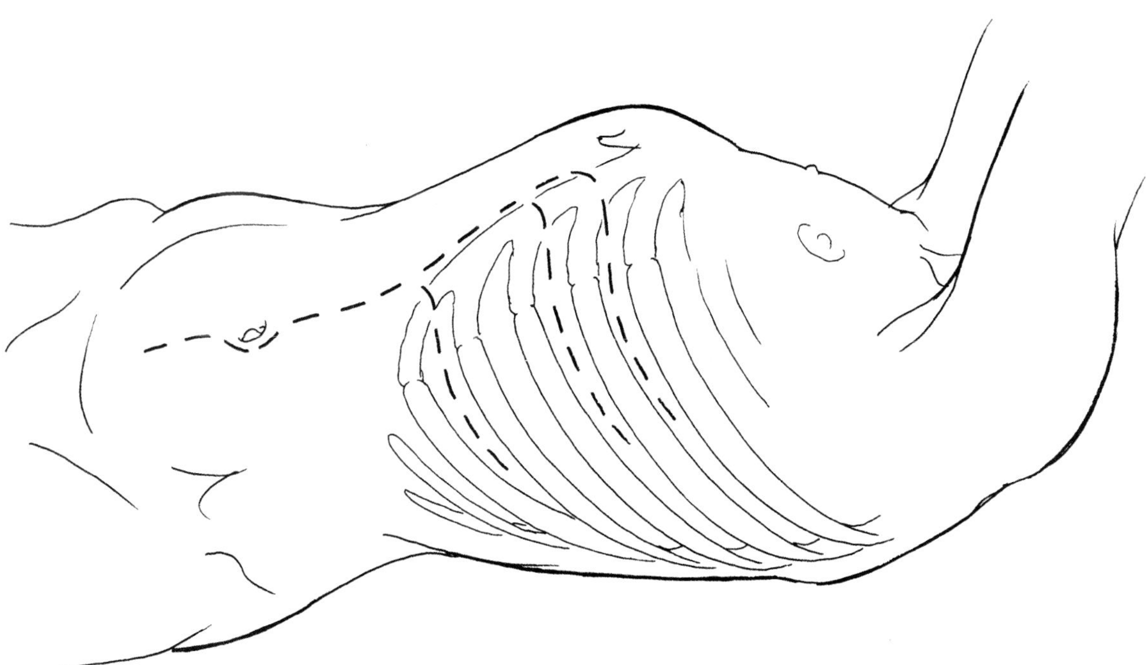

Fig. 9-23 The optimal level for the thoracic portion of the incision is determined by the proximal extent of the aneurysm.

The length and location of the abdominal incision are determined by the distal extent of the aneurysm. If limited exposure of the abdominal aorta below the celiac artery is required (e.g., aneurysm types I and V), then the upper abdominal aorta can be exposed through a modified thoracoabdominal incision[26] (Fig. 9-24A). The incision should be extended to the abdominal midline to expose thoracoabdominal aneurysms involving the visceral aorta (Fig. 9-24B). Type II, III, and IV aneurysms require more extensive exposure of the infrarenal abdominal aorta; a more formal thoracoabdominal incision should be extended down the abdominal midline (Fig. 9-24C).

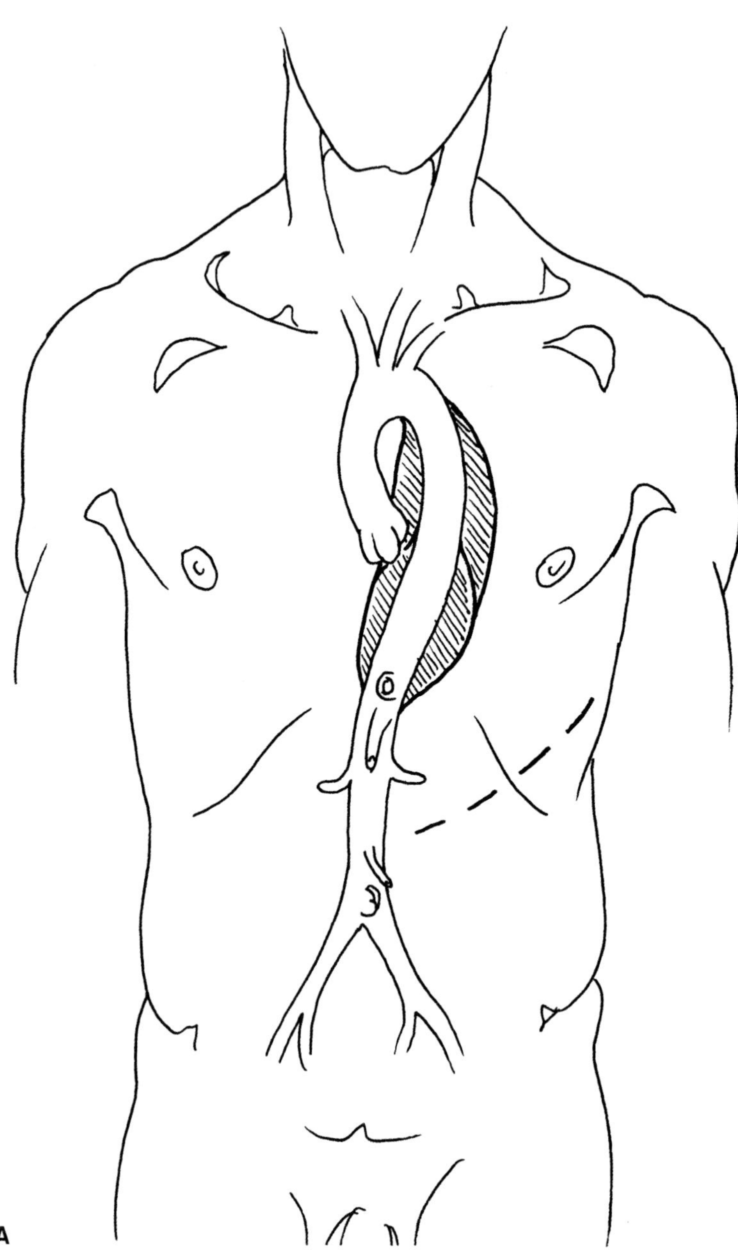

Fig. 9-24 The abdominal portion of the incision is determined by the distal extent of the aneurysm. **A:** The abdominal incision may terminate in the upper abdomen for aneurysms that do not extend distal to the celiac artery. **B:** The incision should be extended to the abdominal midline for aneurysms involving the visceral aortic segment. **C:** An extended abdominal incision is required for aneurysms extending to the infrarenal aorta.

Fig. 9-24 *(continued)*

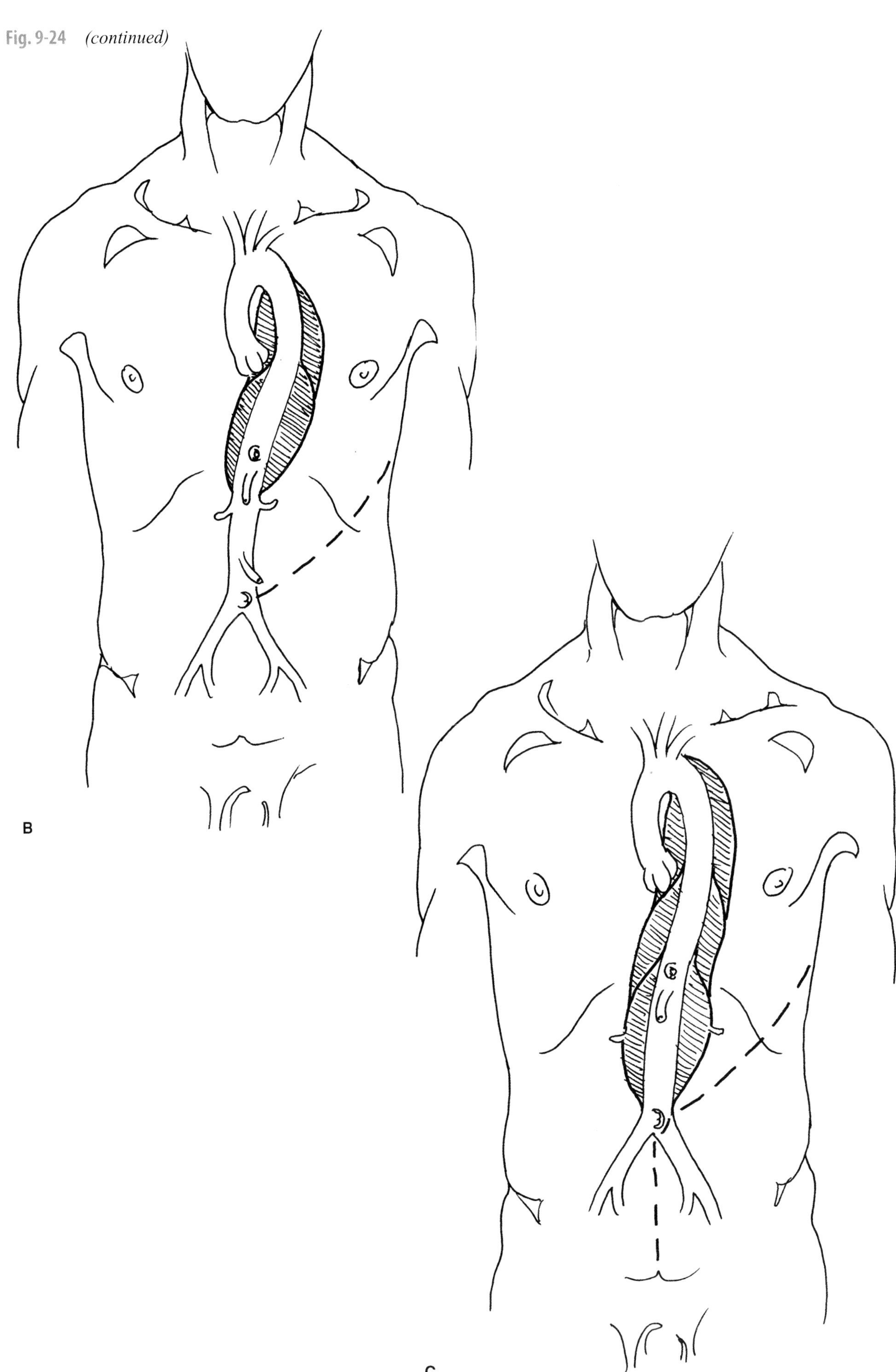

The incision is begun in the appropriate interspace, continued across the costal margin, and extended obliquely to the abdominal midline (Fig. 9-25). More distal exposure can be gained by continuing the abdominal incision in the midline to the level of the symphysis pubis. The abdominal incision is deepened through subcutaneous tissue, the external abdominal oblique aponeurosis, and the anterior rectus sheath. The external abdominal oblique muscle is split in the direction of its fibers, and the underlying internal oblique and transversus abdominus muscles are divided between the costal margin and lateral edge of the rectus sheath. The left rectus muscle is divided, taking care to ligate branches of the epigastric vessels that course posterior to the muscle within the rectus sheath.

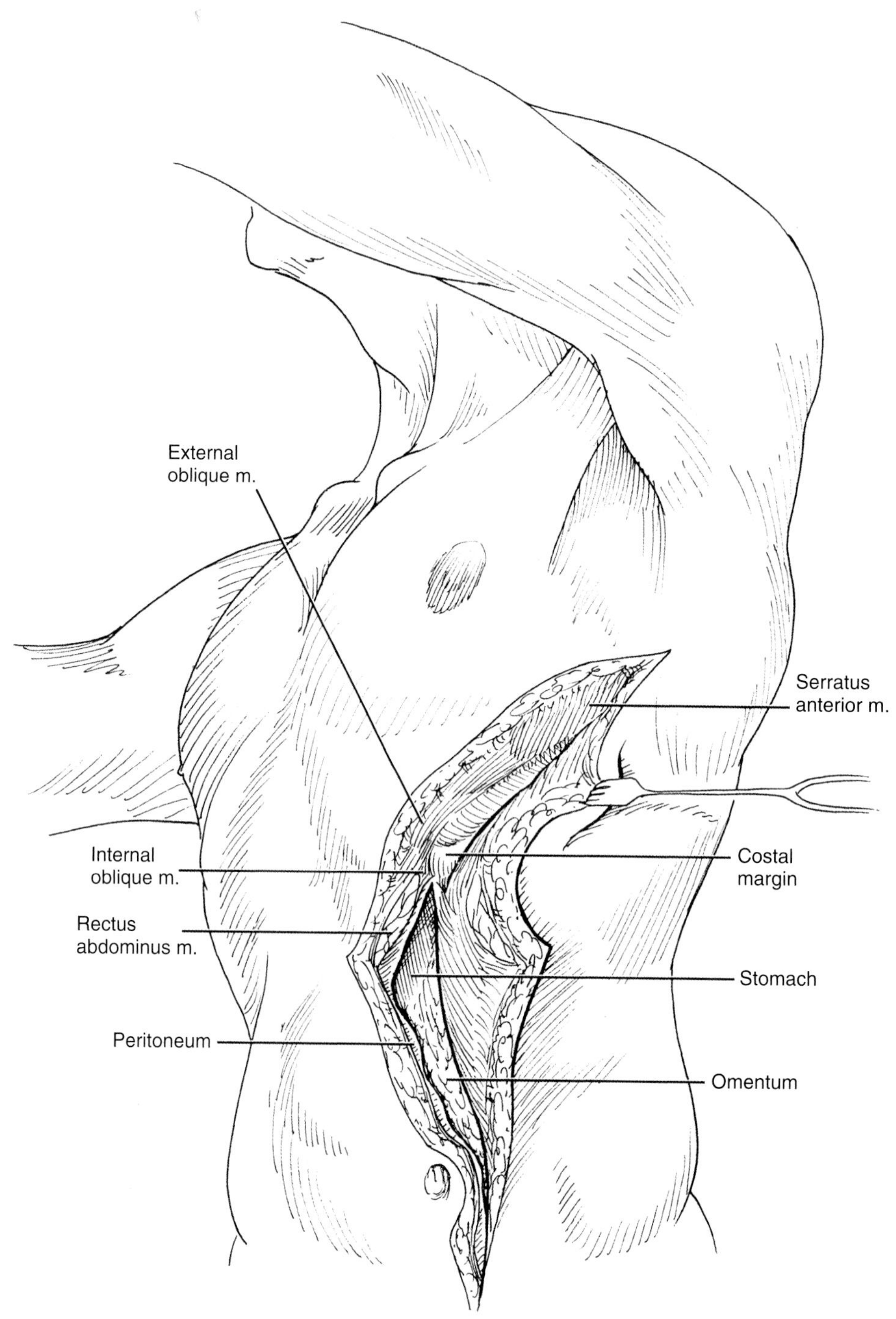

Fig. 9-25 The layers of abdominal and chest walls are divided.

The thoracic portion of the incision should usually extend posteriorly as far as the erector spinae fascia. The incision is deepened through subcutaneous tissue and the external oblique fascia to reach the intercostal muscles over the appropriate interspace. Before entry into the left pleural cavity is attempted, the abdominal portion of the incision is developed. The aorta may be reached by an extraperitoneal or transperitoneal approach. The extraperitoneal technique may be ideal for repairing thoracoabdominal aneurysms, especially those involving the upper abdominal aorta. The transperitoneal approach may be preferred in cases in which visceral artery revascularization is planned, especially bypasses to the right renal artery.

The extraperitoneal approach proceeds by developing the plane between transversalis fascia and parietal peritoneum. The peritoneum is separated from the lateral and posterior abdominal walls and then from the diaphragm superiorly (Fig. 9-26). To assist in the development of the retroperitoneal plane, wider exposure should next be gained by

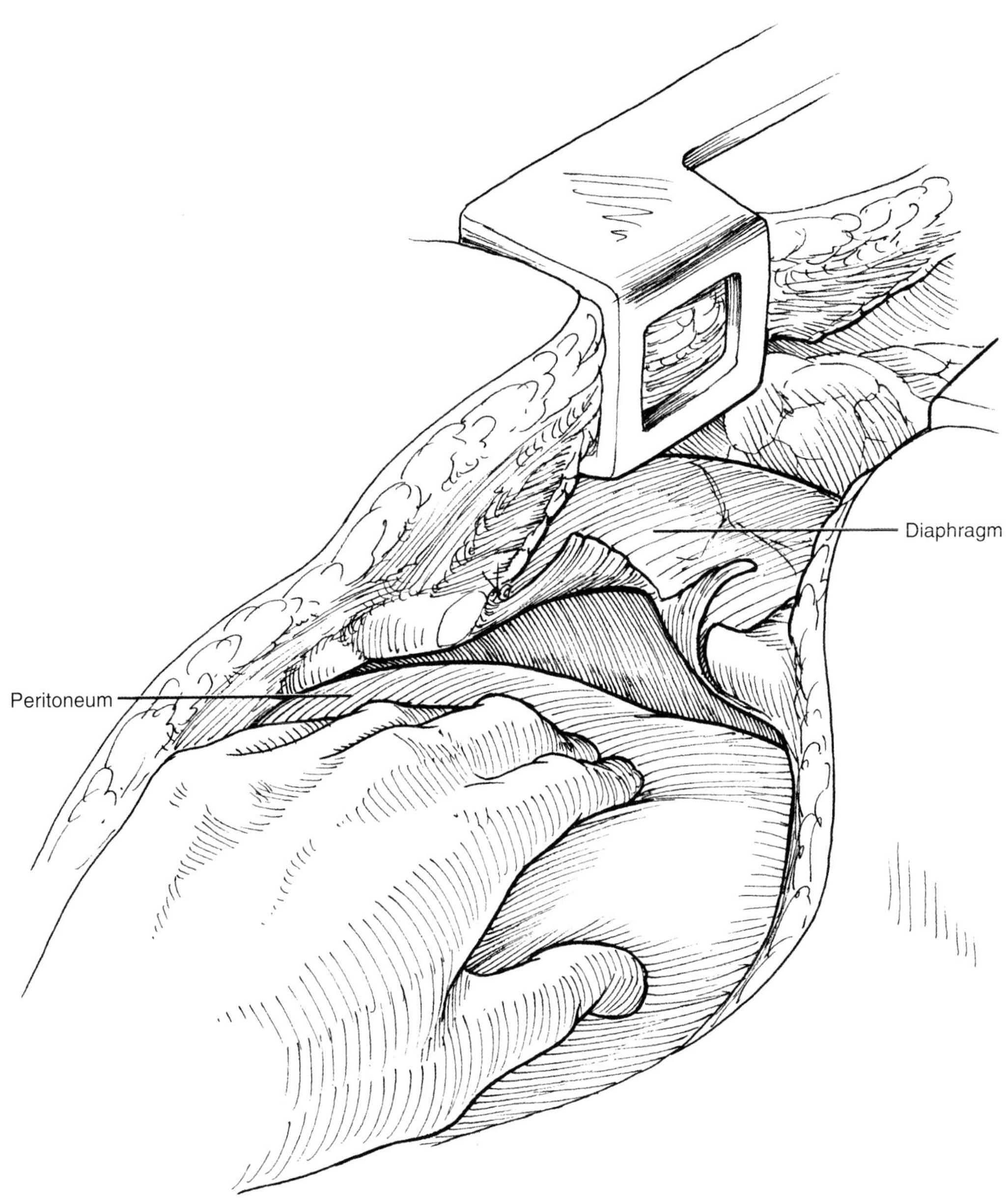

Fig. 9-26 For the extraperitoneal approach to the abdominal aorta, the peritoneum is separated from the undersurface of the diaphragm, and the chest is entered across the costal margin.

opening the left thorax and dividing the diaphragm. The intercostal muscles are divided, and the pleural cavity is entered on the superior border of the ninth (or sixth or seventh) rib. Resection of the lower rib aids in exposure and reduces pain associated with rib fracture from forceful retraction. It is important to locate the intercostal vessels to prevent injury during rib resection. A rib retractor is used to widen the interspace, and the costal margin separating the thoracic and abdominal wounds is divided.

The wound is further widened by incising the diaphragm, either partially or completely (Fig. 9-27). Partial incision through the muscular portion of the diaphragm with preservation of the central tendinous portion has been recommended to minimize respiratory complications.[27] Preservation of the diaphragm has been associated with reduced pulmonary complications; however, additional exposure of the aorta at the hiatus will be required. Complete division proceeds from the divided costal margin to the aortic hiatus. Some surgeons perform the incision radially,[28] while others[29] prefer partial or complete division of the diaphragm in a circumferential fashion approximately 3 cm from the internal costal margin to avoid cutting major branches of the phrenic nerve. The circumferential incision avoids transecting the phrenic nerve branches, theoretically leading to earlier return of diaphragm function. This advantage may prove extremely important because ventilatory failure is one of the most common complications of thoracoabdominal incisions. However, advocates of the radial incision technique have noted that circumferential division is cumbersome, difficult to close, and associated with equivalent results.[28]

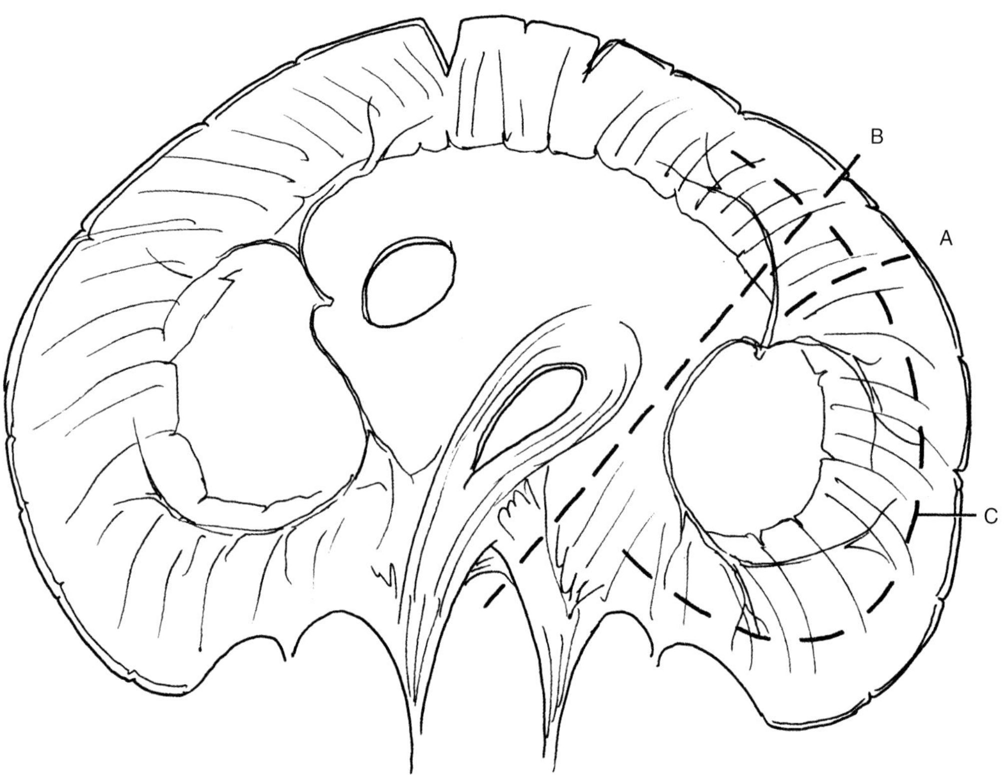

Fig. 9-27 The diaphragm can be divided partially **(A)** or completely using radial **(B)** or circumferential **(C)** incisions.

The retroperitoneal tissue plane in the posterior abdomen can now be easily developed to the aorta. The anterior renal fascia is opened, and the plane posterior to the left kidney is developed. The left kidney is mobilized anteriorly along with the adrenal gland, spleen, and pancreas (Fig. 9-28). The large lumbar branch of the left renal vein should be ligated and divided during this maneuver (Fig. 9-19). The left ureter should be identified and reflected with the mobilized retroperitoneal tissue. As the peritoneum is removed from the undersurface of the diaphragm, the pancreas is reflected anteromedially along with the peritoneal contents. During exposure of the juxtarenal aortic segment, it is important to identify the left renal artery in the areolar tissues overlying the anteromedial surface of the aorta. The left renal artery will be in an unusual location when the left kidney is retracted anteriorly, making it prone to accidental transection as the periaortic tissues are incised. The distal abdominal aorta and proximal left common iliac artery are exposed by reflecting the peritoneal

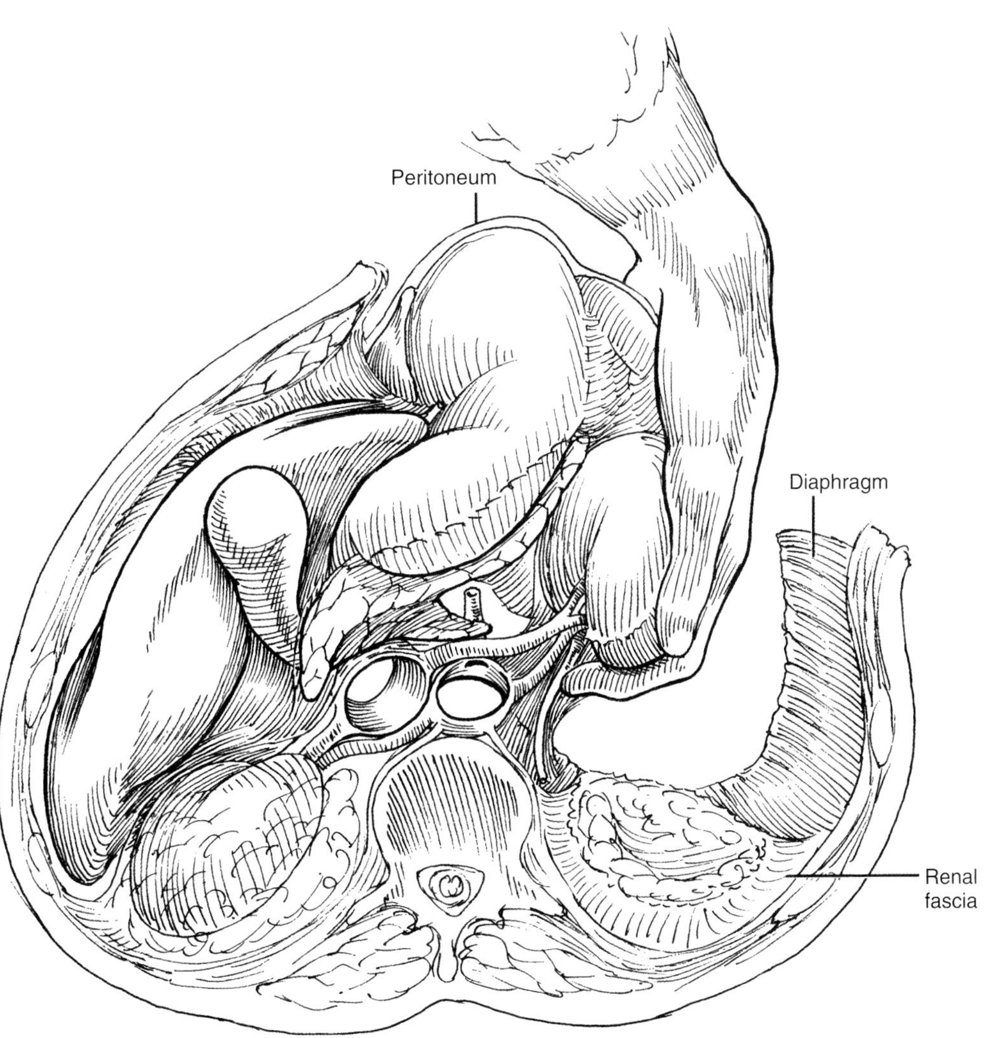

Fig. 9-28 The anterior renal fascia is opened, and the kidney is mobilized along with the upper abdominal organs on the left.

sac in the distal wound and ligating the inferior mesenteric artery at its origin (Fig. 9-29). Exposure of the more distal left iliac artery or any portion of the right iliac artery is technically difficult using the extraperitoneal approach; revascularization of these vessels should be performed at the level of the femoral arteries. Alternatively, the right iliac vessels can be exposed through a separate right flank incision (see Chapter 12).

If the transperitoneal approach to the retroperitoneal tissue plane is chosen, the peritoneum should be opened for the full length of the abdominal wound, up to the costal margin. A relatively avascular plane is developed posterior to the left colon

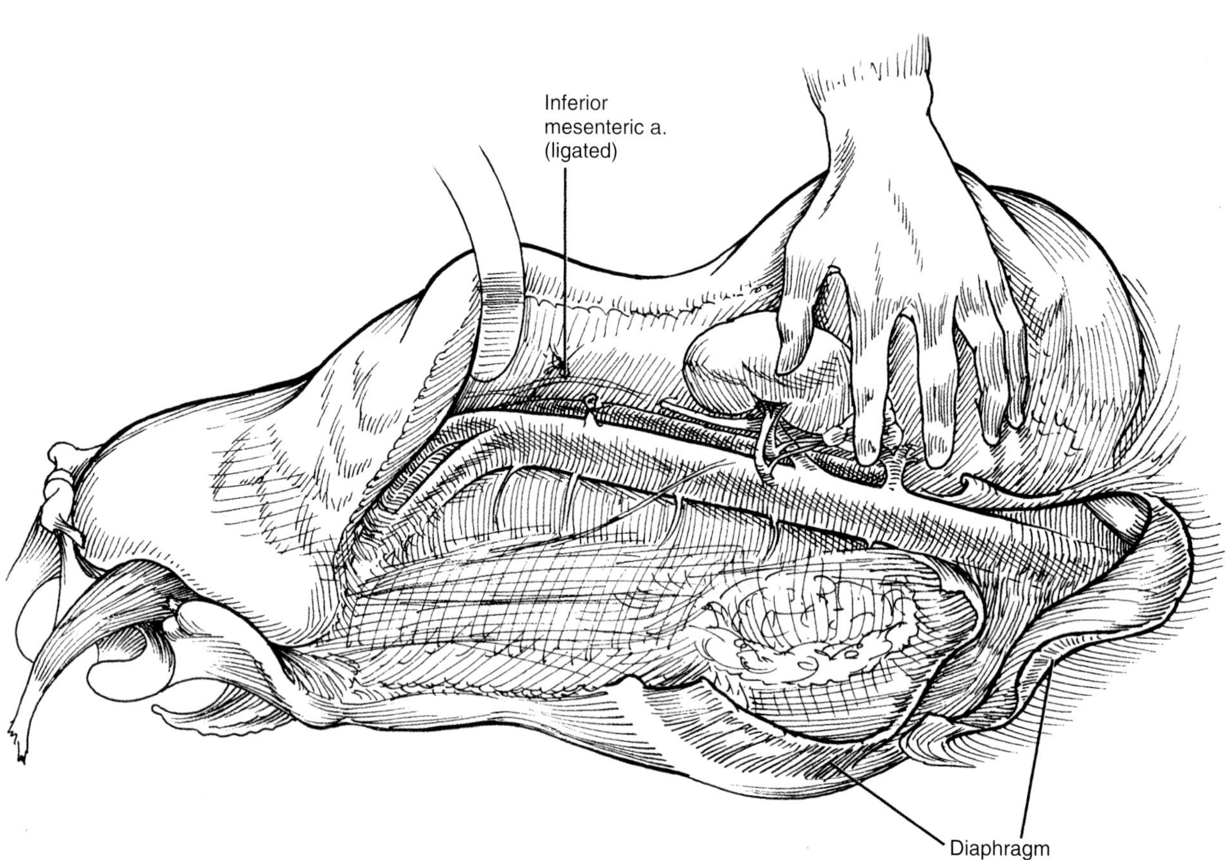

Fig. 9-29 Further mobilization in the extraperitoneal plane along the left gutter exposes the lower abdominal aorta.

mesentery by dividing the lateral peritoneal attachments along the left gutter and mobilizing the left colon medially (Fig. 9-30). Medial reflection of the colon and its mesentery is carried cranially to the level of the spleen. The spleen is mobilized from the posterior peritoneum by dividing the splenorenal and splenophrenic ligaments. Wider exposure is obtained at this juncture by opening the left pleural cavity and incising the diaphragm as described above. The left kidney and adrenal gland are mobilized and reflected anteriorly after dividing lumbar and gonadal branches of the left renal vein. The left kidney, adrenal gland, spleen, pancreas, stomach, colon, and intestines are all reflected to the midline, exposing the abdominal aorta from the bifurcation to the diaphragm. Exposure of the left iliac arteries and right common iliac artery is accomplished by reflection of the sigmoid colon and its mesentery in the distal wound.

To expose the descending thoracic aorta through the thoracoabdominal incision, the inferior pulmonary ligament and any adhesions between the left lung and aorta are incised, allowing the left lung to

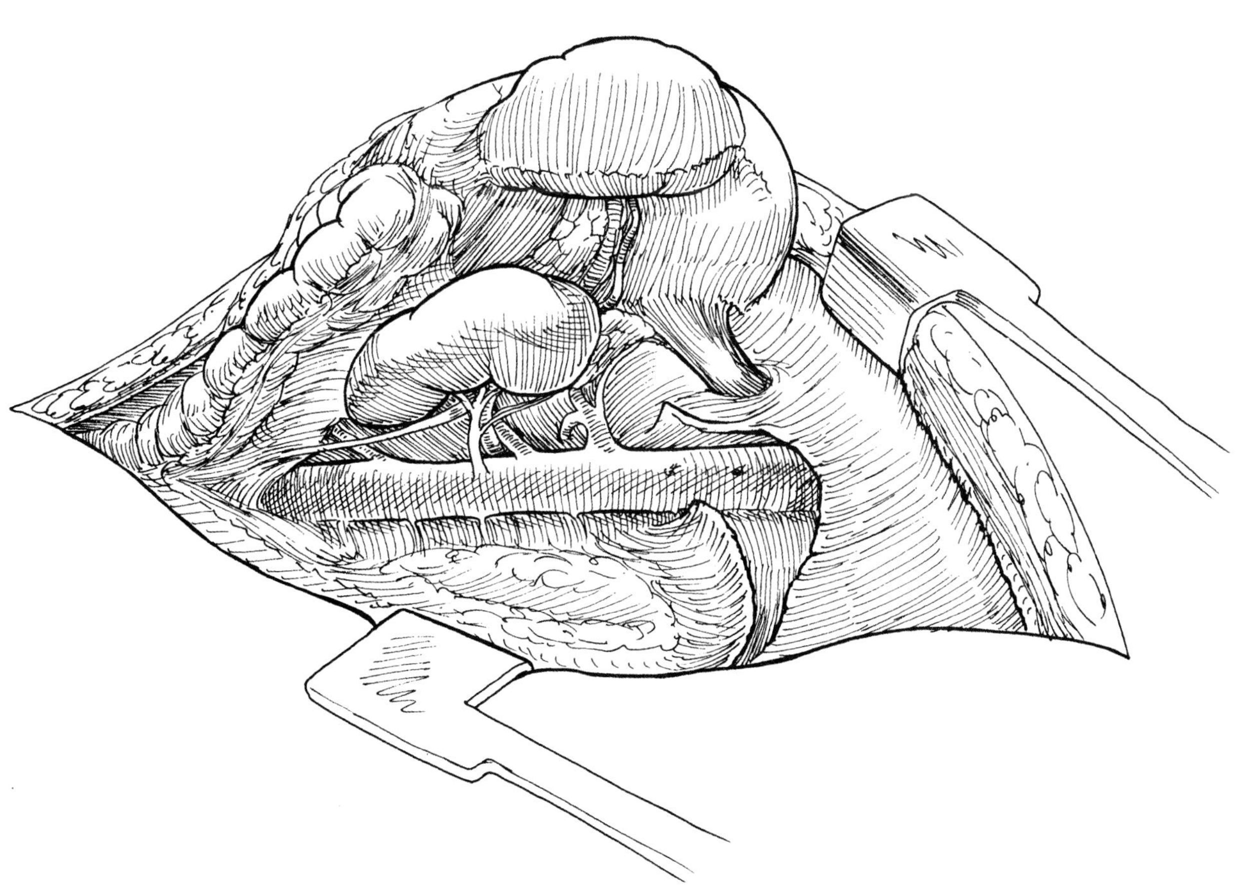

Fig. 9-30 The intraperitoneal approach to organ mobilization is shown.

deflate and be retracted superomedially (Fig. 9-31). The parietal pleura is incised directly over the segment of thoracic aorta to be exposed, gaining access to the lateral periadventitial plane. Using blunt dissection, the aorta is carefully encircled at a level desired for proximal control. This is performed most easily between intercostal arterial branches.

The segment of the aorta immediately proximal to the celiac artery is exposed by dividing the left crus of the diaphragm. By extending the incision from the lateral side of the aortic hiatus through the left crus to the posterior margin of the circumferential incision, the entire thoracoabdominal aorta can be exposed.

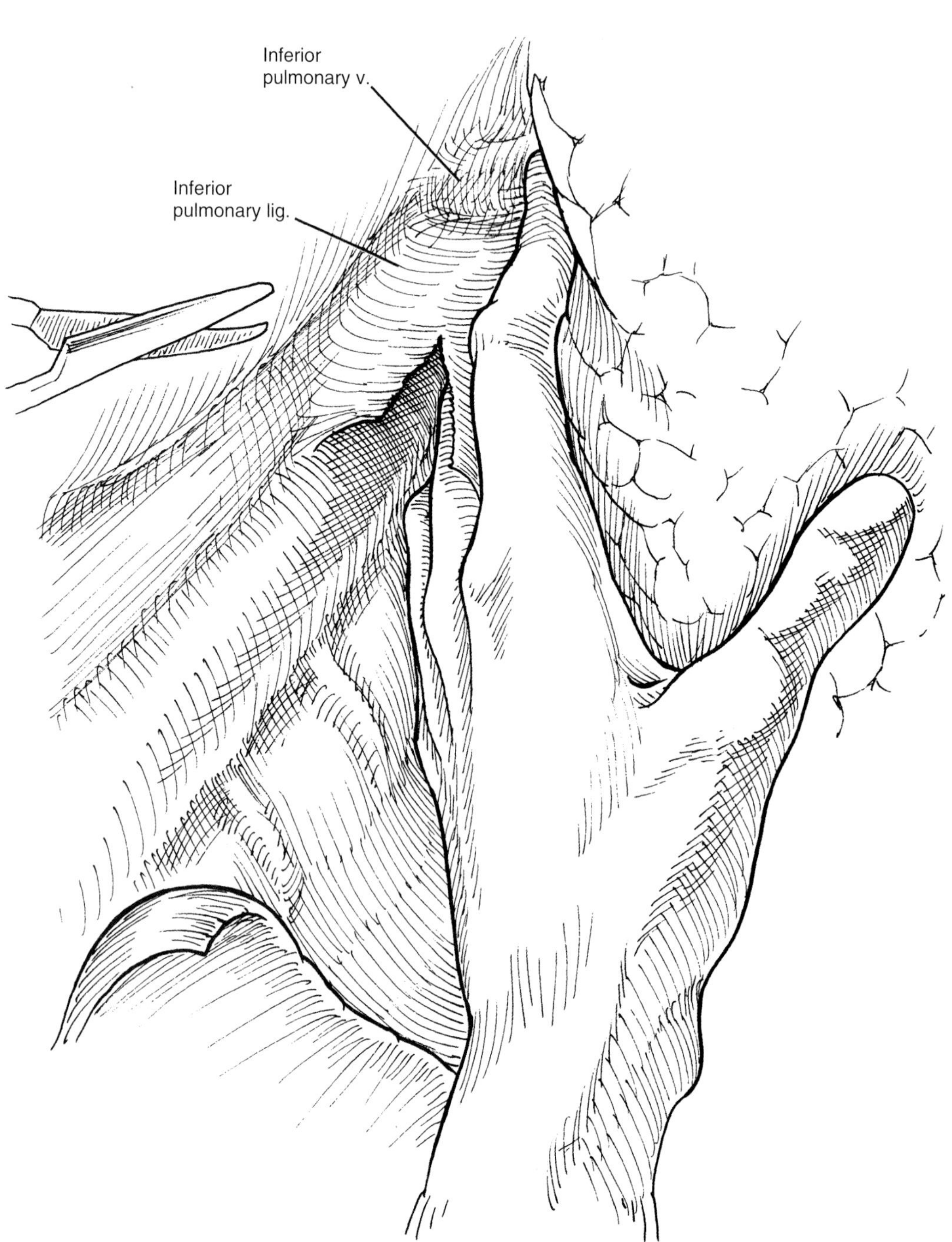

Fig. 9-31 The lower thoracic aorta is exposed by dividing the inferior pulmonary ligament up to the inferior pulmonary vein.

References

1. Lei QF, Marks SC, Touliopoulos P, et al. Fascial planes of the posterior abdomen: the perirenal and pararenal pathways. *Clin Anat.* 1990;3:115.
2. Back MR, Bandyk M, Bradner M, et al. Critical analysis of outcome determinants affecting repair of intact aneurysms involving the visceral aorta. *Ann Vasc Surg.* 2005;19:648–656.
3. Tang T, Boyle JR, Dixon AK, et al. Inflammatory abdominal aortic aneurysms. *Eur J Endovasc Surg.* 2005;29:353–362.
4. Wahlgren CM, Piano G, Desai T, et al. Transperitoneal versus retroperitoneal suprarenal cross-clamping for repair of abdominal aortic aneurysm with a hostile infrarenal aortic neck. *Ann Vasc Surg.* 2007;21:687–694.
5. Mehta M, Paty PSK, Roddy SP, et al. Treatment options for delayed AAA rupture following endovascular repair. *J Vasc Surg.* 2011;53:14–20.
6. Darling RC III, Cordero JA Jr, Chang BB, et al. Advances in the surgical repair of ruptured abdominal aortic aneurysms. *Cardiovasc Surg.* 1996;4:720–723.
7. Schneider JR, Gottner RJ, Golan JF. Supraceliac versus infrarenal aortic cross-clamp for repair of non-ruptured infrarenal abdominal aortic aneurysm. *Cardiovasc Surg.* 1997;5:279–285.
8. Oderich GS, Gloviczki P, Bower TC. Open surgical treatment for chronic mesenteric ischemia in the endovascular era: when is it necessary and what is the preferred technique? *Semin Vasc Surg.* 2010;23:36–46.
9. Borkon MJ, Zaydfudim V, Carey CD, et al. Retroperitoneal repair of abdominal aortic aneurysms offers postoperative benefits to male patients in the Veterans Affairs Health System. *Ann Vasc Surg.* 2010;24:728–732.
10. Arko FR, Bohannon WT, Mettauer M, et al. Retroperitoneal approach for aortic surgery: is it worth it? *Cardiovasc Surg.* 2001;9:20–26.
11. Cambria RP, Brewster DC, Abbott WM, et al. Transperitoneal versus retroperitoneal approach for aortic reconstruction: a randomized prospective study. *J Vase Surg.* 1990;11:314–325.
12. LeMaire SA, Green SY, Kim JH, et al. Thoracic or thoracoabdominal approaches to endovascular device removal and open aortic repair. *Ann Thorac Surg.* 2012;93:726–732.
13. Wong DR, Parenti JL, Green SY, et al. Open repair of thoracoabdominal aortic aneurysms in the modern surgical era: contemporary outcomes in 509 patients. *J Mm Coll Surg.* 2011;212:569–579.
14. Safi HJ, Estrera AL, Azizzadeh A, et al. Progress and future challenges in thoracoabdominal aortic aneurysm management. *World J Surg.* 2008;32:355–360.
15. Martin GH, O'Hara PJ, Hertzer NR, et al. Surgical repair of aneurysms involving the suprarenal, visceral, and lower thoracic aortic segments: early results and late outcome. *J Vase Surg.* 2000;31:851–862.
16. Coselli JS, Bozinovski J, LeMaire SA. Open surgical repair of 2,286 thoracoabdominal aortic aneurysms. *Ann Thorac Surg.* 2007;83:S862–S864.
17. Shepard AD, Tollefson DFJ, Reddy DJ, et al. Left flank retroperitoneal approach: a technical aid to complex aortic reconstruction. *J Vasc Surg.* 1991;14:283–291.
18. Williams GM. Extraperitoneal exposure of the aorta. *Semin Vase Surg.* 1989;2:217–222.
19. Estrera AL, Sheinbaum R, Miller CC, et al. Cerebrospinal fluid drainage during thoracic aortic repair: safety and current management. *Ann Thorac Surg.* 2009;88:9–15.
20. Fedorow CA, Moon MC, Mutch WA, et al. Lumbar cerebrospinal fluid drainage for thoracoabdominal aortic surgery: rationale and practical considerations for management. *Anesth Analg.* 2010;111:46–58.
21. Tabayashi K, Saiki Y, Kokubo H, et al. Protection from postischemic spinal cord injury by perfusion cooling of the epidural space during most or all of a descending thoracic or thoracoabdominal aneurysm repair. *Gen Thorac Cardiovasc Surg.* 2010;58:228–234.
22. Black JH, Davidson JK, Cambria RP. Regional hypothermia with epidural cooling for prevention of spinal cord ischemic complications after thoracoabdominal aortic surgery. *Semin Thorac Cardiovasc Surg.* 2003;15:345–352.
23. Hsu CC, Kwan GN, van Driel ML, et al. Distal aortic perfusion during thoracoabdominal aneurysm repair for prevention of paraplegia. *Cochrane Database Syst Rev.* 2012;3:CD008179.
24. Shimizu H, Yozu R. Current strategies for spinal cord protection during thoracic and thoracoabdominal aortic aneurysm repair. *Gen Thorac Cardiovasc Surg.* 2011;59:155–163.
25. Crawford ES, Crawford JL, Safi HJ, et al. Thoracoabdominal aortic aneurysm: preoperative and intraoperative factors determining immediate and long-term results of operations in 605 patients. *J Vase Surg.* 1986;3:389–409.
26. Safi HJ, Miller CC III, Huynh TTT, et al. Thoracoabdominal aortic aneurysm graft repair. *Contemp Surg.* 2000;56:666–675.
27. Engle J, Safi HJ, Miller CC III, et al. The impact of diaphragm management on prolonged ventilator support after thoracoabdominal aneurysm repair. *J Vase Surg.* 1999;29:150–156.
28. Acher CW, Wynn MM. Technique of thoracoabdominal aneurysm repair. *Ann Vase Surg* 1995;9:585–595.
29. Gilling-Smith GL, Wolfe JHN. Thoracoabdominal aneurysms: which patients should we operate on? *Perspect Vase Surg.* 1995;8:29–53.

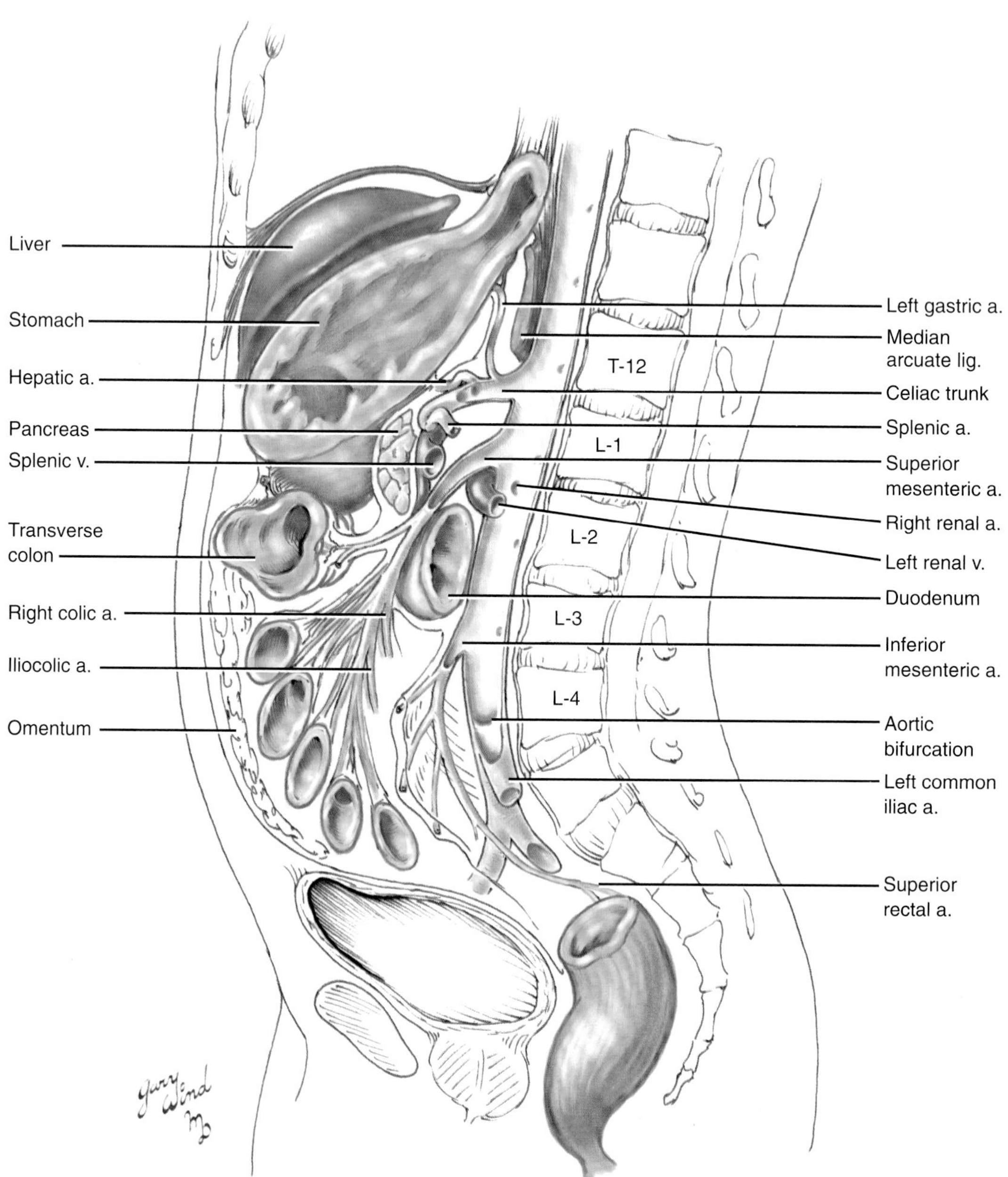

Fig. 10-1 The origins of the major mesenteric vessels are shown in relation to the adjacent vertebral bodies.

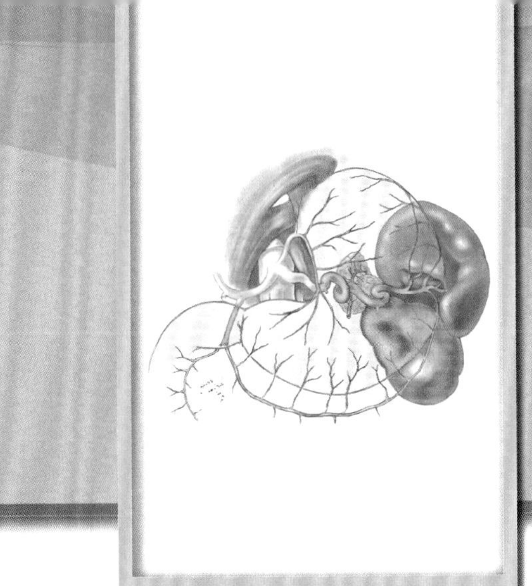

Celiac and Mesenteric Arteries

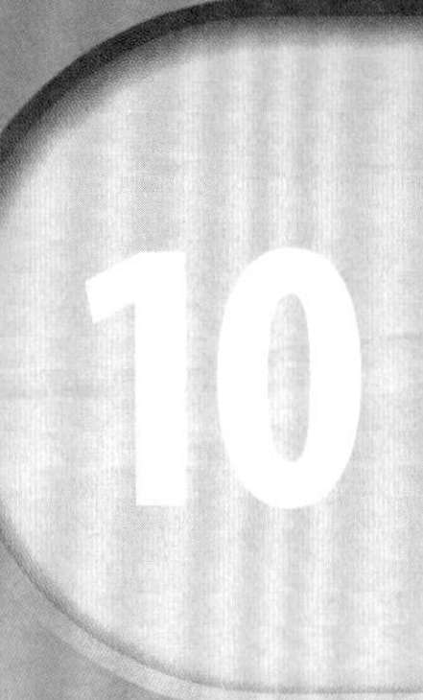

10

Surgical Anatomy of the Mesenteric Vessels

Three large, unpaired midline vessels supply the majority of organs enclosed by the outer envelope of parietal peritoneum. Two of these, the celiac and superior mesenteric arteries, arise within centimeters of each other at the level of the first lumbar vertebra (Fig. 10-1). The third, the inferior mesenteric artery, arises from the anterior wall of the aorta at the level of the third lumbar vertebra.

Celiac Trunk

The celiac trunk is closely flanked by the median arcuate ligament of the aortic hiatus above and the superior border of the pancreas below (Fig. 10-2). Viewed from an anterior perspective, the celiac trunk lies beneath the overlapping edges of the liver and stomach. On separating these two organs, the connecting gastrohepatic ligament, which forms the anterior wall of the omental bursa, is seen overlying the celiac trunk. Inside the omental bursa lies a final covering membrane, the posterior parietal peritoneum. Beneath the peritoneum, the celiac trunk is surrounded by lymphatic and nerve plexuses.

The celiac trunk is almost perpendicular to the aorta. The three branches of the celiac trunk most often form a trifurcation (see variations, Chapter 19). One significant vein, the left gastric (or coronary) vein, crosses over the celiac trunk in its course from the lesser curve of the stomach to the portal vein.

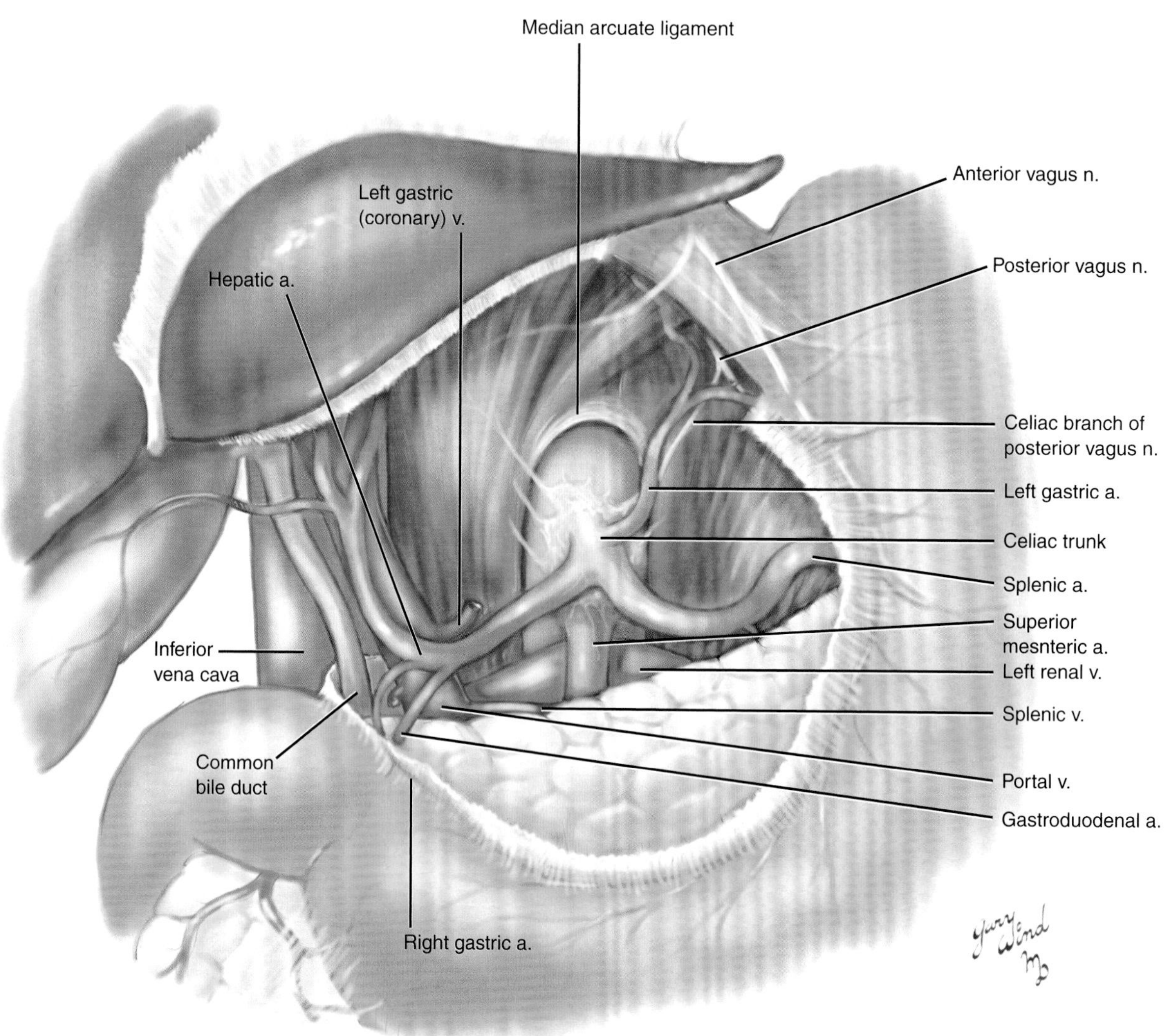

Fig. 10-2 The gastrohepatic omentum and posterior peritoneum of the omental bursa have been removed to expose the celiac trunk.

The hepatic artery passes to the right beneath the posterior peritoneum of the omental bursa, enters the hepatoduodenal ligament just cephalad to the pylorus, and ascends to the hilum of the liver on the left side of the common bile duct. The terminal branching of the hepatic artery is highly variable, and alternate origins of hepatic artery branches are not uncommon.

The splenic artery descends beneath the peritoneum to undulate along the cephalad border of the pancreas where it gives off a significant dorsal pancreatic branch and a few smaller branches. After dividing into four to five branches near the hilum of the spleen, it gives off short gastric branches and the left gastroepiploic artery that run in the gastrosplenic ligament and the gastrocolic ligament, respectively (Fig. 10-3).

The left gastric artery ascends a short distance beneath the peritoneum to reach the lesser curve of the stomach at the gastroesophageal junction. It is accompanied by the left gastric (coronary) vein and the celiac branch of the posterior vagus nerve. When the esophagus is mobilized, the left gastric artery limits the surgeon from sliding a finger further down the posterior wall of the stomach.

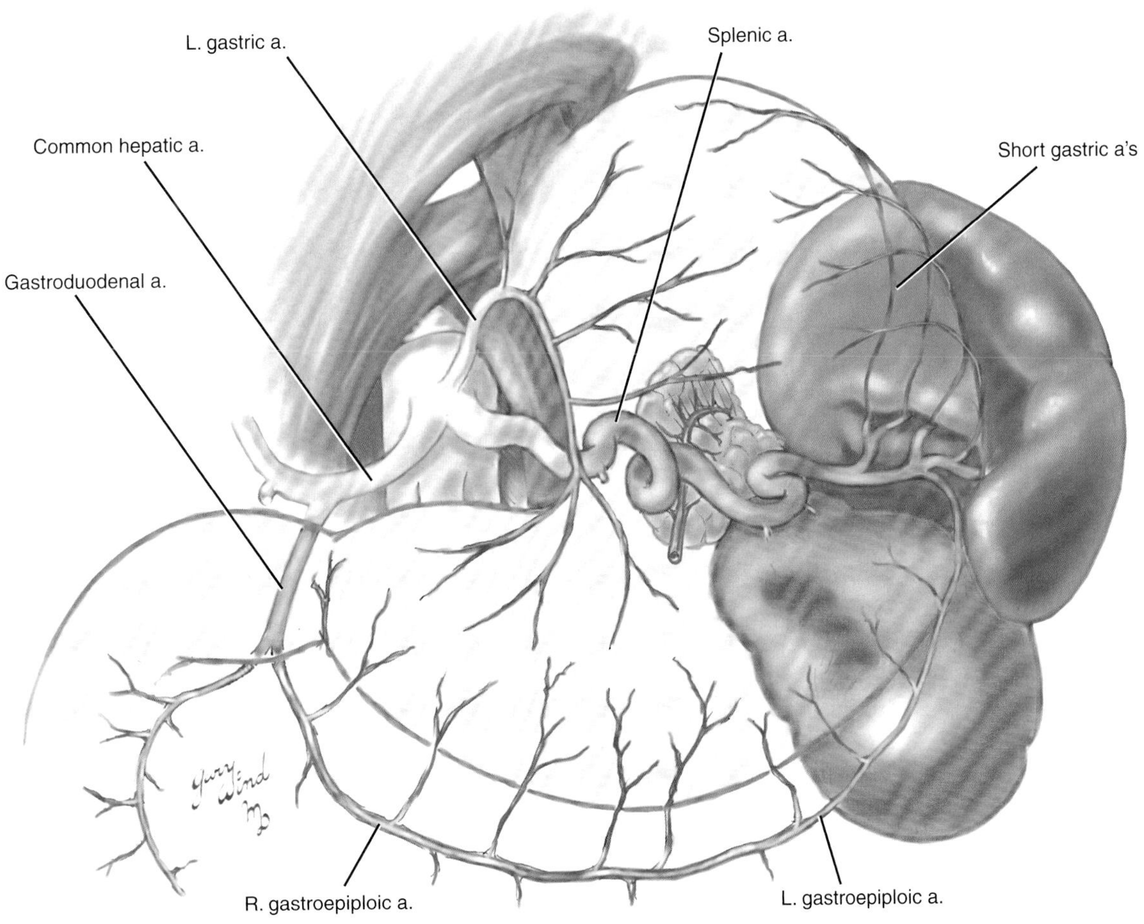

Fig. 10-3 Anastomoses of celiac branches around the stomach are shown.

Superior Mesenteric Artery

The origin of the superior mesenteric artery from the aorta forms a sharp caudal angle. The left renal vein is wedged into the acute angle. The first part of the superior mesenteric is crossed by the neck of the pancreas and the splenic vein. Behind the neck of the pancreas, the artery converges with the superior mesenteric vein so that the two structures are side by side at the lower margin of the pancreatic neck (Fig. 10-4). The vessels then pass over the uncinate process of the pancreas and the third portion of the duodenum to enter the root of the small bowel mesentery.

As soon as the superior mesenteric artery emerges below the pancreas, it sends the middle colic artery into the overlying root of transverse mesocolon. At the level of the uncinate process, the superior mesenteric artery also gives rise to the inferior pancreaticoduodenal artery, which makes a potentially important connection with the celiac circulation through the pancreaticoduodenal arcade.

The continuation of the superior mesenteric artery gives rise to two named branches and numerous vessels supplying the small bowel. Shortly after crossing the duodenum, the superior mesenteric gives off the right colic artery, which lies within the fused mesentery of the right colon. The ileocolic branch arises in common with or distal to the right colic and descends toward the cecum. The root of the small bowel mesentery passes from midline to the right lower quadrant, allowing mobilization of

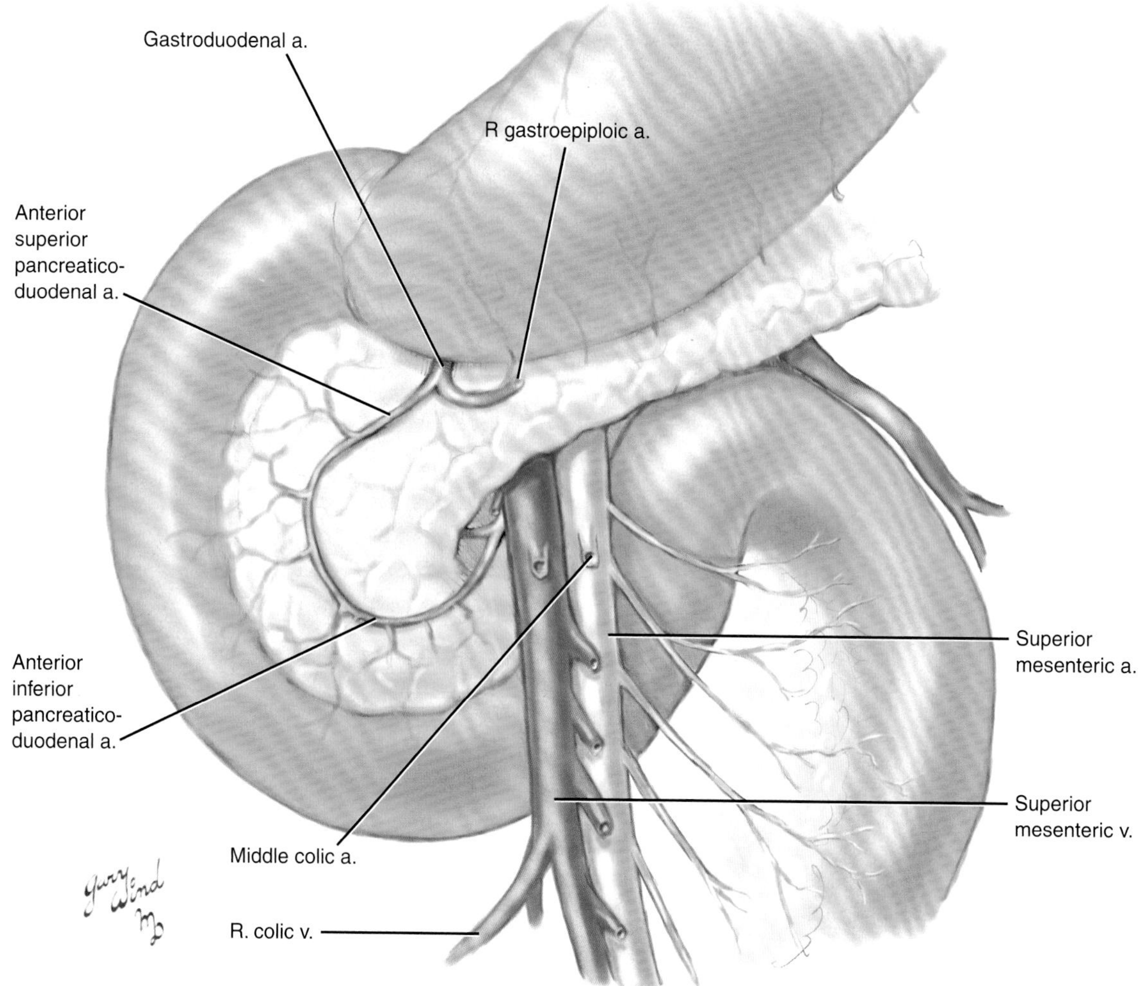

Fig. 10-4 The superior mesenteric artery and vein lie together over the third portion of the duodenum and uncinate process of the pancreas.

this mesentery to the right for exposure of the aorta (Fig. 10-5).

Inferior Mesenteric Artery

The inferior mesenteric artery emerges near the lower border of the third portion of the duodenum where the latter crosses the aorta (Fig. 10-1). It is closely applied to the aorta as it passes to the left into the fused mesentery of the left colon. Within 5 cm of its origin, the artery first gives off a left colic branch and then several sigmoidal branches into the mobile sigmoid mesentery and finally terminates as the superior rectal branch. The latter crosses over the left iliac vessels to reach the posterior wall of the upper rectum (Fig. 10-1). In some cases of superior mesenteric occlusive disease, mesenteric channels between the left colic and middle colic arteries hypertrophy to form a meandering mesenteric artery (described by Riolan, see below),

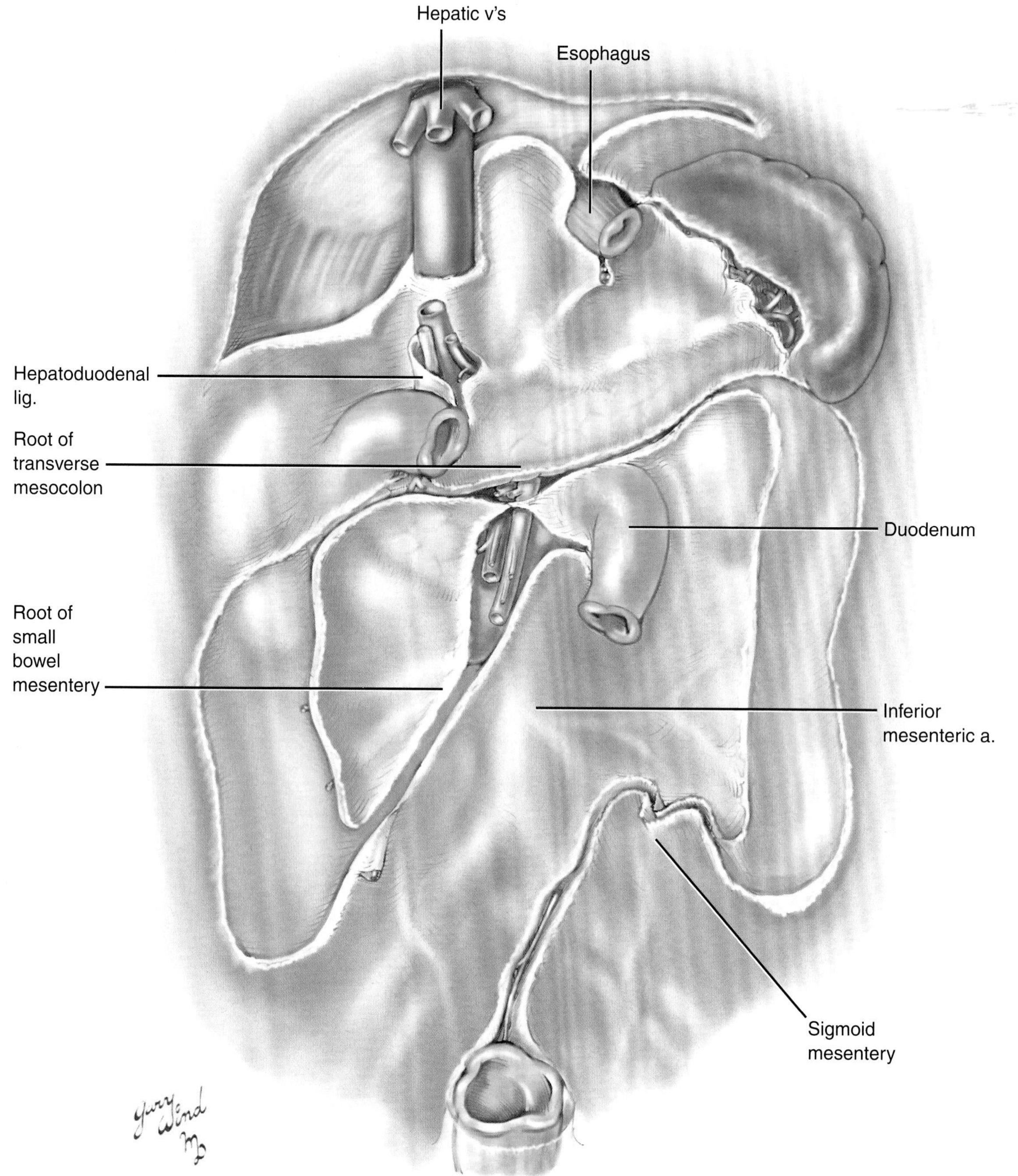

Fig. 10-5 The superior mesenteric artery can be located where the roots of the transverse mesocolon and small bowel mesentery meet.

which supplements the deficient superior mesenteric system.

Collateral Visceral Circulation

Major communications among the three levels of visceral vessels provide collateral circulation in case of segmental occlusion (Fig. 10-6). The pancreaticoduodenal arcade connects the celiac and superior mesenteric circulations. The marginal artery (of Drummond) is composed of the left branch of the middle colic artery and the ascending branch of the left colic artery. If complete across the splenic flexure, the marginal artery may be adequate to maintain visceral perfusion between the superior and inferior mesenteric circulations when one or the other is occluded. Some individuals develop an enlarged accessory collateral between the inferior and superior mesenteric circulations. This so-called meandering mesenteric artery (of Riolan) is named for its tortuous appearance within the transverse mesocolon owing to extensive hypertrophy in patients with occlusive disease of the superior or inferior mesenteric branches. The inferior mesenteric circulation is also supported by collaterals between the superior rectal artery and the inferior rectal branches of the internal iliac artery.

Exposure of the Mesenteric Arteries

The collateral network between the three main arteries of the mesenteric circulation provides a margin of safety for bowel viability when flow to

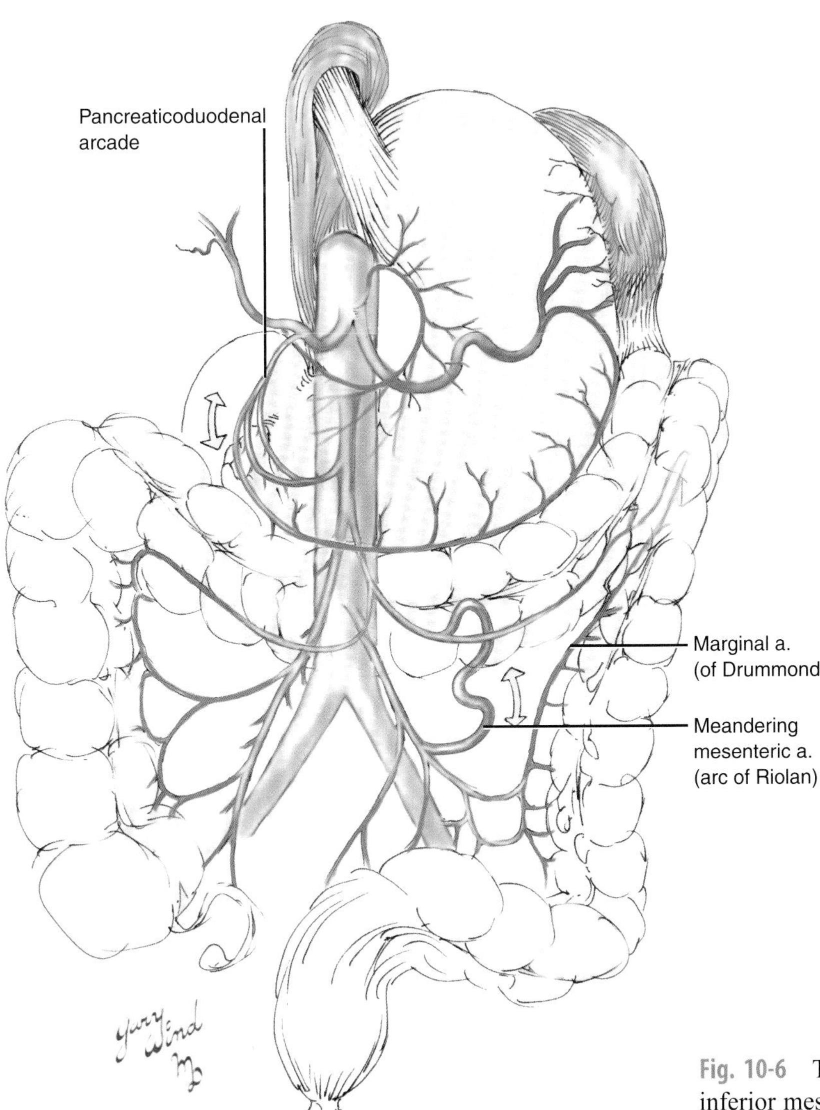

Fig. 10-6 The celiac, superior mesenteric, and inferior mesenteric circulations are connected by collateral vessels.

one or more of the mesenteric arteries is slowly reduced by atherosclerotic occlusive disease. In general, flow in at least two of the three arteries must be reduced to produce symptoms of chronic intestinal ischemia.[1] There appear to be many exceptions to this rule, however. Occlusion of two or even all three of the vessels has been observed in asymptomatic individuals.[2,3] Conversely, the compression of a single mesenteric artery (the celiac axis) by the median arcuate ligament or by abnormal celiac ganglion fibers is believed by many authors to be responsible for symptoms of mesenteric ischemia in the so-called celiac axis compression syndrome.[4,5] This syndrome remains controversial because several authors have shown that release of celiac axis compression may not permanently relieve symptoms in some patients.[6,7] Furthermore, up to 5% of healthy, asymptomatic individuals have evidence of celiac compression on CT.[8]

In contrast to chronic mesenteric arterial insufficiency, acute occlusion of a single mesenteric artery usually produces sudden abdominal symptoms because adequate collateral circulation does not have time to develop. The superior mesenteric artery is the most common site for acute occlusive mesenteric arterial insufficiency,[9,10] and rapid restoration of flow in this artery is necessary if intestinal necrosis is to be avoided. The nonocclusive variety of mesenteric ischemia is adequately summarized elsewhere.[10,11]

The two common causes of acute flow interruption in the proximal superior mesenteric artery are often distinguishable at laparotomy. Thrombosis usually occurs near the superior mesenteric artery origin, leading to gangrene of the entire small bowel and proximal half of the colon. In contrast, emboli usually lodge near the point where the middle colic artery branches from the superior mesenteric artery, maintaining viability of a small segment of proximal jejunum through the first few jejunal branches[9] (Fig. 10-7).

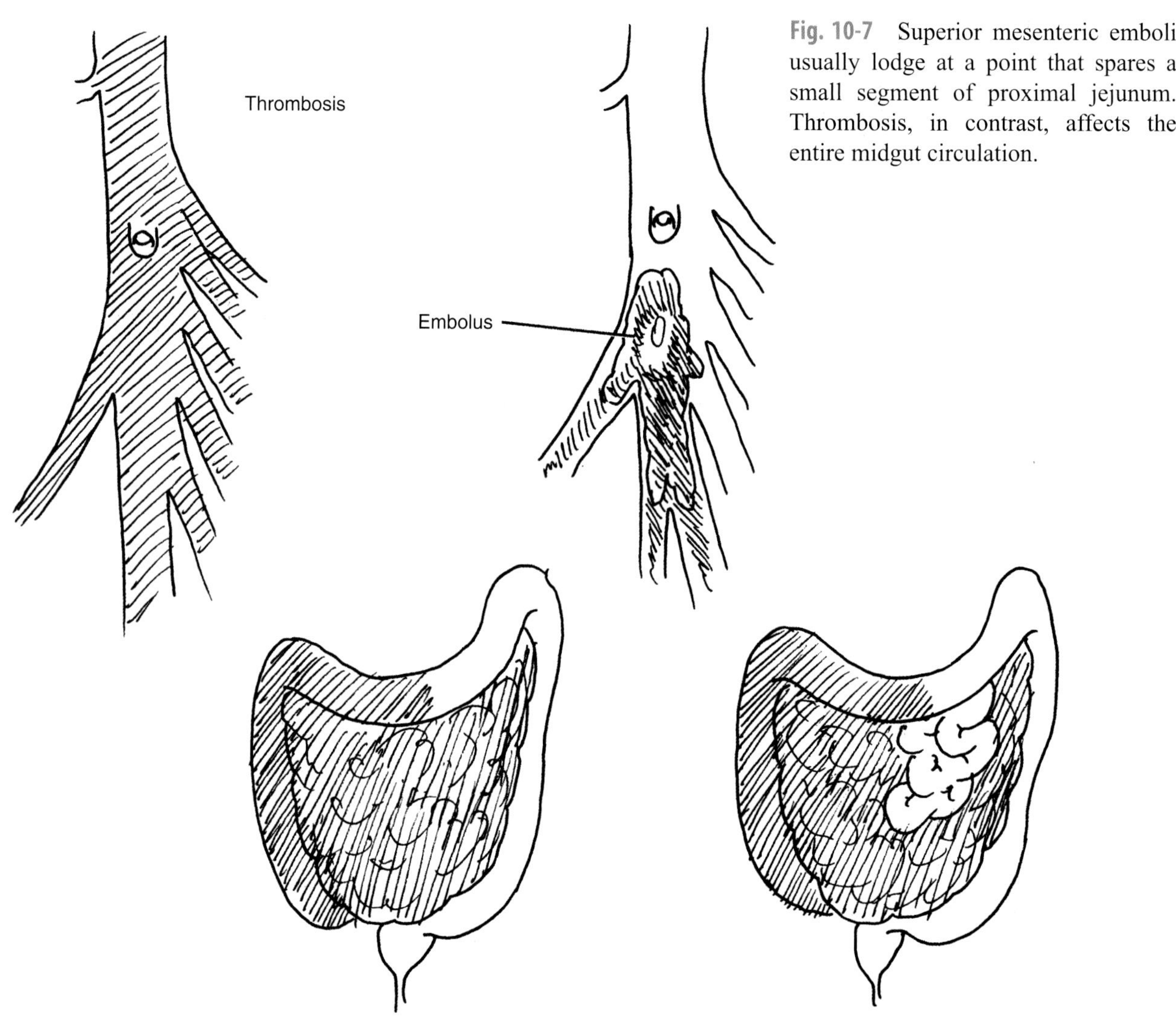

Fig. 10-7 Superior mesenteric emboli usually lodge at a point that spares a small segment of proximal jejunum. Thrombosis, in contrast, affects the entire midgut circulation.

Endovascular techniques are a useful alternative in some patients with chronic mesenteric ischemia, but surgical treatment is still considered the gold standard: surgical revascularization has been associated with a lower incidence of recurrent symptoms compared with percutaneous angioplasty and stenting.[12,13] Open surgical treatment with embolectomy or bypass is also indicated in acute mesenteric ischemia. Although direct infusion of thrombolytic agents through a percutaneous catheter can restore superior mesenteric artery flow,[14] operative intervention for acute mesenteric ischemia affords the opportunity to inspect the intestine for viability.

Superior mesenteric artery embolectomy is a simple and durable operation for the correction of acute embolic occlusions.[9] The best method for restoring mesenteric flow in patients with thrombotic occlusion is controversial and dependent on the underlying disorder. Excellent long-term results have been reported for antegrade bypasses,[15] retrograde bypasses[16] (see Fig. 10-16), and transaortic endarterectomy.[17] As an alternative to bypass, retrograde stenting of the occluded superior mesenteric artery can be performed at the time of operative exploration and may shorten the time of ischemia in an ill patient.[18]

The following discussions concern the exposure of mesenteric arteries using a transperitoneal approach through abdominal incisions. The retroperitoneal approach using thoracoabdominal incisions favored for use in transaortic endarterectomy is discussed in detail in Chapter 9.

Transperitoneal Exposure of the Celiac and Superior Mesenteric Arteries at Their Origins

The patient is placed in the supine position, and the entire abdomen and lower chest are prepped and draped. A longitudinal incision is made in the midline, extending from the xiphoid process to the umbilicus. The wound is deepened through subcutaneous tissue, the linea alba is incised, and the peritoneum is entered under direct vision. After routine

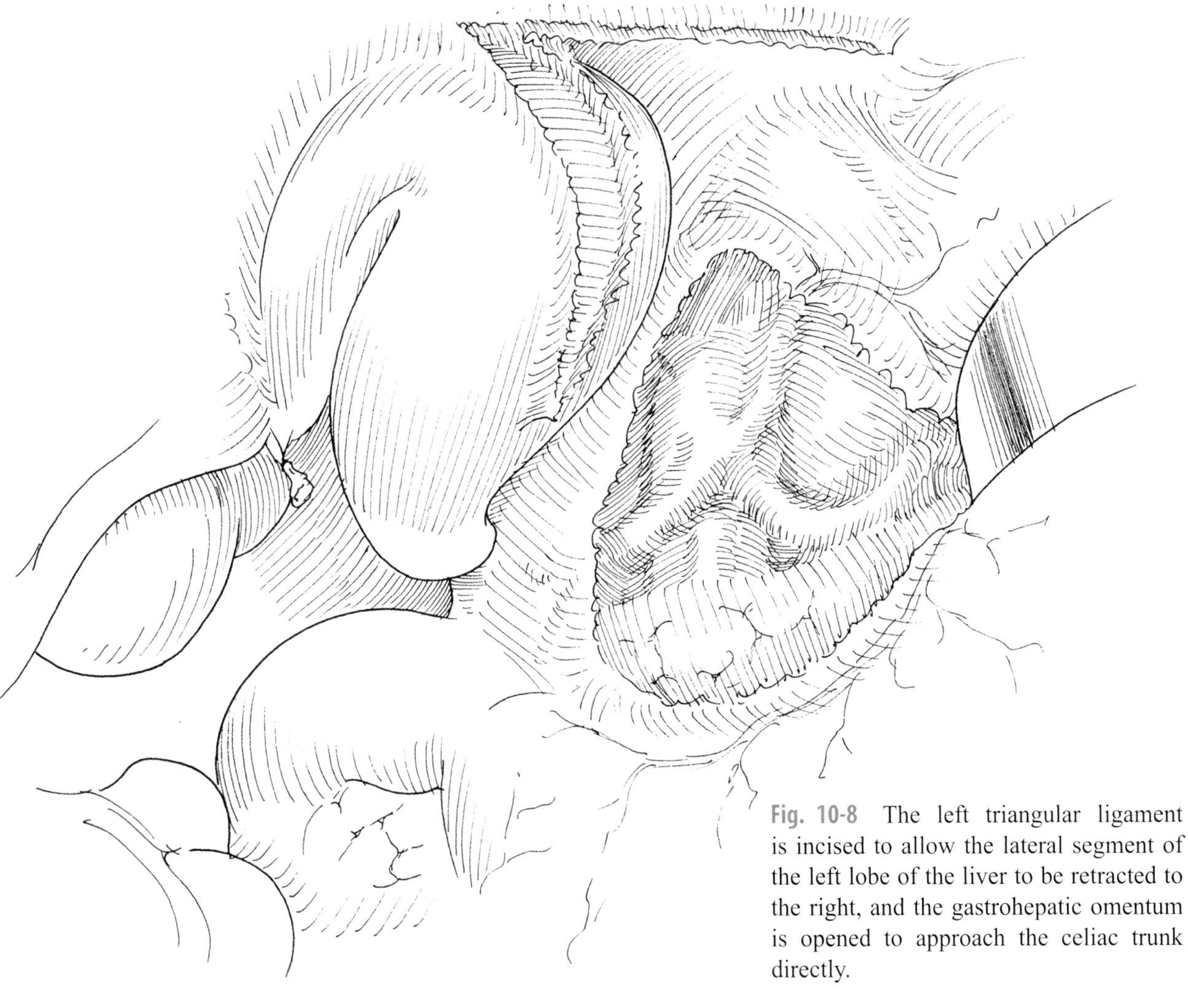

Fig. 10-8 The left triangular ligament is incised to allow the lateral segment of the left lobe of the liver to be retracted to the right, and the gastrohepatic omentum is opened to approach the celiac trunk directly.

examination of the peritoneal contents, the wound edges are retracted with a self-retaining device.

The left triangular ligament is incised, allowing mobilization and retraction to the right of the lateral segment of the left hepatic lobe (Fig. 10-8). The underlying gastrohepatic ligament is opened from the gastroesophageal junction to the pylorus, taking care to preserve the vagus nerve fibers near the lesser curvature of the stomach. Gentle retraction of the lower esophagus and lesser curvature to the patient's left exposes the celiac artery trunk and its major branches lying deep to the posterior parietal peritoneum. The distal thoracic aorta is exposed by opening the posterior peritoneum and vertically dividing the median arcuate ligament and interdigitating fibers of the left and right crura over the anterior aortic surface (Fig. 10-9). Exposure of the celiac artery is accomplished by dividing the celiac ganglion

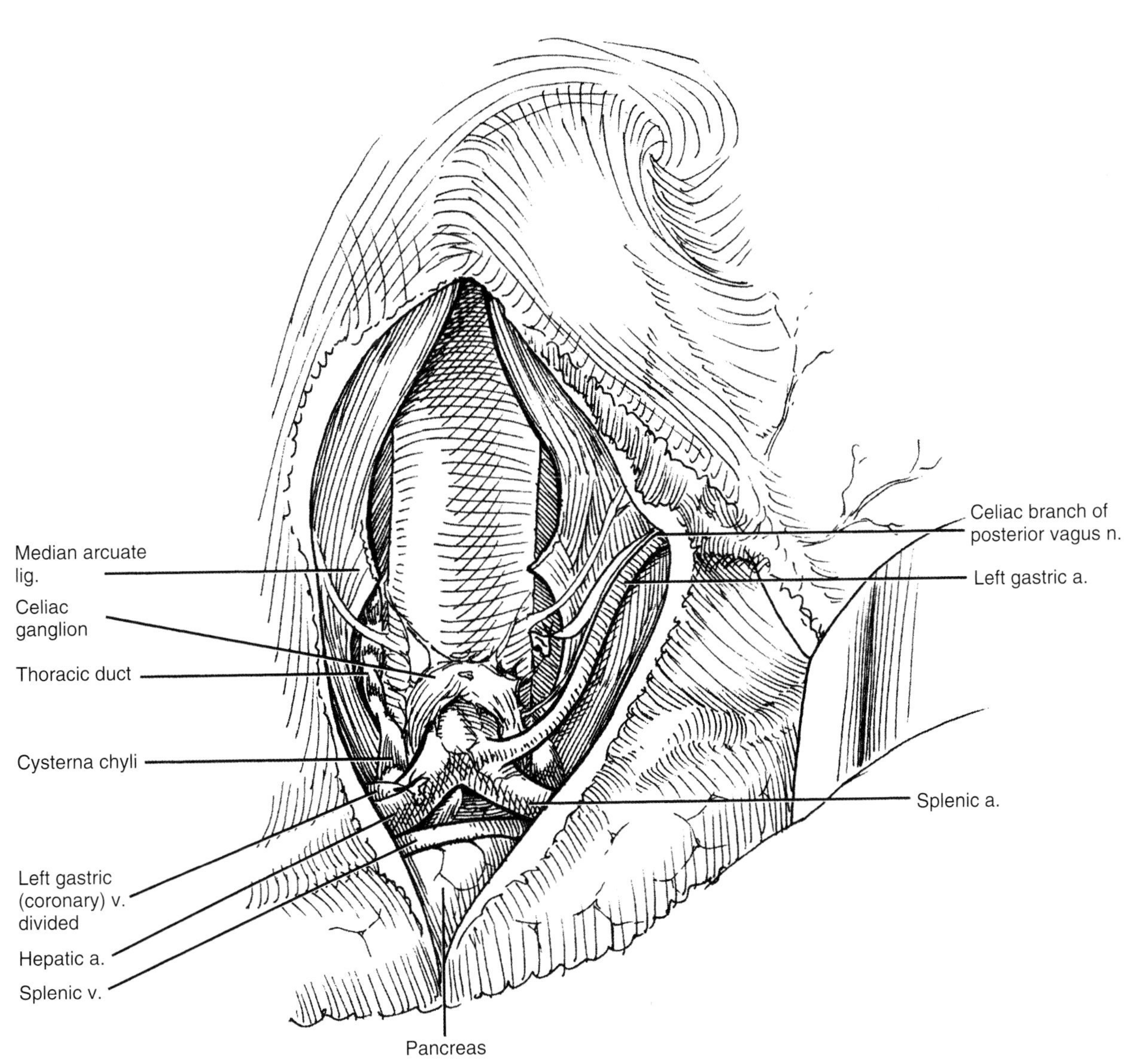

Fig. 10-9 The posterior parietal peritoneum and median arcuate ligament are opened to gain access to the celiac trunk.

(Fig. 10-10), which surrounds the celiac artery 3 to 5 mm from its origin and may be associated with a thick layer of fibrous tissue. The inferior phrenic arteries originate from the celiac artery in 47% of cases[19] and should be controlled during celiac trunk isolation.

The superior mesenteric artery origin is exposed by mobilizing the superior border of the pancreas

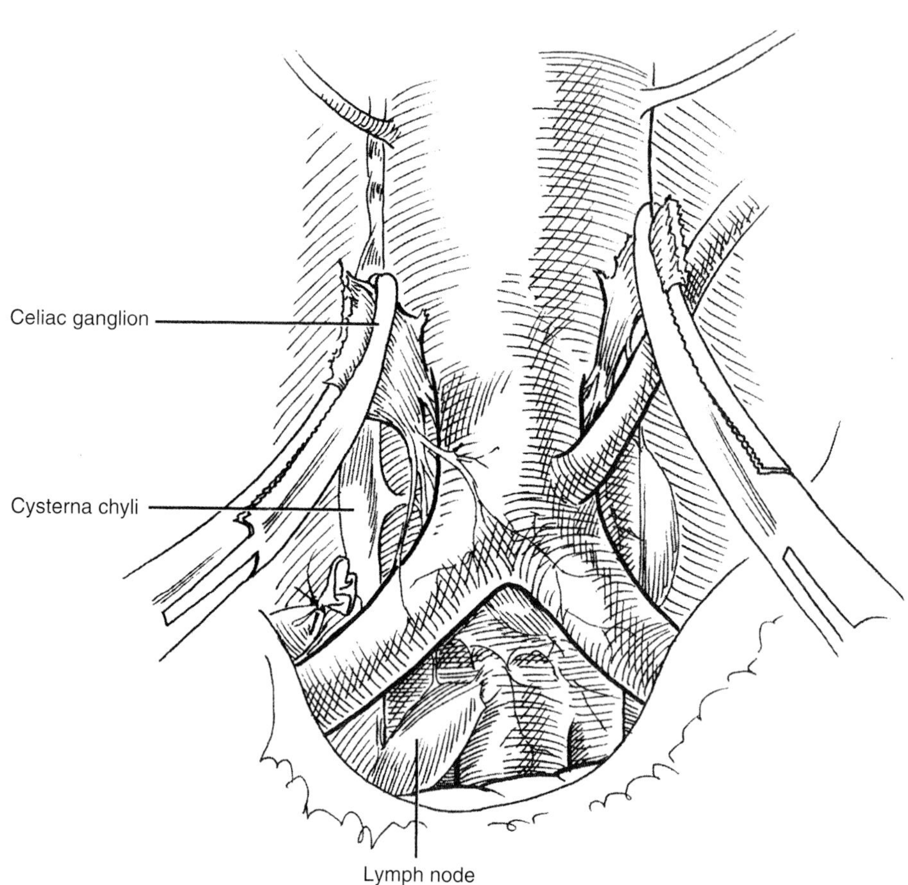

Fig. 10-10 The celiac ganglion must be cleared to fully expose the celiac trunk.

(Fig. 10-11) and continuing the dissection on the anterior surface of the aorta caudal to the celiac trunk.[20] The dissection proceeds between the superior border of the pancreas and the hepatic and splenic artery branches. To prevent avulsing pancreatic branches of the splenic artery, lateral dissection or forceful retraction of the superior pancreatic border to the left of the aorta should be avoided. Fibers of the celiac ganglion caudal to the celiac artery trunk should be cleared to expose the small intervening aortic segment. The origin of the superior mesenteric artery is exposed posterior to the neck of the pancreas, which is mobilized and retracted anteriorly along with the splenic vein. Care should be taken to avoid inadvertent injury to the inferior pancreaticoduodenal arteries during mobilization of the superior mesenteric artery. If peripancreatic inflammation or other local pathology renders exposure of the superior mesenteric artery origin difficult or dangerous, the artery can be isolated in the intestinal mesentery (see below).

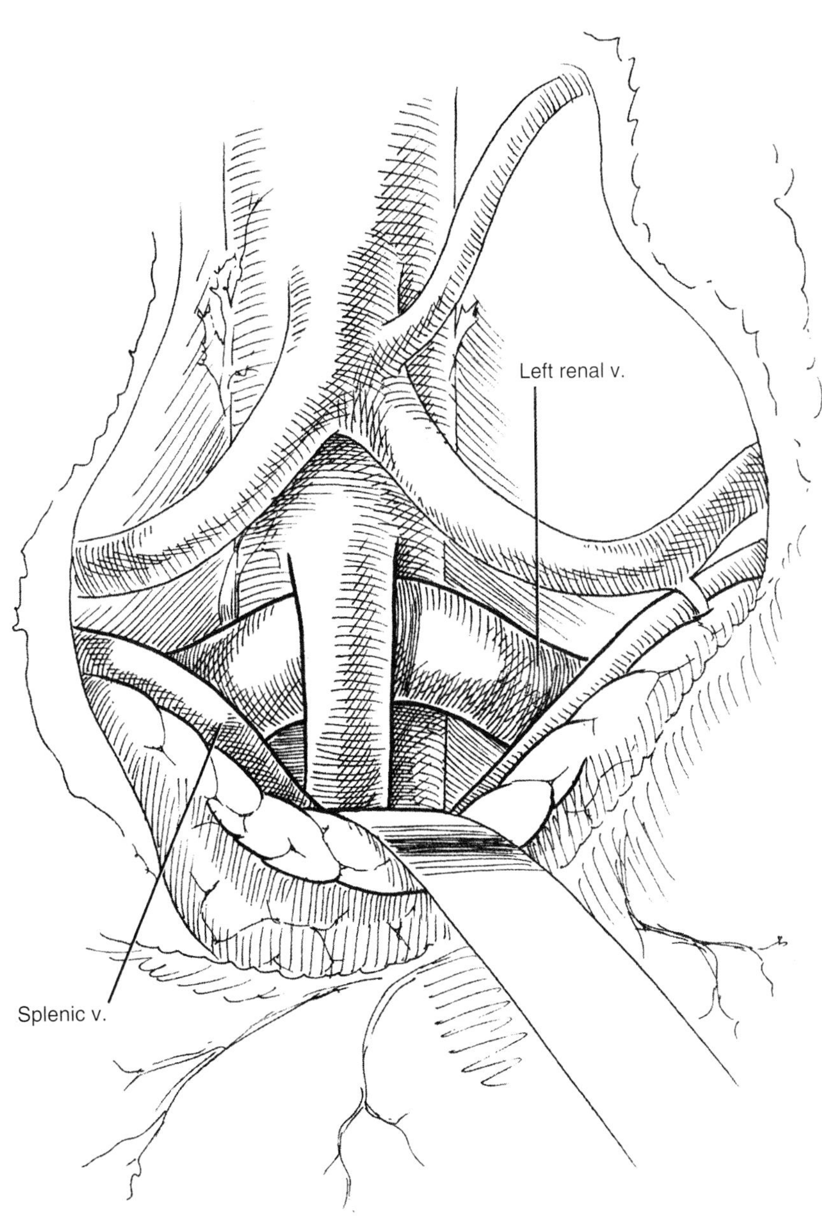

Fig. 10-11 The superior mesenteric artery origin can be exposed by retracting the superior border of the pancreas caudally.

Exposure of the Superior Mesenteric Artery in the Intestinal Mesentery

There are two popular approaches for exposure of the superior mesenteric artery distal to the inferior border of the pancreas. The anterior approach at the base of the transverse mesocolon is rapid and quite adequate for simple embolectomy in cases of acute occlusion. However, retrograde bypasses from the infrarenal aorta cannot be routed to the anteriorly exposed superior mesenteric artery without crossing the duodenum. In these cases, a lateral approach craniad to the fourth portion of the duodenum is necessary.

After the peritoneal cavity is entered under direct vision, the peritoneal contents are rapidly evaluated, noting especially the location and extent of bowel necrosis. To approach the superior mesenteric artery anteriorly, the transverse colon and omentum are elevated, and the intestines are wrapped in moist laparotomy packs and retracted to the right. A horizontal incision is made in the peritoneum at the base of the transverse mesocolon, extending from the duodenal–jejunal junction toward the patient's right. The middle colic artery should be identified in the transverse mesocolon and traced proximally to locate its origin from the superior mesenteric artery (Fig. 10-12).

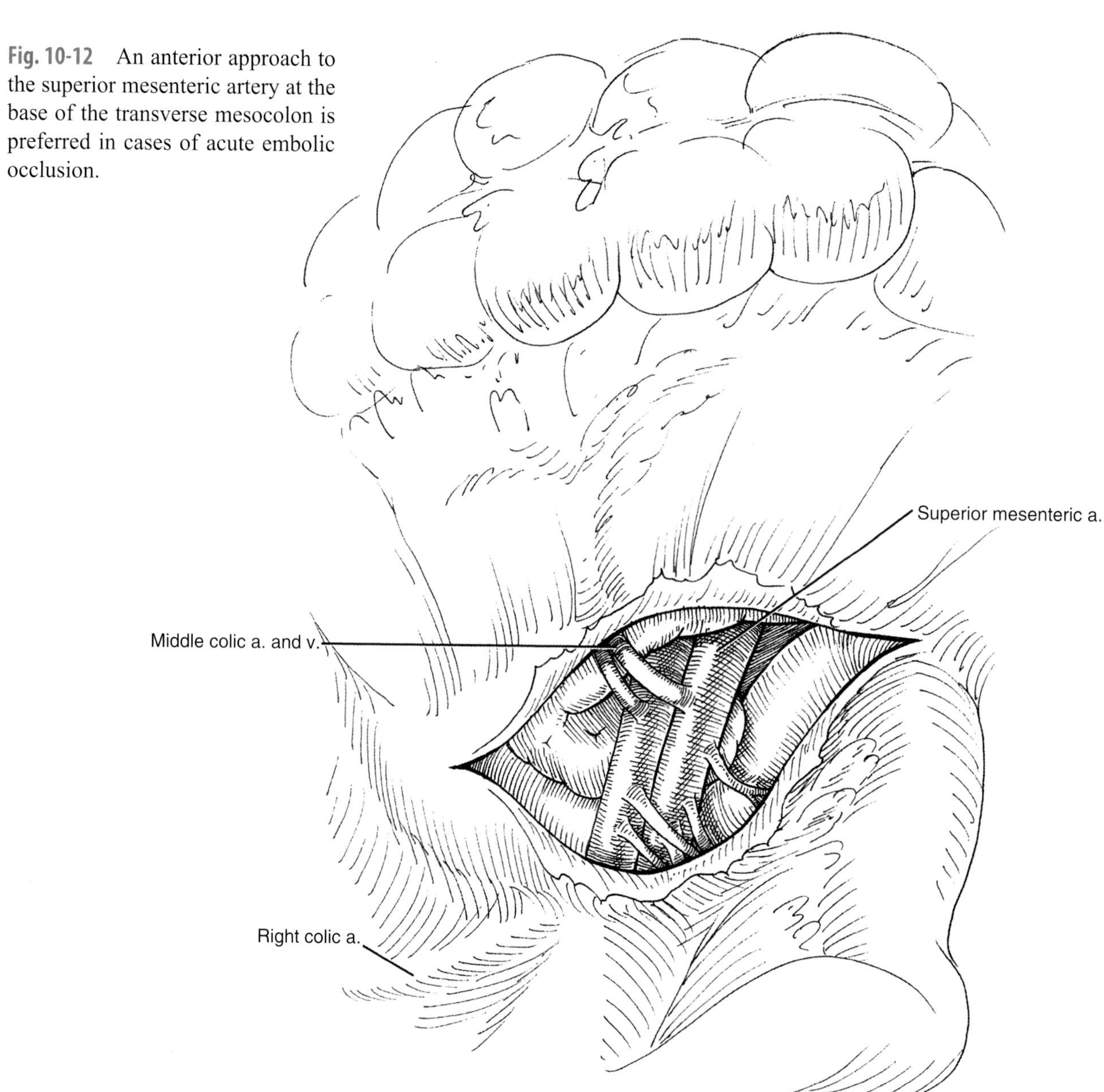

Fig. 10-12 An anterior approach to the superior mesenteric artery at the base of the transverse mesocolon is preferred in cases of acute embolic occlusion.

The segment of superior mesenteric artery between the middle and right colic artery branches is readily isolated from surrounding lymphatics and autonomic nerve fibers. It is important to preserve any jejunal branches seen before proceeding with the embolectomy (Fig. 10-13). Extreme care should be taken not to injure the fragile superior mesenteric artery or its branches during isolation. Exposure of more proximal segments is possible by judicious cephalad retraction of the inferior pancreatic border.

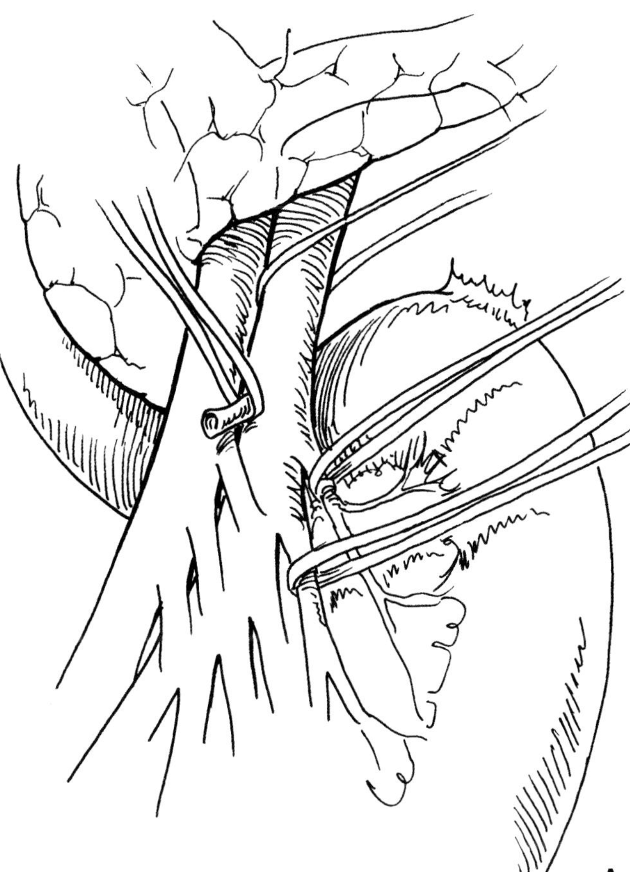

Fig. 10-13 Isolation, arteriotomy, and embolectomy of the superior mesenteric artery are shown.

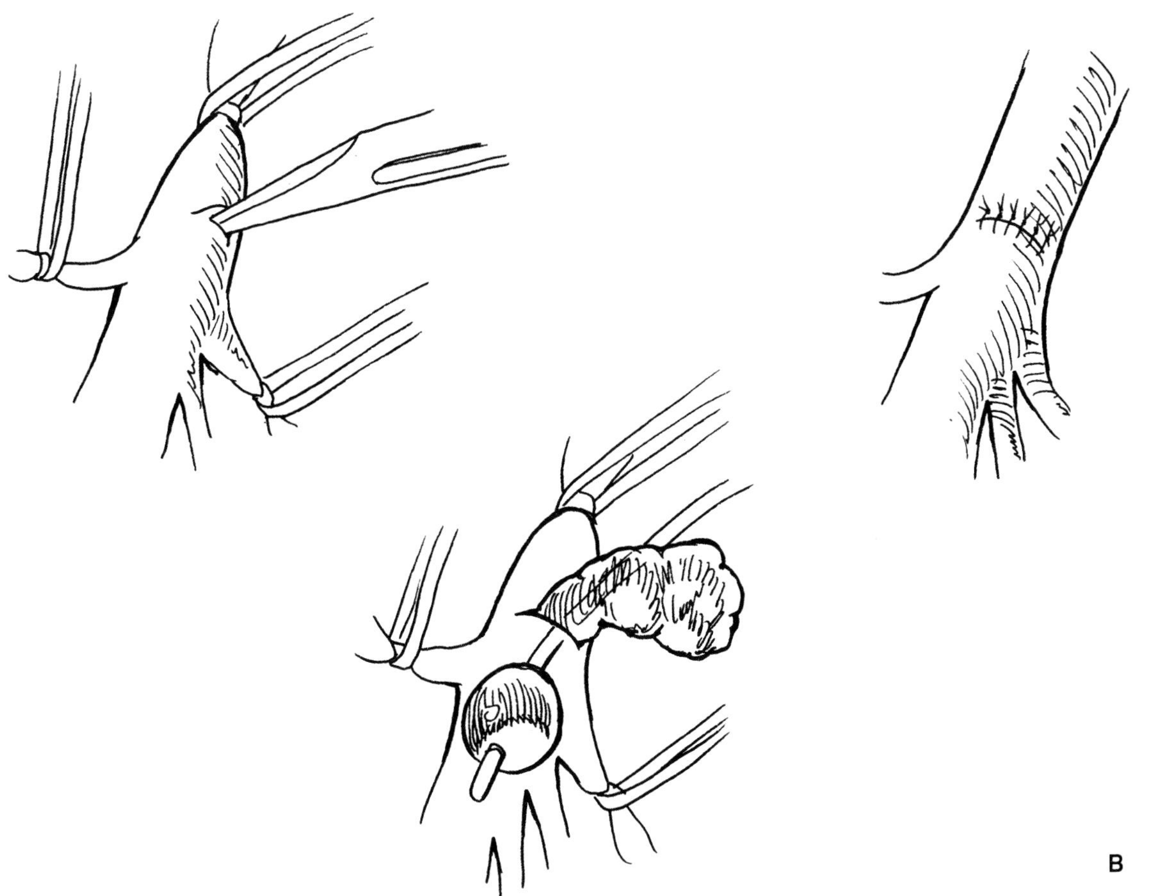

To expose the superior mesenteric artery from a lateral approach, the fourth portion of the duodenum should be mobilized by dividing Treitz's ligament and other peritoneal attachments. The superior mesenteric artery can be isolated in the tissues cephalad to the duodenum (Fig. 10-14). Proximal exposure is enhanced by retracting the inferior border of the pancreas to the level of the left renal vein.

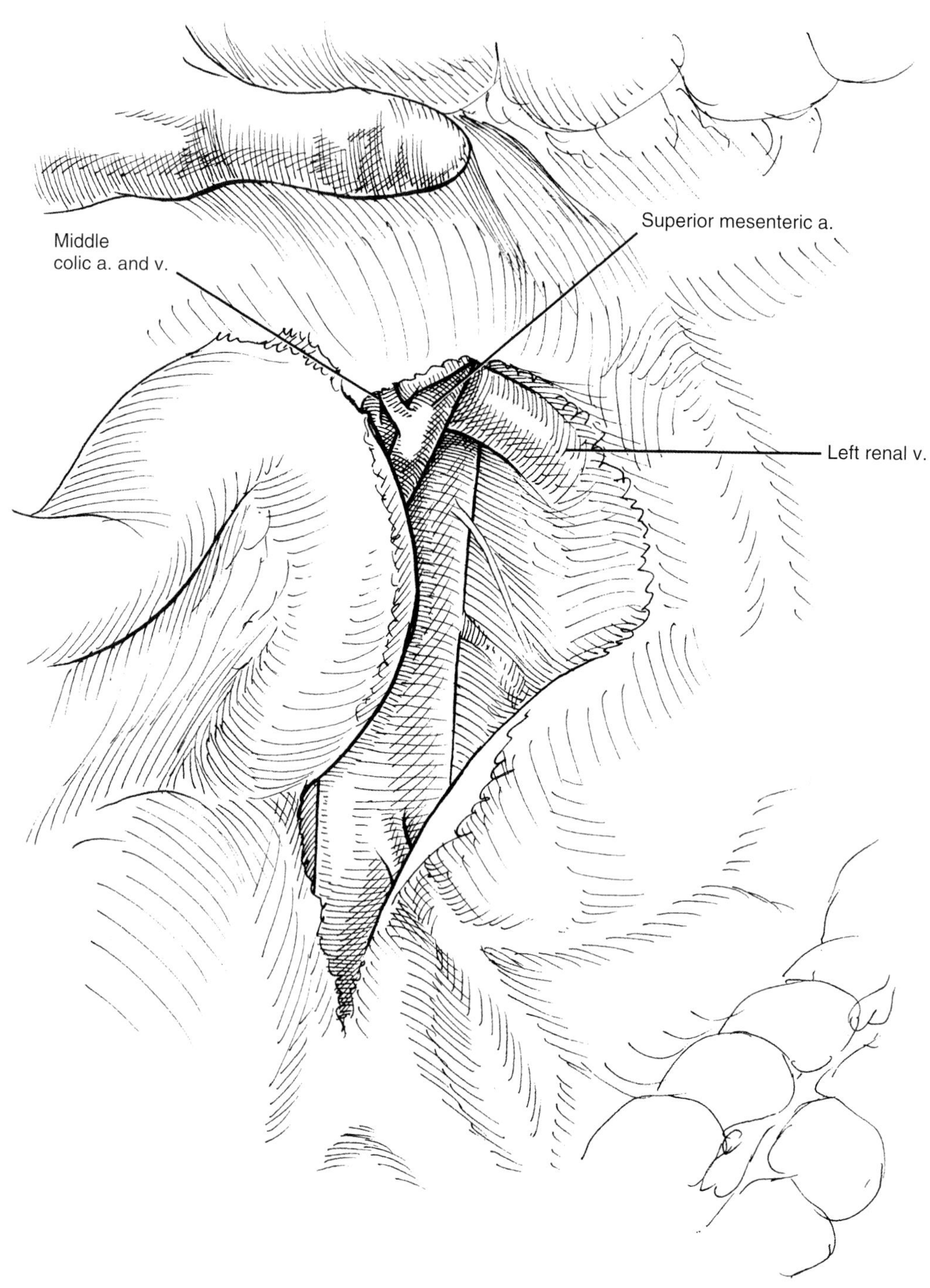

Fig. 10-14 For bypassing a chronic superior mesenteric artery stenosis, the fourth portion of the duodenum is mobilized to expose both the subpancreatic portion of the mesenteric artery and subjacent aorta.

Several alternatives are available for mesenteric reconstruction. Short bypasses to the superior mesenteric artery routed in retrograde fashion directly from the infrarenal aorta can be completed rapidly and with minimal dissection (Fig. 10-15). However, because of the frequent coexistence of atherosclerotic plaque in the infrarenal aorta, other inflow sites are generally preferred. Superior patency rates have

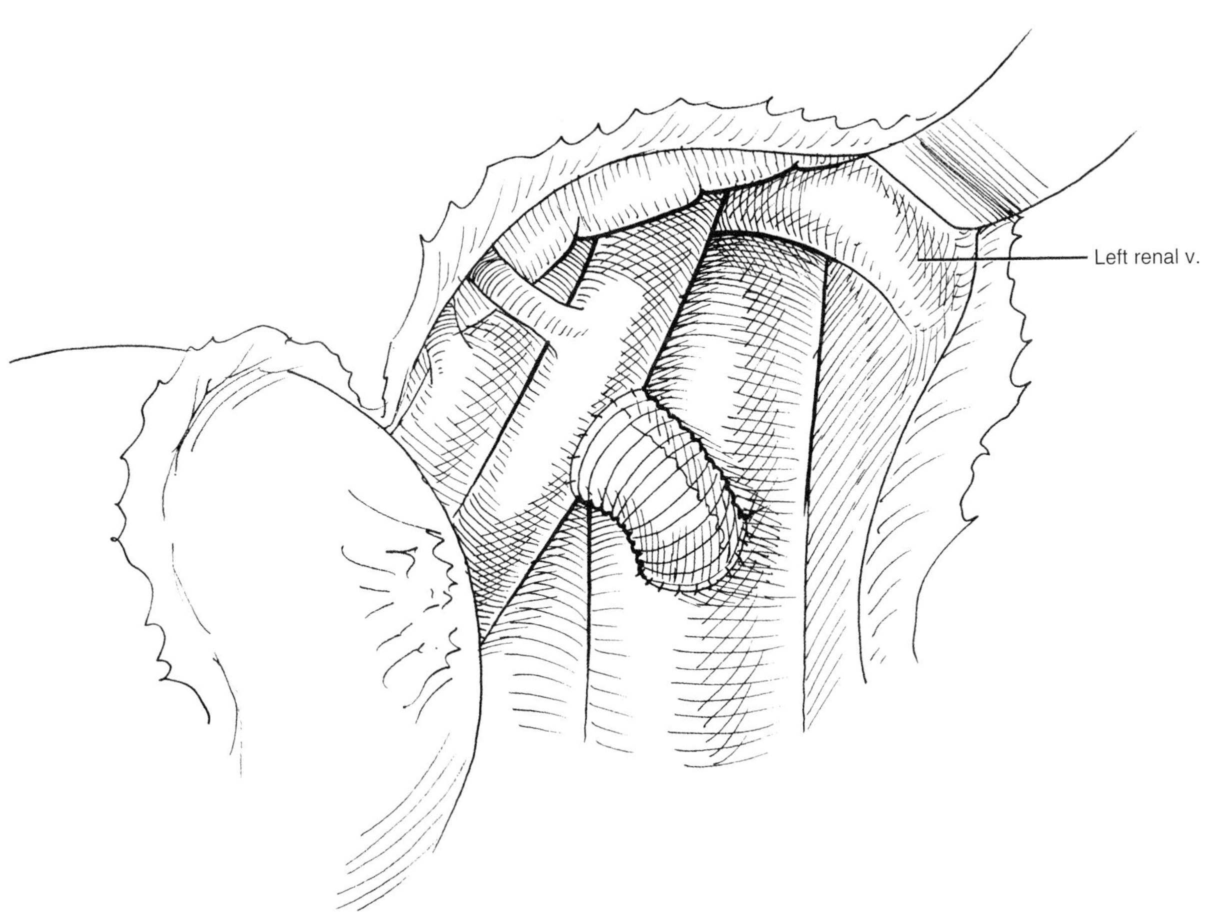

Fig. 10-15 A short, wide synthetic graft from the aorta to the superior mesenteric artery creates a retrograde bypass.

been reported using either long, retrograde C-loop configurations from the right iliac artery (Fig. 10-16) or antegrade bypasses routed posterior to the pancreas from the supraceliac aorta[15,16] (Fig. 10-17).

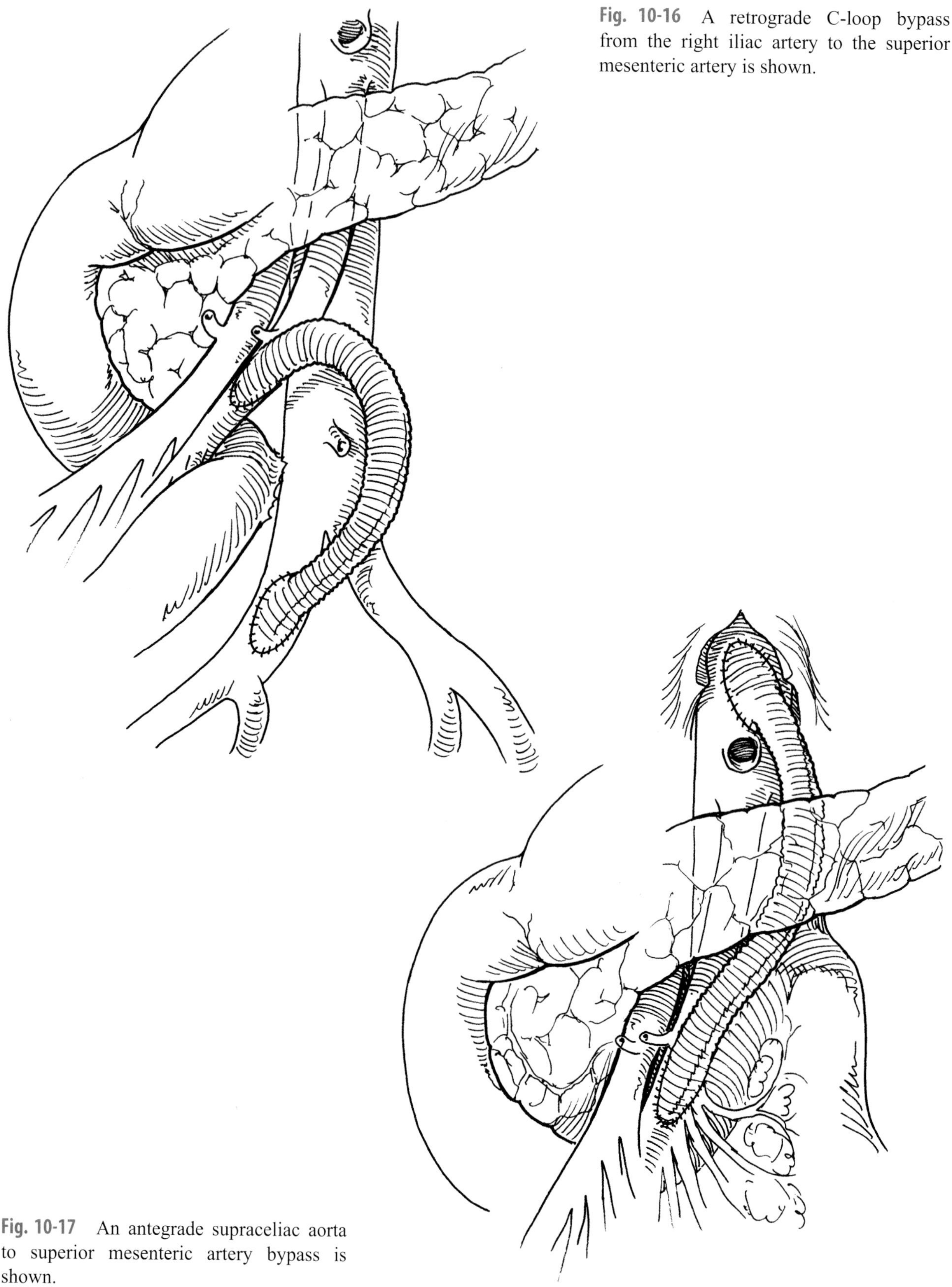

Fig. 10-16 A retrograde C-loop bypass from the right iliac artery to the superior mesenteric artery is shown.

Fig. 10-17 An antegrade supraceliac aorta to superior mesenteric artery bypass is shown.

Exposure of the Inferior Mesenteric Artery

Isolated revascularization of the inferior mesenteric artery may be necessary in rare cases when revascularization of the other major mesenteric arteries is not possible owing to inadequate outflow or extensive intraabdominal adhesions.[21] Evidence of a large, intact collateral circulation with the inferior mesenteric artery must be present.[21]

Patient positioning and surgical preparation are as previously described. Most authors prefer vertical midline incisions, but transverse infraumbilical incisions yield excellent exposure and superior wound healing.[22] After the peritoneal cavity has been entered, the transverse colon is elevated, wrapped in moist laparotomy pads, and placed on the superior abdominal wall. The small intestine is wrapped in moist laparotomy pads or in a bowel bag and gently retracted to the right. After Treitz's ligament and other duodenal adhesions are incised, the duodenum is mobilized to the right with the rest of the small intestine (Fig. 10-18). The abdominal aorta is exposed by incising the posterior parietal peritoneum. It is important to confine the dissection to the right of the aortic midline to avoid inadvertent injury to the inferior mesenteric artery or its branches. Fibrous tissue overlying the anterior wall of the aorta should be ligated and divided to prevent lymphatic leak. The glistening surface of the aortic adventitia is recognized by incising a thin, fibrous sheath, allowing entry into the periadventitial plane. The aorta should be cleared of overlying tissue from the area just proximal to the bifurcation to the level of the left renal vein. The inferior mesenteric artery is recognized arising from the anterior surface of the aorta just to the left of the aortic midline, approximately 3 to 4 cm above the aortic bifurcation. Isolation of the inferior mesenteric artery should be performed as close to its origin as possible to avoid injuring its nearby branches.

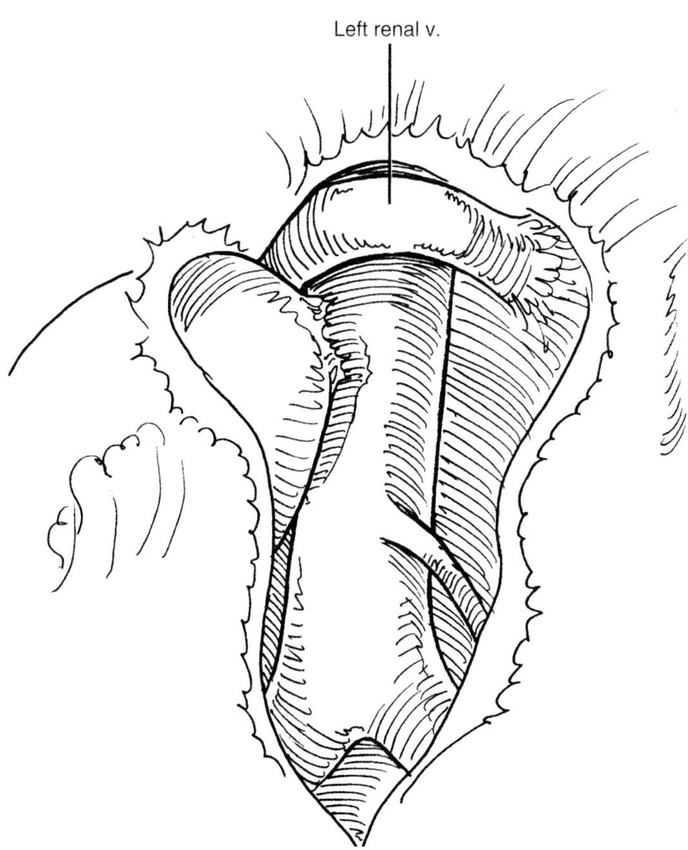

Fig. 10-18 The inferior mesenteric artery is exposed by incising the posterior peritoneum below the mobilized duodenum, staying to the right of midline.

Exposure of the Hepatic Artery

The hepatic artery has been used to revascularize the right renal artery in cases in which aortic pathology or previous retroperitoneal surgery renders aortic exposure difficult or dangerous (see Chapter 11, Fig. 11-14). Although aortorenal bypass is generally preferred, the hepatorenal bypass is considered a safe and durable alternative for revascularization of the right kidney in patients with renovascular hypertension or ischemic nephropathy.[23,24] The hepatorenal bypass is also an excellent option to allow more proximal placement of aortic endografts in patients with unsuitable infrarenal neck anatomy.[25,26] Because of the extreme variability in the anatomy of the hepatic circulation, it is imperative to obtain preoperative imaging with CT, MR, or catheter angiography. To rule out the existence of occlusive disease at the origin of the celiac axis, lateral views should be included in the preoperative studies.[2]

The patient is placed in the supine position with the right flank elevated on a rolled sheet (Fig. 10-19). The lower chest, abdomen, groin, and thighs are prepped and draped. A right subcostal incision is made 4 to 5 cm below and parallel to the inferior costal margin, extending from the midline to a point opposite the tip of the right 11th rib.[27] When necessary in large or obese individuals, the incision may be carried across the midline as a chevron.[28]

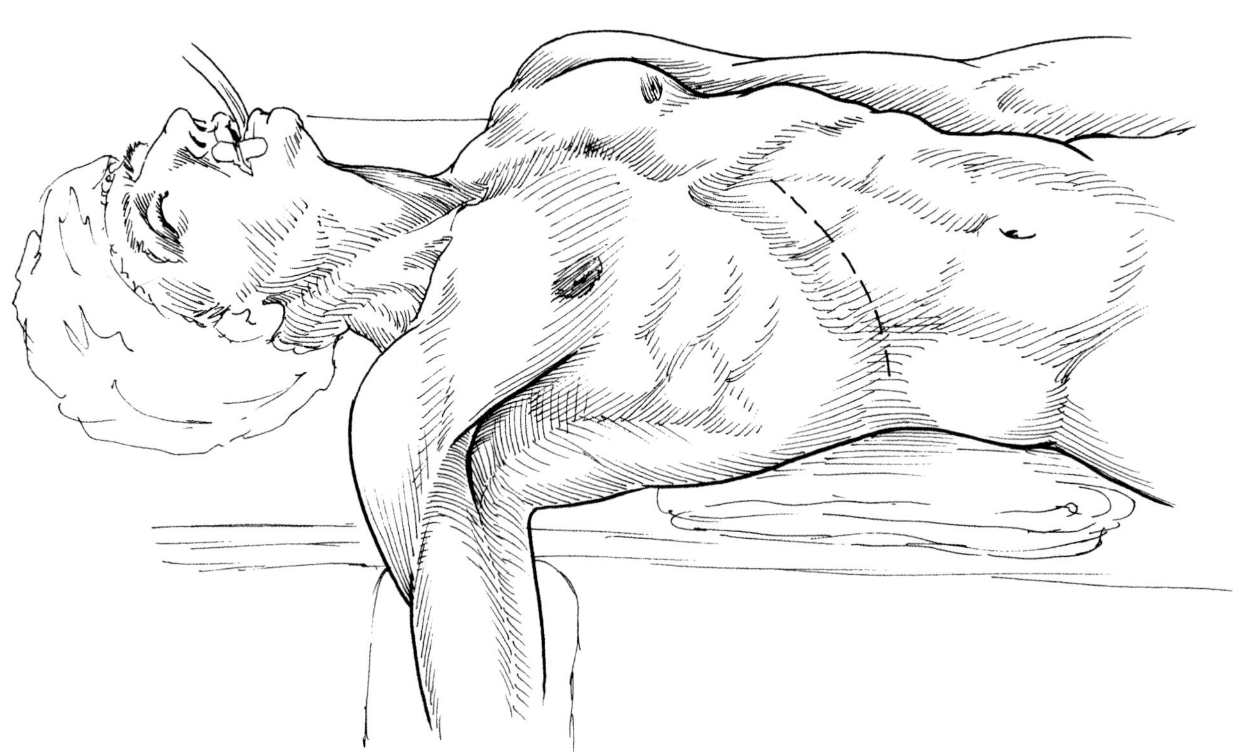

Fig. 10-19 The hepatic artery is approached through a right subcostal incision.

The area of the hepatoduodenal ligament is exposed by retracting the right lobe of the liver superiorly and packing the intestines and right colon into the inferior wound with moist laparotomy packs (Fig. 10-20). The hepatoduodenal ligament is incised transversely near the superior wall of the duodenum, and the hepatic artery is located on the left side of the common duct. The artery should be carefully mobilized and encircled with elastic vessel loops on both sides of the gastroduodenal artery. Bypasses may be anastomosed to the side of the hepatic artery either proximal or distal to the gastroduodenal artery,[27] or the gastroduodenal artery can be sacrificed and used as a direct source of inflow.[29]

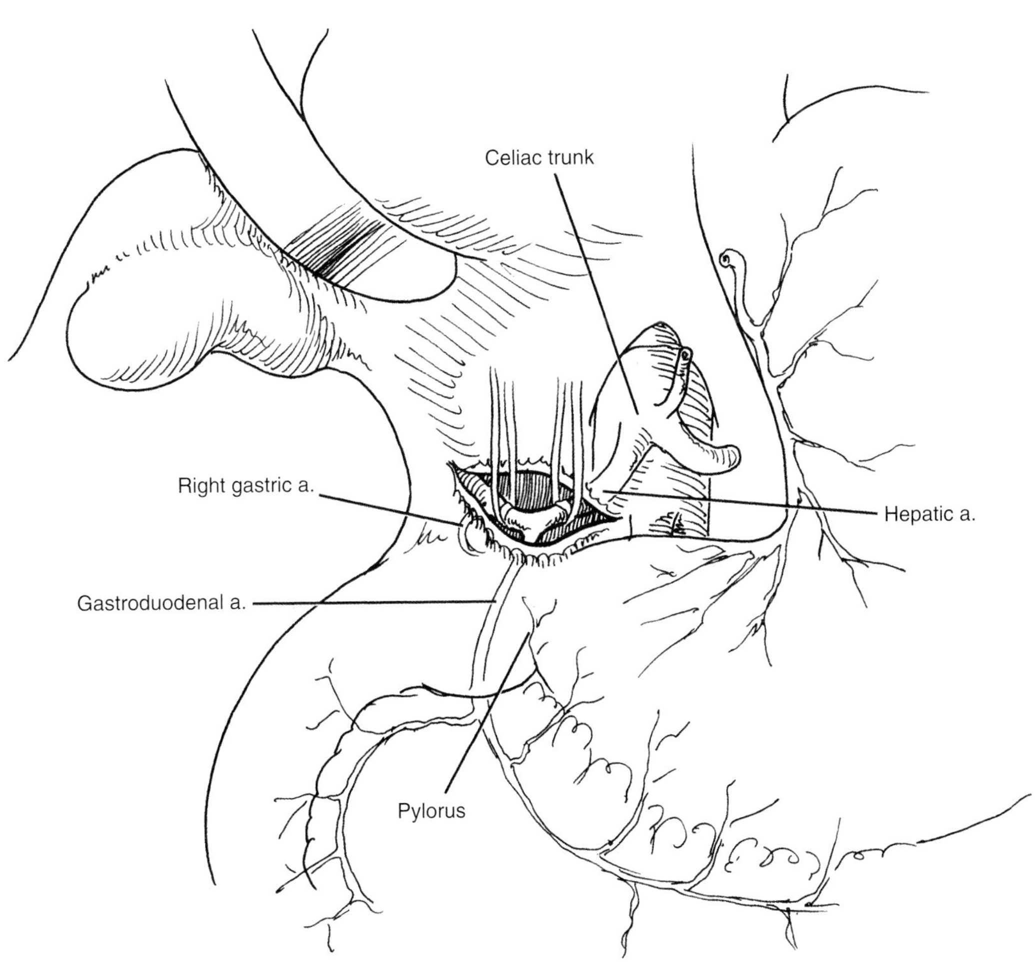

Fig. 10-20 The hepatic artery is exposed by incising the gastroduodenal ligament above the pylorus.

Exposure of the Splenic Artery

The splenic artery has been used as an alternative source of inflow for left renal artery revascularization in cases in which the aorta cannot be used because of previous surgery, local pathology, or severe atherosclerosis[23,24] (see Chapter 11, Fig. 11-14). The splenorenal bypass has also been used to allow more proximal placement of an aortic endograft in patients with unsuitable infrarenal neck anatomy.[26] To document the adequacy of flow, preoperative imaging studies should be obtained to document splenic artery patency and to rule out the existence of occlusive disease at the origin of the celiac artery.[2]

The patient is placed in the supine position with the left flank elevated on a rolled sheet. The lower chest, abdomen, groins, and anterior thighs are prepped and draped. Although Moncure et al.[27] and Brewster and Darling[30] advocate a thoracoabdominal incision for exposure of the splenic artery, Novick et al.[31,32] have achieved excellent visualization and exposure through a bilateral subcostal incision. It is extremely helpful to use self-retaining retractors for cranial elevation of the superior wound.

After routine exploration of the peritoneal cavity has been performed, the transverse colon is elevated and the small intestines are wrapped in warm laparotomy packs and retracted to the right. The left colon is mobilized by incising its lateral peritoneal attachments and developing a relatively bloodless plane between the left colon mesentery and the anterior surface of Gerota's fascia. After the left colon has been reflected to the level of the splenic flexure, the spleen is mobilized by incising the splenophrenic and splenorenal ligaments. A plane between the pancreas and Gerota's fascia is developed bluntly, allowing the spleen and distal pancreas to be reflected anteriorly and medially (Fig.10-21). The splenic artery is easily identified near the superior border of the pancreas. To avoid kinking associated with redundancy, only the central portion of the splenic artery should be dissected and mobilized. The distal portion is often smaller in caliber and should be left undisturbed. Pancreatic branches should be ligated with fine silk sutures before being divided to prevent troublesome bleeding that occurs when hemoclips are dislodged. Sufficient length of the splenic artery should be obtained by proximal mobilization to allow a tension-free anastomosis with the left renal artery. After the splenic artery is clamped and divided, the distal end should be ligated, and the proximal end gently dilated with a balloon embolectomy catheter or graduated probes to overcome spasm.[30,31] The spleen receives sufficient blood supply from the short gastric and gastroepiploic collaterals and should not require removal.[30–32] However, splenic infarction has been reported after a splenorenal arterial bypass.[33]

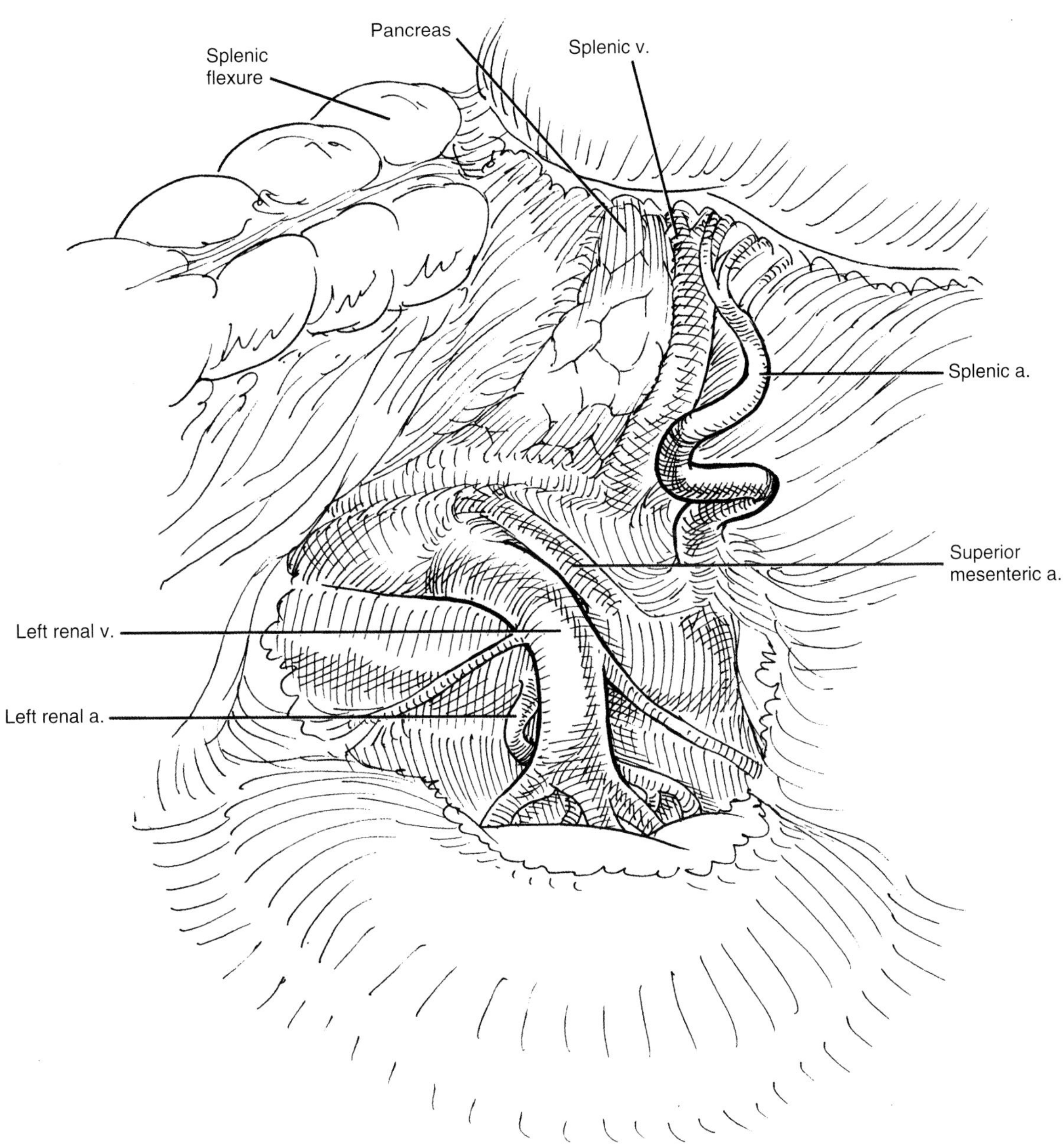

Fig. 10-21 When it is to be used for splenorenal bypass, the splenic artery is exposed retroperitoneally by mobilizing spleen and left colon.

References

1. Zeller T, Macharzina R. Management of chronic atherosclerotic mesenteric ischemia. *Vasa*. 2011;40;99–107.
2. Valentine RJ, Martin JD, Myers SI, et al. Asymptomatic celiac and superior mesenteric artery stenoses are more prevalent among patients with unsuspected renal artery stenoses. *J Vasc Surg*. 1991;14:195–199.
3. Thomas JH, Blake K, Pierce GE, et al. The clinical course of asymptomatic mesenteric arterial stenosis. *J Vasc Surg*. 1998;27:840–844.
4. Grotemeyer D, Duran M, Iskandar F, et al. Median arcuate ligament syndrome: vascular surgical therapy and follow-up of 18 patients. *Langenbechs Arch Surg*. 2009;394:1085–1092.
5. Duffy AJ, Panail L, Eisenberg D, et al. Management of median arcuate ligament syndrome: a new paradigm. *Ann Vasc Surg*. 2009;23:778–784.
6. Gloviczi P, Duncan AA. Treatment of celiac artery compression syndrome: does it really exist? *Perspect Vasc Surg Endovasc Ther*. 2007;19:259–263.
7. Tulloch AW, Jiminez JC, Lawrence PF, et al. Laparoscopic versus open celiac ganglionectomy in patients with median arcuate syndrome. *J Vasc Surg*. 2010;52:1283–1289.
8. Soman S, Sudhakar SV, Keshava SN. Celiac axis compression by median arcuate ligament on computed tomography among asymptomatic patients. *Indian J Gastroenterol*. 2010;29:121–123.
9. Wyers MC. Acute mesenteric ischemia: diagnostic approach and surgical treatment. *Semin Vasc Surg*. 2010;23:9–20.
10. Berland T, Oldenburg WA. Acute mesenteric ischemia. *Curr Gastroenterol Rep*. 2008;10:341–346.
11. Trompeter M, Brazda T, Remy CT, et al. Non-occlusive mesenteric ischemia: etiology, diagnosis, and interventional therapy. *Eur Radiol*. 2002;12:1179–1187.
12. Brown DJ, Schemerhorn ML, Powell RJ, et al. Mesenteric stenting foe chronic mesenteric ischemia. *J Vasc Surg*. 2005;42:268–274.
13. Biebl, Oldenburg WA, Paz-Fumagalli R, et al. Endovascular treatment as a bridge to successful revascularization for chronic mesenteric ischemia. *Am Surg*. 2004;70:994–998.
14. Savassi-Rocha PR, Veloso LF. Treatment of superior mesenteric artery embolism with a fibrinolytic agent: case report and literature review. *Hepatogastroenterology*. 2002;49:1307–1310.
15. Jiminez JG, Huber TS, Ozaki CK, et al. Durability of antegrade synthetic aortomesenteric bypass for chronic mesenteric ischemia. *J Vasc Surg*. 2002;35:1078–1084.
16. Park WM, Cherry KJ Jr., Cua HK, et al. Current results of open revascularization for chronic mesenteric ischemia: a standard for comparison. *J Vasc Surg*. 2002;35:853–859.
17. Mell MW, Archer CW, Hoch JR, et al. Outcomes after endarterectomy for chronic mesenteric ischemia. *J Vasc Surg*. 2008;48:32–38.
18. Wyers MC, Powell RJ, Nolan BW, et al. Retrograde mesenteric stenting during laparotomy for acute occlusive mesenteric ischemia. *J Vasc Surg*. 2007;45:269–275.
19. McVay CB. Thoracic walls. In: McVay CB, ed. *Anson and McVay's Surgical Anatomy*. Philadelphia, PA: WB Saunders; 1984:343–384.
20. Stoney RJ, Schneider PA. Technical aspects of visceral artery revascularization. In: Bergan JJ, Yao JST, eds. *Techniques in Arterial Surgery*. Philadelphia, PA: WB Saunders; 1990:271–283.
21. Schneider DB, Nelken NA, Messina LM, et al. Isolated inferior mesenteric artery revascularization for chronic visceral ischemia. *J Vasc Surg*. 1999;30:51–58.
22. Fry WJ. Occlusive arterial disease: upper aortic branches. In: Nora PF, ed. *Operative Surgery: Principles and Techniques*. Philadelphia, PA: Lea & Febiger; 1980:763–777.
23. Cambria RP, Brewster DC, L'Italien GJ, et al. The durability of different reconstructive techniques for atherosclerotic renal artery disease. *J Vasc Surg*. 1994;20:76–87.
24. Geroulakos G, Wright JG, Tober JC, et al. Use of the splenic and hepatic artery for renal revascularization in patients with atherosclerotic renal artery disease. *Ann Vasc Surg*. 1997;11:85–89.
25. Lerussi G, O'Brien N, Sessa C, et al. Hepatorenal bypass allowing fenestrated endovascular repair of juxtarenal aortic aneurysm: a case report. *Eur J Vasc Endovasc Surg*. 2010;39:529–536.
26. Hanish M, Geroulakos G, Hughes DA, et al. Delayed hepato-renal-splenal bypass for renal salvage following malposition of an infrarenal aortic endograft. *J Endovasc Ther*. 2010;178:326–331.
27. Moncure AC, Brewster DC, Darling RC, et al. Use of the splenic and hepatic arteries for renal revascularization. *J Vasc Surg*. 1986;3:196–203.
28. Chibara EA, Libertino JA, Novick AC. Use of the hepatic circulation for renal revascularization. *Ann Surg*. 1984;199:406–412.
29. Moncure AC, Brewster DC, Darling RC, et al. Use of the gastroduodenal artery in right renal artery revascularization. *J Vasc Surg*. 1988;8:154–159.
30. Brewster DC, Darling RC. Splenorenal anastomosis for renovascular hypertension. *Ann Surg*. 1979;189:353–358.
31. Novick AC, Banowsky LHW, Stewart BH, et al. Splenorenal bypass in the treatment of stenosis of the renal artery. *Surg Gynecol Obstet*. 1977;144:891–898.
32. Khauli RB, Novick AC, Ziegelbaum M. Splenorenal bypass in the treatment of renal artery stenosis: experience with sixty-nine cases. *J Vasc Surg*. 1985;2:547–551.
33. Valentine RJ, Rossi MB, Myers SI, et al. Splenic infarction after splenorenal arterial bypass. *J Vasc Surg*. 1993;17:602–606.

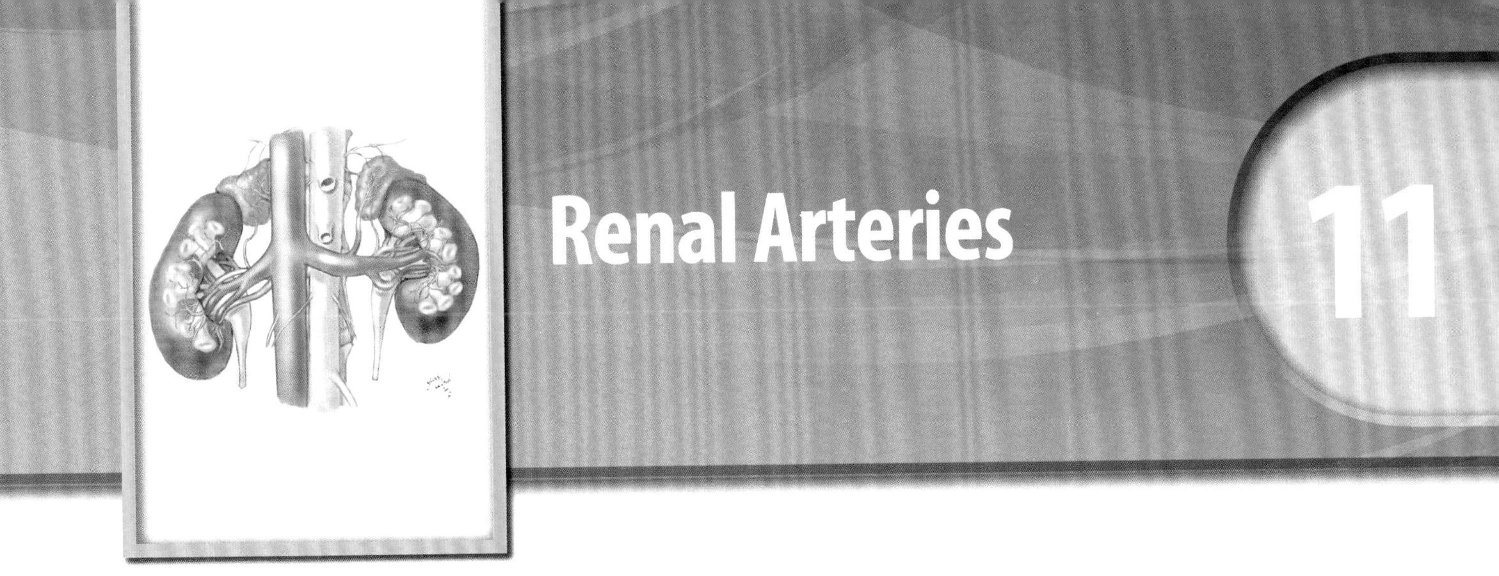

11 Renal Arteries

Surgical Anatomy of the Renal Arteries

The renal arteries arise from the abdominal aorta at approximately the level of the disc between the first two lumbar vertebrae (Fig. 11-1). The left is usually slightly more cephalad than the right, and supernumerary vessels are not uncommon. Because the aorta is elevated on the promontory of the spinal

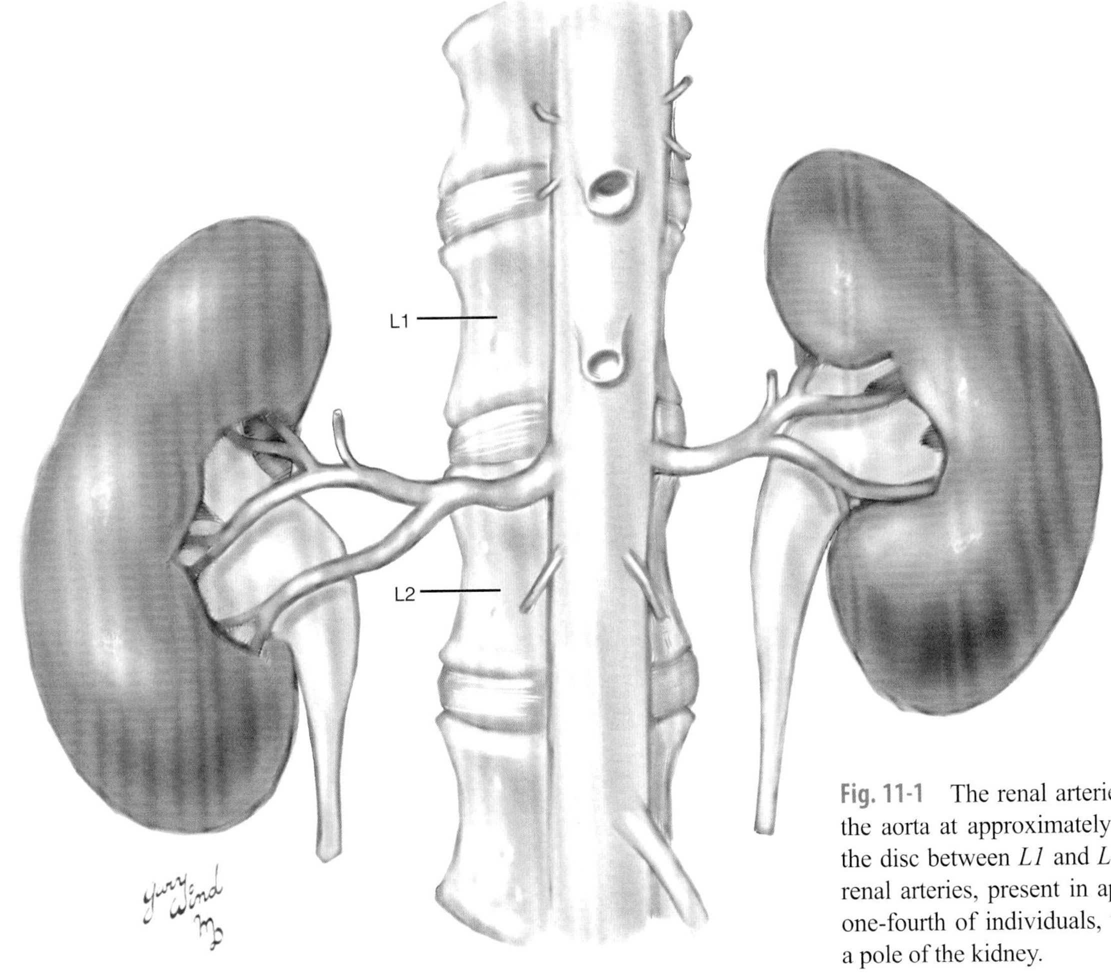

L1
L2

Fig. 11-1 The renal arteries arise from the aorta at approximately the level of the disc between *L1* and *L2*. Accessory renal arteries, present in approximately one-fourth of individuals, usually enter a pole of the kidney.

column and the kidneys rest in the adjacent gutters, the angle formed by the renal vessels with the aorta is almost 90° (Fig. 11-2). The position of the aorta to the left of midline makes the right renal artery longer than the left.

Fasciae

The kidneys are embedded in a layer of fat and enclosed by fascial layers in front and back. These anterior and posterior renal fasciae fuse laterally with

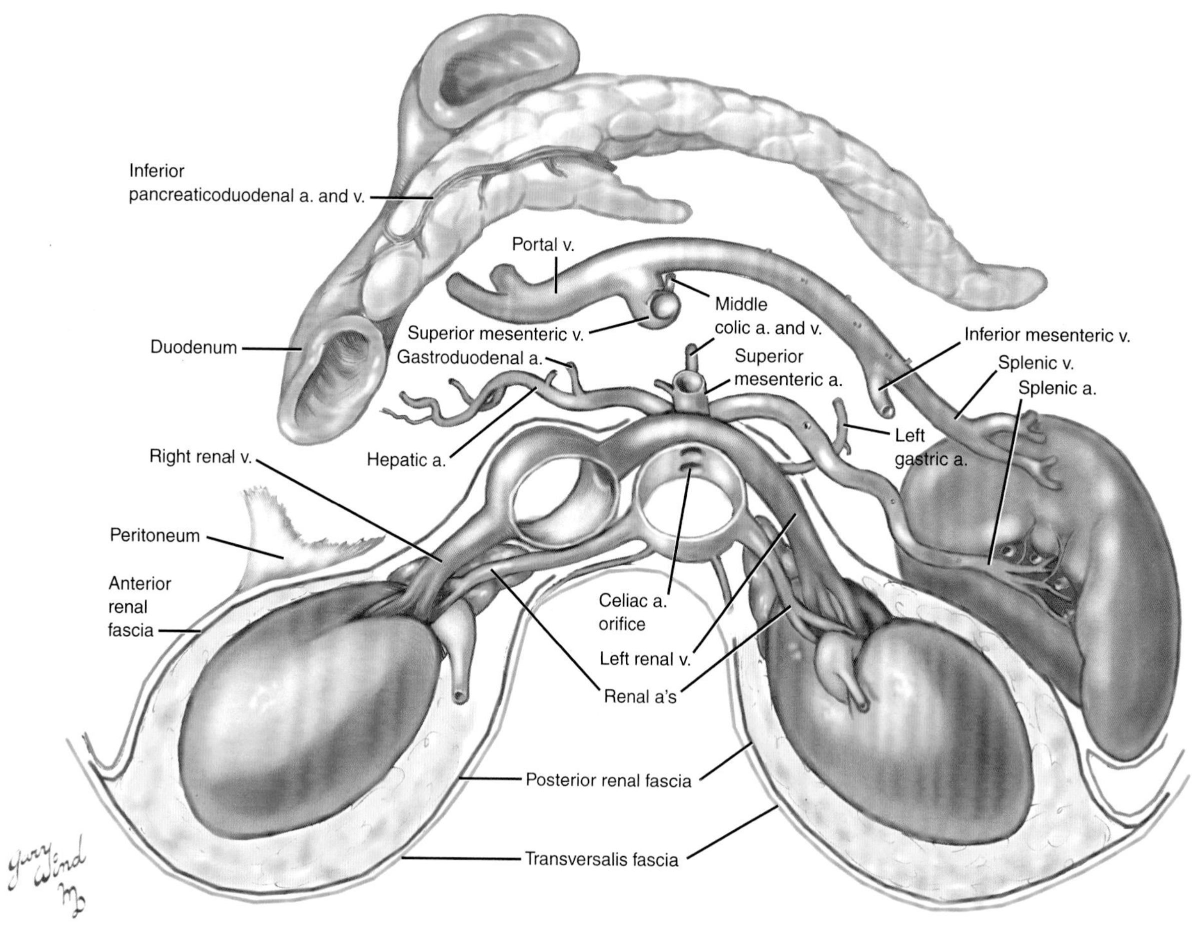

Fig. 11-2 The renal arteries drape posteriorly over the spinal column. The right renal artery often divides behind the inferior vena cava.

each other and with the posterior parietal peritoneum. The anterior and posterior renal fasciae continue loosely across the midline ventral and dorsal to the great vessels, respectively. The posterior layer lies on the transversalis fascia.

The layers of the renal fascia taper above to enclose the adrenal glands on each side and taper below to ensheath the proximal ureters (Fig. 11-3). The anterior renal fascia is partly covered by the posterior parietal peritoneum. The remaining part of

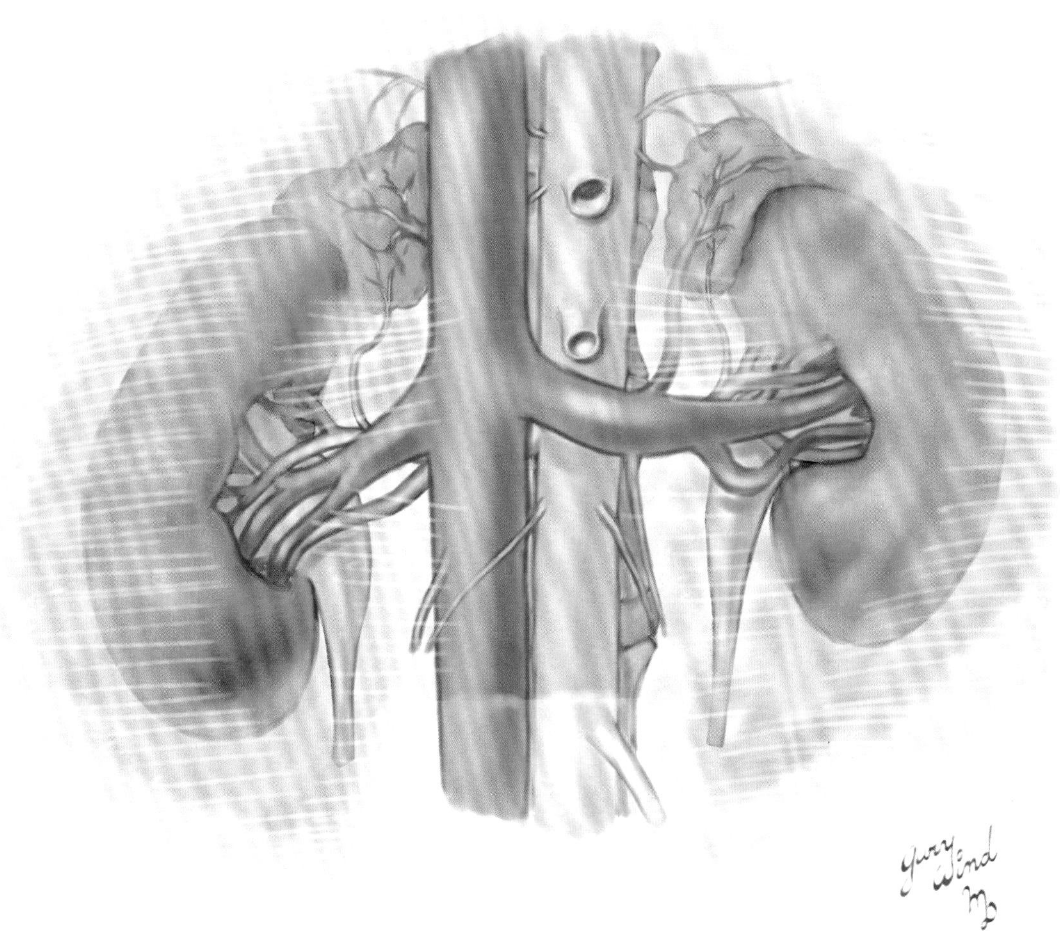

Fig. 11-3 The kidneys and perinephric fat are enclosed by an envelope of renal fascia that tapers around the adrenals above and the ureters below.

the fascia over the right kidney is covered by the second portion of the duodenum and the hepatic flexure of the colon (Fig. 11-4). On the left, the part of the anterior renal fascia not in contact with the peritoneum is covered by the tail of the pancreas, the spleen, and the splenic flexure of the colon.

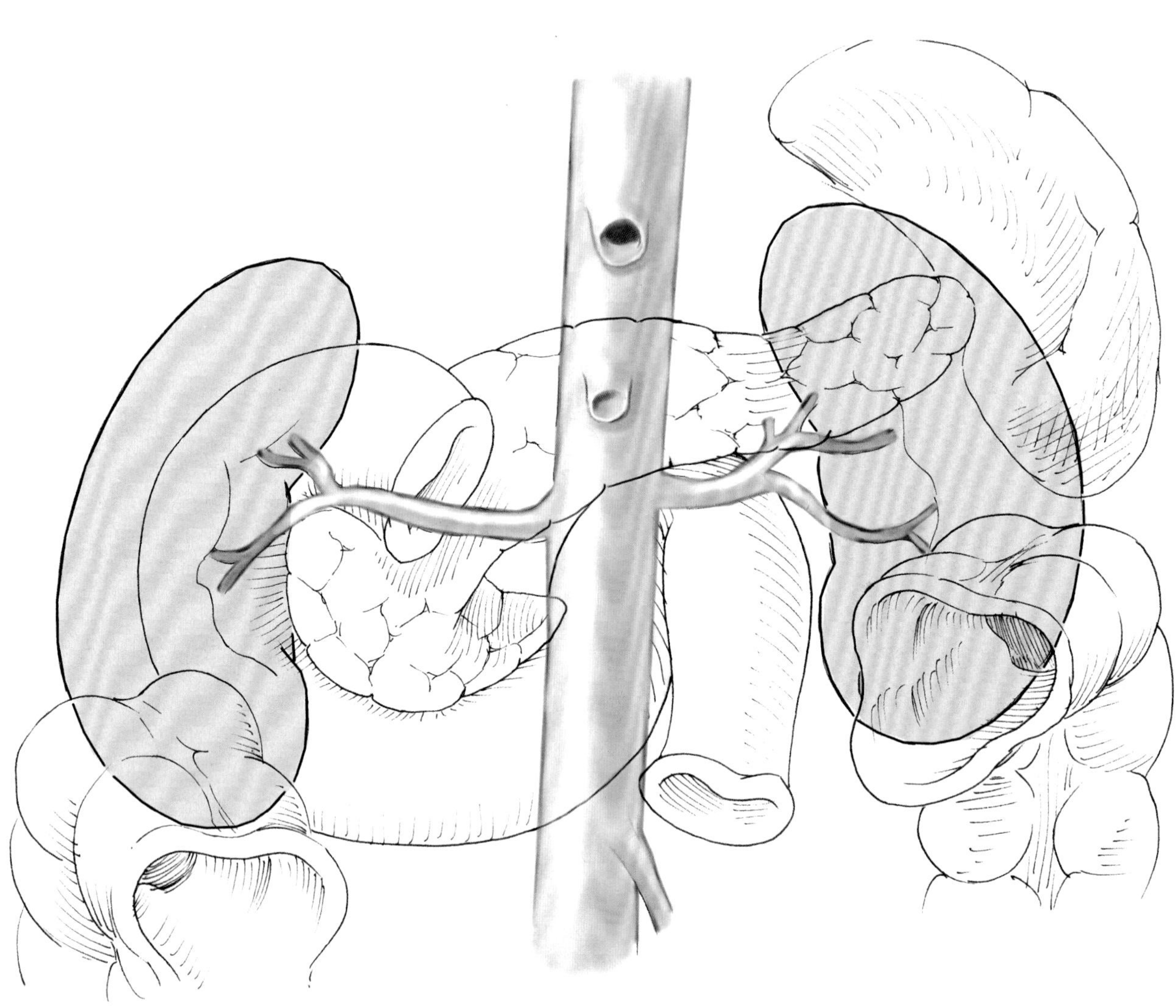

Fig. 11-4 The relationships of the renal arteries and kidneys to overlying organs are shown.

Vessels

The renal arteries lie posterior to the corresponding renal veins on each side, and the right renal artery passes behind the inferior vena cava where the first branch points are commonly found (Fig. 11-5). The left renal artery is most commonly found near the cephalad border of the long left renal vein. Each renal artery usually sends a small branch to the ipsilateral adrenal gland, complementing the aortic and inferior phrenic artery branches to those organs. Near the hilum of each kidney, the renal artery divides into four or five branches that enter the kidney between the vein branches anteriorly and the calyces posteriorly.

The left renal vein serves as a landmark for locating the level of the renal artery origins. The left renal artery is usually found beneath the left renal vein near the cephalad margin of the vein. The right renal vein and artery junctions with the inferior vena cava and aorta are slightly caudal to the left. Both renal veins may receive a lumbar vein. In addition, the left renal vein receives the left adrenal and left gonadal veins.

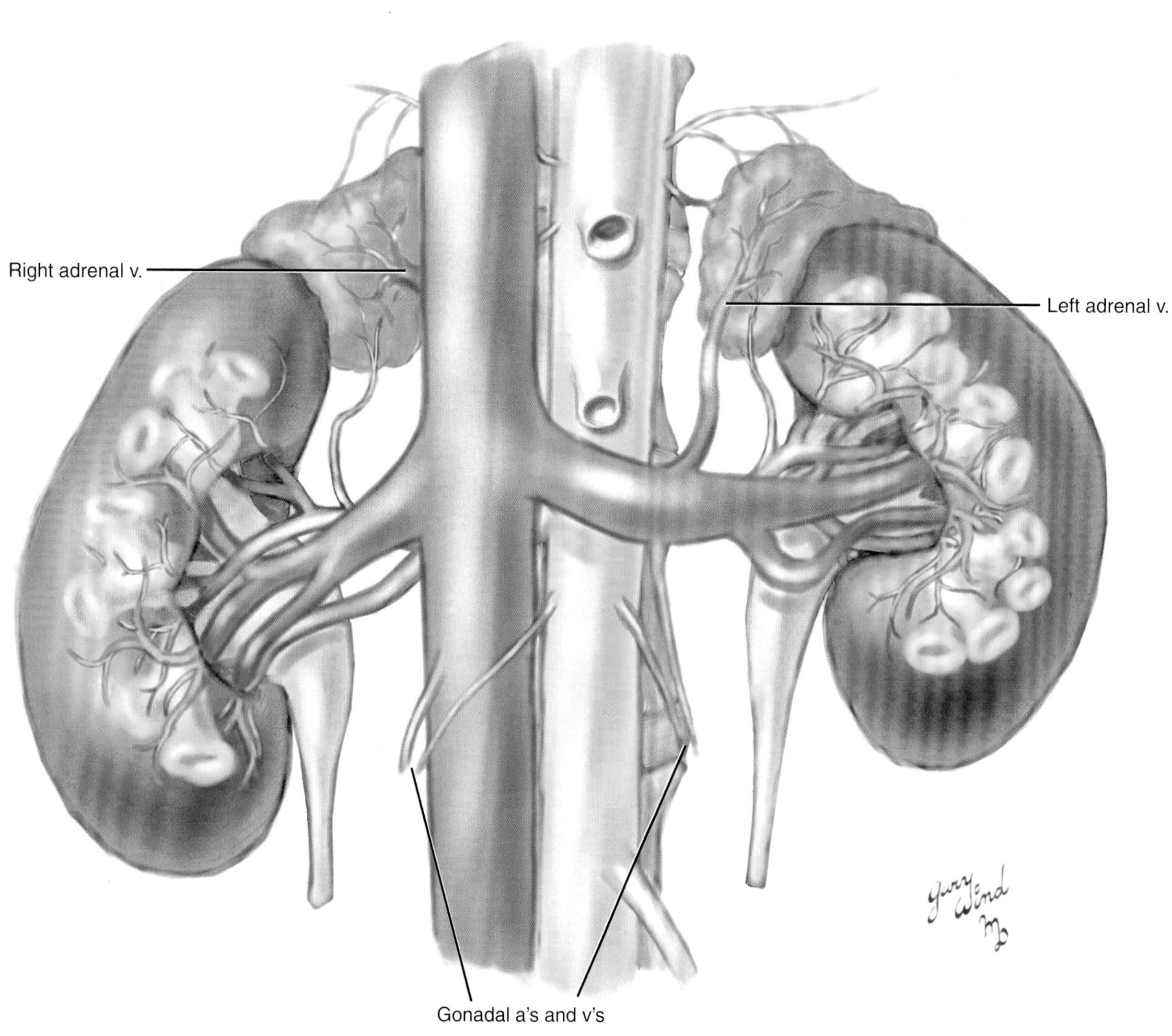

Fig. 11-5 The branches of the renal arteries and veins are shown.

Exposure of the Renal Arteries

Surgical exposure of the renal arteries may be necessary to treat traumatic injuries, aneurysms, or chronic stenoses. A common indication for isolation of the renal artery in the traumatized patient is to obtain vascular control before exploring a parenchymal injury. Vascular repair of a renal artery injury is indicated only for pseudoaneurysms or dissection with preserved flow. Because most injuries result in thrombosis and irreversible ischemia, reported outcomes for vascular repair are similar to nephrectomy.[1,2] The indications for repair of renal artery aneurysms are detailed elsewhere.[3,4] These lesions are often located in the distal arterial branches or the renal hilum; therefore, advanced techniques such as extracorporeal repair should be available when surgery is indicated.[5] Chronic renal artery stenoses may be due to fibromuscular dysplasia (10%) or atherosclerosis (90%). Percutaneous balloon angioplasty without a stent is considered the treatment of choice for renovascular hypertension due to fibromuscular dysplasia.[6] Regardless of the type of intervention, long-term cure rates are lower for atherosclerotic lesions. The clinical evidence summarizing the effectiveness of angioplasty versus medical therapy for treating atherosclerotic renal artery stenosis is published elsewhere.[7] Many surgeons favor open renal artery revascularization over angioplasty and stenting, especially after failed percutaneous therapy.[8,9] The following discussions concern exposure of the renal arteries using midline and lateral approaches. As sources of inflow, exposure of the aorta and iliac arteries is considered in Chapter 12. Exposure of the splenic and hepatic arteries for extraanatomic bypass is discussed in Chapter 10.

Midline Exposure of the Renal Arteries at Their Origins

The patient is placed in the supine position with the entire abdomen, lower chest, and both groins prepped and draped. The abdomen is entered through a long, vertical midline incision made from the xiphoid process to a point 5 to 7 cm below the umbilicus. As an alternative approach, some surgeons prefer to use a transverse supraumbilical incision that extends into both flanks.

After routine exploration of the peritoneal cavity, the transverse colon and omentum are packed in moist laparotomy pads and lifted onto the anterior abdominal wall at the superior end of the incision. The small intestine is eviscerated and packed in moist laparotomy pads or placed in a bowel bag and mobilized to the right side of the incision. The infrarenal aorta is exposed by incising the ligament of Treitz and other duodenal attachments, allowing mobilization of the distal duodenum and proximal jejunum to the right side. The posterior parietal peritoneum overlying the aorta is opened, and intervening lymphatics are ligated to prevent the development of lymphoceles or chylous ascites.[10,11] When the anterior periadventitial plane is reached, exposure proceeds superior to the level of the left renal vein (Fig. 11-6). The left renal vein crosses anterior to the aorta in approximately 97% of cases,[12] and its superior border is nearly always superimposed on the origin of the left renal artery.[13] It is important to recognize several venous anomalies that occur in this area, including circumaortic left renal veins (up to 8.7%), retroaortic left renal veins (up to 3.4%), left-sided venae cavae (0.2% to 0.5%), and double inferior venae cavae (1% to 3%) (see also Chapter 19).[12] To expose the left renal vein as far as the left renal hilum, the posterior peritoneal incision can be extended to the left along the inferior border of the pancreas (Fig. 11-7). The inferior mesenteric vein should be ligated during this maneuver.

Mobilization of the left renal vein is necessary to expose the origins of both renal arteries. The inferior border of the pancreas is retracted cranially, allowing exposure and dissection of the superior border of the left renal vein. The vein should be carefully encircled with a vascular tape for retraction. The left gonadal and left adrenal branches should be ligated and divided to prevent avulsion during the retraction. A large lumbar vein branch often enters the posterior wall of the left renal vein and requires ligation to prevent injury during renal vein retraction. The left renal vein can now be retracted either superiorly or inferiorly to expose the origins of the left renal artery. In some cases, it may be necessary to divide the left renal vein. Many surgeons have stressed the importance of restoration of vein continuity[14] at the completion of the procedure to

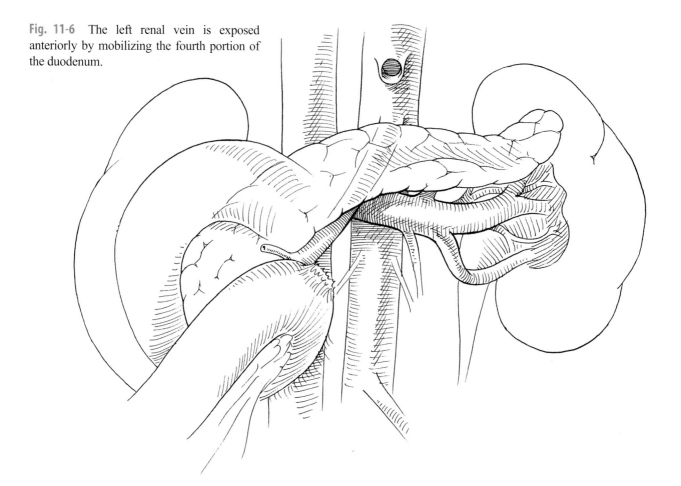

Fig. 11-6 The left renal vein is exposed anteriorly by mobilizing the fourth portion of the duodenum.

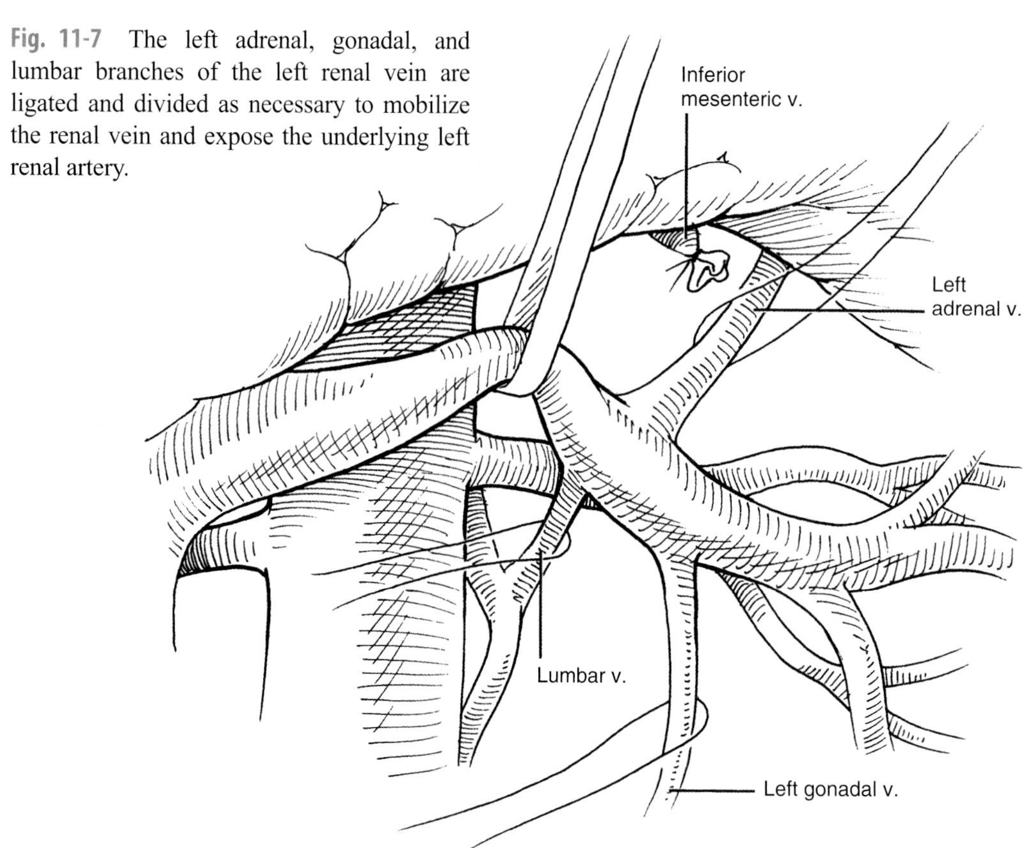

Fig. 11-7 The left adrenal, gonadal, and lumbar branches of the left renal vein are ligated and divided as necessary to mobilize the renal vein and expose the underlying left renal artery.

reduce the risk of renal compromise and hematuria, but at least one recent series suggests that this may be unnecessary.[15]

To isolate the right renal artery at its origin, the medial wall of the vena cava should be mobilized. Lateral retraction of the vena cava above or below the left renal artery, combined with respective inferior or superior retraction of the left renal vein, exposes the proximal right renal artery at the aortic junction (Fig. 11-8).

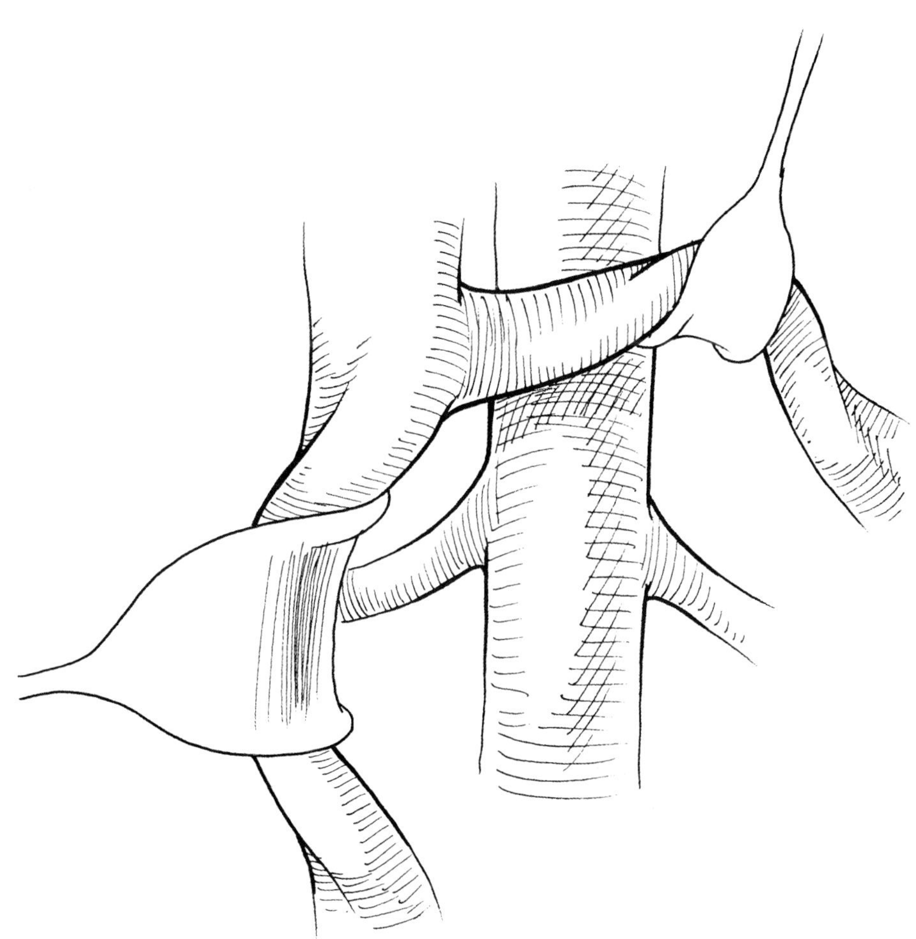

Fig. 11-8 The origins of both renal arteries can be approached between the left renal vein and inferior vena cava.

Exposure of the Left Renal Artery

The patient is placed in the supine position with the left flank elevated on a rolled sheet. The lower chest, abdomen, both groins, and anterior thighs are prepped and draped. The incision may be midline or transverse. If the latter is chosen, the abdomen is opened through a transverse supraumbilical incision extending from the right midclavicular line to the left posterior axillary line between the costal margin and superior iliac crest (Fig. 11-9). After routine exploration of the peritoneal cavity, the abdominal viscera are wrapped in warm, moist laparotomy pads and retracted to the right. Exposure of the left renal vessels proceeds in the relatively bloodless retroperitoneal plane between the left colon mesentery and the anterior surface of Gerota's fascia. This plane is developed by incising the lateral peritoneal attachments of the left colon from the level of the sigmoid to the splenic flexure, allowing

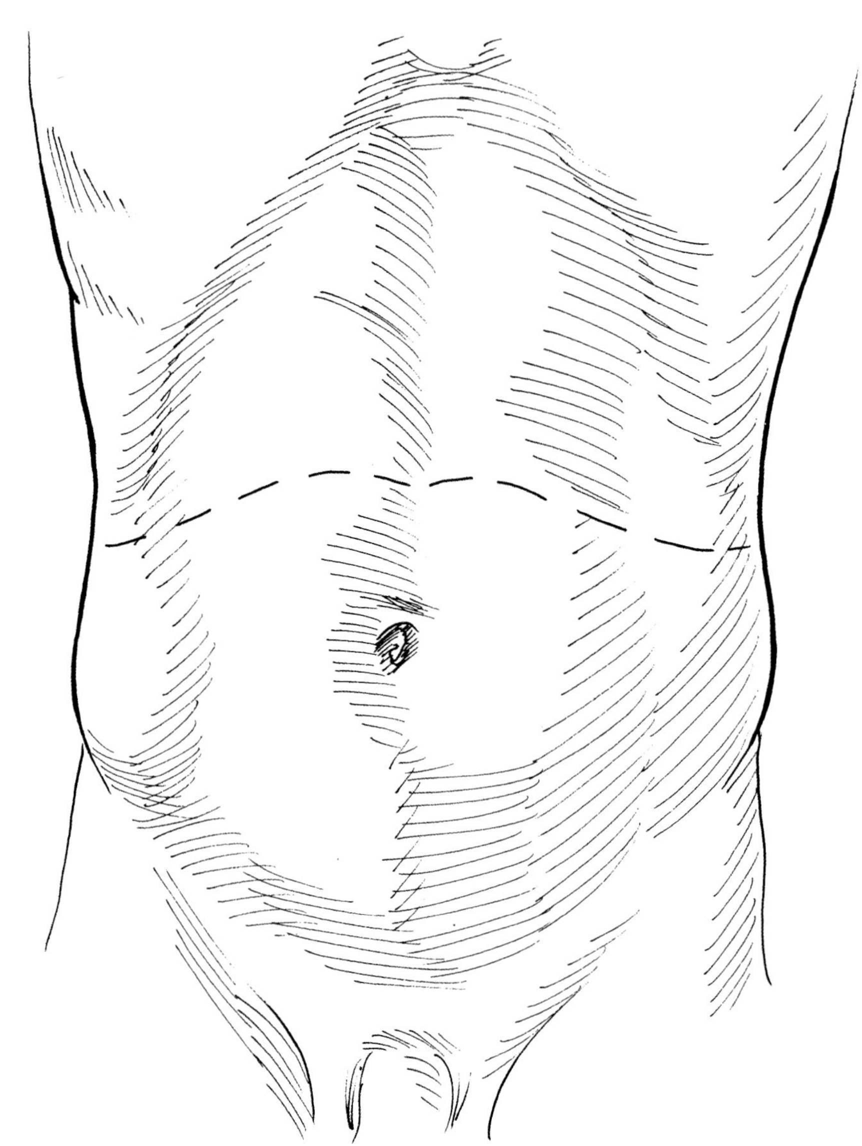

Fig. 11-9 A transverse supraumbilical incision affords good exposure of the renal artery on each side.

medial reflection of the colon with its mesentery. The spleen is mobilized in the superior wound by dividing the splenophrenic and splenorenal ligaments. A plane between the posterior surface of the pancreas and the anterior surface of Gerota's fascia is developed bluntly, and the spleen, pancreas, left colon, and mesocolon are reflected to the midline over the aorta (Fig. 11-10).

The left renal vein can be located easily as it crosses anterior to the aorta. The vein is encircled with a vascular tape and mobilized by ligating gonadal, adrenal, and lumbar branches to permit wide

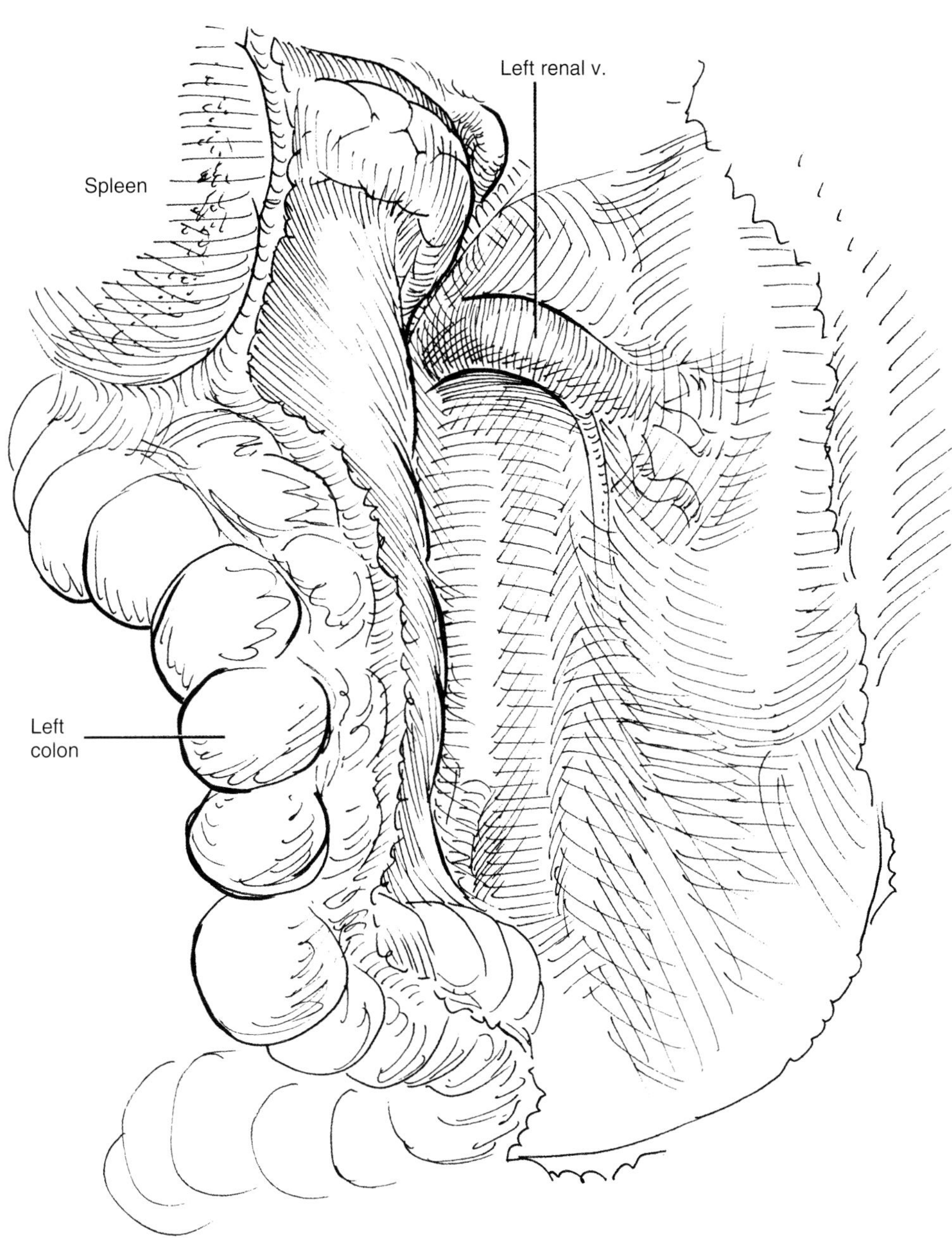

Fig. 11-10 Mobilization of the spleen, tail of the pancreas, and splenic flexure of the colon provides retroperitoneal exposure of the left renal vessels.

retraction (Fig. 11-11). The left renal artery lies directly beneath the cephalad border of the left renal vein in most cases.[13] The artery is readily dissected from surrounding lymphatics and encircled with a vascular tape. To ensure that the main trunk of the left renal artery is isolated rather than a distal branch, proximal exposure of the artery should proceed to its aortic origin.

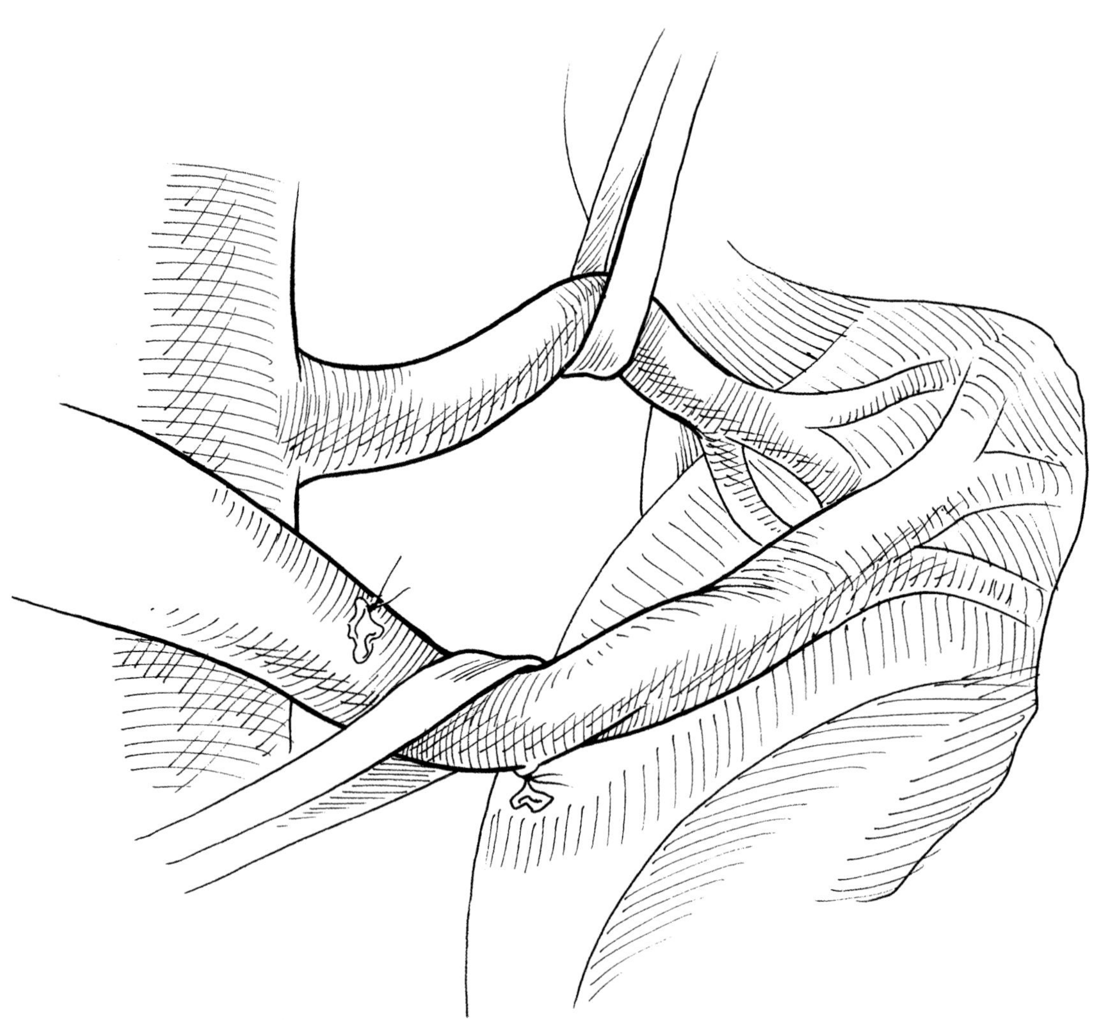

Fig. 11-11 The left renal vein is mobilized to expose the renal artery.

Exposure of the Right Renal Artery

The patient is placed supine, with the right flank elevated on a rolled sheet. The lower chest, abdomen, both groins, and anterior thighs are prepped and draped. As noted above, the incision may be midline or transverse. The transverse supraumbilical incision is begun at the left midclavicular line and extended to the right posterior axillary line between the costal margin and the superior iliac crest, crossing the midline 3 to 5 cm above the umbilicus.

After routine peritoneal exploration is completed, the small intestines are wrapped in moist laparotomy pads and retracted to the left. Lateral peritoneal attachments of the right colon are incised from the cecum to the hepatic flexure, and the right colon and mesentery are reflected medially. The duodenum is similarly mobilized by incising retroperitoneal attachments to the level of the hepatoduodenal ligament superiorly (Kocher maneuver), permitting extensive medial reflection of the duodenum and pancreas to the left (Fig. 11-12).

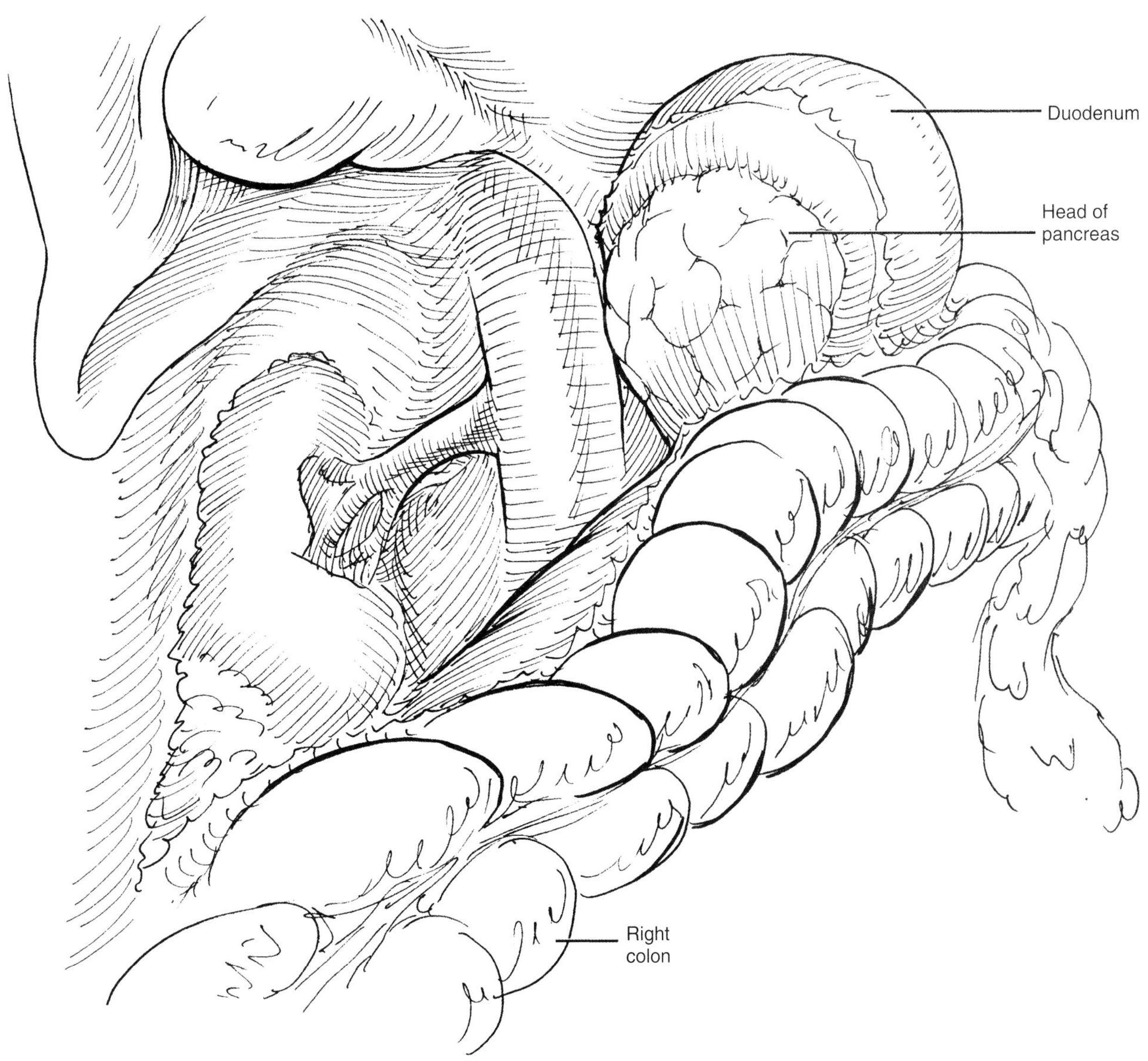

Fig. 11-12 Retroperitoneal exposure of the right renal vessels is accomplished by mobilizing the duodenum, head of the pancreas, and hepatic flexure of the colon.

This maneuver exposes the inferior vena cava. The right renal vein is easily identified and encircled with a vascular tape. The right renal artery can be dissected and isolated in the retroperitoneal tissues behind the right renal vein just lateral to the vena cava. To ensure that the main renal artery trunk is exposed, proximal isolation of the right renal artery should be carried out to its aortic origin. This requires careful leftward retraction of the lateral wall of the vena cava, either directly above or directly below the junction of the right renal vein (Fig. 11-13). Lumbar veins entering the vena cava just below the

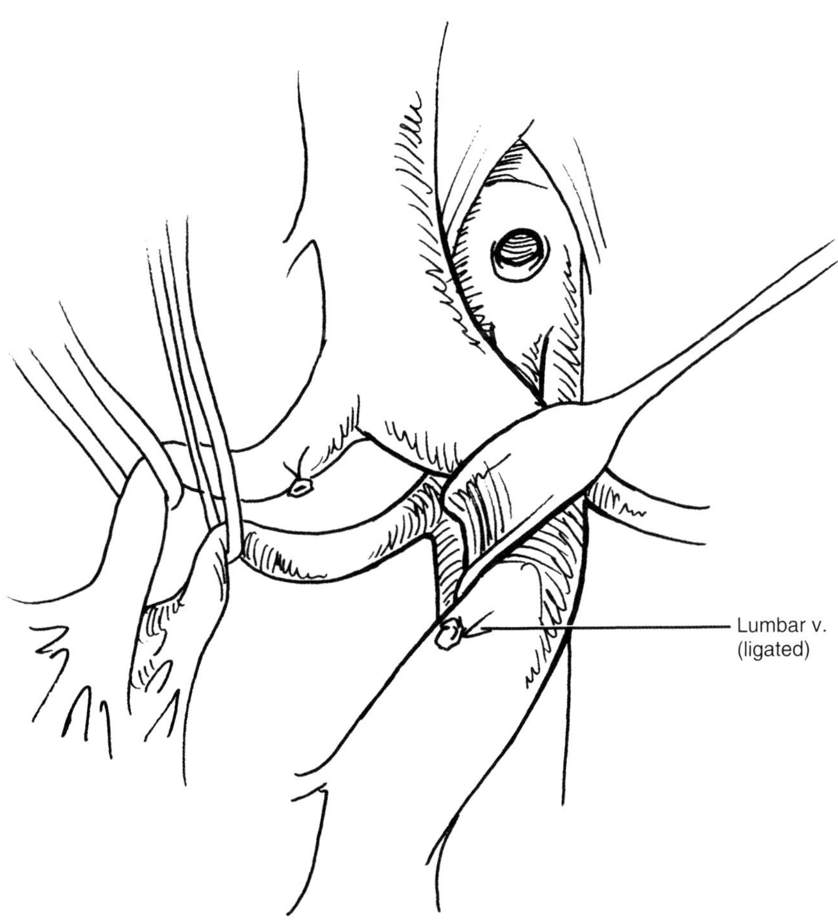

Fig. 11-13 The right renal vein is mobilized, and the vena cava is retracted to the left to expose the right renal artery to its origin. Lumbar branches of the vena cava are ligated as necessary.

renal veins should be carefully ligated. Bypasses to the right renal artery most often lie best when routed behind the vena cava from the aorta or right iliac artery. In some situations, the graft lies better in front of the vena cava, routed posteriorly to the right renal artery beneath the caudal border of the overlying renal vein (Fig. 11-14).

In cases involving correction of ostial lesions, the right renal artery can be isolated in the small space between the inferior vena cava and the aorta. This can be accomplished through either a midline transperitoneal approach (see above) or the right retroperitoneal approach described in this section.

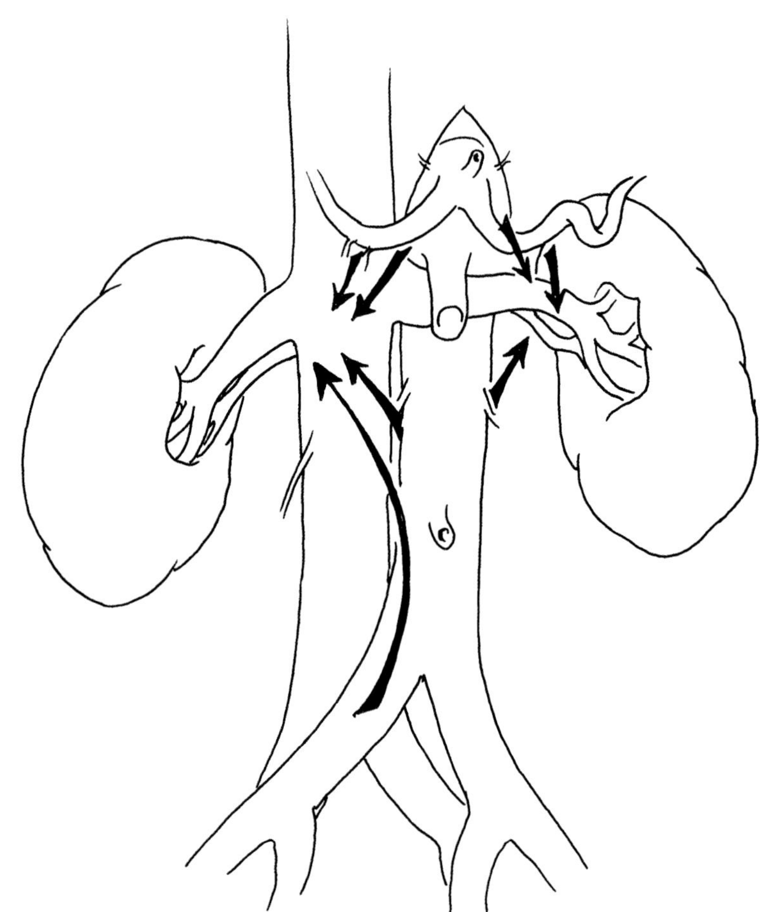

Fig. 11-14 Several bypass options are available for renal artery revascularization. Bypass grafts may originate from the aortoiliac system **(A–E)** or from branches of the celiac artery **(F–H)** if significant aortic disease is present.

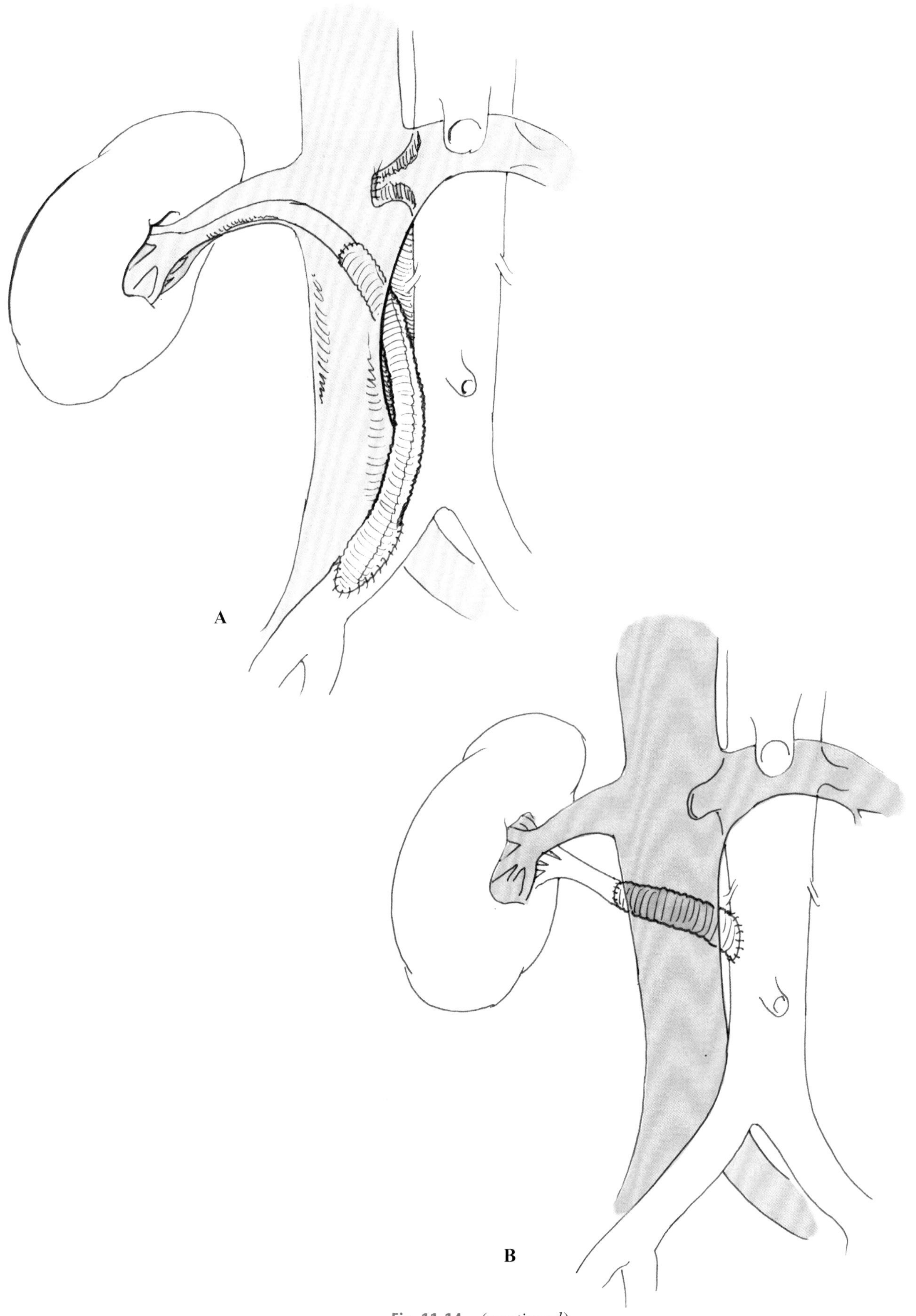

Fig. 11-14 *(continued)*

Fig. 11-14 (*continued*)

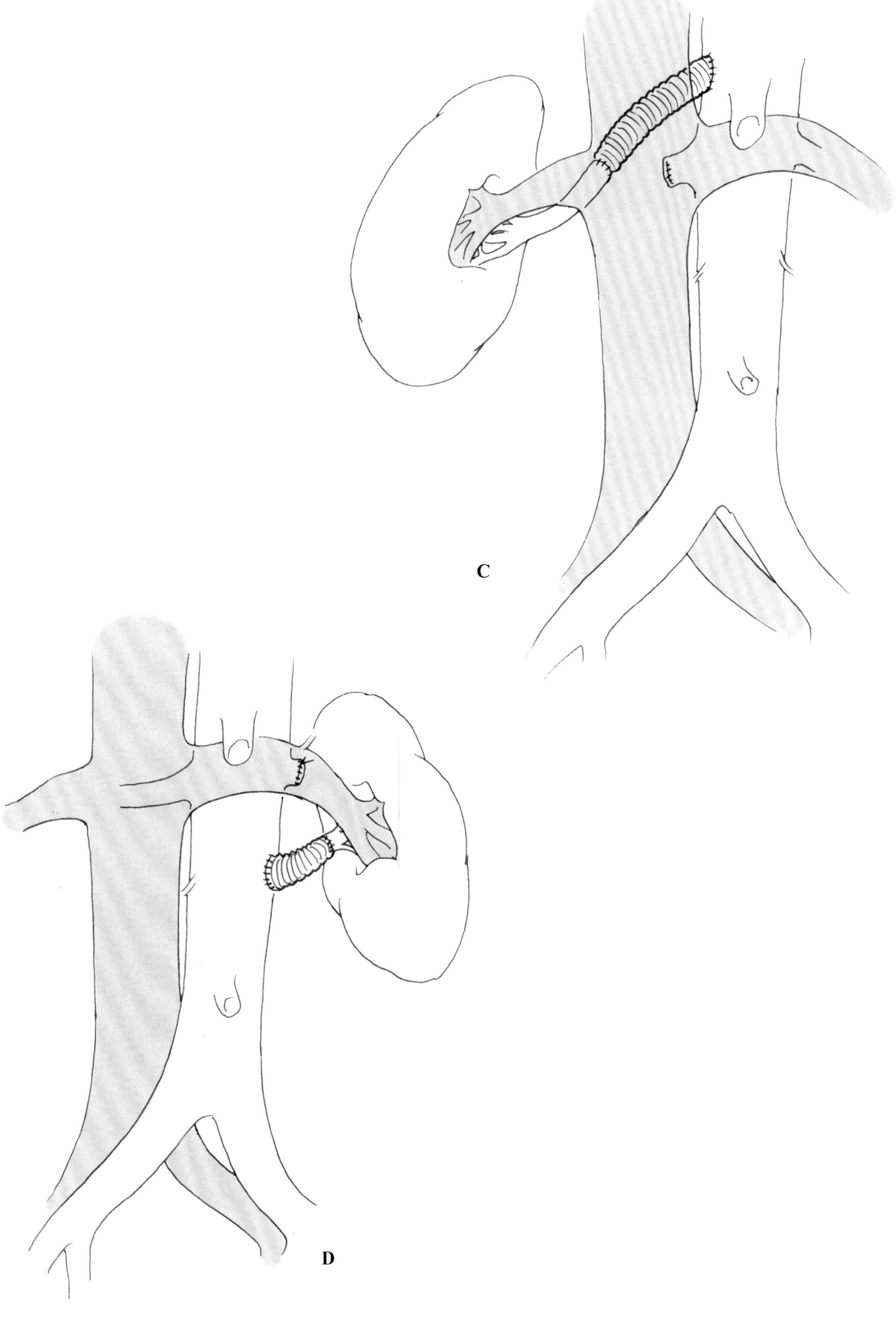

C

D

Fig. 11-14 (*continued*)

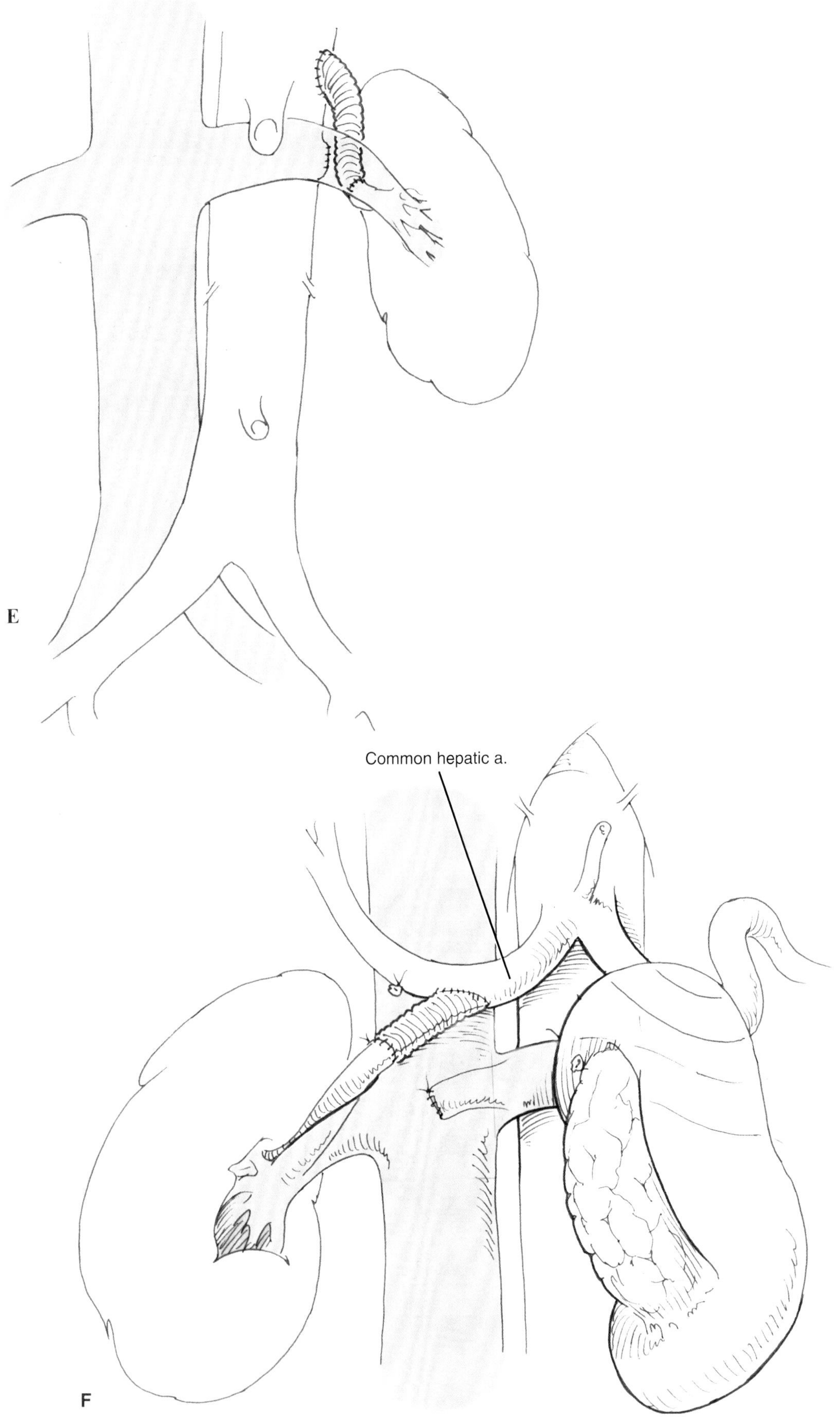

Fig. 11-14 (*continued*)

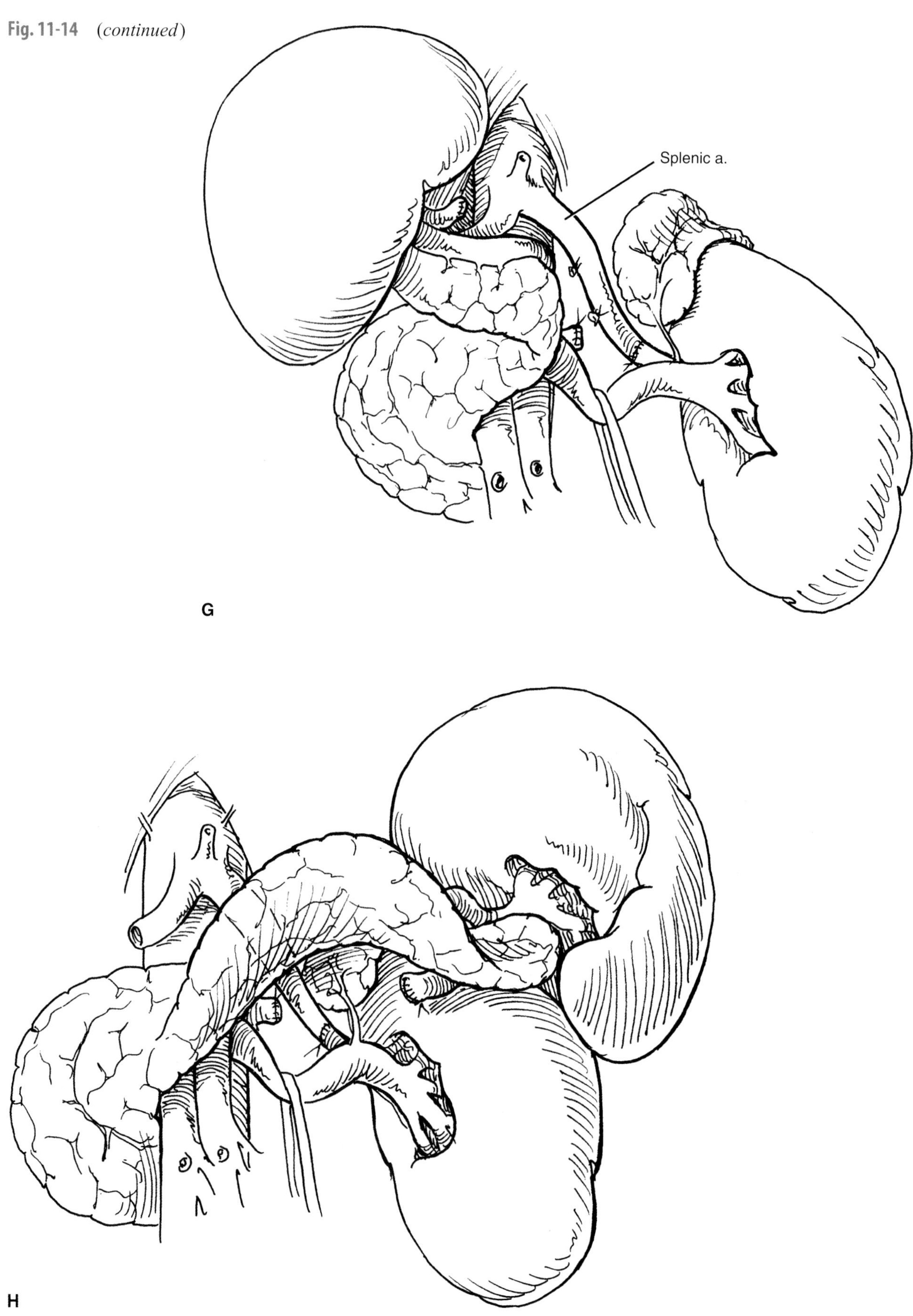

References

1. Sangthong B, Demetriades D, Martin M, et al. Management and hospital outcomes of blunt renal artery injuries: analysis of 517 patients from the National Trauma Data Bank. *J Am Coll Surg.* 2006;203:612–617.
2. Elliott SP, Olweny EO, McAninch JW. Renal artery injuries: a single center analysis of management strategies and outcomes. *J Urol.* 2007;178:2451–2455.
3. Pfieffrer T, Reiher L, Grabitz K, et al. Reconstruction for renal artery aneurysm: operative techniques and long-term results. *J Vasc Surg.* 2003;37:293–300.
4. Henke PK, Cardneau JD, Welling TH III, et al. Renal artery aneurysms: a 35-year clinical experience with 252 aneurysms in 168 patients. *Ann Surg.* 2001;234:454–462.
5. Crutchley TA, Pearce JD, Craven TE, et al. Branch renal artery repair with cold perfusion protection. *J Vasc Surg.* 2007;46:405–412.
6. Olin JW. Recognizing and managing fibromuscular dysplasia. *Cleve Clin Med.* 2007;74:273–274, 277–282.
7. Eisenberg Center at Oregon Health & Sciences University. *Management of Atherosclerotic Renal Artery Stenosis. Comparative Effectiveness Review Summary Guides for Clinicians.* Rockville, MD: AHRQ Comparative Effectiveness Reviews; 2007.
8. Balzer KM, Pfeiffer T, Rossbach S, et al. Prospective randomized trial of operative vs interventional treatment for renal artery ostial occlusive disease (RAODD). *J Vasc Surg.* 2009;49:667–674.
9. Balzer KM, Neuschafer S, Sagban TA, et al. Renal artery revascularization after unsuccessful percutaneous therapy: a single center experience. *Langenbecks Arch Surg.* 2012;397:111–115.
10. Garrett HE Jr, Richardson JW, Howard HS, et al. Retroperitoneal lymphocele after abdominal aortic surgery. *J Vasc Surg.* 1989;10:245–253.
11. Williams RA, Vetto J, Quinones-Baldrich W, et al. Chylous ascites following abdominal aortic surgery. *Ann Vasc Surg.* 1991;5:247–252.
12. Malaki M, Willis AP, Jones RG. Congenital anomalies of the inferior vena cava. *Clin Radiol.* 2012;67:165–171.
13. Valentine RJ, MacGillivray DC, Blankenship CL, et al. Variations in the anatomic relationship of the left renal vein to the left renal artery at the aorta. *Clin Anat.* 1990;3:249–255.
14. AbuRahma AF, Robinson PA, Boland JP, et al. The risk of ligation of the left renal vein in resection of the abdominal aortic aneurysm. *Surg Gynecol Obstet.* 1991;173:33–36.
15. Samson RH, Lepore MR, Showalter DP, et al. Long-term safety of left renal vein division and ligation to expedite complex abdominal aortic surgery. *J Vasc Surg.* 2009;50:500–504.

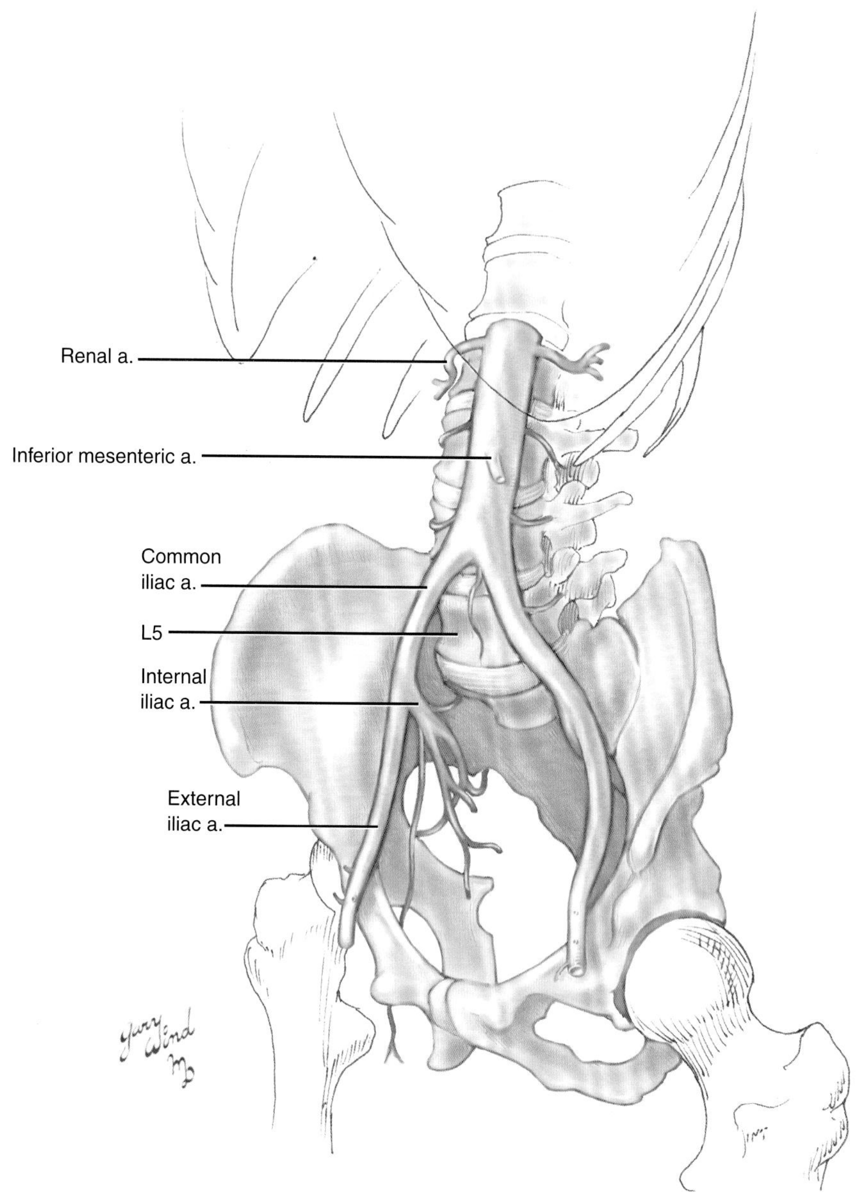

Fig. 12-1 The lower aortic segment rides the crest of the lumbar vertebrae.

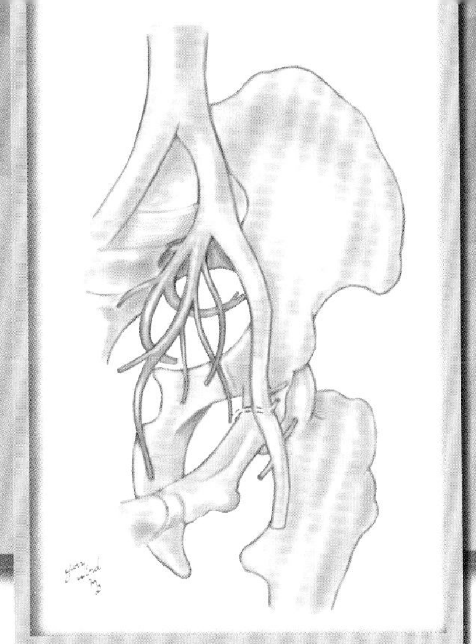

Infrarenal Abdominal Aorta, Pelvic Arteries, and Lumbar Sympathetic Chain

12

Surgical Anatomy of the Infrarenal Aorta and Iliac Arteries

The lower aortic segment between the renal artery origins at the cephalad end of the second lumbar vertebra and the bifurcation at the fourth lumbar vertebra lies slightly to the left of midline (Fig. 12-1). Paired lumbar arteries arise from the back wall of the aorta and girdle the first through fourth vertebral bodies. The fifth lumbar arteries lie below the bifurcation and may arise from the common iliac arteries or the middle sacral artery. The inferior mesenteric artery is the only visceral branch arising in this segment of aorta (see Chapter 10).

The common iliac arteries diverge from the aorta and descend a short distance to the lip of the true pelvis where they bifurcate into internal and external branches (Fig. 12-2). The internal iliac arteries dive into the bowl of the true pelvis where they immediately divide in a highly variable pattern, sending branches to the pelvic viscera and the external pelvic muscles (see Chapter 19, Figs. 19-20 and 19-21). The external iliac arteries hug the pelvic brim medial to the psoas muscles and give off only the small inferior epigastric and deep circumflex iliac branches near the inguinal ligament.

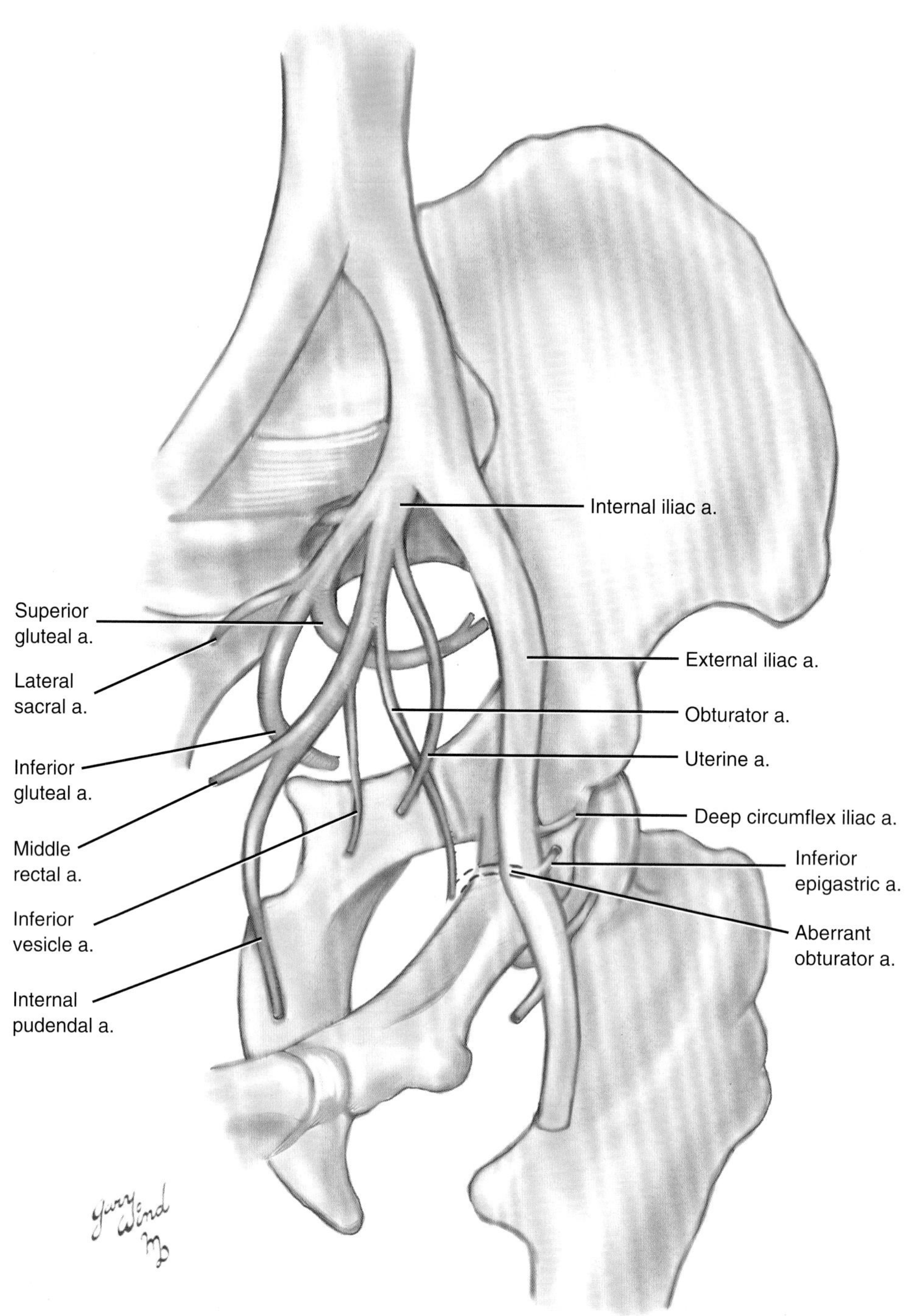

Fig. 12-2 The iliac vessels lie around the lip and in the bowl of the true pelvis.

Iliac Veins

The bifurcation of the aorta is separated from the fourth lumbar vertebra by the left common iliac vein. The vein crosses beneath the right iliac artery and joins the right iliac vein to form the vena cava on the right side of L5 (Fig. 12-3). Left common iliac vein compression from the overlying right common iliac artery can lead to venous hypertension and increased potential for thrombosis (May–Thurner syndrome), an anatomic variant that has been well described elsewhere.[1] Adhesion between the bifurcations of the aorta and vena cava is not uncommon, making manipulation of these vessel segments hazardous. These vessel segments are also vulnerable to injury during posterior lumbar disc surgery when the rongeur inadvertently bites through the anterior longitudinal ligament. Arterial, venous, and combined injury resulting in arteriovenous fistulae have been reported.[2] The iliac veins lie medial and deep to the common and external iliac arteries, occupying a position deep in the groove between the psoas muscle and pelvic brim.

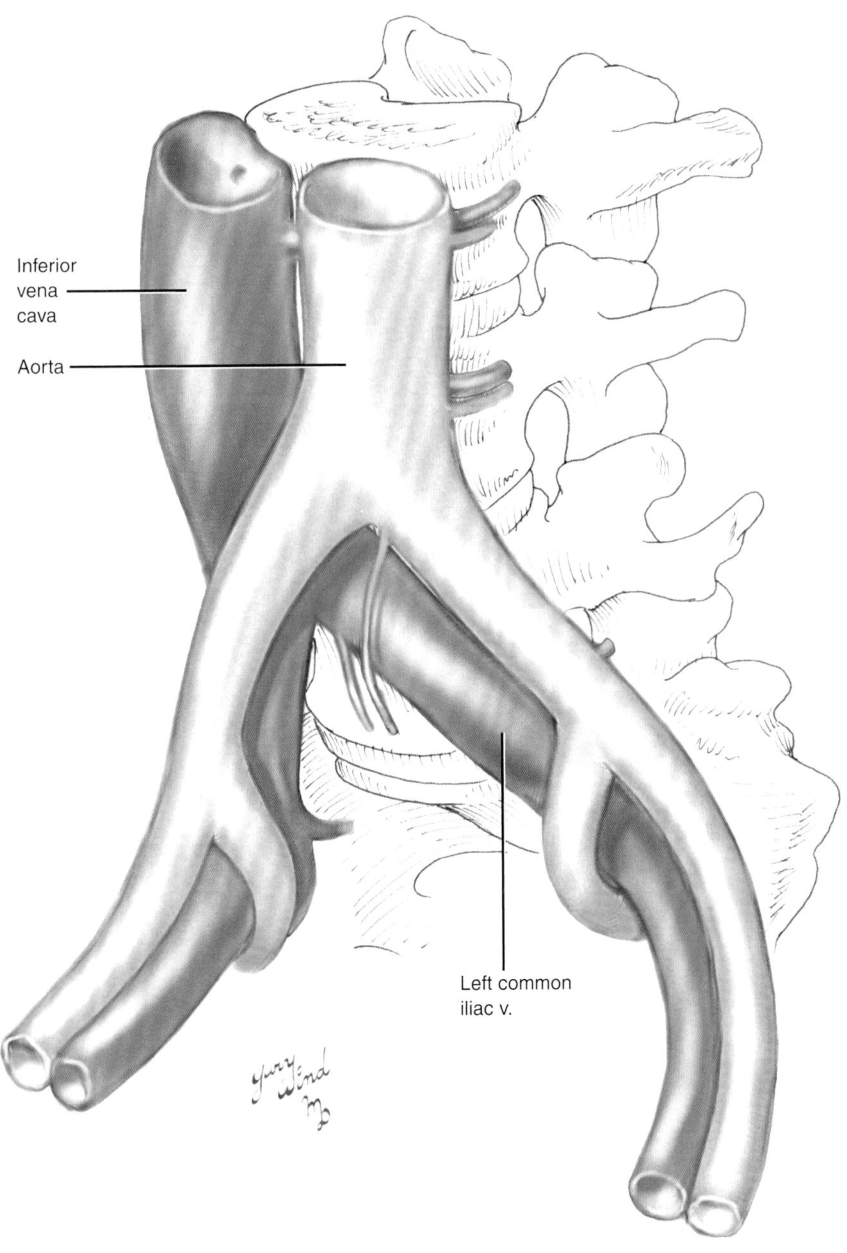

Fig. 12-3 The more proximal aortic bifurcation overrides the bifurcation of the vena cava and may be adherent.

Retroperitoneal Relationships

The gonadal vessels and ureters lie along the psoas muscles in the paravertebral gutters and cross anterior to the iliac vessels in the pelvis (Fig. 12-4). The root of the sigmoid mesocolon crosses the left iliac vessels, and the right iliac vessels lie directly beneath the peritoneum.

The lumbar branches of the aorta and vena cava pass beneath the sympathetic chains and the

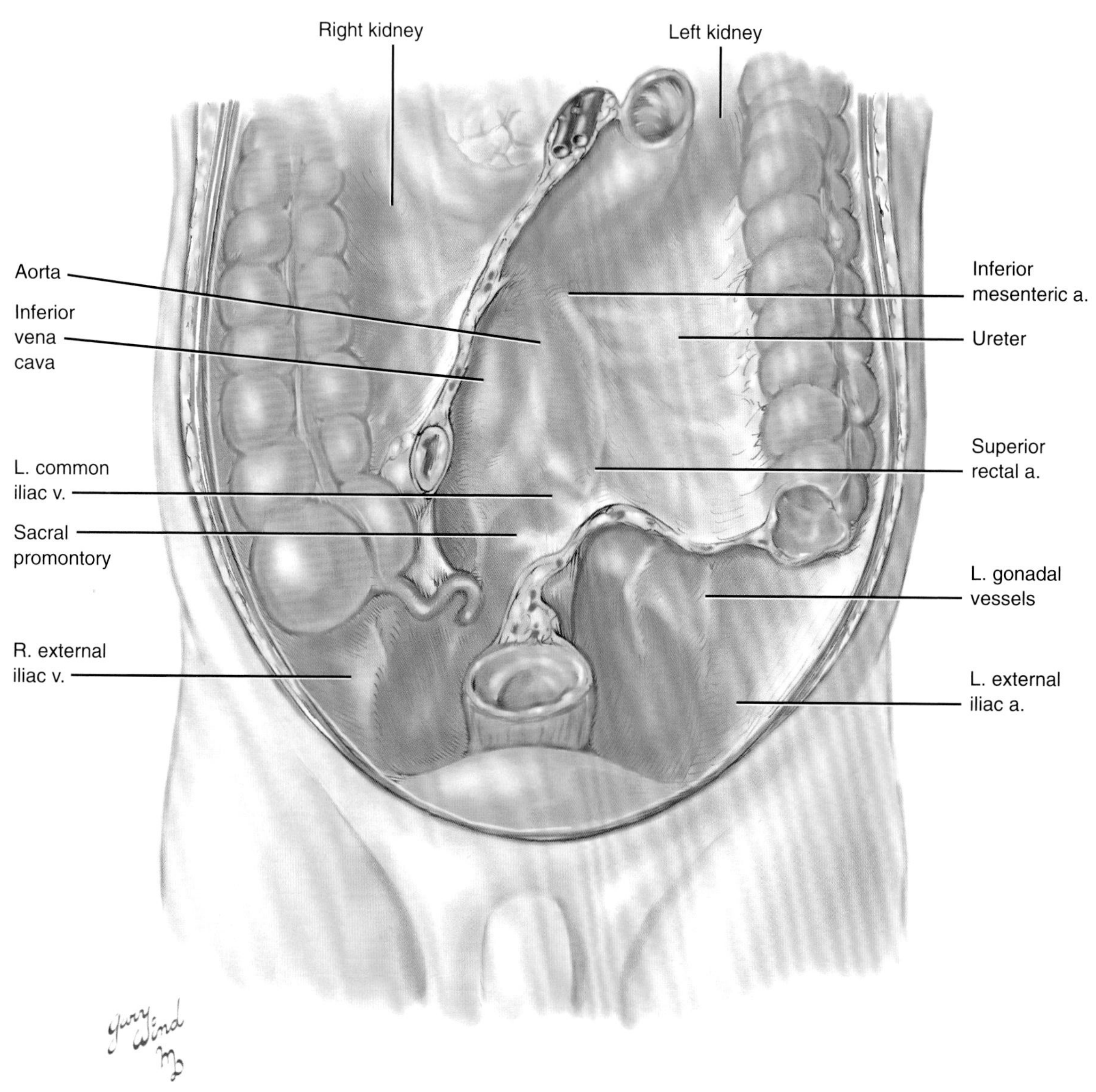

Fig. 12-4 Peritoneal relationships of the aorta are shown.

fibrous arches between slips of psoas origin and hug the vertebral bodies deep to the psoas muscles (Fig. 12-5). Occasional venous tributaries may overlie the sympathetic trunks. The lumbar sympathetic trunks lie more anteriorly on the vertebral bodies than do their thoracic counterparts. The lumbar trunks occupy a position between the anterior edges of the psoas muscles and the great vessels. Because of the offset arrangement of the great vessels toward the right, there is a slightly greater space between the lateral border of the aorta and psoas on the left than between the lateral border of the vena cava and psoas on the right. The sympathetic trunks pass behind the common iliac vessels into the sacral hollow of the pelvis.

The paired lumbar veins are interconnected. The major communications are the large ascending lumbar veins that lie far posterior in the angle between the vertebral bodies and the transverse processes, deep to the psoas muscles. Smaller anterior venous interconnections may lie superficial to the sympathetic trunks and make access to the trunks and ganglia more difficult.

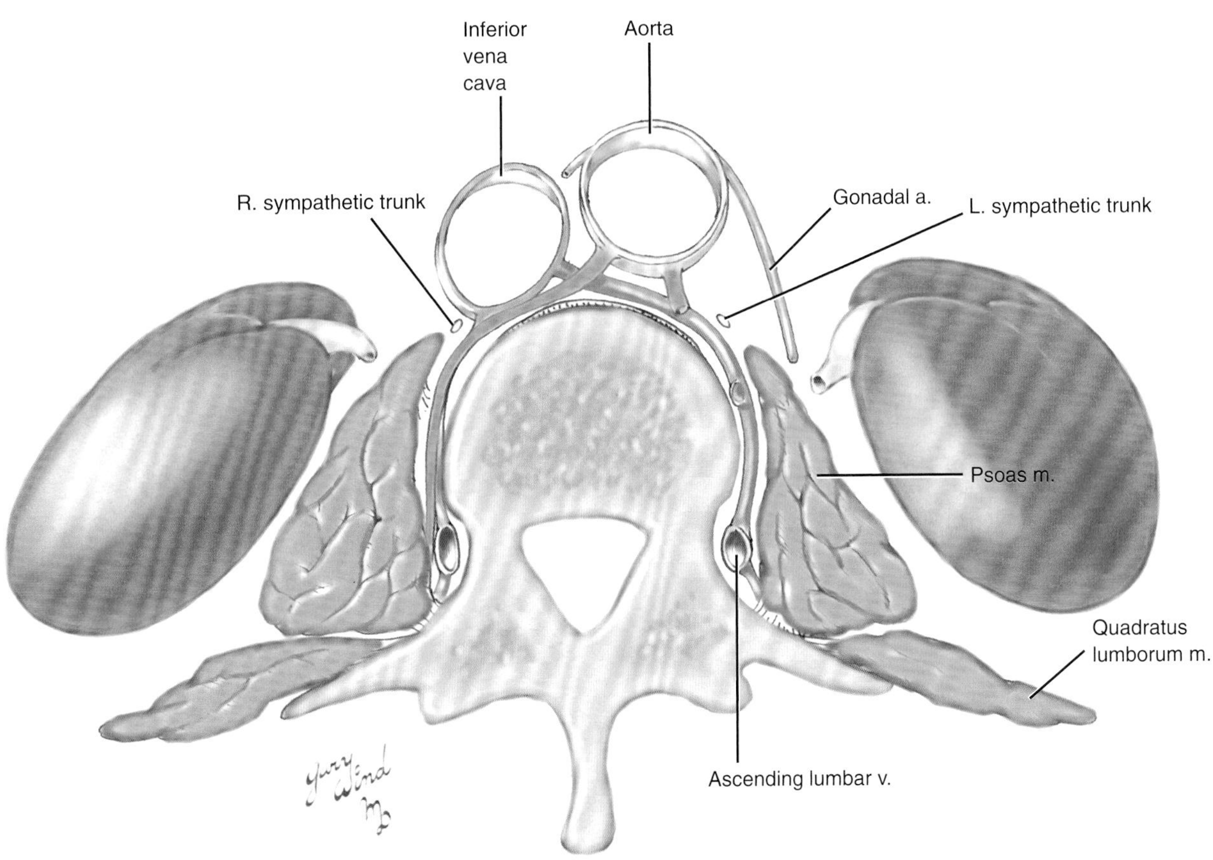

Fig. 12-5 The lumbar vessels lie between the vertebral bodies and the psoas muscles.

Nerves

The lumbar spinal nerves emerge from the vertebral foramina posterior to the ascending lumbar veins and enter the posterior portion of the psoas muscle (Fig. 12-6). There they interconnect to form the lumbar plexus (Fig. 12-7). The ventral rami of the first three and part of the fourth lumbar nerves contribute to the lumbar plexus. The two major motor nerves derived from the lumbar plexus are the femoral nerve to the quadriceps of the thigh and the obturator nerve to the adductor group.

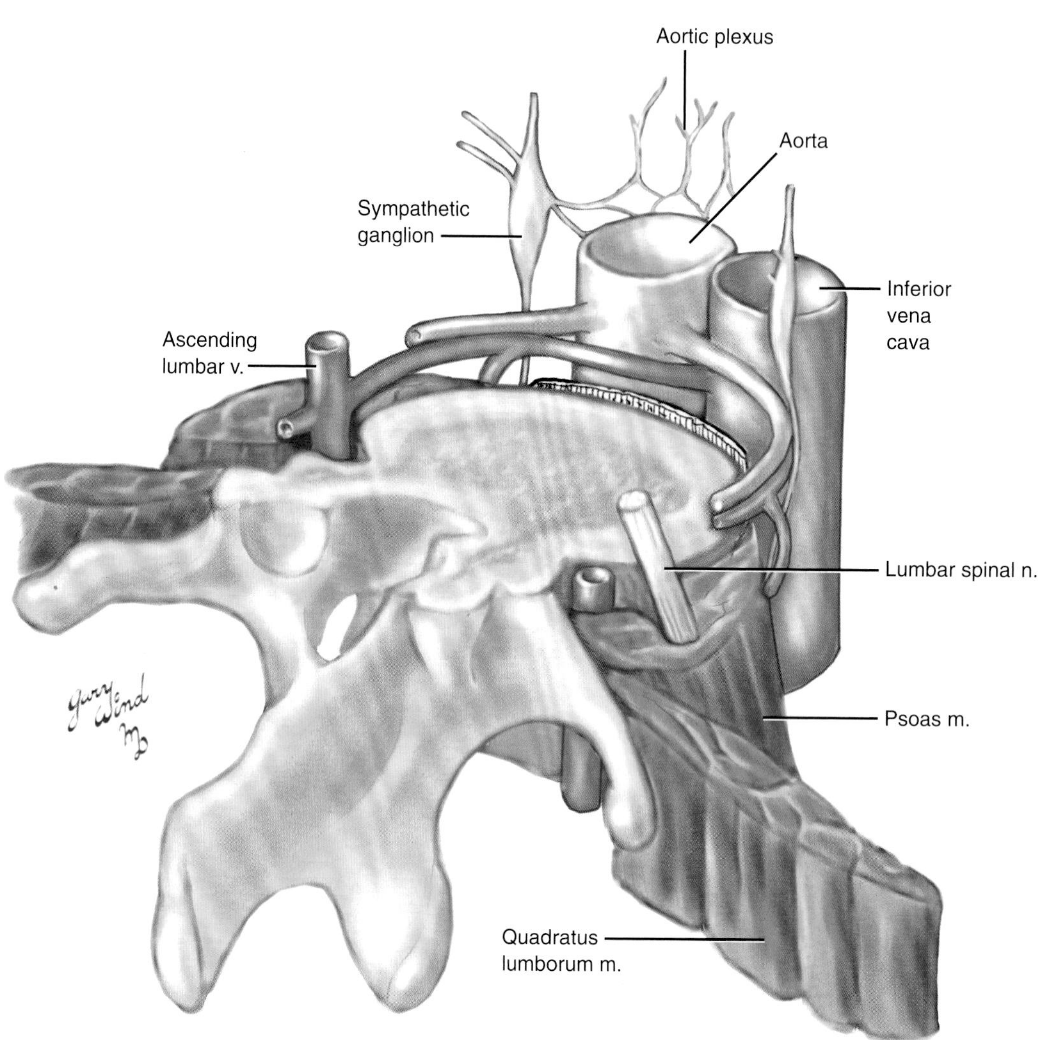

Fig. 12-6 The spinal nerves pass behind the ascending lumbar veins and pass through the psoas muscle.

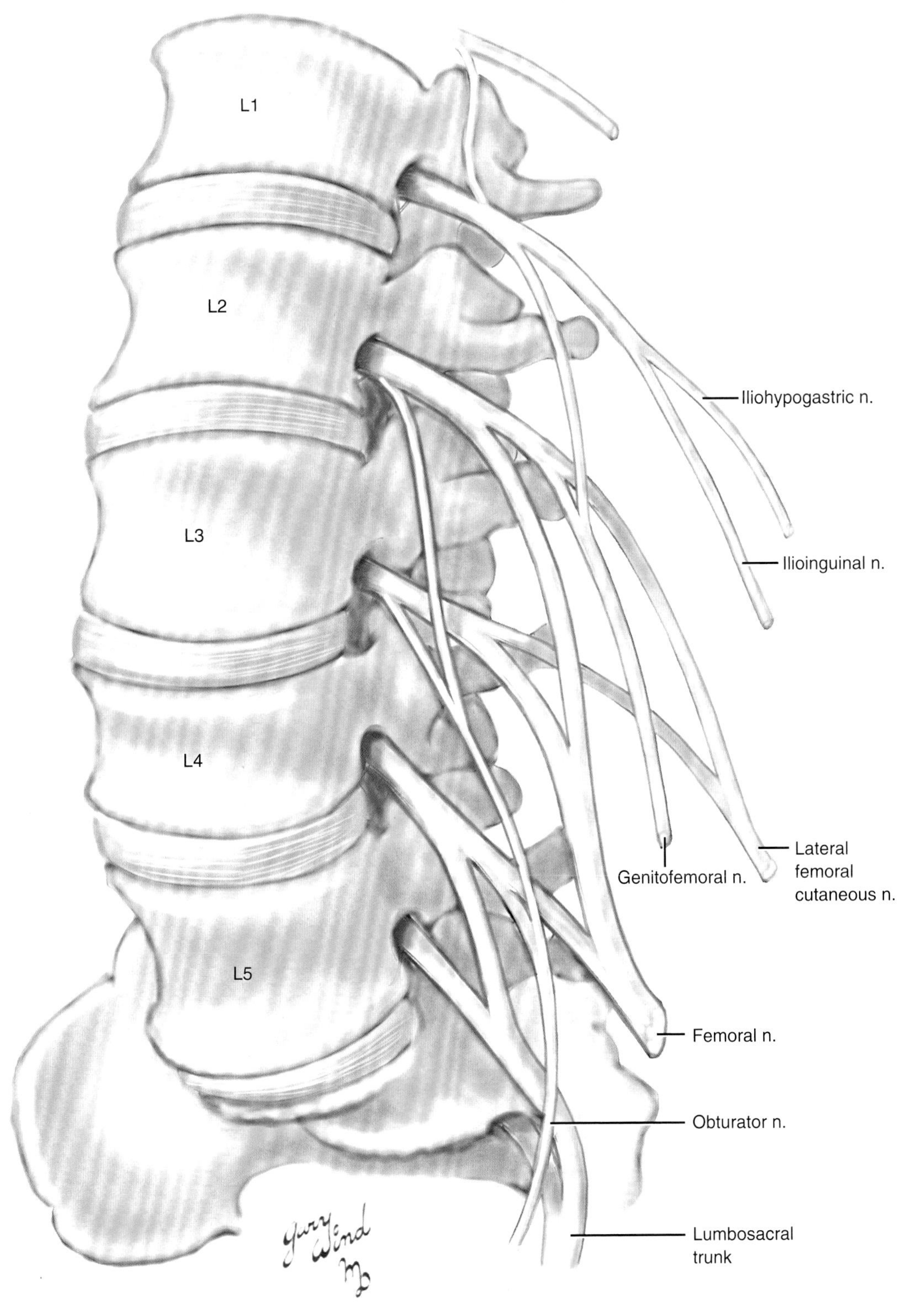

Fig. 12-7 The lumbar plexus lies within the psoas muscle.

The lumbar sympathetic chain consists of two to six ganglia in a variable pattern (Fig. 12-8). The ganglia receive sympathetic efferents from the first two lumbar nerves and send afferent gray rami to all the lumbar nerves. Lumbar splanchnic branches travel from the sympathetic chain to the aortic plexus where they are joined by postganglionic fibers from the celiac plexus. An additional plexus

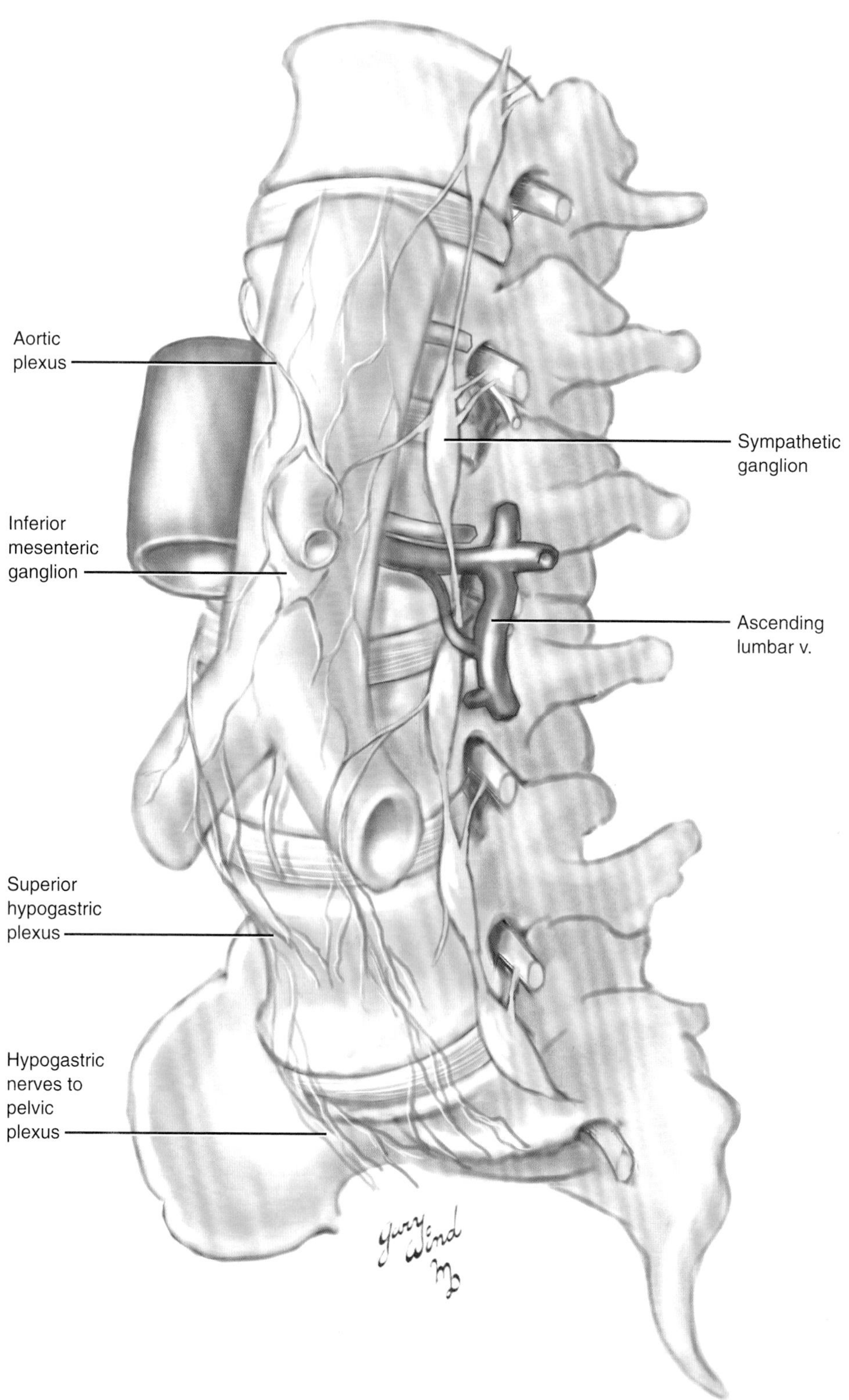

Fig. 12-8 The lumbar sympathetic chains lie on the anteromedial portions of the vertebral bodies.

is formed around the inferior mesenteric artery. Visceral branches from the plexus travel along the inferior mesenteric artery to the structures supplied by the artery. A variable number of hypogastric nerves coalesce from fibers caudal to the inferior mesenteric plexus. These nerves pass over the aortic bifurcation to form the superior hypogastric plexus in the sacral hollow. Autonomic fibers then pass to the inferior hypogastric plexus and from there join the pelvic plexus.

Interruption of sympathetic outflow from the first two lumbar ganglia through the hypogastric nerves and plexuses impairs ejaculation in males.

Exposure of the Aorta below the Renal Arteries

Most aortic pathology is confined to the infrarenal segment, allowing placement of proximal occluding clamps below the renal arteries during operative repair. Infrarenal aortic occlusion has significant physiologic advantages over occlusion proximal to the renal arteries. Exposure of the infrarenal aorta is eminently easier than exposure of the aorta above the renal arteries, which usually requires extensive dissection (see Chapter 9).

Infrarenal aortic exposure can be obtained through simple abdominal or flank incisions. There are two popular approaches: transperitoneal (i.e., intraperitoneal) and retroperitoneal. The transperitoneal approach has been popular for many years and is still favored by many surgeons. Compared with the retroperitoneal approach, it is simpler, requires less retraction, and allows examination of the intraabdominal cavity for unsuspected pathology.[3] Because the transperitoneal approach is more rapidly performed by most surgeons, it is the approach of choice for ruptured abdominal aortic aneurysms. However, gastrointestinal complications are prevalent after transperitoneal aortic operations.[4] The retroperitoneal approach has been associated with shorter duration of intestinal ileus, fewer pulmonary complications, and shorter hospital stays than the transperitoneal approach.[5,6] Retroperitoneal exposure is particularly useful in patients with complex aortic problems such as juxtarenal aneurysms, inflammatory aneurysms, and horseshoe kidneys.[7,8] Although visceral arteries can be readily repaired using left retroperitoneal incisions, the right external iliac and renal arteries are difficult to isolate. Aortic operations involving concomitant repair of aortic and right external iliac lesions should be performed transperitoneally or through separate left flank and right lower quadrant retroperitoneal incisions. Left retroperitoneal incisions are inappropriate for right renal artery reconstruction.

Transperitoneal Exposure of the Infrarenal Aorta

There are two commonly used incisions that provide adequate transperitoneal exposure of the abdominal aorta below the renal arteries: the longitudinal midline and the transverse infraumbilical approaches (Fig. 12-9). The midline incision is more rapidly made and is less likely to cause superficial nerve damage. However, transverse incisions may be associated with decreased postoperative pain in the upper abdomen, permitting increased ventilation and a more effective cough mechanism in patients with chronic pulmonary disease. Reported hernia rates are similar for both incisions at 1 to 6 years of follow-up.[9]

After the peritoneal cavity has been entered, the transverse colon and greater omentum are displaced from the abdomen, wrapped in moistened laparotomy pads, and reflected onto the superior abdominal wall. The small intestine is eviscerated and placed in a sterile plastic sac or wrapped in

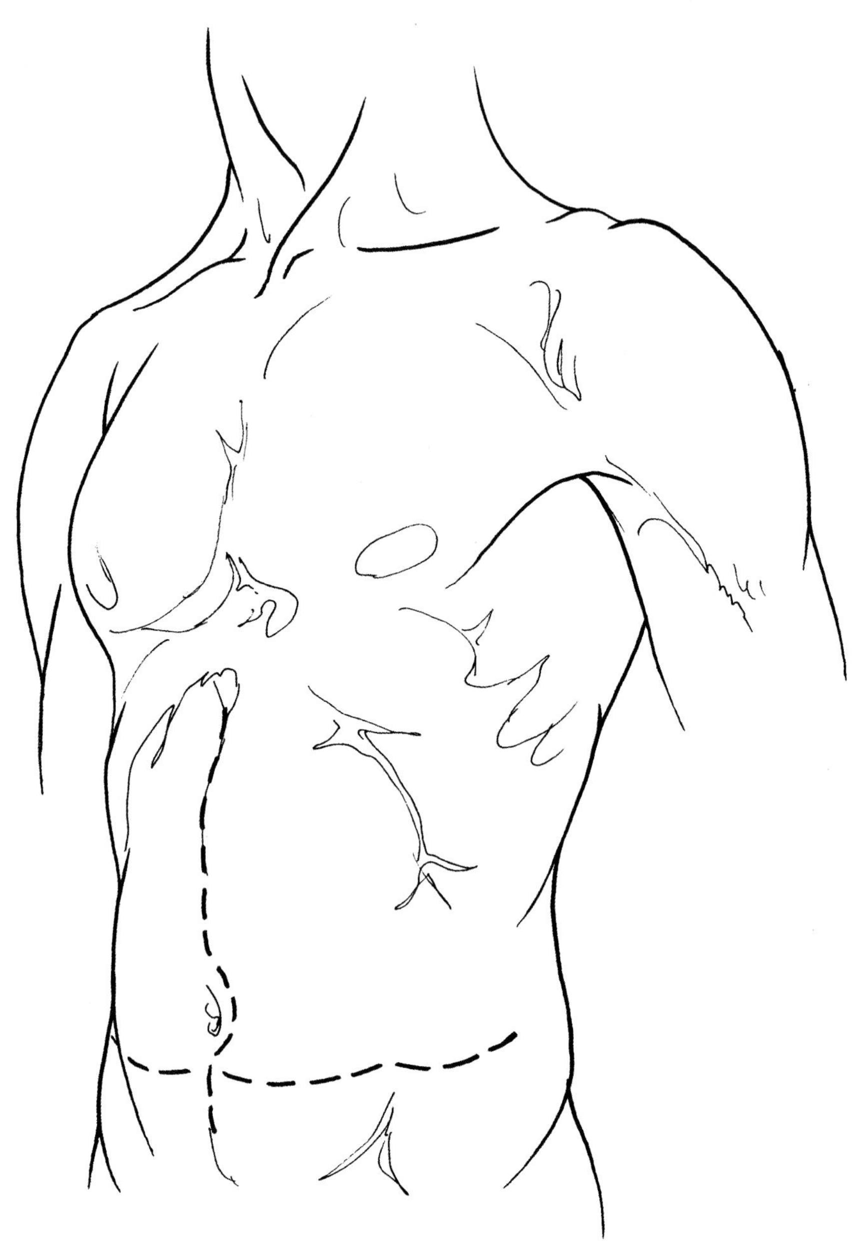

Fig. 12-9 Midline and transverse infraumbilical incisions provide adequate transperitoneal exposure of the infrarenal abdominal aorta.

moistened laparotomy pads and retracted into the right side of the abdomen. The retroperitoneal space is entered through an incision in the posterior parietal peritoneum near the duodenum (Fig. 12-10). This incision is carried superiorly to include division of the ligament of Treitz, allowing the third and fourth portions of the duodenum to be reflected toward the right side. Any identifiable lymphatic tissue overlying the anterior surface of the aorta should be ligated to prevent chylous leaks.[10] The periadventitial plane over the glistening surface of the anterior aorta is exposed by incising a thin layer of fibrous tissue. The incision is continued superiorly to the level of the left renal vein, which crosses anterior to the aorta in 97% of cases[11] and is a useful landmark for identifying the juxtarenal aorta (see Chapter 11).

The incision through the posterior peritoneum and preaortic tissue is continued inferiorly near the

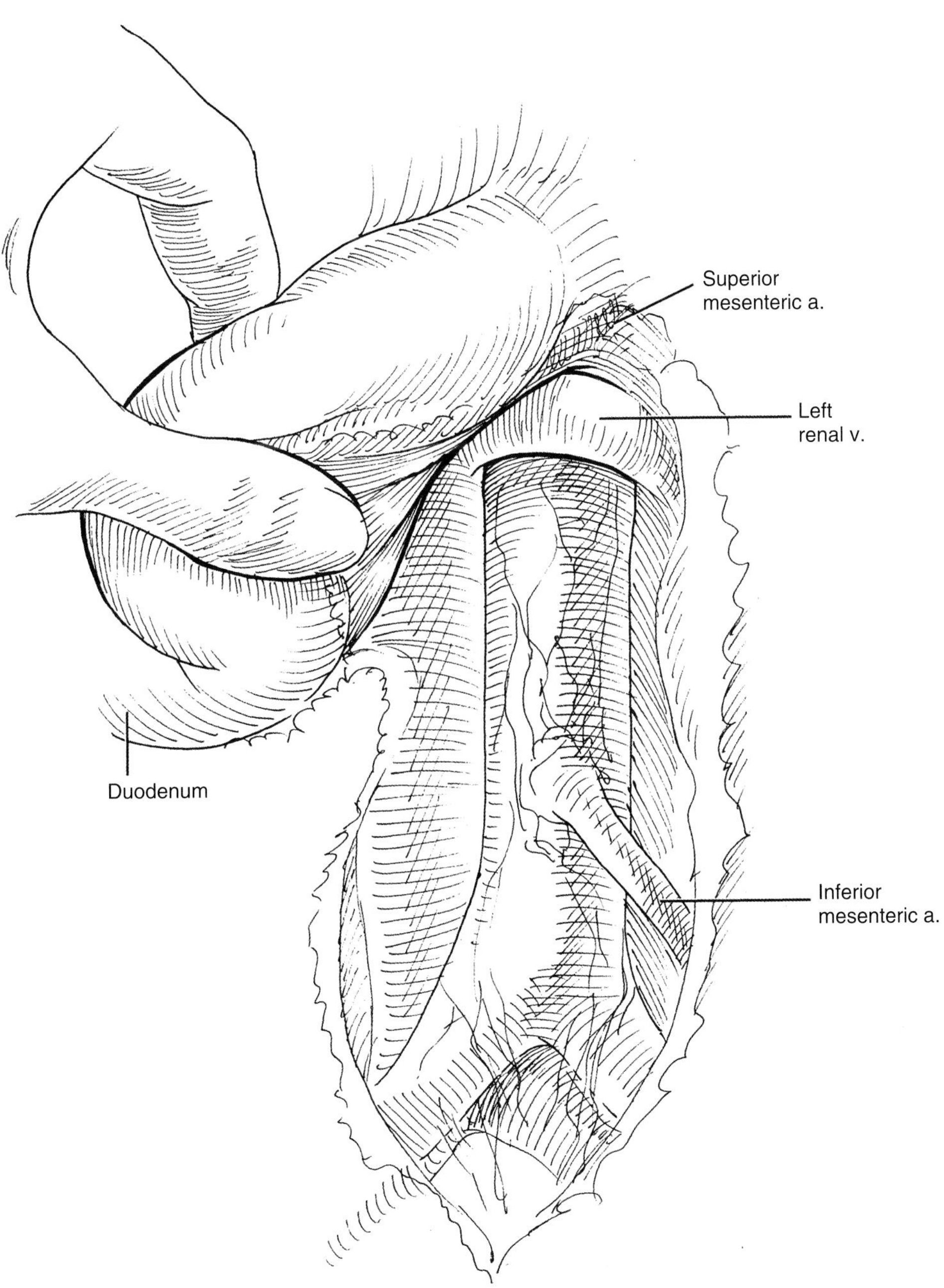

Fig. 12-10 The fourth portion of the duodenum is mobilized, and the aorta is exposed from the left renal vein to the bifurcation.

base of the small bowel mesentery to the level of the aortic bifurcation. The incision should be made to the right side of the aortic midline to avoid injuring the inferior mesenteric artery and other vessels in the sigmoid mesentery. Confining division of preaortic tissues to the right side also reduces the risk of injuring the preaortic autonomic plexus with the resulting sexual dysfunction.[12] Mobilization of the posterior wall of the aorta should be performed with great care to avoid injury to venous structures. Aortic mobilization just below the renal arteries requires careful finger dissection close to the posterior aortic wall, avoiding lumbar arterial branches. A lumbar venous plexus lies in the retroaortic tissues near the vertebral column and is prone to rapid hemorrhage when injured.[13] Retroaortic left renal veins and renal collars (i.e., circumaortic left renal veins) are especially prone to injury if unrecognized.[14] Mobilization of the aortic bifurcation is dangerous because the iliac vein confluence is often adherent to the posterior wall of the aorta from periaortic fibrosis. Control of the distal aorta is best carried out at the level of the common iliac arteries (see below).

Retroperitoneal Exposure of the Infrarenal Aorta

The patient is placed in a modified thoracotomy position with the left shoulder angled approximately 60° from the operating table and the hips rotated posteriorly as far as possible toward the horizontal position (Fig. 12-11). Posterior hip rotation is important to expose the groins for possible femoral

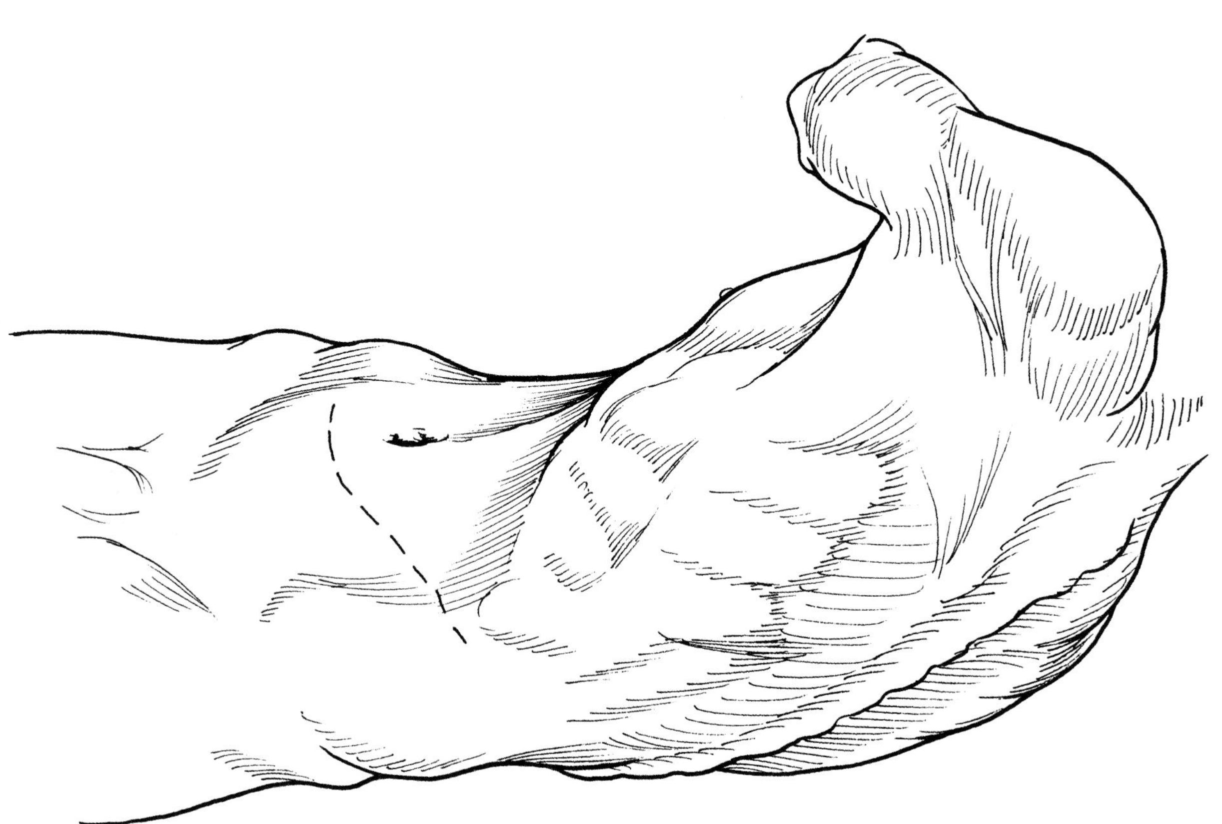

Fig. 12-11 Torsion of the trunk facilitates the retroperitoneal approach to the infrarenal aorta.

anastomoses, and the axial alignment lessens retraction requirements. The chest should be secured with wide tape, and a vacuum beanbag apparatus may be of value in maintaining the axial alignment.

An oblique left flank incision is made from the tip of the 11th or 12th rib to the abdominal midline 4 to 5 cm below the level of the umbilicus. The incision can be extended across the right rectus sheath in patients who require exposure of the right common iliac artery or in whom passage of a graft to the right femoral space is necessary. The incision is deepened through subcutaneous tissue, and the external oblique muscle, aponeurosis, and left anterior rectus sheath are divided. The left rectus is divided next, taking care to ligate branches of the inferior epigastric artery lying on the posterior surface of the muscle. After dividing the internal oblique and transversus abdominus muscle layers, the retroperitoneal space is entered in the lateral wound. The transversalis fascia lateral to the rectus sheath is opened, and the underlying peritoneal surface is stripped away from the transversalis fascia as the latter is divided for the length of the wound (Fig. 12-12). The posterior rectus sheath is incised medially, and the peritoneum is stripped from its posterior surface. As the peritoneum is often adherent to the posterior rectus

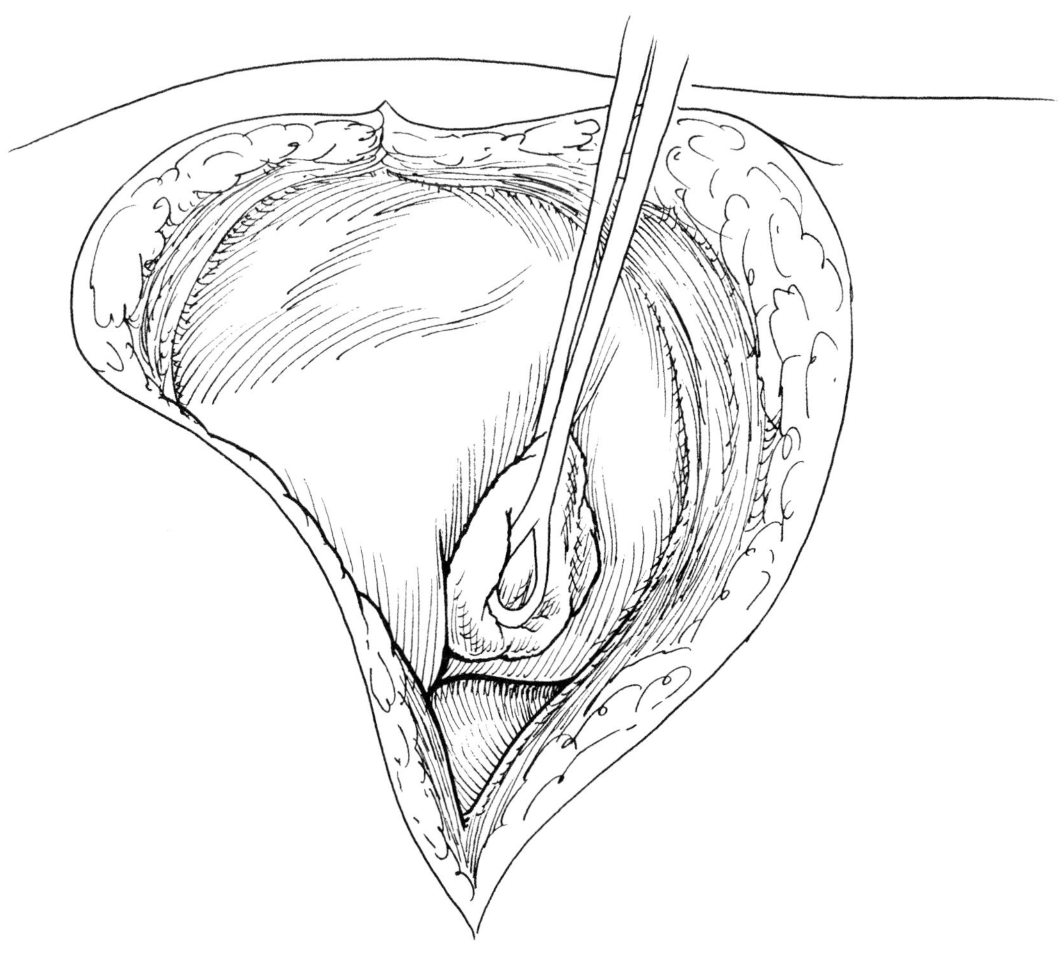

Fig. 12-12 The retroperitoneal dissection is begun in the lateral wound.

sheath, it may be necessary to stop the incision 2 to 5 cm from the linea alba to avoid inadvertent peritoneal entry. Any small tears inadvertently made in the peritoneum should be closed.

A retroperitoneal plane is developed by stripping the peritoneum from the abdominal wall laterally and posteriorly, staying anterior to Gerota's fascia over the left kidney. Extension of the plane behind Gerota's fascia with anterior mobilization of the left kidney should be performed in cases when suprarenal exposure of the aorta is desired (see Chapter 9). When the plane is developed anterior to the left kidney, the ureter is best left in the posterior retroperitoneal tissues as the posterior peritoneal surface is retracted forward. Mobilizing the left ureter forward with the peritoneum brings the proximal ureter directly in front of the juxtarenal aorta and renders exposure inconvenient.

The peritoneal sac is mobilized medially and cephalad until the aorta is exposed from the left renal vein to the left iliac artery bifurcation (Fig. 12-13). This requires that the inferior mesenteric artery be ligated and divided near the anterior aortic wall. The left gonadal vein should be ligated and divided near

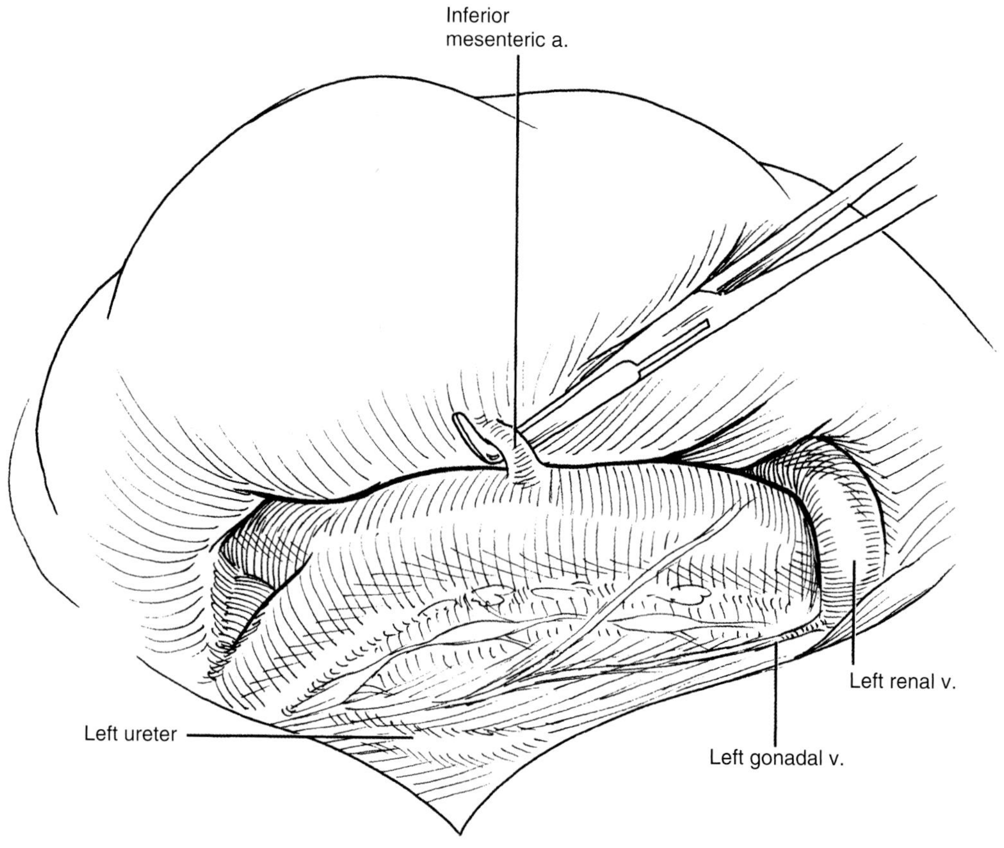

Fig. 12-13 The inferior mesenteric artery and left gonadal vessels are divided to complete retroperitoneal exposure of the aorta.

its junction with the renal vein to prevent avulsion injury. The peritoneum can be mobilized far to the patient's right side to expose the origin of the right common iliac artery. Vascular control of the left iliac artery is easily obtained, but the right iliac artery is often obscured from view by large aneurysms or other local pathology. In these cases, it may be easier to obtain vascular control from within the lumen of the aorta using Fogarty catheters.[15] Retroperitoneal exposure of the right external iliac artery should be obtained through a separate transverse incision in the right lower quadrant (see below).

Transperitoneal Exposure of the Iliac Arteries

Patient positioning, abdominal incision, and visceral displacement proceed as described for transperitoneal exposure of the aorta. The posterior peritoneum is incised over the anterior aortic surface just to the left of the fourth portion of the duodenum. The peritoneal incision is continued caudally on the right side of the aortic midline and extended over the anterior surface of the right common iliac artery (Fig. 12-14). Using blunt dissection, the anterior periadventitial plane of the

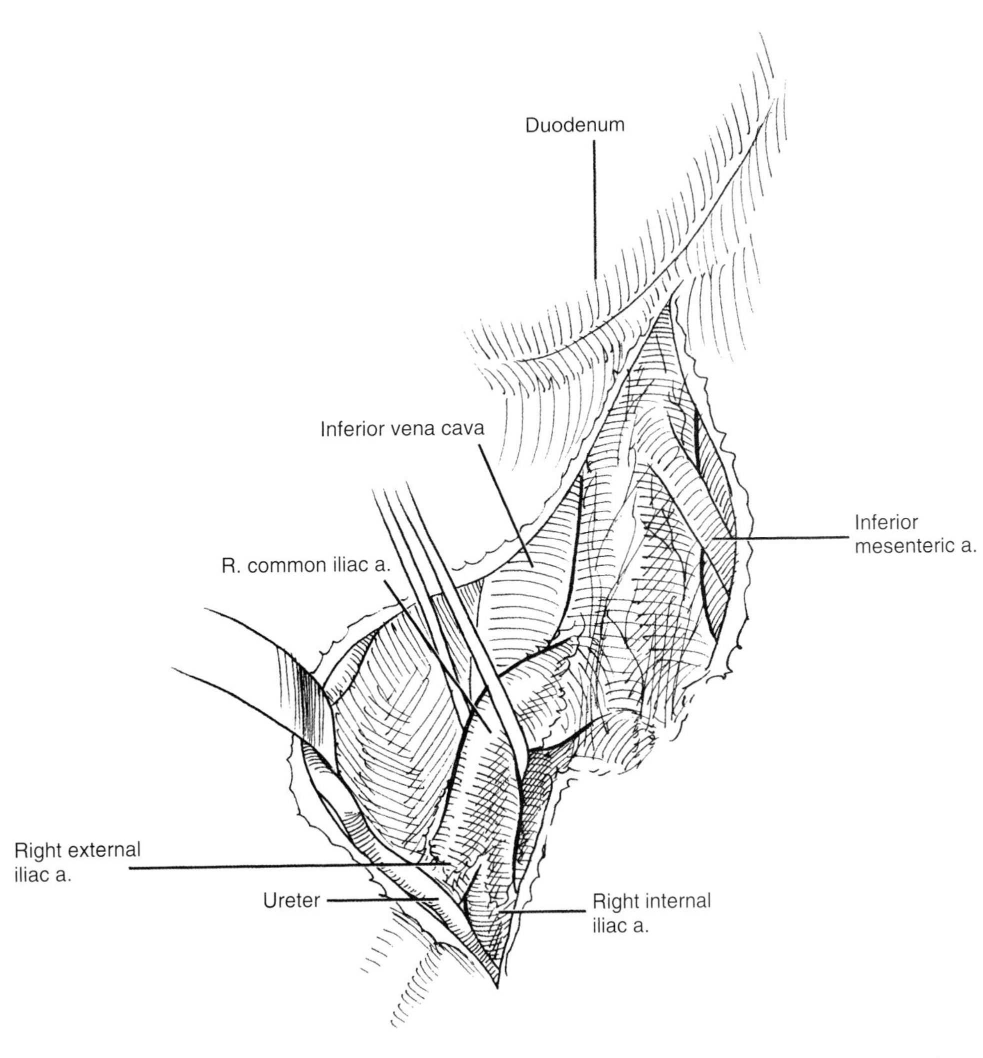

Fig. 12-14 The peritoneal incision is extended to expose and control the right iliac vessels.

common iliac artery is located and opened to the level of the aortic bifurcation. The artery is next encircled with a vascular tape, taking care to avoid injury to the common iliac vein that lies on its posterolateral surface. Distal exposure of the common iliac artery proceeds to its bifurcation. The right ureter courses in the periadventitial tissues over the common iliac artery adjacent to the bifurcation; it should be identified and retracted laterally with the associated periadventitial tissues. When mobilization of the ureter away from the bifurcation is difficult, it may be encircled with a vessel loop and retracted laterally. The internal and external iliac arteries are then isolated and encircled with vessel tapes. The corresponding internal and external iliac veins lie on the posteromedial surfaces of their respective arteries.

The left common iliac artery and its branches are exposed by laterally retracting the left side of the incised posterior peritoneum (Fig. 12-15). The posterior peritoneum and associated periadventitial tissues should not be incised over the aortic bifurcation or the left common iliac artery in males because sympathetic nerve disruption leading to ejaculatory dysfunction can result. The left side of the posterior peritoneal incision is retracted laterally to identify

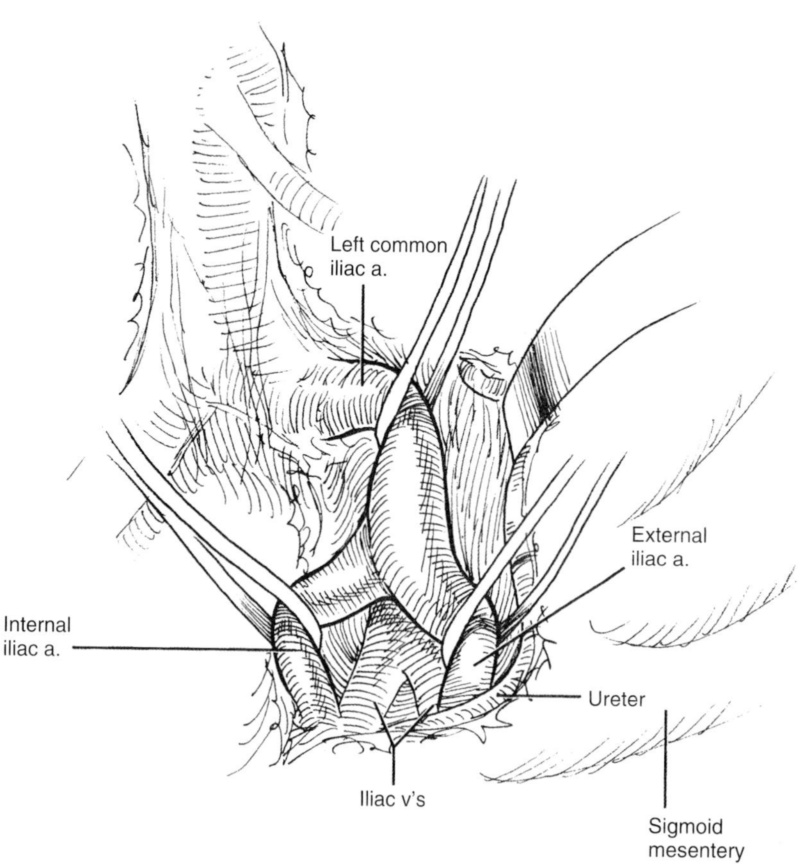

Fig. 12-15 Peritoneal retraction on the left side permits isolation of the left iliac vessels.

the common iliac artery and its branches, taking care to identify the left ureter. If posterior peritoneal retraction from the midline does not permit adequate exposure, a lateral approach will be required. The sigmoid colon is mobilized along its lateral surface by incising peritoneal attachments. A relatively avascular plane is developed posterior to the sigmoid and its mesentery, which are reflected medially to expose the left common iliac artery and its branches (Fig. 12-16).

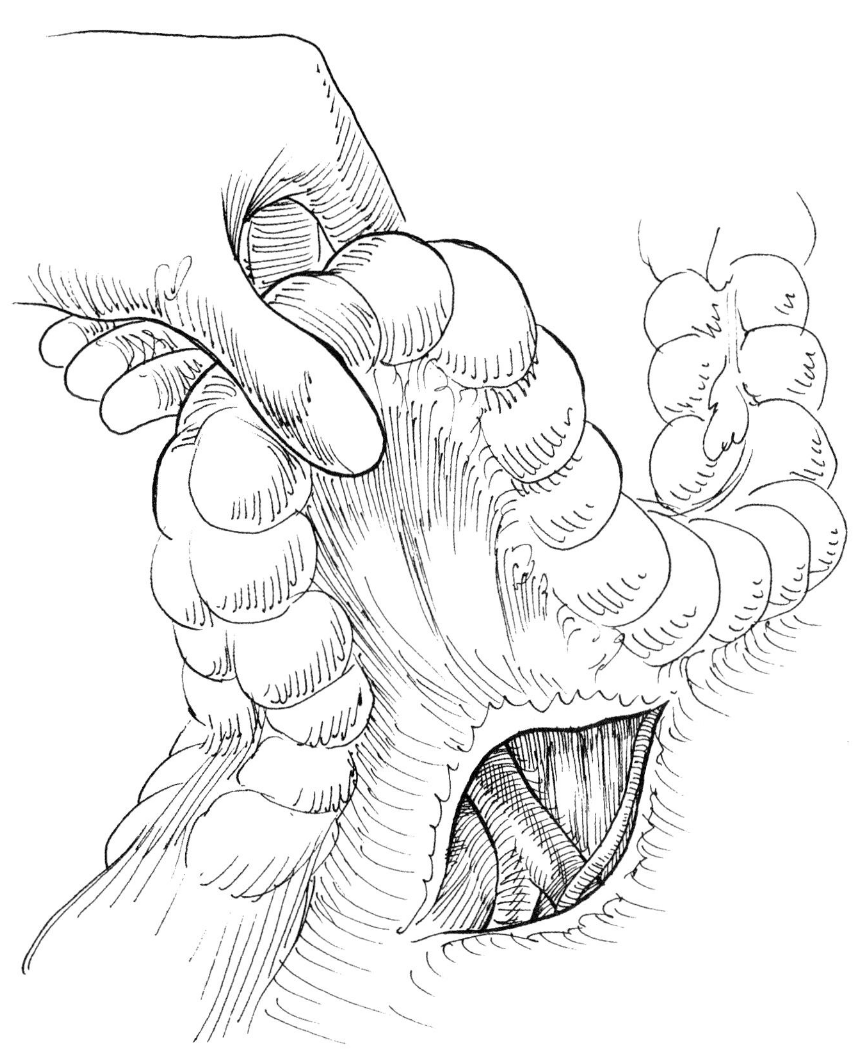

Fig. 12-16 The left iliac vessels may also be approached by opening the lateral side of the root of the sigmoid mesocolon.

Retroperitoneal Exposure of the Iliac Arteries

The patient is placed in the supine position with the ipsilateral hip elevated 10° on a rolled sheet. The entire abdomen and flank are prepped and draped. An oblique skin incision is begun at the lateral border of the rectus muscle approximately 3 cm above the inguinal ligament and extended to the midaxillary line halfway between the subcostal margin and iliac crest (Fig. 12-17). As the wound is deepened through subcutaneous tissues, ligation of the superficial epigastric and superficial circumflex iliac arteries should be performed to prevent troublesome hemorrhage from the wound edges.

The aponeuroses of the external oblique and internal oblique muscles are next divided parallel to the wound axis. Laterally, the internal oblique muscle should be bluntly split apart in the direction of its fibers. The transversus abdominus and transversalis fascia are opened in the lateral half of the

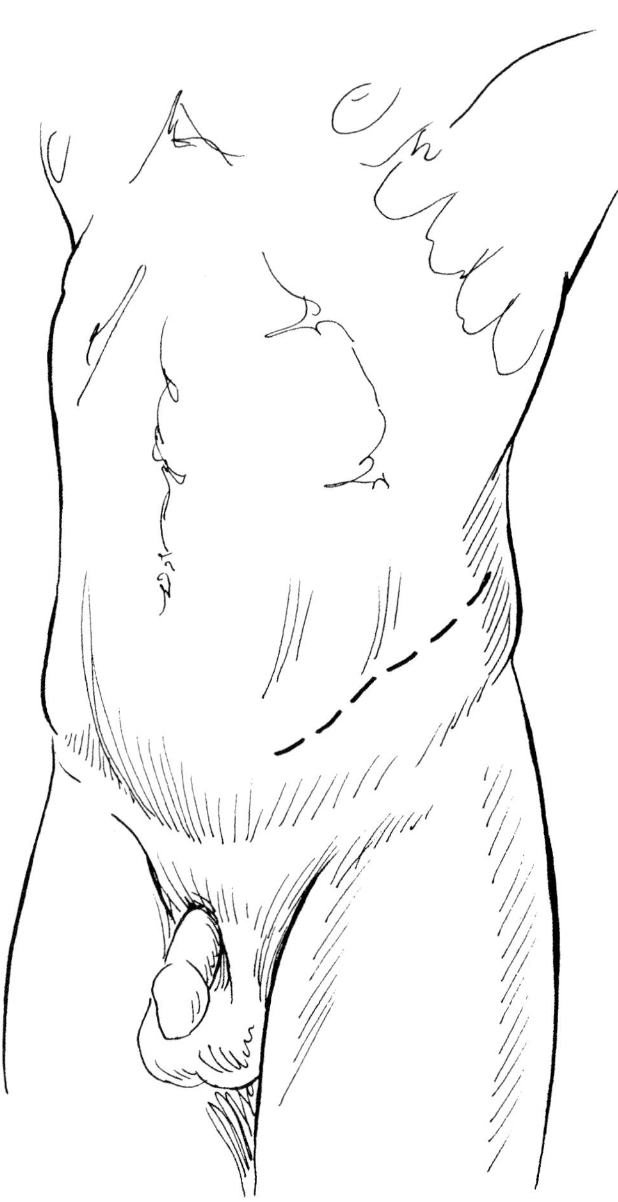

Fig. 12-17 A low, oblique anterior flank incision is used for extraperitoneal exposure of the iliac arteries.

wound, gaining access to the retroperitoneal space (Fig. 12-18). The retroperitoneal space is most easily entered in the wound's lateral aspect because the peritoneum may be fused to the transversalis fascia near the midline. The peritoneum is carefully stripped from the lateral pelvic wall and retracted medially to expose the psoas muscle and iliac vessels on the medial side of the psoas muscle. The ureter is best left attached to the posterior peritoneal surface, where it is safely retracted along with the peritoneal sac into the medial wound. The external iliac artery can be identified in the lower wound and traced proximally to identify the common and internal iliac segments. Proximal exposure can be accomplished to the level of the terminal abdominal aorta with further medial retraction of the peritoneum.

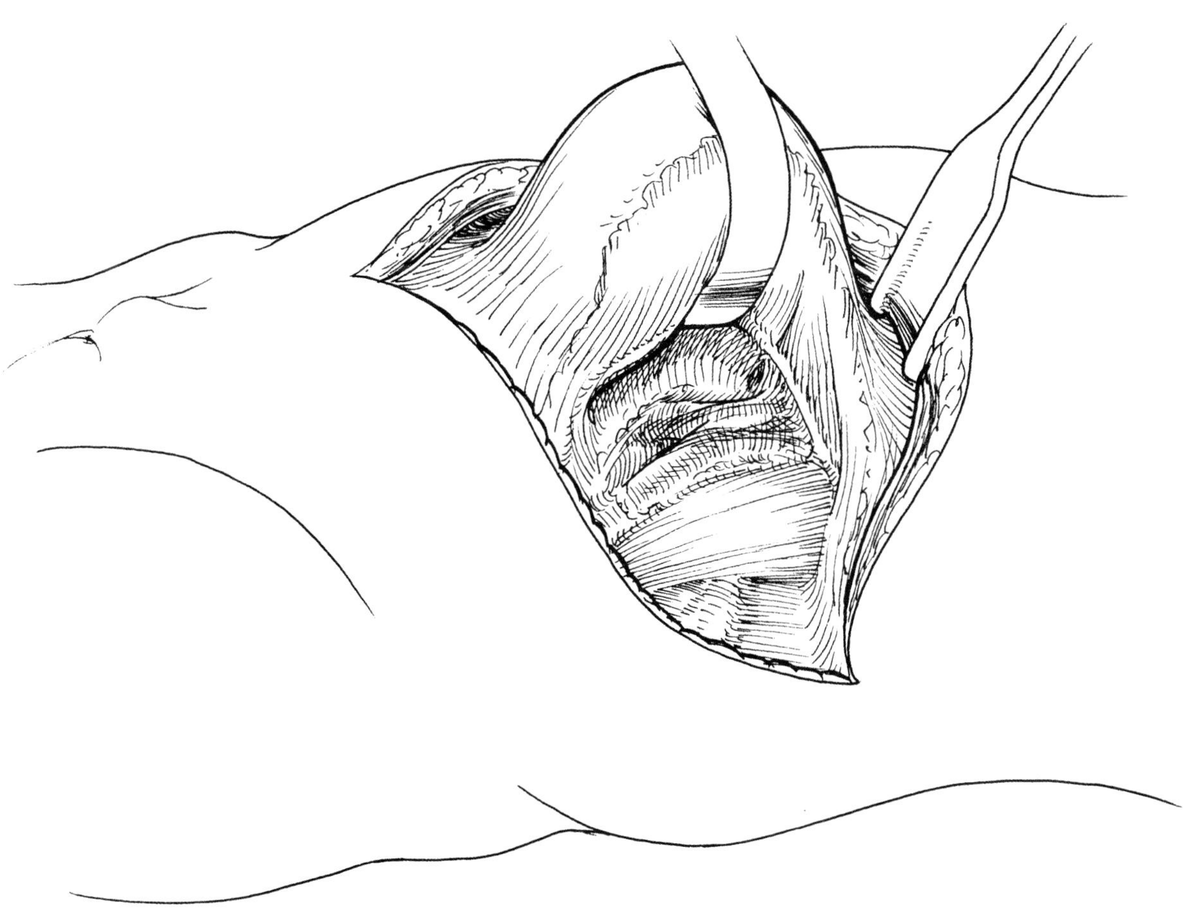

Fig. 12-18 The retroperitoneal space is entered laterally.

Extraperitoneal Exposure of the External Iliac Artery

The patient is positioned and prepped as previously described. The incision is made 2 cm above and parallel to the inguinal ligament, extending from the lateral rectus sheath to a point 2 cm cephalad to the anterior superior iliac spine (Fig. 12-19). Again, proper hemostasis requires that the superficial epigastric and superficial circumflex iliac vessels be ligated in the subcutaneous layer.

The external and internal oblique aponeuroses are divided, and the fibers of the internal oblique muscle in the lateral wound are split apart. The transversus muscle and transversalis fascia are opened in the lateral wound, where separation of the peritoneum from the anterior abdominal wall is easier. Entry into the

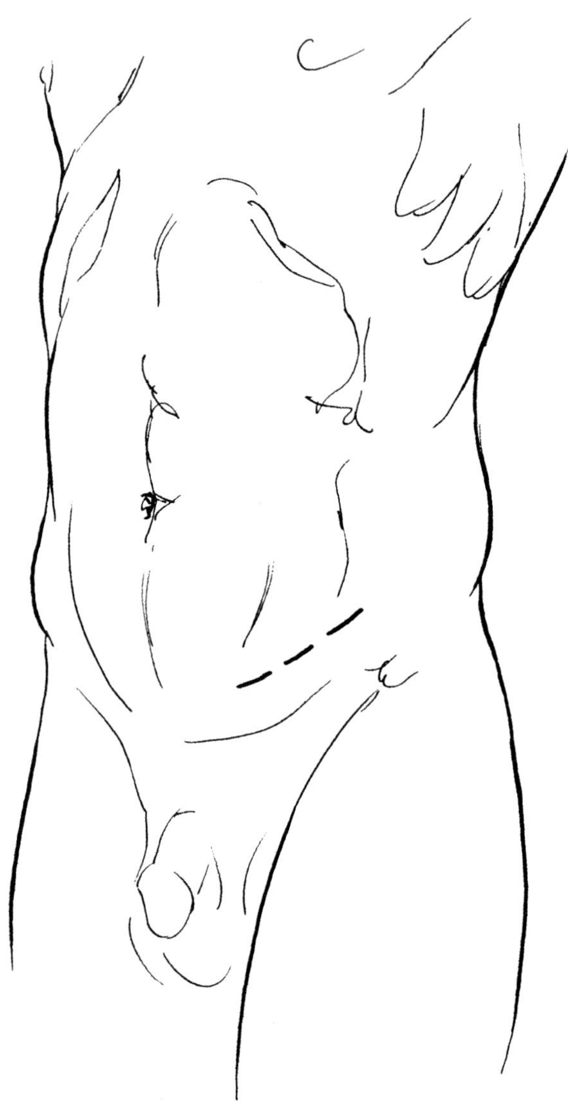

Fig. 12-19 The external iliac artery can be exposed through a more limited suprainguinal incision.

retroperitoneal space is gained laterally, and the peritoneum is carefully stripped away from the anterior abdominal wall in the inferior wound (Fig. 12-20). Superior retraction of the peritoneum reveals the external iliac artery in the center of the wound; the external iliac vein lies on the artery's posteromedial surface. Proximal exposure of the external iliac artery can be gained all the way to its origin by retracting the peritoneal sac superomedially. Distal exposure to the level of the inguinal ligament can be obtained by caudal retraction of the inferior wound margin. Care should be taken to avoid injuring the deep circumflex iliac and inferior epigastric vessels during distal dissection. Exposure of arterial segments below the inguinal ligament should be performed through a separate vertical groin incision (see Chapter 15).

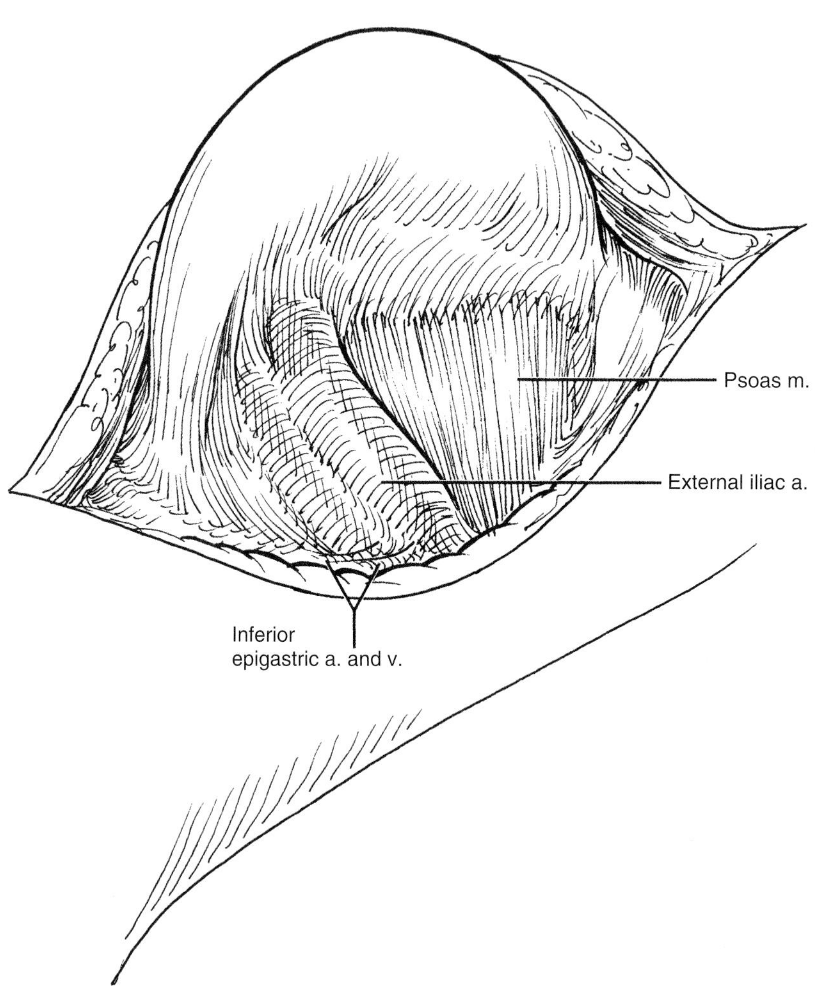

Fig. 12-20 Care is taken to avoid the small distal abdominal wall branches of the external iliac artery during peritoneal retraction.

Exposure of the Lumbar Sympathetic Chain

Sympathetic denervation procedures were first advocated for treatment of lower extremity vascular disorders more than a century ago.[16] The improved results obtained with modern revascularization procedures have relegated lumbar sympathectomy to a limited secondary role in the treatment of a small subgroup of patients with a particular pattern of vascular occlusive disease.[17] Other currently accepted indications include causalgia, reflex sympathetic dystrophy, and hyperhidrosis.[18–20] It is not indicated as a routine adjunctive procedure after aortic bypass. Lumbar sympathectomy is currently performed using minimally invasive techniques such as retroperitoneoscopy; the following discussion of open lumbar sympathectomy is included for the sake of completion.

The patient is placed in the supine position with the ipsilateral flank elevated 15° to 20° on a rolled sheet. A transverse skin incision is made midway between the costal margin and the superior iliac crest and extended to the lateral border of the rectus sheath (Fig. 12-21). In large or obese individuals, the incision can be extended to the 12th rib laterally or across the rectus sheath medially.

After the wound is deepened through the subcutaneous tissues, a muscle-splitting technique, as originally described by Pearl,[21] is employed. The retroperitoneal space is most easily entered in the lateral wound, and the peritoneum is bluntly stripped away from the lateral and posterior abdominal walls. The peritoneal sac and its contents are retracted medially, while retroperitoneal exposure continues along the posterior abdominal wall. The psoas muscle is readily identified, as are the ilioinguinal and genitofemoral nerves that course downward along the lateral side of the psoas. Identification of these nerves is important so that they may be distinguished from the lumbar sympathetic chain. The ureter should also be identified and protected; this is most easily accomplished by allowing it to be gently retracted with the peritoneal sac.

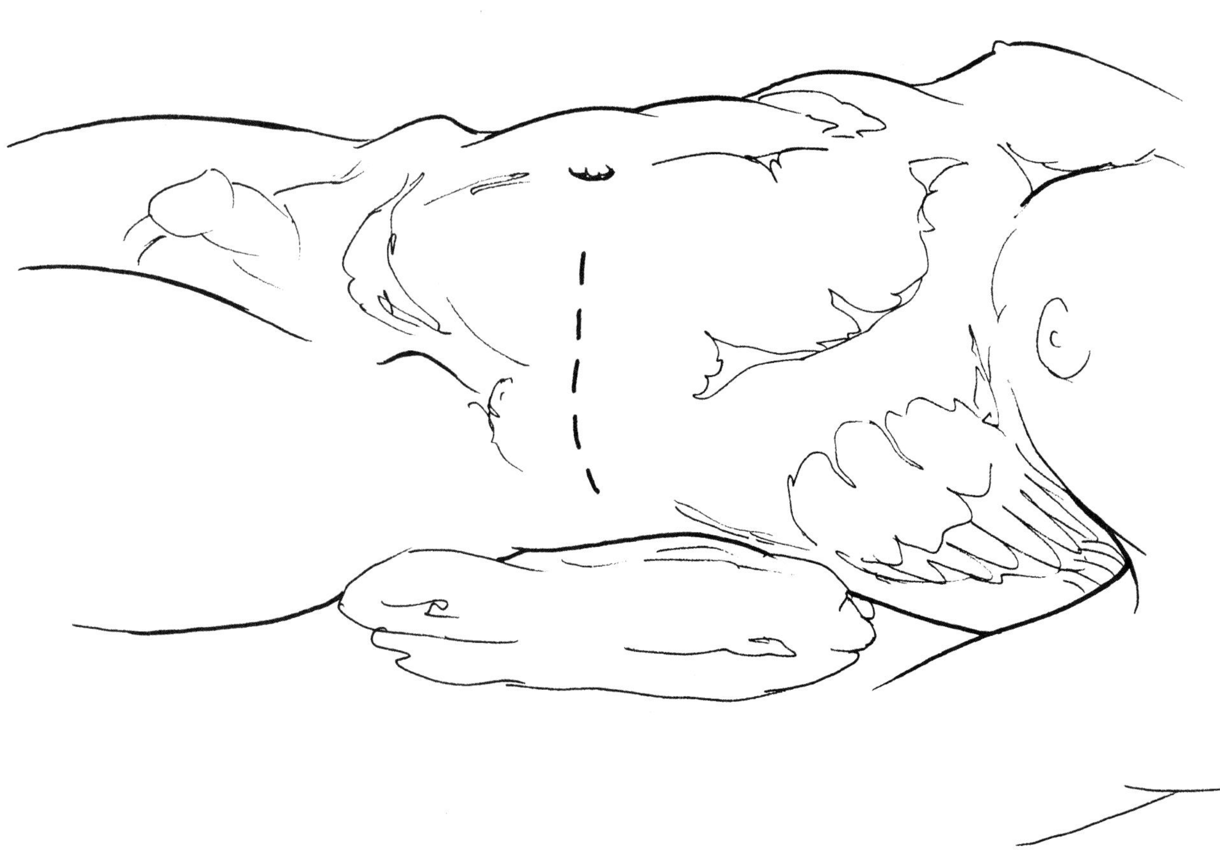

Fig. 12-21 A transverse midflank incision provides access to the lumbar sympathetic chain.

The sympathetic chain is exposed medial to the psoas muscle, along the bodies of the lumbar vertebrae (Fig. 12-22). The chain lies just under the lateral border of the inferior vena cava on the right side and is adjacent to the lateral border of the aorta on the left. It is identified most easily by palpation of a nodular string that gives a characteristic "snap" as it is plucked.[18] Overlying fatty tissue should be gently swept away to achieve adequate visualization. Lumbar vessels that course anterior to the sympathetic chain should be meticulously ligated and divided to prevent troublesome hemorrhage in the retroperitoneal tissues. The lateral edge of the inferior vena cava may require medial retraction for adequate visualization of the right sympathetic chain. The most distal lumbar ganglion is easily identified as the last accessible distal ganglion near the iliac crest. It is useful to identify all other lumbar ganglia by following the sympathetic trunk retrograde. The first lumbar ganglion may be partly concealed by the medial lumbocostal arch; exposure may be gained by vertically incising the overlying diaphragmatic tissues.

Vascular Exposure of the Lumbar Spine

Improvement of vertebral stabilization devices for anterior disc replacement or fusion (anterior lumbar interbody fusion/ALIF) has led to a resurgence of interest in the anterior approach for treatment of degenerative or malignant spine disease. Used alone or in combination with posterior fusion, the anterior approach has been used for spinal decompression

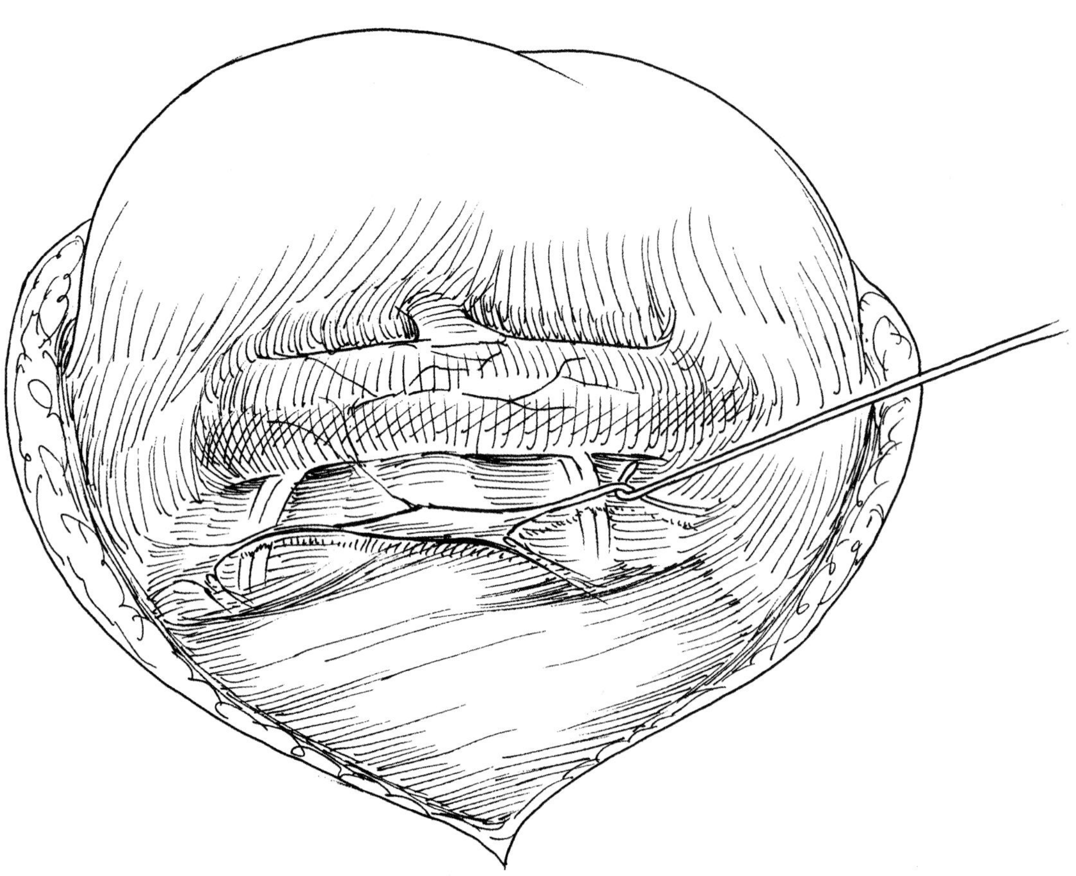

Fig. 12-22 The sympathetic chain is identified on the vertebral bodies between the anterior edge of the psoas muscle and the aorta (or vena cava).

or tumor resection from T11 to S1.[22] Although the anterior retroperitoneal approach affords excellent visualization of the anterior spine and vertebral discs, operative exposure often requires extensive dissection and mobilization of the aorta, iliac arteries, inferior vena cava, and iliac veins (Fig. 12-23). The vascular surgeon may be called upon to provide safe exposure for the spine surgeon and be available in the event of injury to the great vessels. The L4/L5 and L5/S1 disc spaces are common sites of exposure, and the vascular surgeon should be intimately aware of the anatomic peculiarities and the vascular structures at risk for injury at these levels. The following discussion considers anatomic exposure of the anterior spine at the L5/S1 and L4/5 levels.

L5/S1 Exposure

The patient is positioned supine on a radiolucent table, and the left flank is elevated on a lumbar back roll. The L5/S1 disc space is localized with fluoroscopy, and a radio opaque skin marker may help determine the extent of incision, level of dissection, and angle of instrumentation in coordination with the spine surgeon. Although a number of incisions have been

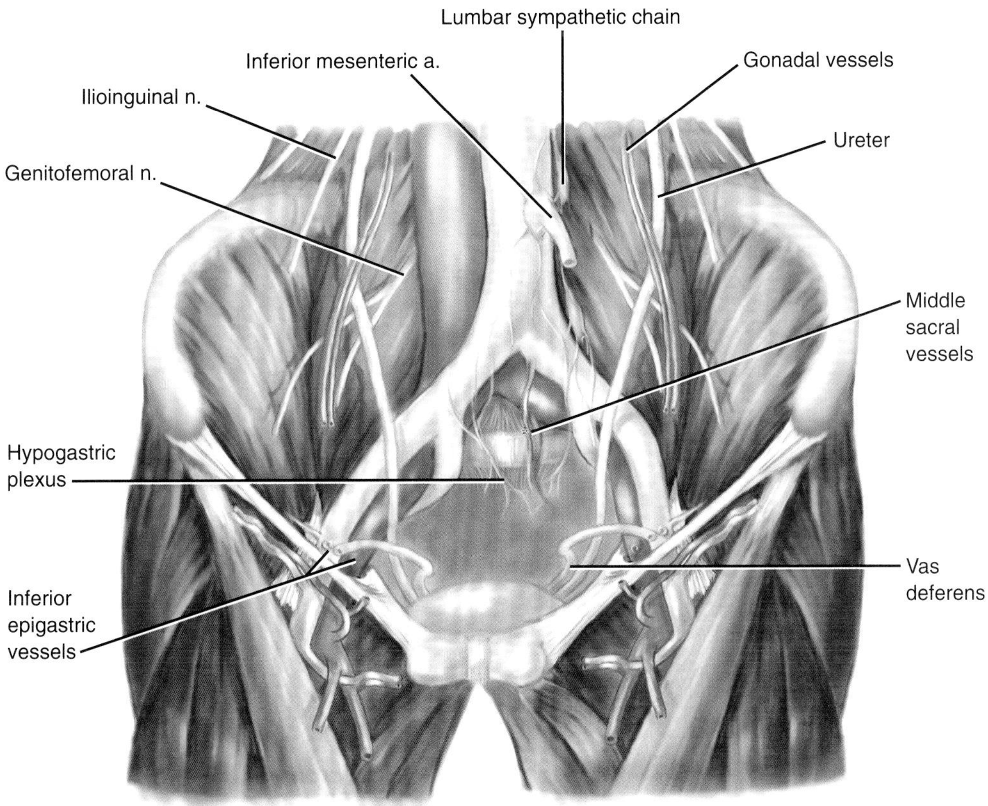

Fig. 12-23 The anatomy related to the lower lumbar spine is shown.

described, our experience suggests that the left paramedian incision is the most direct anterior approach that best accommodates modern stabilization devices (Fig. 12-24). The incision is extended from the level of the umbilicus to the pubis. The underlying anterior rectus sheath is incised longitudinally leaving wide flaps for closure. The rectus abdominis muscle is mobilized from its medial attachments the length of the incision and retracted laterally (Fig. 12-25). Small feeding vessels, encountered at the junction of

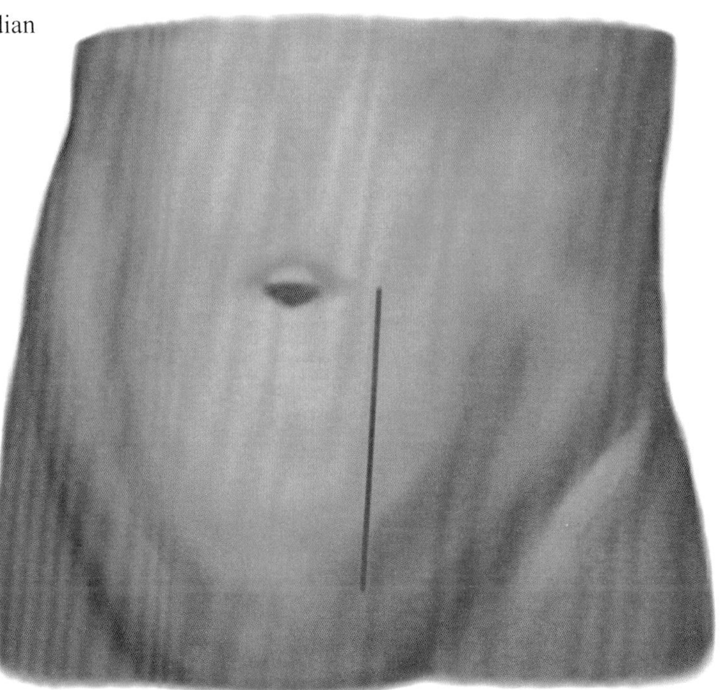

Fig. 12-24 The position of the lower left paramedian incision is shown.

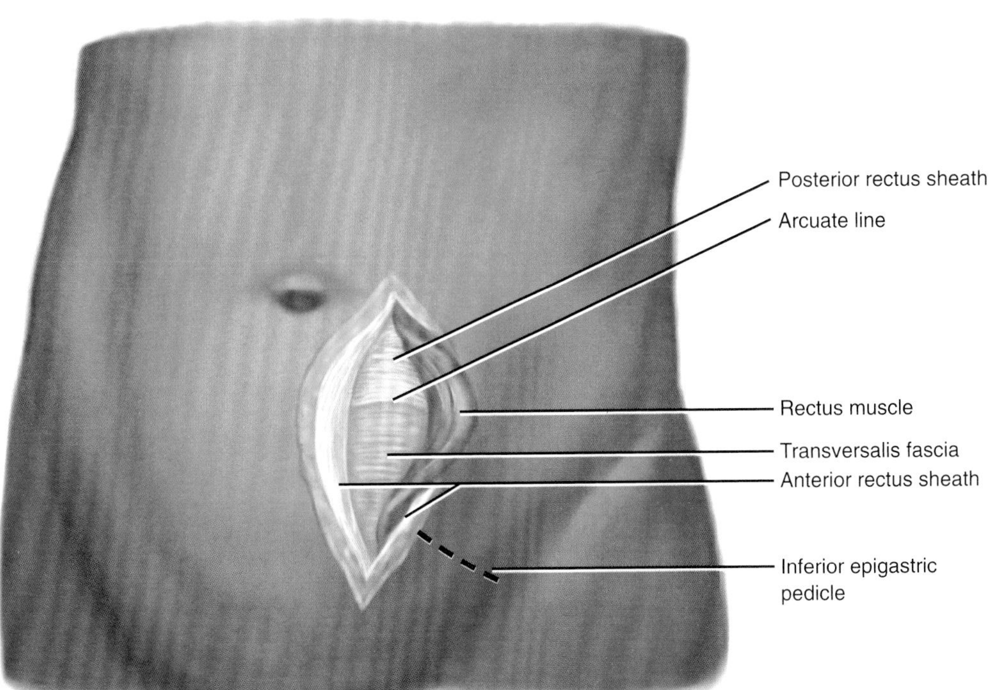

Fig. 12-25 Lateral mobilization of the left rectus muscle exposes the arcuate line at the termination of the posterior rectus sheath. Caudal to the arcuate line, only transversalis fascia covers the preperitoneal fat plane. The inferior epigastric pedicle lies deep to the caudal end of the rectus muscle.

tendinous inscriptions and midline should be meticulously ligated.

The transversalis fascia is delicately entered at the caudal end of the incision and opened up to the arcuate line, exposing the preperitoneal fat plane (Fig.12-26). The posterior rectus sheath and underlying transversalis fascia are opened to the cephalad end of the incision. The retroperitoneal plane is developed under the retracted left rectus muscle, with a combination of blunt and sharp dissection. The envelope of parietal peritoneum including the left colon is mobilized from lateral to medial to expose the retroperitoneal space in the midline as far as the great vessels of the abdomen (Fig. 12-27). As the

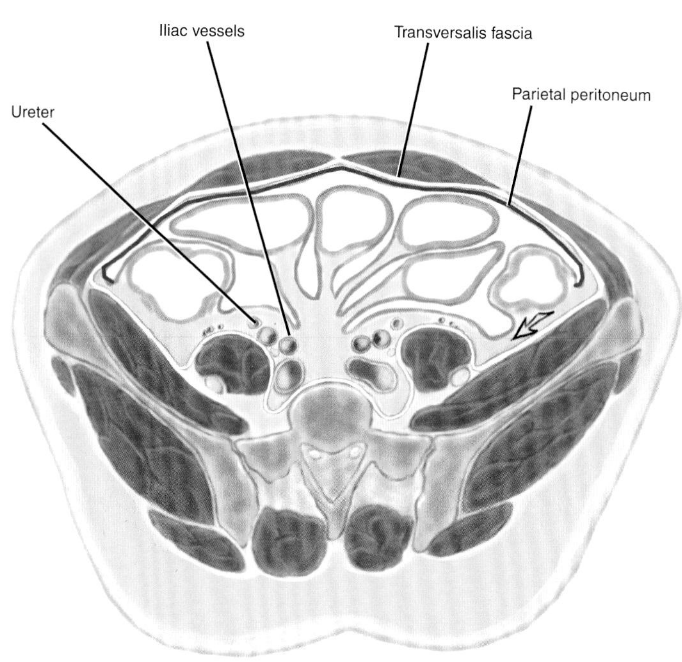

Fig. 12-26 The relationships of the preperitoneal plane are shown.

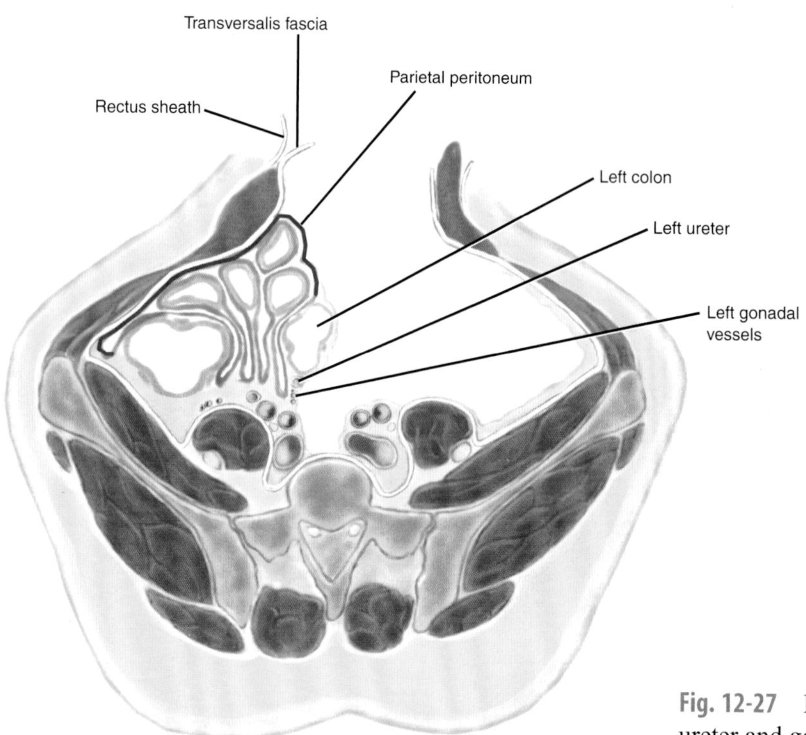

Fig. 12-27 Retraction of the peritoneal envelope, ureter and gonadal vessels is shown.

peritoneal mobilization progresses, the inferior epigastric vessels are gently retracted laterally with the rectus muscle. Deep in the wound, the psoas muscle is exposed, and the overlying genitofemoral and ilioinguinal nerves are left in situ on the muscle's anterior surface. The ureter is carefully identified as it crosses the junction of external and internal iliac arteries and is mobilized with the peritoneum. The gonadal vessels are similarly elevated with the peritoneum. Care is taken to protect the nerve elements that cross the external iliac artery origin, to prevent retrograde ejaculation. Using bipolar cautery to control bleeding from small paraspinous bleeding vessels may reduce the risk of inadvertent nerve injury in this area. In women, the round ligament can be divided as necessary to improve exposure.

A self-retaining retractor such as the Omni or Bookwalter retractor is placed for optimal exposure of the L5/S1 disc space. The space is easily exposed between the left common iliac vein and right common iliac artery. Mobilization of the left common iliac vein requires ligation and division of the left medial iliosacral vein (Fig. 12-28) that is often encountered on the medial border just distal to

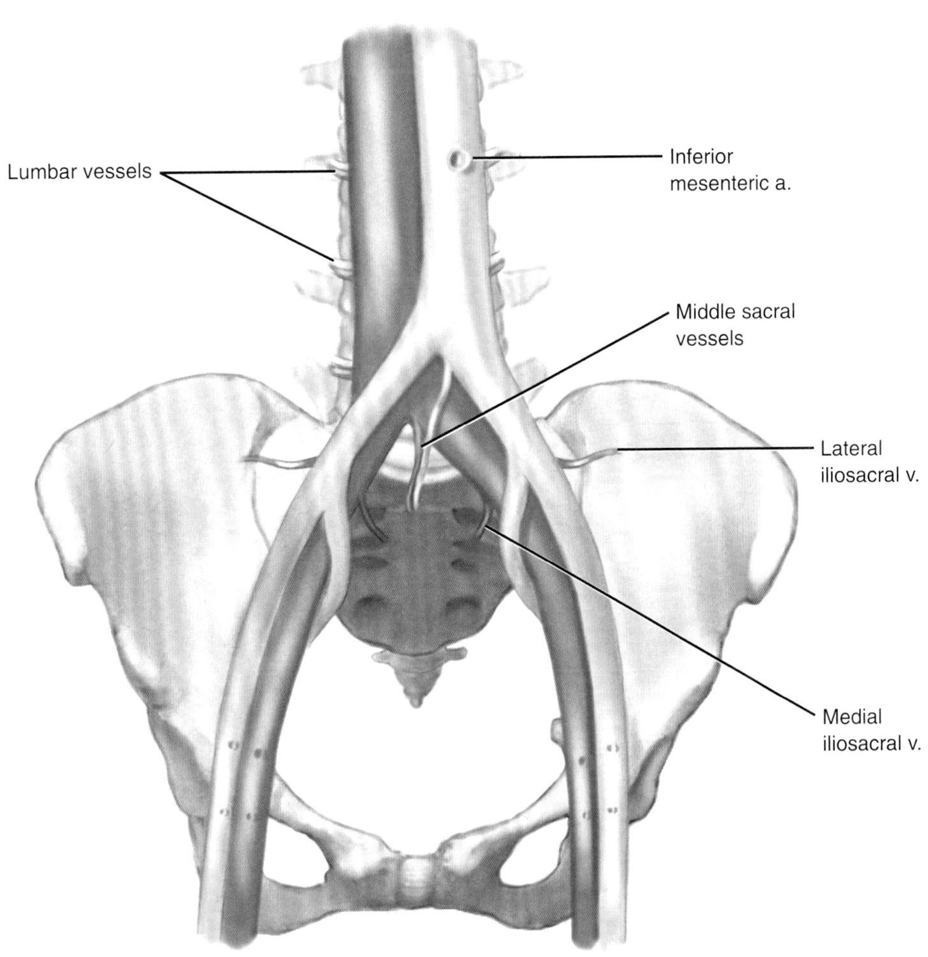

Fig. 12-28 The common position of the aortic and vena caval bifurcations bracketing the L4/L5 disc space is shown.

the iliac vein bifurcation. To complete mobilization of the right common iliac artery, the middle sacral artery and vein should be divided with a combination of bipolar electrocautery, surgical clips, and/or silk ligatures. The remaining soft tissue covering the L5/S1 disc is carefully mobilized with the use of a Cobb elevator. Inflammatory changes associated with degenerative disc disease can cause adherence of the vessels to the underlying vertebrae and make mobilization difficult and hazardous. In these cases, more extensive mobilization including the aorta and distal iliac vessels may be required. Lumbar arteries and unnamed venous tributaries should be carefully controlled and ligated in these circumstances.

After the right common iliac artery and left common iliac vein have been adequately mobilized, positive identification of the L5/S1 interspace should be confirmed radiologically. The spine surgeon places a radio-opaque marker in the disc space, and the spinal level is assessed using a straight lateral fluoroscopic view (Fig.12-29).

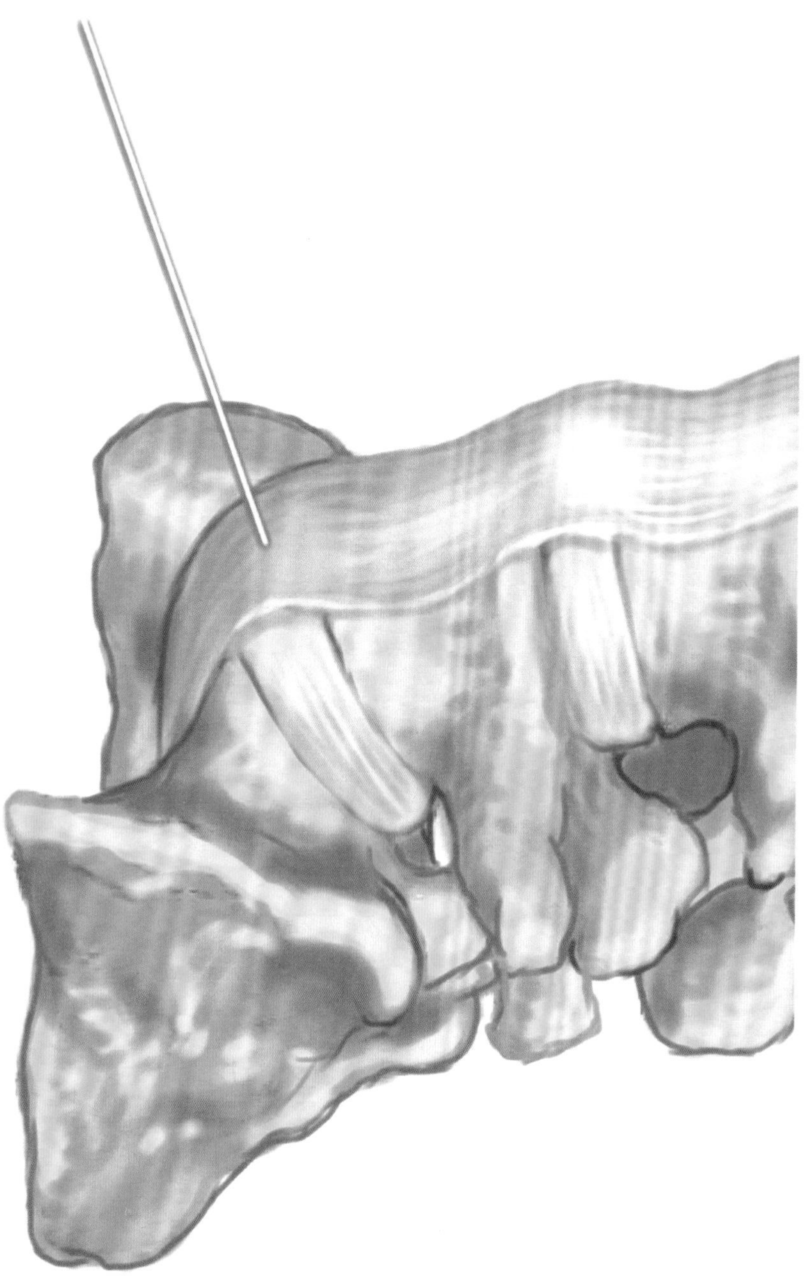

Fig. 12-29 Pin marker placement for fluoroscopic confirmation of the L5/S1 disc space is shown.

After confirmation of the disc space, a combination of ring retractors and/or Steinmann pins (Fig. 12-30) are secured with the assistance of the spine surgeon to secure a stable view for the discectomy and implant placement. The retractors elevate and widen the space between the common iliac vessels, exposing the L5/S1 disc. The Steinmann pin must be sheathed with a red rubber catheter to prevent injury to the vessels by direct contact with the metal. Care must be exercised to avoid unnecessary traction/compression of the iliac vessels to prevent injury or potential stasis and thrombosis.

Upon completion of the discectomy and fusion by the spine team, the retraction system is carefully removed. If a Steinmann pin was used for the retraction, the catheter is held against the vertebral body as the point is withdrawn to prevent laceration of the left iliac vein as it returns to its normal location. After hemostasis is secured, the peritoneal envelope is allowed to gently fall back into position. Any peritoneal tears can be carefully closed. Distal pulses are confirmed. It is not necessary to reconstruct the posterior sheath or arcuate line, although, if possible, it does help facilitate closure of the anterior rectus sheath. Anterior rectus sheath and skin are closed in standard fashion.

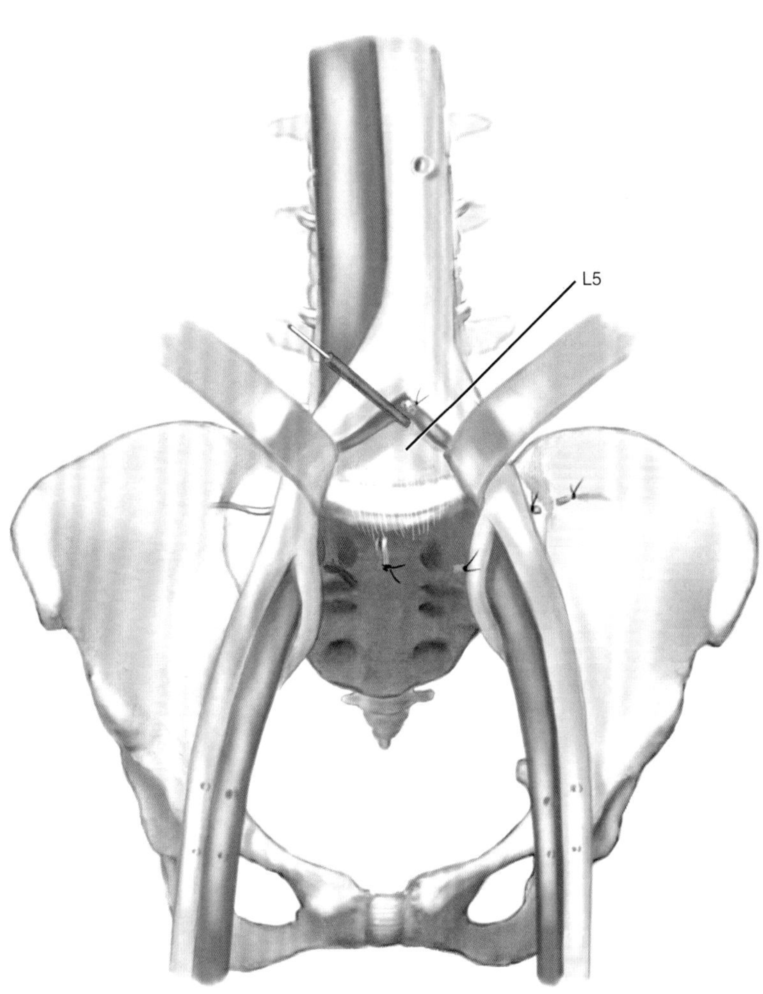

Fig. 12-30 Exposure of the L5/S1 disc is shown.

L4/L5 Exposure

Anterior retroperitoneal exposure of the L4/L5 disc space proceeds in the same manner as for the L5/S1 exposure described above. The L4/L5 exposure requires mobilization of the distal aorta and left iliac vessels from left to right. The left lateral iliosacral vein branch (Fig. 12-28) tends to pin the iliac vein tightly to the lumbosacral structures and should be carefully suture ligated and clipped to facilitate adequate mobilization of the iliac vein. This is an area of frequent anomalies, and the surgeon must be alert for additional branches. A left medial iliosacral vein is often encountered just distal to the confluence of the iliac veins. This vein should be carefully controlled and suture ligated, which may be difficult due to chronic surrounding inflammation. Failure to control this vessel can lead to injury during medial retraction of the left iliac vein. The challenge of controlling hemorrhage from this injury cannot be overstated. Other tributaries, especially the L4/L5 lumbar artery and vein also require ligation as the iliac vessels are mobilized.

The optimal exposure of the L4/L5 disc space depends on the degree of surrounding inflammation and the location of the aortic and caval bifurcations. With the bifurcations in their most common position bracketing the L4-5 disk level, the vessels may be retracted to the right (Fig. 12-31A). When the bifurcations ride higher, the left common iliac vessels can be retracted to the patient's left to an almost horizontal position (Fig. 12-31B), or can be separated apart (Fig. 12-31C). Regardless of the retraction configuration, flow in the distal external iliac artery should be confirmed by pulse or with a Doppler probe after the retractors are set. To complete the exposure of the disc space, the remaining soft tissue covering the L4/L5 disc space can be mobilized with the use of a Cobb elevator.

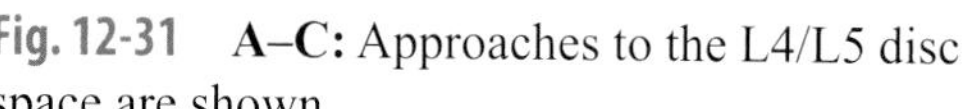

Fig. 12-31 **A–C:** Approaches to the L4/L5 disc space are shown.

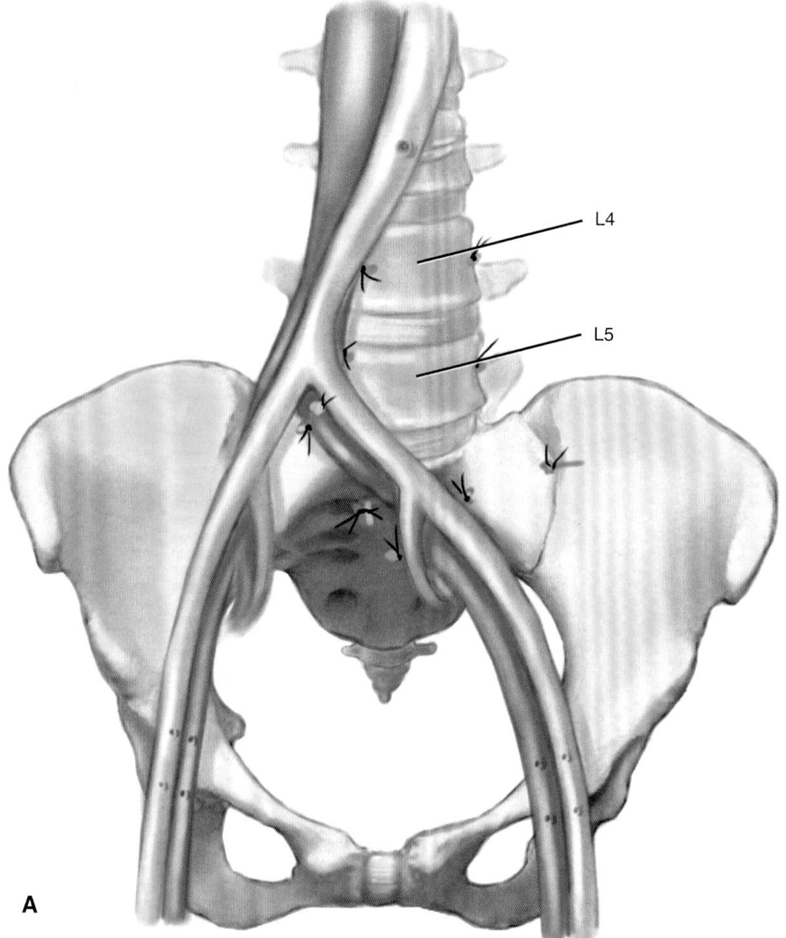

Fig. 12-31 *(continued)*

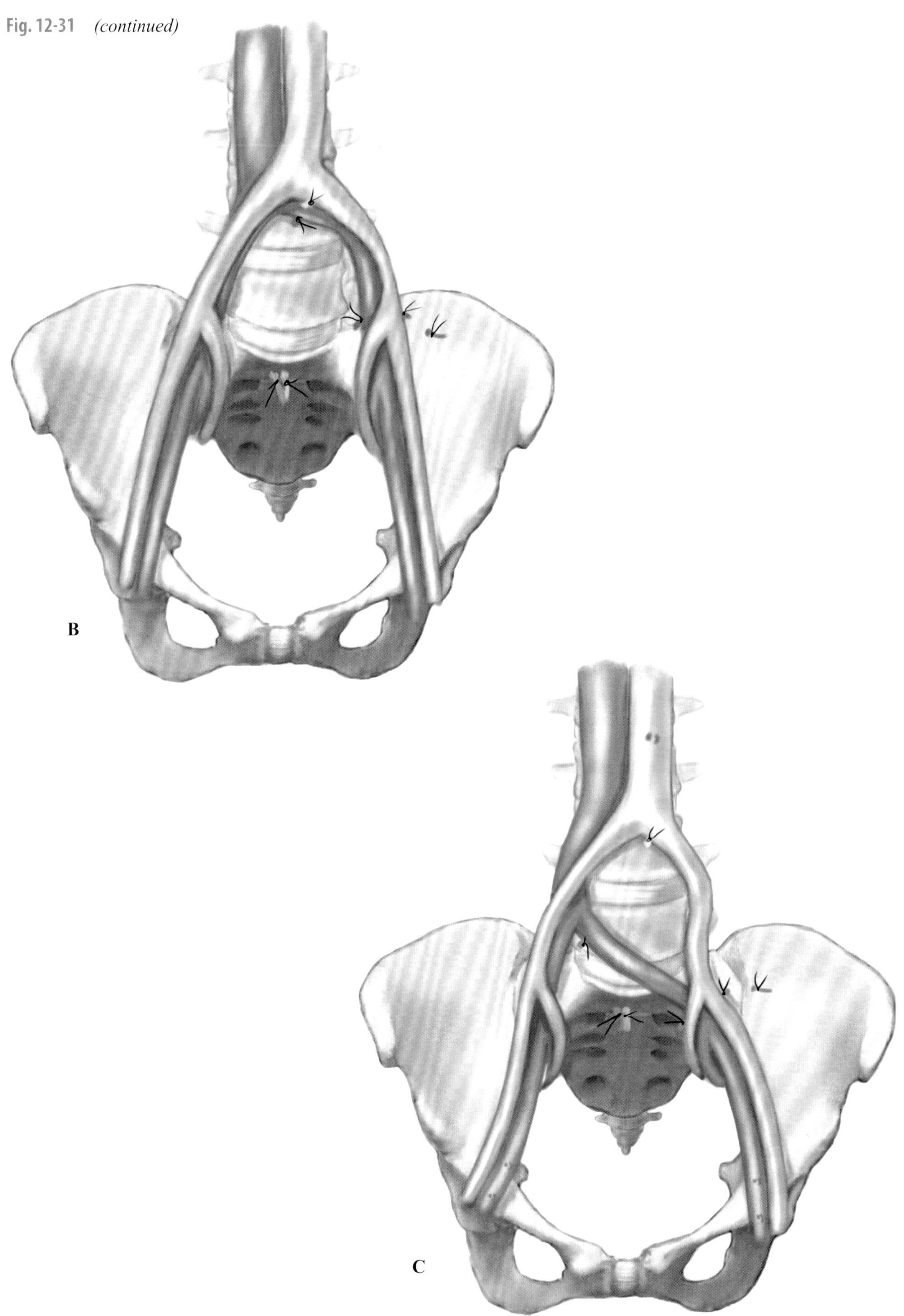

Positive identification of the L4/L5 disc space is made by placing a radio-opaque marker into the disc space and confirming with a lateral fluoroscopic view. After confirmation, a combination of ring retractors and Steinmann pins are carefully secured with the assistance of the spine surgeon to create a stable view for discectomy and implant placement. Any further manipulation of the vascular retractors should be performed by the vascular team as the potential for vascular injury in this case is even greater than the exposure for the L5/S1 disc space.

Steinmann pins are removed with the same precautions noted above, and closure is the same as above.

References

1. Suwanabol PA, Tefera G, Schwarze ML. Syndromes associated with the deep veins: phlegmasia cerulea dolens, May-Thurner syndrome, and nutcracker syndrome. *Perspect Vasc Surg Endovasc Ther*. 2010;22:223–230.
2. Seeley SF, Hughes CW, Jahnke EJ Jr. Major vessel damage in lumbar disk operations. *Surgery*. 1954;35:421–429.
3. Wachenfeld-Wahl C, Engelhardt M, Gengenbach B, et al. Transperitoneal versus retroperitoneal approach for treatment of infrarenal aortic aneurysms: is one superior? *Vasa*. 2004;33:72–76.
4. Valentine RJ, Hagino RT, Jackson MR, et al. Gastrointestinal complications after aortic surgery. *J Vasc Surg*. 1998;28:404–412.
5. Borkon MJ, Zaydfudim V, Carey CD, et al. Retroperitoneal repair of abdominal aortic aneurysms offers postoperative benefits to male patients in the Veterans Affairs Health System. *Ann Vasc Surg*. 2010;24:728–732.
6. Kalko Y, Ugurlucan M, Basaran M, et al. Comparison of transperitoneal and retroperitoneal approaches in abdominal aortic surgery. *Acta Chir Belg*. 2008;108:557–562.
7. Shepard AD, Tollefson DFJ, Reddy DJ, et al. Left flank retroperitoneal exposure: a technical aid to complex aortic reconstruction. *J Vasc Surg*. 1991;14:283–291.
8. Todd GJ, DeRose JJ Jr. Retroperitoneal approach for repair of inflammatory aneurysms. *Ann Vasc Surg*. 1995;9:525–534.
9. Seiler CM, Deckert A, Diener MK, et al. Midline versus transverse incision in major abdominal surgery: a randomized, double-blind equivalence trial (POVATI: ISRCTN60734227). *Ann Surg*. 2009;249:913–920.
10. Aalami OO, Organ CH Jr. Chylous ascites: a collective review. *Surgery*. 2000;128:761–768.
11. Valentine RJ, MacGillivray DC, Blankenship CL, et al. Variations in the anatomic relationship of the left renal vein to the left renal artery at the aorta. *Clin Anat*. 1990;3:249–255.
12. van Schaik J, van Baalen JM, Visser MJT, et al. Nerve-preserving aortoiliac reconstruction surgery: anatomical study and surgical approach. *J Vasc Surg*. 2001;33:983–989.
13. Davis RA, Milloy FJ, Anson BJ. Lumbar, renal, and associated parietal and visceral veins based upon a study of 100 specimens. *Surg Gynecol Obstet*. 1958;107:1–22.
14. Malaki M, Willis AP, Jones RG. Congenital anomalies of the inferior vena cava. *Clin Radiol*. 2012;67:165–171.
15. Williams GM, Ricotta J, Zinner M, et al. The extended retroperitoneal approach for treatment of extensive atherosclerosis of the aorta and renal vessels. *Surgery*. 1980;88:846–855.
16. Jaboulay M. Le traitement de quelques troubles trophiques du pied et de la jambe par la dénudation de l'artère fémorale et de la distension des nerfs vasculaires. *Lyon Med*. 1899;91:467.
17. Collins GJ, Rich NM, Clagett GP, et al. Clinical results of lumbar sympathectomy. *Am Surg*. 1981;47:31–35.
18. Haimovici H. Lumbar sympathectomy. In: Haimovici H, ed. *Vascular Surgery: Principles and Techniques*. Norwalk, CT: Appleton-Centuy-Crofts; 1984:925–939.
19. Rieger R, Pedevilla S, Pochlauer S. Endoscopic lumbar sympathectomy for plantar hyperhidrosis. *Br J Surg*. 2009;96:1422–1428.
20. Bandyk DF, Johnson BL, Kirkpatrick AF, et al. Surgical sympathectomy for reflex sympathetic dystrophy syndromes. *J Vasc Surg*. 2002;35:269–277.
21. Pearl FL. Muscle-splitting extraperitoneal lumbar ganglionectomy. *Surg Gynecol Obstet*. 1937;65:107–112.
22. Bianchi C, Ballard JL, Abou-Zamzam Jr AM, Teruya TH: Anterior retroperitoneal lumbosacral spine exposure: operative technique and results. *Ann Vasc Surg*. 2003;17:137–142.

Bibliography for Lumbar Spine Exposure

Garg J, Woo K, Hirsch J, et al., Vascular complications of exposure for anterior lumbar interbody fusion. *J Vasc Surg*. 2010;51(4):946–950.

Gumbs AA, Shah RV, Yue JJ, et al. The open anterior paramedian retroperitoneal approach for spine procedures. *Arch Surg*. 2005;140(4):339–343.

Hamdan AD, Malek JY, Schermerhorn ML, et al. Vascular injury during anterior exposure of the spine. *J Vasc Surg*. 2008;48(3):650–654.

Jarrett CD, Heller JG, Tsai L. Anterior exposure of the lumbar spine with and without an "access surgeon": morbidity analysis of 265 consecutive cases. *J Spinal Siord Tech*. 2009;22(8):559–564.

Lindley EM, McBeth ZL, Henry SE, et al. Retrograde ejaculation following anterior lumbar spine surgery. *Spine*. 2012;37(20):1785–1789.

Pomposelli F. Vascular injury during spine exposure. In: Eskandari MK, Morasch MD, Pearce WH, Yao JST (eds.) *Vascular Surgery: Therapeutic Strategies*. Shelton, CT: People's Medical Publishing House; 2010:219–231.

Than KD, Wang AC, Rahman SU, et al. Complication avoidance and management in anterior lumbar interbody fusion. *Neurosurg Focus*. 2011;31(4):E6.

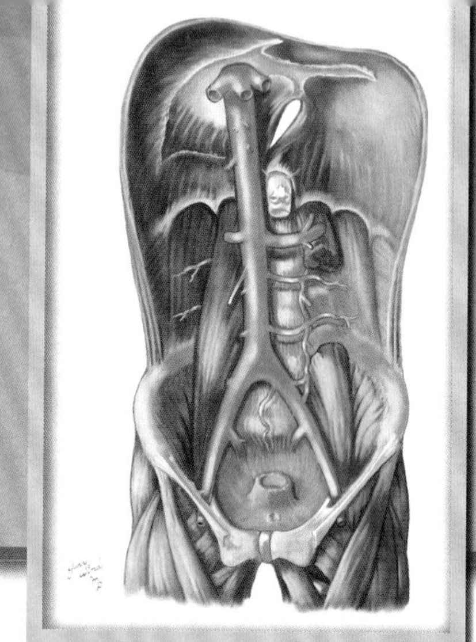

Inferior Vena Cava

13

Surgical Anatomy of the Inferior Vena Cava

The distal inferior vena cava begins at the confluence of the common iliac veins anterior to the fifth lumbar vertebra to the right of the midline (Fig. 13-1). It penetrates the membranous portion of the diaphragm at the level of T8 and immediately drains into the right atrium. The vena cava is crossed by the root of the small bowel mesentery, the first and third portions of the duodenum, and the head of the pancreas (see Figs. 10-5 and 12-4). The vena cava is separated from the portal vein anteriorly by the cleft of the epiploic foramen. The position of the vena caval trunk deviates slightly more to the right above the renal veins as the vessel traverses the liver, partially embedded between the caudate and right lobes.

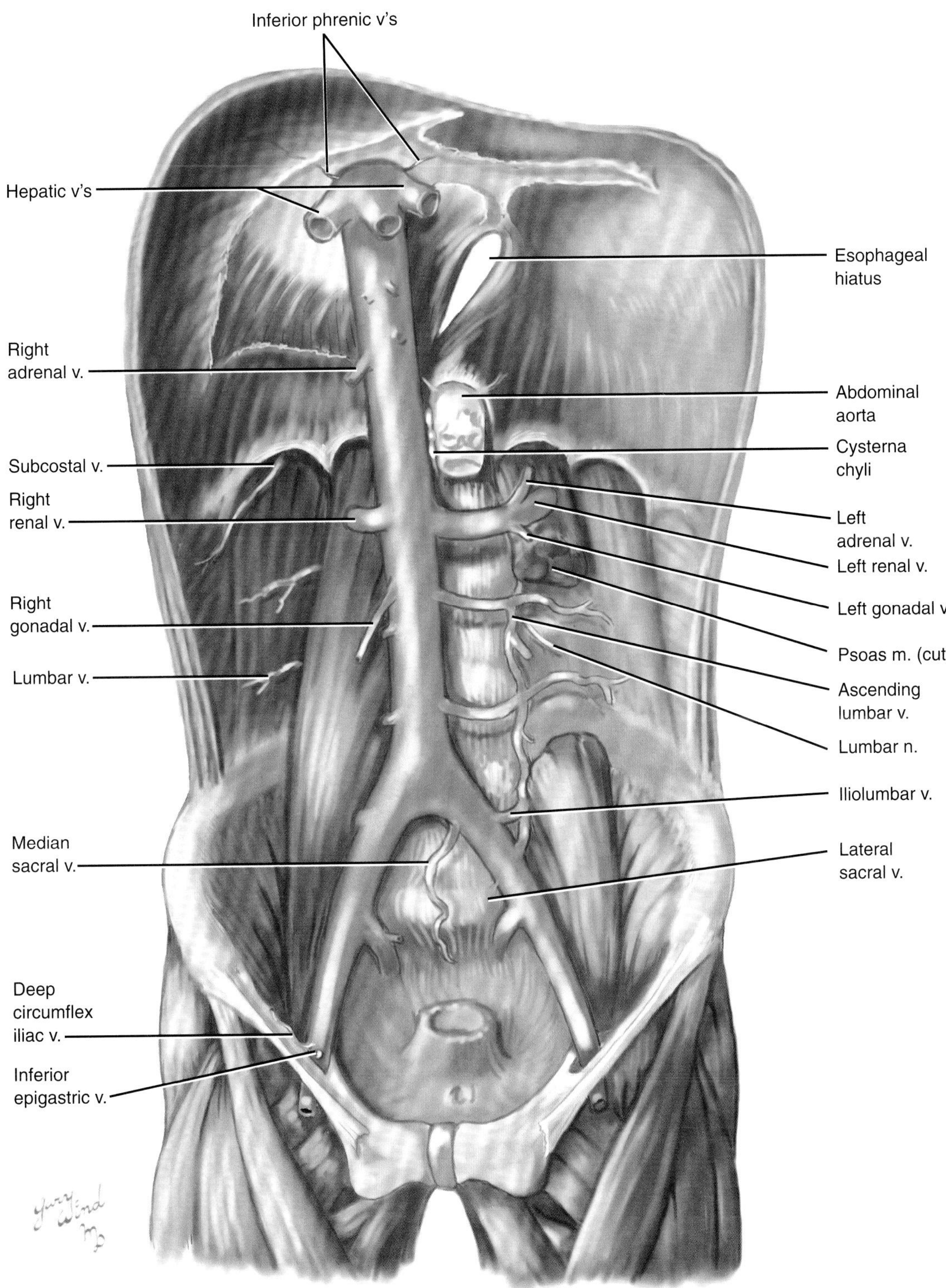

Fig. 13-1 The inferior vena cava lies to the right of midline between the levels of the eighth thoracic and fifth lumbar vertebrae.

Iliac Veins

The external iliac veins draining the lower extremities begin behind the inguinal ligaments and run around the brim of the true pelvis medial to the psoas muscles. The internal iliac veins, which drain all the pelvic viscera except the rectosigmoid area, join the external iliac veins adjacent to the sacroiliac joints to form the common iliac veins. The common iliac veins ascend to unite in front of L5. The ureter, ductus deferens (male), and round ligament of the uterus and ovarian vessels (female) cross the external iliac vessels. The sympathetic trunk and obturator nerve from the lumbar plexus pass beneath the common iliac veins. The aortic bifurcation is slightly more cephalad than that of the vena cava. The iliac arteries cross the iliac veins in such a way that the arteries end up straddling and embracing the veins (Fig. 13-2). The bifurcation of the inferior vena cava is crossed anteriorly by the

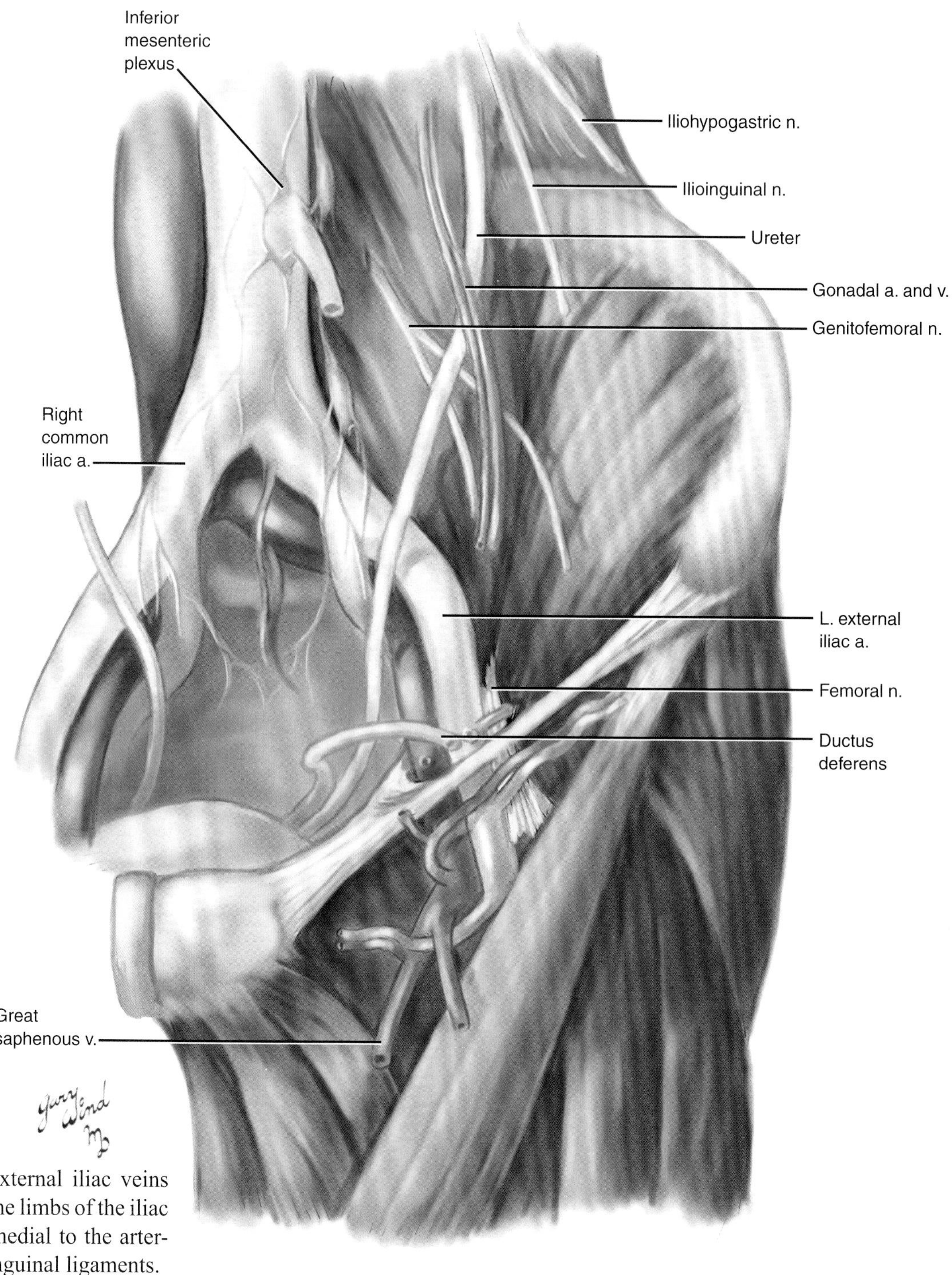

Fig. 13-2 The external iliac veins are enfolded by the limbs of the iliac arteries and lie medial to the arteries beneath the inguinal ligaments.

right common iliac artery. Thus, the arteries are always lateral to the veins at the groin. Where the bifurcations overlap, there is often dense adherence between the arteries and veins.

Infrarenal Vena Cava

The only anterior branch of the infrarenal vena cava is the small right gonadal vein. The paired lumbar veins are situated posteriorly and contribute to an extensive paravertebral venous plexus (Fig. 13-3). Longitudinal ascending lumbar veins within this plexus connect with the lateral sacral veins of the pelvis and with the azygous and hemiazygous veins of the chest. There are other variable connections between this system and veins of the posterior body wall as well as occasional connections with renal and adrenal veins. In addition, vein branches draining the spinal canal anastomose with the paravertebral plexus via the intervertebral foramina. These spinal vein branches extend along the length of the spinal canal as an extensive valveless plexus draining both bone and neural structures. This complex, described by Batson, is thought to facilitate metastasis and spread of infection to the spinal column and brain.

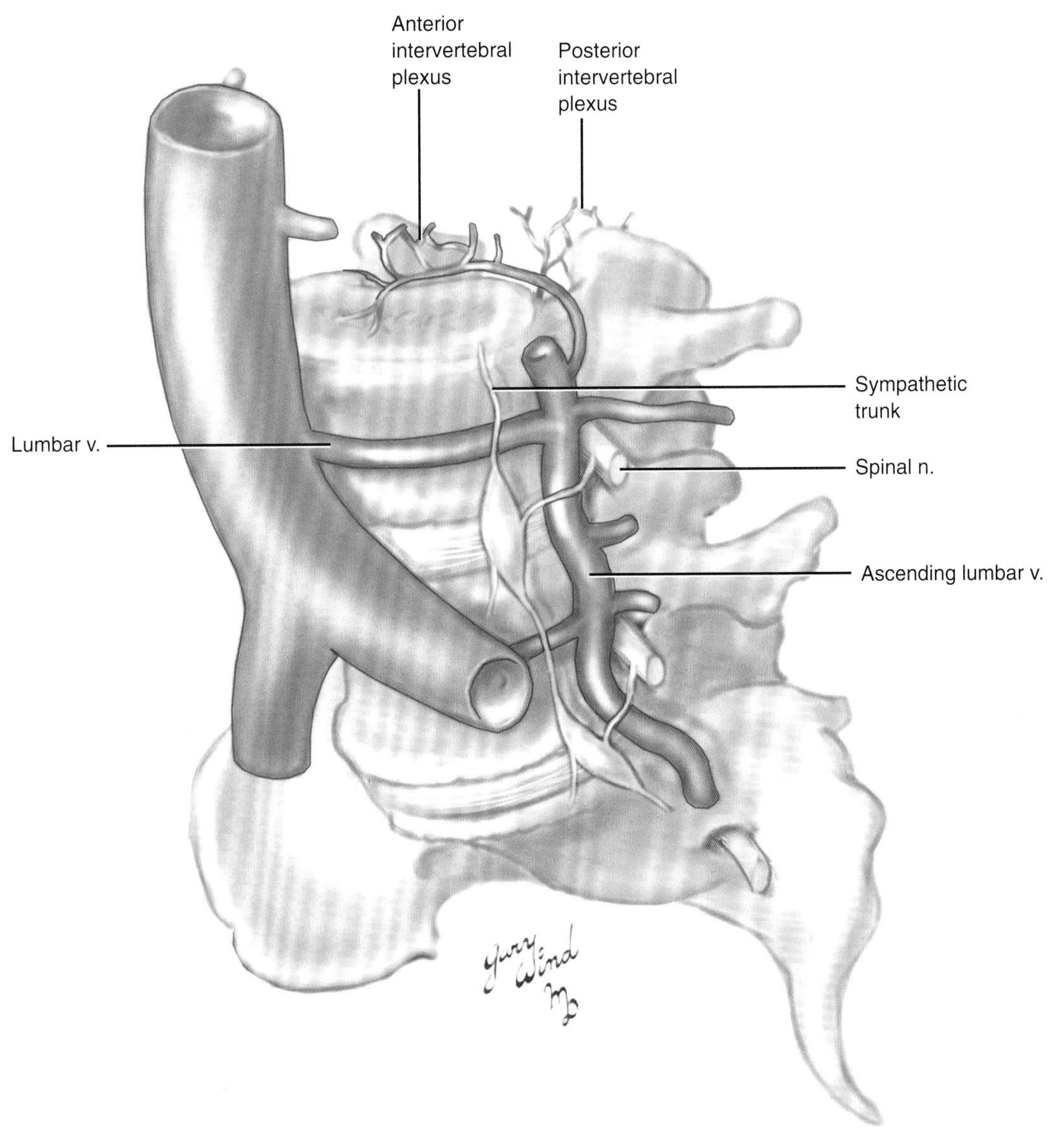

Fig. 13-3 The lumbar veins communicate with an extensive paravertebral network of veins.

Perirenal Vena Cava

The renal veins enter the vena cava at the level of L2 and are usually single. The right renal vein follows a short path anteromedially (see Fig. 11-2) from the renal hilum. The left renal vein arches across the aorta in the acute angle formed by the takeoff of the superior mesenteric artery and joins the vena cava at a 90° angle. The anterior relationships of this segment of vena cava are described in Chapter 11.

Retrohepatic Vena Cava

The portion of inferior vena cava traversing the liver is enfolded on three sides by liver substance (Fig. 13-4). There are several small branches draining from the caudate lobe directly into the vena cava. At the dome of the liver, the vena cava receives the large hepatic veins, usually three in number. The hepatic vein–vena cava junction is located at the anterior angle of the diamond-shaped bare area bounded by the coronary

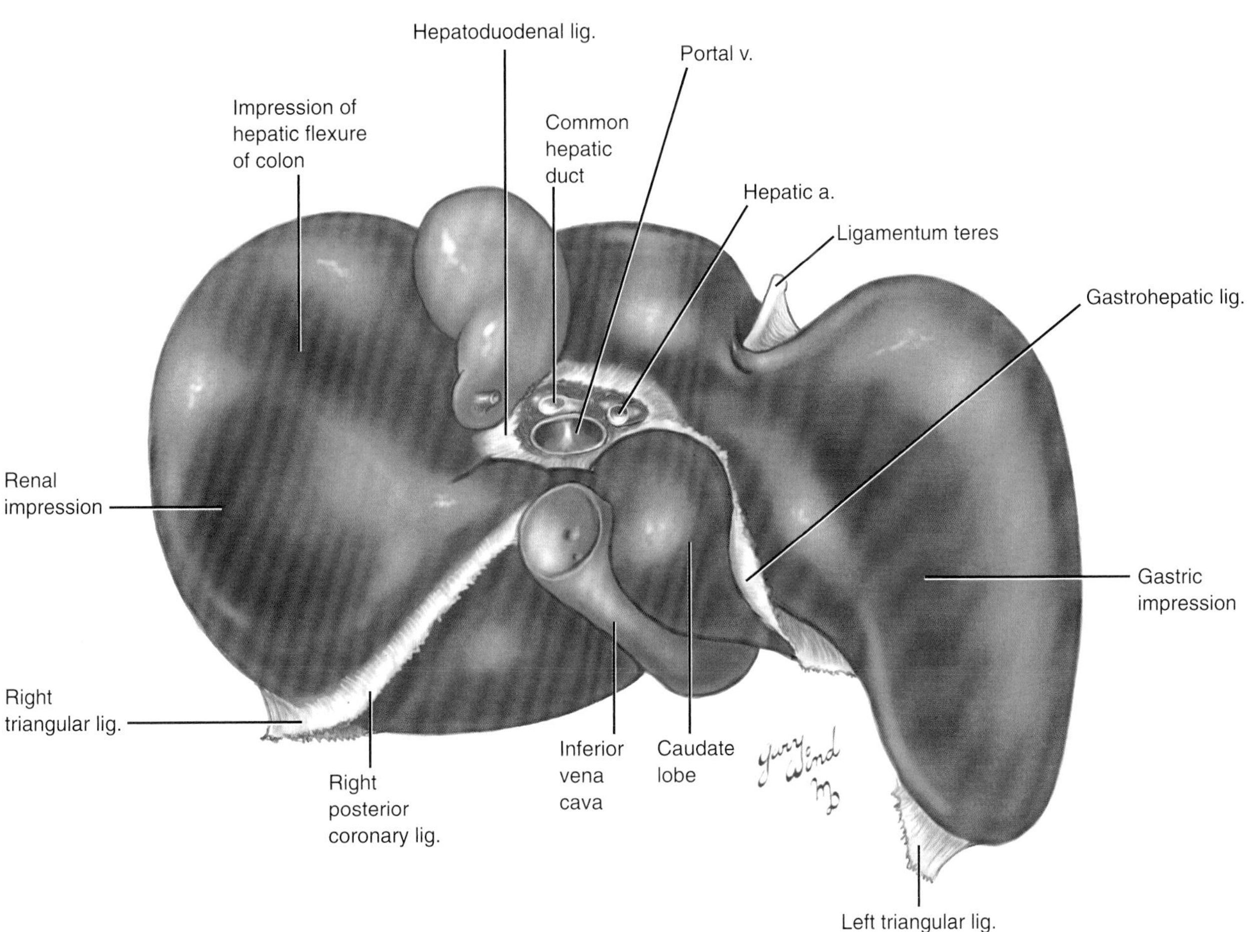

Fig. 13-4 The retrohepatic segment of vena cava is partially embedded in the liver.

ligaments (see Fig. 10-5). The proximity of these structures must be kept in mind when dividing the left triangular ligament and falciform ligament lest the veins be entered.

Exposure of the Infrahepatic Vena Cava

The popularity of intraluminal devices for the treatment of venous thrombosis has rendered elective surgical exposure of the inferior vena cava virtually obsolete. These devices are effective and extremely convenient as they can be inserted percutaneously through the jugular or femoral vein with low associated morbidity.[1] Modern filter devices can be placed permanently or on a temporary basis; indications and outcomes are well described elsewhere.[1,2] Despite the ease of placement, complications have been described from filter migration, including filter embolization, strut fracture, and vena cava perforation.[3] Open extraction has become necessary in some cases involving retroperitoneal bleeding, bowel perforation, or aortic puncture.[3,4] The retroperitoneal approach to the inferior vena cava may provide adequate exposure in these circumstances; however, due to the possibility of associated bowel and/or aortic injury, the midline transabdominal approach is generally preferred.

Exposure of the inferior vena cava is also indicated in the extraction of intraluminal renal carcinoma extensions,[5,6] in the management of traumatic injuries,[7] and, rarely, in reconstructive venous operations.[8,9] Midline transperitoneal approaches are most appropriate in these circumstances.

Extraperitoneal Approach

The patient is placed in the supine position with the right flank elevated 15° to 20° on rolled sheets. The lower chest, abdomen, and right flank are prepped and draped. General anesthesia is recommended because complete muscle paralysis greatly enhances this approach.

A transverse incision is made from the lateral border of the right rectus muscle just above the level of the umbilicus and is extended laterally to the tip of the 11th rib (Fig. 13-5). The

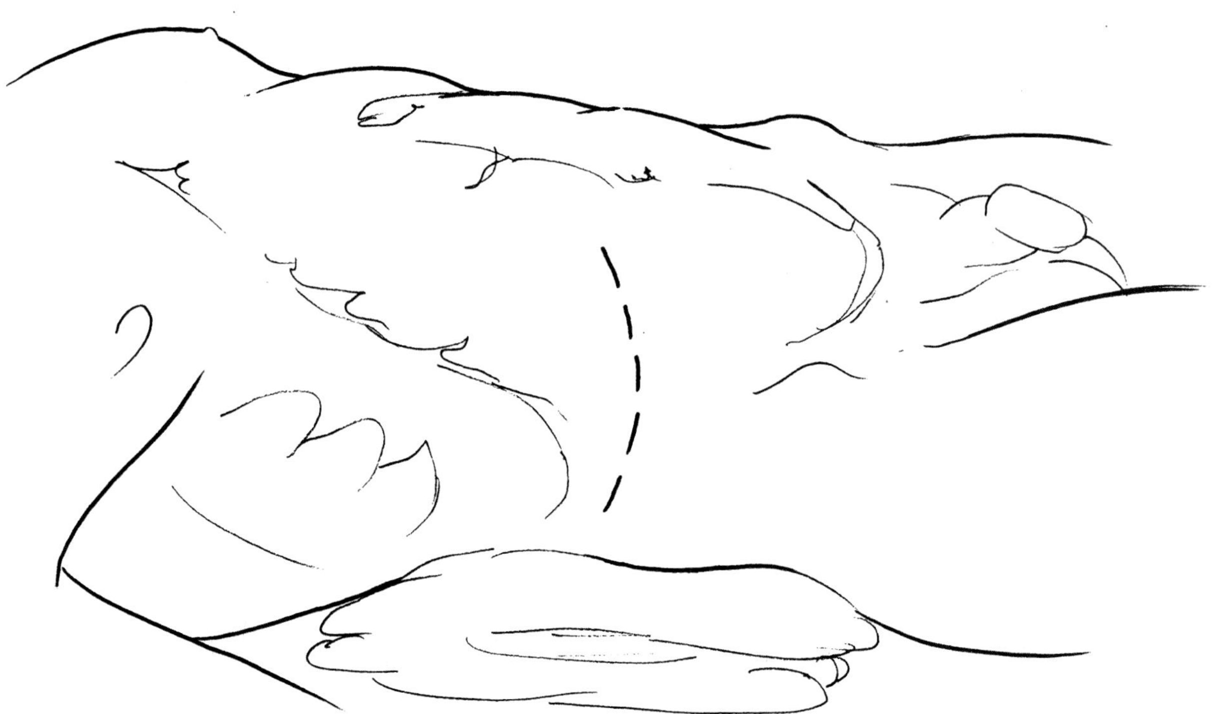

Fig. 13-5 The vena cava is accessible through a right flank approach.

external oblique aponeurosis is incised, and fibers of the external oblique muscle are divided in the lateral wound. The underlying internal oblique muscle is split in the direction of its fibers and freed on its undersurface to permit wide retraction. The transversus abdominis muscle and transversalis fascia are opened in the lateral portion of the incision where separation of the peritoneum from the overlying fascia is relatively simple. These layers can then be opened medially to the rectus muscle as the peritoneum is bluntly separated away. Any peritoneal rents should be sutured closed.

The retroperitoneal plane is developed to the inferior vena cava by bluntly dissecting the right colon and peritoneum away from the transversalis fascia and underlying psoas muscle posteriorly (Fig. 13-6). The ureter is allowed to remain attached to the peritoneal surface, which is retracted anteriorly and to the left.

The inferior vena cava is located anteromedial to the right psoas muscle in the deep wound. With good retraction, complete exposure of a 6-cm segment of vena cava is possible using this approach. Vascular control of the vena cava should be obtained just cephalad to the highest lumbar veins.

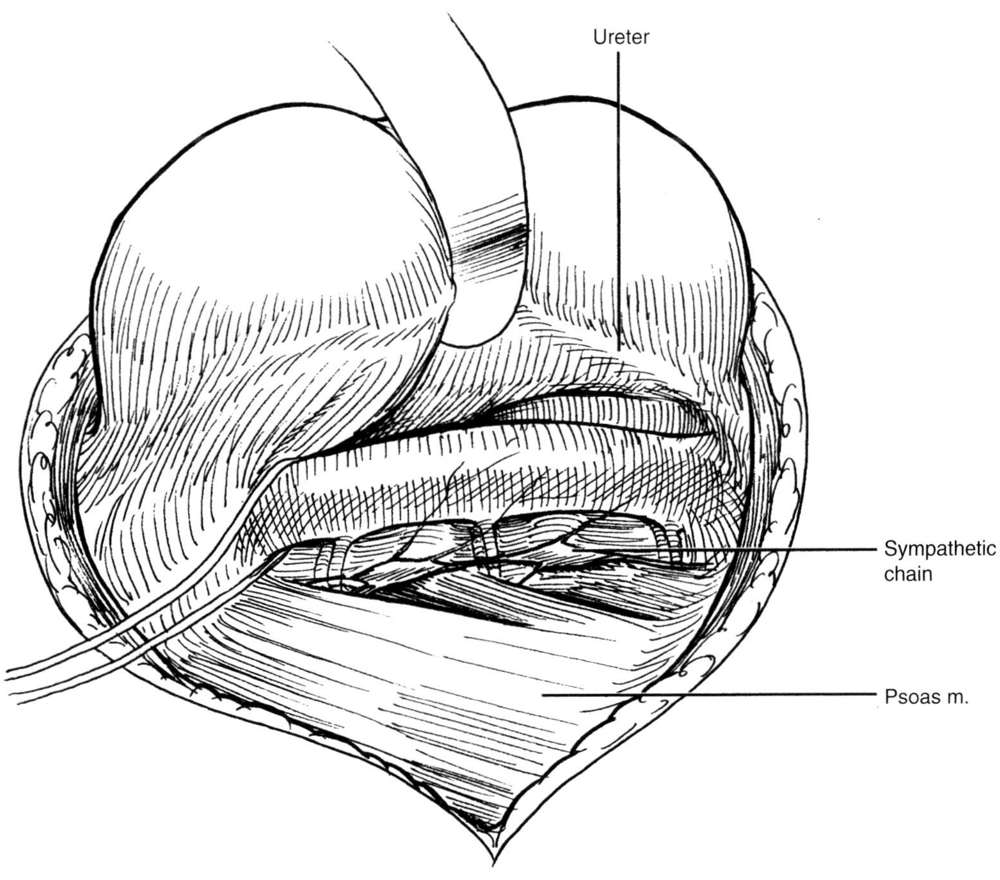

Fig. 13-6 The peritoneum with the ureter attached is elevated to expose the vena cava.

Intraperitoneal Approach

The patient is placed in the supine position, and the lower chest and abdomen are prepped and draped. A vertical midline incision is preferred in trauma cases;[10] in elective cases, a subcostal incision may be used.

After the peritoneal cavity is entered and routine exploration has been completed, the small intestines are retracted to the patient's left. Lateral peritoneal attachments of the right colon are incised, allowing medial reflection of the right colon and its mesentery. The second and third portions of the duodenum are also mobilized by incising retroperitoneal attachments. The underlying inferior vena cava is exposed from the iliac bifurcation to the level of the caudate lobe by reflecting the duodenum and head of the pancreas medially (Fig. 13-7). Before mobilization of the infrarenal vena cava is attempted, areolar tissue and lymphatics should be cleared from the anterior and lateral caval surfaces. The infrarenal vena cava can then be encircled with a vascular tape just below the renal veins in preparation for more extensive mobilization.

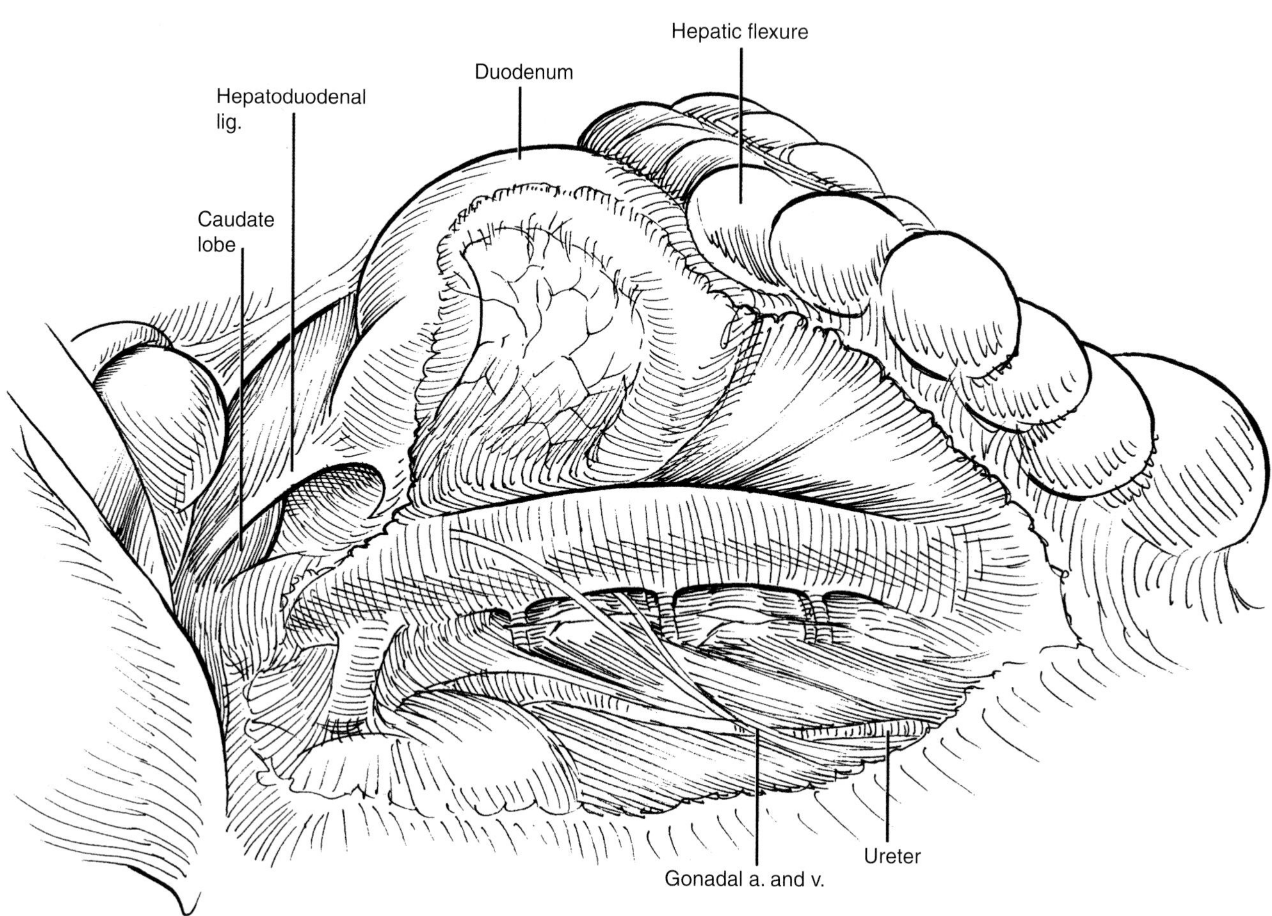

Fig. 13-7 The perirenal vena cava is unroofed by mobilizing the right colon, duodenum, and head of the pancreas.

In elective circumstances, the posterior wall of the infrarenal vena cava can be exposed by rolling the lateral surface anteriorly (Fig. 13-8). Care should be taken to control the lumbar veins draining into the posterior caval wall; ligation and division of these vein branches permit full mobilization of the infrarenal vena cava. This maneuver is not recommended for control of injuries to the posterior vena cava wall because avulsion of lumbar veins is likely. Such injuries may be repaired by enlarging

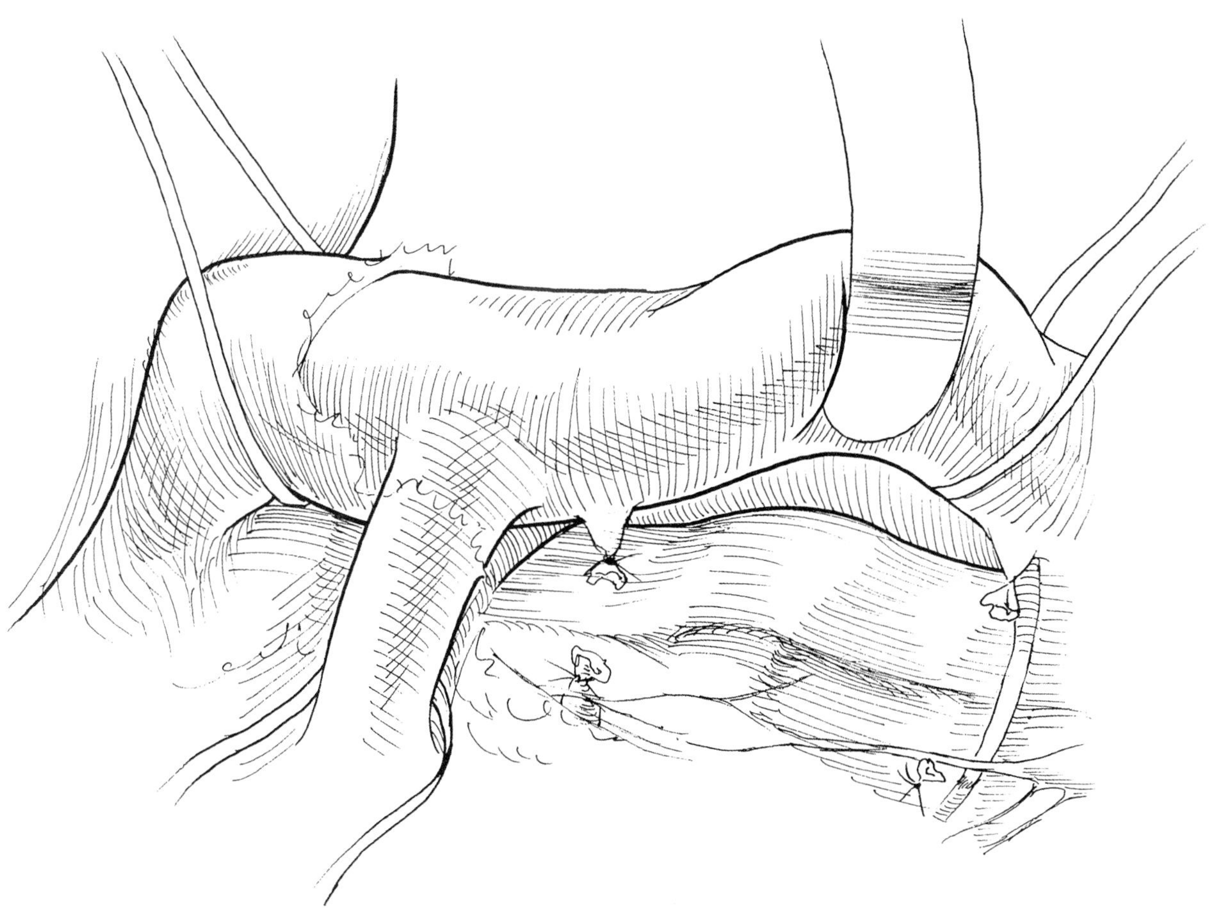

Fig. 13-8 Ligating adjacent lumbar veins allows a segment of the back wall of the vena cava to be visualized.

the anterior wound and closing the posterior wound from within the vena cava (Fig. 13-9).[10]

The vena cava cephalad to the renal veins and inferior to the caudate lobe of the liver can be encircled with a vascular tape. The right adrenal vein should be identified and controlled to prevent avulsion during this maneuver. Because this short segment of vena cava is tethered by the renal veins below and by the liver above, extensive mobilization is not possible.

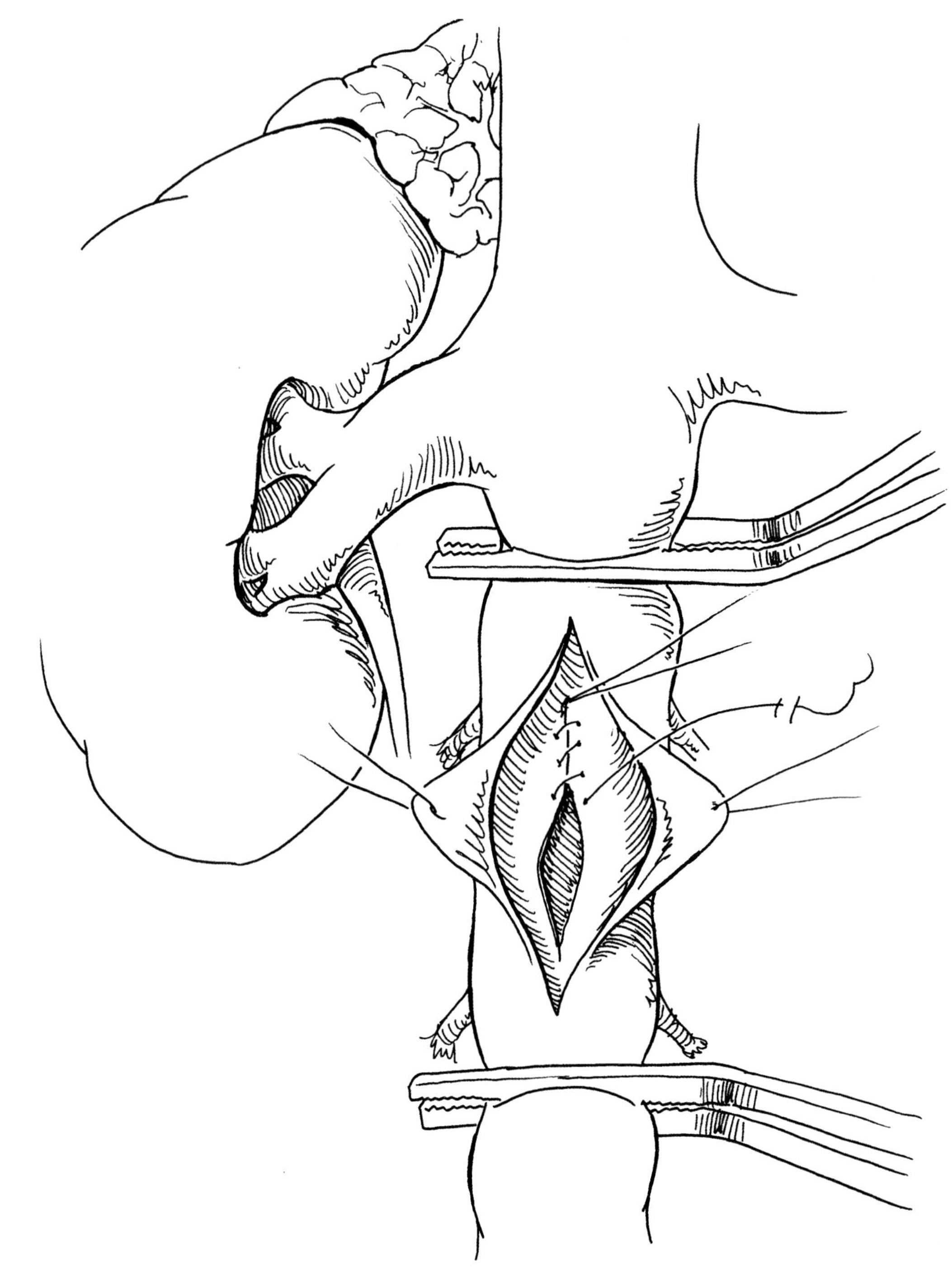

Fig. 13-9 Posterior wounds of the inferior vena cava can be repaired from inside the vessel.

Exposure of the Retrohepatic Inferior Vena Cava

The patient is placed in the supine position, and the entire abdomen, anterior chest, and lower neck are prepped and draped. Some surgeons prefer a thoracoabdominal incision to expose this portion of the vena cava,[11] but others recommend a midline abdominal approach with superior extension into a median sternotomy, if necessary.[12] The median sternotomy greatly enhances exposure of the area posterior to the right lobe of the liver and allows rapid control of the supradiaphragmatic inferior vena cava within the pericardium should this become necessary (see below).

A vertical midline incision is made from the xiphoid process to the pubis. After the peritoneal cavity is entered, self-retaining retractors should be placed in the upper wound margins on both sides to elevate the costal margins superiorly (Fig. 13-10).

The right triangular ligament is divided to expose the bare area of the liver. Peritoneal

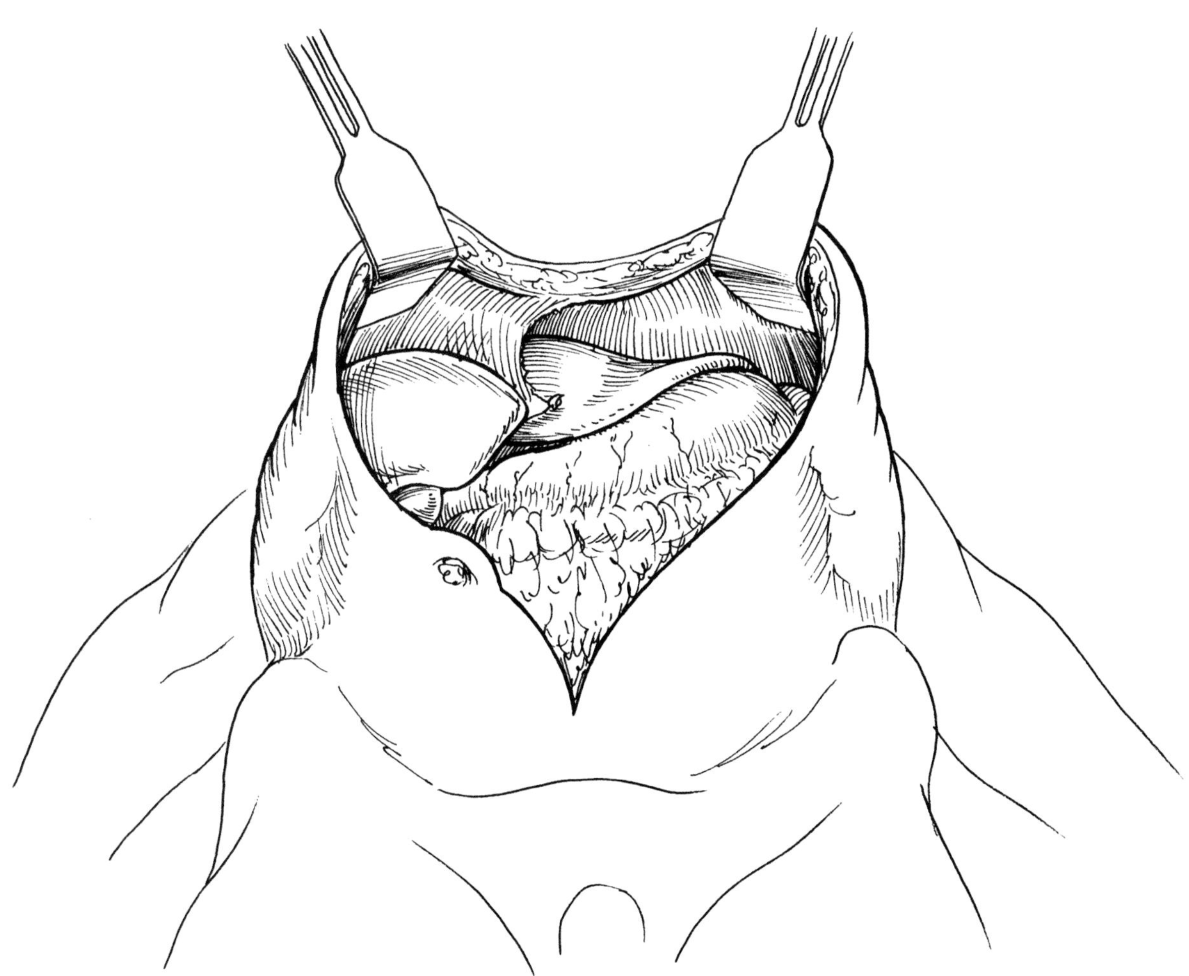

Fig. 13-10 Firm retraction of the lower rib cage is necessary for exposure of the perihepatic vena cava.

attachments of the lateral and posterior surfaces of the right hepatic lobe are divided as the right lobe is retracted medially by an assistant (Fig. 13-11). If the retroperitoneal portion of the liver is difficult to visualize using these maneuvers, a median sternotomy should be performed at this time (see Chapter 3).

The retrohepatic vena cava is visualized by completely mobilizing the right hepatic lobe and retracting it medially. A variable number (three to eight) of small hepatic vein branches enters the inferior vena cava from the posterior surface of the right and caudate lobes; these should be carefully ligated and divided to prevent troublesome bleeding. Three large hepatic veins enter the vena cava from the posterior surface of the upper liver. Exposure and control of these larger veins are discussed in the following section.

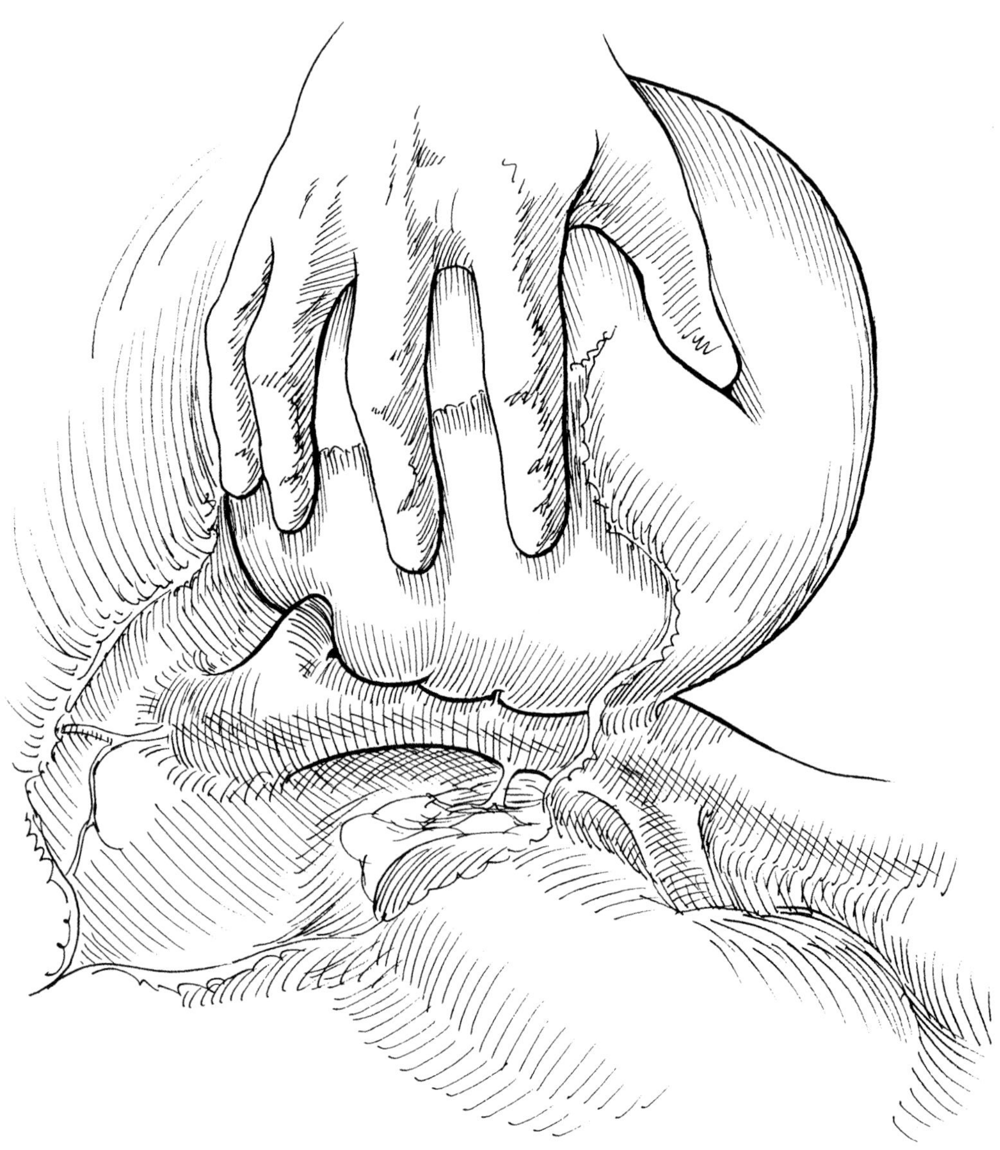

Fig. 13-11 The right triangular and coronary ligaments of the liver are divided, and the right lobe of the liver is gently rotated to the left to visualize the retrohepatic vena cava.

Exposure of the Hepatic Veins

Exposure of hepatic veins is indicated in emergency control of exsanguinating injuries and in elective liver resections. In emergency situations, consideration should be given to surgically isolating the retrohepatic vena cava using the Schrock technique[13] or temporarily occluding the vena cava with large balloons. The Shrock shunt is time consuming, technically difficult and seldom successful. In unstable patients, it may be prudent to pack the abdomen to allow a brief period of resuscitation before proceeding with vena cava exposure. For major hepatic trauma, damage control packing, ICU resuscitation, followed by return to the OR for liver resection is often the safest strategy. In elective circumstances, resection of the right hepatic lobe necessitates concomitant exposure of the retrohepatic vena cava (see above).

Patient preparation and incision options are described in the above section. After the peritoneal cavity has been entered and anterior vena cava exposure has been adequately obtained, the round ligament of the liver is divided, and the cut ends are ligated. The falciform and coronary ligaments above the liver are widely incised, exposing the bare area. The liver should be retracted caudally, allowing identification of two or three large hepatic veins within the areolar tissues of the bare area (Fig. 13-12). These veins should be carefully dissected and encircled near their junctions with the suprahepatic vena cava.

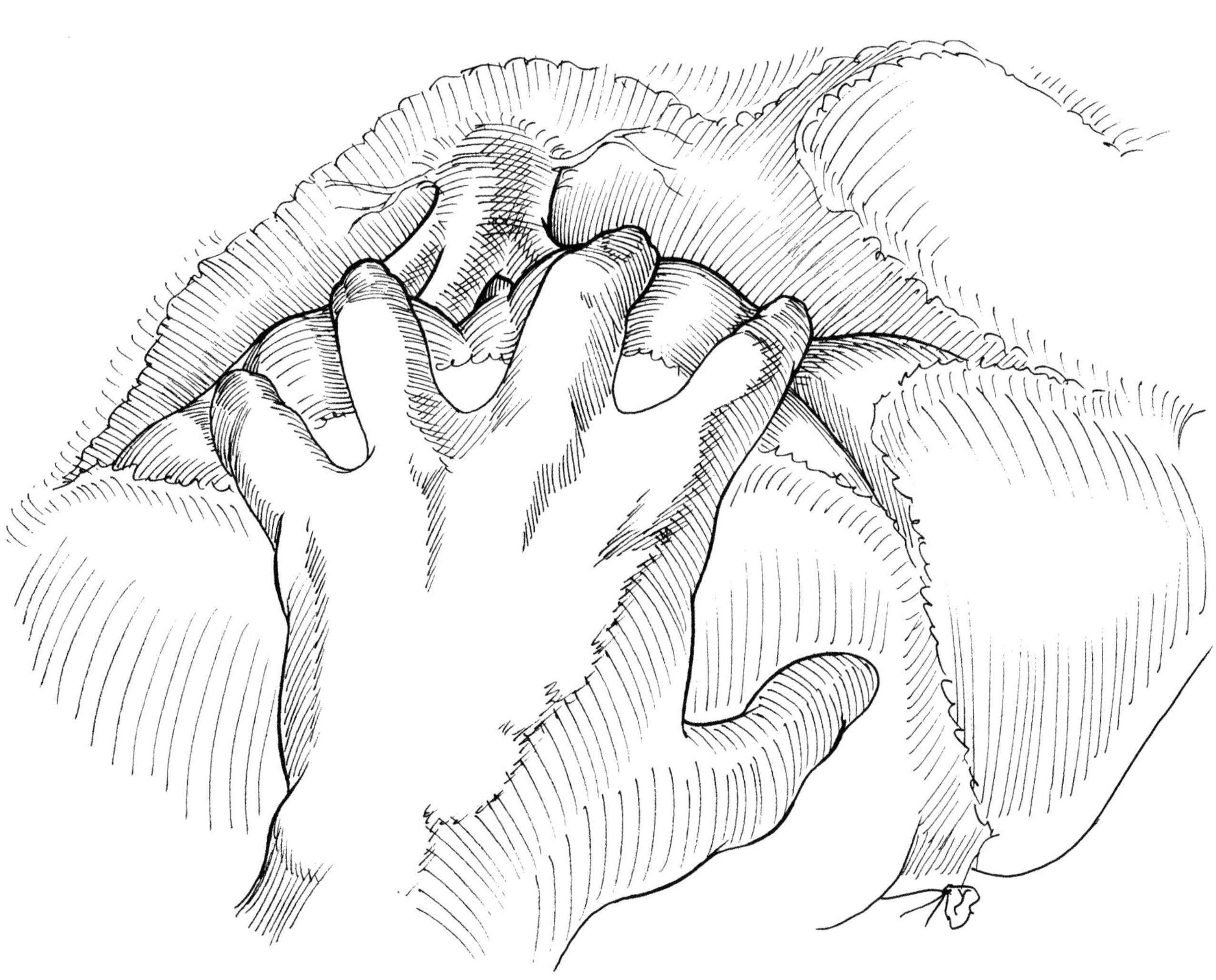

Fig. 13-12 The falciform and anterior coronary ligaments are opened, and the dome of the liver is gently retracted downward to expose the hepatic veins and suprahepatic vena cava.

Exposure of the Suprahepatic Vena Cava within the Pericardial Sac

Isolation of the inferior vena cava above the liver is hampered by the presence of hepatic veins below the diaphragm and the close proximity of the pericardium above the diaphragm. Although the short supradiaphragmatic segment can be isolated inferior to the pericardial sac by incising the central tendon of the diaphragm, control is easier and more rapid within the pericardial sac.

Adequate exposure requires a median sternotomy (see Chapter 3). After the sternal edges are separated, the glistening pericardial sac is opened vertically in the midline. To enhance exposure, the divided pericardial edges can be retracted laterally with sutures (Fig. 13-13). The terminal portion of the inferior vena cava can be identified as it enters the right atrium near the inferior corner of the pericardial space on the patient's right side. Loose areolar tissue within Gibbon's space behind the vena cava is easily separated using blunt dissection, permitting passage of a vascular tape.

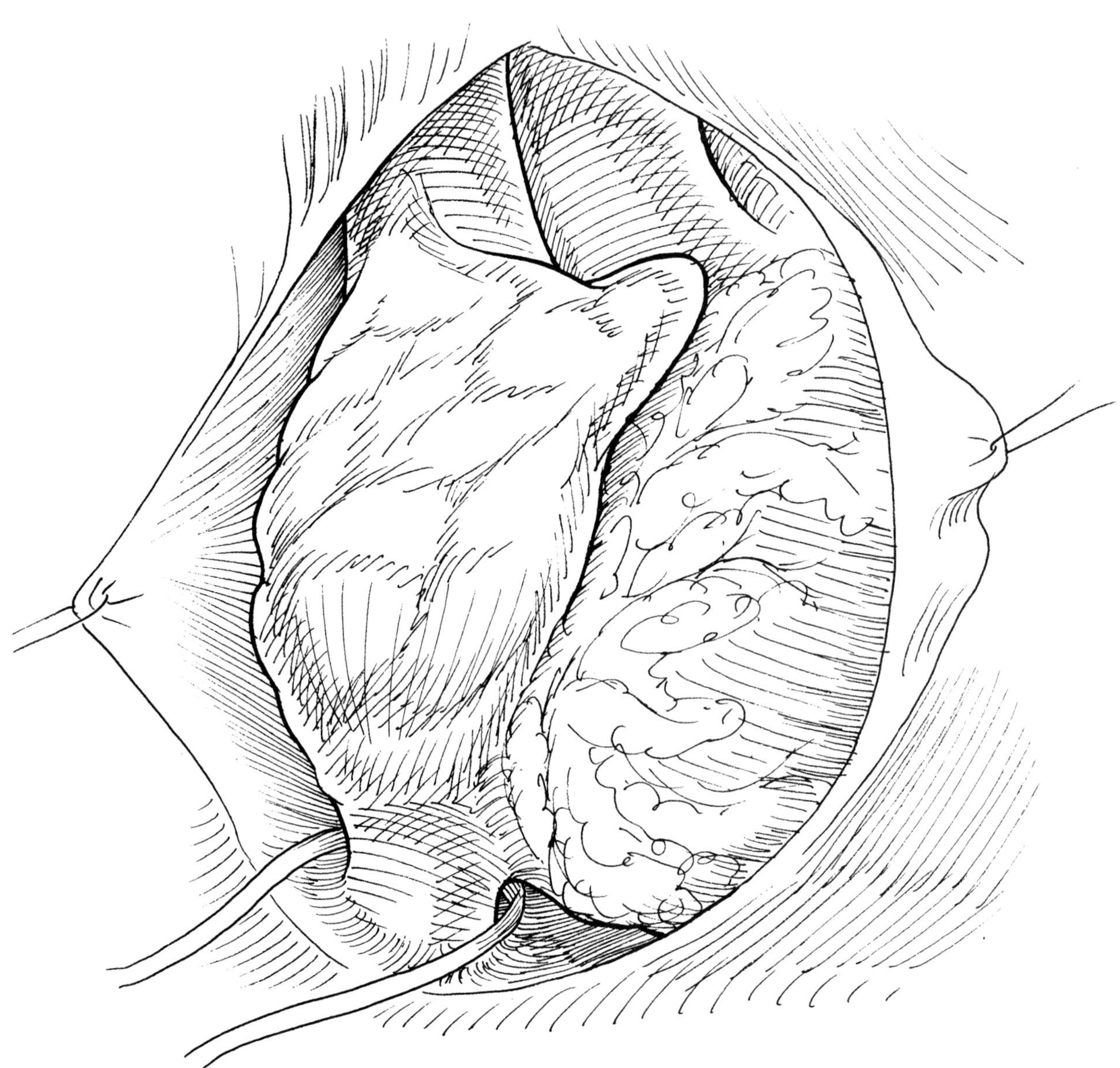

Fig. 13-13 The intrapericardial portion of the inferior vena cava can be isolated at its junction with the right atrium through a median sternotomy.

References

1. Fairfax LM, Sing RF. Vena cava interruption. *Crit Care Clin.* 2011;27:781–804.
2. Angel LF, Tapson V, Galgon RE, et al. Systematic review of the use of retrievable inferior vena cava filters. *J Vasc Interv Radiol.* 2011;22:1522–1530.
3. Belenotti P, Sarlon-Bartoli G, Bartoli MA, et al. Vena cava filter migration: an underappreciated complication. About four cases and review of the literature. *Ann Vasc Surg.* 2011;25:1141. e9–e14.
4. Shang EK, Nathan DP, Carpenter JP, et al. Delayed complications of inferior vena cava filters: case report and literature review. *Vasc Endovascular Surg.* 2011;45:290–294.
5. Wang GJ, Carpenter JP, Fairman RM, et al. Single-center experience of caval thrombectomy in patients with renal cell carcinoma with tumor thrombus extension into the inferior vena cava. *Vasc Endovascular Surg.* 2008;42:335–340.
6. Helfand BT, Smith ND, Kozlowski JM, et al. Vena cava thrombectomy and primary repair after radical nephrectomy for renal cell carcinoma: single-center experience. *Ann Vasc Surg.* 2011;25:39–43.
7. Pappas PJ, Haser PB, Teehan EP, et al. Outcome of complex venous reconstructions in patients with trauma. *J Vasc Surg.* 1997;25:398–404.
8. Quinones-Baldrich W, Alktaifi A, Eilber F, et al. Inferior vena cava resection and reconstruction for retroperitoneal tumor excision. *J Vasc Surg.* 2012;55:1386–1393.
9. Caso J, Seigne J, Back M, et al. Circumferential resection of the inferior vena cava for primary and recurrent malignant tumors. *J Urol.* 2009;182:887–893.
10. Perry MO. Injuries to the inferior vena cava. In: Thal ER, Weigelt JA, Carrico CJ, eds. *Operative Trauma Management: An Atlas*, 2nd ed. New York, NY: McGraw-Hill, 2002:316–321.
11. Bower TC, Nagorney DM, Cherry KJ Jr, et al. Replacement of the inferior vena cava for malignancy: an update. *J Vasc Surg.* 2000;31:270–281.
12. Fullen WD, McDonough JJ, Popp MJ, et al. Sternal splitting approach for major hepatic or retrohepatic vena cava injury. *J Trauma.* 1974;14:903–911.
13. Schrock T, Blaisdell FW, Mathewson C Jr. Management of blunt trauma to the liver and hepatic veins. *Arch Surg.* 1968;96:698–704.

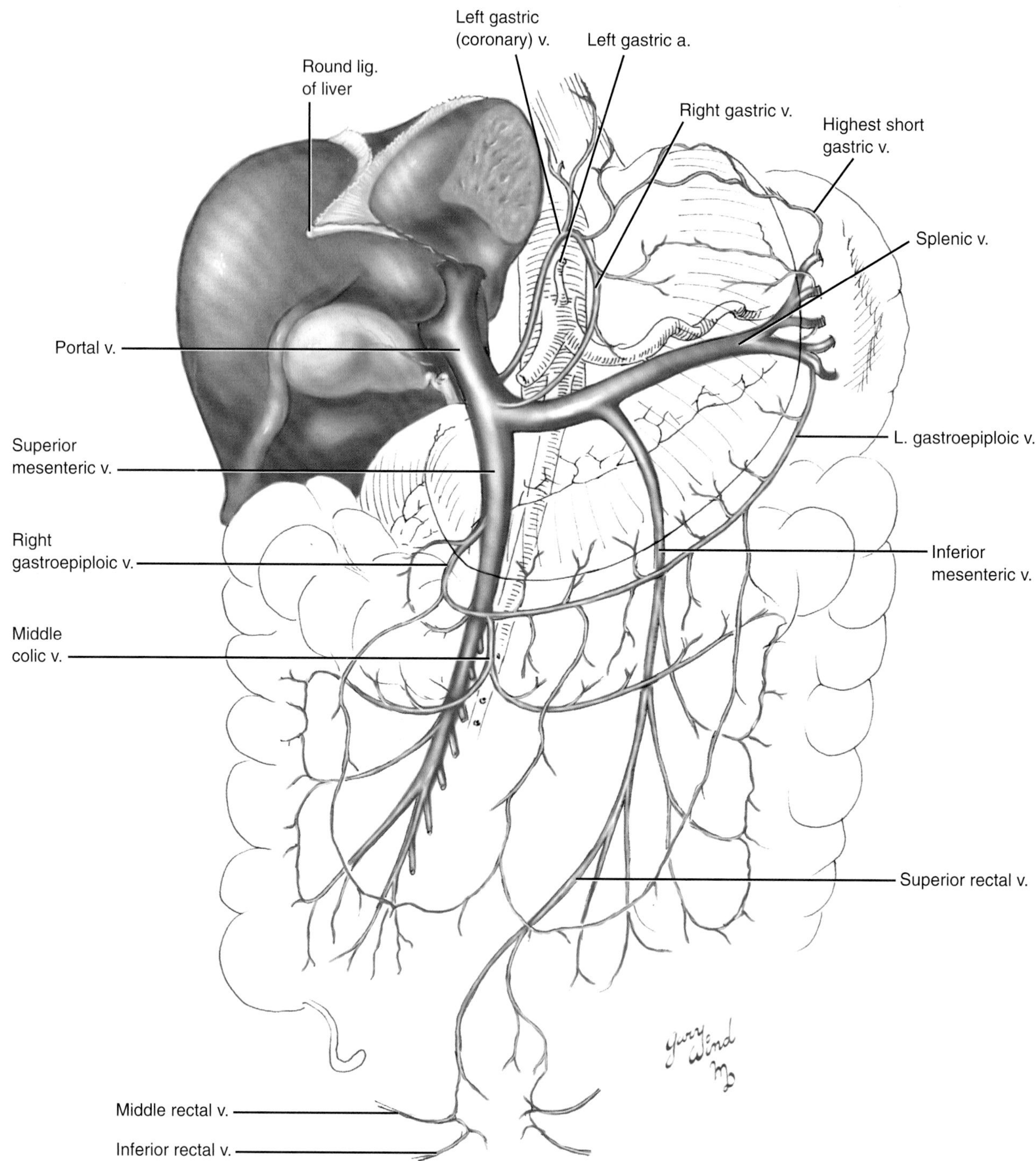

Fig. 14-1 The main venous trunks feeding into the portal vein are the superior and inferior mesenteric veins and the splenic vein.

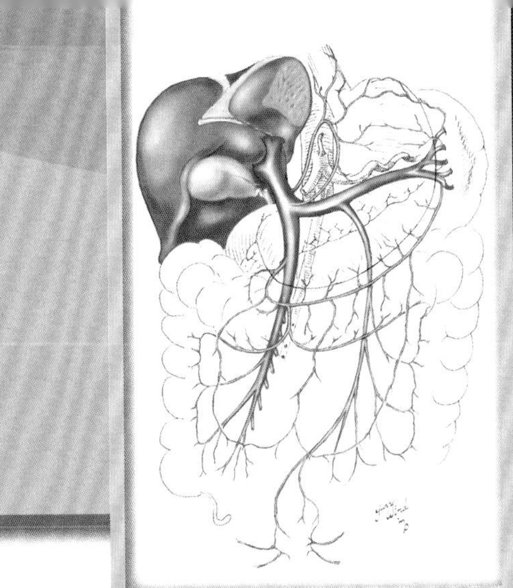

Portal Venous System

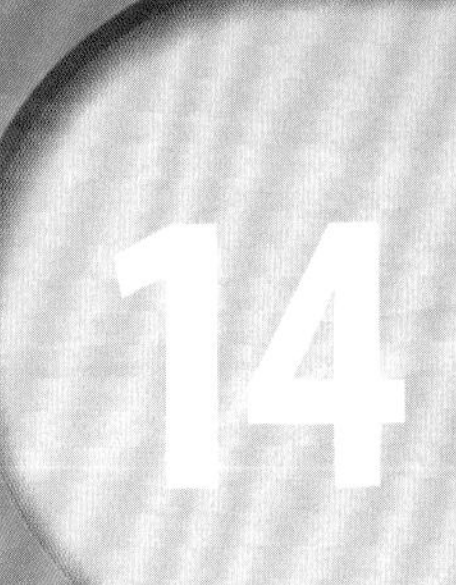

14

Surgical Anatomy of the Portal Vein

The portal venous system drains the viscera supplied by the celiac, superior, and inferior mesenteric arteries and normally carries the blood to the liver (Fig. 14-1). The portal vein is formed by the confluence of splenic and superior mesenteric veins at the level of the second lumbar vertebra. Most commonly, the inferior mesenteric vein joins the proximal splenic vein, but it may alternatively join the superior mesenteric vein or form a common junction with the other two veins. These three veins drain the areas supplied by their corresponding named arteries.

Anatomically, the superior mesenteric and splenic veins lie close to their corresponding arteries (Fig. 14-2). The superior mesenteric vein lies to the right of the artery in the root of the small bowel mesentery and ascends over the third portion of the duodenum and uncinate process of the pancreas. The vein passes behind the neck of the pancreas and is joined by the splenic vein near the cephalad border of the gland. The splenic vein is cradled in a groove running the length of the upper border of the posterior surface of the pancreas (inset). Numerous small branches drain from the tail and body of the pancreas into the apposed surface of the vein.

The inferior mesenteric vein lies deep to the left posterior parietal peritoneum and ascends in close proximity to the underlying infrarenal aorta.

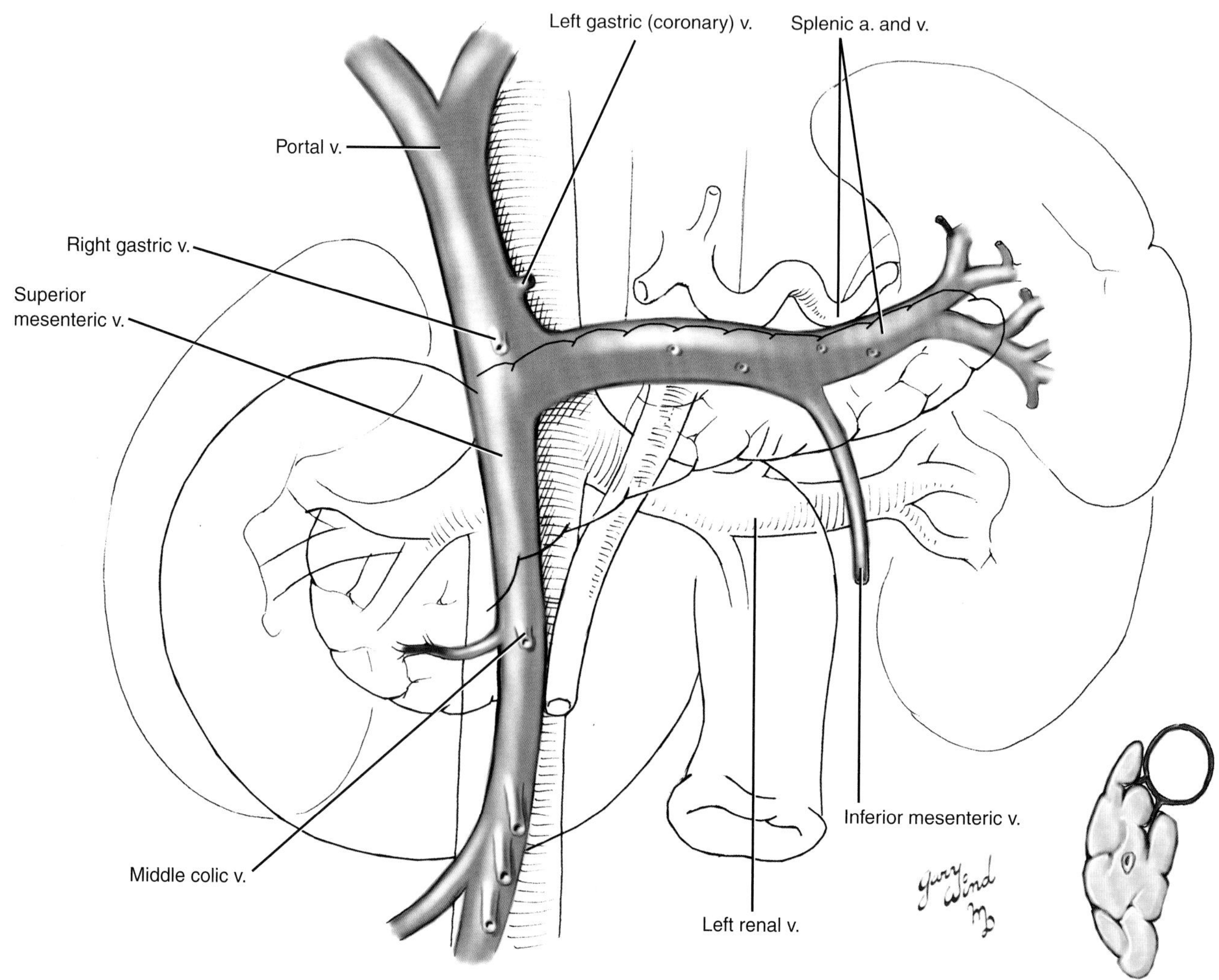

Fig. 14-2 The relationships of the main trunks of the portal system to the surrounding structures are shown.

It courses beneath the root of the transverse mesocolon and dives under the inferior border of the pancreas where it joins the splenic or superior mesenteric vein or their junction. From the confluence of these branches, the portal vein ascends within the thickened edge of the gastrohepatic ligament accompanied by the hepatic artery and common bile duct.

Another component of the portal system is the circuit formed by the left (coronary) and right gastric veins that empty into the left side of the portal vein just proximal to the junction of splenic and superior mesenteric veins (Fig. 14-3). The right gastric vein lies along the lesser curvature of the stomach beneath the gastric root of the gastrohepatic omentum. The left gastric vein spans the distance between the esophagogastric junction and the posterior wall of the omental bursa lying alongside the left gastric artery. It descends diagonally over the celiac trunk beneath the posterior peritoneum of the omental bursa to reach the portal vein. The apex of this loop receives drainage from the lower esophageal veins. Small pyloric and duodenal veins also enter the portal vein near the gastric veins.

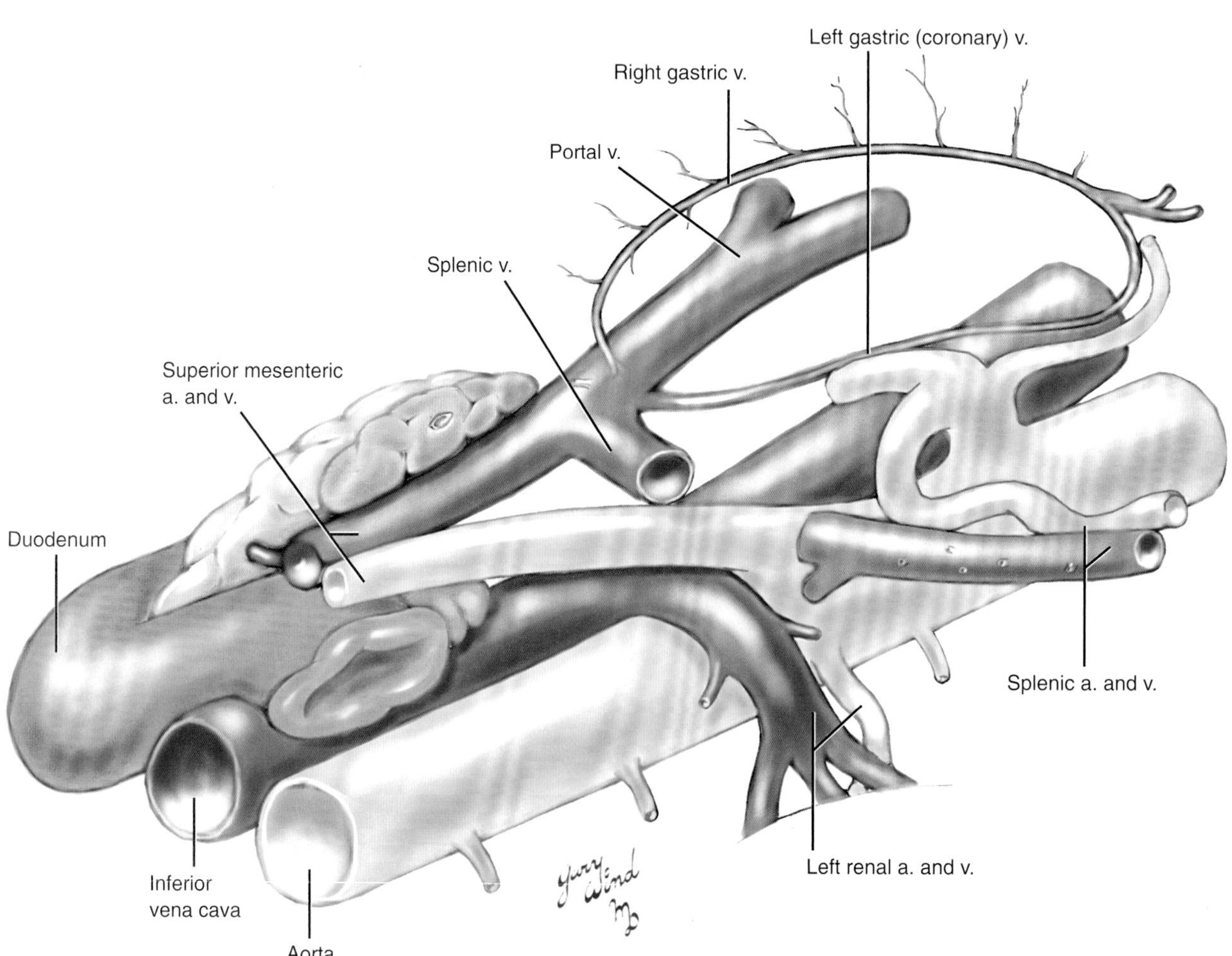

Fig. 14-3 The gastric vein circuit consists of the right gastric vein along the lesser curve of the stomach and the left gastric or coronary vein beneath the posterior peritoneum of the lesser sac.

Secondary Portal Venous Connections

There are three more peripheral circuits through which major branches of the portal system communicate (Fig. 14-4). The gastroepiploic arch connects the terminal splenic vein with the superior mesenteric vein and runs in the gastrocolic omentum where it receives drainage from the omentum and greater curvature of the stomach. The second of these circuits is formed by connections between peripheral branches of the superior mesenteric, inferior mesenteric, and middle colic veins around the mesenteric margin of the colon. The final connection is between the short gastric branches of the terminal splenic vein and branches of the gastric circuit across the cardia of the stomach.

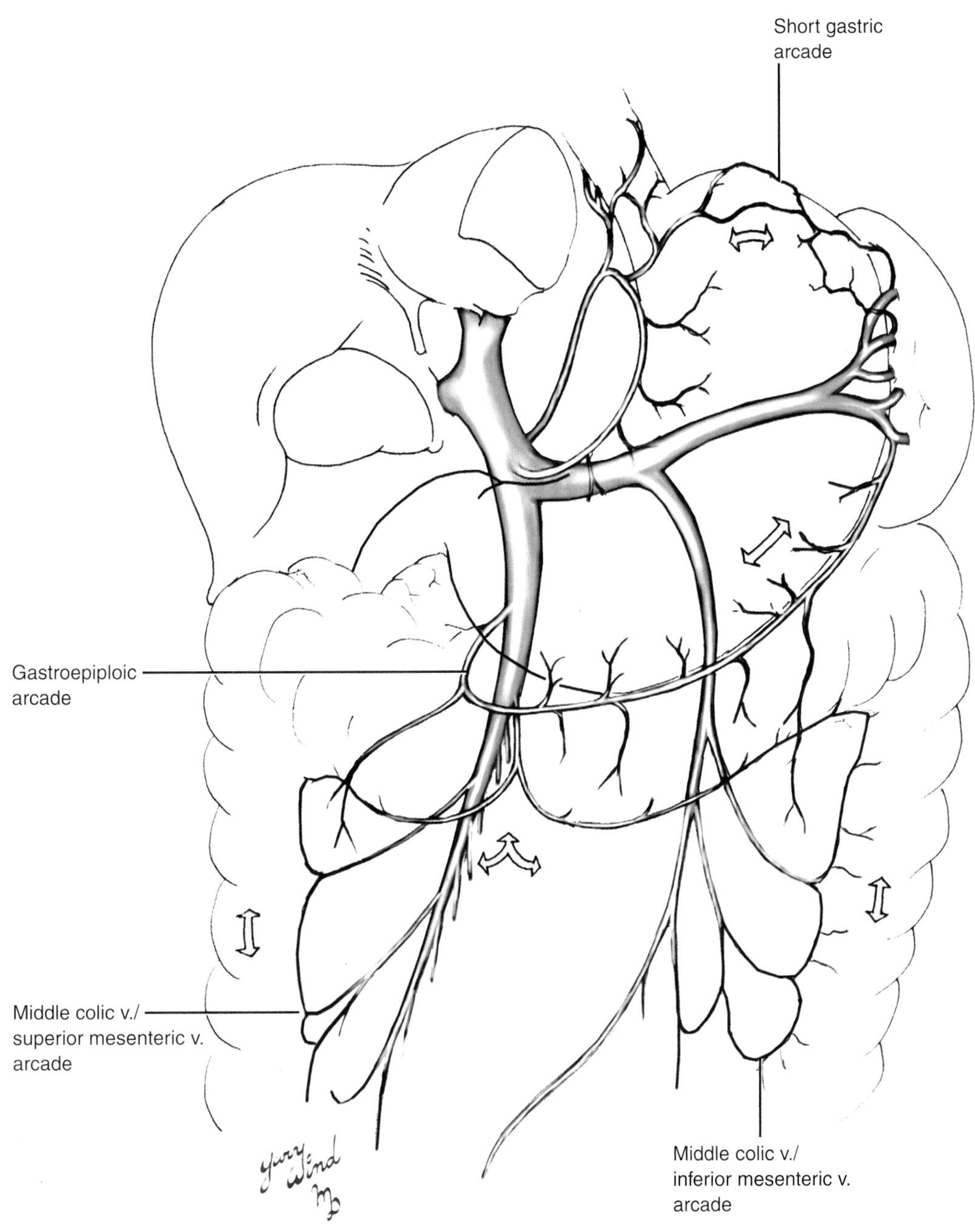

Fig. 14-4 Peripheral links between limbs of the portal system are shown.

Portosystemic Venous Connections

Portal hypertension occurs as a result of increased portal vein resistance or, on rare occasions, from increased portal vein flow. It is associated with a number of hepatic and extrahepatic disorders that have been well described elsewhere.[1] Among other consequences of increased pressure in the portal system, the thin-walled veins become engorged. Normally small connections between the portal and systemic venous circulations often become clinically apparent.

There are several peripheral connections between the portal system and the systemic circulation that become enlarged as a result of abnormally elevated portal pressure (Fig. 14-5). Peripheral dilation is most dangerous in the submucosal esophageal plexus connecting the portal circulation to the azygous system. Resultant esophageal varicosities are in danger of erosion and massive hemorrhage.

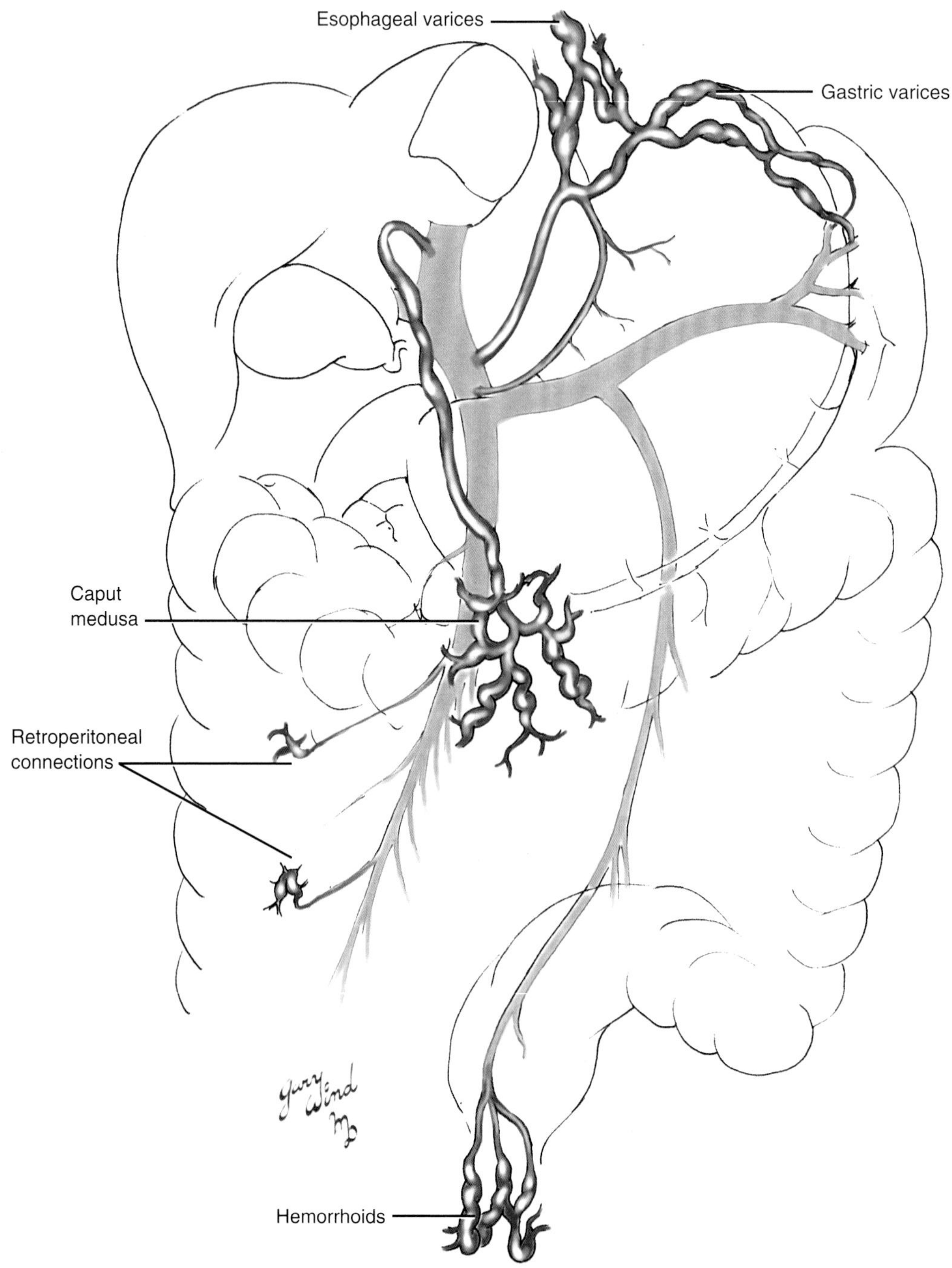

Fig. 14-5 Important portosystemic connections are found in the esophageal, periumbilical, and rectal veins. Multiple small retroperitoneal communications are also found when portal pressure is elevated.

Hemorrhoids are visible manifestations of the connection between superior rectal veins and middle and inferior rectal veins. Caput medusae results from engorgement of connections between the paraumbilical veins and veins of the anterior abdominal wall, connecting to the portal system via the recanalized umbilical vein in the edge of the falciform ligament. Multiple small retroperitoneal connections between the two systems (veins of Retzius) may lead to increased bleeding during retroperitoneal dissection and tissue mobilization.

Exposure of the Portal Circulation

Historically, the main indication for exposure of the portal circulation was to create a portosystemic shunt for surgical decompression of portal hypertension. The management of patients with bleeding esophageal varices has evolved significantly in the past two decades, however. Liver transplant is now considered definitive therapy for portal hypertension, and there are numerous temporizing options that can achieve hemostasis and prevent rebleeding, including endoscopic variceal sclerotherapy or banding, transjugular intrahepatic portosystemic shunts (TIPs), and devascularization procedures.[1–3] Operative shunts are rarely performed in the modern era, and may be contraindicated because they interfere with the anatomy in patients who may be eligible for liver transplant. However, some surgeons believe that surgical shunts represent a reasonable alternative in patients who are not candidates for liver transplant or who fail attempts at TIPs.[1,3] A wide variety of surgical options is available for the treatment of patients who have had one or more variceal bleeds[3] (Fig. 14-6). Surgical outcome is better when operations are performed

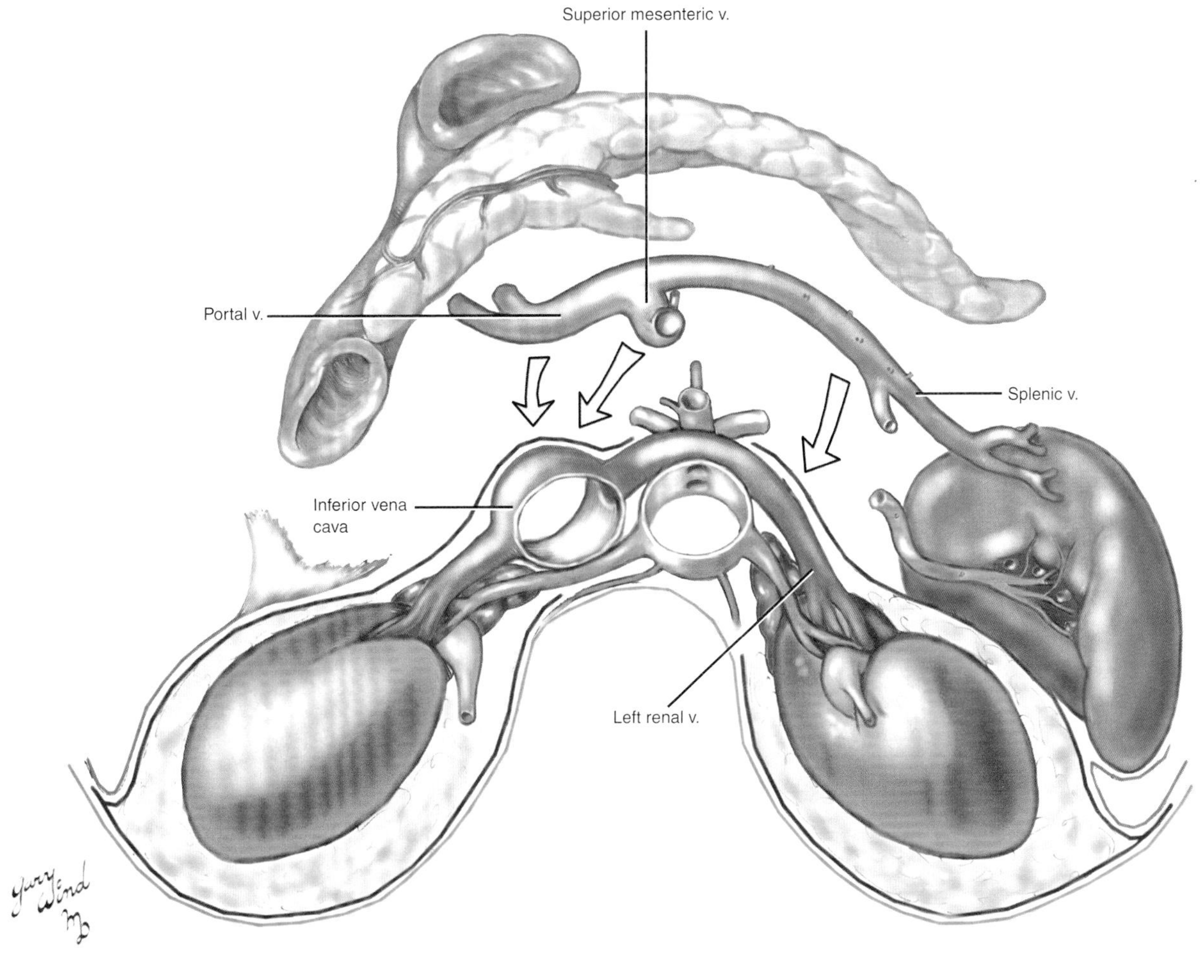

Fig. 14-6 Surgical decompression of the portal system into the systemic venous system is accomplished by connecting the portal or superior mesenteric veins to the inferior vena cava or the splenic vein to the left renal vein.

electively in patients with less advanced liver disease.

Therapeutic portal decompression shunts can generally be divided into two categories: nonselective and selective. Nonselective shunts include portacaval (both end-to-side and side-to-side), mesocaval, and proximal splenorenal anastomoses (Fig. 14-7). These shunts prevent recurrent bleeding if they remain patent but do not improve survival rates or quality of life because of the high associated rates of hepatic encephalopathy.[1,3] Selective shunts include the Warren distal splenorenal shunt[4]

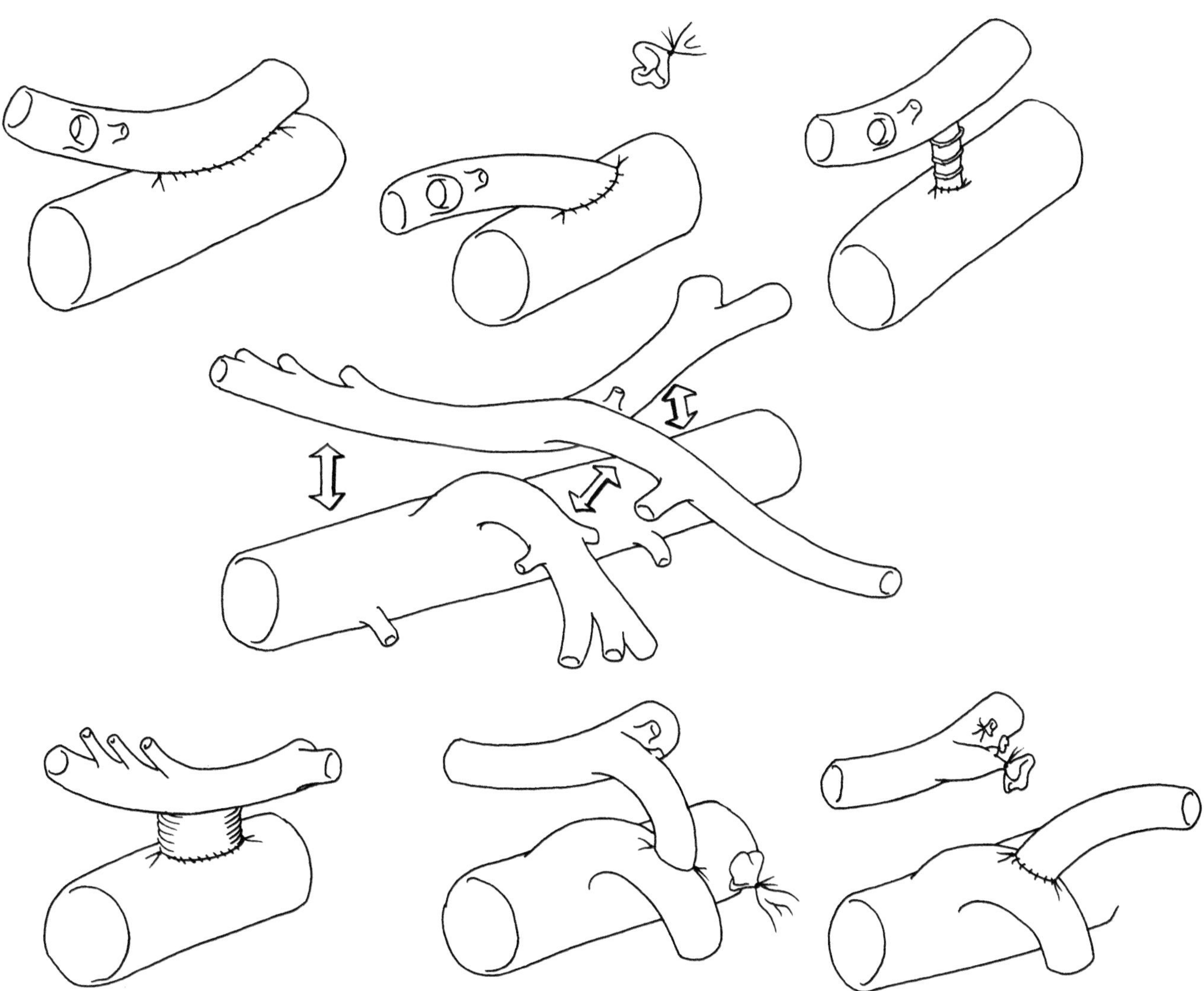

Fig. 14-7 Nonselective portacaval shunts are shown in the top row of three drawings, and nonselective mesocaval and central splenorenal shunts are shown in the two drawings on the lower left. Selective shunts include small-caliber variations of nonselective shunts and the distal splenorenal shunt shown on the lower right.

(Fig. 14-8) and variations of the nonselective shunts (e.g., Sarfeh small-diameter portacaval H graft[5] and Johansen small-diameter portacaval anastomosis[6]).

Beyond portal decompression surgery, there are two modern indications for exposure of the portal venous system: repair of traumatic injuries[7,8] and resection and reconstruction of the portal and superior mesenteric veins in patients with invasive pancreatic tumors.[9,10] The following discussion concerns exposure of the portal vein and its tributaries in consideration of performing decompression procedures, repair of traumatic injuries, or reconstruction in patients with invasive pancreatic cancer.

Exposure of the Portal Vein

The patient is placed in the supine position with the right flank elevated 15° to 20° on rolled sheets. The entire abdomen, lower chest, and right flank are prepped and draped. An extended right subcostal

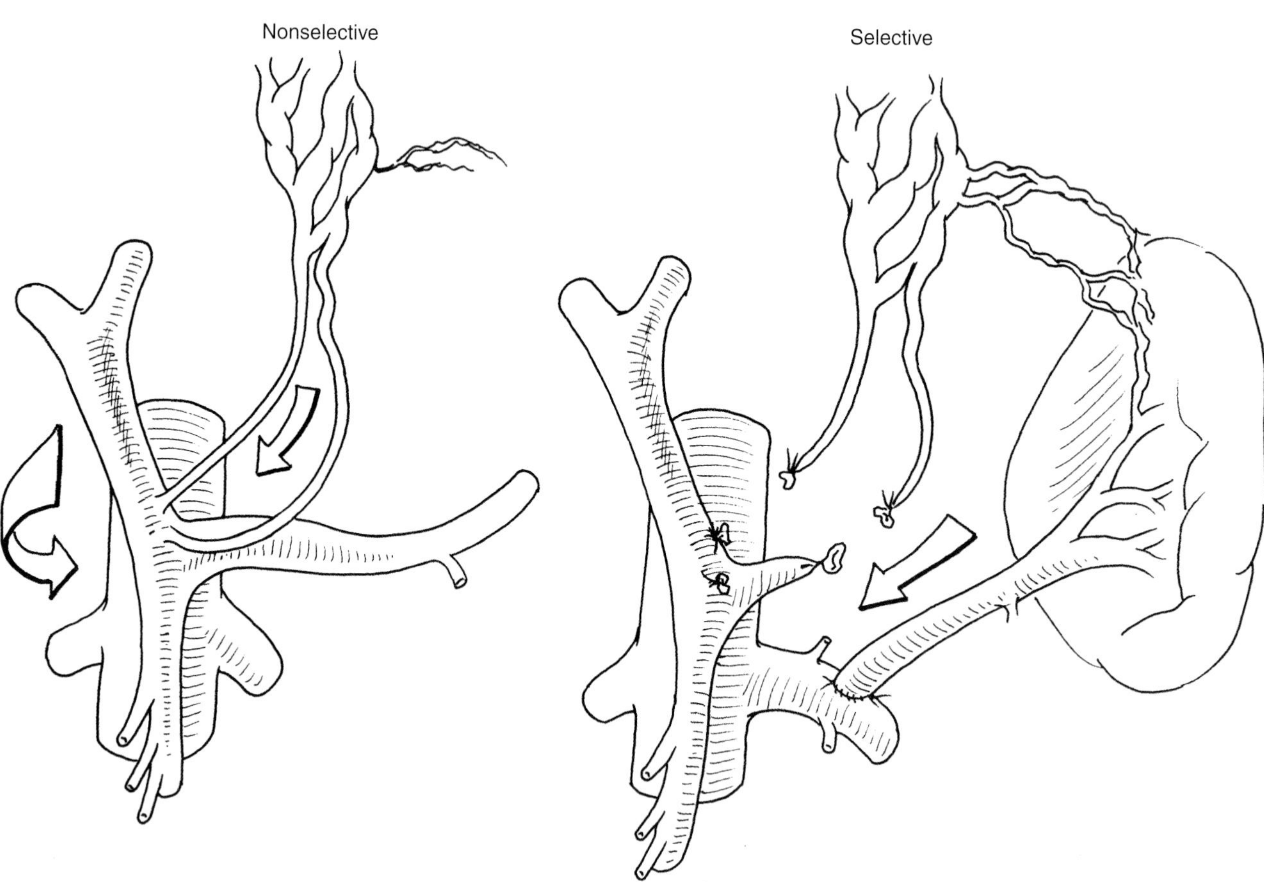

Fig. 14-8 The selective distal splenorenal shunt isolates the drainage of the esophageal venous plexus from the portal system, preserving portal flow to the liver undisturbed.

incision is made 2 to 3 cm below the right costal margin, extending across both rectus muscles and into the right flank (Fig. 14-9). The incision should not be placed below this level in patients who have hepatomegaly because exposure of the porta hepatis is more difficult through lower incisions. Alternatively, a midline incision may be more appropriate in patients undergoing exploratory laparotomy for trauma or pancreaticoduodenectomy for cancer.

After the peritoneal cavity is entered, routine exploration of the abdominal contents is carefully performed. In patients with portal hypertension, the umbilical vein and falciform ligament are divided to interrupt an important source of collateral flow between the portal and systemic venous circulations. The portal pressure can be determined manometrically at this time through a mesenteric vein branch.

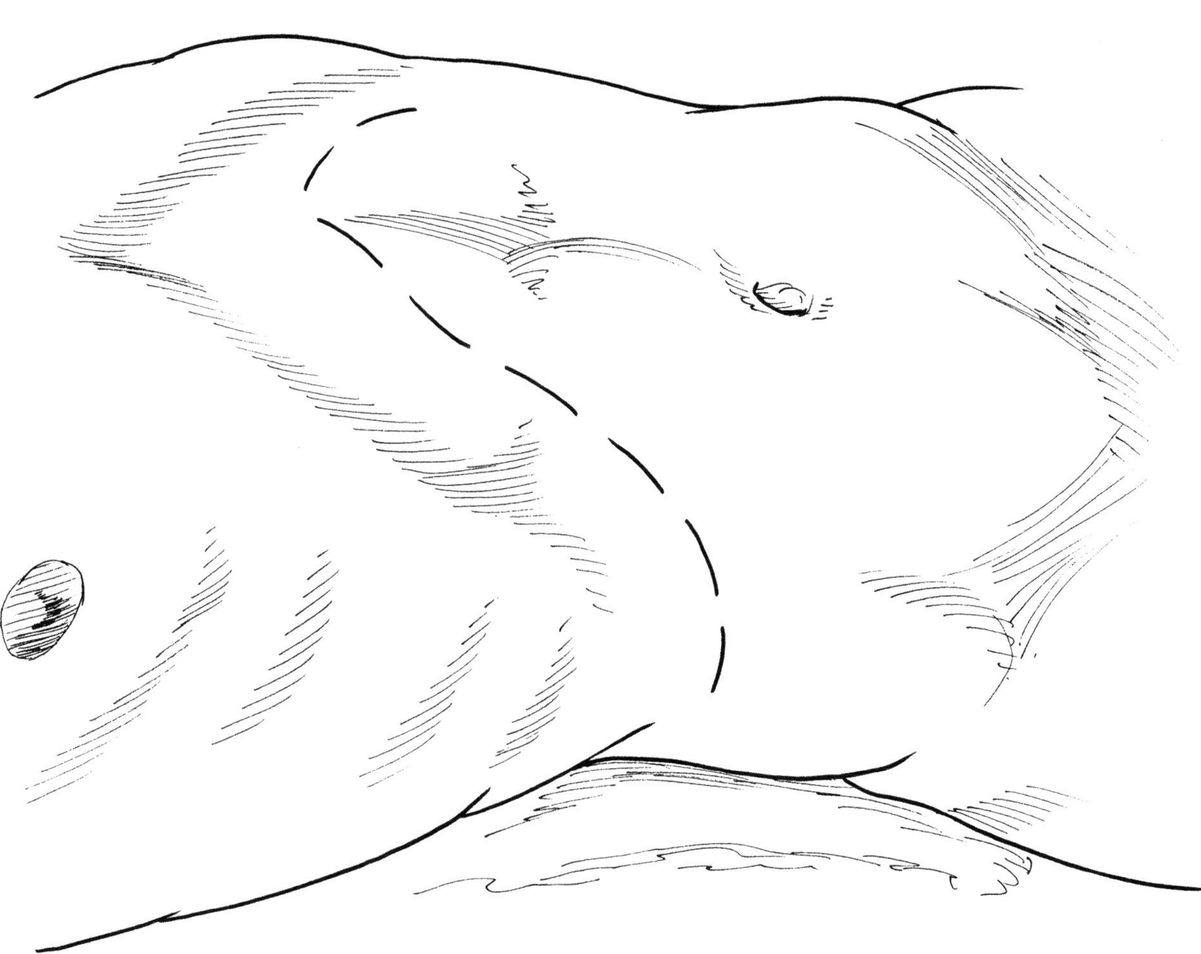

Fig. 14-9 An extended right subcostal incision provides good exposure of the portal vein.

The porta hepatis is exposed by retracting the right lobe of the liver cephalad and the hepatic flexure downward (Fig. 14-10). The hepatic flexure of the colon may occasionally require mobilization to enhance exposure, but unnecessary dissection should be avoided to minimize blood loss. The first and second portions of the duodenum are mobilized next by dividing lateral and posterior peritoneal attachments up to the right edge of the gastrohepatic ligament. Downward traction of the mobilized duodenum greatly enhances exposure of porta hepatis structures.

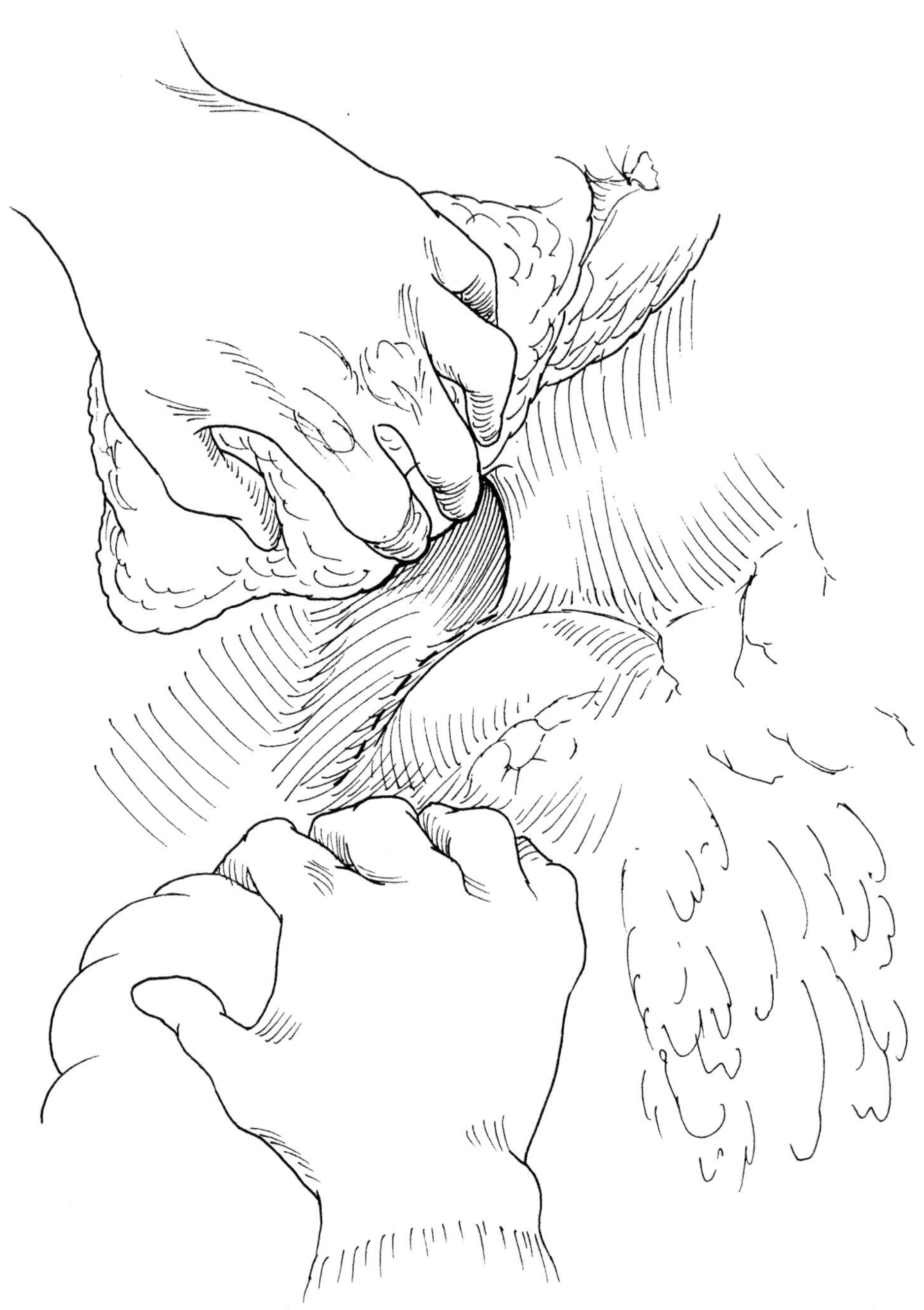

Fig. 14-10 Elevation of the right lobe of the liver and caudal retraction of the hepatic flexure of the colon expose the hepatoduodenal ligament. The line of the peritoneal incision for mobilizing the duodenum is shown.

The portal vein is best exposed along the right posterior border of the hepatoduodenal ligament, away from the anterior aspect where distended lymphatics with large blood vessels are commonly present[11] (Fig. 14-11). It is not necessary to expose the common duct using this approach. The portal vein is usually distended and easily palpable as the most posterior structure in the hepatoduodenal ligament.[11] A longitudinal incision is made in the peritoneum over the posterior wall of the portal vein where it forms the anterior margin of the foramen of Winslow. It is important to place the incision posteriorly and not too close to the free margin of the hepatoduodenal ligament.[11] The incision is carefully extended superiorly as far as the liver hilum and inferiorly as far as the head of the pancreas. Using careful blunt dissection, the portal vein is encircled with a vessel tape in the midpoint

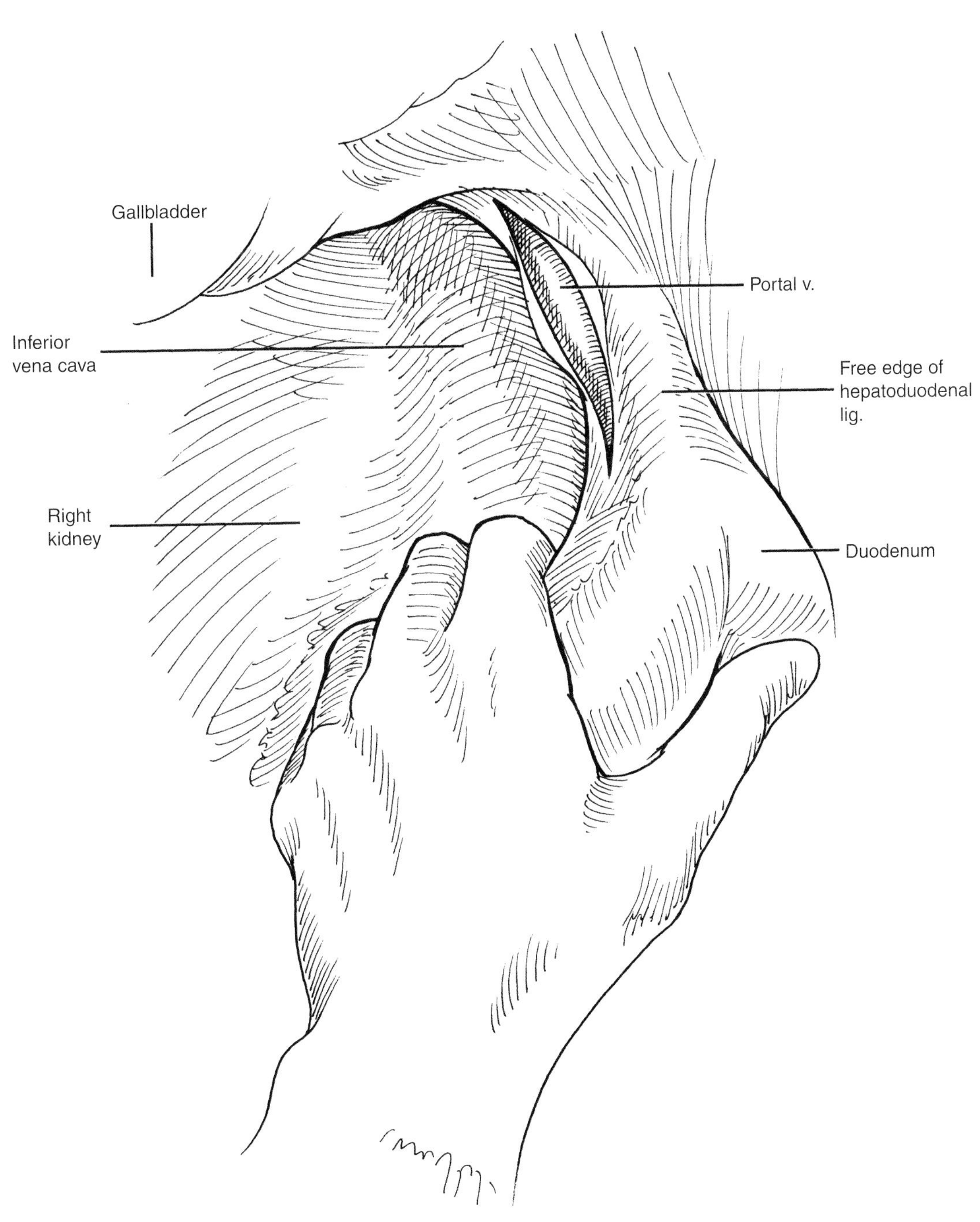

Fig. 14-11 The portal vein is exposed on the posterolateral surface of the hepatoduodenal ligament.

of the hepatoduodenal ligament. Gentle traction placed on the portal vein exposes major branches, including the pyloric, duodenal, right gastric, and coronary veins, that drain into its medial surfaces (Fig. 14-12). Inferiorly, the large coronary vein can often be found at the portal vein's medial surface near its intersection with the splenic vein. After meticulous ligation and division of all portal vein tributaries are ensured, the portal vein can be exposed and completely mobilized from the level of the pancreas to its bifurcation at the liver hilum. Dissection of the portal vein behind the pancreas is difficult because of dense vascular, lymphatic, and connective tissues located in the area.[11] In patients with invasive pancreatic cancer, separate exposure of the superior mesenteric and splenic veins below the pancreas allows vascular control during tumor resection.[9] It is important to bear in mind that anomalous right hepatic arteries pass near the portal vein (see Chapter 19).

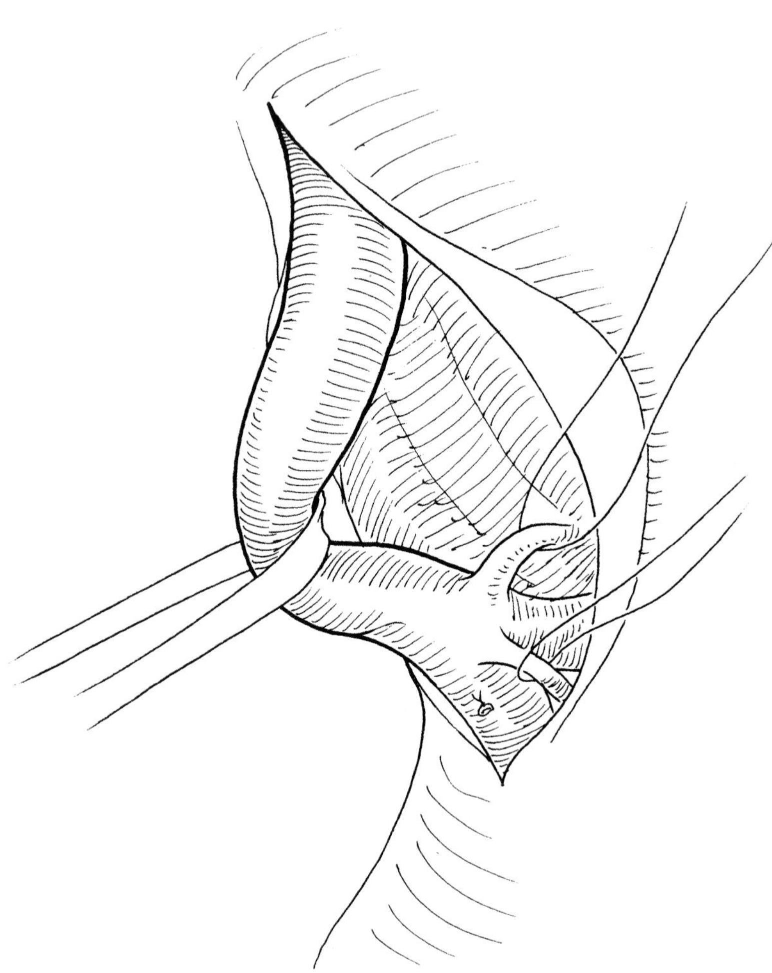

Fig. 14-12 The portal vein is isolated, and venous tributaries draining into the origin of the portal vein are ligated and divided.

Exposure of the Superior Mesenteric Vein

The patient is placed in the supine position, and the entire abdomen and lower chest are prepped and draped. A midline abdominal incision made from a point halfway between the umbilicus and xiphoid process to the top of the pubis provides excellent exposure and can be extended superiorly as necessary. The incision should be carried to the left of the umbilicus to prevent entry into the engorged umbilical vein. A transverse midabdominal incision is a useful alternative but may be associated with increased blood loss from venous collaterals in the abdominal wall.

After the peritoneal cavity has been entered and carefully examined, the transverse colon is elevated and retracted superiorly to expose the root of the mesocolon (Fig. 14-13). The small intestine is retracted inferiorly, placing the intestinal mesentery

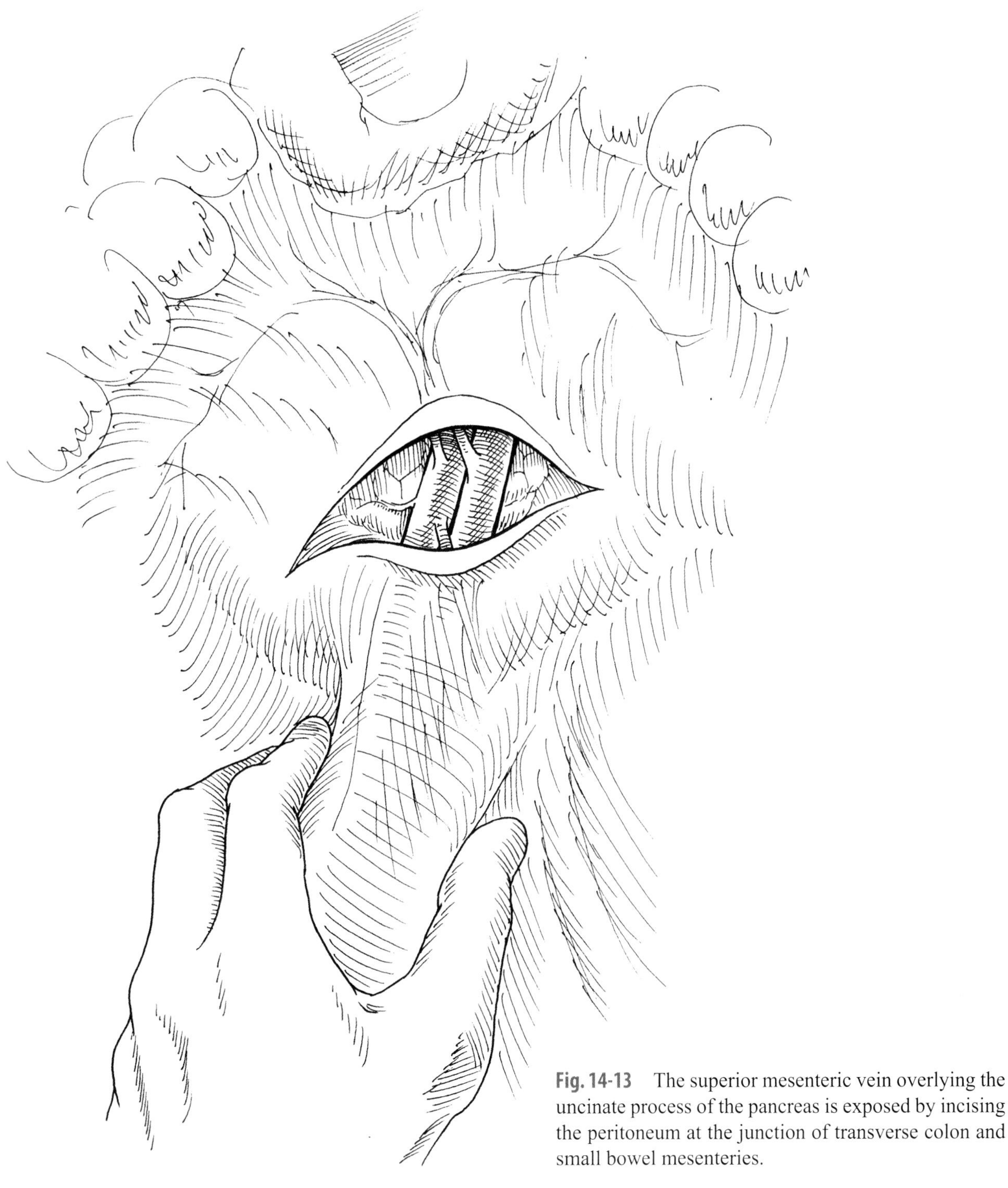

Fig. 14-13 The superior mesenteric vein overlying the uncinate process of the pancreas is exposed by incising the peritoneum at the junction of transverse colon and small bowel mesenteries.

under slight tension. The superior mesenteric artery can be palpated at the base of the transverse mesocolon; the vein lies to the right of the artery near the midline. A 7-cm transverse incision is made in the peritoneum at the root of the transverse mesocolon, and the superior mesenteric vein is carefully exposed. If necessary, a superior T extension can be made onto the transverse mesocolon for additional exposure. Multiple well-vascularized lymphatics overlying the vein require careful dissection and meticulous control to avoid hemorrhage.[11] After the vein is freed on all sides, it is carefully encircled with a vessel tape (Fig. 14-14). Dissection should proceed superiorly to the point where the middle colic vein enters the superior mesenteric vein as the latter courses over the uncinate process.[11] Numerous tributaries entering the vein on the anterior and left lateral surfaces must be ligated and divided. To gain more proximal exposure, the superior mesenteric vein can be further isolated to the point where it disappears under the inferior border of the pancreatic neck by dividing the middle colic branch. Distally, the vein can be isolated for only a short distance before it branches into tributaries too small

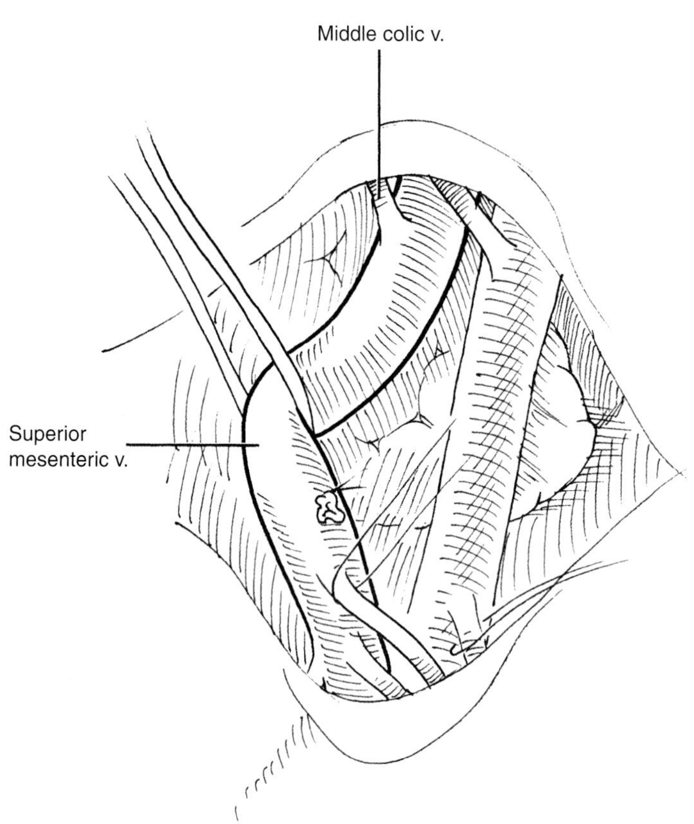

Fig. 14-14 The superior mesenteric vein is controlled, and branches are ligated to provide space for the anastomosis. The right colic vein may be divided, if necessary.

for bypass construction. Still, enough of the superior mesenteric vein can usually be isolated over the uncinate process to permit creation of a large anastomosis.[11]

In the patient undergoing a portosystemic shunt, direct access to the inferior vena cava can be obtained by opening the posterior peritoneum over the third part of the duodenum to the right of the mesenteric vein. Careful upward mobilization of the duodenum exposes the underlying vena cava (Fig. 14-15). Grafts brought from the anterior surface of the vena cava should curve beneath the duodenum to reach the anterolateral surface of the large, single trunk of the superior mesenteric vein over the uncinate process, assuming a C shape. Alternatively, a short H-graft configuration can be brought more directly from the vena cava to the posterior surface of the superior mesenteric vein. The latter is less desirable because the superior mesenteric anastomosis is made at a more distal location where the vein is of smaller caliber and has multiple branches.

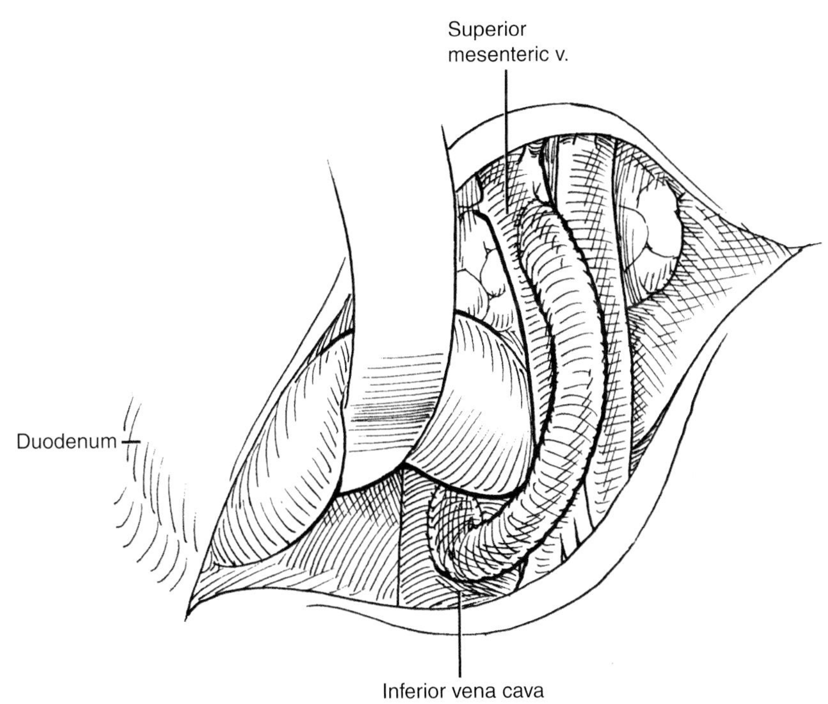

Fig. 14-15 Mobilization of the duodenum to the right of the superior mesenteric vein provides direct access to the underlying inferior vena cava.

Alternate exposure of the inferior vena cava can be obtained by mobilizing the right colon (see Chapter 13). A tunnel from the vena cava to the superior mesenteric vein should be carefully created in the base of the right colon mesentery to the right of the superior mesenteric vein (Fig. 14-16). Grafts brought to the mesenteric vein from the vena cava in this fashion are routed around the third portion of the duodenum and again anastomosed to the anterior surface of the superior mesenteric vein over the uncinate process.

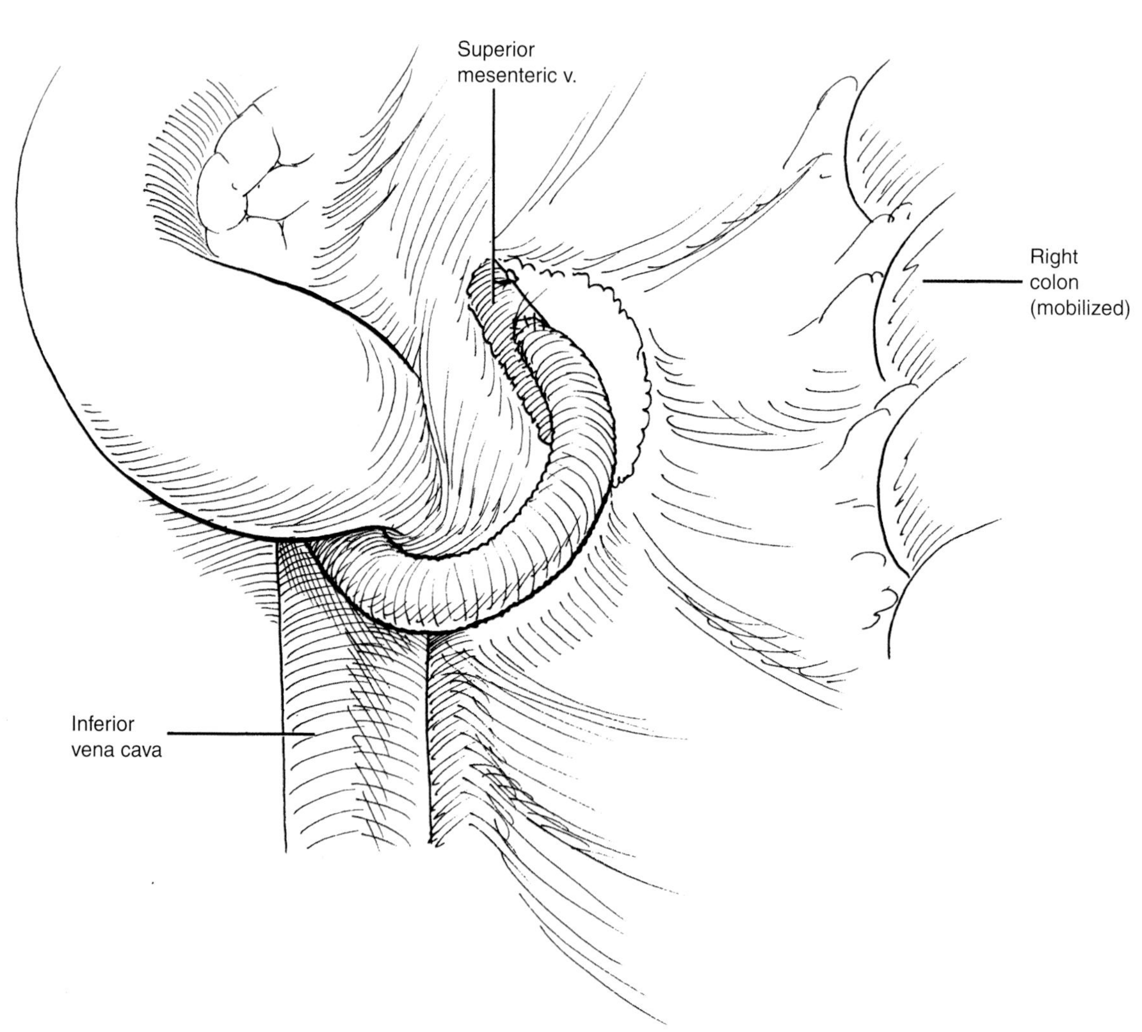

Fig. 14-16 The alternative approach of mobilizing the right colon provides wider exposure of the inferior vena cava. The graft is then brought through a tunnel in the mobilized right colon mesentery to reach the superior mesenteric vein over the uncinate process.

Exposure of the Splenic Vein

There are two popular approaches to the splenic vein: a direct approach through the lesser sac[12] and an inferior approach beneath the root of the mesocolon.[13] The former approach offers the advantages of simultaneous gastric venous devascularization and complete exposure of the pancreatic body and tail, but dissection is often carried out through a deep, narrow hole into the retroperitoneum. The latter approach is associated with reduced retraction requirements and a more central approach to the splenic vein, but isolation of the entire splenic vein to effect a complete splenopancreatic disconnection[12] is more difficult.

Approach through the Lesser Sac

The patient is placed in the supine position with the lower chest and abdomen prepped and draped. Warren and Millikan[12] advocate a "hockey stick" incision 1 to 2 cm below the left costal margin, extending across the midline to the lateral border of the right rectus muscle (Fig. 14-17). An alternative is the upper midline approach; thoracoabdominal incisions are too extensive and associated with needless morbidity. On entering the abdominal cavity, the falciform ligament and the umbilical vein are ligated and divided. The lesser sac is entered by dividing the gastrocolic ligament between the gastroepiploic arcade and the greater curvature

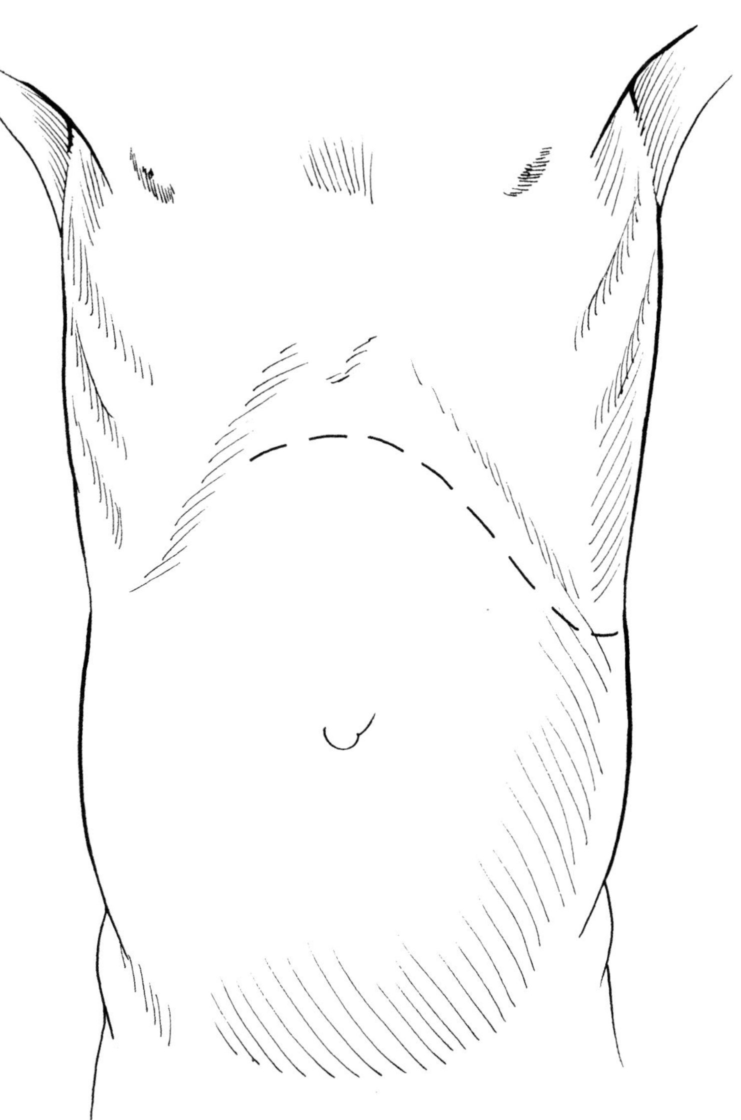

Fig. 14-17 An extended left subcostal incision provides good exposure of the splenic vein.

of the stomach, taking care to ligate all gastric branches (Fig. 14-18). The gastrocolic ligament should be divided from the pylorus to the lowest short gastric vein, and the right gastroepiploic vessels should be ligated. This reduces portosystemic collateralization without compromising the blood supply of the stomach.[12] It is crucial to leave the short gastric veins intact because they represent the principal conduit for decompression of esophageal varices. After dividing adhesions between the posterior wall of the stomach and the pancreas, the greater curvature of the stomach is elevated, allowing cephalad retraction of the posterior stomach.

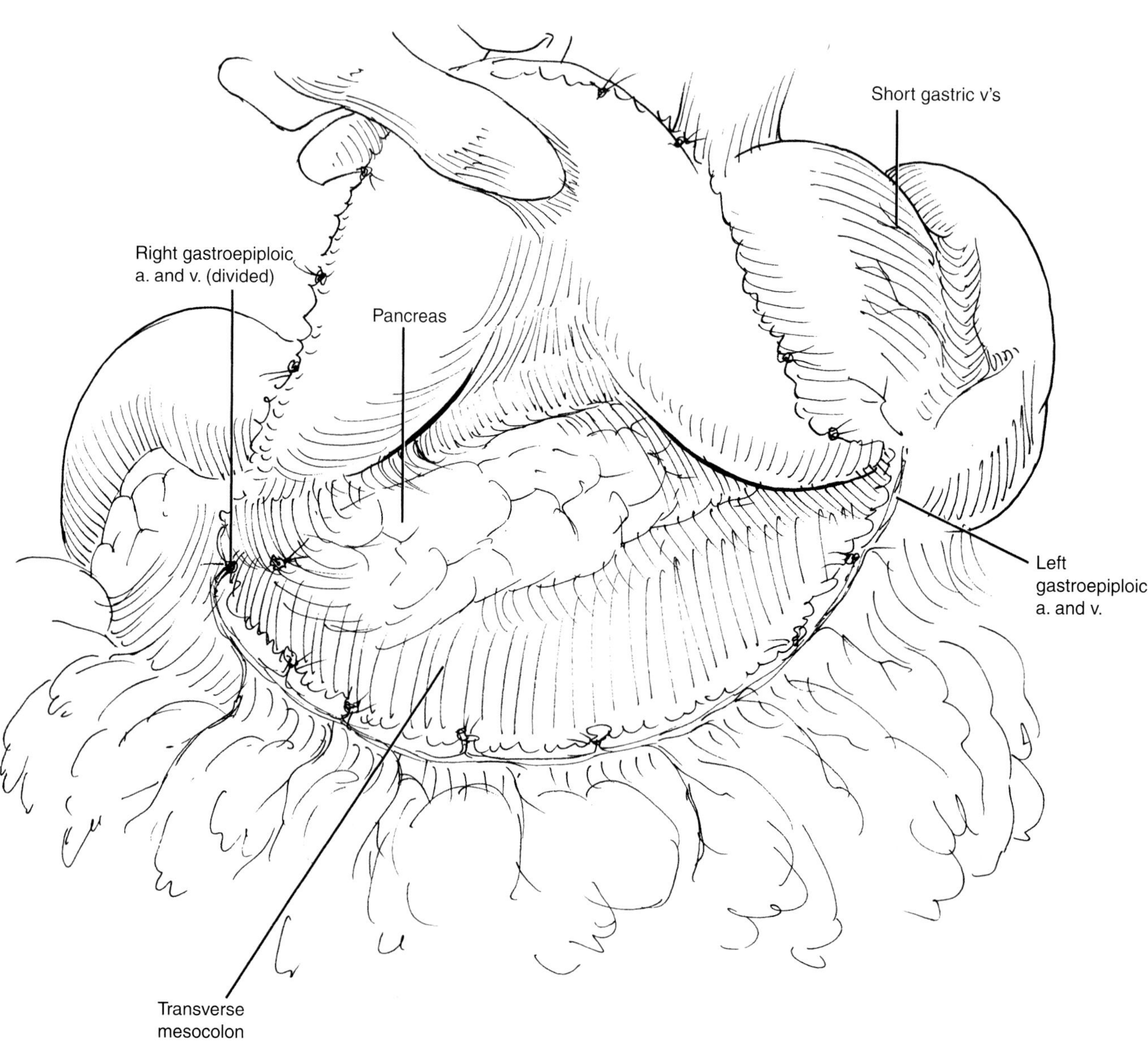

Fig. 14-18 The gastroepiploic arcade is disconnected from the stomach, and the right gastric artery and vein are divided to approach the splenic vein through the lesser sac.

The inferior border of the pancreas is mobilized next (Fig. 14-19). The posterior parietal peritoneum between the pancreas and the duodenum is relatively avascular and should be incised from the level of the superior mesenteric vessels to the tail of the pancreas.[12] Elevation and cephalad retraction of the inferior border of the pancreas allow palpation of the splenic vein along the posterior aspect of the gland. Dissection of the vein commences by incising the adventitial tissues directly overlying the vein's posterior surface. After the posterior surface has been exposed for its entire length, dissection proceeds medially along the vein's inferior border to its superior mesenteric junction. A cluster of vein branches frequently drains into this area, and meticulous ligation and division are necessary for safe isolation of the splenic–mesenteric–portal vein juncture.[12] The splenic vein should be completely isolated and encircled at its junction with the portal vein. The coronary and right gastric veins should be sought near the upper angle of the junction and carefully ligated. The inferior mesenteric vein should also be ligated and divided near its termination at the splenic or superior mesenteric vein.

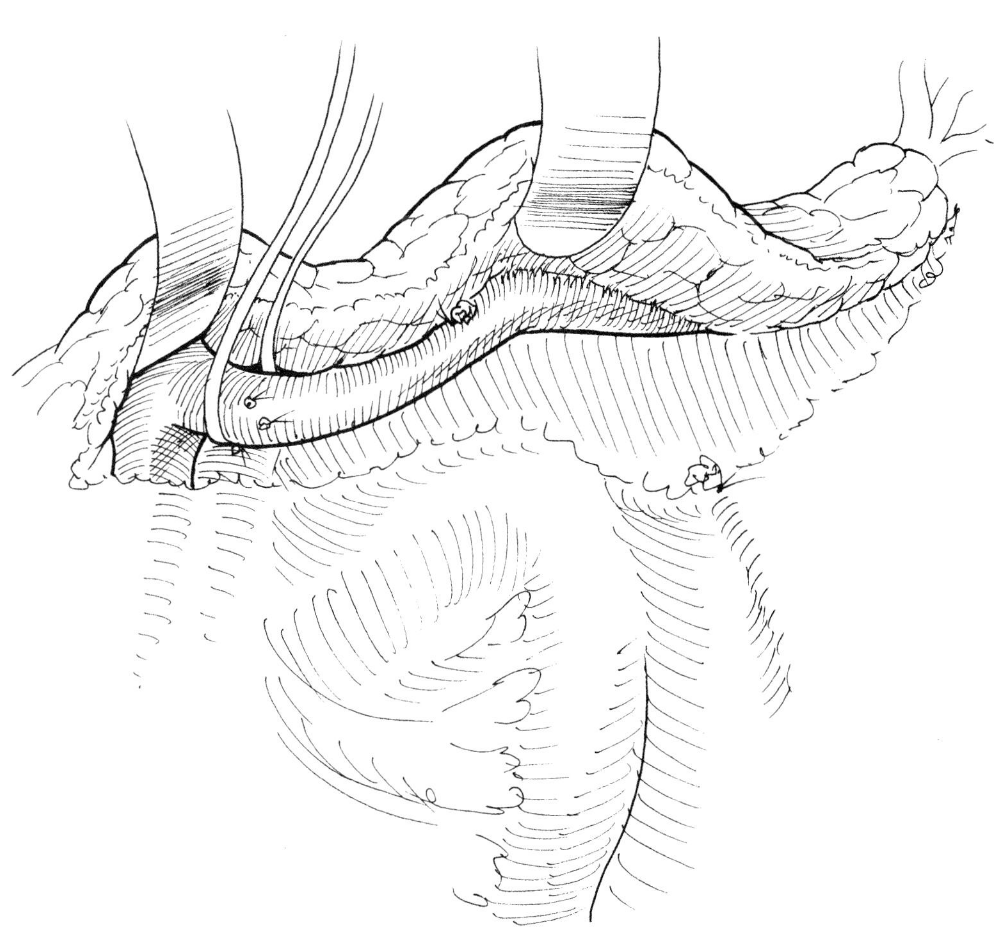

Fig. 14-19 The lower border of the pancreas is mobilized to expose the splenic vein.

Lateral dissection of the splenic vein can now be performed along its superior margin, taking great care to control and ligate the multiple small branches that drain directly from the posterior wall of the pancreas (Fig. 14-20). Meticulous, unhurried dissection is required to prevent branch avulsion and rapid associated blood loss. The splenic vein should be dissected totally free of the pancreas.[12]

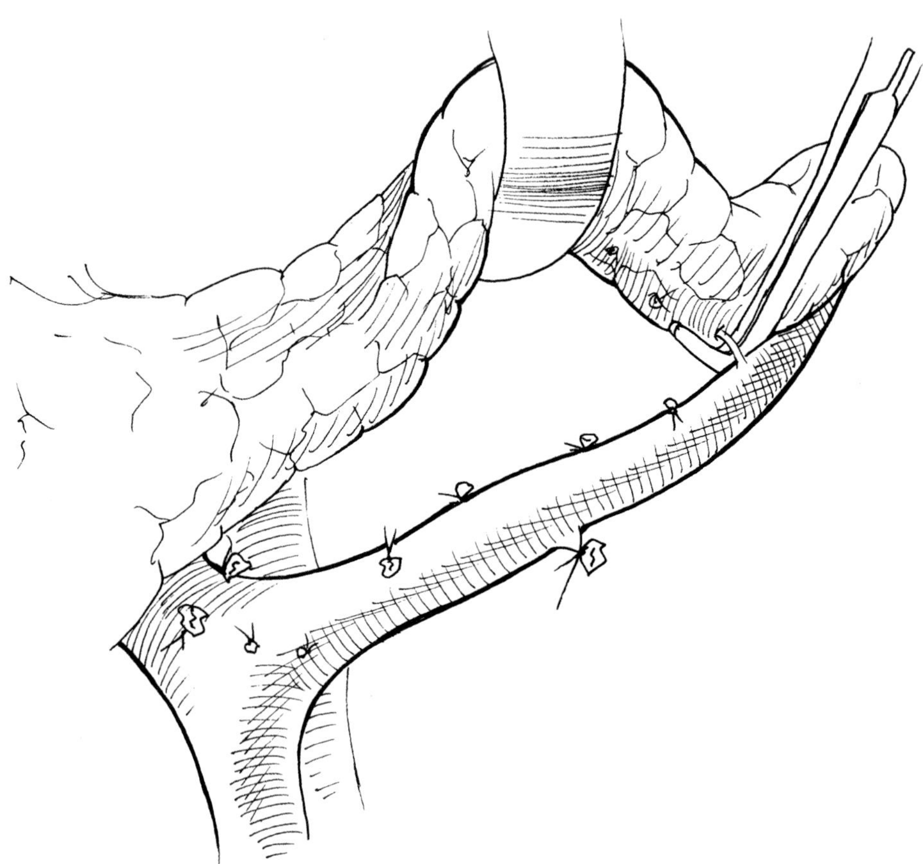

Fig. 14-20 Multiple small pancreatic branches are divided to free the splenic vein.

To create a distal splenorenal (Warren) shunt, the left renal vein is isolated in the retroperitoneal tissues inferior and deep to the splenic vein. The left adrenal and gonadal branches should be divided close to the renal vein to permit wide mobilization. In preparation for anastomosis, the splenic vein should be divided as close to the splenic–portal–mesenteric junction as possible and brought directly to the left renal vein (Fig. 14-21).

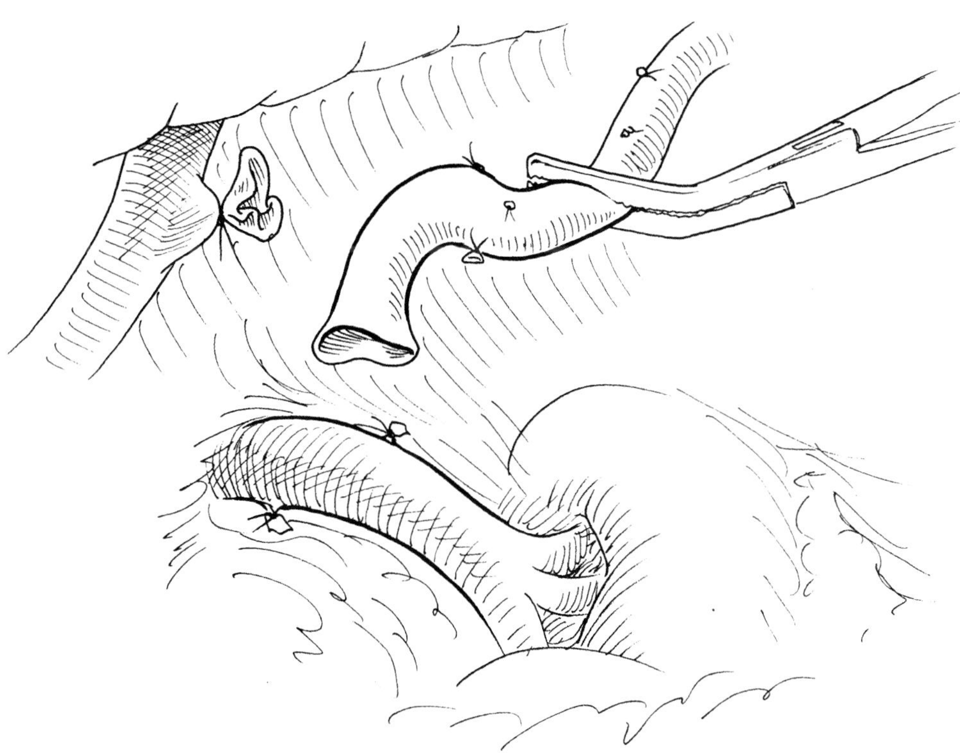

Fig. 14-21 The left renal vein is exposed, and the splenic vein is ligated and divided as proximally as possible.

Approach beneath the Mesocolon

The patient is positioned and prepped as previously described. An upper midline incision provides excellent exposure, although a supraumbilical transverse incision may be used instead.

After entry into the peritoneal cavity, the transverse mesocolon is elevated, and the small intestines are wrapped in moist laparotomy pads and retracted to the patient's right side. The retroperitoneal space is entered through a vertical incision in the posterior peritoneum over the infrarenal aorta. The incision is carried superiorly to include division of the ligament of Treitz, allowing rightward reflection of the third and fourth portions of the duodenum. The left renal vein is identified as it crosses the aorta in the superior incision. The vein is encircled, and its gonadal and adrenal branches are divided to permit wide mobilization.

To locate the splenic vein, the posterior parietal incision is extended to the left along the root of the mesocolon, parallel to the inferior border of the pancreas (Fig. 14-22). The inferior mesenteric vein should be identified as it courses along beneath the posterior parietal peritoneum to the left of the aorta and traced superiorly to locate the splenic vein. Anterior and cephalad retraction of the inferior border of the pancreas exposes the splenic vein coursing along the posterior pancreatic surface. The remainder of the dissection proceeds as previously described.

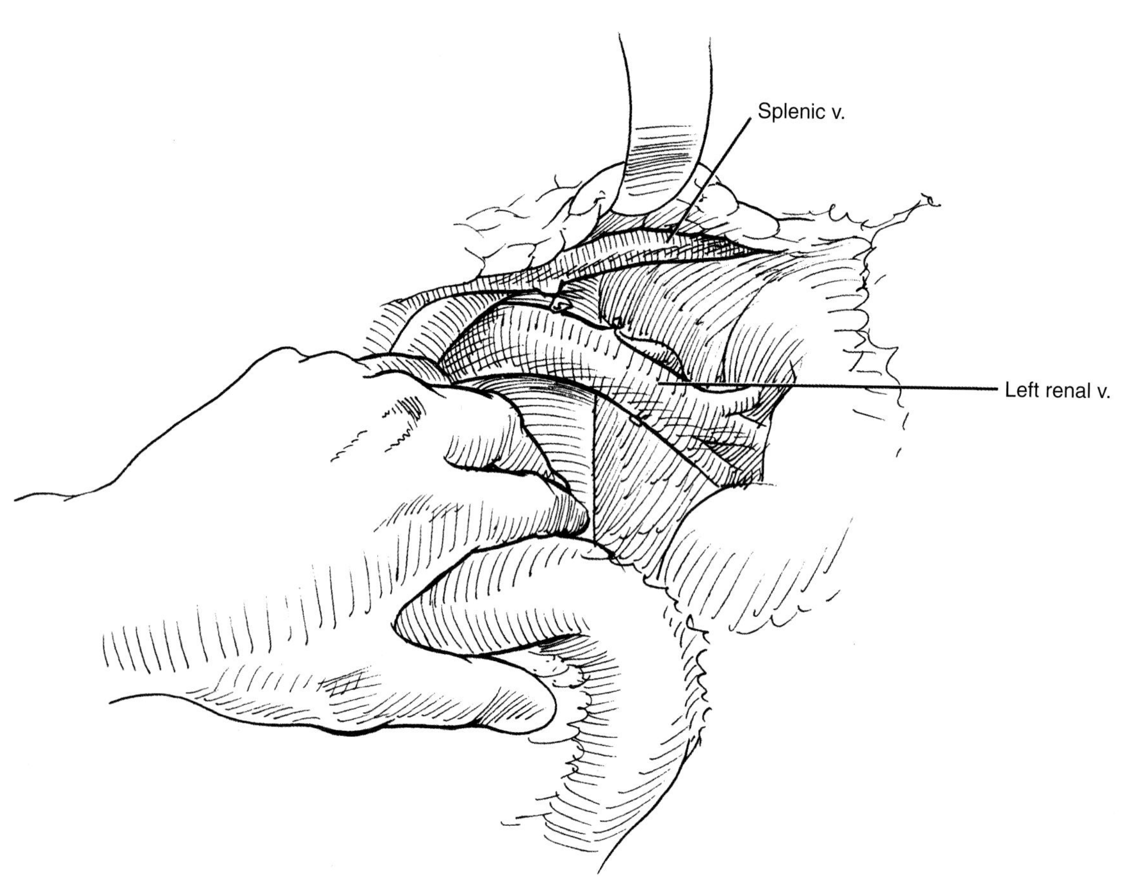

Fig. 14-22 The splenic and renal veins may also be reached through the root of the transverse mesocolon.

References

1. Rosemurgy AS, Zorros EE. Management of variceal hemorrhage. *Curr Prob Surg*. 2003;40:255–343.
2. Rana SS, Bjasin DK. Gastrointestinal bleeding: from conventional to nonconventional. *Endoscopy*. 2008;40:40–44.
3. Wright AS, Rikkers LF. Current management of portal hypertension. *J Gastrointest Surg*. 2005;9: 992–1005.
4. Livingstone AS, Koniaris LG, Perez EA, et al. 507 Warren-Zeppa distal splenorenal shunts: a 34-year experience. *Ann Surg*. 2006;243:884–892.
5. Sarfeh IJ, Rypins EB, Fardi M, et al. Clinical implications of portal hemodynamics after small-diameter portacaval H graft. *Surgery*. 1984;96:223–229.
6. Johansen K, Eide B, Carrico CJ. Enhanced survival in patients with variceal bleeding after elective portal decompression. *Am J Surg*. 1983;145:596–598.
7. Asensio JA, Petrone P, Garcia-Nunez L, et al. Superior mesenteric venous injuries: to ligate or to repair remains the question. *J Trauma*. 2007;62(3):668–675.
8. Fraga GP, Bansal V, Fortlage D, et al. A 20-year experience with portal and superior mesenteric venous injuries: has anything changed? *Eur J Vasc Endovasc Surg*. 2009;37(1):87–91.
9. Lee DY, Mitchell EL, Jones MA, et al. Techniques and results of portal vein/superior mesenteric vein reconstruction using femoral and saphenous vein during pancreaticoduodenectomy. *J Vasc Surg*. 2010;51:662–666.
10. Fleming JB, Barnett CC, Clagett GP. Superficial femoral vein as a conduit for portal vein reconstruction during pancreaticoduodenectomy. *Arch Surg*. 2005;140:698–701.
11. Smith GW. Portal hypertension. In: Shackelford RT, Zuidema GD, eds. *Surgery of the Alimentary Tract*. Philadelphia, PA: WB Saunders; 1983: 513–604.
12. Warren WD, Millikan WJ. Selective transsplenic decompression procedure: changes in technique after 300 cases. *Contemp Surg*. 1981;18:11–26.
13. Zapolanski A, Siminovitch J, Cooperman AM. A simplified method and approach to the distal splenorenal shunt. *Surg Gynecol Obstet*. 1980;150:405–406.

VESSELS OF THE LOWER EXTREMITY

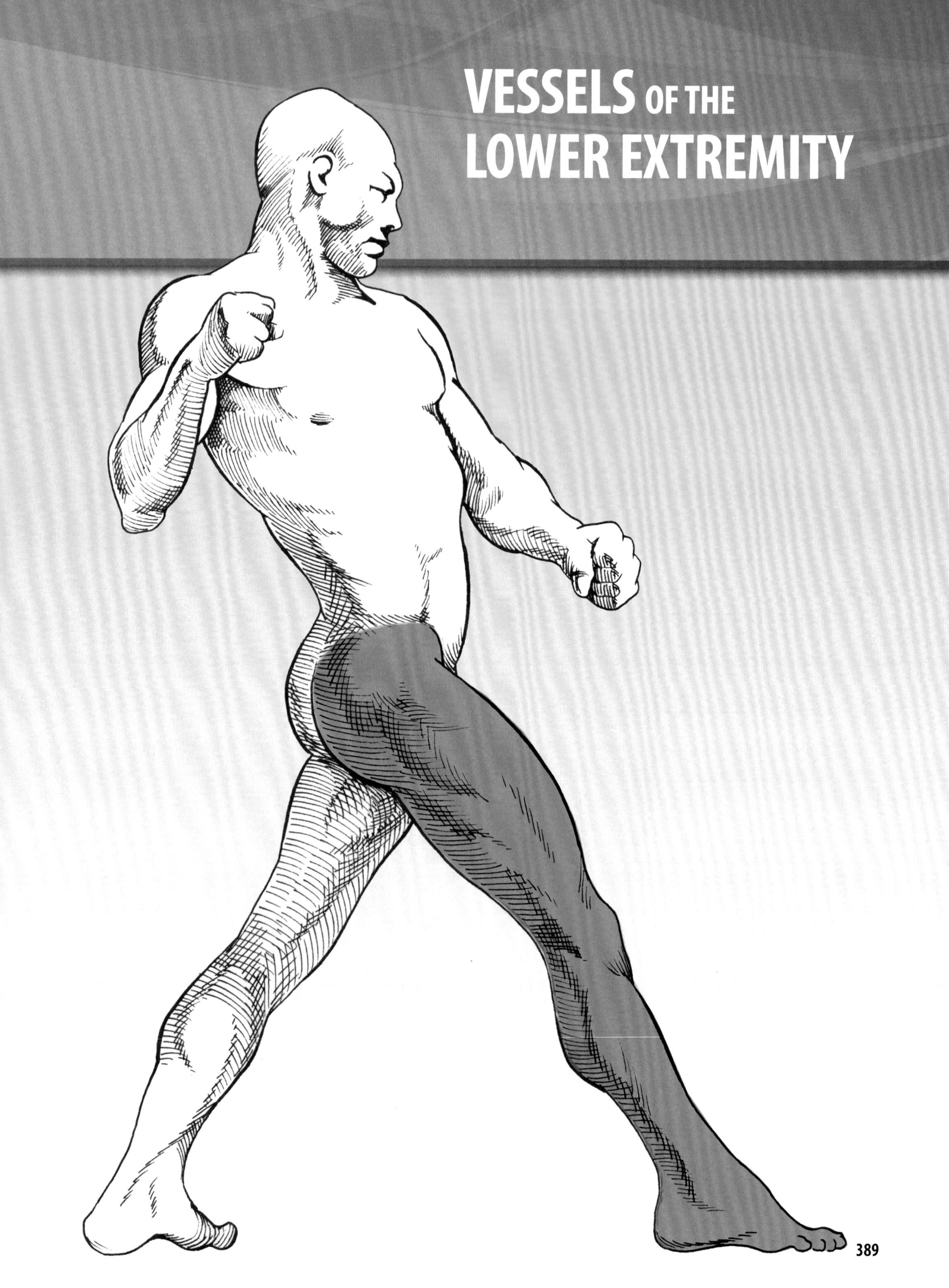

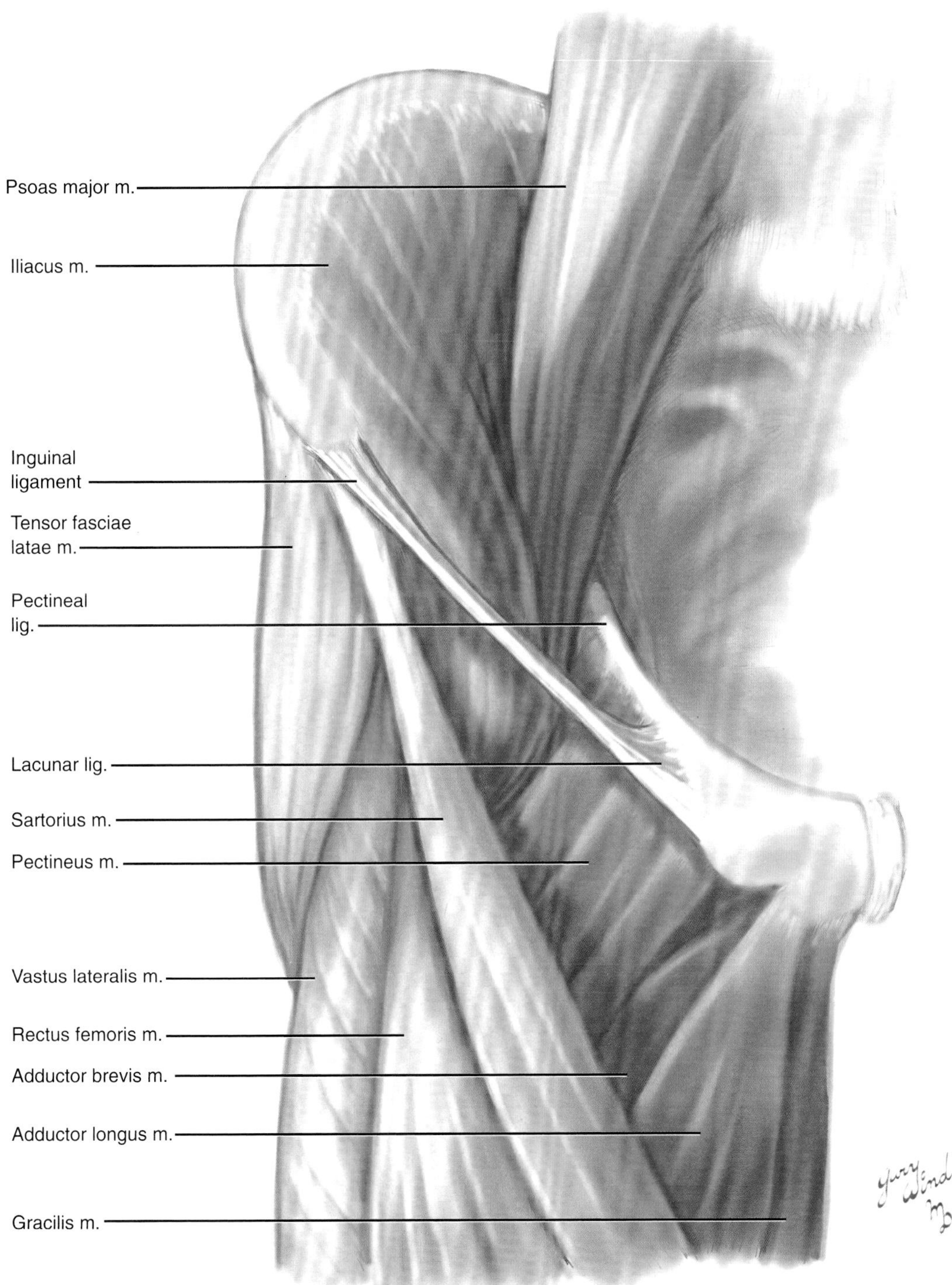

Fig. 15-1 The femoral vessels pass beneath the inguinal ligament medial to the bulk of the iliopsoas muscle. After crossing the pectineal line of the pubis, the vessels cross the pectineus muscle en route to the subsartorial femoral canal.

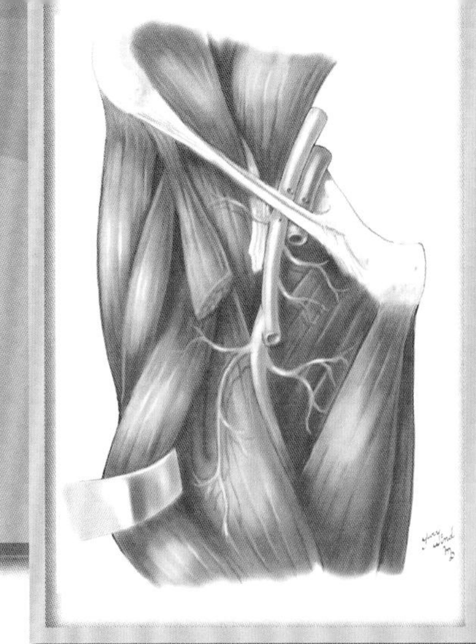

Common Femoral Artery

15

Surgical Anatomy of the Femoral Region

The femoral artery is the principal channel supplying blood to the lower extremity. The boundary marking the transition between the external iliac and common femoral arteries is the inguinal ligament. The artery lies just medial to the midpoint of the inguinal ligament, within a triangular passage between the pelvis and thigh. This femoral vascular aperture is bounded laterally by the iliopsoas muscles, medially by the reflected fibers of the inguinal ligament (forming the lacunar ligament), and posteriorly by the superior ramus of the pubis (Fig. 15-1).

The proximal femoral artery and vein are wrapped in a fibrous covering called the femoral sheath. This sheath is made up of several components (Fig. 15-2). The lateral part of the sheath adjacent to the femoral nerve is the continuation of the iliac fascia covering the iliopsoas muscle. The posterior portion of the sheath is the fascia covering the pectineus muscle. Anteriorly and medially, the sheath is a tubular extension of the transversalis endoabdominal fascia lining the anterior abdominal wall. Within the sheath, there is a well-developed septum separating the artery from the vein. The sheath fits snugly around the vessels except on the medial side, where a narrow channel (femoral canal)

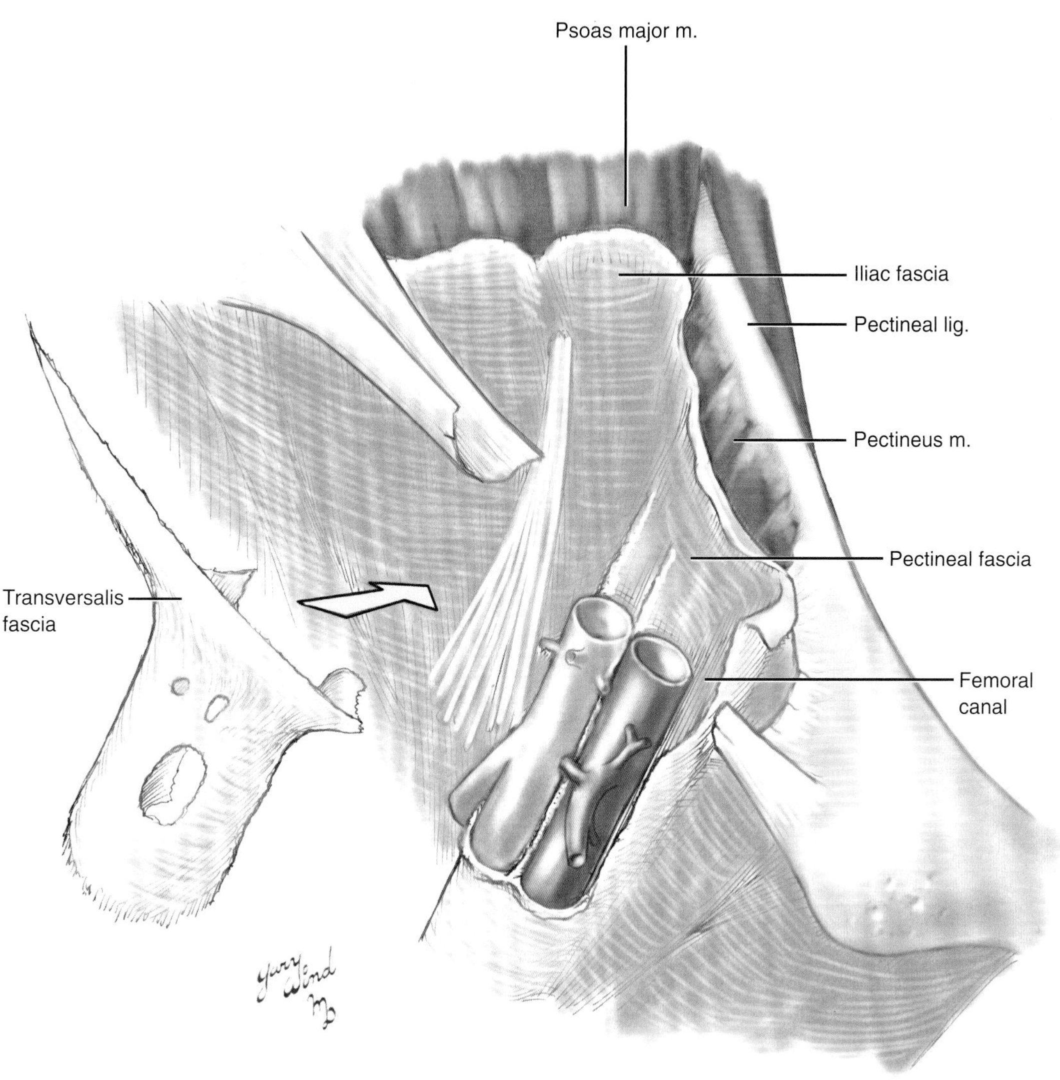

Fig. 15-2 The femoral sheath enclosing the vessels is a continuation of the endoabdominal fascia. The components of this fascia contributing to the sheath are named transversalis, iliac, and pectineal fascia. The femoral canal is the space within the sheath medial to the femoral vein.

accommodates the passage of lymphatics. The pelvic end of this channel is covered with weak fascia and is the site through which a femoral hernia passes (Fig. 15-3). The femoral sheath becomes continuous with the adventitia of the vessels at the origin of the deep femoral artery and vein. The sheath is perforated by small arterial branches and the great saphenous vein.

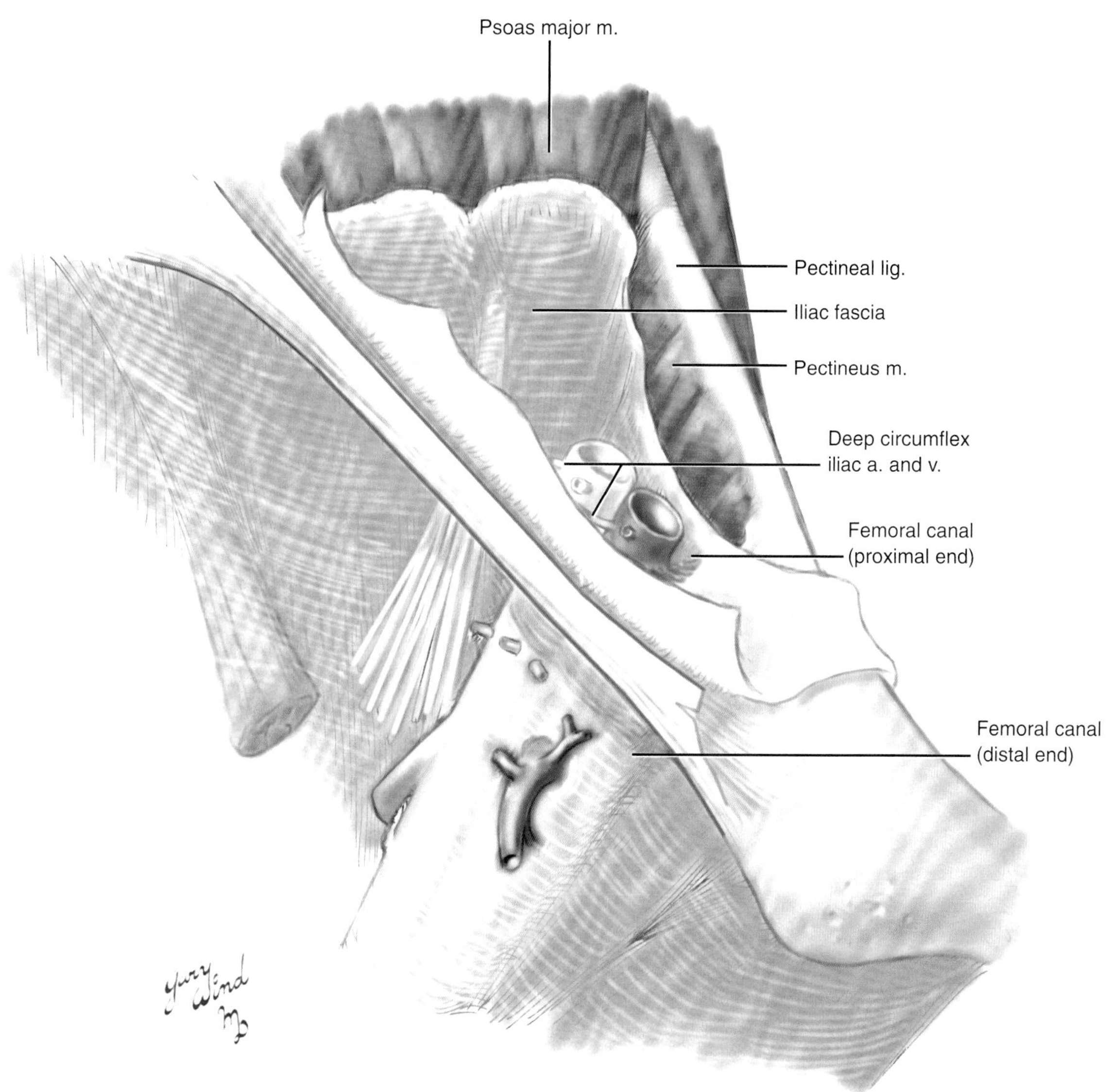

Fig. 15-3 The proximal end of the femoral canal is covered with loose fascia, which is violated when a femoral hernia forms. The hernia dissects and breaches the medial femoral sheath below the inguinal ligament to protrude. Peritoneum overlies both the vessels and the endoabdominal fascia.

Wrapped in their sheath, the femoral vessels lie cradled in a bed of muscles (Fig. 15-4). The course of the vessels in the proximal third of the thigh lies within another triangular space defined by muscular boundaries (Scarpa's triangle). The lateral margin of the triangle is formed by the sartorius muscle, the medial margin by the adductor longus muscle, and the cephalad base of the

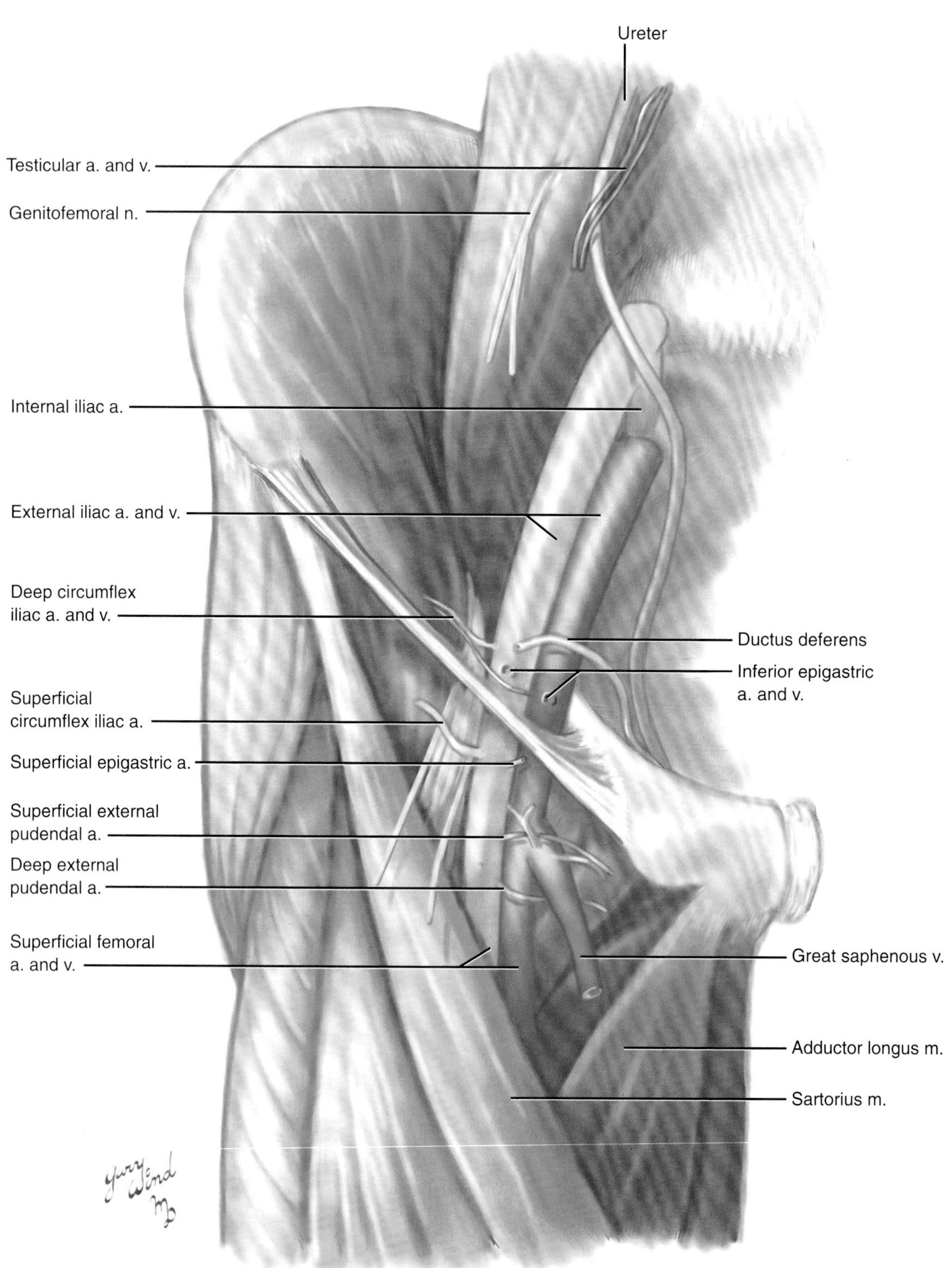

Fig. 15-4 Removing the pelvic fascia and femoral sheath reveals the relationships of other retroperitoneal structures to the vessels and exposes the small external iliac and common femoral branches above and below the inguinal ligament, respectively.

triangle by the inguinal ligament. Between these boundaries, the triangle appears as a depressed plane when the thigh is flexed in external rotation (Fig. 15-5).

The fascia lata forms an anterior roof over the femoral triangle and attaches to the inguinal ligament. It is breached by an oval opening (fossa ovalis) through which lymphatics and the great saphenous

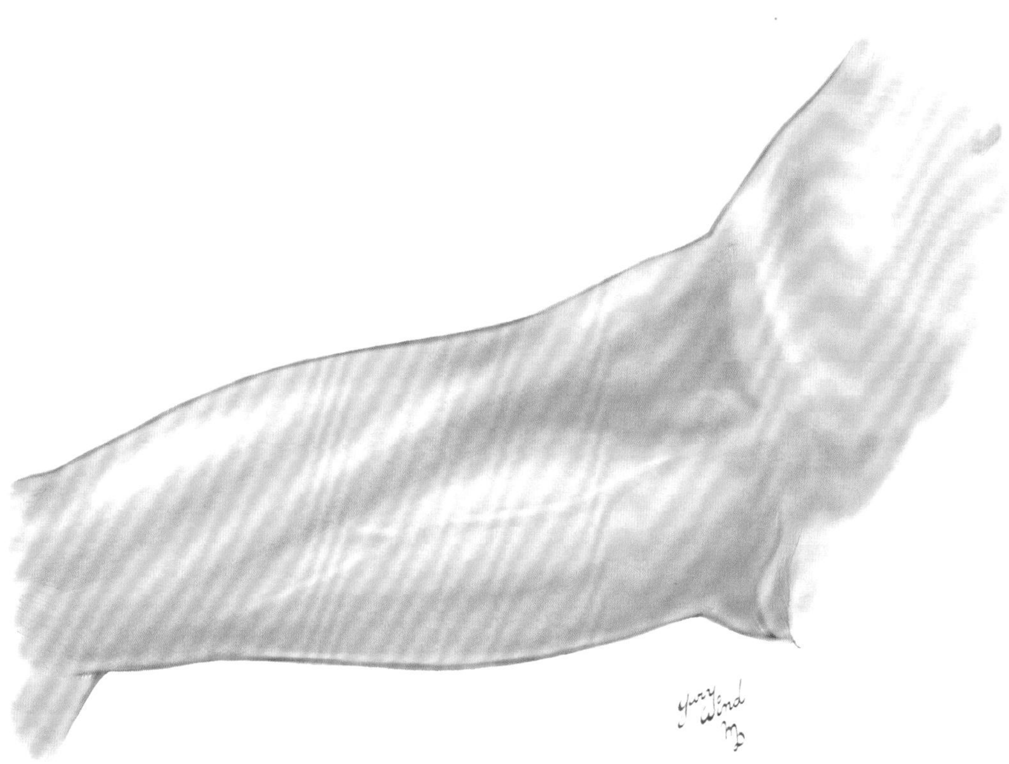

Fig. 15-5 Flexion and external rotation of the thigh make the muscular margins of the femoral triangle stand out. The sartorius muscle forms the lateral boundary, and the adductor longus muscle forms the medial border.

vein pass (Fig. 15-6). The fossa ovalis is covered by the poorly defined cribriform fascia, which supports one of two groups of superficial subinguinal lymph nodes (Fig. 15-7). The more cephalad group of nodes parallels the inguinal ligament. These nodes lie in the path of an anterior groin incision onto the femoral artery, and the rich plexus of lymphatic channels surrounding these nodes increases the

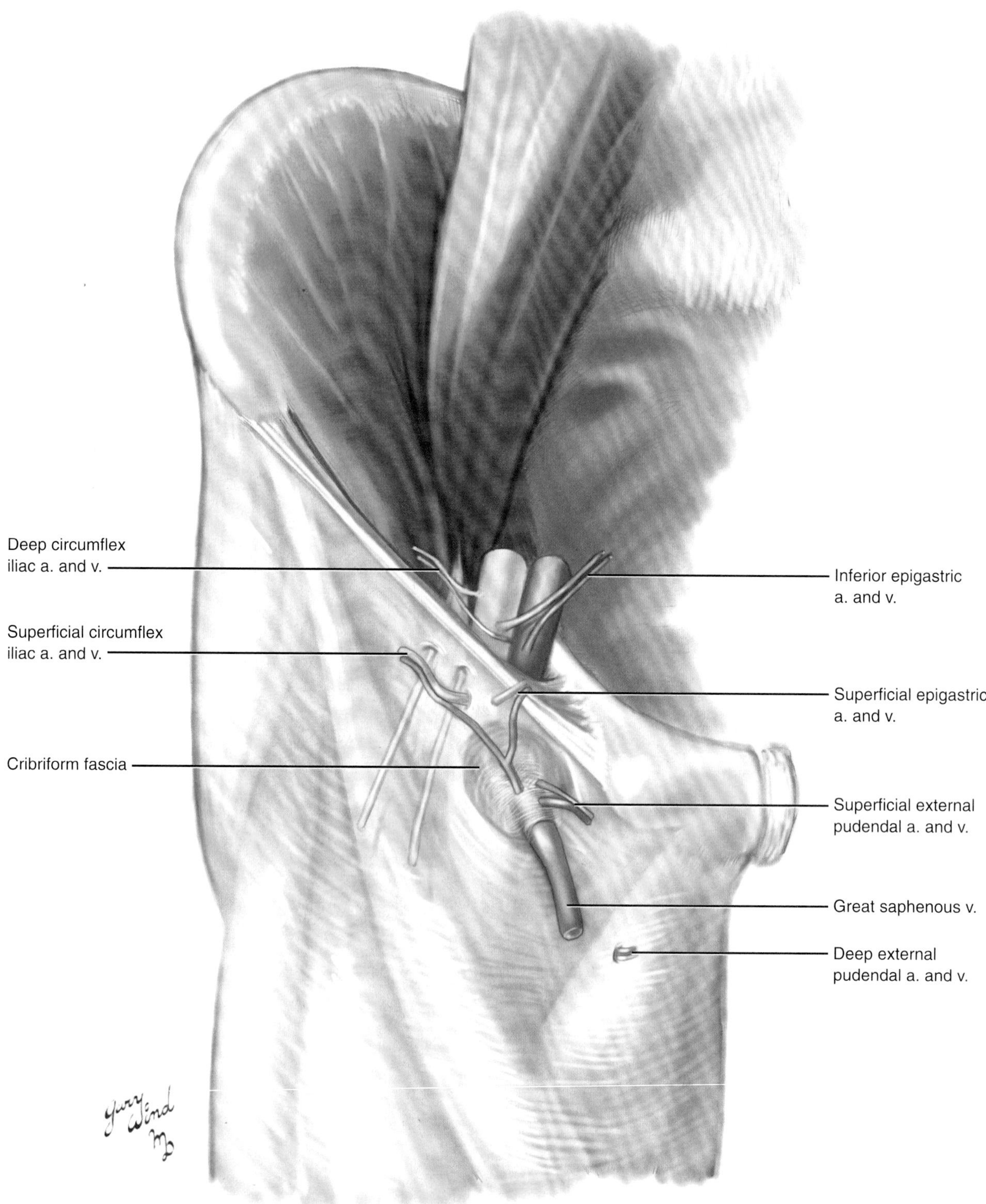

Fig. 15-6 Anteriorly, the fascia lata attaches to the inguinal ligament. It is perforated by branches of the femoral artery and by cutaneous nerves. Venous channels reach the femoral vein through the loosely capped fossa ovalis.

risk of lymphocele after incisions in this area. Both groups of nodes drain to the deep subinguinal nodes found in the fatty areolar tissue within the femoral triangle, and from there lymph drains through the femoral canal to the external iliac chain.

Three superficial branches of the femoral artery arise just distal to the inguinal ligament and penetrate both the femoral sheath and fascia lata to reach the subcutaneous tissue of the lower abdomen and upper thigh. These are the superficial external pudendal, superficial circumflex iliac, and superficial epigastric arteries. Their accompanying veins converge on the great saphenous vein near its junction with the femoral vein. These vessels should be

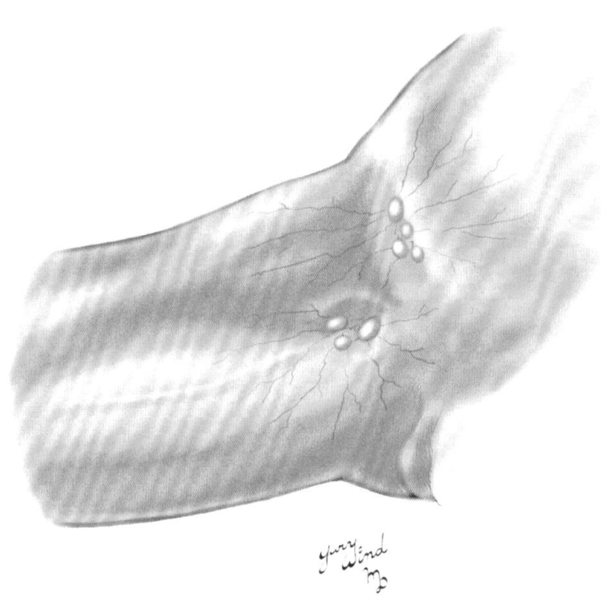

Fig. 15-7 The superficial inguinal lymph nodes are clustered beneath the inguinal ligament and around the fossa ovalis.

protected if possible when incising directly down to the femoral artery. The superficial epigastric pedicle has long been used to support an axial lower abdominal skin flap. The superficial external pudendal artery crosses the femoral vein immediately adjacent to the saphenofemoral junction.

Before peeling back the fascia lata to examine the deeper structures of the femoral triangle, we should briefly look at the relationships of the external iliac artery just inside the abdominal wall to anticipate the major route through which bypass grafts to the femoral artery must pass.

Just inside the abdominal wall, the external iliac artery gives off two small branches that run in the plane between the peritoneum and the transversalis fascia (Fig. 15-8). The inferior epigastric artery runs

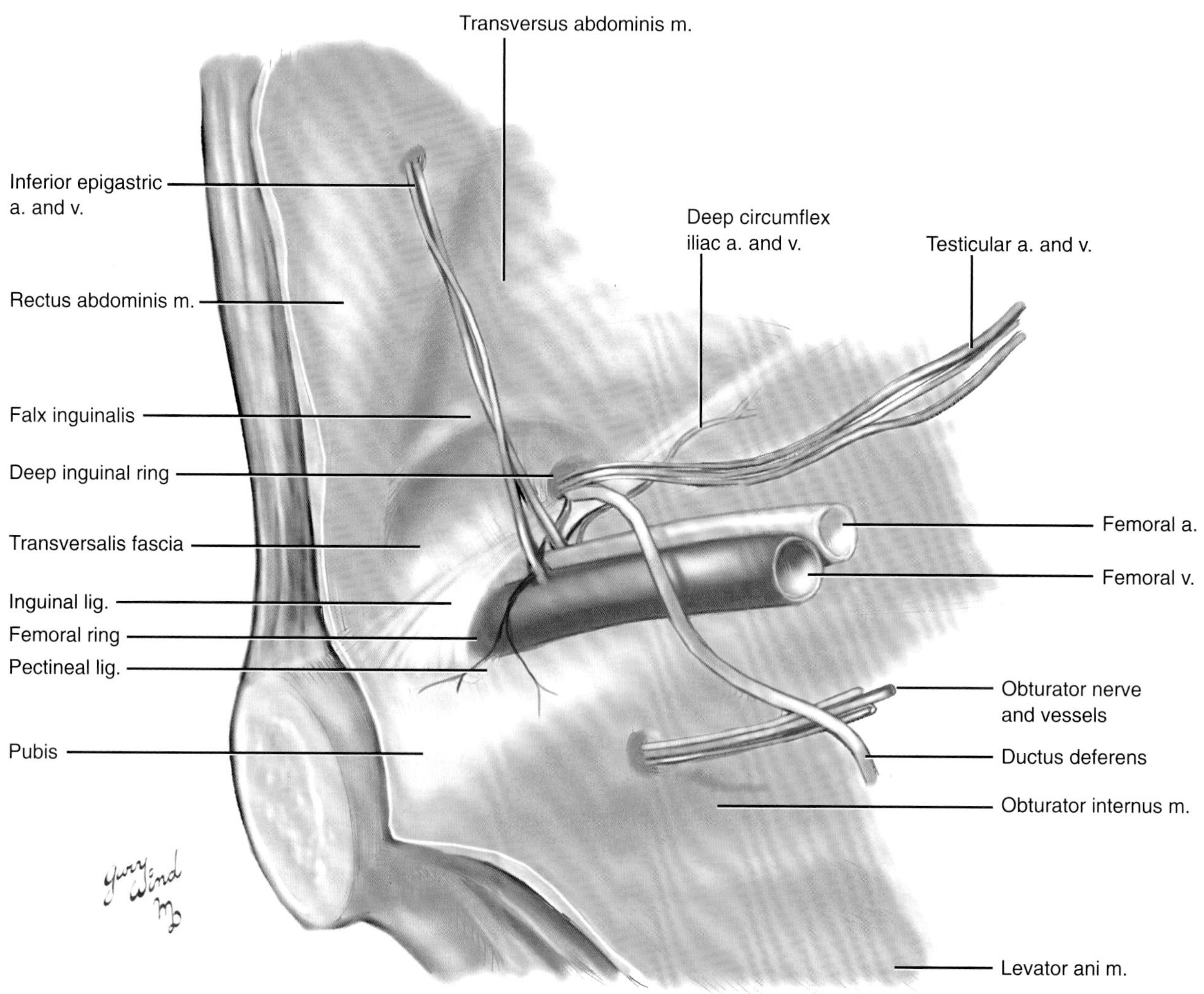

Fig. 15-8 A medial view of the right superior pubic ramus stripped of peritoneum shows the relationships of the femoral and obturator vessels.

toward the umbilicus, penetrating the transversalis fascia below the arcuate line of the posterior rectus sheath to reach the lower third of the rectus abdominis muscle. Immediately after its origin, the inferior epigastric sends a small branch with the internal oblique fibers that form the cremasteric covering of the spermatic cord in the male. The second small branch of the terminal external iliac artery is the deep circumflex iliac artery, which runs behind the lateral portion of the inguinal ligament. Any of these small arteries and especially their accompanying veins may be injured in creating the tunnel for the bypass graft. The resultant bleeding is annoying and increases the risk of infection. In addition, approximately 20% of patients have an obturator artery that arises from the inferior epigastric rather than from the internal iliac artery (Fig. 15-9 and see Fig. 19-21). This aberrant vessel descends across the pelvic end of the femoral canal and across the pectinate line of the pubis to reach the obturator canal. There is a potential for injury of this vessel during graft tunneling, a lesson learned from repair of femoral and inguinal hernias.

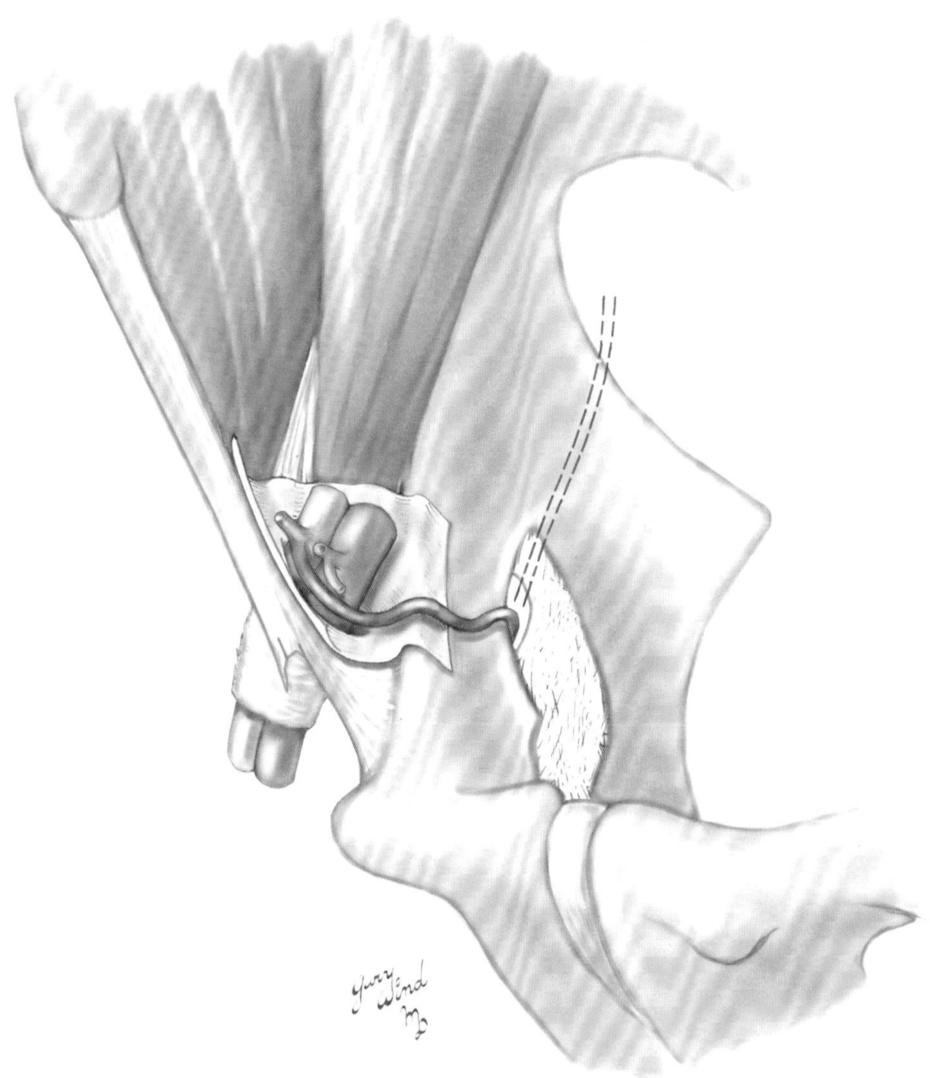

Fig. 15-9 A surgically treacherous origin of the obturator artery from the inferior epigastric artery is found in nearly one-fifth of individuals.

The floor of the femoral triangle beneath the femoral vessels consists of the pectineus muscle medially and the iliopsoas muscle arching over the anterior aspect of the hip joint laterally (see Fig. 15-1). The proximity of the underlying hip joint is demonstrated by the occasional joint infection after femoral arteriography when sterile technique is broken. Deep to the pectineus muscle lies the obturator foramen, covered by a dense membrane in all but its cephalad portion (Fig. 15-10).

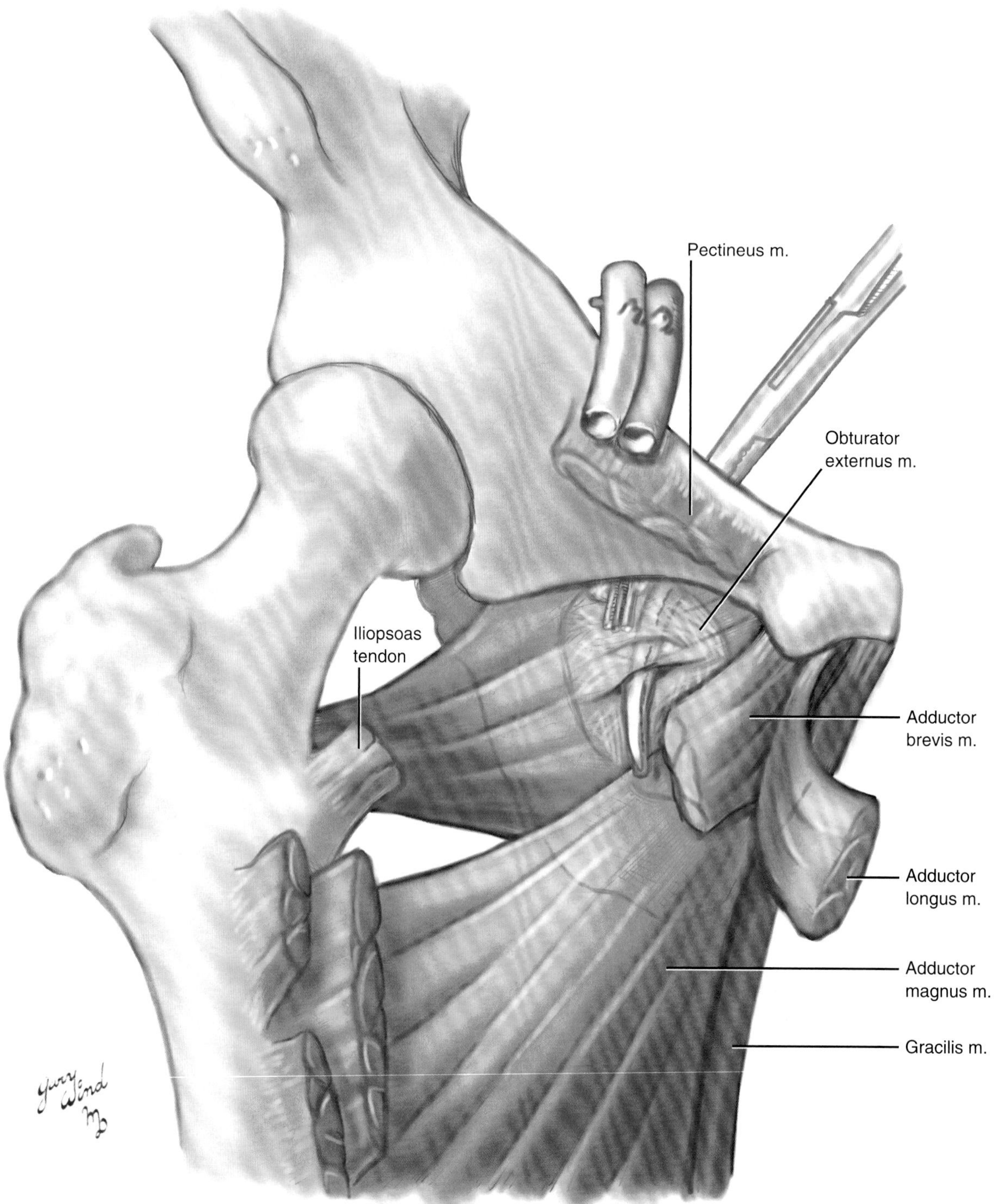

Fig. 15-10 The relationships of obturator membrane, obturator canal, obturator externus muscle, and surrounding adductor muscle origins make the obturator membrane a practical route for bypass grafts.

The attachments of the adductor muscles around the bony margins of the obturator foramen form the rim of a cone, with the obturator membrane as its base. Within this cone, the obturator externus muscle has its broad origin from the lower part of the membrane, and the obturator nerve and vessels pass from the pelvis to the thigh through the more cephalad obturator canal. The obturator membrane provides an alternate route for bypass grafts to the femoral artery (Fig. 15-11).

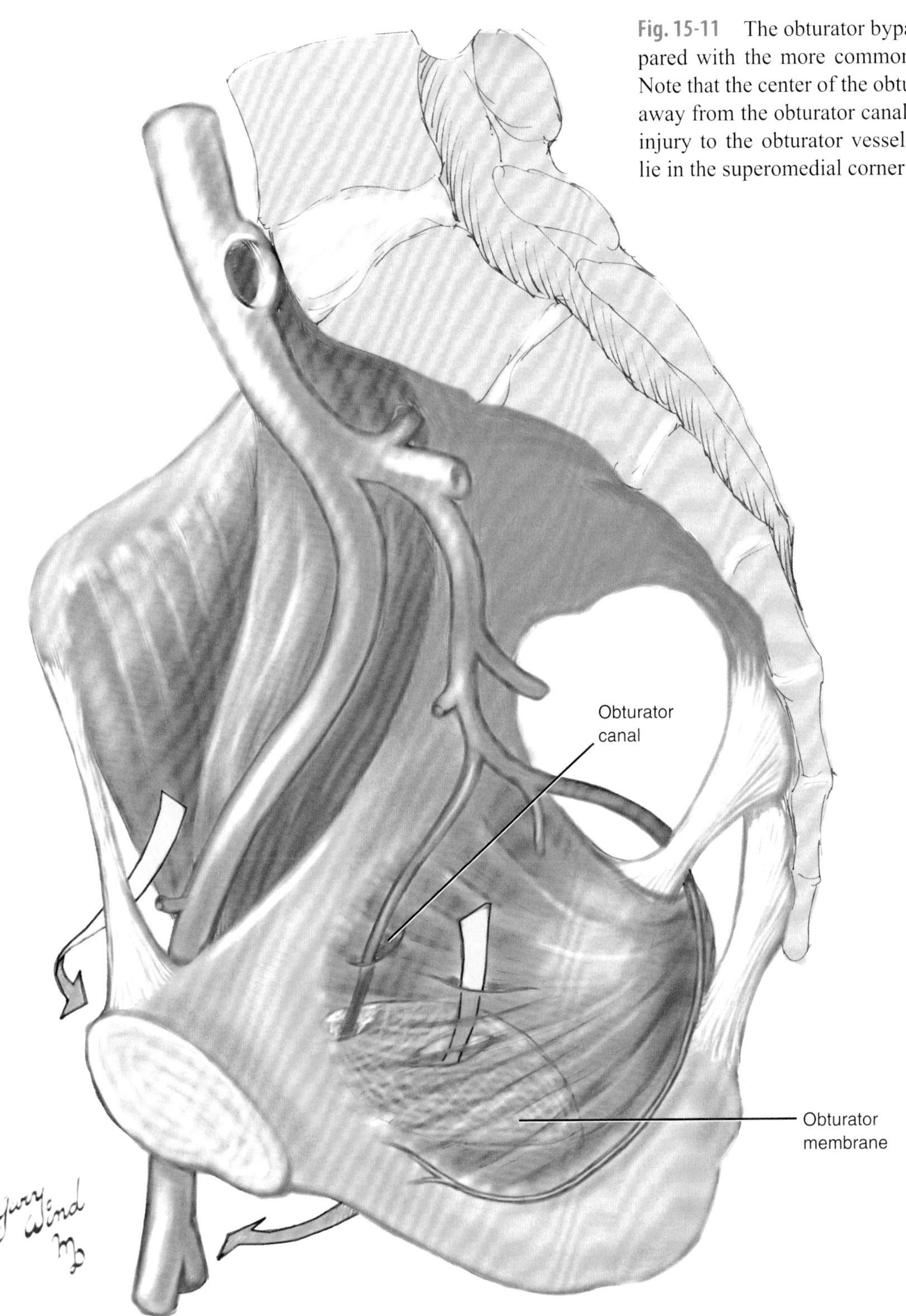

Fig. 15-11 The obturator bypass route is compared with the more common inguinal route. Note that the center of the obturator membrane away from the obturator canal is used to avoid injury to the obturator vessels and nerve that lie in the superomedial corner of the foramen.

The common femoral artery crosses the pectineus muscle diagonally and divides into the superficial and deep femoral arteries. The deep femoral (profunda femoris) artery provides the majority of blood flow to the thigh muscles, supplemented by the obturator artery and descending branches of the superior and inferior gluteal arteries (Fig. 15-12). The superficial femoral artery reaches the inverted apex of the femoral triangle and then traverses the thigh in the adductor canal (Hunter's canal) between the quadriceps and adductor muscles, giving off only minor muscular branches (see Fig. 15-4).

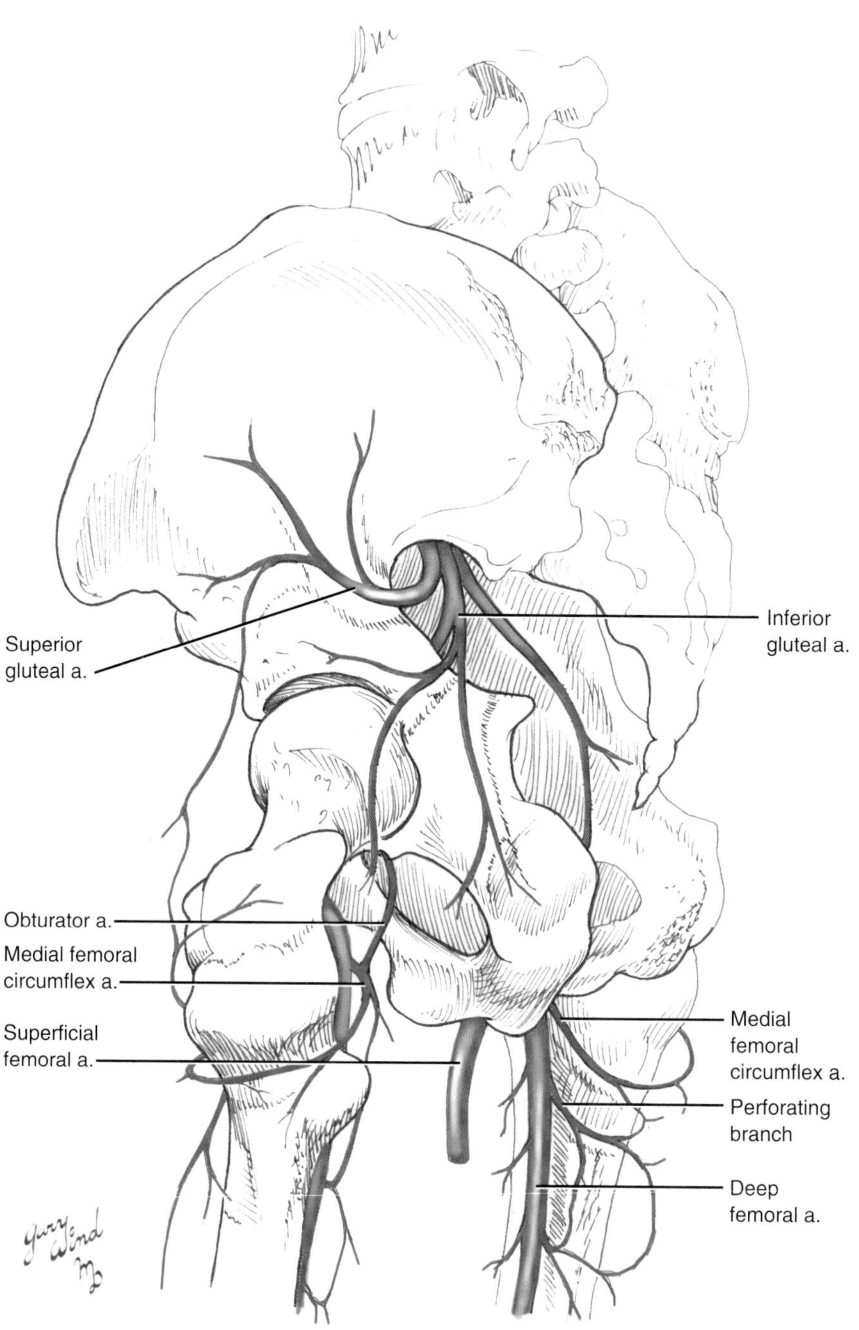

Fig. 15-12 Branches of the gluteal arteries and the obturator artery supplement the deep femoral in providing blood supply to the thigh.

Near the adductor hiatus, the superficial femoral artery gives off the highest genicular artery that may assume importance as a collateral channel in femoral occlusive disease (see Chapter 17).

The common femoral artery gives off the small deep external pudendal artery before giving rise to the large deep femoral branch approximately 4 cm distal to the inguinal ligament. The deep femoral artery usually arises on the lateral side of the parent vessel. Shortly after its origin, the deep femoral artery gives rise to the lateral and medial femoral circumflex vessels (Fig. 15-13). Either of these vessels may less commonly arise from the common femoral artery and be confused with the deep femoral trunk.

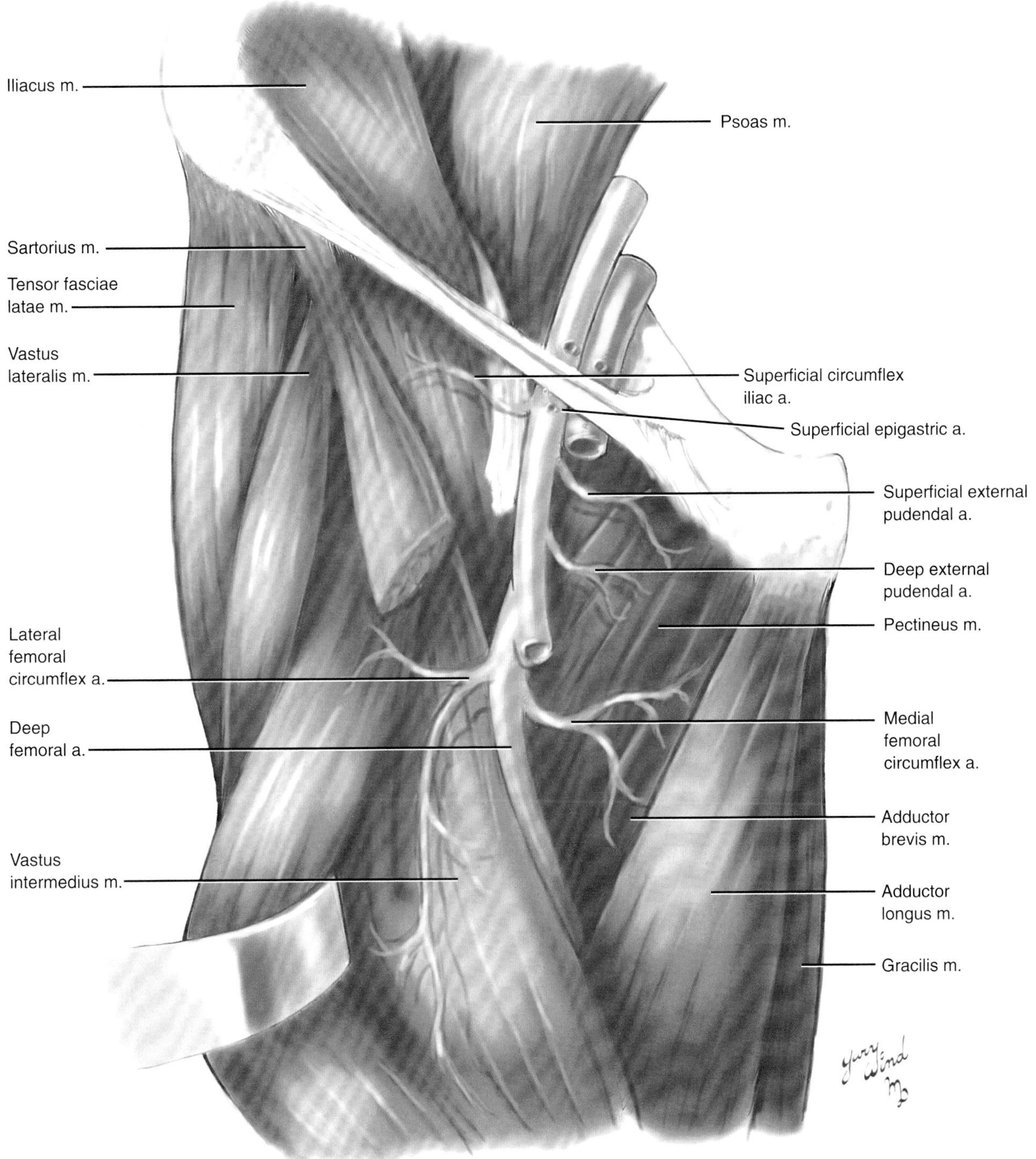

Fig. 15-13 In this medial view, the posterolateral origin of the deep femoral artery gives rise to the medial and lateral femoral circumflex arteries to the surrounding muscles. Either or both may at times arise from the common femoral artery.

Such variant branches must be identified to obtain control of this segment for anastomosis.

The origin of the deep femoral artery is crossed by the lateral femoral circumflex vein (Fig. 15-14). Branches of the lateral femoral circumflex artery supply the proximal quadriceps muscle. The descending branch of the lateral femoral circumflex artery enters the substance of the vastus lateralis where it anastomoses with genicular collaterals. Branches of the medial femoral circumflex artery supply the proximal adductor compartment. These vessels anastomose with each other, with the inferior gluteal artery, and with the first perforating branch of the deep femoral artery.

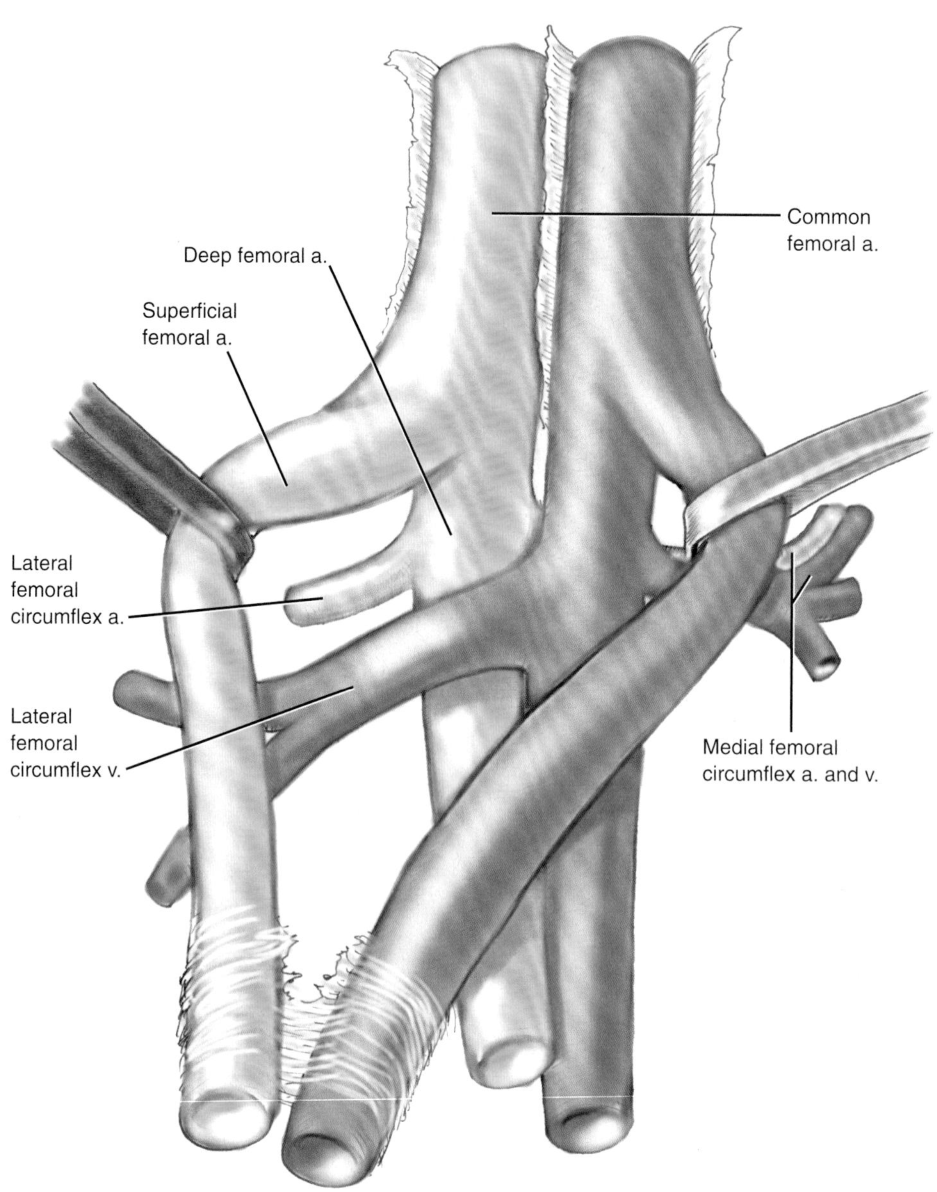

Fig. 15-14 The origin of the deep femoral artery is crossed by the lateral femoral circumflex vein that may be divided for exposure.

The continuation of the deep femoral artery turns posteromedially toward the femur and enters the plane posterior to the adductor longus where it closely parallels the femoral shaft (Fig. 15-15A, B). It supplies the bodies of the adductor muscles and sends four perforating vessels through openings in the adductor brevis and magnus muscles. The first two branches usually perforate both muscles, whereas the lower branches penetrate only the tendinous attachment

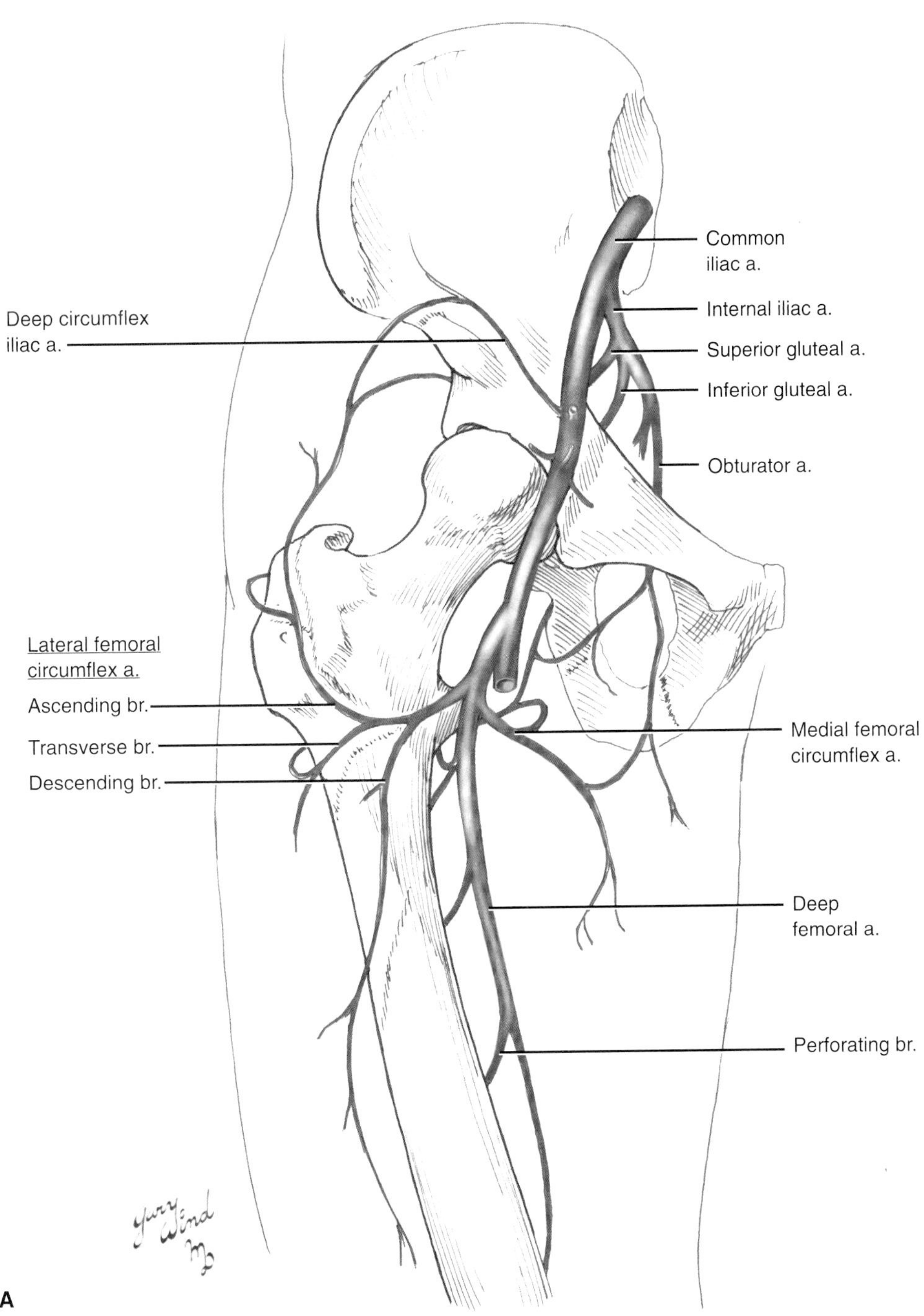

Fig. 15-15 **A:** Anterior view of the rich collateral circulation around the hip joint and proximal femur.

of the adductor magnus muscle along the medial lip of the linea aspera of the femur. The last perforator is the termination of the deep femoral artery. The perforators anastomose with each other along the posterior side of the adductor magnus muscle and provide blood to the hamstring muscles of the flexor compartment. The second perforator usually provides a major nutrient vessel to the femur, and the distal perforators anastomose with branches of the popliteal artery.

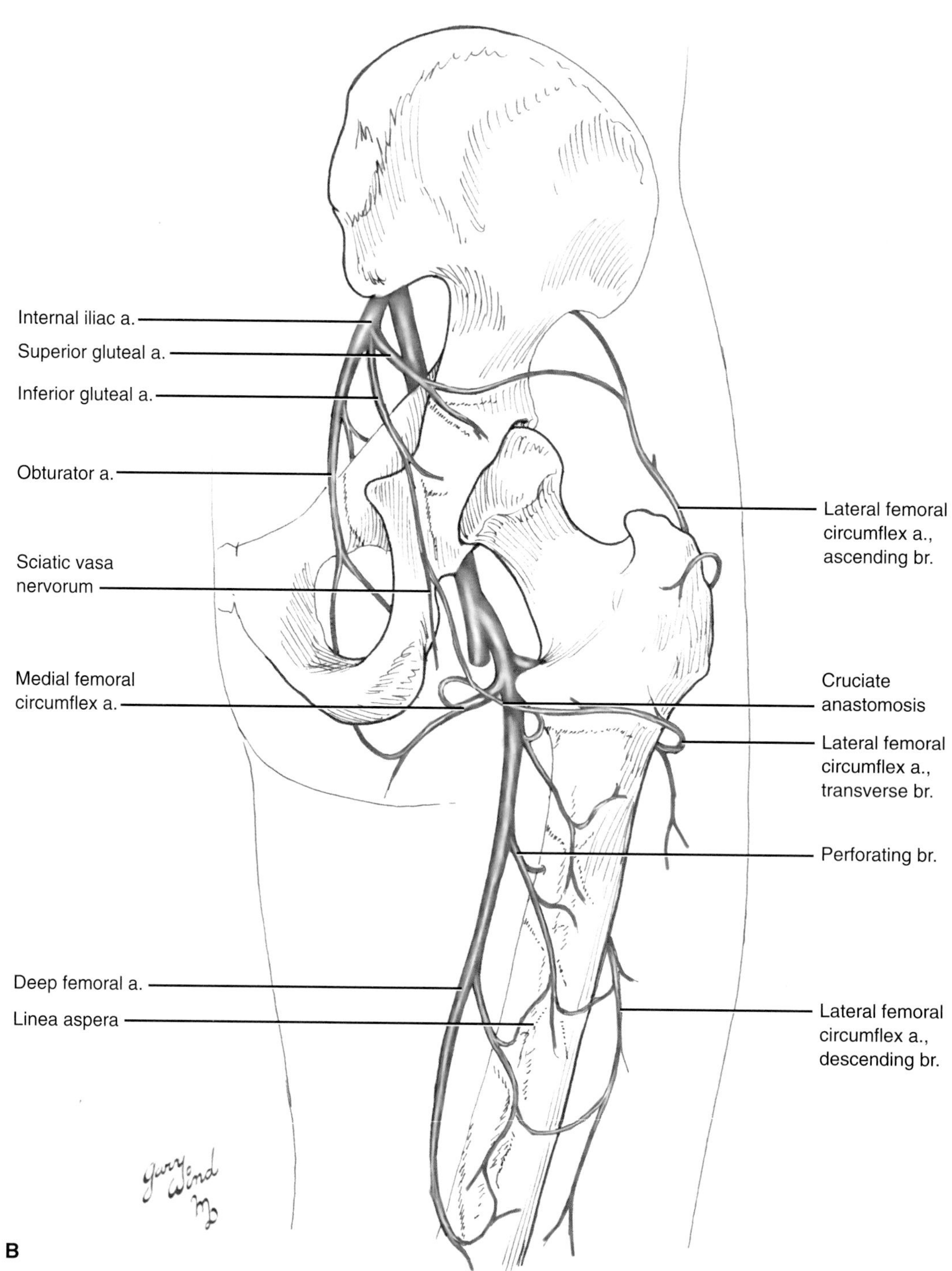

Fig. 15-15 B: Posterior view of the rich collateral circulation around the hip joint and proximal femur.

Exposure of the Femoral Artery in the Groin

The segmental nature of atherosclerosis has been recognized for many years.[1,2] Although the pathologic factors leading to atherosclerosis probably affect all arteries equally in a given individual, some arteries tend to remain patent until proximal occlusive disease is far advanced. The common femoral artery is one such vessel. Because of a rich network of collateral branches anastomosing with the distal iliac and deep femoral arteries, the common femoral and deep femoral arteries remain patent in all but the most advanced cases of aortoiliac occlusive disease, embolic occlusion, or trauma. Surgeons have learned to take advantage of this tendency by using the easily accessible femoral artery for bypass anastomosis.

The femoral artery is also an important access site for percutaneous peripheral and coronary interventions. Although improved catheter and wire design also permit safe access through the radial, brachial, and axillary arteries, the femoral artery is preferred in most cases due to its relatively large size and the ability to compress the artery against the underlying femoral head. Retrograde puncture of the common femoral artery is simple and affords direct catheter access to the aorta and most branches, including the arteries of the head and neck. Antegrade puncture is more difficult, but permits direct access to arteries of the ipsilateral extremity using shorter catheter lengths and reduced radiation doses. The prevalence and risk factors for local complications related to access site have been detailed elsewhere.[3]

Exposure of the Common Femoral Artery

The patient is placed in the supine position, and the leg and lower abdomen are prepped and draped from the level of the umbilicus to the knee. The entire abdomen and chest should be prepped in cases involving concomitant exposure of more proximal arteries. Wide exposure of the femoral vessels and their branches is most readily obtained through a vertical incision. For endovascular procedures requiring limited exposure of the common femoral artery above its bifurcation, an oblique incision may be associated with fewer wound complications.[4,5]

The vertical skin incision is made directly over the femoral pulse and extended above the groin crease such that one-third of the incision is above the inguinal ligament, and two-thirds are below it.[6] When there is no palpable pulse in the femoral artery, the incision should extend vertically from a point slightly medial to the midpoint of the inguinal ligament[7] (Fig. 15-16). The oblique incision is made parallel to the inguinal ligament just above the groin crease (Fig. 15-17A). In obese patients, the oblique incision allows placement of the endovascular device through an additional incision for tunneling to the arteriotomy (Fig 15-17B).

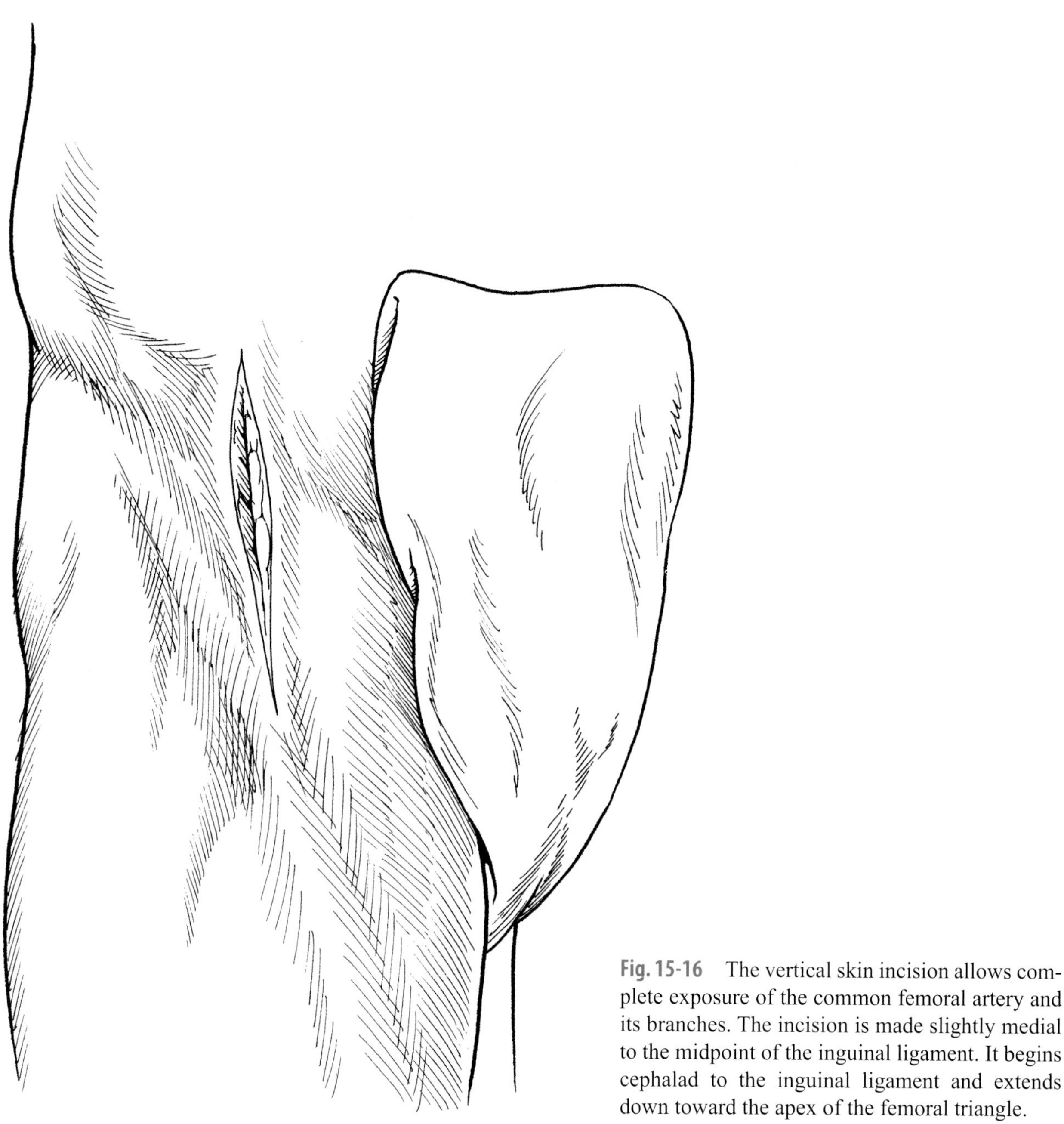

Fig. 15-16 The vertical skin incision allows complete exposure of the common femoral artery and its branches. The incision is made slightly medial to the midpoint of the inguinal ligament. It begins cephalad to the inguinal ligament and extends down toward the apex of the femoral triangle.

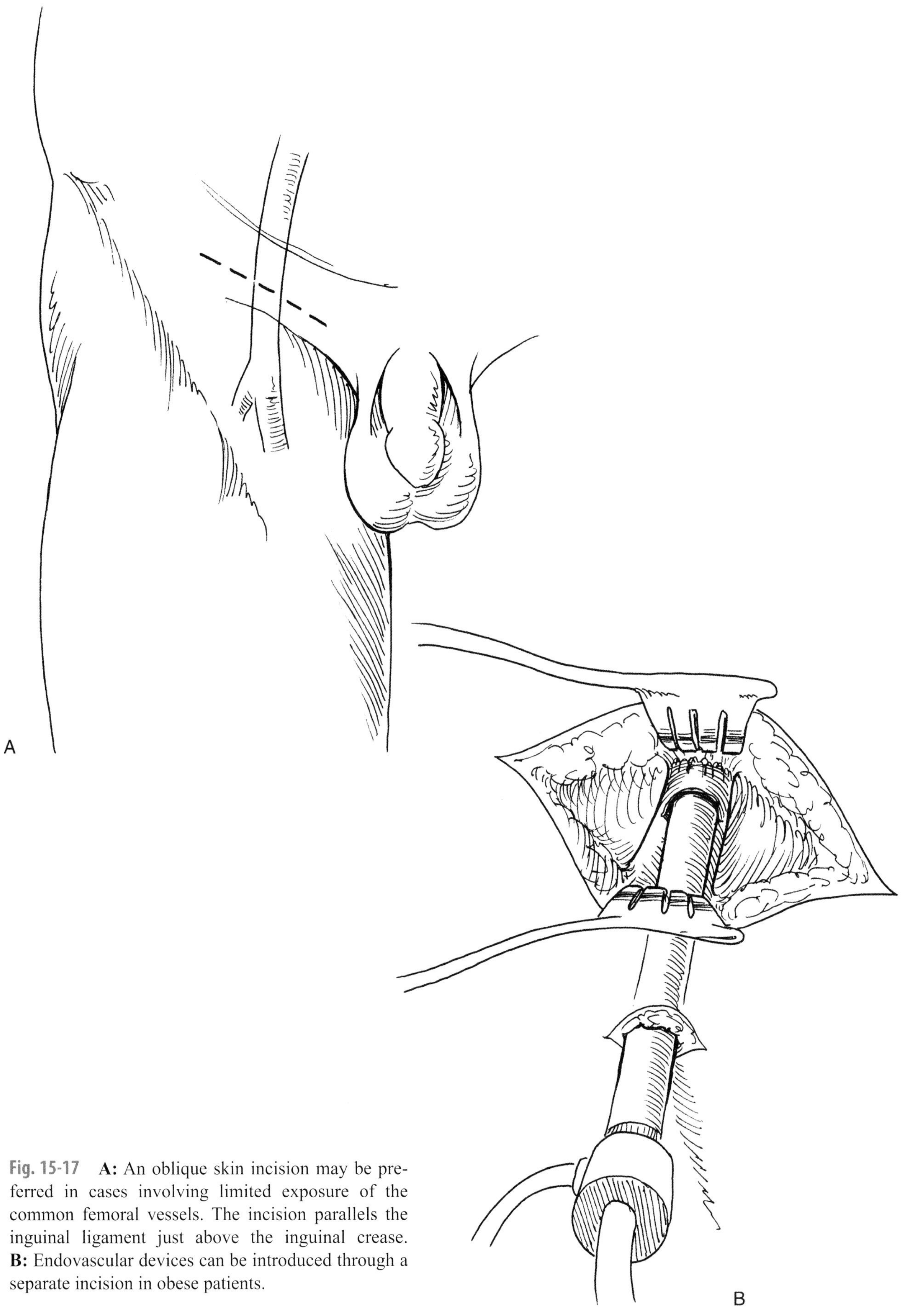

Fig. 15-17 **A:** An oblique skin incision may be preferred in cases involving limited exposure of the common femoral vessels. The incision parallels the inguinal ligament just above the inguinal crease. **B:** Endovascular devices can be introduced through a separate incision in obese patients.

On deepening the incision, one encounters the small superficial epigastric and superficial circumflex iliac branches of the femoral vessels in the subcutaneous tissue. These branches should be divided and ligated to gain access to deeper structures. In addition, time spent in ligating all lymphatics associated with the superficial inguinal nodes reduces the risk of a lymphocele developing postoperatively[8] (Fig. 15-18). The fascia lata is opened along the medial margin of the sartorius muscle, and the incision is extended proximally to the level of the inguinal ligament. Lateral retraction of the sartorius muscle exposes the underlying femoral triangle and vessels within the funnel-shaped femoral sheath (Fig. 15-19).

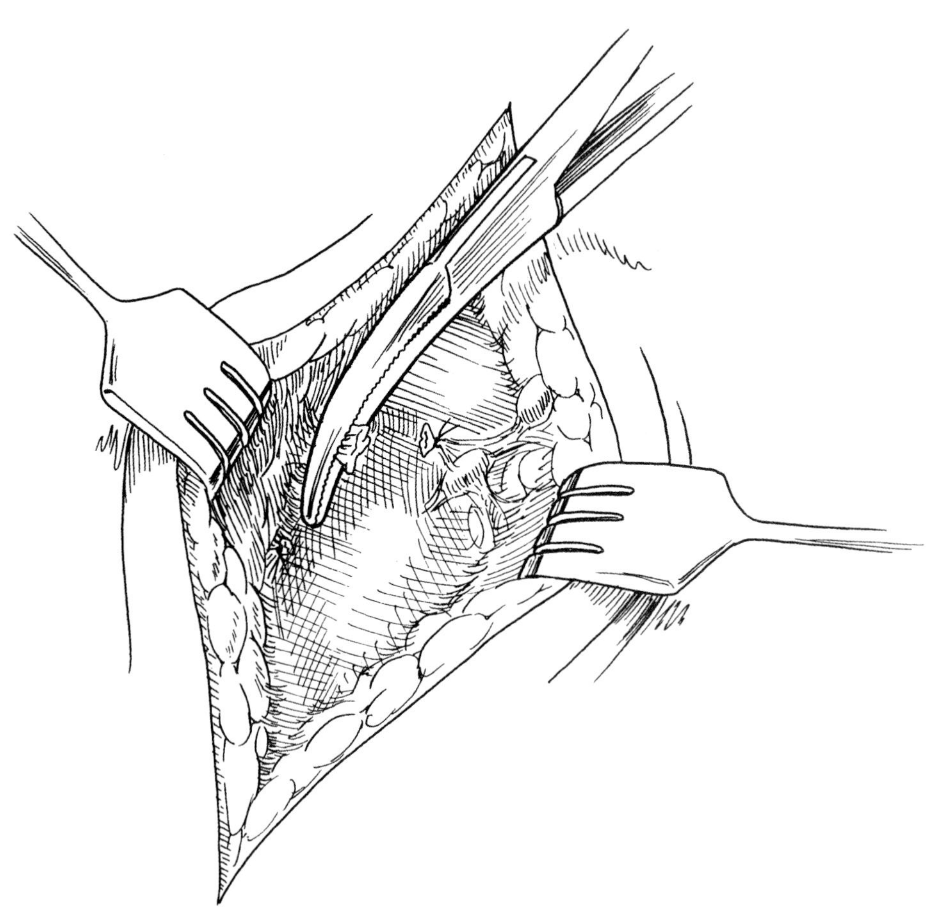

Fig. 15-18 Careful ligation of inguinal lymphatics helps to prevent postoperative lymphocele.

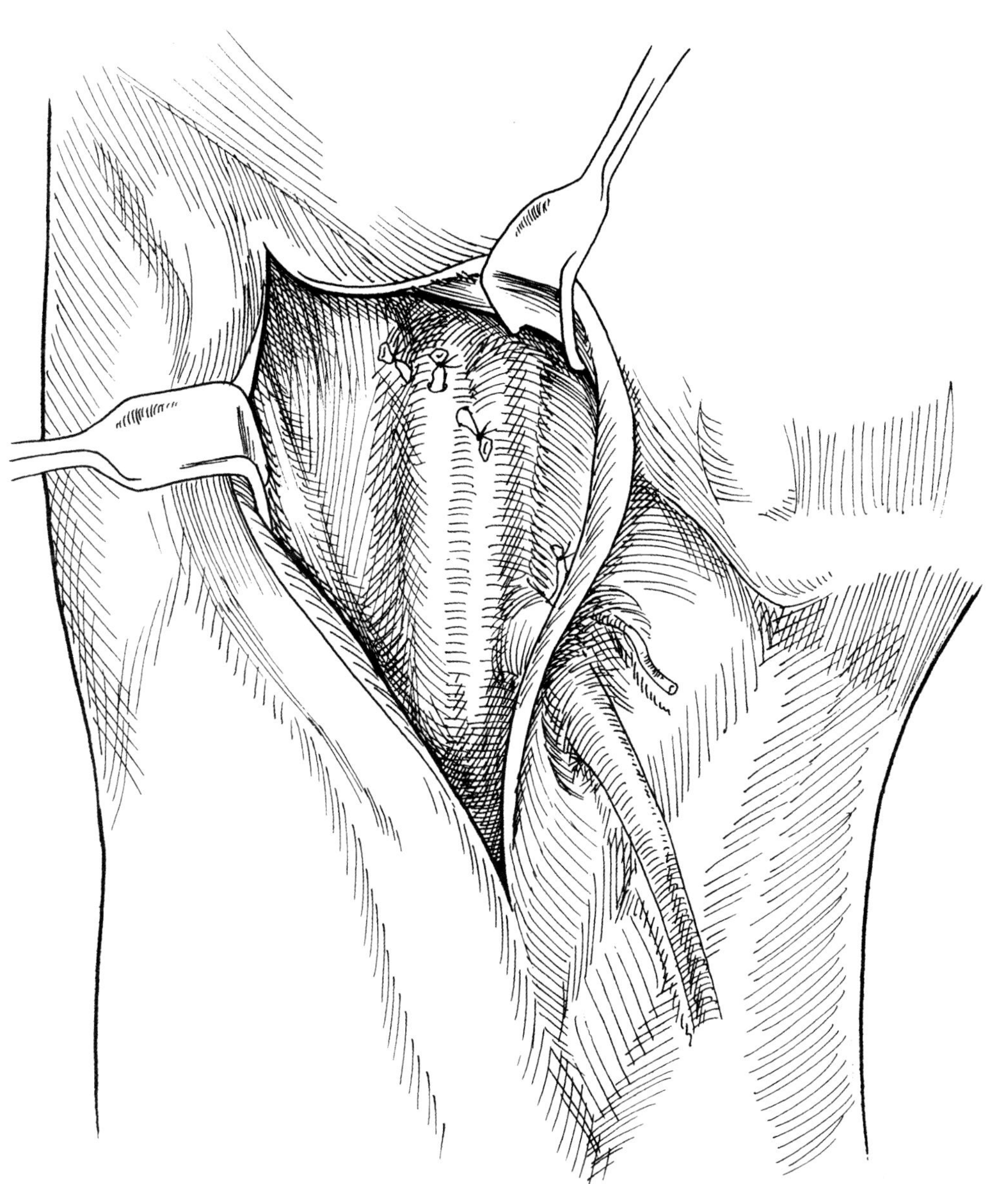

Fig. 15-19 In this view, the skin and subcutaneous fat have been removed to show the incision in the fascia lata along the medial border of the sartorius muscle.

Further proximal exposure can be obtained by cephalad retraction of the inguinal ligament.

Direct access to the common femoral artery is gained by opening the femoral sheath (Fig. 15-20). Separation of areolar tissue is all that is necessary to encircle this vessel. One should take great care to avoid entry into the femoral vein that lies medial to the artery in the femoral sheath. On occasion, there may be inflammatory changes within the femoral sheath that render the vessels difficult to separate.

The common femoral artery divides into two major trunks, the deep (profunda) and superficial femoral arteries, which are best exposed by dissecting distally on the anterior surface of the parent trunk. Few branches will be encountered on the anterior surface of the artery, and the deep femoral artery will not be injured using this approach. The superficial femoral artery is easily isolated in the distal wound. The origin of the deep femoral artery is most often found laterally about 3.5 cm below the

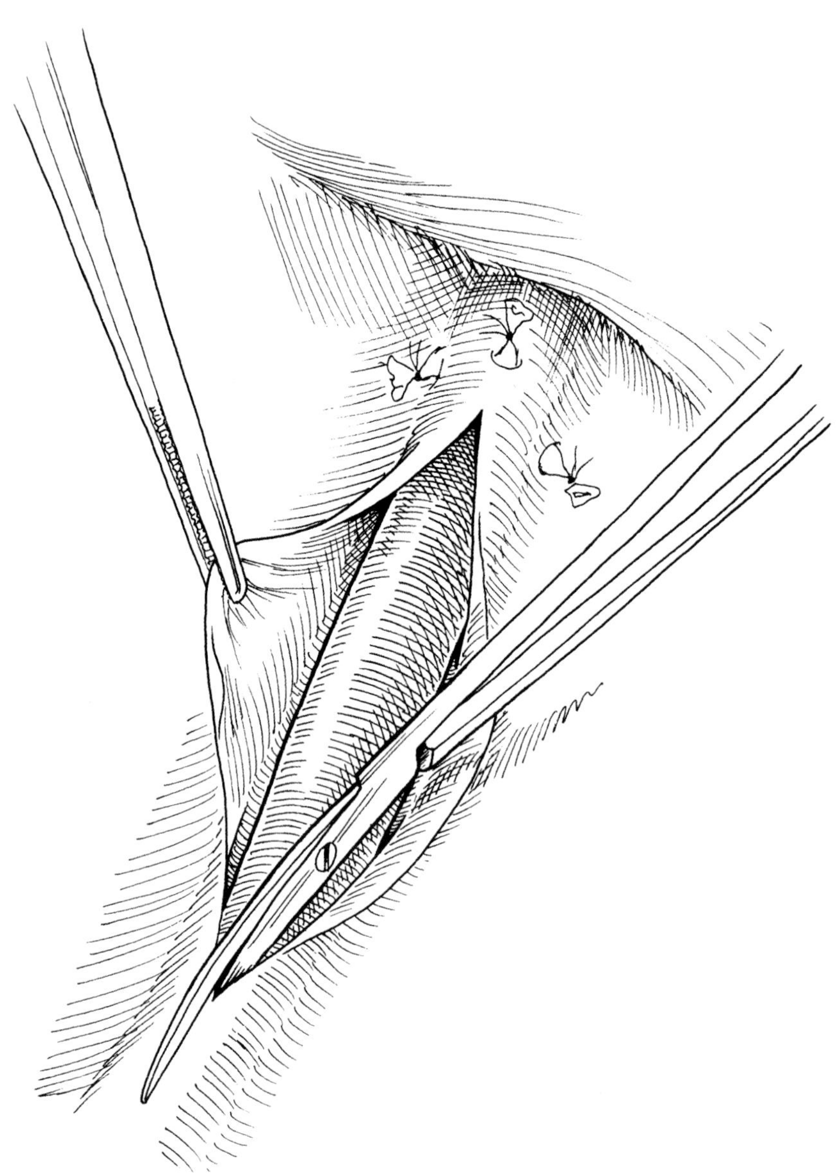

Fig. 15-20 The femoral sheath is opened directly over the artery; the artery is mobilized by blunt dissection and encircled for control.

inguinal ligament, although it may occasionally be more proximal or more distal[7] (Fig. 15-21). The lateral femoral circumflex vein crosses anterior to the deep femoral artery at this level and should be identified during dissection. Injury to this vein can occur during dissection at the "crotch" formed by the origins of the deep and superficial femoral arteries. The vein should be divided when more extensive exposure of the deep femoral artery is necessary.

In 25% of cases, the medial femoral circumflex artery arises directly from the common femoral trunk, as does the lateral femoral circumflex

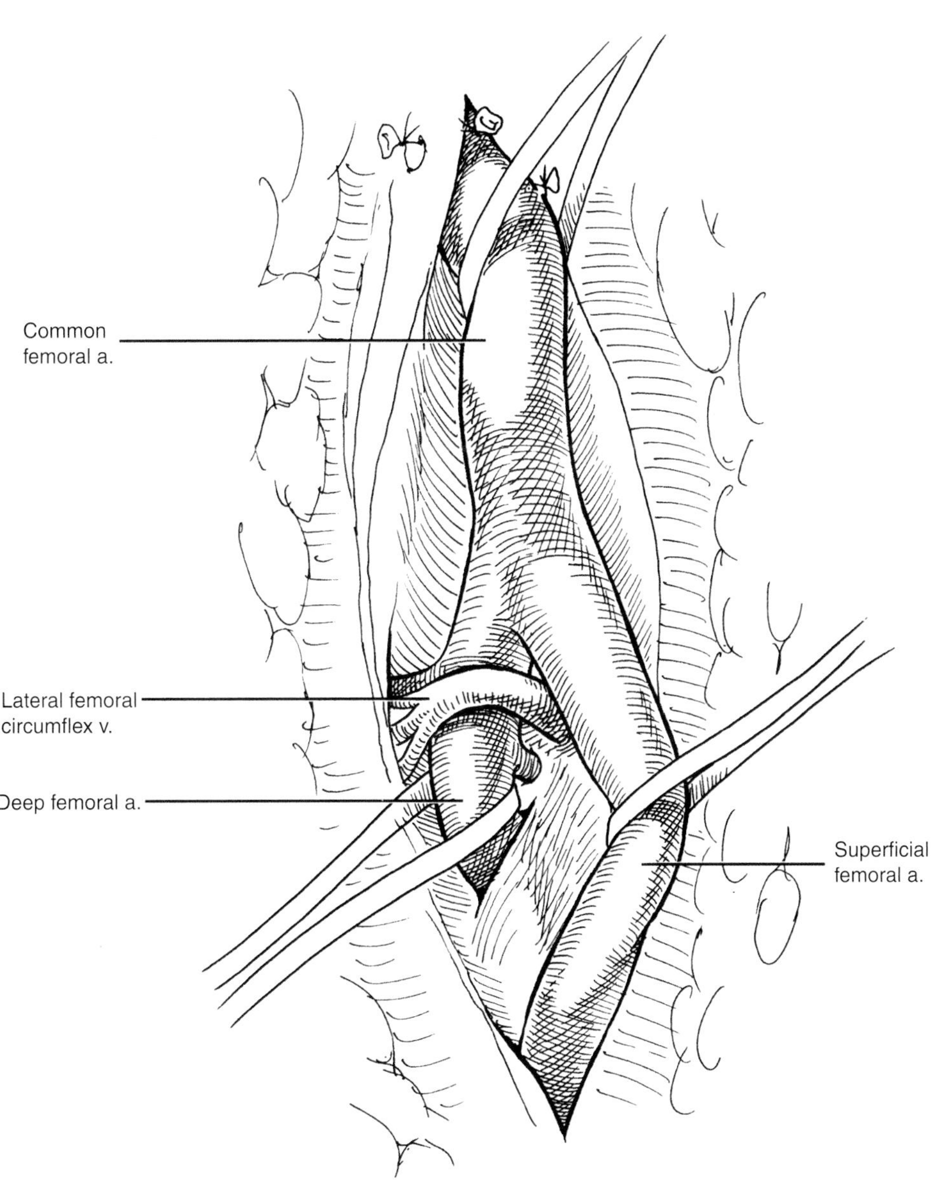

Fig. 15-21 The deep femoral artery normally arises laterally off the common femoral trunk about 3.5 cm distal to the inguinal ligament. Its origin is crossed by the lateral femoral circumflex vein.

artery in 20% of cases[7] (Fig. 15-22). It is important to identify and control these anomalous branches before opening the femoral artery: significant backbleeding that occurs from the opened, cross-clamped femoral artery is usually from one of these branches.

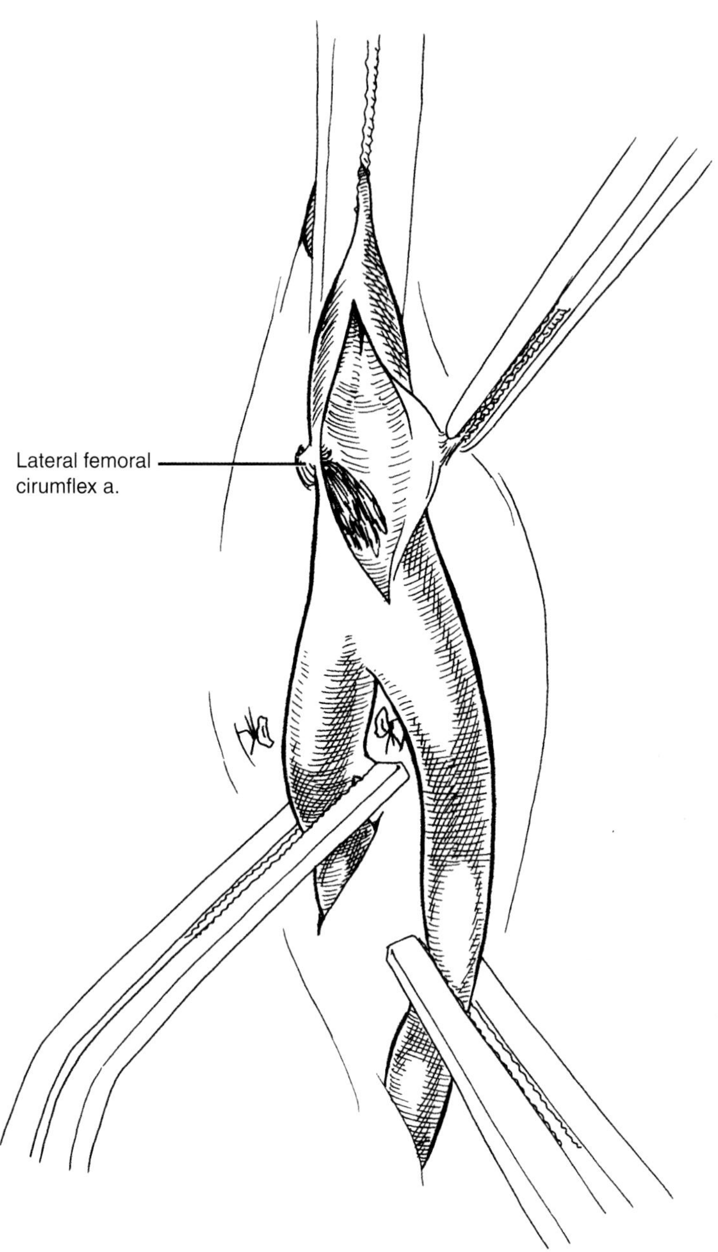

Fig. 15-22 The lateral or medial femoral circumflex arteries may arise from the common femoral trunk and cause troublesome backbleeding if unrecognized.

Anatomy of Inflow to the Femoral Artery

Atherosclerotic occlusive disease is commonly found in the infrarenal aorta and iliac arteries. Bypasses around flow-limiting stenoses or occlusions of these arteries can be accomplished with a variety of procedures that use the femoral artery as the outflow vessel to the leg. Concomitant occlusive lesions in the common or superficial femoral arteries do not necessarily contraindicate the use of any of these procedures because the deep femoral artery (which is often devoid of stenoses) has been shown to be an adequate recipient vessel in these situations.[9]

The aortofemoral bypass is the most popular inflow procedure to the femoral artery. Suitable extraanatomic alternatives include the femorofemoral bypass, the axillofemoral bypass, and the obturator foramen bypass to the femoral or popliteal artery (Fig. 15-23). The following discussion concerns the

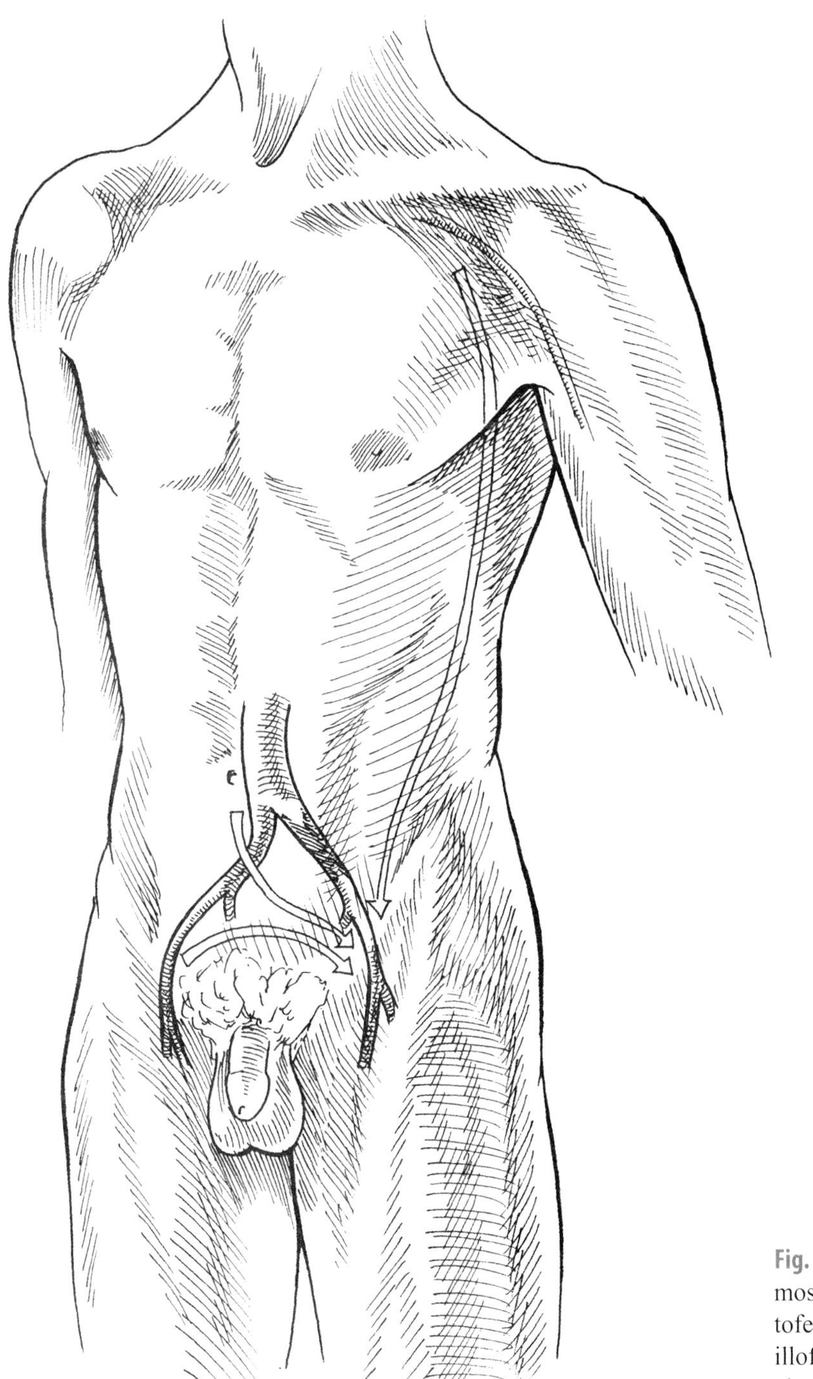

Fig. 15-23 Aortoiliac occlusive disease is most commonly revascularized by the aortofemoral route, but femorofemoral and axillofemoral routes are useful extraanatomic alternatives.

anatomy of tunnels to the femoral artery; exposures for proximal anastomoses at the aorta and axillary artery are covered in other chapters.

Anatomy of the Aortofemoral Bypass Tunnel

This tunnel connects the incisions used to expose the abdominal aorta and the femoral artery. The most popular route follows the natural course of the iliac and femoral arteries, allowing the graft to remain protected in the retroperitoneal tissues. Tunneling is begun with finger dissection on the anterior aspect of the femoral artery in the periadventitial plane (Fig. 15-24). Alternatively, the tunnel may begin in the empty space medial to the femoral vein. Grafts brought through the latter tunnel are routed across the vein for anastomosis with the femoral artery. Either tunnel passes deep to the inguinal ligament and enters the pelvis on the anterior aspect of the external iliac artery. The inferior epigastric and deep circumflex iliac veins cross anterior to the external iliac artery and may be injured during this blind dissection. Direct vision under the retracted inguinal ligament may aid in identifying these vessels when they are injured.

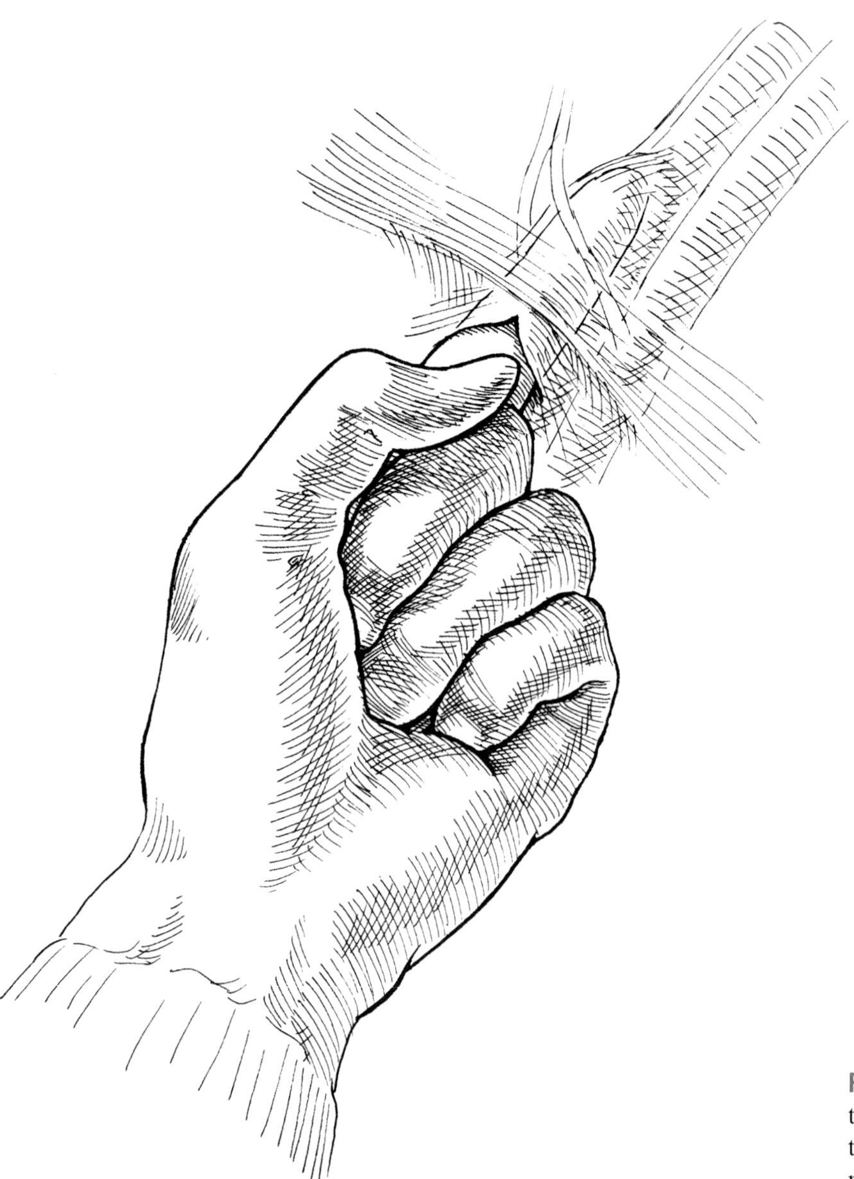

Fig. 15-24 The aortofemoral bypass tunnel is begun with finger dissection in the periadventitial plane beneath the inguinal ligament.

The proximal tunnel is begun in the abdomen on the anterior surface of the common iliac artery. The correct plane is found by opening the peritoneum overlying the distal aorta and aortic bifurcation. This maneuver may be aided by reflecting the duodenum off the aorta as described elsewhere. The tissues overlying the ventral surface of the aorta are incised down to the periadventitial plane, and the incision is carried distally to the level of the aortic bifurcation.

Finger dissection begins in the periadventitial plane near the aortic bifurcation and continues on the anterior surface of the common iliac artery. The dissecting finger should be advanced blindly on the anterior surface of the external iliac artery to meet the finger passing upward from the groin incision (Fig. 15-25). Care should be taken to ensure that the tunnel passes posterior to the ureter to prevent compression between the native iliac artery and the graft.

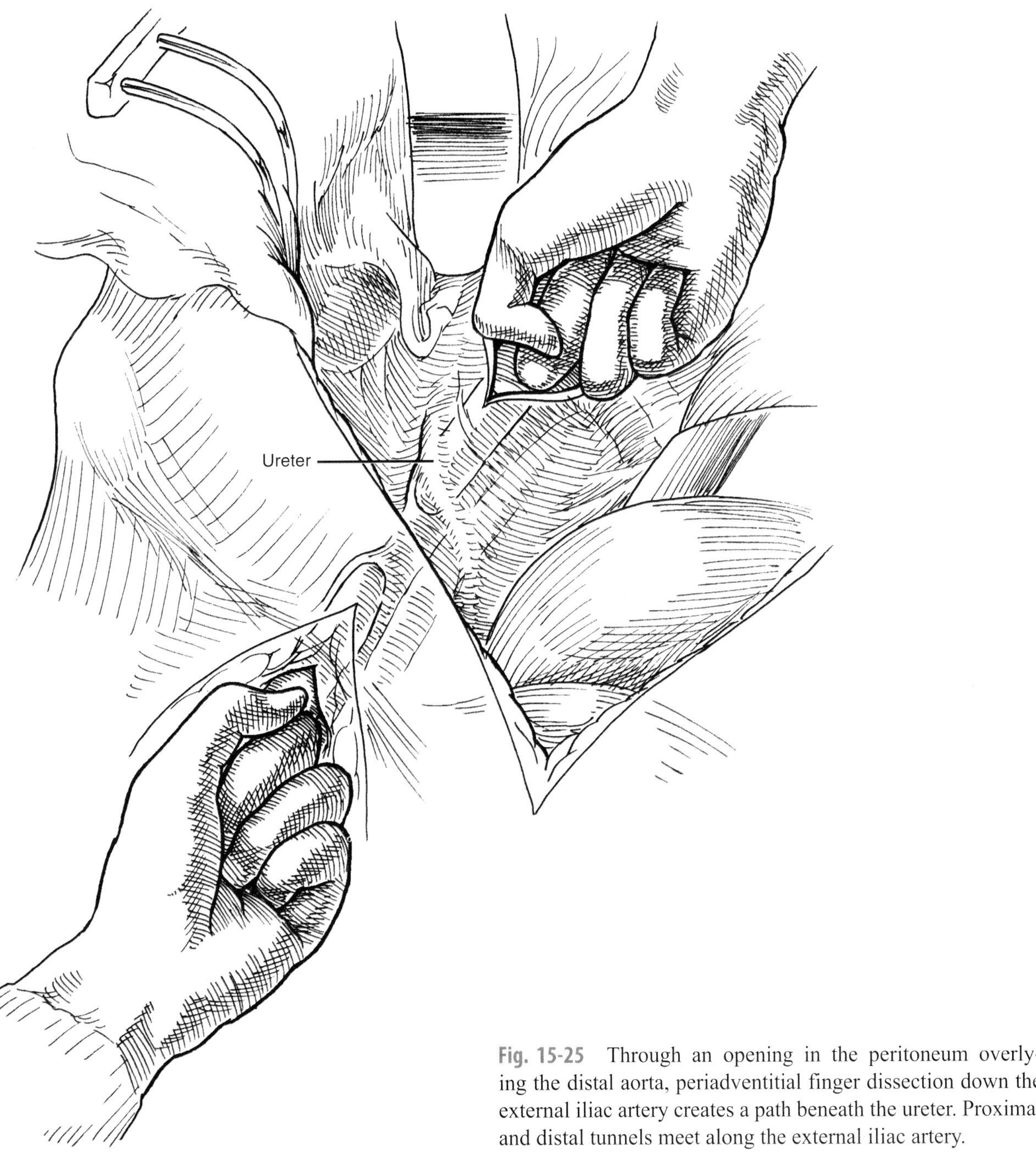

Fig. 15-25 Through an opening in the peritoneum overlying the distal aorta, periadventitial finger dissection down the external iliac artery creates a path beneath the ureter. Proximal and distal tunnels meet along the external iliac artery.

Anatomy of the Axillofemoral Bypass Tunnel

The route from the axillary artery to the ipsilateral femoral artery is a long subcutaneous tunnel that traverses the lateral trunk.[10] Exposure of the axillary artery is considered in more detail in Chapter 5. Tunneling is best begun near the axillary artery and routed beneath the pectoralis major muscle with a long tunneling instrument (Fig. 15-26). The tunneling instrument should be guided so that it reaches the inferior border of the pectoralis major muscle anterior to the midaxillary line, where it is pushed through the axillary fascia into the subcutaneous tissue of the lateral chest wall. An intermediate incision may be needed just below the costal margin in cases in which the tunneling instrument does not reach the

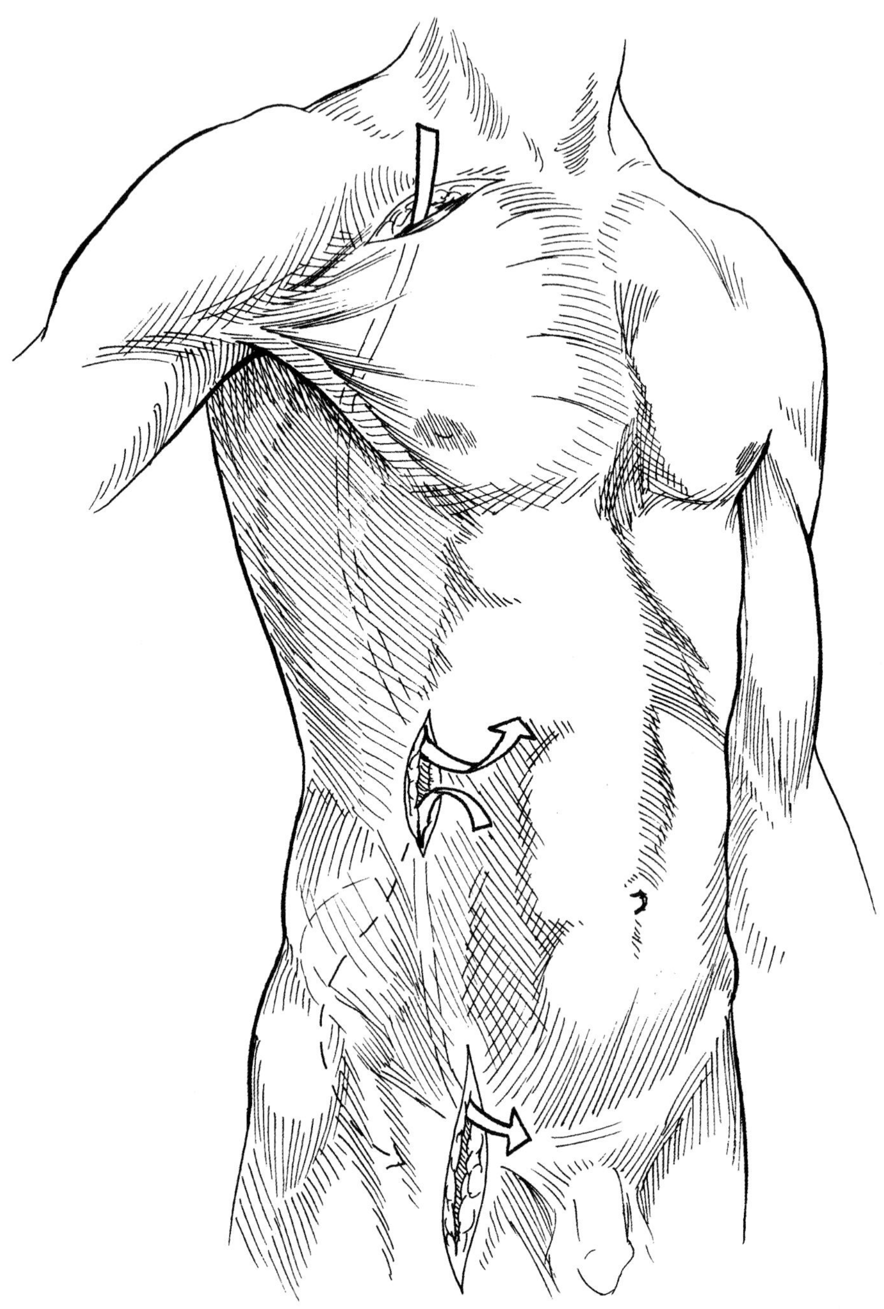

Fig. 15-26 The axillofemoral bypass runs deep to the pectoralis major muscle proximally and then in the subcutaneous plane to reach the groin. An intermediate incision between costal margin and iliac crest facilitates formation of the tunnel. Many surgeons use a transverse jump incision. The graft may be brought laterally over the iliac crest when the midgroin must be avoided (dashed line).

groin from the axillary incision. The distal tunnel continues down the lateral abdominal wall anterior to the midaxillary line. It terminates in a gentle curve toward the groin by passing medial to the anterior superior iliac spine. The tunnel should enter the superolateral aspect of the open groin wound. In cases of groin wound infection, when the anastomotic site must be created away from the groin, tunnels can be routed more laterally. These tunnels can cross over the iliac crest with little concern for undue pressure on grafts[11] to reach the deep femoral artery away from the femoral sheath (see above).

Because of the long distances involved with this bypass technique, synthetic grafts (8 to 10 mm) are preferred over autogenous saphenous veins. Use of grafts supported with external rings may provide additional protection against kinking. These grafts are introduced through the tunnel described above and routed into the deeper tissues of the femoral triangle for anastomosis with the respective femoral artery.

Anatomy of the Femorofemoral Bypass

A patent femoral artery may serve as the source of blood flow to the contralateral vessel. Cross-femoral bypass is an attractive option for revascularization because it avoids laparotomy and potential damage to autonomic genital supply, which are associated with aortofemoral bypass. However, the long-term success of this technique is inferior to that of aortofemoral reconstruction.[12] A steal phenomenon may occur if the donor iliac artery system is compromised and the recipient arterial system has a lower resistance than the donor limb. Proof of the adequacy of inflow to the donor femoral artery is necessary; angiography is often unreliable. Physiologic tests to determine the significance of inflow lesions are considered in detail elsewhere.[13] Transluminal angioplasty of the donor artery can be used to correct inflow stenoses without compromising long-term patency of the femoral bypass graft.[14]

The femoral arteries are exposed through bilateral groin incisions as described above. The femorofemoral bypass can be constructed with prosthetic or autogenous tissue.[15,16] The graft tunnel is begun in the subcutaneous tissue just superficial to the medial part of the inguinal ligament of one incision and passed subcutaneously in an inverted U fashion cephalad to the pubis. It is introduced into the superomedial aspect of the contralateral groin incision by passing over the inguinal ligament on that side. The graft is routed from the subcutaneous tunnel directly into the deep tissues of both incisions for femoral anastomoses (Fig. 15-27). Alternatively,

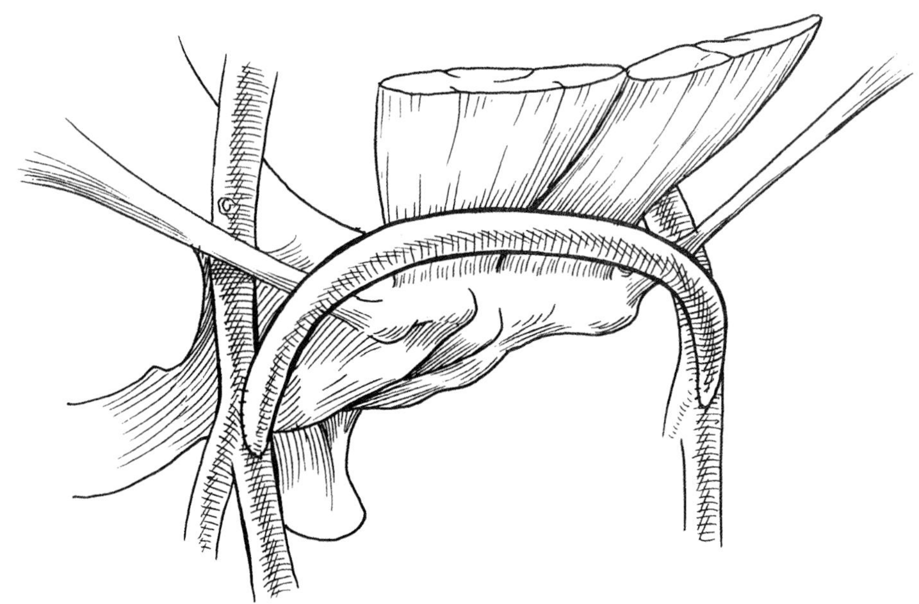

Fig. 15-27 The femorofemoral bypass is usually brought subcutaneously over the pubis.

the graft may be tunneled posterior to the rectus abdominis sheath, offering a less awkward trajectory through several tissue layers and possibly improved graft protection. The tunnel is begun medial to the femoral vein (in the empty space) and introduced under the inguinal ligament. The tunnel is routed in the properitoneal space cephalad to the dome of the bladder and reaches the opposite incision under the contralateral inguinal ligament (Fig. 15-28). Graft ends are brought across the respective femoral veins for femoral artery anastomoses.

The precise site of femoral artery anastomosis has been shown to be a determining factor in long-term patency of femorofemoral bypasses. A superior patency rate has been demonstrated when both anastomoses are created at the bifurcation of the common

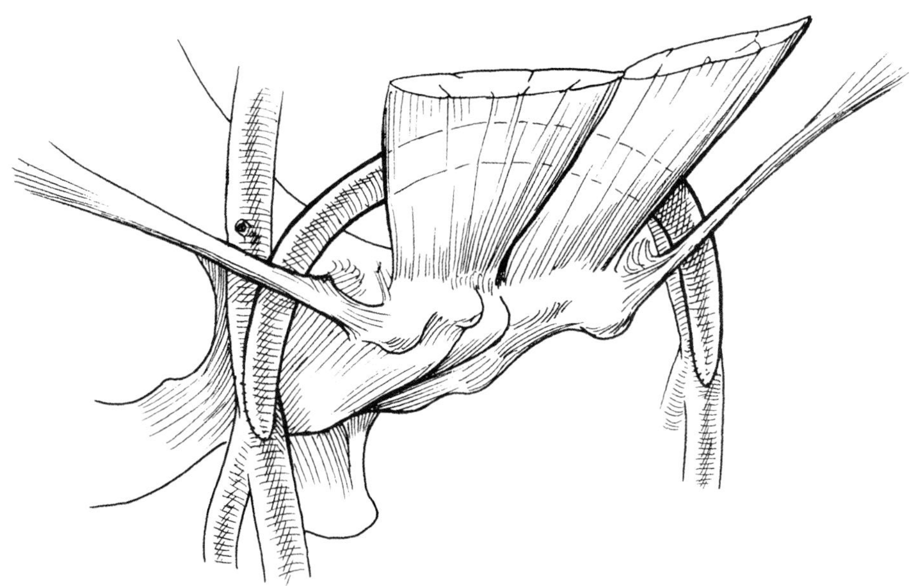

Fig. 15-28 The bypass may also be placed deep to the rectus abdominis muscle for added protection.

femoral arteries rather than at the iliac level.[17,18] The ends of the graft are best anastomosed to respective common-superficial femoral artery junctions on the side opposite the orifices of the deep femoral branches (Fig. 15-29). In cases involving occlusion of the superficial femoral artery, the anastomosis may be created directly with the deep femoral artery trunk (Fig. 15-30).

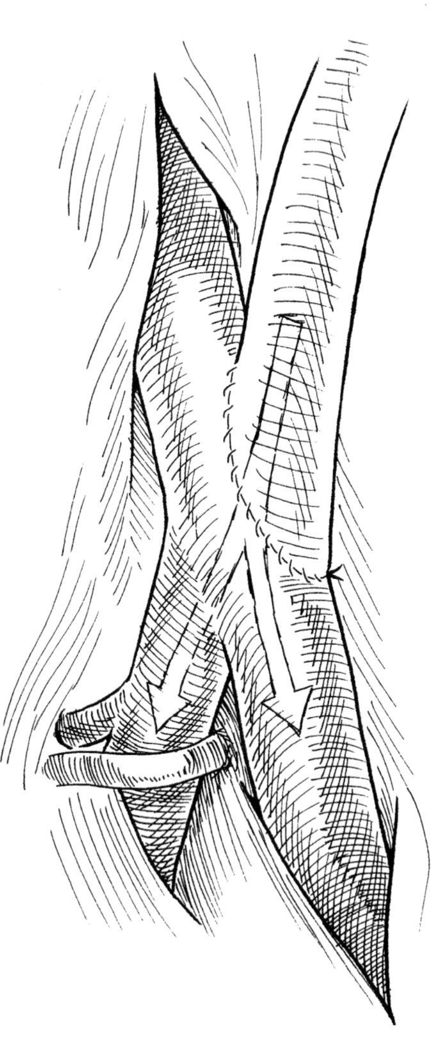

Fig. 15-29 The femoral graft anastomosis is placed opposite the orifice of the deep femoral artery for optimal outflow hemodynamics into both the deep and superficial branches.

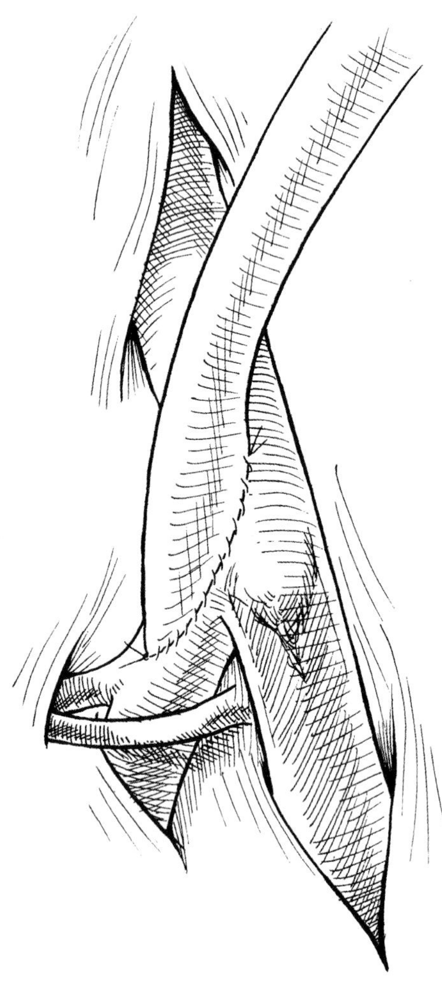

Fig. 15-30 When the superficial femoral artery is occluded, the anastomosis is made directly over the origin of the deep femoral artery.

Anatomy of the Obturator Foramen Bypass

The obturator bypass brings direct blood flow to the femoral artery from the ipsilateral iliac system. This extraanatomic procedure is an excellent option for managing septic complications of the femoral artery, such as localized graft infections or mycotic aneurysms of the femoral artery in substance abusers. The technique has also been championed in cases of suppurative groin lymphadenopathy, radiation necrosis, and severe scar tissue in the groin after previous surgery. If an ipsilateral aortofemoral limb proximal to the affected groin is proposed as the inflow source for the obturator bypass, it is important to establish that the infection does not extend to this portion of the graft.

The patient is placed in the supine position with a rolled sheet under the flank on the side of the intended incision. If infected, the groin area should be carefully isolated from the sterile field using barrier drapes. The patient should then be prepped and draped from the upper abdomen to the lower leg.

Exposure of the recipient vessel is performed first. Surgeons have performed successful bypasses to a variety of arteries with this technique, including the superficial femoral, deep femoral, suprageniculate popliteal, and infrageniculate popliteal arteries. Exposure of these vessels is discussed in detail in other sections.

A retroperitoneal approach is preferred for exposure of the inflow artery or graft. A curvilinear transverse incision is made approximately 4 cm above and parallel to the inguinal ligament (Fig. 15-31). The muscles of the anterior abdominal wall are next divided. The external oblique is split in the direction of its fibers, and the internal

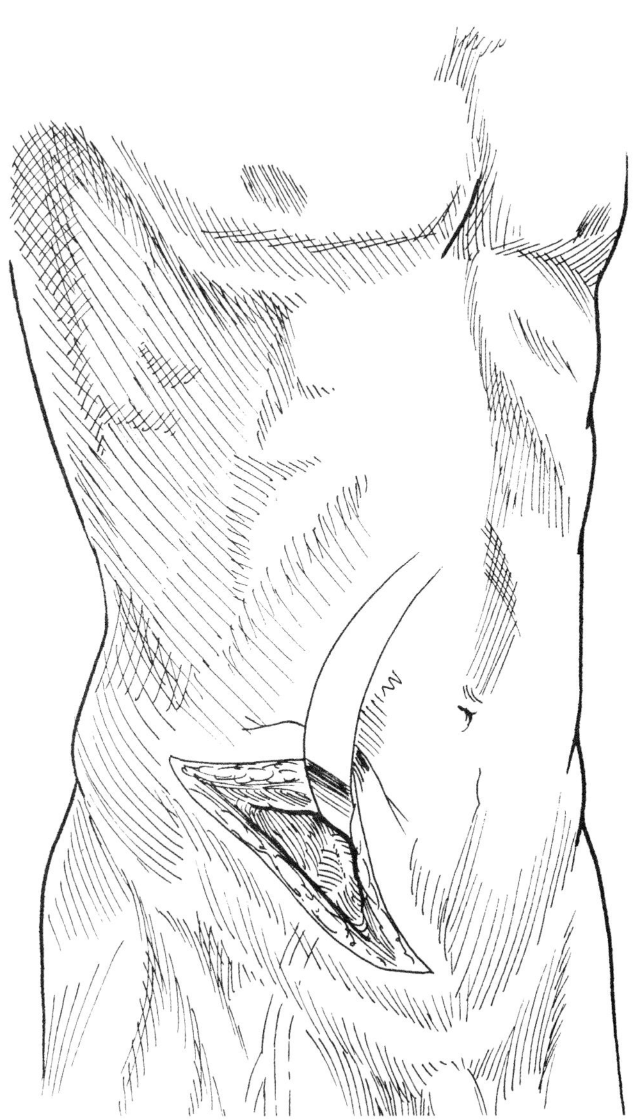

Fig. 15-31 The iliac vessels can be approached retroperitoneally through a lower quadrant incision proximal and parallel to the inguinal ligament. The peritoneal envelope is best elevated from lateral to medial.

oblique, transversus abdominus, and transversalis fascia are divided up to the edge of the rectus sheath. Division of a few centimeters of lateral rectus sheath may occasionally enhance medial wound exposure. Access to the retroperitoneal tissues is most easily gained in the lateral wound, where abundant extraperitoneal fat permits easy separation of the peritoneum from the transversalis fascia. The peritoneum and its contents should be retracted medially along with the ureter.

The iliac vessels are found along the medial prominence of the psoas muscle at this level (Fig. 15-32). Grafts usually lie most comfortably just anterior to the external iliac artery. The obturator

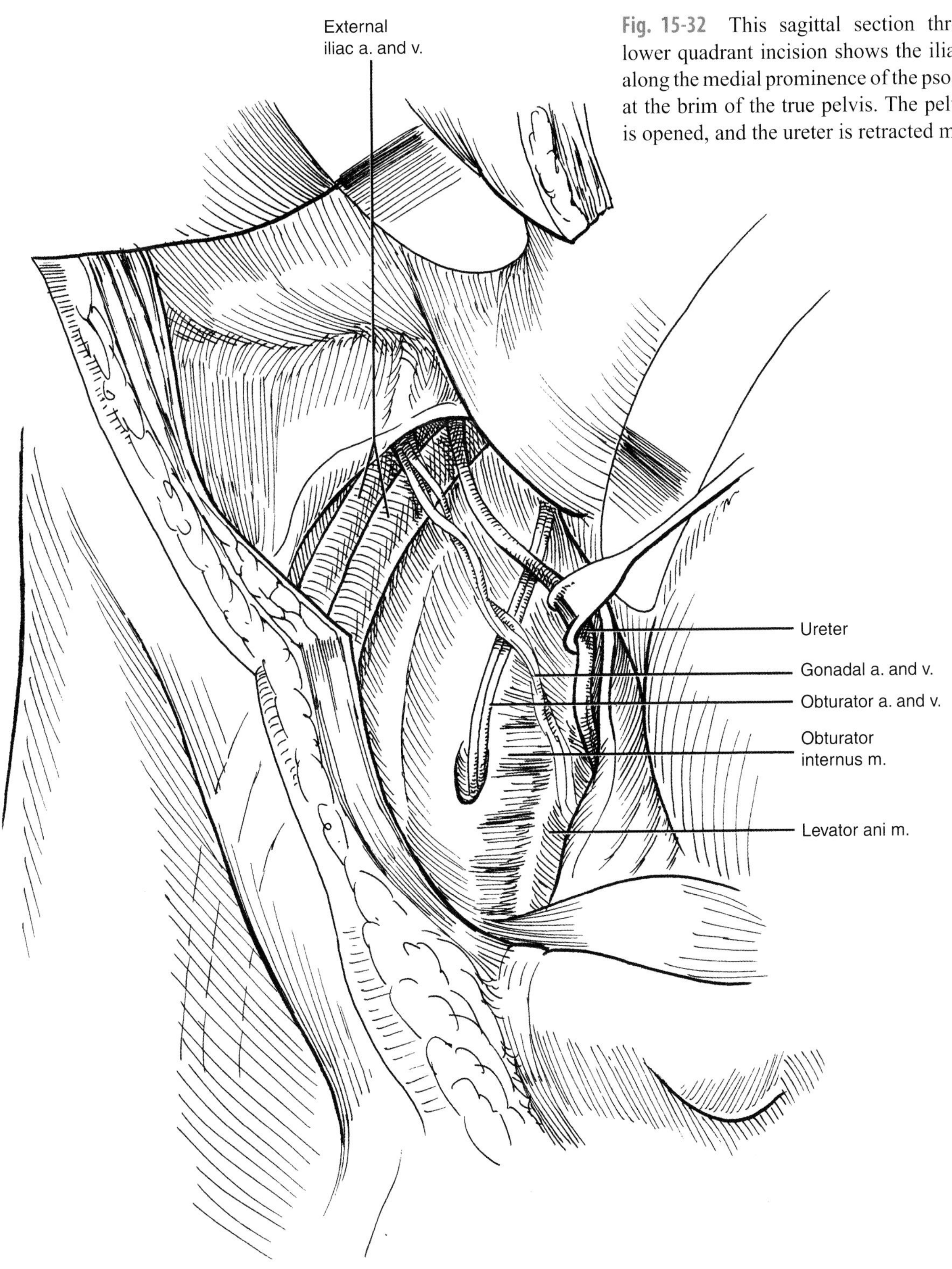

Fig. 15-32 This sagittal section through the lower quadrant incision shows the iliac vessels along the medial prominence of the psoas muscle at the brim of the true pelvis. The pelvic fascia is opened, and the ureter is retracted medially.

foramen is palpated under the superior ramus of the pubic bone. The obturator vessels and nerve traverse the obturator canal superolaterally; the bypass tunnel should be created centrally to avoid these structures. The medial portion of the obturator membrane is reached by incising the endopelvic fascia and bluntly separating a portion of the underlying obturator internus and levator ani muscle fibers (Fig. 15-33). An opening is made on the medial aspect of the tough obturator membrane. A curved tunneling instrument

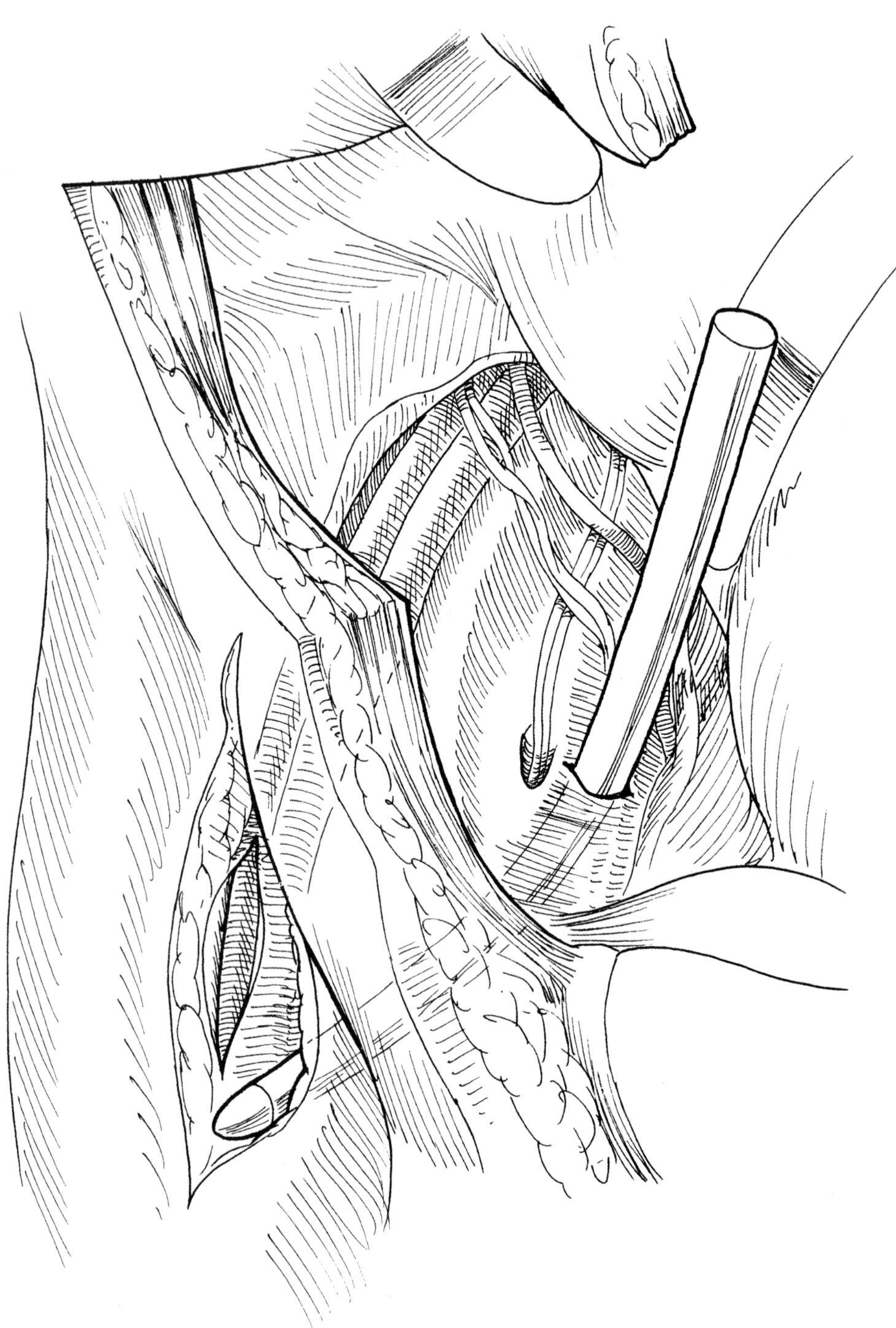

Fig. 15-33 A tunnel is made through the obturator internus muscle to reach the center of the obturator membrane for the obturator bypass.

is passed through the opening and routed behind the pectineus and adductor muscles into the midthigh. There it may be brought through the adductor longus muscle to reach the superficial femoral artery in Hunter's canal (exposure, see Chapter 16) or directed through the adductor magnus muscle to reach the vicinity of the adductor hiatus for anastomosis with the suprageniculate popliteal artery (Fig. 15-34).

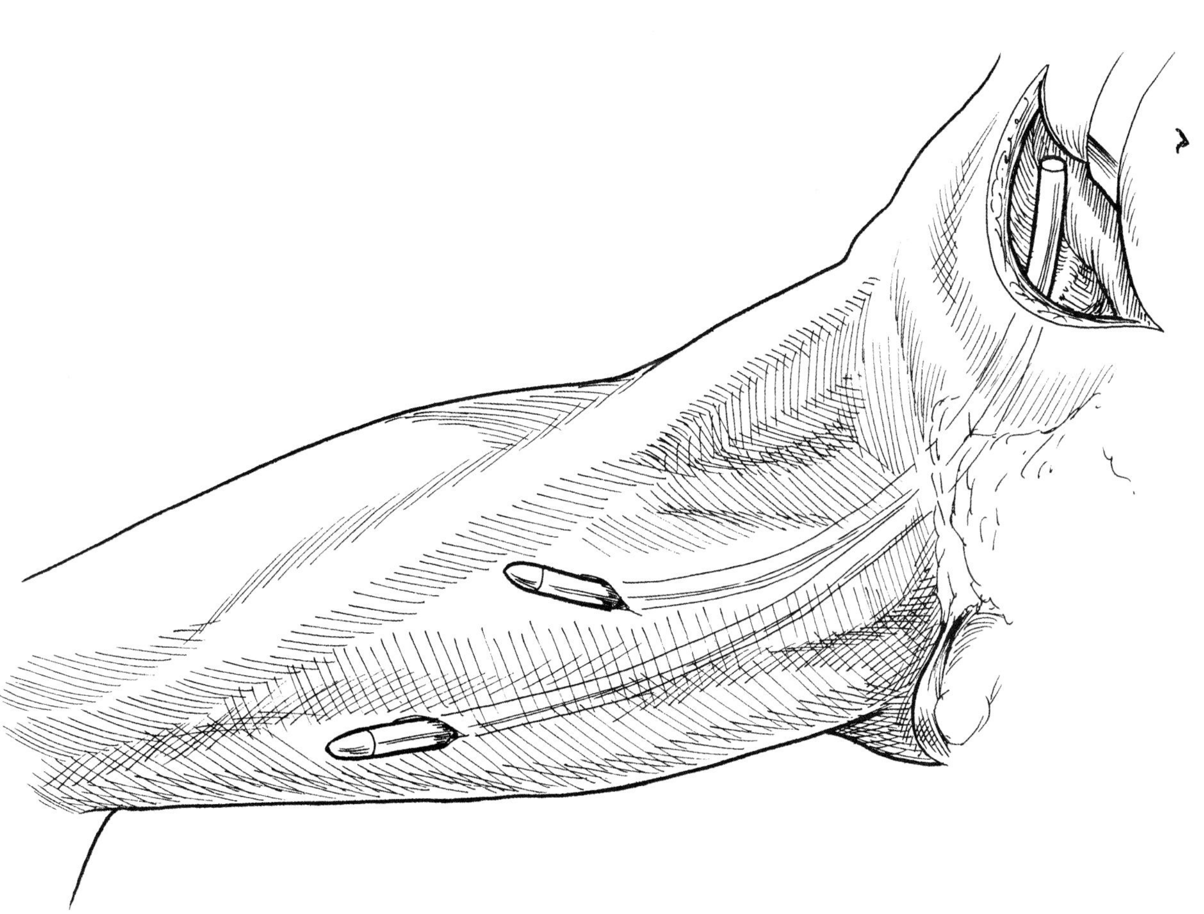

Fig. 15-34 The obturator bypass graft may be brought through the adductor longus muscle to reach the superficial femoral artery in midthigh or through the adductor magnus muscle to reach the popliteal artery.

Bypasses to the deep femoral artery can be brought through tunnels that pierce the surface of the adductor brevis muscle to reach clean lateral groin incisions (see above) (Fig. 15-35).

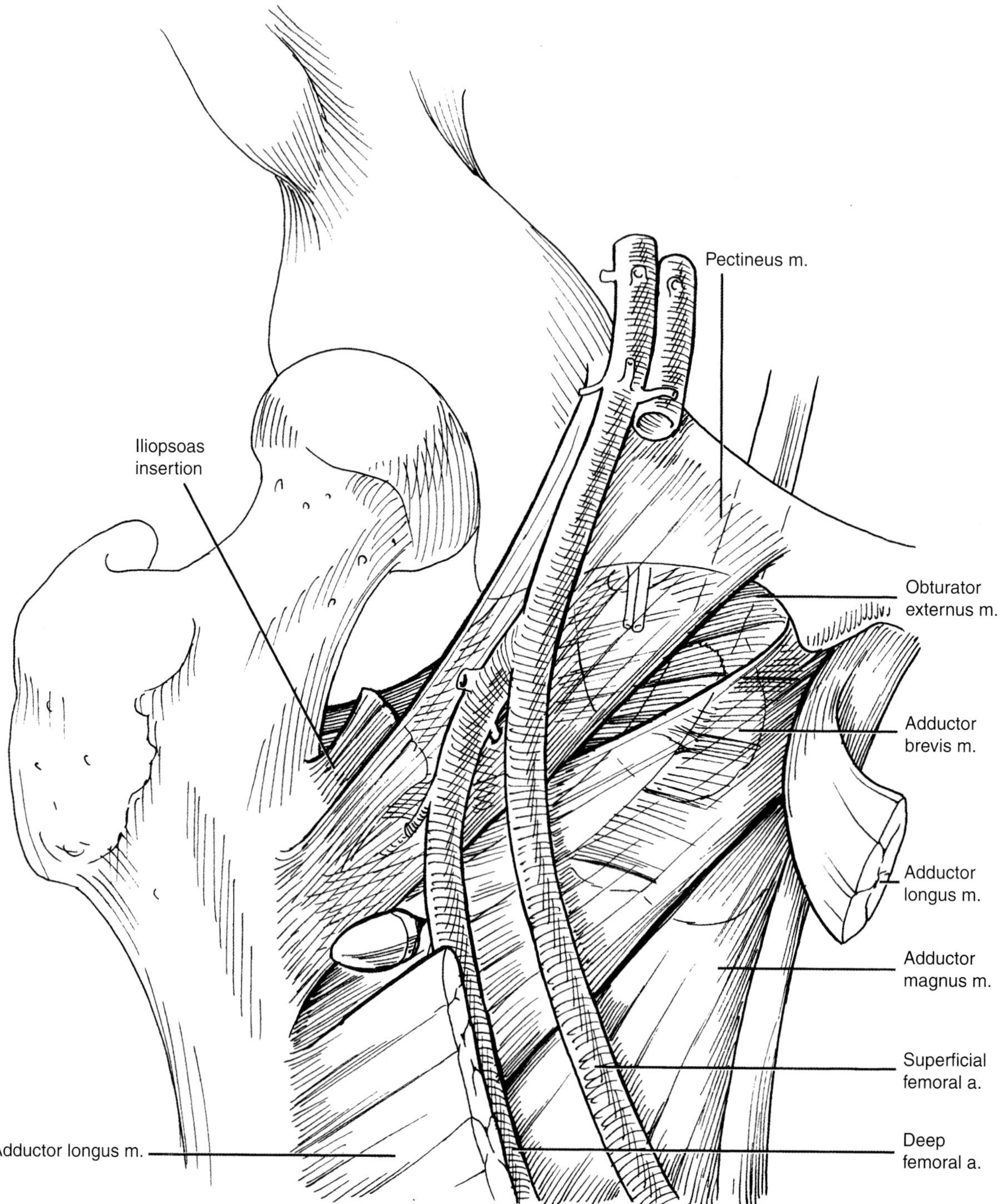

Fig. 15-35 The obturator pathway may also be used to bring a graft laterally to avoid a contaminated medial groin field. The deep femoral artery is exposed and kept under direct vision to avoid injury as the tunneler is passed through the adductor brevis muscle.

References

1. Haimovici H. Patterns of arteriosclerotic lesions of the lower extremity. *Arch Surg.* 1967;95:918–933.
2. Darling RC, Brewster DC, Hallett JW, et al. Aortoiliac reconstruction. *Surg Clin North Am.* 1979;59:565–579.
3. Sambol EB, McKinsey JF. Local complications: endovascular. In: Cronenwett JL, Johnston KW, eds. *Rutherford's Vascular Surgery,* 7th ed. Philadelphia, PA: Saunders Elsevier; 2010:697–715.
4. Beirne C, Martin F, Hynes N, et al. Five years' experience of transverse groin incision for femoral artery access in arterial reconstructive surgery: parallel observational longitudinal group comparison study. *Vascular*. 2008;16:207–212.
5. Swinnen J, Chao A, Tiwari A, et al. Vertical or transverse incisions for access to the femoral artery: a randomized control study. *Ann Vasc Surg.* 2010;24:336–341.
6. Bergan JJ. Occlusive arterial disease—femoral and popliteal. In: Nora PF, ed. *Operative Surgery: Principles and Techniques*. Philadelphia, PA: Lea & Febiger; 1980:788–800.
7. Gabella G. Arteries of the lower limb. In: Bannister LH, Berry MM, Collins P, et al., eds. *Gray's Anatomy: The Anatomic Basis of Medicine and Surgery*, 38th ed. New York, NY: Churchill Livingstone; 1995:1564–1574.
8. Schwartz MA, Schanzer H, Skladany M, et al. A comparison of conservative therapy and early selective ligation in the treatment of lymphatic complications following vascular procedures. *Am J Surg.* 1995;170:206–208.
9. Pearce WH, Kempczinski RF. Extended autogenous profundaplasty and aortofemoral grafting: an alternative to distal synchronous bypass. *J Vasc Surg.* 1984;1:455–458.
10. Landy GL, Moneta GL, Taylor LM Jr, et al. Axillofemoral bypass. *Ann Vasc Surg.* 2000;14:296–305.
11. Connoly JE, Kwaan JHM, Brownell D, et al. Newer developments of extra-anatomic bypass. *Surg Gynecol Obstet.* 1984;159:415–418.
12. Schneider JR, Besso SR, Walsh DB, et al. Femorofemoral versus aortofemoral bypass: outcome and hemodynamic results. *J Vasc Surg.* 1994;19:43–57.
13. Schneider JR. Aortoiliac disease: extra-anatomic bypass. In: Cronenwett JL, Johnston KW, eds. *Rutherford's Vascular Surgery,* 7th ed. Philadelphia, PA: Saunders Elsevier; 2010:1633–1652.
14. Perler BA, Williams GM. Does donor iliac artery percutaneous transluminal angioplasty or stent placement influence the results of femorofemoral bypass? Analysis of 70 consecutive cases with long-term follow-up. *J Vasc Surg.* 1996;24:363–370.
15. Rinckenbach S, Guelle N, Lillaz J, et al. Femorofemoral bypass as an alternative to a direct aortic approach in daily practice: appraisal of its current indications and midterm results. *Ann Vasc Surg.* 2012;26:359–364.
16. D'Addio V, Ali A, Timaran C, et al. Femorofemoral bypass with femoral popliteal vein. *J Vasc Surg.* 2005;42:35–39.
17. Lamerton AJ, Nicolaides AN, Eastcott HHG. The femorofemoral graft: hemodynamic improvement and patency rate. *Arch Surg.* 1985;120:1247–1278.
18. Plecha FR, Plecha FM. Femorofemoral bypass grafts: ten-year experience. *J Vasc Surg.* 1984;1:555–561.

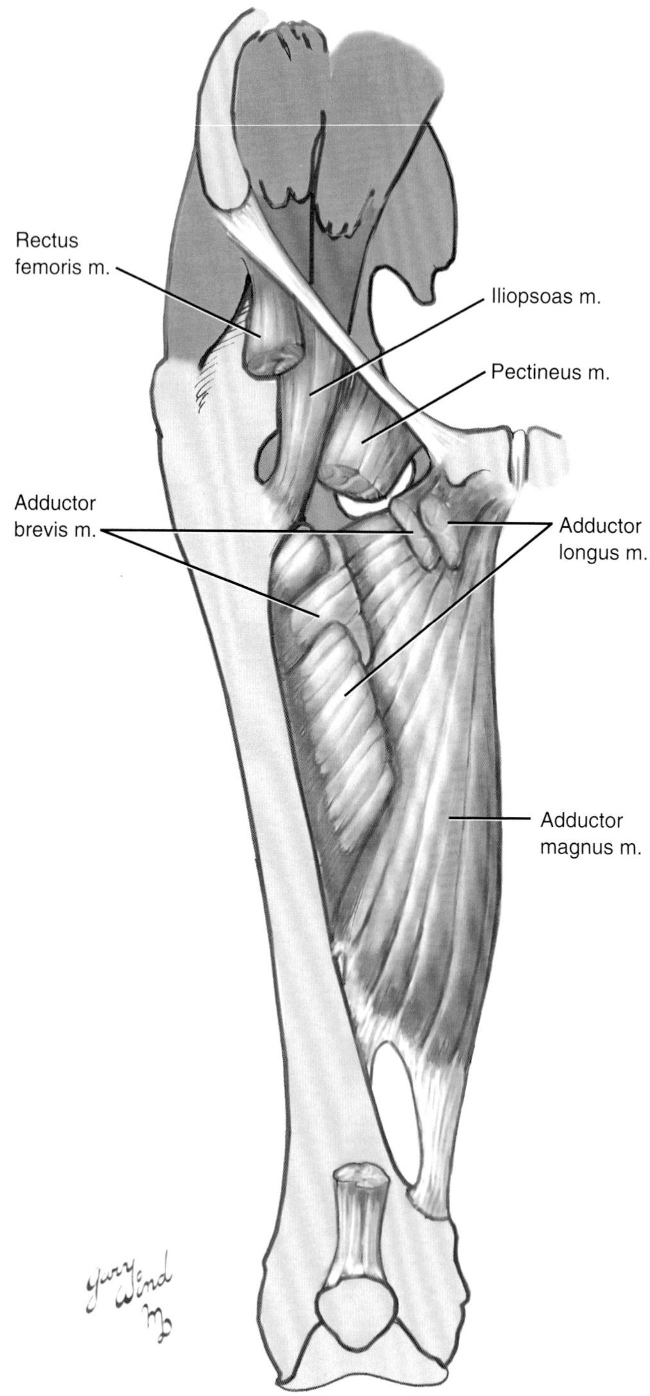

Fig. 16-1 The adductor muscles of the thigh fan out to attach along the linea aspera of the femur.

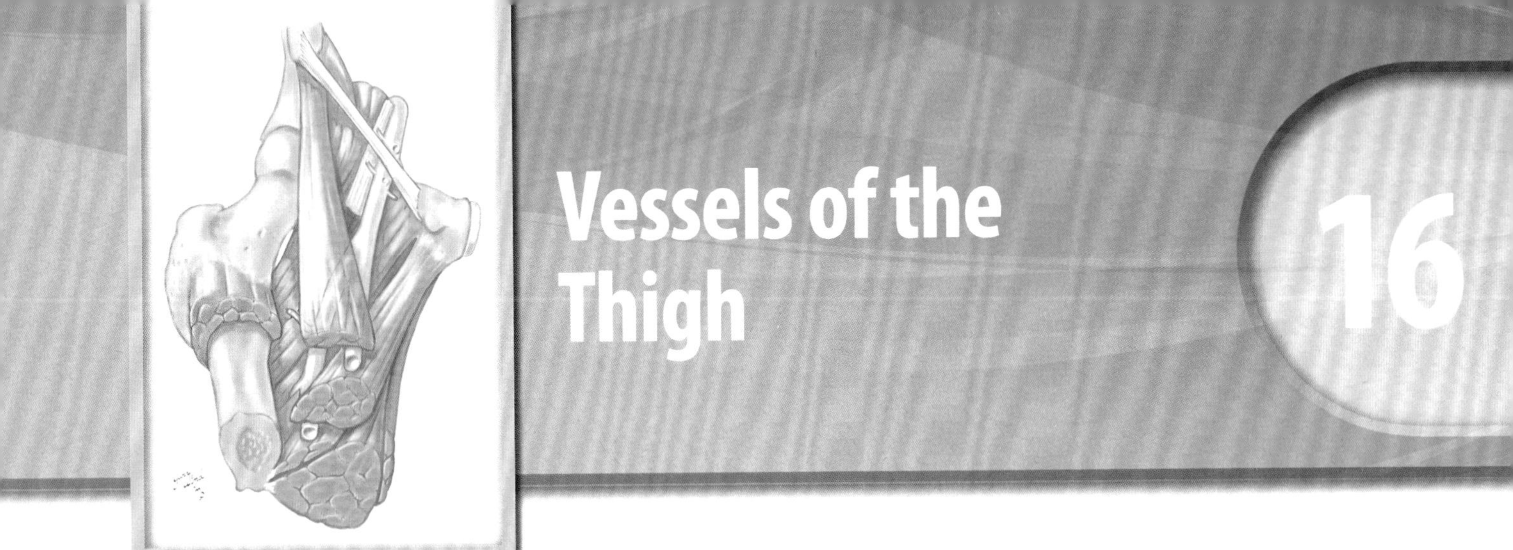

Vessels of the Thigh

Surgical Anatomy of the Thigh

Muscles

Between the bifurcation of the common femoral artery in the femoral triangle and the beginning of the popliteal artery at the adductor hiatus, the deep and superficial divisions of the femoral artery traverse the thigh anteromedial to the femoral shaft, in intimate contact with the adductor muscles. The adductor muscles (Fig. 16-1) originate from the inferior ramus of the pubis and ischium and fan out to attach to the linea aspera along the posterior side of the femur. The deepest of these muscles, the adductor magnus, attaches to the full length of the linea aspera beginning below the lesser trochanter and ending at the adductor tubercle. It is interrupted by four small apertures through which perforating branches of the deep femoral artery reach the posterior compartment, and by the large adductor hiatus at the lower third of the femur through which the superficial femoral artery passes. The lower part of the adductor brevis muscle is located between the magnus and the adductor longus muscles. The pectineus muscle, from the superior pubic ramus, covers the superior part of the adductor brevis muscle.

The posterior view of the adductor magnus muscle (Fig. 16-2) shows the more horizontal direction of the pubic fibers and the predominantly longitudinal ischial fibers. The tendinous openings can be seen along the linea aspera.

The anterior compartment of the thigh consists of the quadratus femoris muscle, which is made up of four heads: rectus femoris, vastus medialis, vastus lateralis, and vastus intermedius (Fig. 16-3). These muscles enlarge from tapered origins proximally to

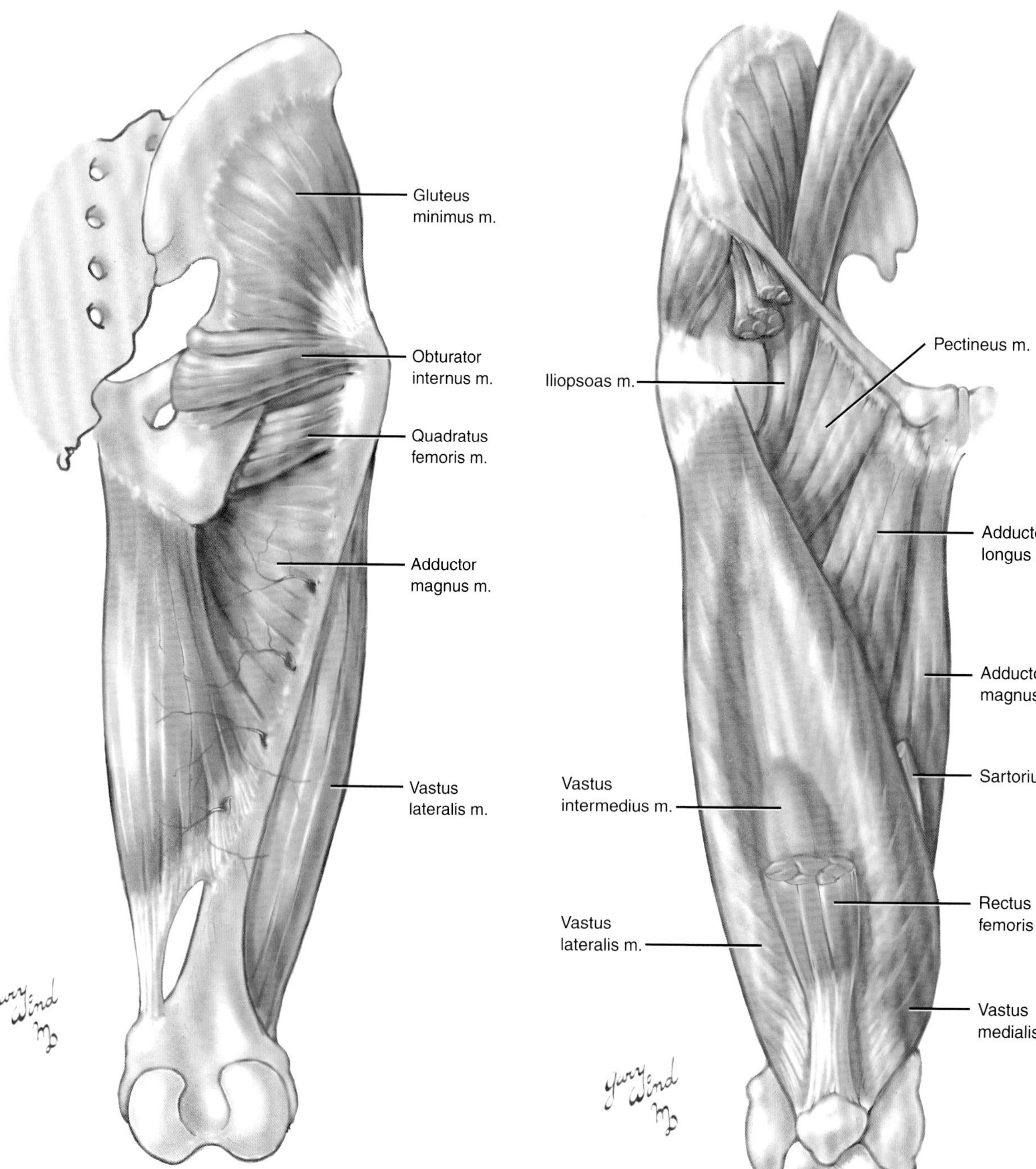

Fig. 16-2 In this posterior view, perforating branches of the deep femoral artery can be seen passing through openings in the tendinous portion of the adductor magnus muscle.

Fig. 16-3 The anterior compartment of the thigh consists of the bulky quadratus femoris muscle.

a bulky teardrop form distally. The deep and superficial femoral vessels lie in the cleft between the vastus medialis and adductor muscles.

Posteriorly, the long hamstrings, the biceps femoris, semimembranosus, and semitendinosus muscles run the length of the thigh from the ischial tuberosity to the tibia and fibula. They lie across the lower portion of the posterior surface of adductor magnus muscle. The upper portion of the adductor magnus muscle is covered by the insertion of the gluteus maximus muscle into the upper part of the linea aspera (Fig. 16-4).

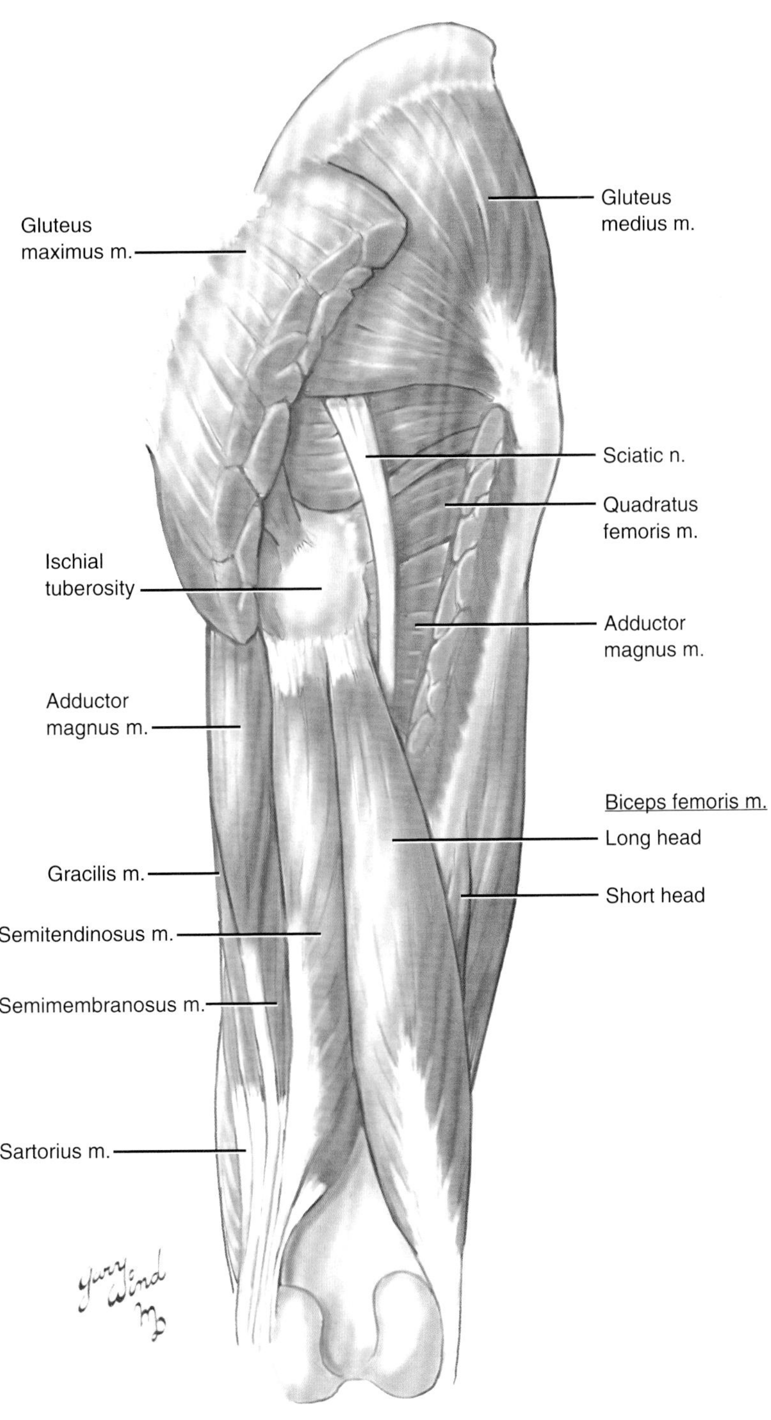

Fig. 16-4 The posterior thigh musculature is shown.

The medial adductor compartment forms a superiorly based pyramid between the quadriceps muscle and the hamstrings (Fig. 16-5). In cross section (Fig. 16-6), the bulky adductor magnus muscle has a roughly triangular profile, with a narrow linear medial attachment along the medial lip of the linea aspera.

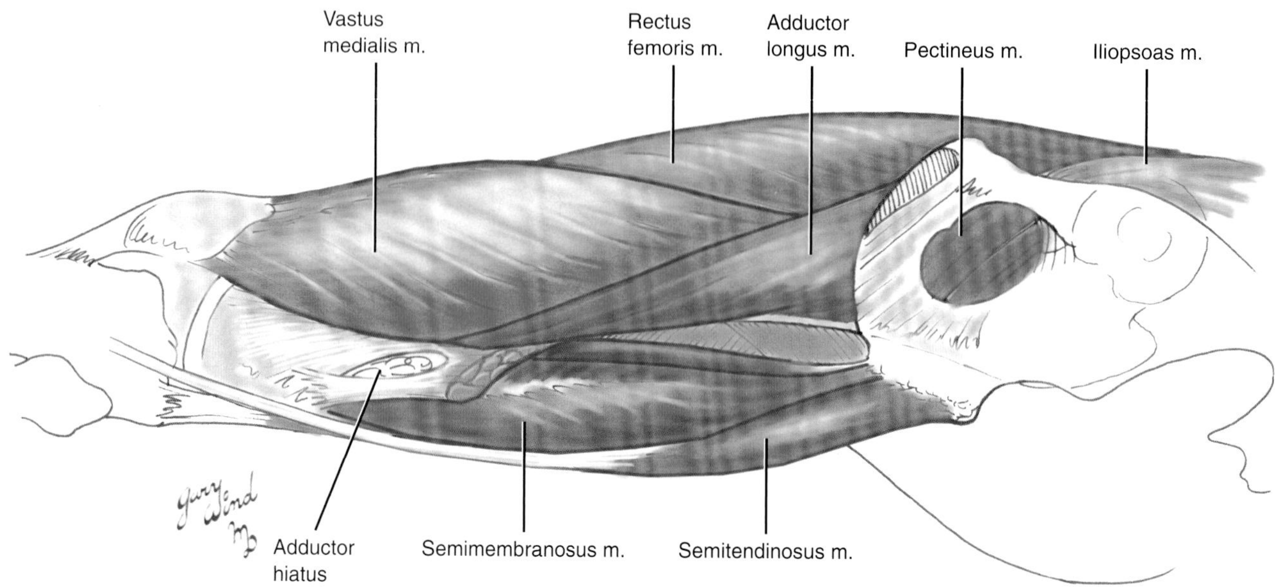

Fig. 16-5 The medial adductor compartment is interposed between the quadratus femoris and hamstring muscles. The body of the adductor magnus has been resected in this view.

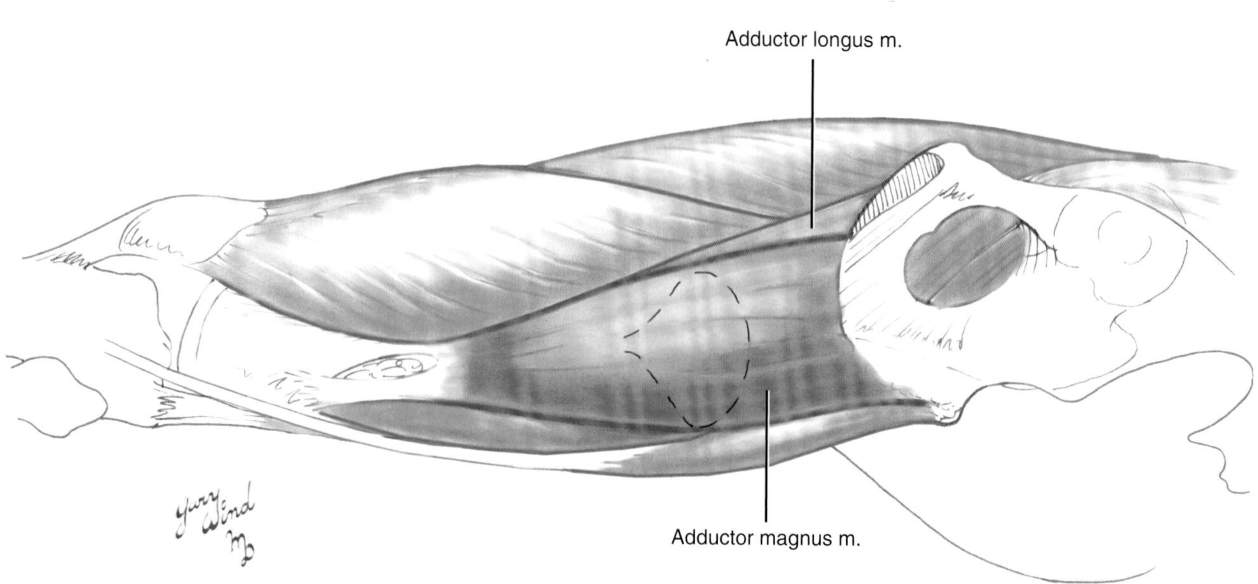

Fig. 16-6 The adductor magnus muscle tapers medially to form a narrow linear attachment along the linea aspera of the femur.

Vessels

The common femoral artery enters the femoral triangle beneath and slightly medial to the midpoint of the inguinal ligament (Fig. 16-7). Within the femoral triangle it divides into deep and superficial branches. The superficial branch crosses the adductor longus muscle to lie beneath the sartorius muscle. The deep (profunda) branch passes between the pectineus and adductor longus muscles to lie beneath the latter muscle.

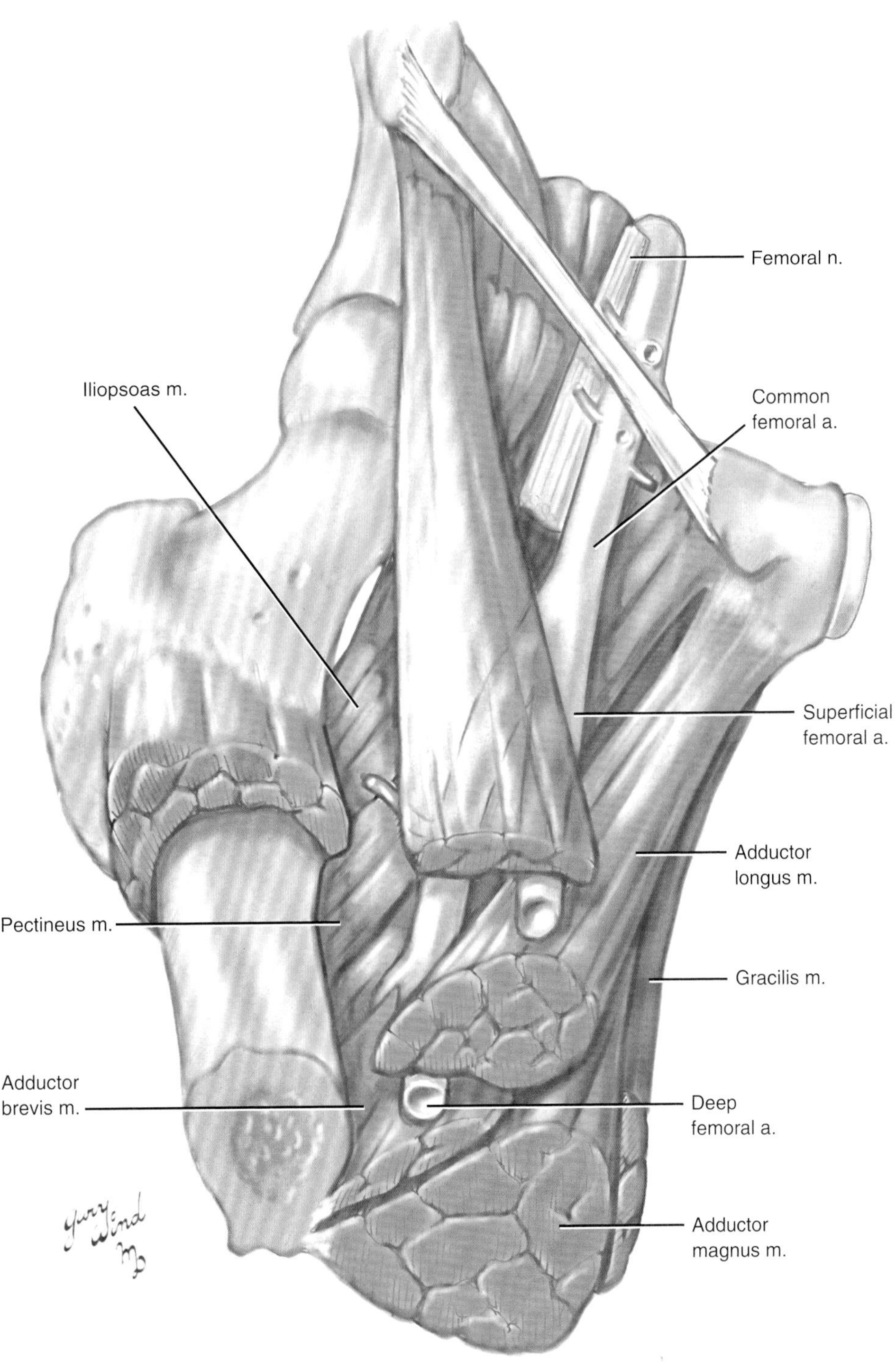

Fig. 16-7 The relationship between the branches of the femoral artery and thigh musculature is shown.

The superficial femoral artery supplies the adjacent adductor muscles and the quadriceps muscle (Fig. 16-8). The deep femoral branch supplies the adjacent adductor muscles and sends three perforating branches and its termination through the tendon of the adductor magnus muscle to supply the hamstrings in the posterior compartment.

At the apex of the femoral triangle, the superficial femoral artery enters a triangular fascia-lined cleft, the adductor (Hunter's) canal, between the vastus medialis, the sartorius, and the adductor longus (upper portion) and adductor magnus (lower portion) muscles. The canal takes a 90° twist as it descends toward the knee (Fig. 16-9). The roof of

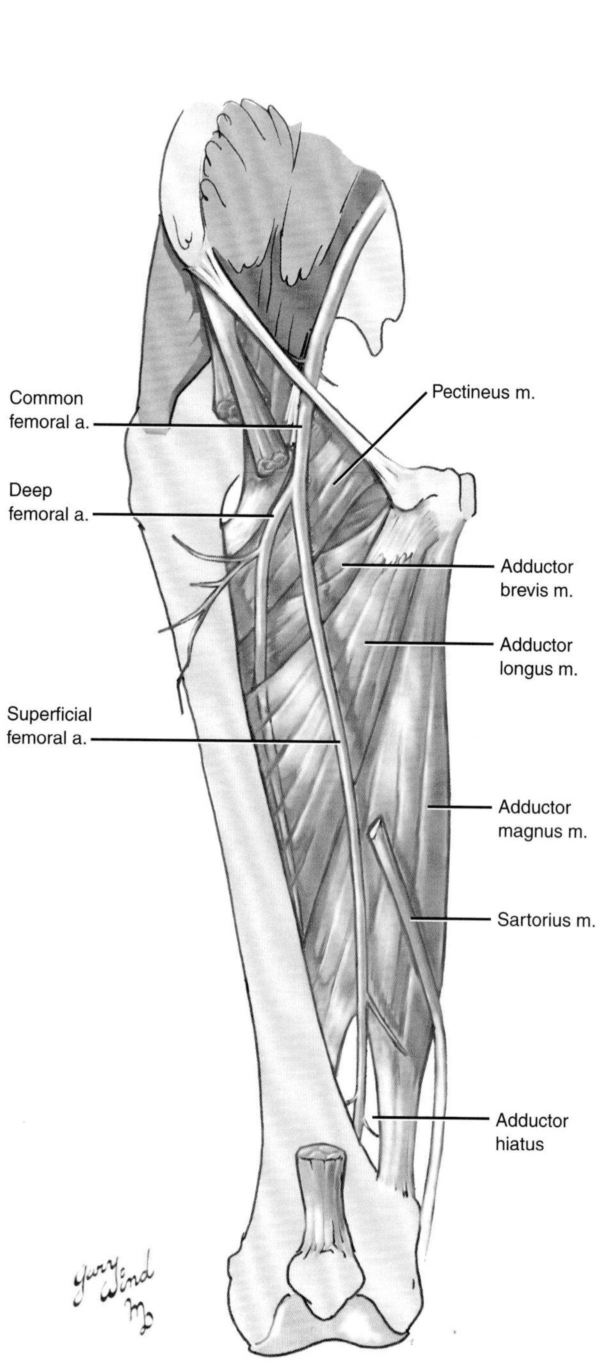

Fig. 16-8 The deep and superficial femoral branches are separated by the adductor longus muscle.

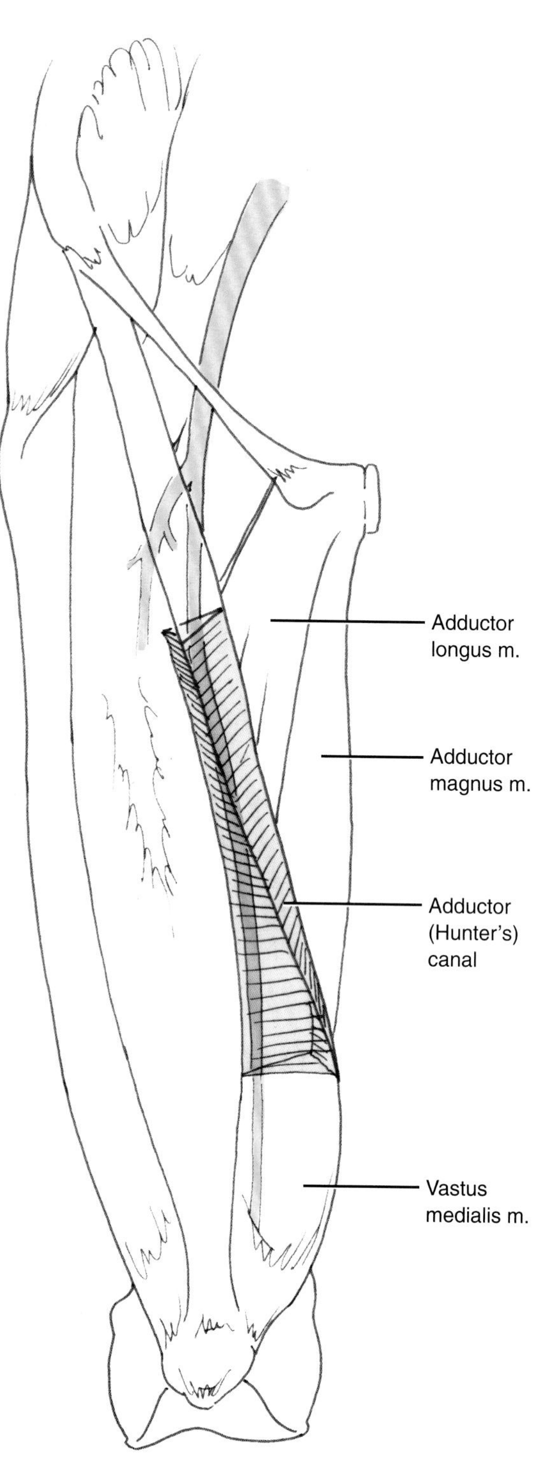

Fig. 16-9 Hunter's canal twists 90° as it descends toward the knee.

the adductor canal is a sling of tough fascia crossing from the vastus medialis to adductor muscles lying just deep to the sartorius muscle. The superficial femoral artery lies superficial to the robust accompanying superficial femoral vein. Two branches of the femoral nerve, the sensory saphenous nerve and the motor nerve to the vastus medialis muscle, accompany the superficial femoral vessels in the canal.

The deep femoral vessels (Fig. 16-10) lie close to the femur beneath the adductor longus muscle. They first lie on the adductor brevis muscle, then directly on the adductor magnus muscle. Its upper perforating branch or two transverse both deeper adductor muscles, whereas the lower branches penetrate only the tendon of the magnus to reach the posterior compartment.

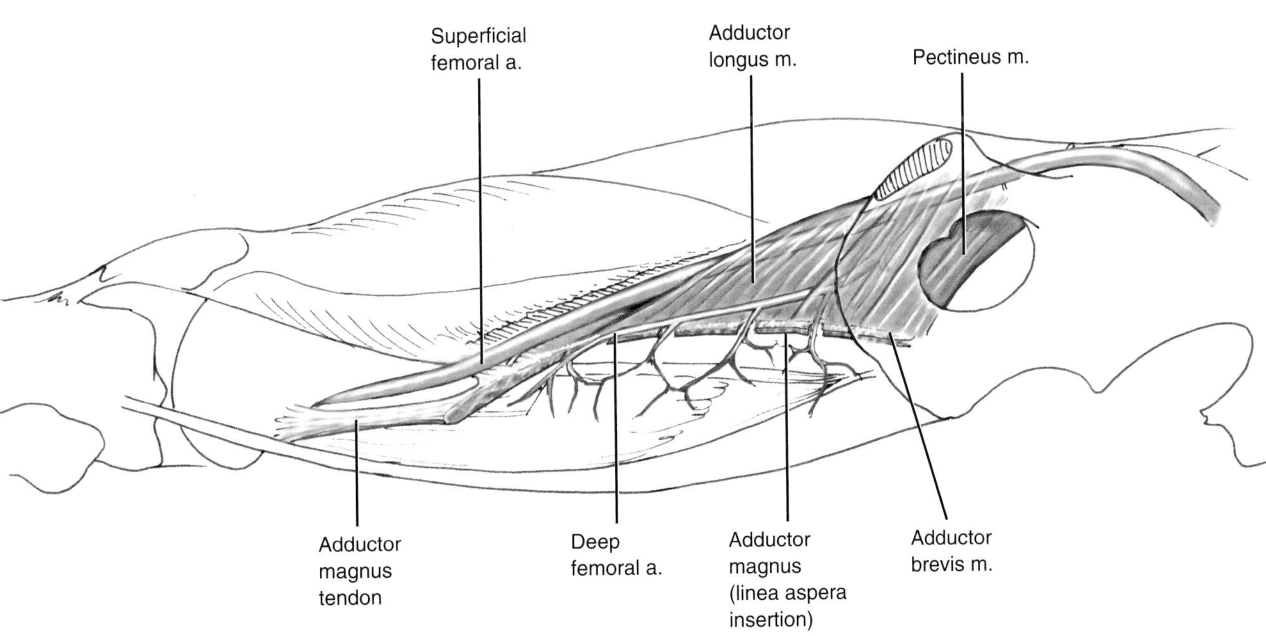

Fig. 16-10 The relationship of the deep femoral vessels to the adductor muscles is shown.

Cross sections of the thigh show the relationships of the vessels to the muscular compartments (Fig. 16-11). The lateral intermuscular septum of the thigh between the vastus lateralis and biceps femoris muscles is dense and well developed. There is firm adhesion between the surface of the adductor longus muscle and the adjacent vastus medialis muscle that requires sharp dissection to separate. The remaining interfaces between muscle groups are less well defined.

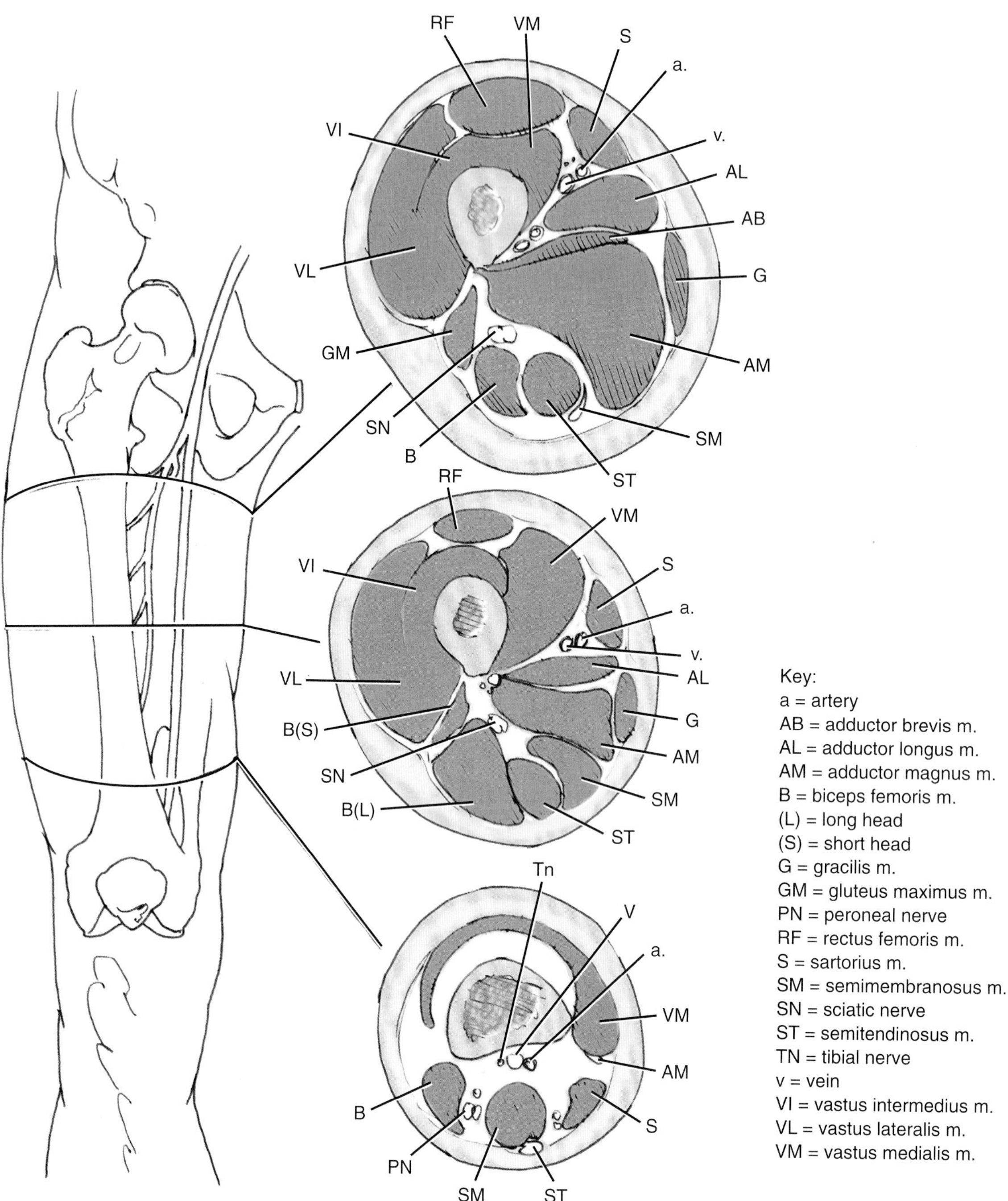

Fig. 16-11 Cross-sectional (caudal) views of the thigh demonstrate the relationship of the femoral vessels to the surrounding musculature.

The superficial femoral-popliteal vein (SFPV) begins on the medial side of the popliteal artery below the knee, passes posterior to the popliteal artery at the knee joint, and comes to lie on the lateral side of the superficial femoral artery at the adductor hiatus (Fig. 16-12). Within the adductor canal, it lies deep to the artery before assuming a medial position again at the groin. Multiple branches drain the adductor and quadriceps muscles along its course.

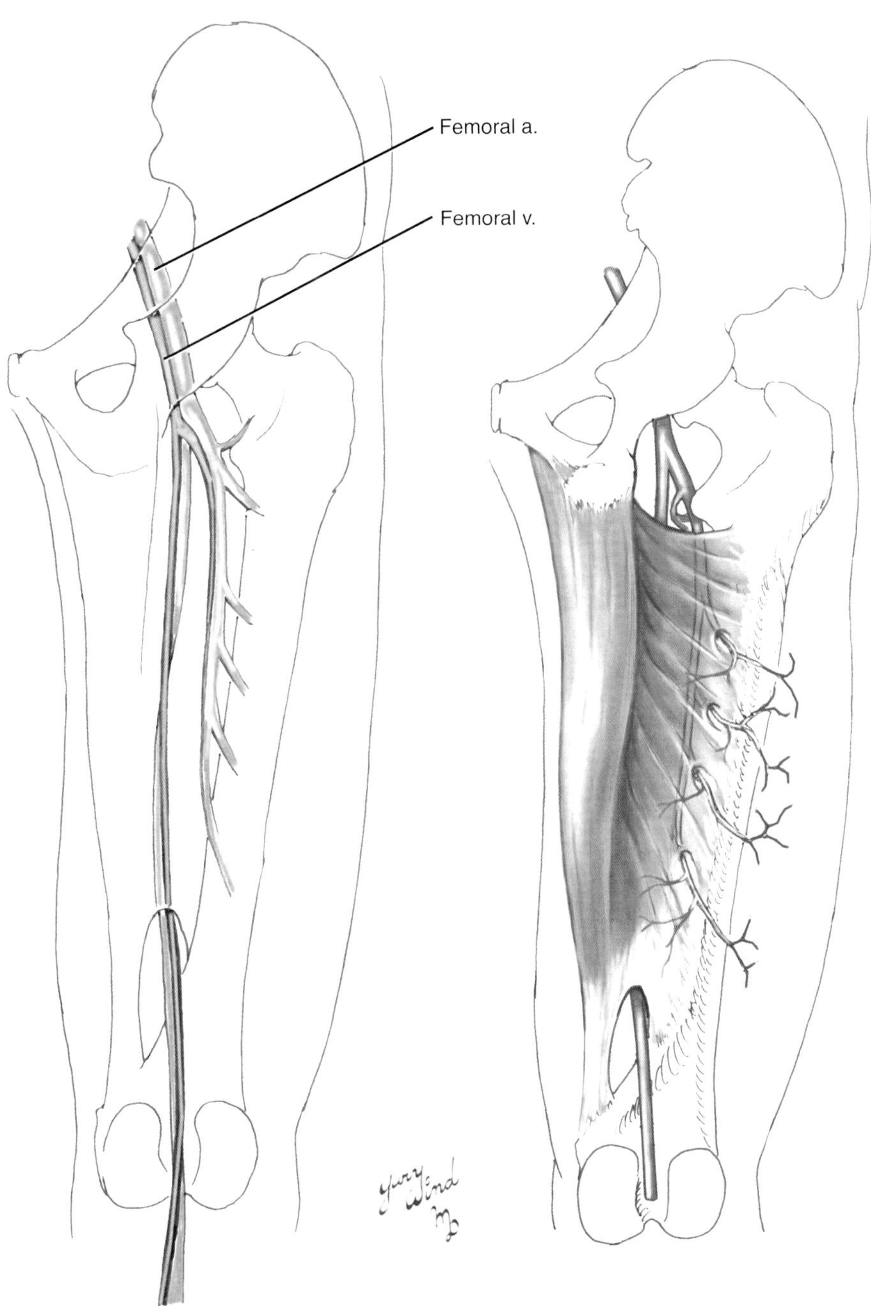

Fig. 16-12 The posterior view shows the relationship between the femoral veins and their accompanying arteries.

For purposes of clarification, Veith[1] described three anatomic subdivisions of the deep femoral artery (Fig. 16-13). The proximal zone extends from the artery's origin to the portion just distal to the lateral circumflex femoral artery. The middle zone includes the segment extending to the second perforating branch, and the distal zone extends from the second perforating branch to the artery's termination. The sartorius muscle overlies the middle and distal zones of the artery.

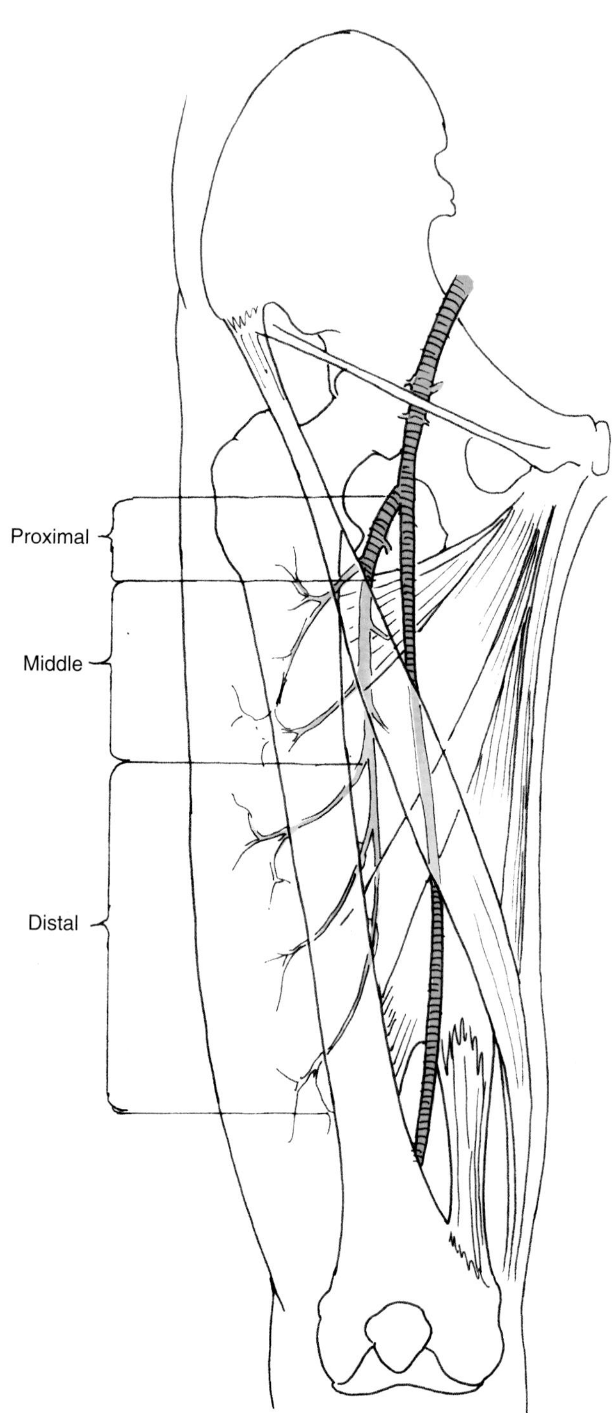

Fig. 16-13 The deep femoral artery can be divided into three anatomic zones. The middle and distal zones lie beneath the sartorius muscle and require rotation of the sartorius muscle for exposure.

Exposure of the Superficial Femoral Vessels in the Thigh

The SFPV is an excellent conduit for large artery bypasses. This graft has proven to be durable for in situ replacement of infected aortic grafts,[2] femoral arterial bypass,[3] central venous reconstruction, thigh arteriovenous fistula, carotid artery reconstruction, and mesenteric artery revascularization.[4] The SFPV creates an excellent size match with the infrarenal abdominal aorta, and we have used it for primary aortofemoral revascularization in young patients with small aortas.[5] SFPV harvest has been associated with surprisingly minimal sequelae.[6] However, the large size of the SFPV makes it unsuitable for bypass to the infrageniculate arteries. The following discussion involves exposure of the entire SFPV for the purpose of vein harvest. More localized exposure of the superficial femoral vessels can be gained through a more limited thigh incision.

The patient is placed in the supine position with the leg externally rotated and the knee flexed 30°. When bilateral vein harvest is anticipated, the legs should be placed in a "frog-leg" position, with the knees flexed as close to 90° as possible. Full exposure of the superficial femoral vessels is most easily achieved through a longitudinal thigh incision that parallels the lateral border of the sartorius muscle. The incision should extend from the lateral groin to the knee (Fig. 16-14). Lateral placement of the incision is necessary to avoid interrupting the segmental blood supply to the sartorius muscle, which enters

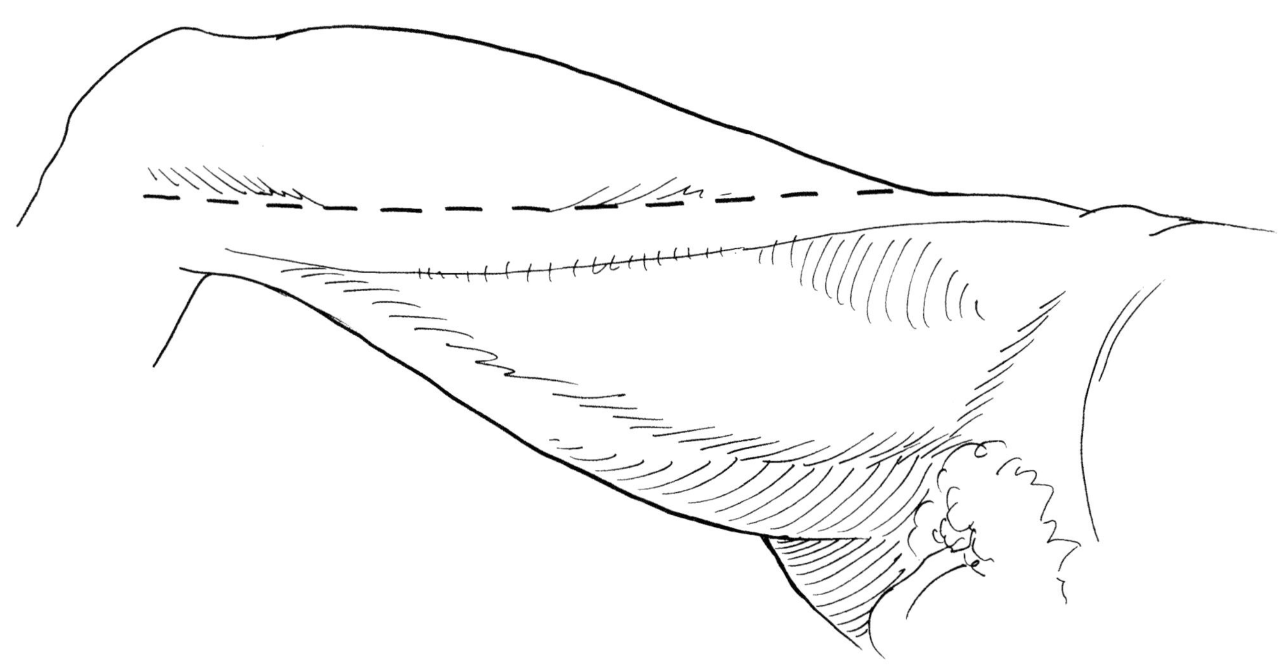

Fig. 16-14 The incision is made parallel to the lateral border of the sartorius muscle.

the muscle on its inferomedial edge.[7] The incision is deepened through the fascia lata, and the sartorius muscle is reflected medially to expose the underlying roof of the adductor canal (Fig. 16-15). Entry into this overlying fascia exposes the superficial femoral vessels. The vein and artery can be carefully separated using sharp dissection to incise loose areolar tissue. The superficial femoral vein has multiple large branches that require secure ligation with double ligatures or transfixing sutures to prevent disastrous bleeding complications when used in the arterial circulation.[8] The saphenous nerve is easily recognized within the adductor canal and should be carefully protected during dissection to prevent saphenous neuralgia (Fig. 16-16).

The superficial femoral vein should always be mobilized proximally to the level of the common femoral vein confluence. If the vein is to be harvested for use as a bypass graft, it is critically important to transect and oversew the vein flush with the deep femoral vein so that there is no residual stump of superficial femoral vein that may serve as a nidus for a pulmonary embolus (Fig. 16-17). The vein can be mobilized distally to the level of the knee joint and transected just proximal to the popliteal vein confluence.

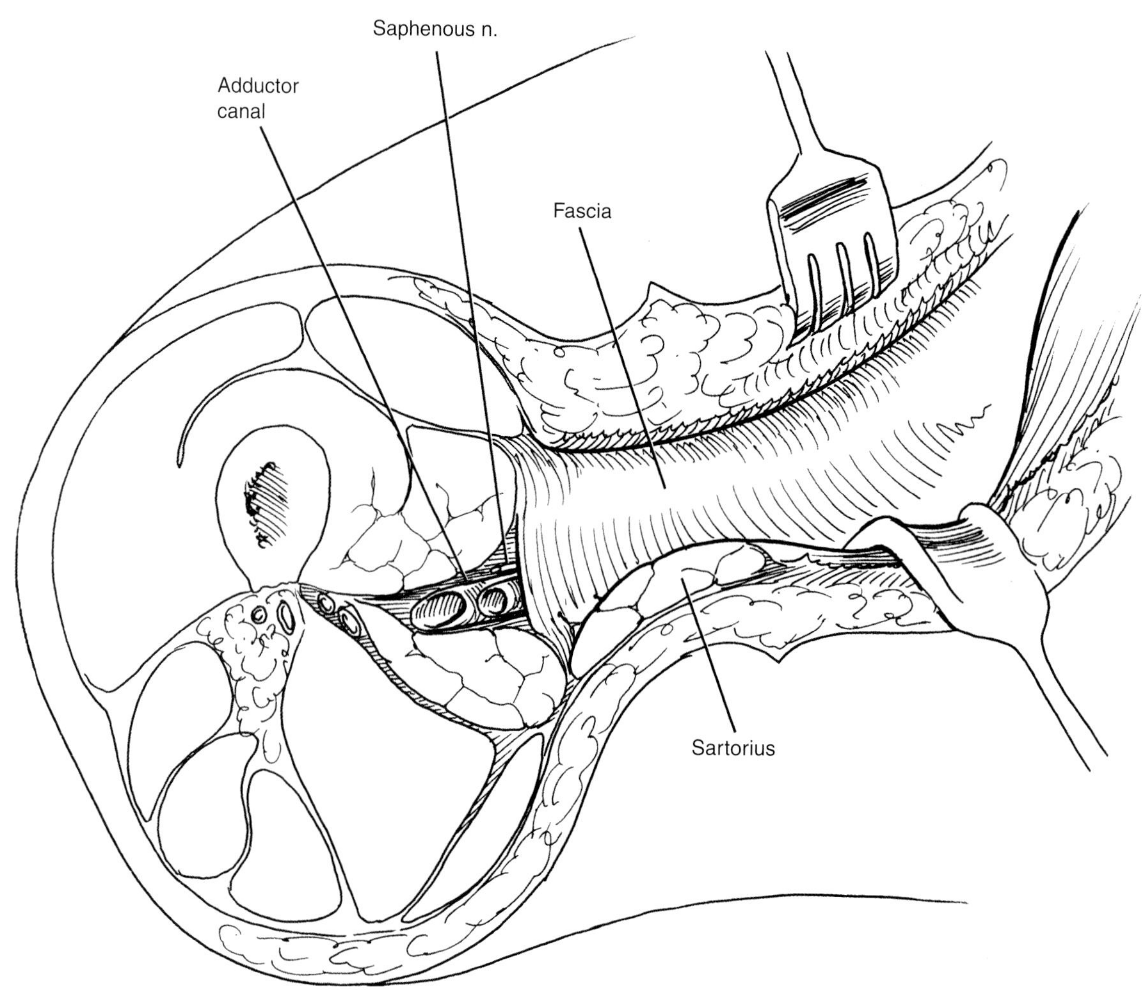

Fig. 16-15 Medial retraction of the sartorius exposes the fascial roof overlying the adductor canal.

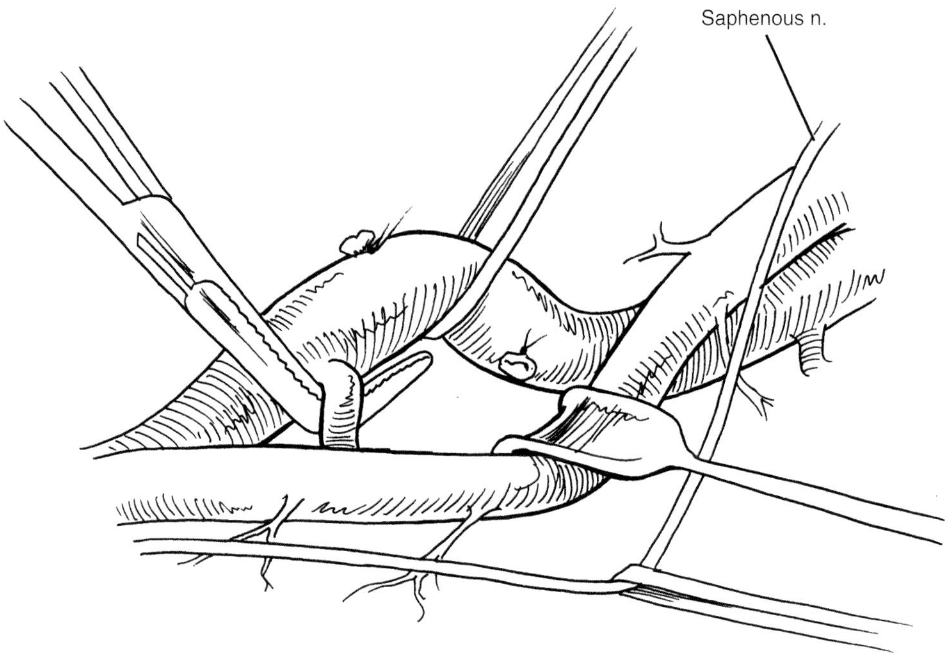

Fig. 16-16 The saphenous nerve traverses the adductor canal alongside the superficial femoral vessels.

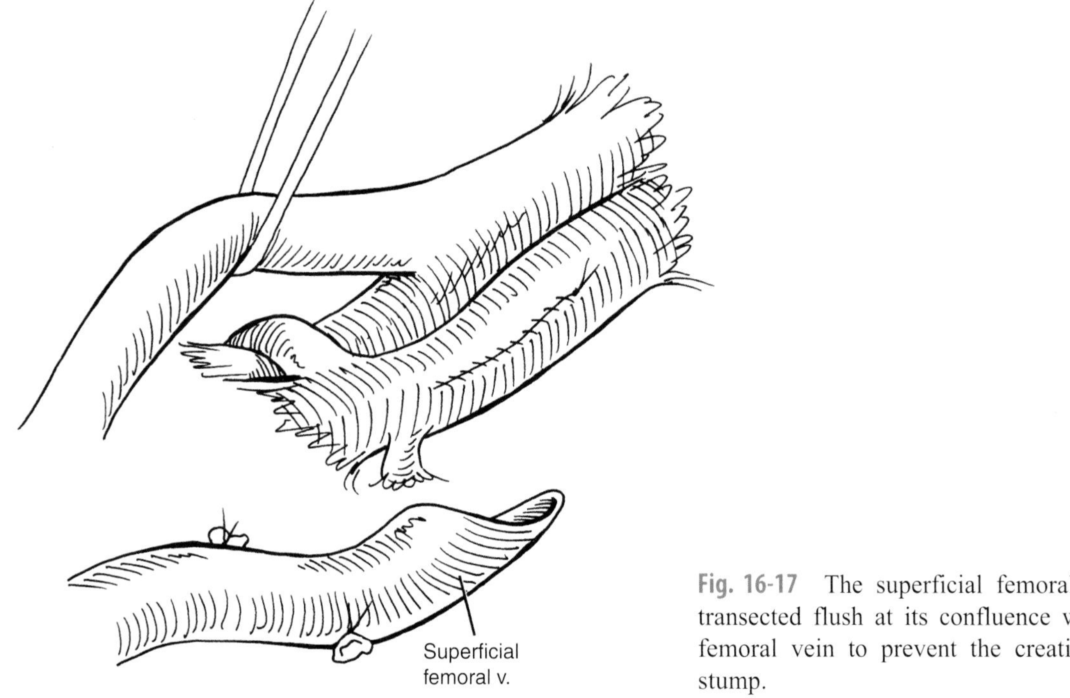

Fig. 16-17 The superficial femoral vein should be transected flush at its confluence with the common femoral vein to prevent the creation of a residual stump.

Lateral Approach to the Middle and Distal Segments of the Deep Femoral Artery

Each of the three segments of the deep femoral artery can serve as an excellent source of inflow for infrainguinal bypass procedures.[9] Locating the proximal anastomosis in the middle or distal segments allows the bypass length to be shortened in patients whose saphenous veins are inadequate to reach the groin. Direct exposure of the proximal segment of the deep femoral artery is best obtained through a vertical groin incision (see Chapter 15). A vertical incision along the lateral border of the sartorius muscle provides access to the deep femoral artery distal to the femoral sheath. This technique may also be preferred to the direct approach through the femoral sheath in vascular procedures involving graft infection, excessive postoperative scarring, or previous radiation to the groin.[10,11]

The patient is placed in the supine position, and the lower abdomen and entire leg are prepped and draped. A vertical incision is made parallel to the lateral border of the sartorius muscle at the lower end of the femoral triangle (Fig. 16-18). After the wound is deepened through the fascia lata,

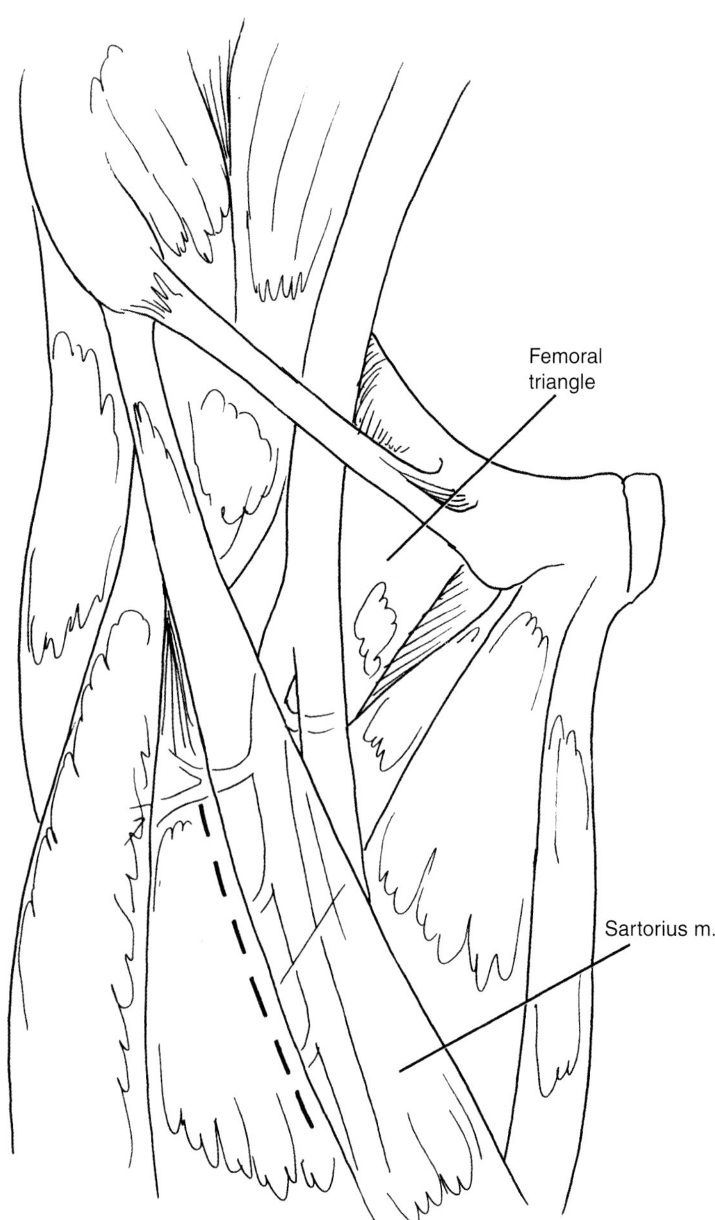

Fig. 16-18 The incision is made lateral to the border of the sartorius muscle at the lower end of the femoral triangle.

the sartorius muscle is mobilized along its lateral border and reflected medially. The incision is further deepened through a tough fascia that extends between the vastus medialis and adductor longus muscles. Lateral retraction of the rectus femoris muscle allows exposure of the lateral circumflex branches of the deep femoral vessels (Fig. 16-19). One or two branches of the femoral nerve will be seen coursing over the lateral femoral circumflex vessels; the nerves should be identified and moved

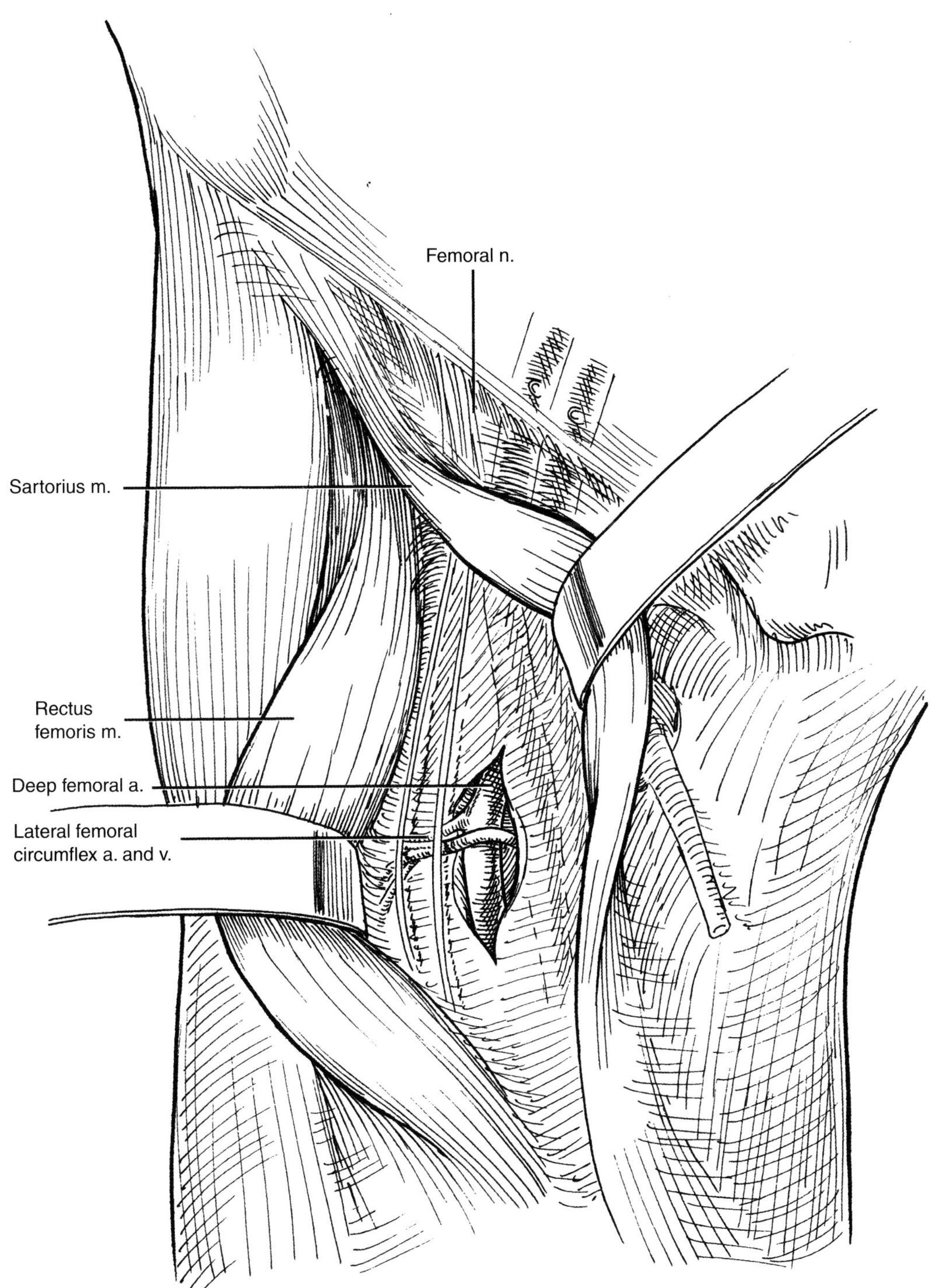

Fig. 16-19 The deep femoral artery may be approached laterally between the sartorius and rectus femoris muscles when a surgically compromised groin must be avoided.

laterally in the wound (Fig. 16-20). Division of the lateral femoral circumflex vein provides exposure of the trunk of the deep femoral artery. Medial dissection exposes the origin of the deep femoral artery at its junction with the common femoral artery. Dissection distal to the lateral femoral circumflex vein exposes the trunk of the deep femoral artery to the level of the second perforating branch, where the artery dives posterior to the adductor longus muscle. Exposure of the artery between the level of the second perforating branch and its termination as the fourth perforator requires division of the adductor longus insertion on the linea aspera (Figs. 16-21 and 16-22).

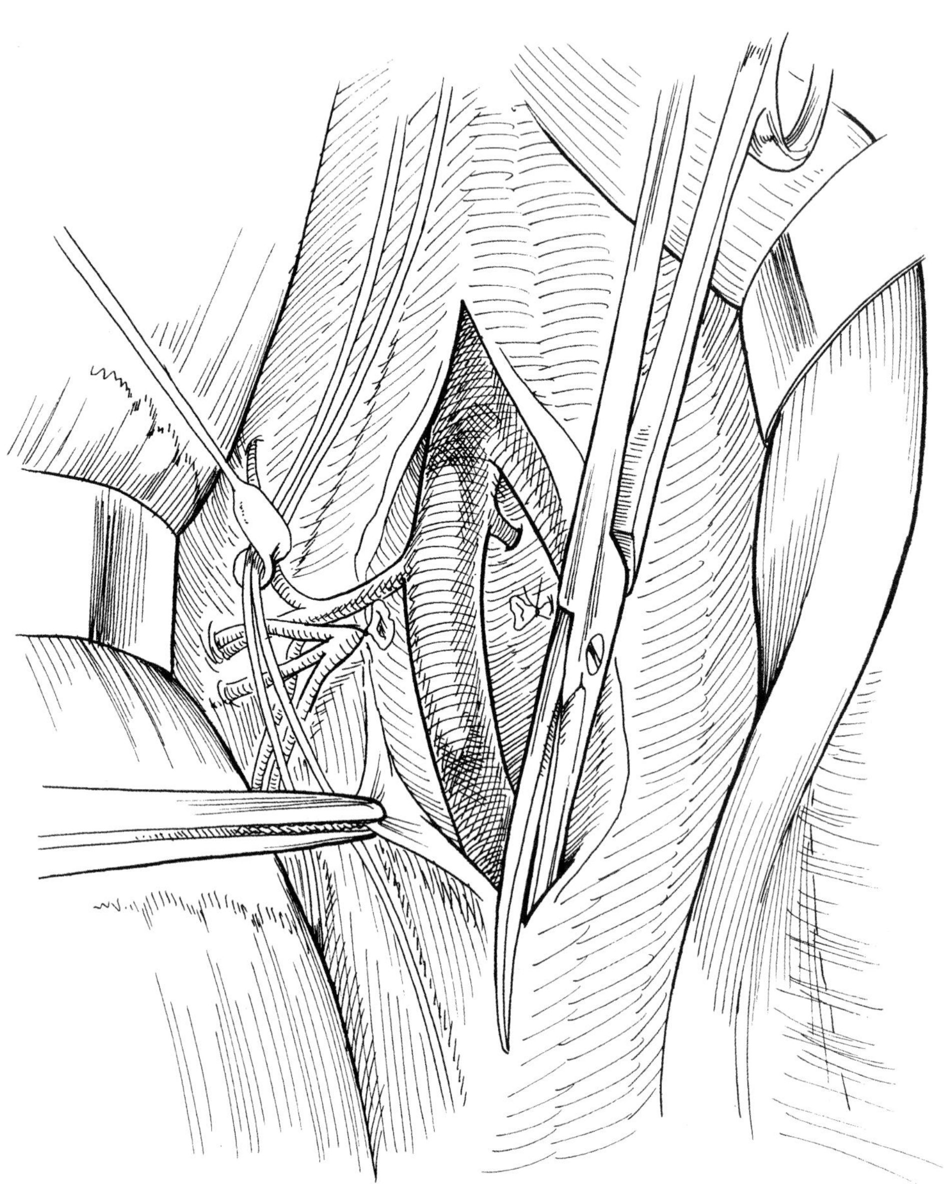

Fig. 16-20 Retraction of femoral nerve branches and division of the lateral femoral circumflex vein expose the deep femoral artery.

Fig. 16-21 Exposure of the deep femoral artery distal to the second perforating branch (distal zone) requires division of the adductor longus muscle.

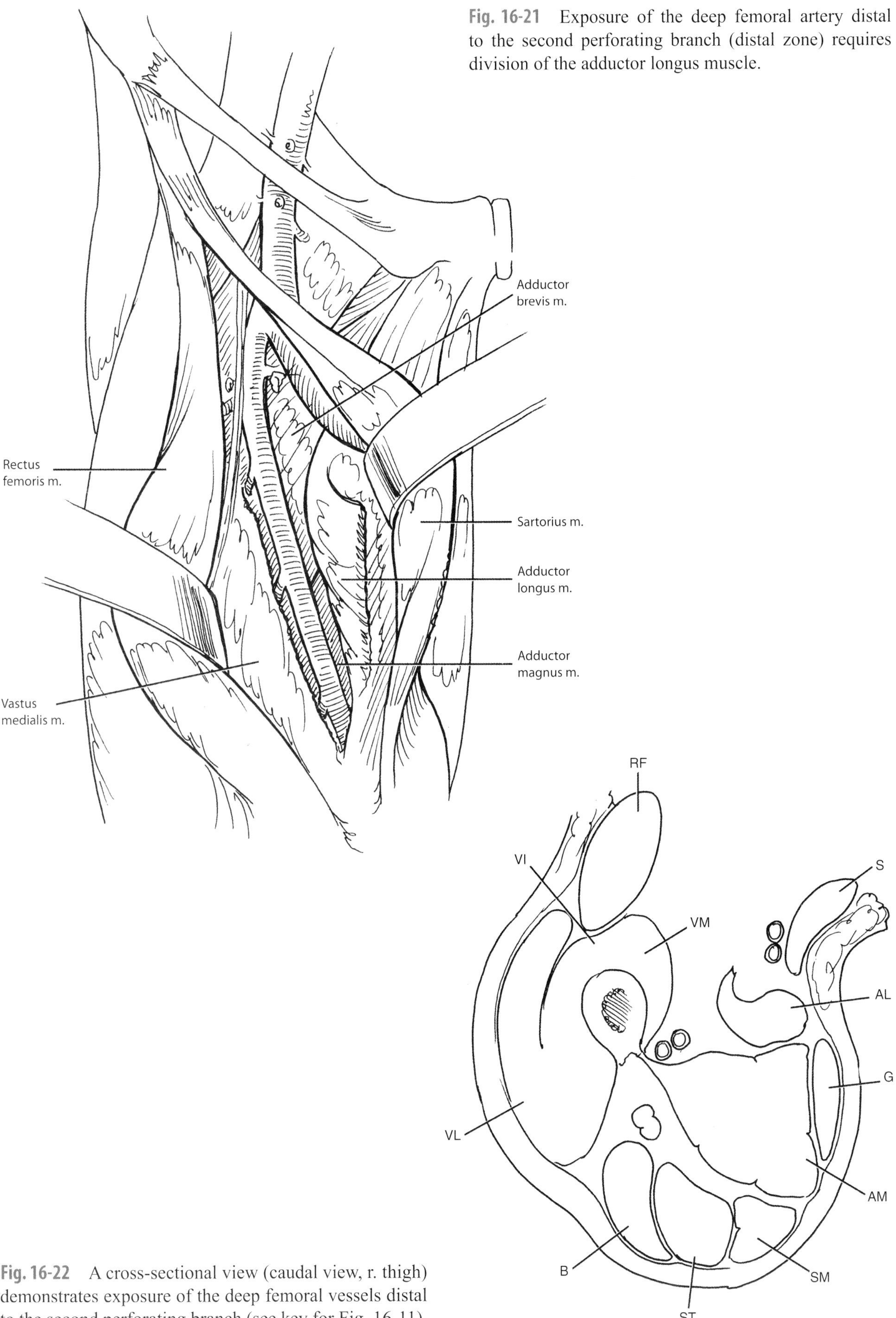

Fig. 16-22 A cross-sectional view (caudal view, r. thigh) demonstrates exposure of the deep femoral vessels distal to the second perforating branch (see key for Fig. 16-11).

Posterior Approach to the Deep Femoral Artery

Secondary revascularizations are often required for limb salvage in patients who have developed bypass graft thrombosis. These procedures are complicated by the presence of scarring or infection, making novel bypass routes attractive. Bertucci et al.[12] described a direct posterior approach to the middle and distal zones of the deep femoral artery. This technique can be combined with posterior exposure of the popliteal (see Chapter 17) or infrageniculate arteries (see Chapter 18) for creation of an all-posterior bypass.

The patient is placed in the prone position, and the entire leg and ipsilateral buttock are prepped and draped. The hamstring muscle group constitutes the important landmark for this approach. A long vertical incision is made parallel to the lateral edge of the biceps femoris muscle, the most lateral muscle in the hamstring group. The incision should extend approximately 6 cm superior to and 10 cm inferior to the gluteal crease[12] (Fig. 16-23). The gluteus maximus muscle is mobilized extensively along its inferior border and retracted superomedially. This maneuver exposes the proximal portion of the biceps femoris muscle and the sciatic nerve. The adductor magnus muscle is exposed in the deep wound by retracting the biceps femoris muscle medially. Gentle medial retraction of the sciatic nerve may be required to improve visualization of the adductor magnus muscle at this level.[12] The distal segments of the deep femoral artery are exposed by making a longitudinal incision in the adductor magnus muscle, using the muscular openings for the perforating branches as a guide (Fig. 16-24). Full exposure requires longitudinal division of the adductor brevis muscle lying just beneath the adductor magnus muscle in this approach (Fig. 16-25).

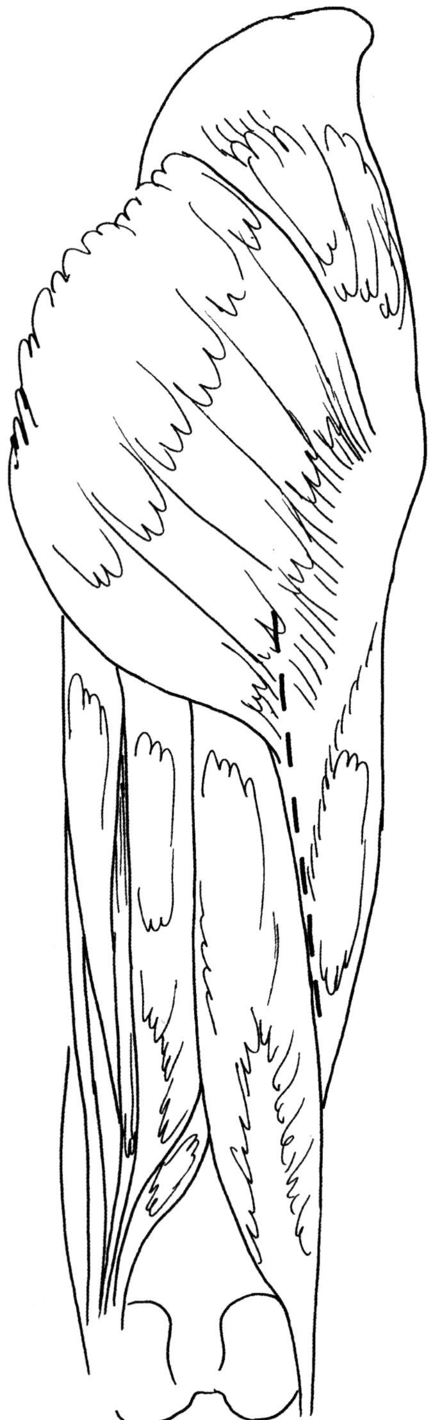

Fig. 16-23 The incision for posterior exposure of the deep femoral artery is shown.

Fig. 16-24 The gluteus maximus muscle is retracted superomedially, and the biceps femoris muscle is retracted medially to expose the adductor magnus muscle. The deep femoral vessels are exposed by incising the adductor magnus muscle near its insertion on the linea aspera.

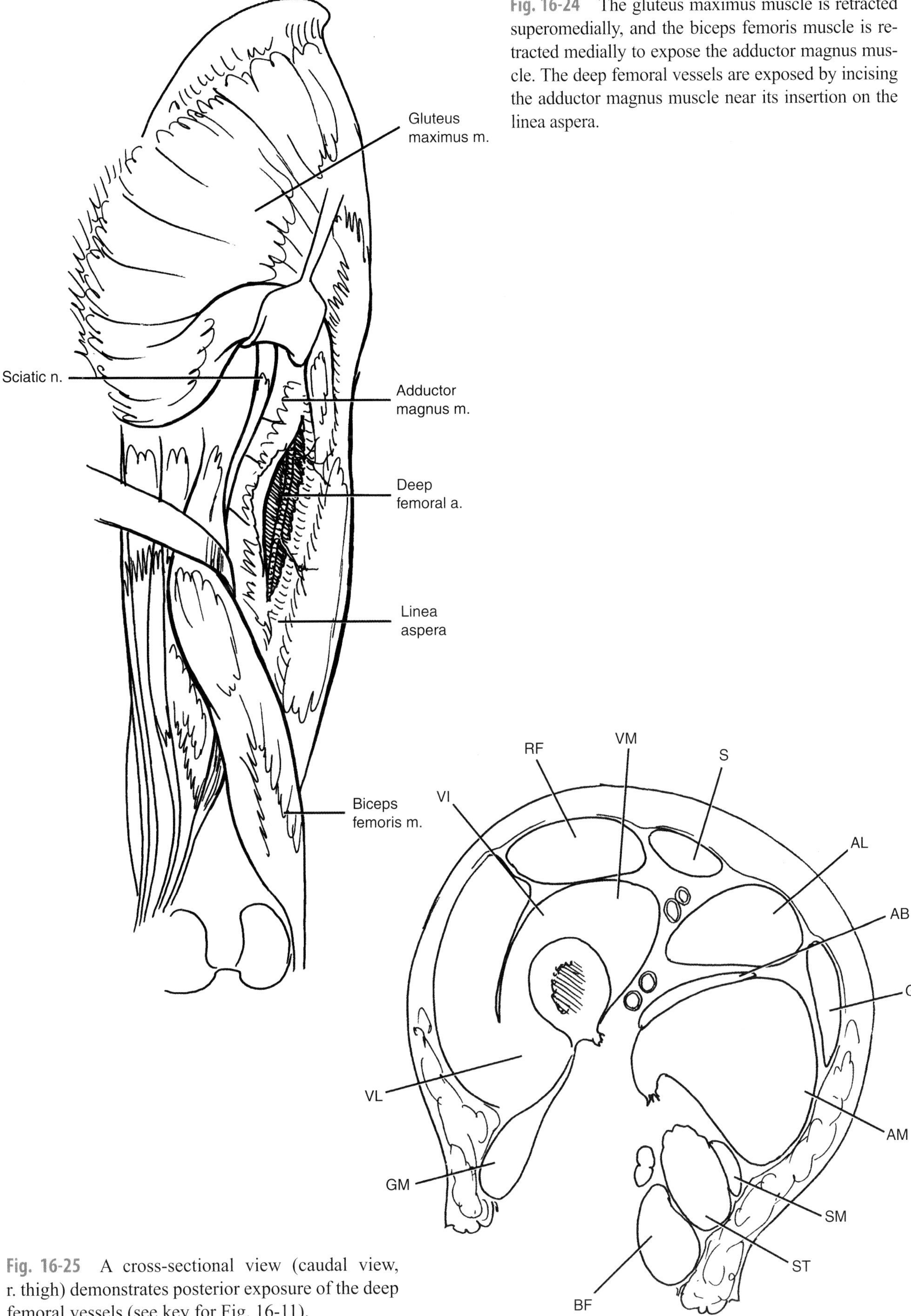

Fig. 16-25 A cross-sectional view (caudal view, r. thigh) demonstrates posterior exposure of the deep femoral vessels (see key for Fig. 16-11).

References

1. Veith FJ. Alternative approaches to the deep femoral, popliteal, and infrapopliteal arteries in the leg and foot: part I. *Ann Vasc Surg*. 1994;8:514–522.
2. Chung J, Clagett GP. Neoaortoiliac system (NAIS) procedures for the treatment of infected aortic graft. *Semin Vasc Surg*. 2011;24:220–226.
3. D'Addio V, Ali A, Timaran C, et al. Femorofemoral bypass with femoropopliteal vein. *J Vasc Surg*. 2005;42:35–39.
4. Brahmanandam S, Clair D, Benja J, et al. Adjunctive use of the superficial femoral vein for vascular reconstructions. *J Vasc Surg*. 2012;55:1355–1366.
5. Jackson MR, Ali AT, Bell C, et al. Aortofemoral bypass in young patients with premature atherosclerosis: is superficial femoral vein superior to Dacron? *J Vasc Surg*. 2004;40:17–23.
6. Modrall JG, Hocking JA, Timaran CH, et al. Late incidence of chronic venous insufficiency after deep vein harvest. *J Vasc Surg*. 2007;46:520–525.
7. Valentine RJ. Harvesting the superficial femoral vein as an autograft. *Semin Vasc Surg*. 2000;13:27–31.
8. Smith ST, Clagett GP. Femoral vein harvest for vascular reconstructions: pitfalls and tips for success. *Semin Vasc Surg*. 2008;21:35–40.
9. Darling RC III, Shah DM, Chang BB, et al. Can the deep femoral artery be used reliably as an inflow source for infrainguinal reconstruction? Long-term results in 563 procedures. *J Vasc Surg*. 1994;20:889–895.
10. Naraysingh V, Karmody AM, Leather RP, et al. Lateral approach to the profunda femoris artery. *Am J Surg*. 1984;147:813–814.
11. Nunez AA, Veith FJ, Collier P, et al. Direct approaches to the distal portions of the deep femoral artery for limb salvage bypasses. *J Vasc Surg*. 1988;8:576–581.
12. Bertucci WR, Mairn ML, Veith FJ, et al. Posterior approach to the deep femoral artery. *J Vasc Surg*. 1999;29:741–744.

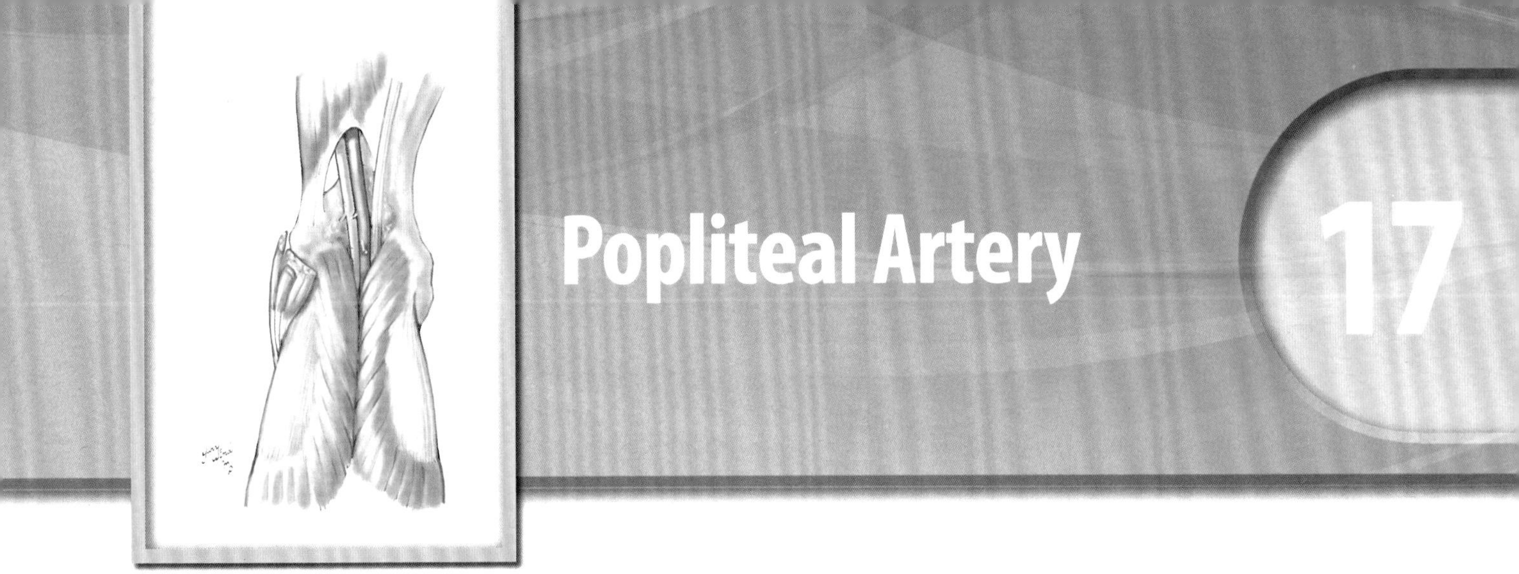

Popliteal Artery

17

Surgical Anatomy of the Popliteal Vessels

The popliteal artery is a short but vital segment of the major arterial conduit of the leg situated between the adductor hiatus and the lower border of the popliteus muscle posterior to the knee joint (Fig. 17-1).

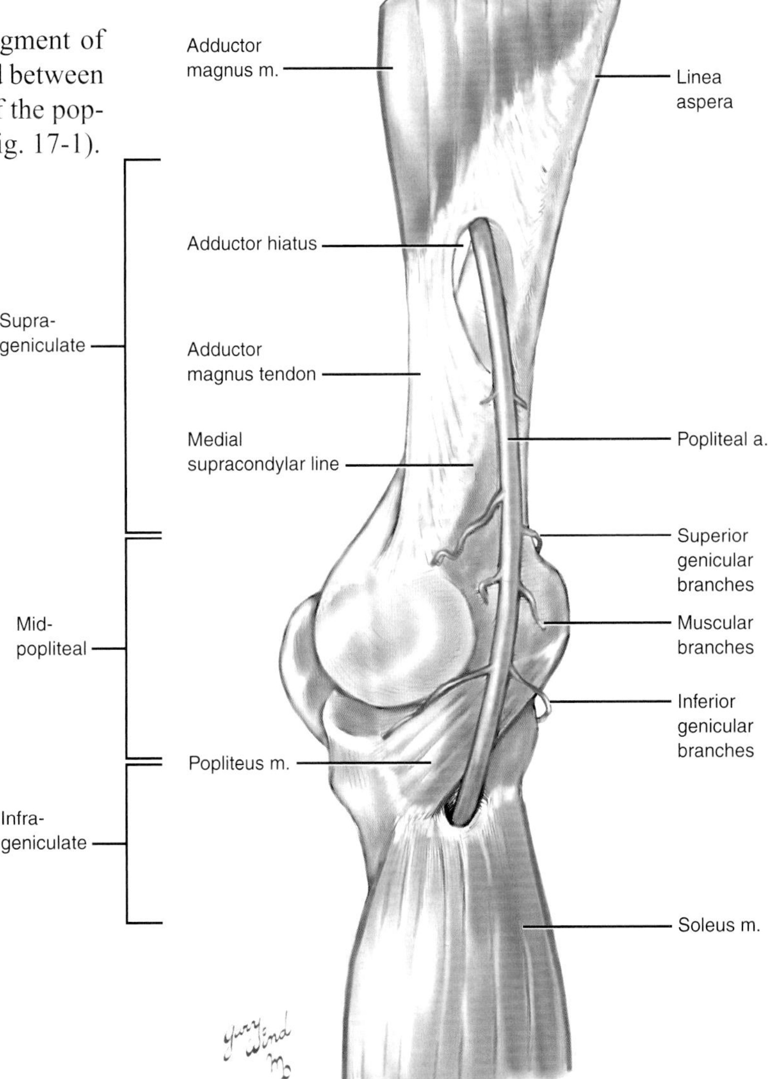

Fig. 17-1 The popliteal artery extends from the adductor hiatus to the lower border of the popliteus muscle.

Because the relationships of the adjoining segments of artery and the muscle groups attaching around the knee are vital to understanding the approaches to the popliteal artery, they are included as an integral part of the following anatomic description.

Fasciae

Beneath skin and superficial fascia, the lower extremity is wrapped in an aponeurotic girdle of varying thickness known as the fascia lata (Fig. 17-2). It is particularly thick along the iliotibial band of the lateral thigh and around the knee joint, where it serves as a retinaculum holding the hamstring tendons and the origins of the gastrocnemius muscle snugly around the popliteal neurovascular bundle.

Two prominent septa connecting the fascia lata to the supracondylar lines of the femur divide the quadriceps muscle of the thigh from the adductor muscles medially and from the hamstring muscles

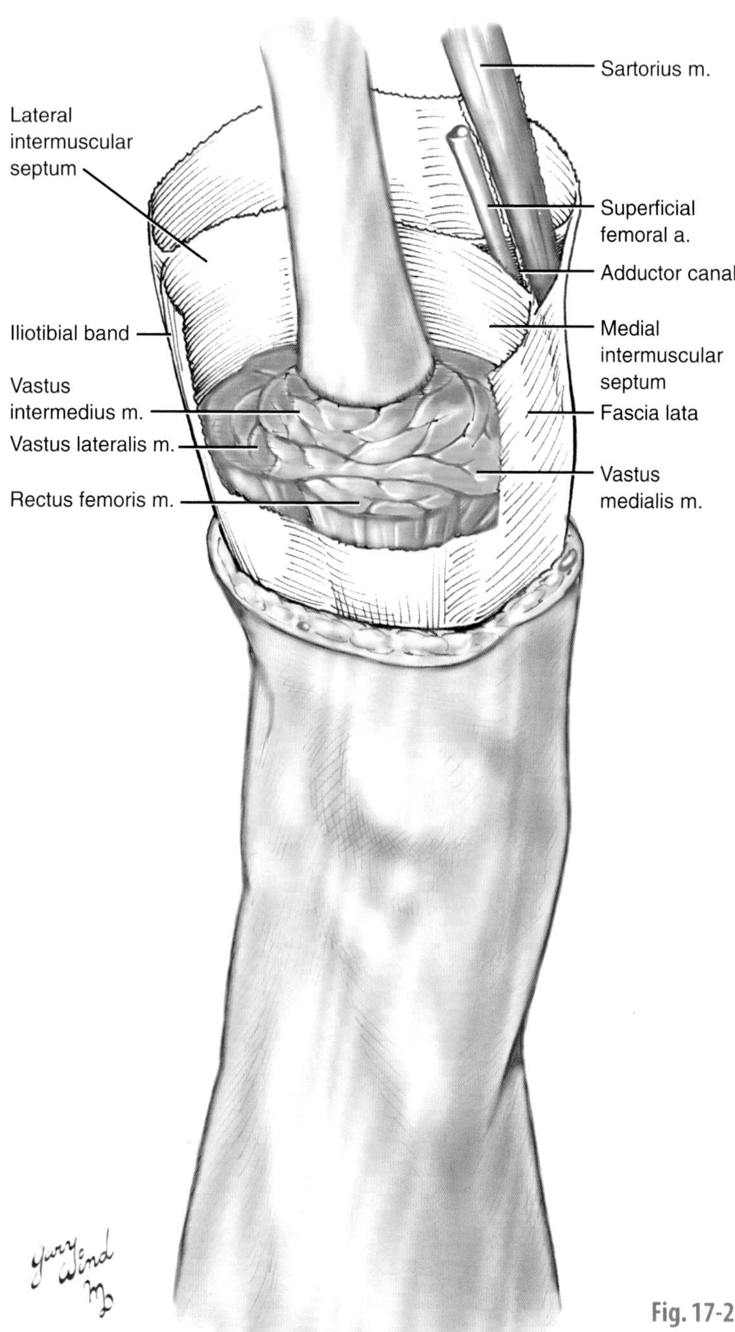

Fig. 17-2 The fascia lata forms a complete sheath around the thigh and attaches to septa that extend to the femur and divide the muscle mass into compartments.

posteriorly. These septa are closely applied to the vastus medialis and vastus lateralis muscles near the femur. There is an additional sling of fascia bridging the cleft between the vastus medialis and adductor muscles. The sartorius muscle lies superficial to this sling, and the superficial femoral vessels occupy the cleft beneath the sling. This passage is known as the adductor canal (Hunter's canal).

Muscle Groups Attaching at the Knee

The bulky quadriceps muscles of the anterior thigh insert into the superior aspect of the patella (Fig. 17-3). The wedge-shaped adductor group fans out from its origins on the inferior pubic ramus to the medial edge of the linea aspera, medial supracondylar ridge, and adductor tubercle of the femur.

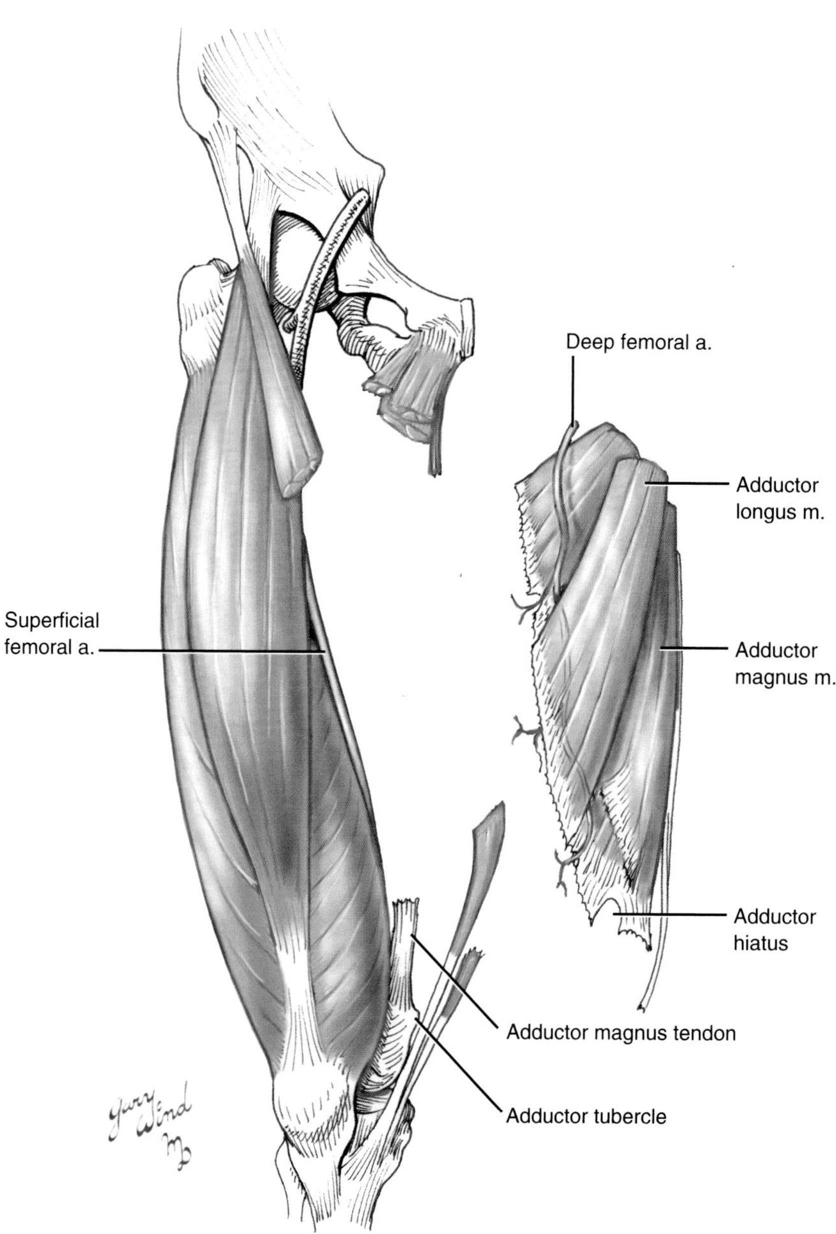

Fig. 17-3 The anterior quadriceps muscle group and the medial adductor muscles of the thigh cradle the superficial femoral artery at their common border.

Several centimeters above the adductor tubercle, the tendon of the adductor magnus splits to form the adductor hiatus through which the superficial femoral artery and vein pass to become the popliteal vessels.

The hamstring muscles of the posterior thigh originate at the ischial tuberosity and separate into the medial semimembranosus and semitendinosus and the lateral biceps femoris muscles (Fig. 17-4). The deep head of the biceps muscle originates from the lower third of the lateral lip of the linea aspera and joins the superficial head to insert on the head of the fibula. The semimembranosus muscle inserts into the posterior lip of the medial tibial condyle. The semitendinosus muscle, along with the gracilis and sartorius muscles, insert on the anterior aspect of the medial tibial condyle.

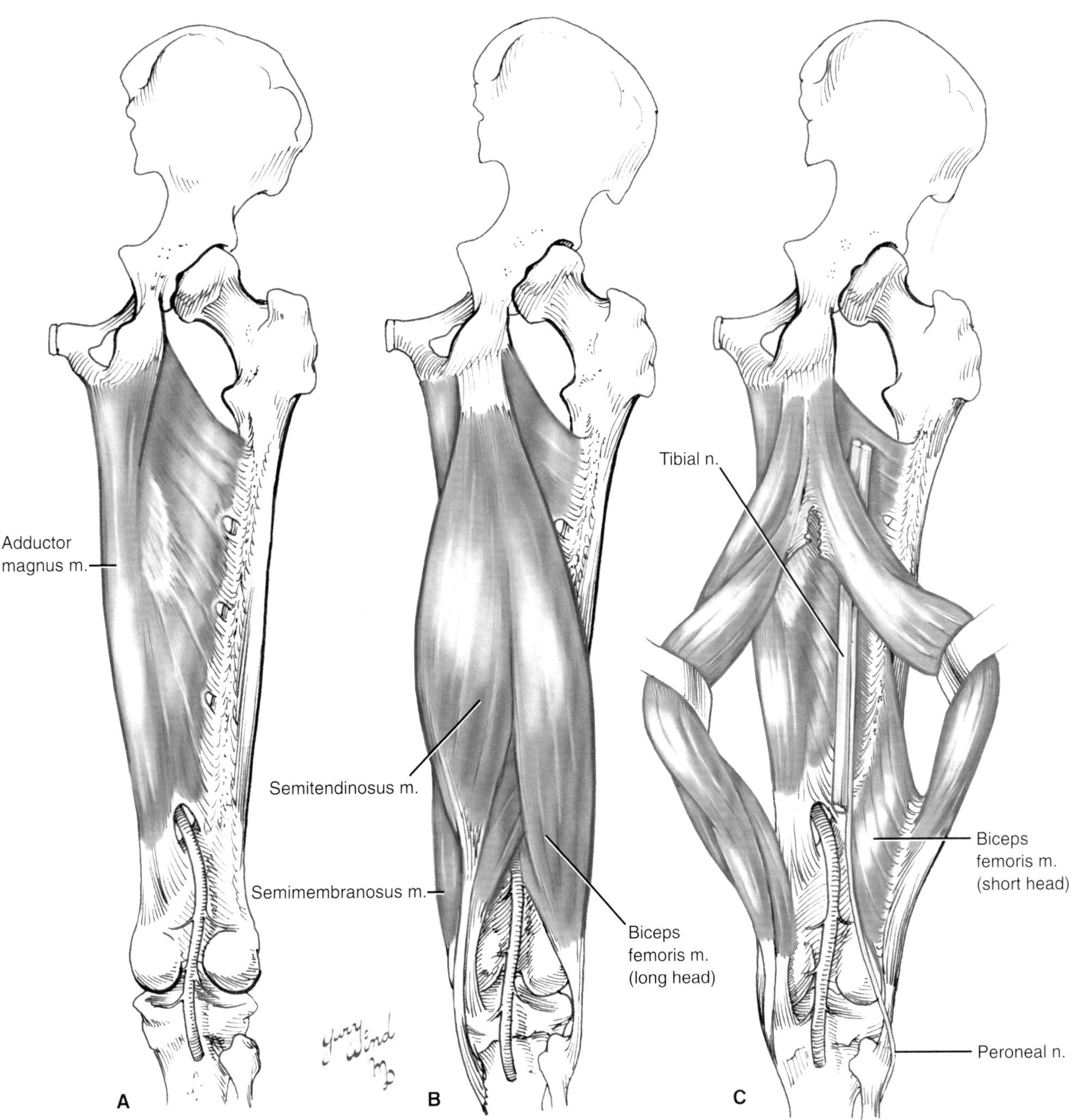

Fig. 17-4 The hamstring muscles of the posterior thigh frame the upper borders of the popliteal fossa.

The tibial and peroneal nerves lie between the hamstring and the adductor magnus muscles. The peroneal nerve spirals around the biceps insertion to reach the lateral aspect of the leg, and the tibial nerve descends to the popliteal space where it is loosely associated with the popliteal artery and vein.

The gastrocnemius muscle's origins from the medial and lateral supracondylar flare of the femur interdigitate with the insertions of the hamstring muscles (Fig. 17-5). The confluence of these two sets of muscle attachments results in the deep, diamond-shaped popliteal fossa.

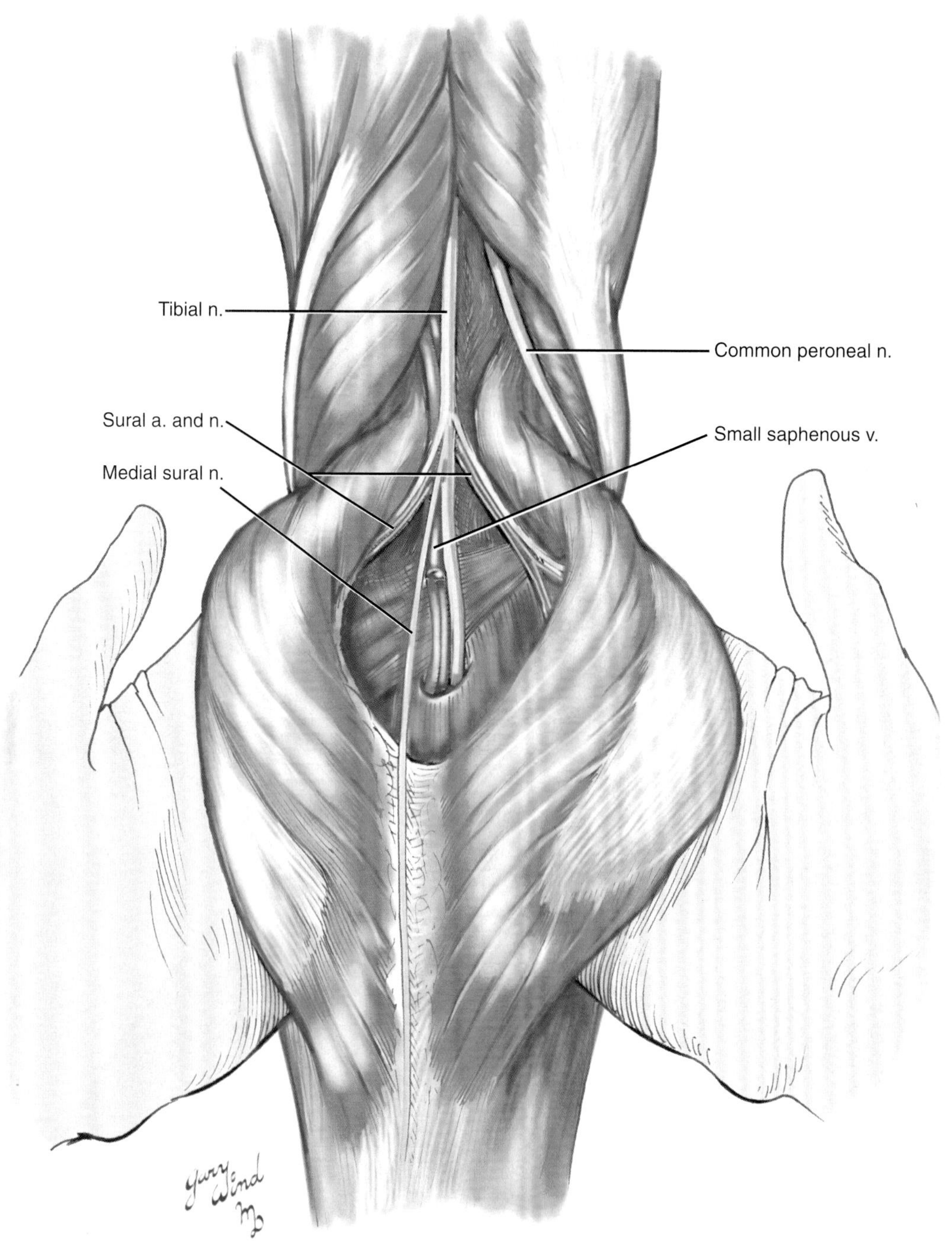

Fig. 17-5 The heads of the gastrocnemius muscle interdigitate with the insertions of the hamstring muscles and form the lower borders of the popliteal fossa. The gastrocnemius muscle is supplied by sural branches from the midpopliteal artery.

Popliteal Artery

At the distal end of the adductor canal, the superficial femoral artery gives off the highest genicular artery, which pierces the subsartorial fascial sling along with the saphenous nerve (Fig. 17-6). The superficial femoral vessels pass through the adductor hiatus to reach the popliteal space.

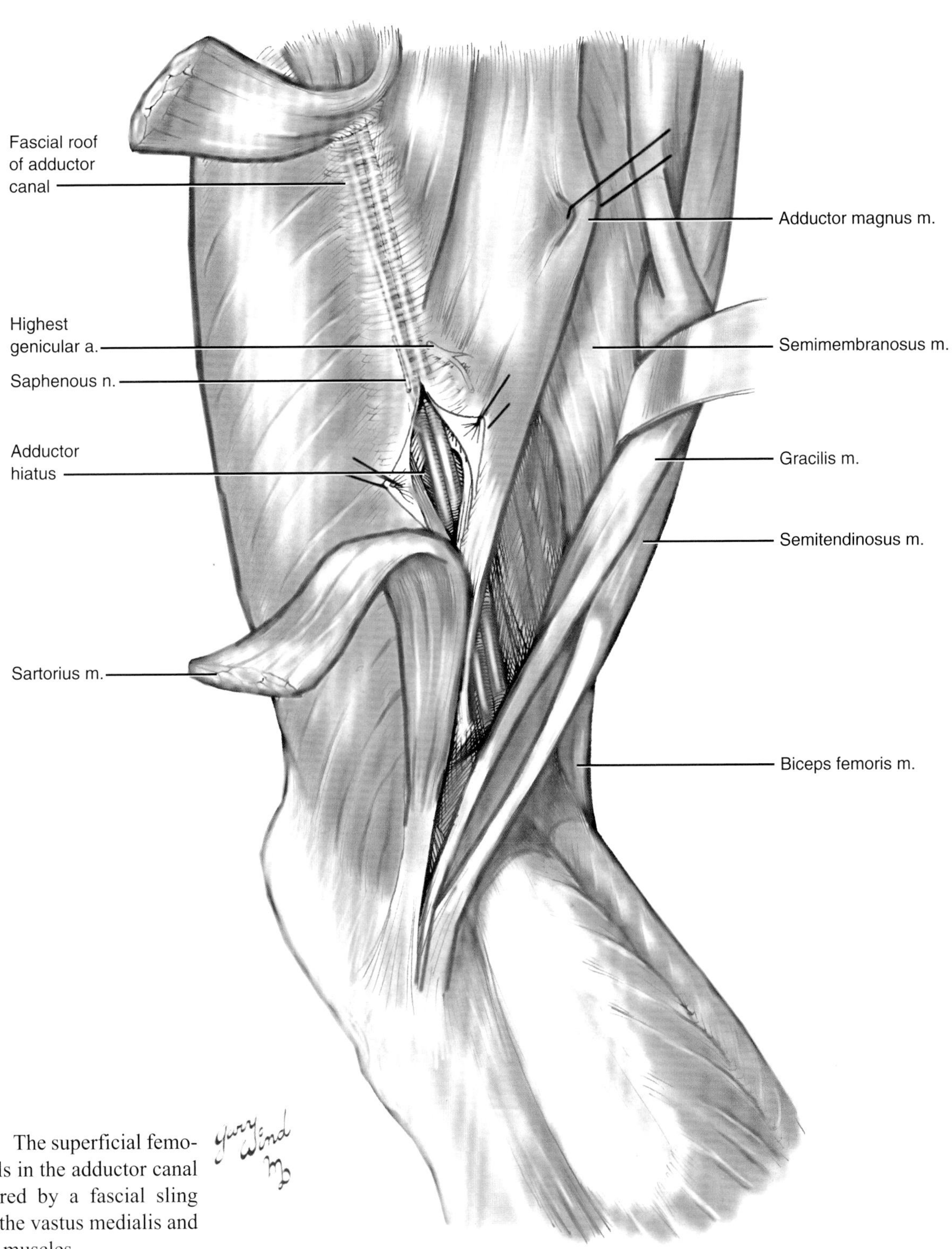

Fig. 17-6 The superficial femoral vessels in the adductor canal are covered by a fascial sling between the vastus medialis and adductor muscles.

The popliteal vessels are enclosed in a firm connective tissue sheath to which the tibial nerve is loosely attached (Fig. 17-7). This sheath is separated from the supracondylar hollow of the popliteal fossa by a small fat pad that facilitates surgical mobilization.

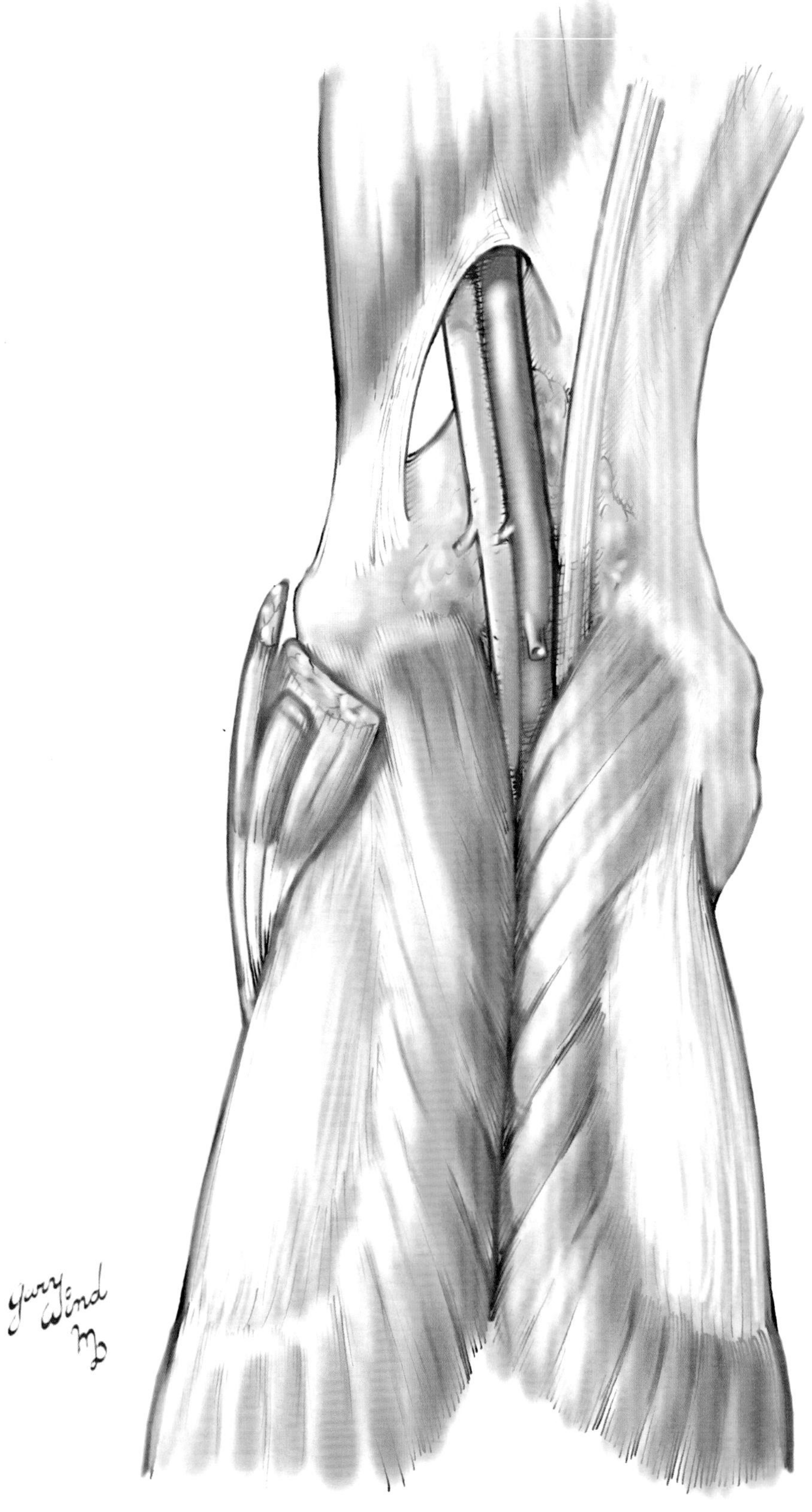

Fig. 17-7 The popliteal vessels are enclosed in a firm fibrous sheath and are separated by a fat pad from the posterior face of the femur.

Muscular branches of the proximal popliteal artery to the lower hamstring muscles anastomose with terminal branches of the profunda femoris artery (Fig. 17-8). Additional muscular branches, the sural vessels, arise from the midpopliteal artery and pass to the heads of the gastrocnemius muscle with the sural branches of the tibial nerve.

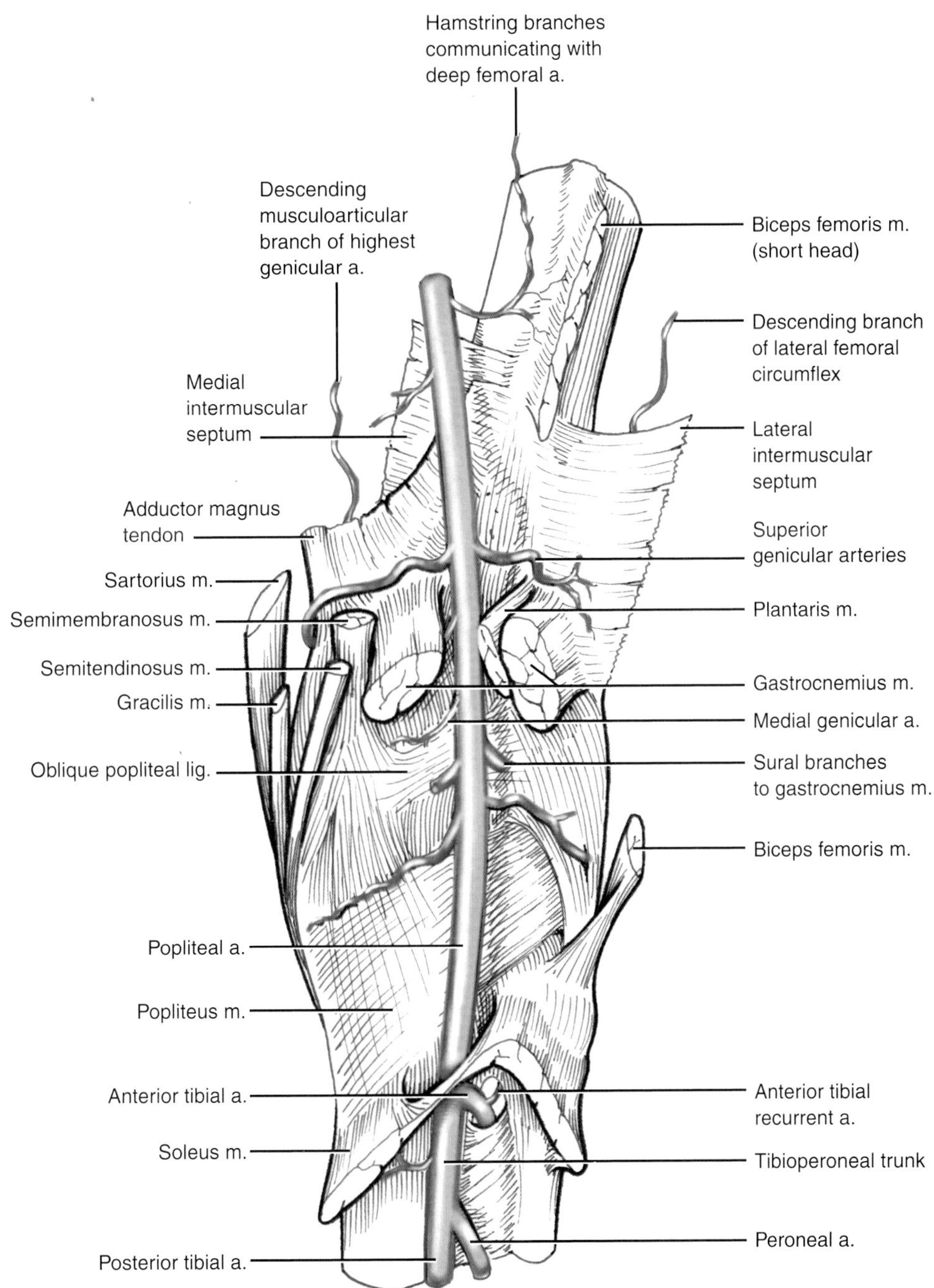

Fig. 17-8 The popliteal artery gives rise to muscular and articular branches.

In addition to the muscular branches, the popliteal artery gives rise to several vessels surrounding and supplying the knee joint (Fig. 17-9).

This network is linked with important collateral channels. It consists of paired superior and inferior genicular arteries and a middle genicular artery.

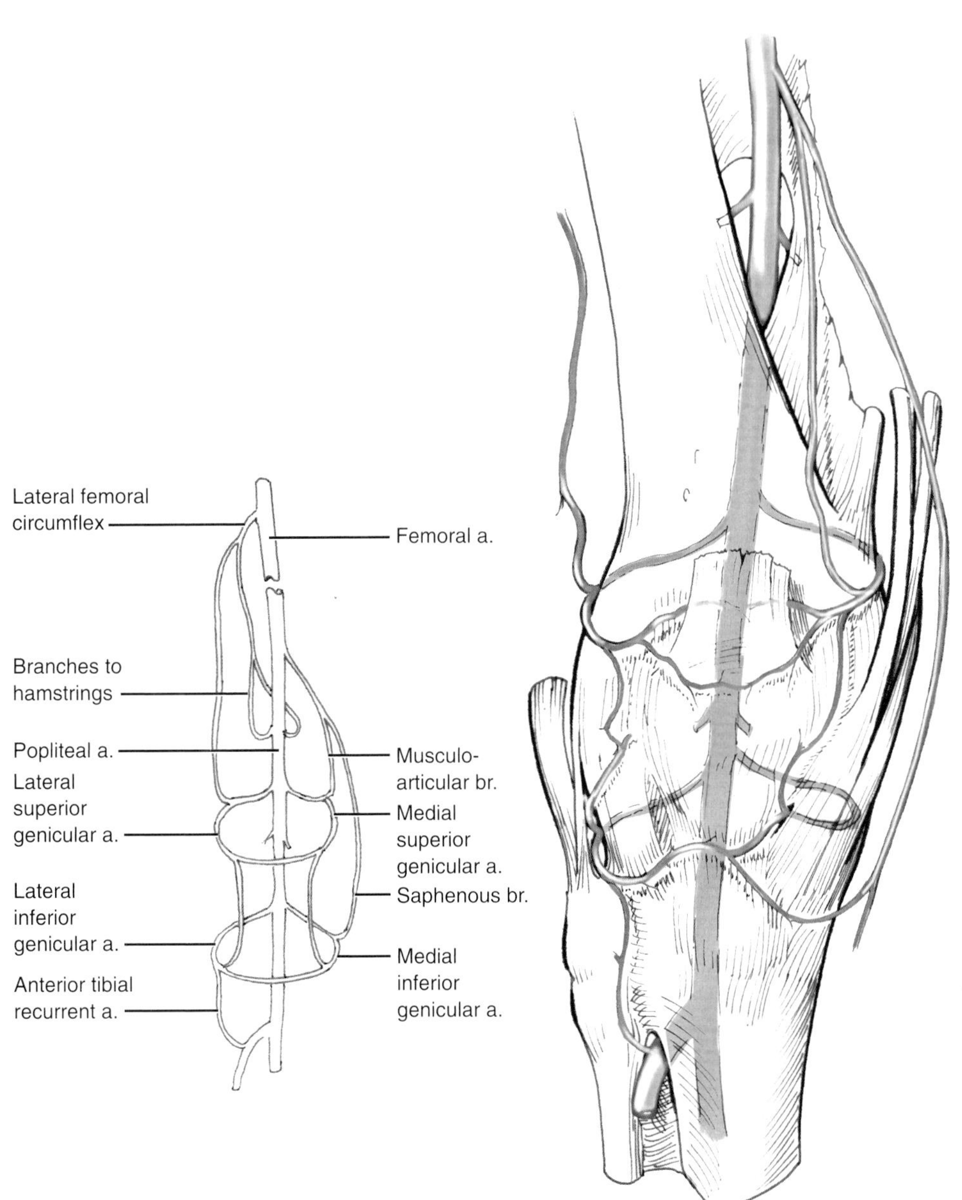

Fig. 17-9 The network of popliteal branches around the knee makes important collateral connections proximally and distally.

The short distal segment of the popliteal artery lies between the heads of the gastrocnemius and popliteus muscles (Fig. 17-8). There are no major branches from this segment, and it is approachable from both the medial and lateral sides of the leg. The popliteal artery disappears through a hiatus in the origin of the soleus muscle.

The path of the popliteal vessels behind the knee can be visualized by dividing and reflecting the posteromedial thigh muscles and the medial head of the gastrocnemius muscle (Fig. 17-10).

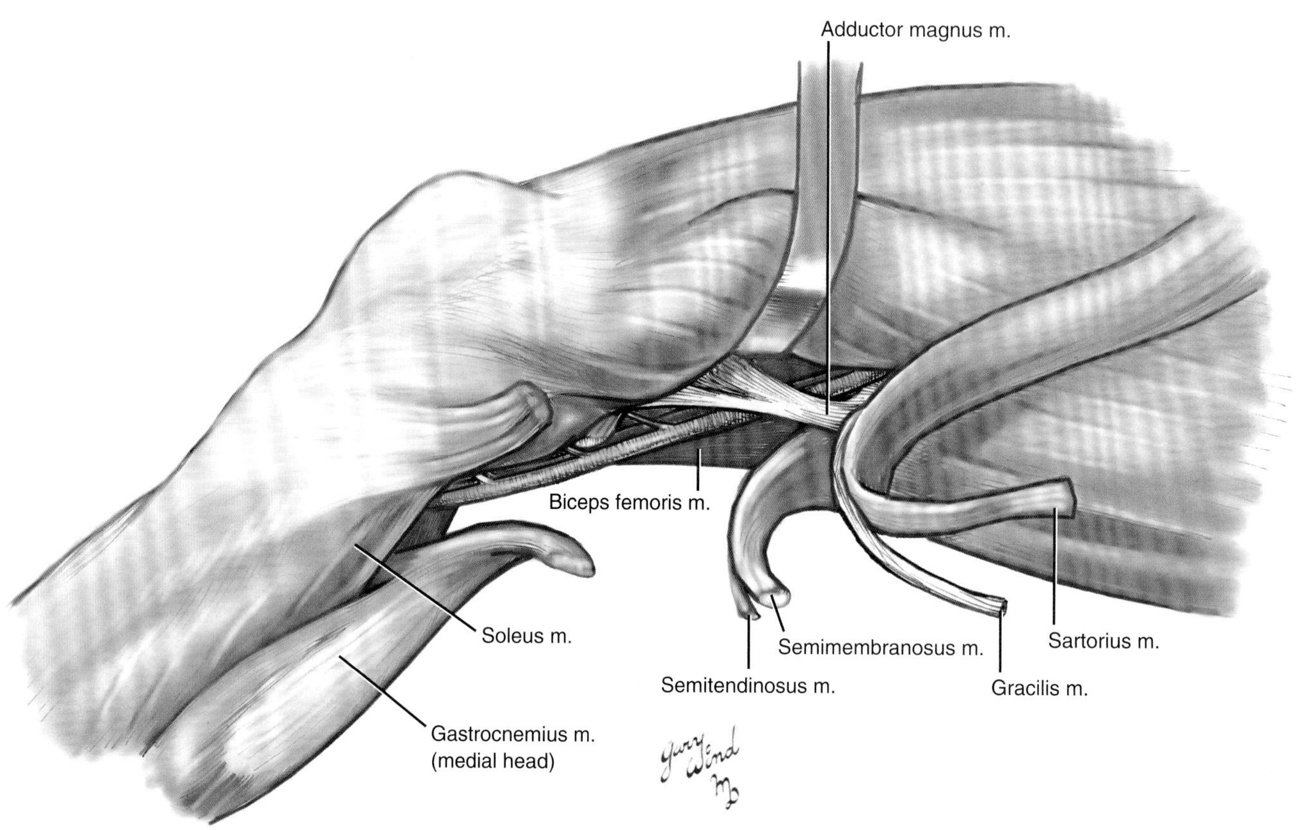

Fig. 17-10 Division of muscular attachments on the medial side of the knee exposes the full length of the popliteal artery.

Surgical Approaches to the Popliteal Artery

The various options for surgical access to the popliteal artery can be considered in terms of three anatomic sections (Fig. 17-1): suprageniculate, infrageniculate, and midpopliteal. The suprageniculate and infrageniculate sections are used in bypassing obstructions of more proximal vessels, usually the superficial femoral artery. Access to these sections of the popliteal artery is usually gained through medial incisions, although lateral approaches have been described (Fig. 17-11). A direct posterior approach is used to expose the midpopliteal section. This classic approach has virtually been abandoned for use in bypass surgery, but it is ideal for surgery involving correction of intrinsic pathology of the midpopliteal artery, such as entrapment, cystic adventitial disease, and localized aneurysms or intimal flaps.

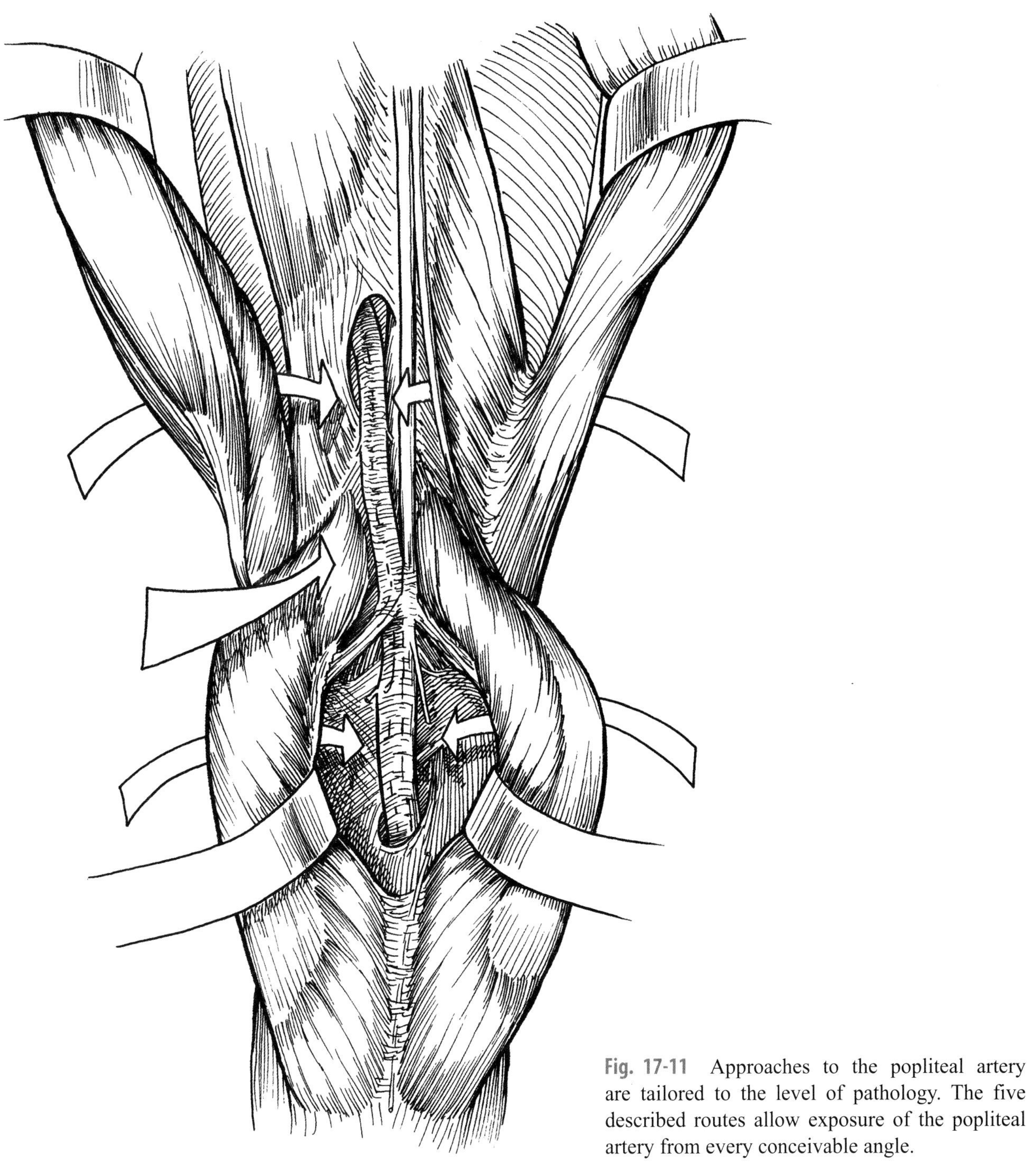

Fig. 17-11 Approaches to the popliteal artery are tailored to the level of pathology. The five described routes allow exposure of the popliteal artery from every conceivable angle.

Exposure of the Suprageniculate Popliteal Artery

This section of the popliteal artery is the preferred position for the distal anastomosis of a femoropopliteal bypass, providing that the arterial tree below this level is devoid of flow-limiting stenoses. Surgeons generally favor autogenous tissue, such as the saphenous vein, for the bypass graft. The use of synthetic graft material for bypasses to the popliteal artery above the knee is also acceptable,[1–3] but the ischemic consequences of a failed bypass are worse with prosthetic graft than with autogenous vein.[4]

The suprageniculate popliteal artery is most easily approached through a medial incision. Veith et al.[5] popularized a lateral approach to the suprageniculate popliteal artery for patients who are undergoing secondary vascular operations, when infection or surgical scarring render the medial approach inconvenient.

Technique of Medial Suprageniculate Exposure

The patient is placed in the supine position with the leg externally rotated and the knee flexed 30° (Fig. 17-12). The entire leg should be shaved and prepped to facilitate movement during the dissection and to ensure that other areas are available for dissection should the popliteal artery prove inadequate. An incision is made in the distal third of the medial thigh along the anterior border of the sartorius muscle.

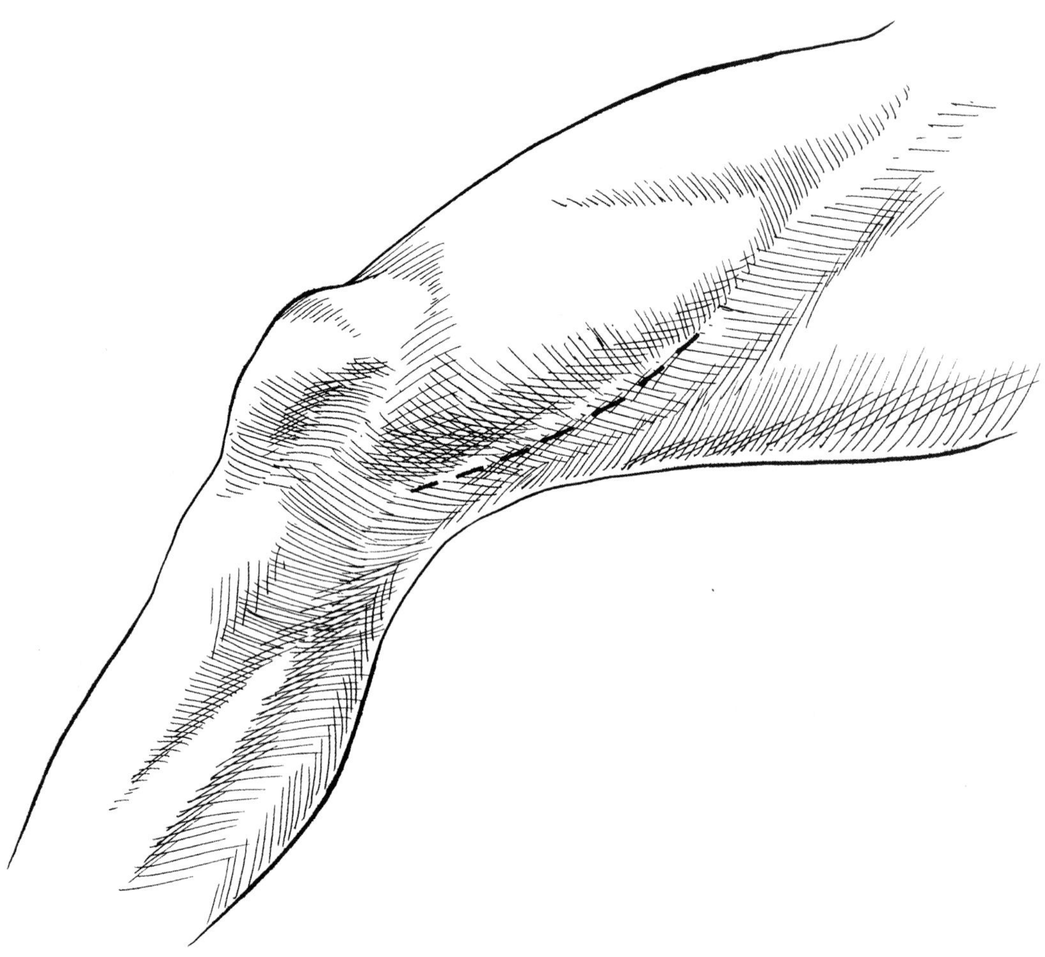

Fig. 17-12 The incision for medial suprageniculate exposure lies along the anterior border of the sartorius muscle.

The fascia over the sartorius muscle is incised, and the muscle is retracted posteriorly (Fig. 17-13). The popliteal vessels are identified by retracting the vastus medialis muscle anteriorly. A fascial bridge of varying thickness between the adductor tendon and semimembranosus muscles may require division to expose the underlying vessels. Additional exposure of the popliteal artery can be obtained by dividing the thickened adductor magnus tendon forming the border of the adductor

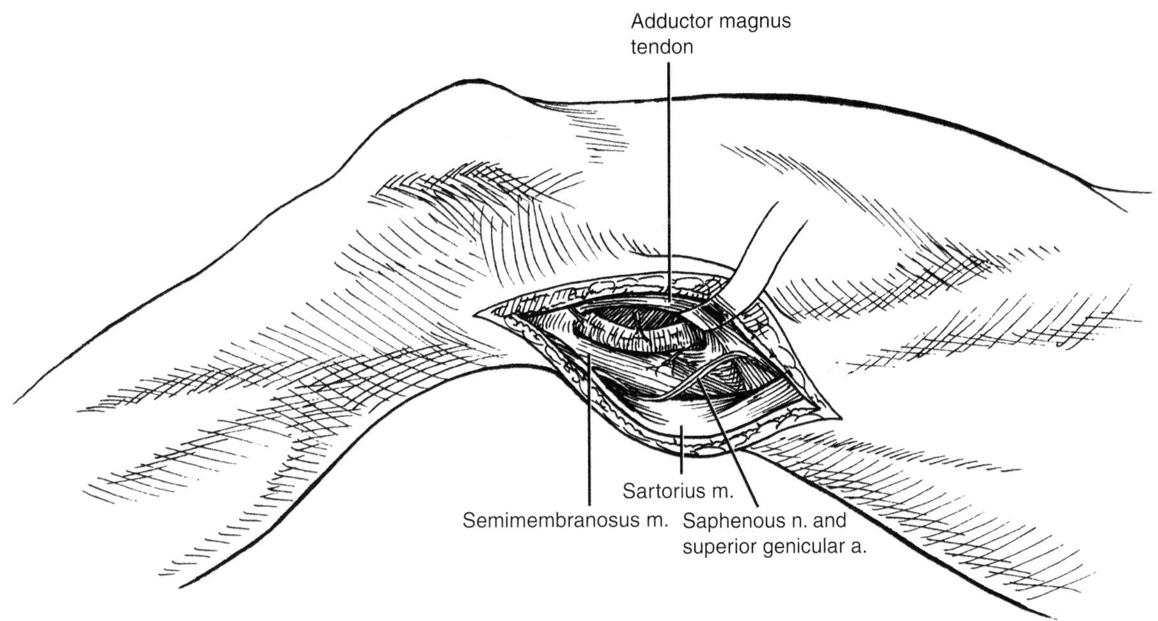

Fig. 17-13 With the sartorius and gracilis muscles retracted posteriorly, the adductor magnus tendon is separated from the semimembranosus muscle to expose the popliteal vessels as they emerge through the adductor hiatus. The saphenous nerve and superior genicular artery emerge through the roof of the adductor canal and cross the edge of the adductor magnus muscle to reach the cleft between the sartorius and gracilis muscles.

hiatus (Fig. 17-14). Fascial connections between the adductor magnus tendon and the medial intermuscular septum anterior to it may require division to expose the anterior surface of the adductor hiatus. Care should be taken to preserve the highest genicular artery and the saphenous branch of the femoral nerve. A tough fibrous sheath envelops the popliteal artery and vein.

The artery is situated medial to the vein at this level and therefore is encountered first on opening the sheath. The vein is often paired, and connecting channels that bridge the artery must be carefully divided to obtain exposure (Fig. 17-15).

Grafts to the suprageniculate popliteal artery are best brought through the adductor canal with a blunt tunneling instrument (Fig. 17-16). The graft is thus situated in a natural anatomic plane where it is protected by the sartorius muscle and overlying fascia lata.

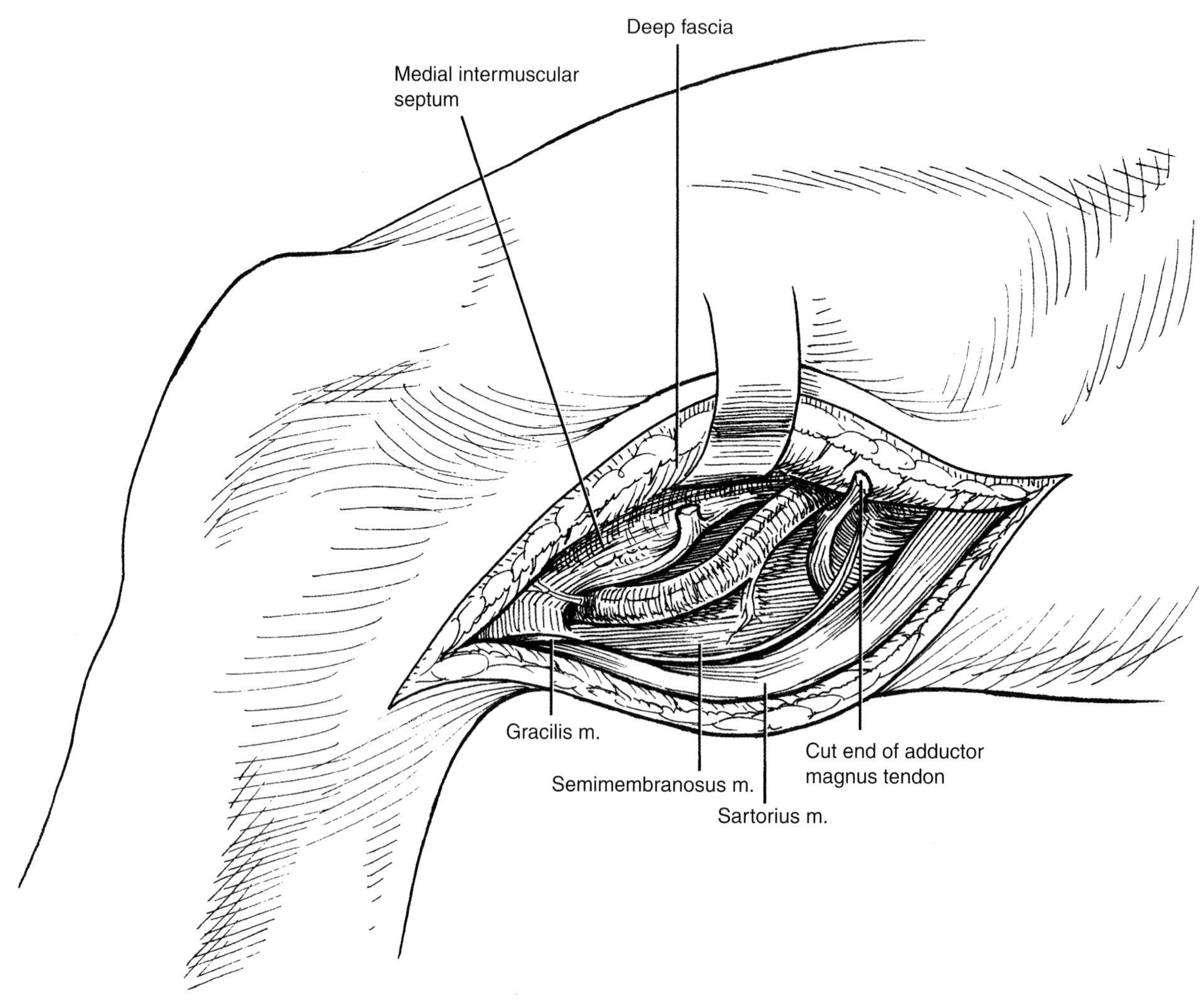

Fig. 17-14 The adductor magnus tendon can be divided to expose the proximal popliteal vessels more completely. There is a fascial connection between the distal adductor tendon and the medial intramuscular septum that must be divided to obtain the exposure shown.

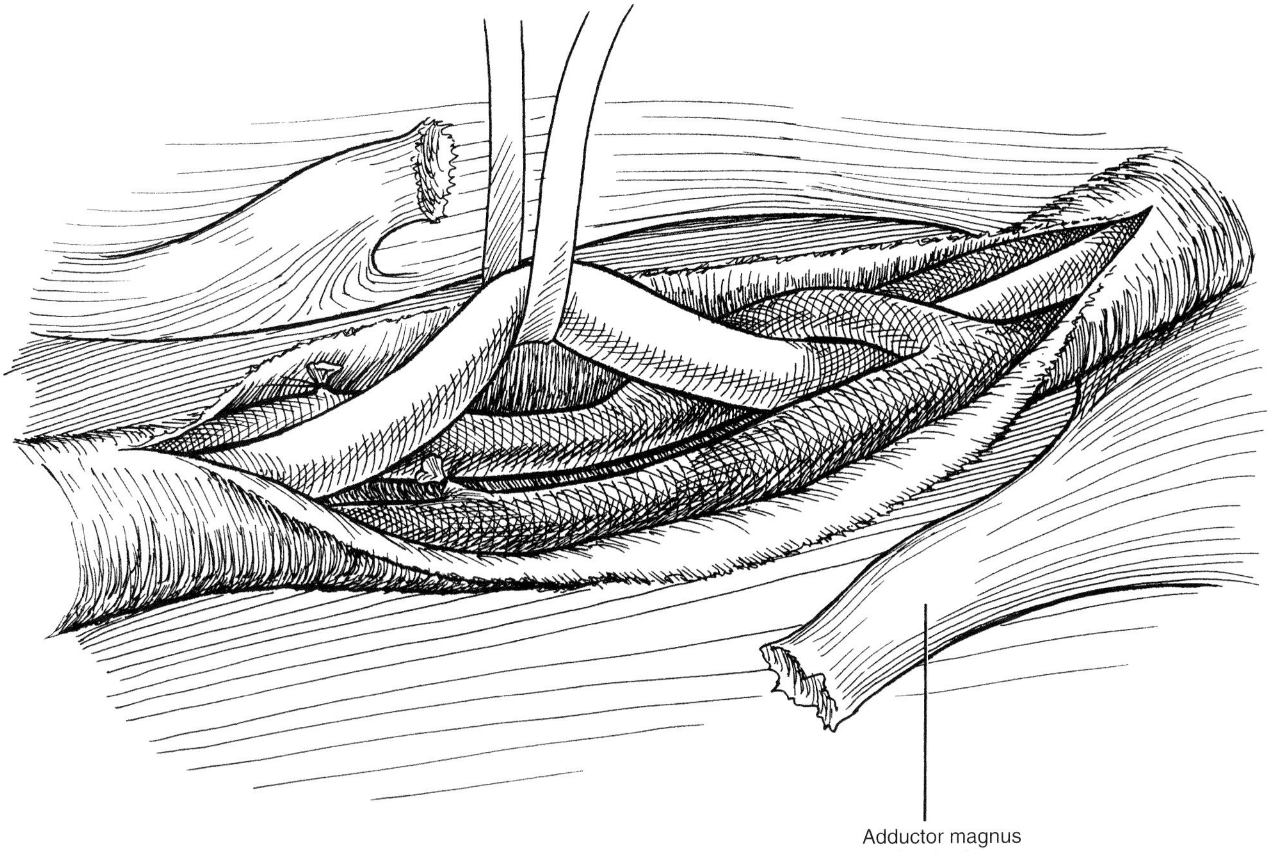

Adductor magnus
tendon (cut)

Fig. 17-15 Within the vascular sheath, the artery must be carefully separated from surrounding veins. Mobilization must be adequate for safe exposure and may be aided by the use of soft vessel tapes.

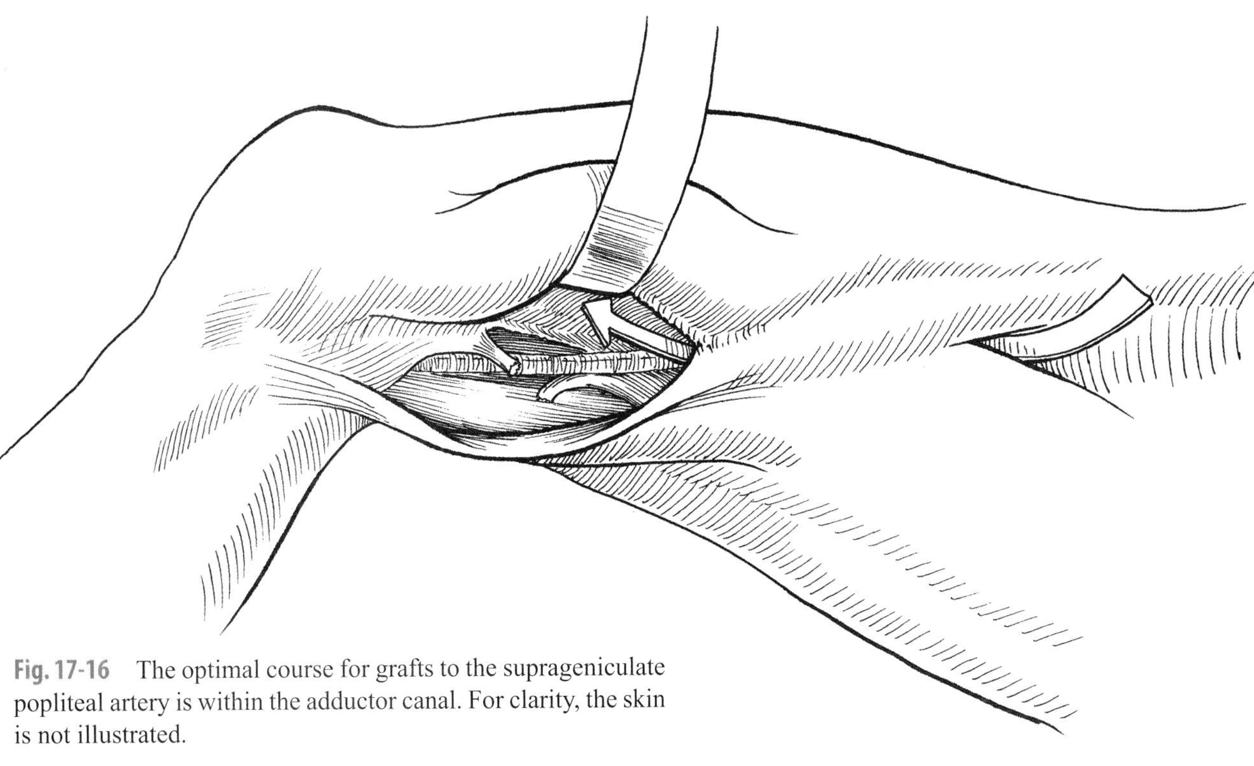

Fig. 17-16 The optimal course for grafts to the suprageniculate popliteal artery is within the adductor canal. For clarity, the skin is not illustrated.

Technique of Lateral Suprageniculate Approach

The leg is internally rotated and flexed at the knee (Fig. 17-17). A longitudinal incision is made in the distal third of the thigh between the biceps femoris muscle and the iliotibial tract. The fascia lata is incised posterior to the junction of iliotibial tract and lateral intermuscular septum. An incision that is too anterior leads into the vastus lateralis muscle in front of the lateral intermuscular septum (Fig. 17-18). The origin of the short head of the biceps femoris muscle ends several centimeters above the lateral femoral condyle, leaving a loophole[6] between muscle and bone through which the vessels may be reached (Fig. 17-19).

When this space is opened, the tibial and peroneal nerves remain in a posterior plane bound to the hamstring muscles by loose fascia, and the vessels are found directly beneath the femur (Fig. 17-20).

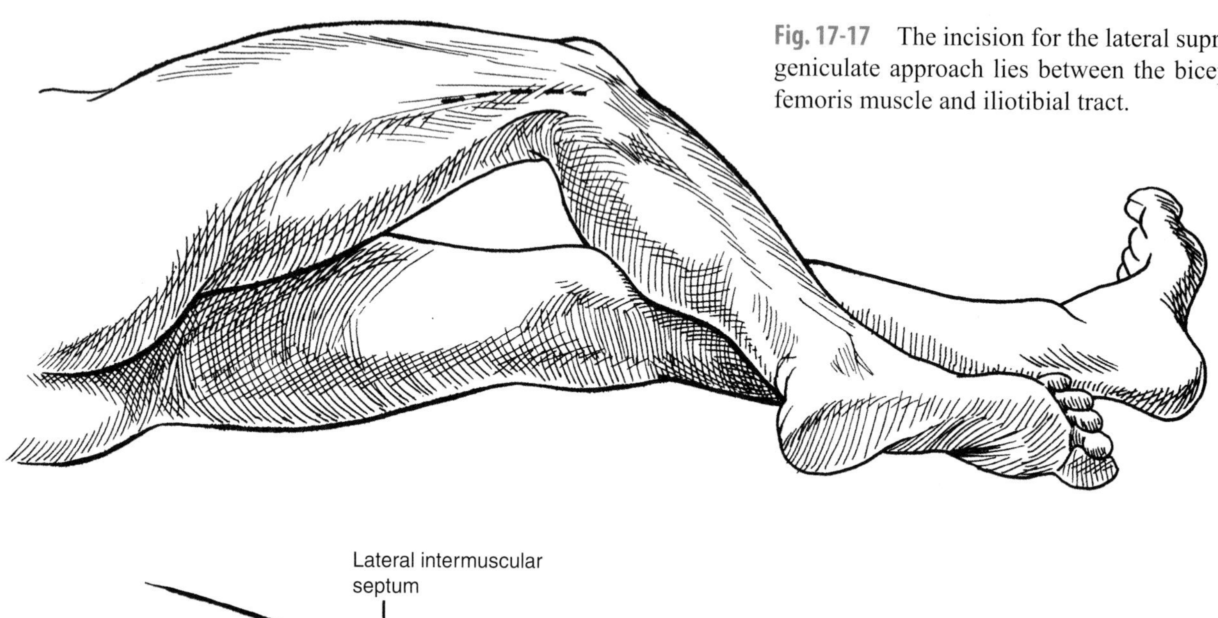

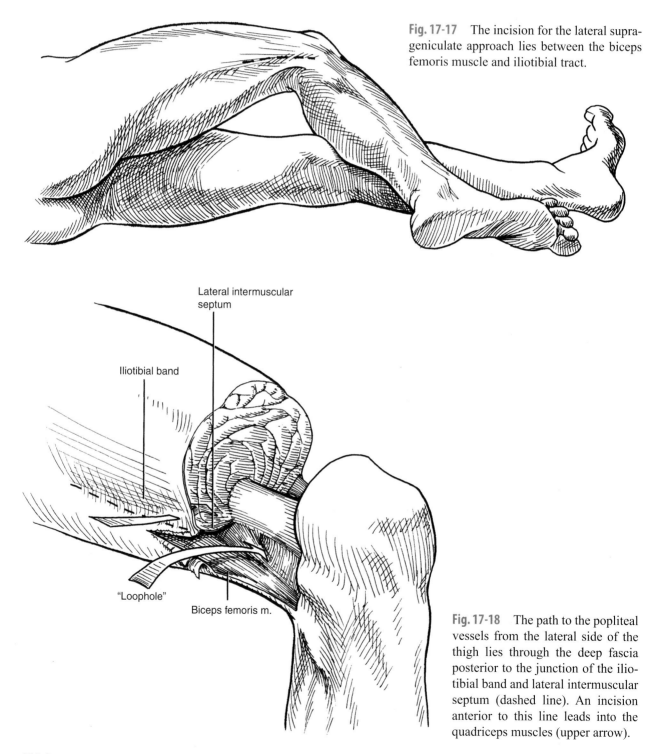

Fig. 17-17 The incision for the lateral suprageniculate approach lies between the biceps femoris muscle and iliotibial tract.

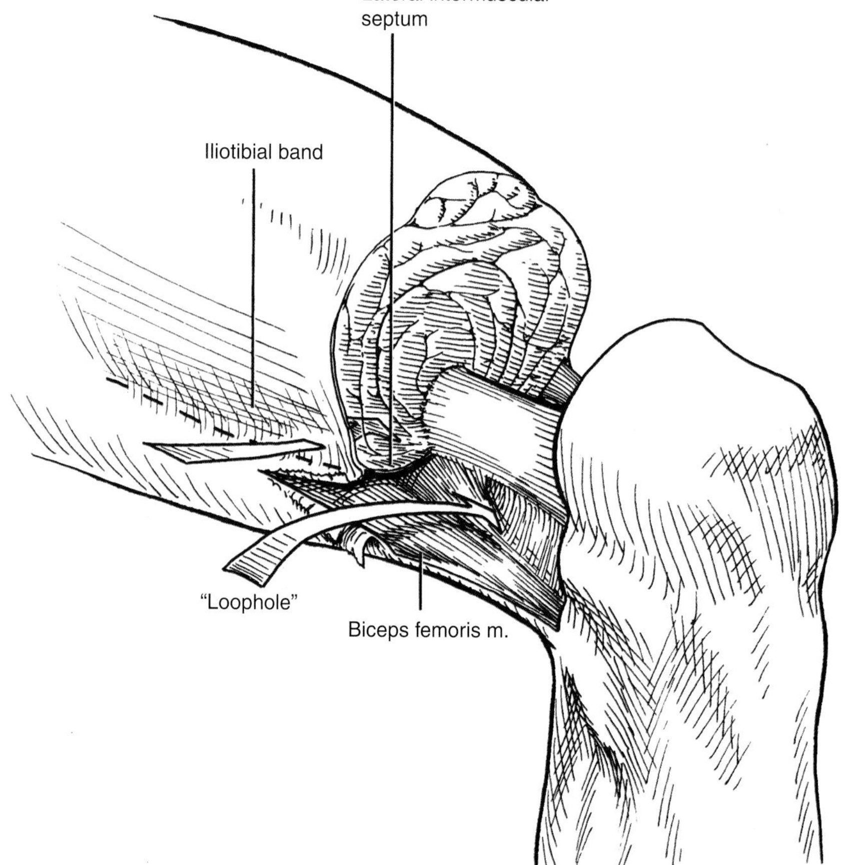

Fig. 17-18 The path to the popliteal vessels from the lateral side of the thigh lies through the deep fascia posterior to the junction of the iliotibial band and lateral intermuscular septum (dashed line). An incision anterior to this line leads into the quadriceps muscles (upper arrow).

Fig. 17-19 The origin of the short head of the biceps muscle ends several centimeters above the femoral condyle. The distal part of the short head is connected to the femur by a thin sheet of fascia. Opening this thin fascia exposes the popliteal vessels.

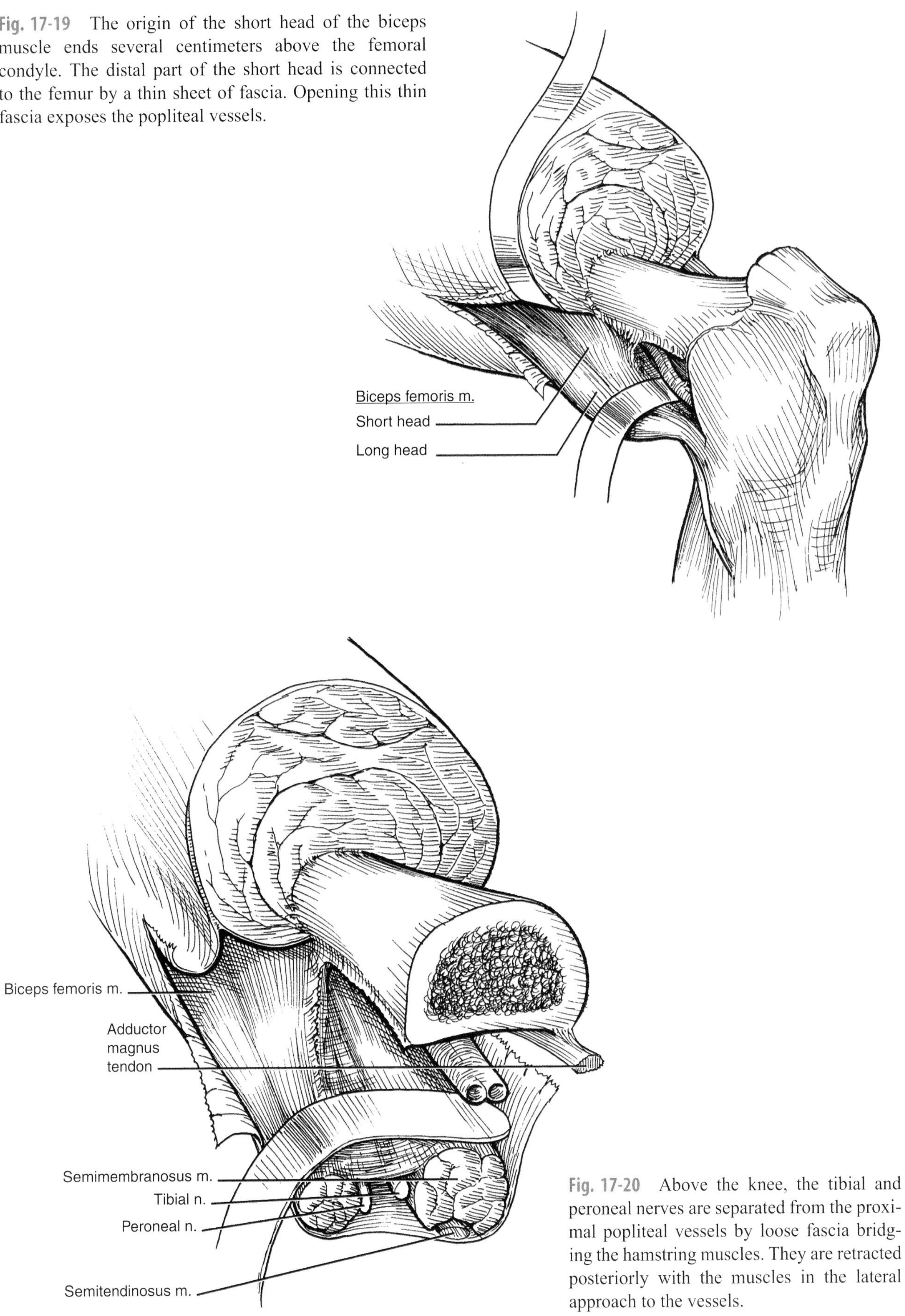

Fig. 17-20 Above the knee, the tibial and peroneal nerves are separated from the proximal popliteal vessels by loose fascia bridging the hamstring muscles. They are retracted posteriorly with the muscles in the lateral approach to the vessels.

The popliteal vein (which may be paired) is encountered first in the vascular sheath. It is mobilized and retracted posteriorly with the biceps femoris muscle (Fig. 17-21).

Exposure of the Infrageniculate Popliteal Artery

The infrageniculate popliteal artery is used more commonly in bypass surgery than the proximal popliteal segments because it is less likely to be involved with atherosclerotic plaque. The preferred conduit is ipsilateral saphenous vein, which has superior long-term patency compared with prosthetic graft.[7] When ipsilateral saphenous vein is unavailable, suitable alternatives include contralateral great saphenous vein, arm vein, or spliced small saphenous vein segments. In the rare patient without suitable autogenous vein, use of prosthetic graft or endovascular options may be preferable to amputation, even for TASC IID lesions.[8–10]

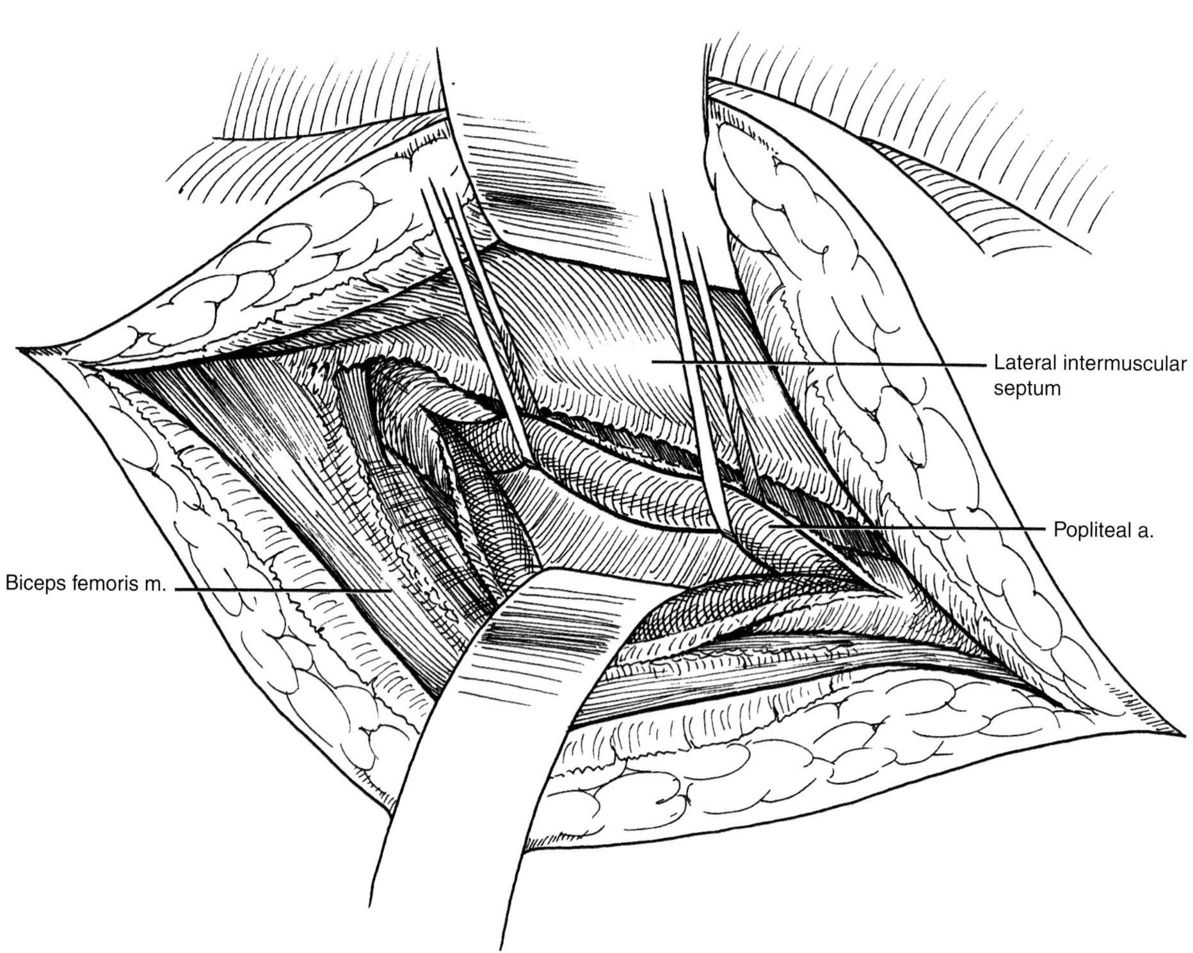

Fig. 17-21 The popliteal vein is encountered first in the vascular sheath and is best retracted posteriorly with the biceps muscle.

Exposure of the infrageniculate popliteal artery is most easily carried out through a medial incision. For some patients undergoing complex secondary vascular procedures, the lateral approach popularized by Veith et al.[5] may be appropriate.

Technique of Medial Infrageniculate Approach

The patient is placed in the supine position with the leg externally rotated and the knee flexed 30° (Fig. 17-22). The entire leg is shaved and prepped as in the previous exposures. A longitudinal incision is made approximately 1 cm behind the posterior border of the tibia, extending a third of the way down the calf from the lower posterior edge of the medial tibial condyle. Care should be exercised to avoid injuring the great saphenous vein, which may course directly through this area. The great saphenous vein is found 1 to 2 cm posterior to the medial border of

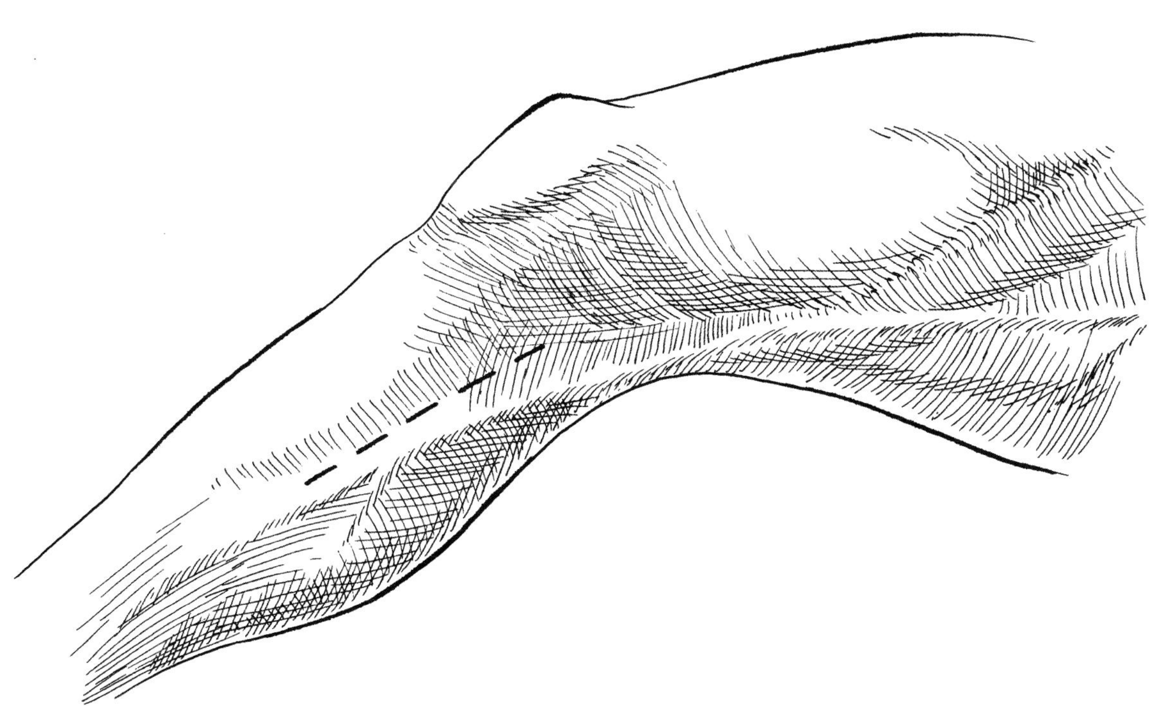

Fig. 17-22 The incision for the medial infrageniculate approach lies approximately 1 cm behind the posterior border of the tibia. The proximity of the saphenous vein requires careful dissection. The vein usually remains with the posterior flap.

the tibia and is most conveniently retracted with the posterior wound edge. Anterior perforating branches from the saphenous vein may require ligation to ensure safe retraction.

The crural fascia is incised 1 cm posterior to the tibia, and the fascial incision is extended proximally to the level of the semitendinosus tendon (Fig. 17-23). The underlying medial head of the gastrocnemius muscle is retracted posteriorly, exposing the neurovascular bundle in the proximal aspect of the incision (Fig. 17-24). More proximal exposure can be obtained by dividing the tendons of the semitendinosus, gracilis, and sartorius muscles, but the divided ends should routinely be marked with suture tags and reapproximated at the end of the procedure to preserve knee stability. More distal exposure can be obtained by dividing the tibial attachments of the soleus muscle, which lies deep to the gastrocnemius muscle in the incision (Fig. 17-25).

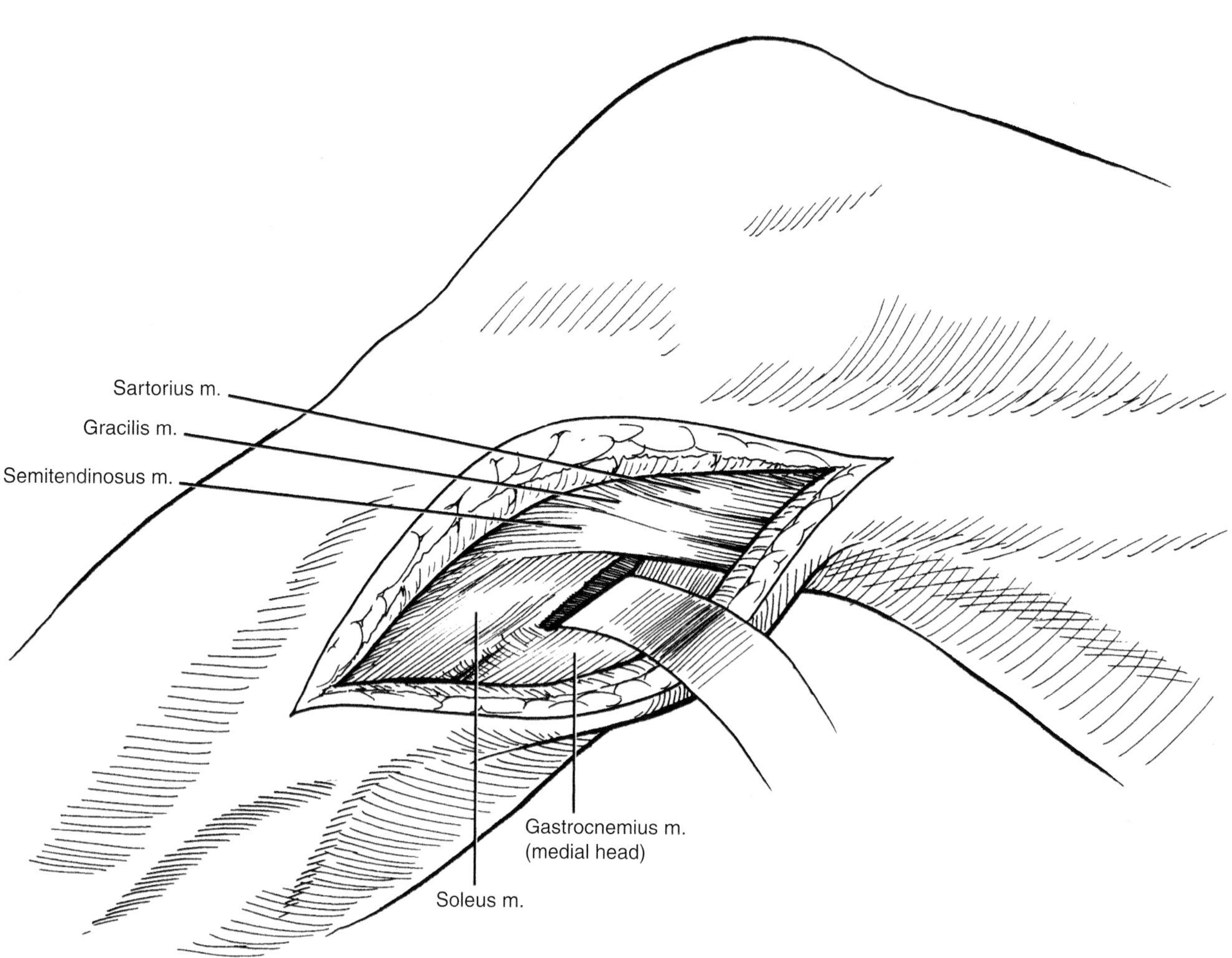

Fig. 17-23 After the crural fascia is incised, the underlying medial head of the gastrocnemius muscle is retracted posteriorly.

Fig. 17-24 The neurovascular bundle can be located deep in the proximal aspect of the incision.

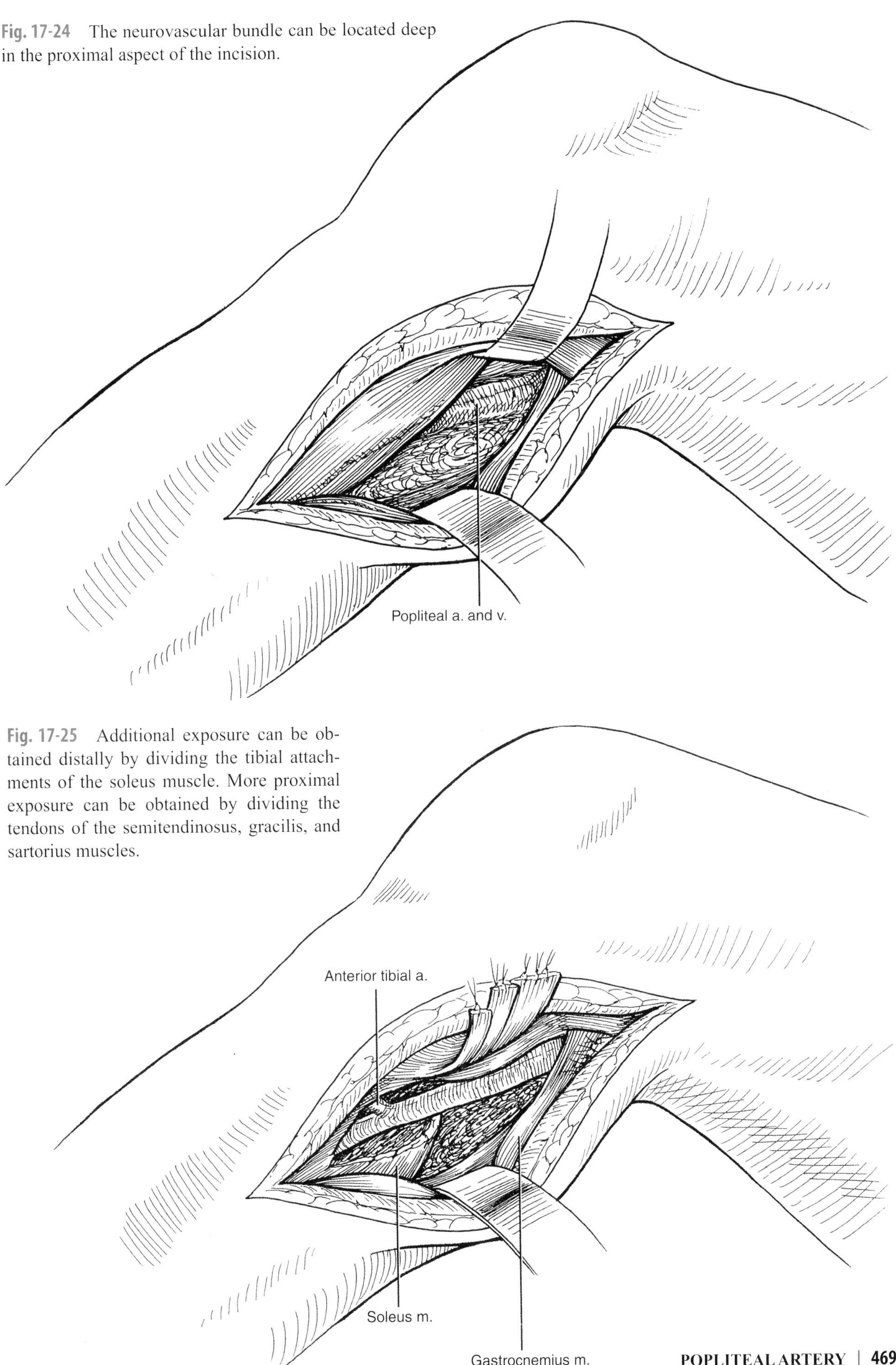

Fig. 17-25 Additional exposure can be obtained distally by dividing the tibial attachments of the soleus muscle. More proximal exposure can be obtained by dividing the tendons of the semitendinosus, gracilis, and sartorius muscles.

The first structure encountered on entering the neurovascular sheath is the popliteal vein (Fig. 17-26). This structure is more often paired than single, and bridging veins must be divided to gain access to the underlying popliteal artery. Few important collateral vessels occur at this level of the popliteal artery, and any small arterial branches can be ligated with impunity. Exposure of the artery is facilitated by the use of vessel tapes to elevate the artery above the vein into the incision. The tibial nerve lies posteromedially and should be carefully protected during arterial dissection.

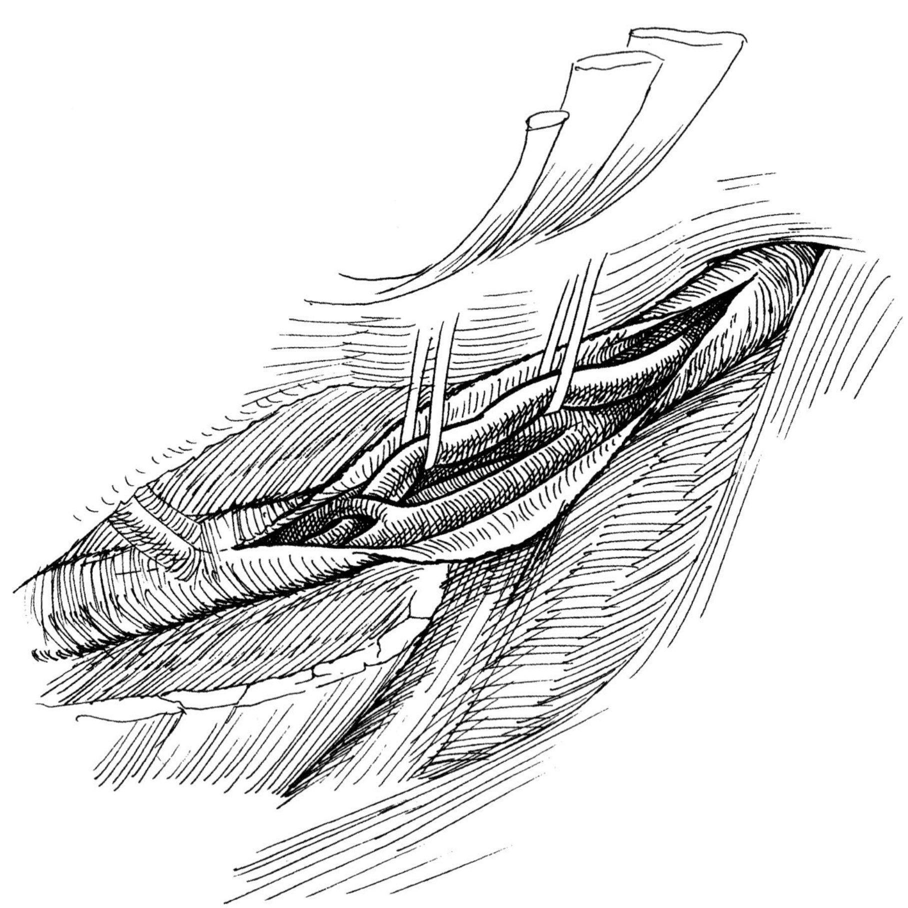

Fig. 17-26 The first structure encountered on entering the neurovascular sheath is one of the paired popliteal veins. After careful dissection, the artery is elevated into the incision using soft vessel tapes.

Grafts to the infrageniculate popliteal artery are best routed through the adductor canal, then tunneled posterior to the knee between the femoral condyles (Fig. 17-27). Because the tunnel is created blindly, the actual pathway through the musculature of the thigh can only be estimated. Care should be taken to ensure that the graft is brought between the heads of the gastrocnemius muscle at the level of the knee joint; grafts routed through this muscle tissue may be compressed during muscle contraction. The distal anastomosis is created in a plaque-free segment of the popliteal artery.

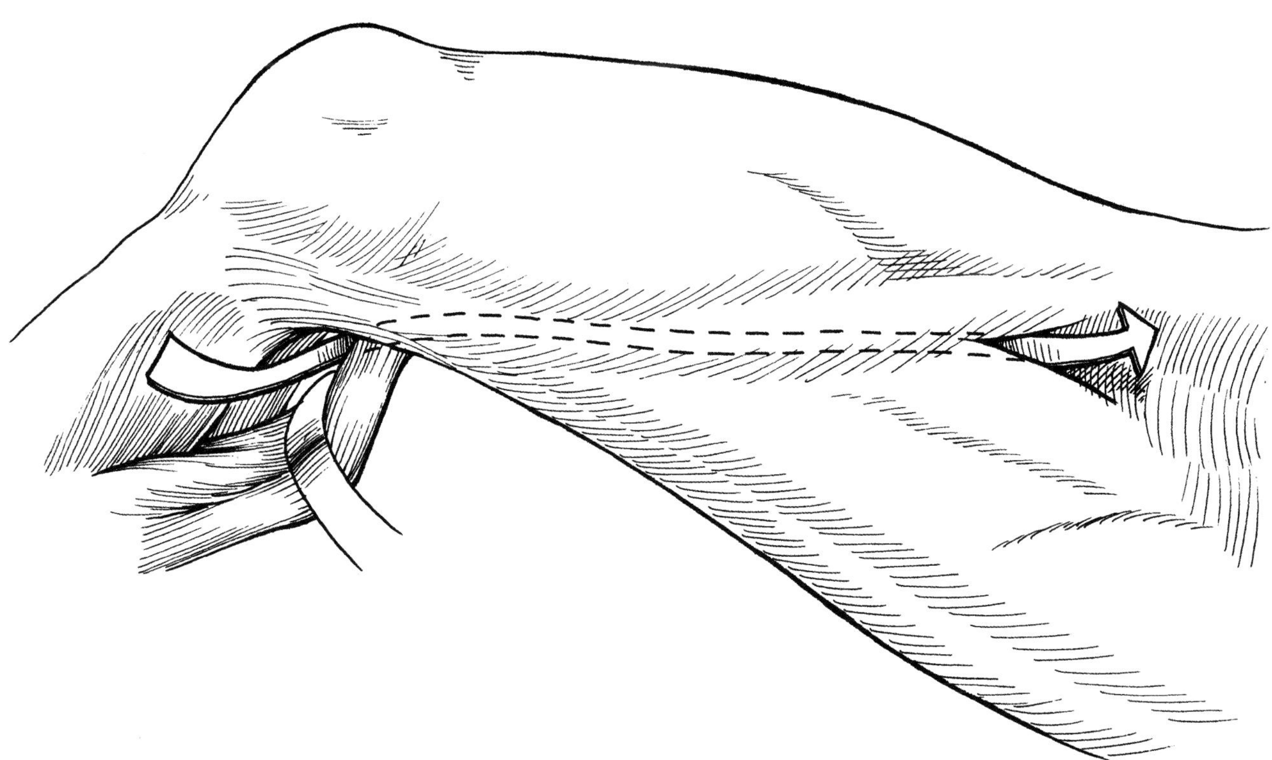

Fig. 17-27 Grafts to the infrageniculate popliteal artery should be routed through the adductor canal and tunneled posterior to the knee between the femoral condyles and heads of the gastrocnemius muscle.

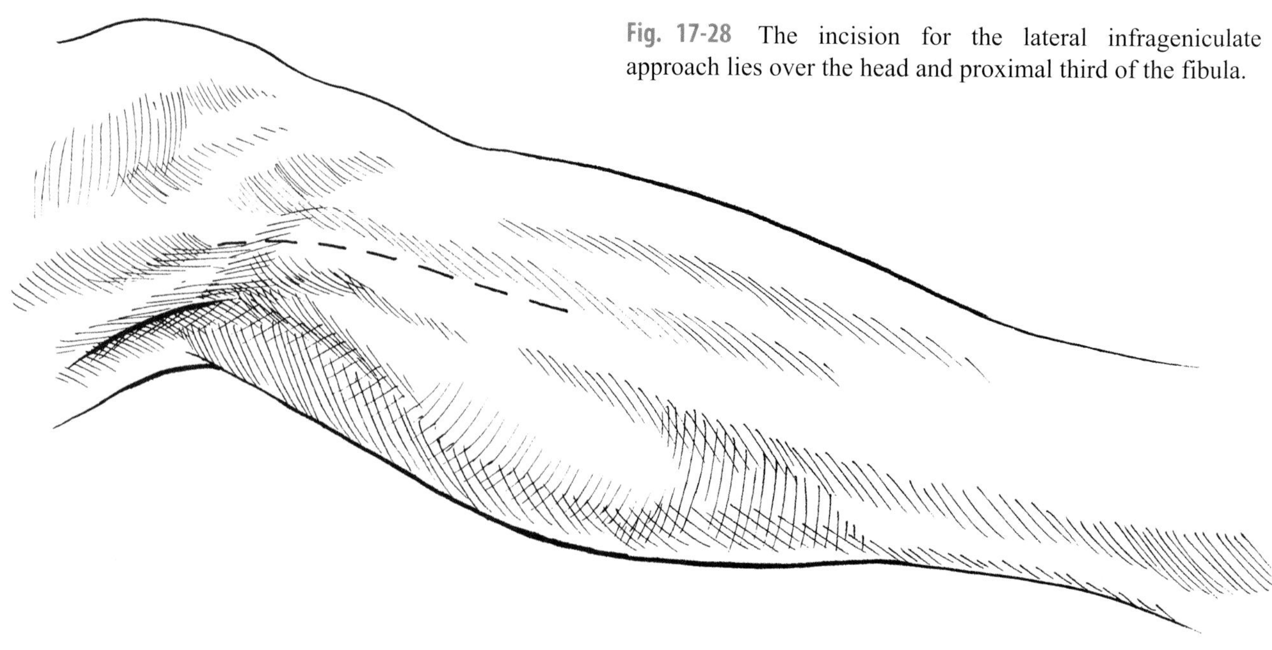

Fig. 17-28 The incision for the lateral infrageniculate approach lies over the head and proximal third of the fibula.

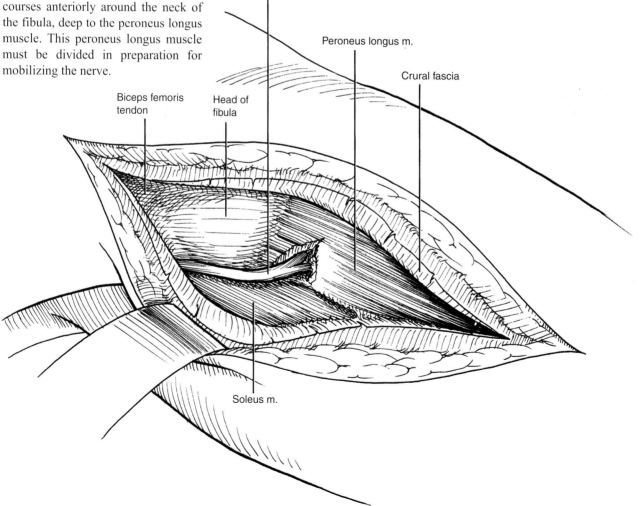

Fig. 17-29 The common peroneal nerve should be identified as it emerges posterior to the biceps tendon and courses anteriorly around the neck of the fibula, deep to the peroneus longus muscle. This peroneus longus muscle must be divided in preparation for mobilizing the nerve.

Technique of Lateral Infrageniculate Approach

The patient is placed in the supine position with the leg internally rotated and flexed at the knee. A vertical incision is made over the fibular head and extended distally over the proximal third of the fibula (Fig. 17-28). On deepening the incision, one notes the tendon of the biceps femoris muscle inserting on the superior aspect of the fibular head (Fig. 17-29). The common peroneal nerve should be identified as it emerges posterior to the biceps tendon and courses anteriorly around the neck of the fibula. The biceps tendon is divided, and the common peroneal nerve with its deep and superficial branches is carefully dissected and retracted anteriorly (Fig. 17-30).

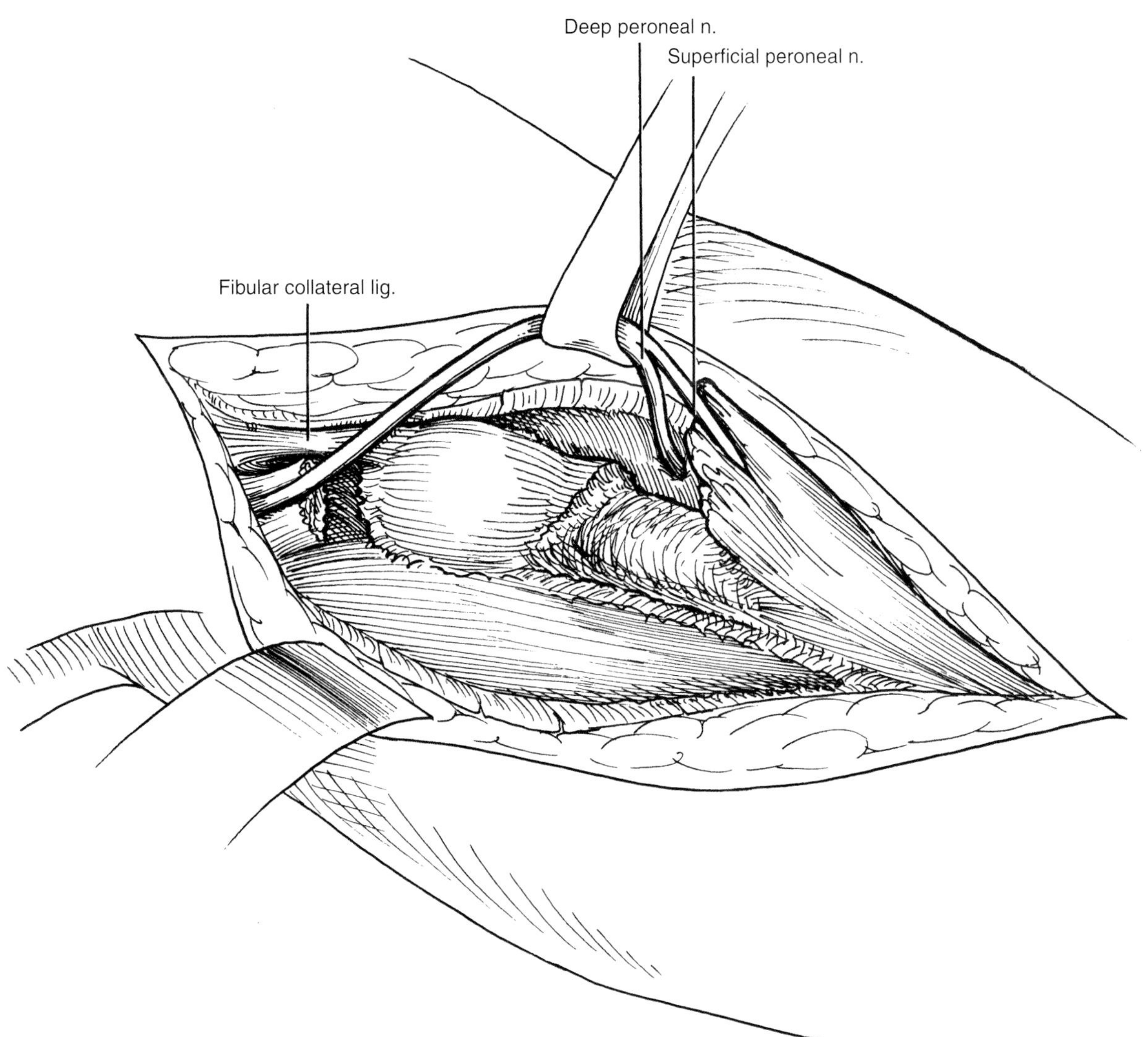

Fig. 17-30 The peroneal nerve with its deep and superficial branches is carefully retracted away from the fibula. The biceps tendon and fibular collateral ligament are divided to begin mobilization of the head of the fibula.

The upper third of the fibula is then removed from its bed. This is most easily accomplished by dividing the ligamentous attachments of the fibular head and shaft, staying close to the bone. Blunt dissection of the muscular and ligamentous attachments deep to the fibula is enhanced by retracting the freed fibular head into the wound (Fig. 17-31). The fibular shaft can then be transected with rib shears and the bone removed from its bed. The popliteal artery is encountered just deep to the fibular bed (Fig. 17-32),

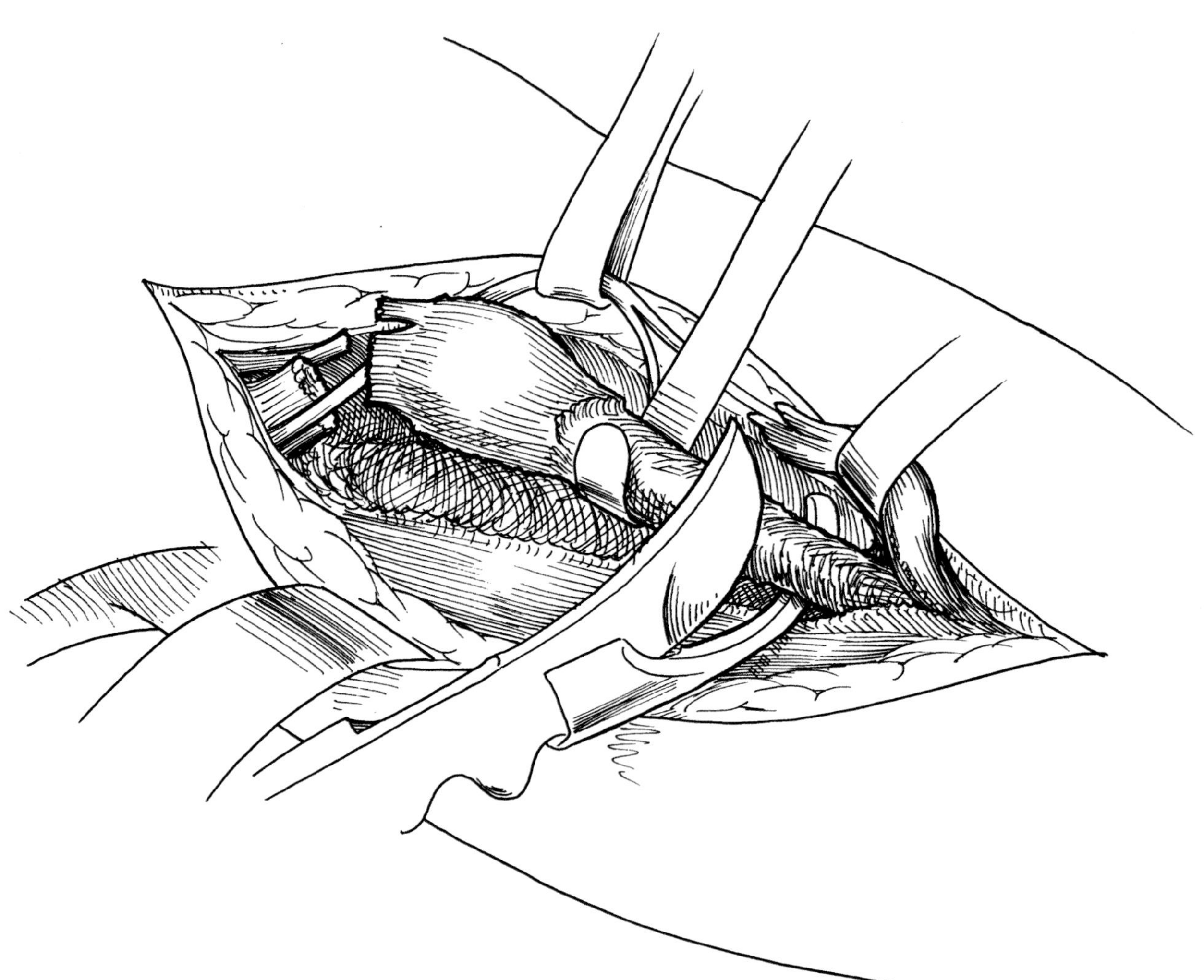

Fig. 17-31 The proximal third of the fibula is stripped of attachments to the soleus and peroneus longus muscles. A periosteal elevator may aid in the disarticulation of the tibiofibular joint. Transsection of the fibular shaft with rib shears is aided by elevation of the proximal fibula.

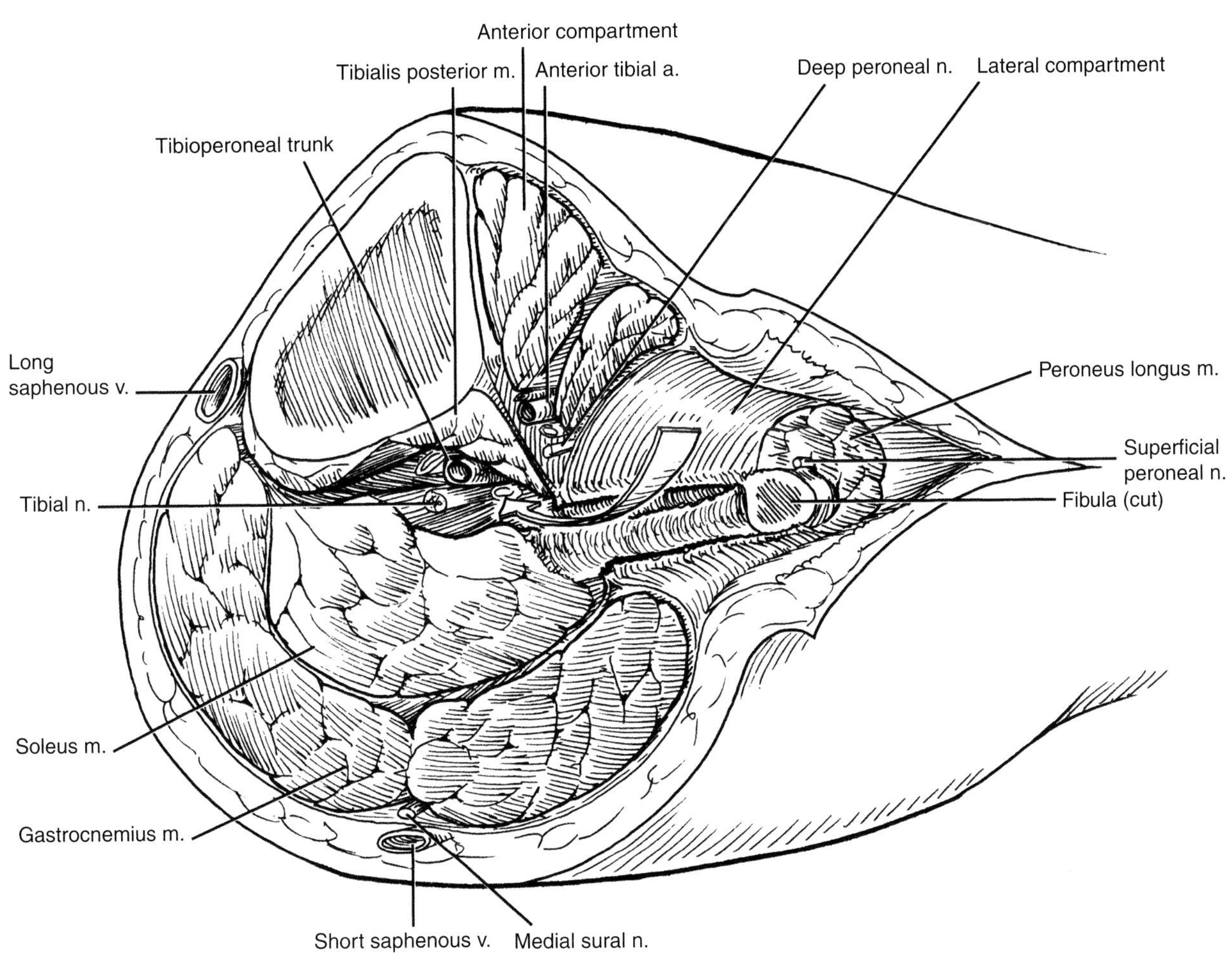

Fig. 17-32 The lateral infrageniculate approach exposes the distal popliteal artery and its branches.

and its superficial location facilitates separation from the adjacent vein (Fig. 17-33).

Grafts brought to the popliteal artery using this approach are best routed subcutaneously.[5] Bypasses from the femoral artery are brought across the anterior thigh (Fig. 17-34). To prevent kinking, grafts should be routed such that they cross the knee at the midpoint of the lateral femoral condyle.[11]

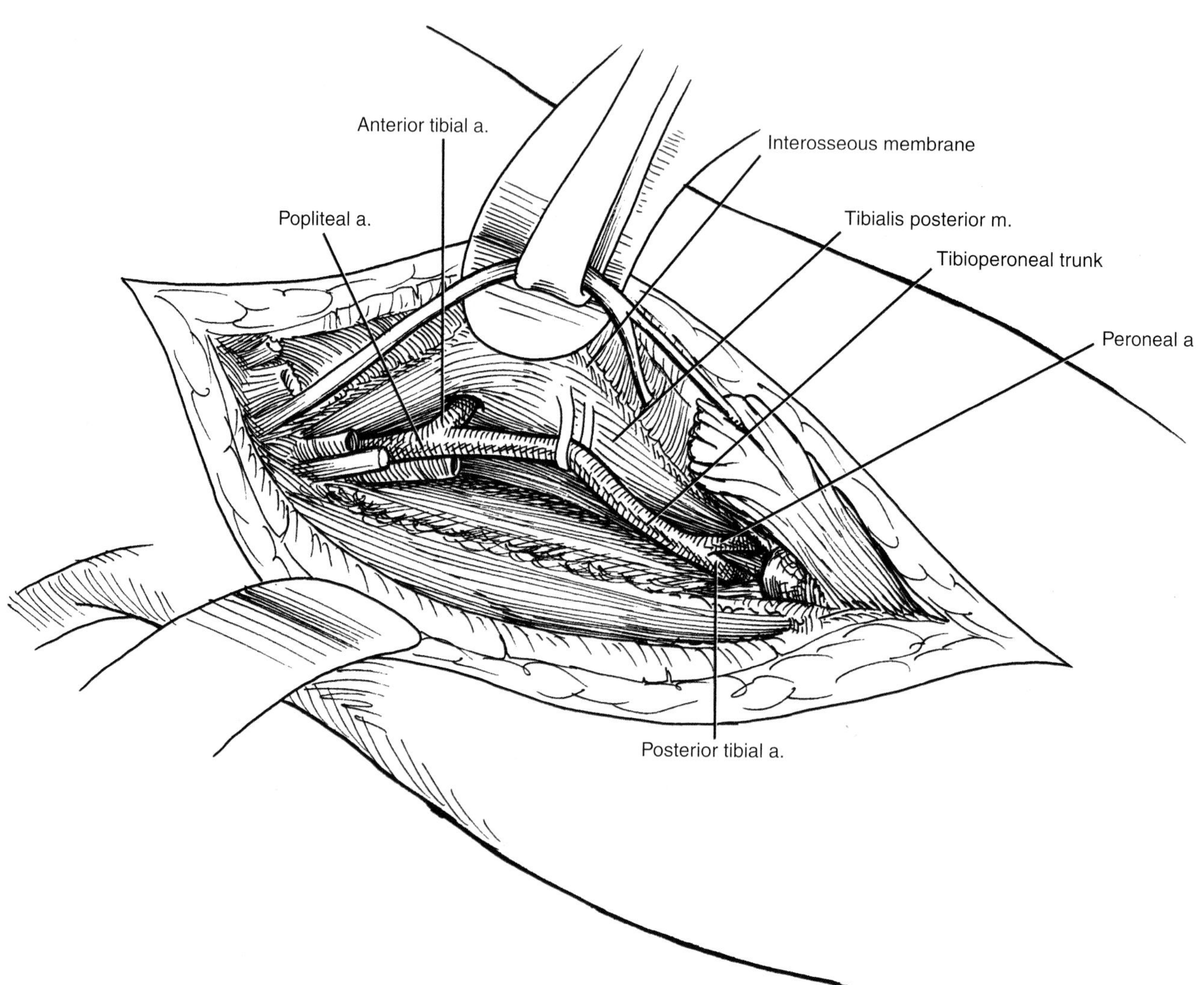

Fig. 17-33 The vessels are found deep to the fibular bed and posterior to the interosseous membrane.

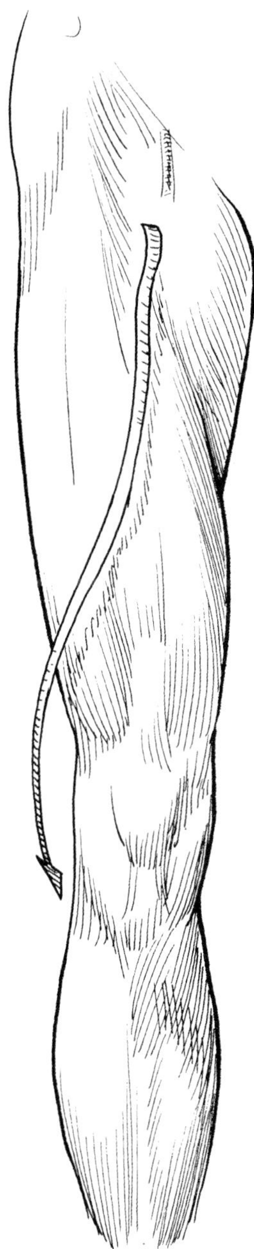

Fig. 17-34 The most direct route between the femoral vessels and the lateral infrageniculate incision is a subcutaneous path across the anterior thigh.

Exposure of the Midpopliteal Artery

There is a group of disorders peculiar to the section of the popliteal artery that traverses the knee joint (midpopliteal artery). These disorders include popliteal entrapment syndrome, cystic adventitial disease, and traumatic intimal flaps from posterior knee dislocations. Aneurysms may sometimes be confined to the midpopliteal artery, allowing a relatively limited dissection for correction of the pathology. The posterior approach may also be useful in cases of reoperative arterial surgery.[12]

The use of the posterior approach is contraindicated in procedures designed to correct more diffuse vessel pathology. Exposure of the suprageniculate and infrageniculate arteries is hampered by the muscle boundaries of the popliteal fossa. The need to reposition patients intraoperatively adds to the inconvenience of this approach for procedures involving arterial bypasses.

Technique of Posterior Approach

The patient is placed in the prone position with the knee slightly flexed. An S-shaped incision is preferred to avoid the deforming scar contractures associated with simple vertical incisions across the posterior knee (Fig. 17-35). The superior longitudinal portion of the incision is made on the

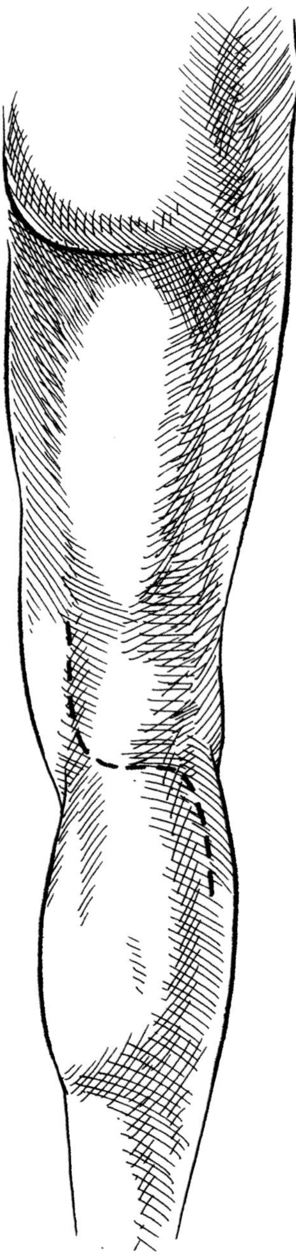

Fig. 17-35 The incision for posterior exposure of the popliteal vessels is S shaped to minimize scar contractures associated with simple vertical incisions.

posteromedial aspect of the lower thigh, and the horizontal portion is brought across the flexion crease. The inferior longitudinal extension of the incision is made laterally, for a distance of 6 to 8 cm.

The first structure to be identified in the subcutaneous tissue is the small saphenous vein, which should be ligated and divided (Fig. 17-36). The deep fascia is incised vertically, and the underlying

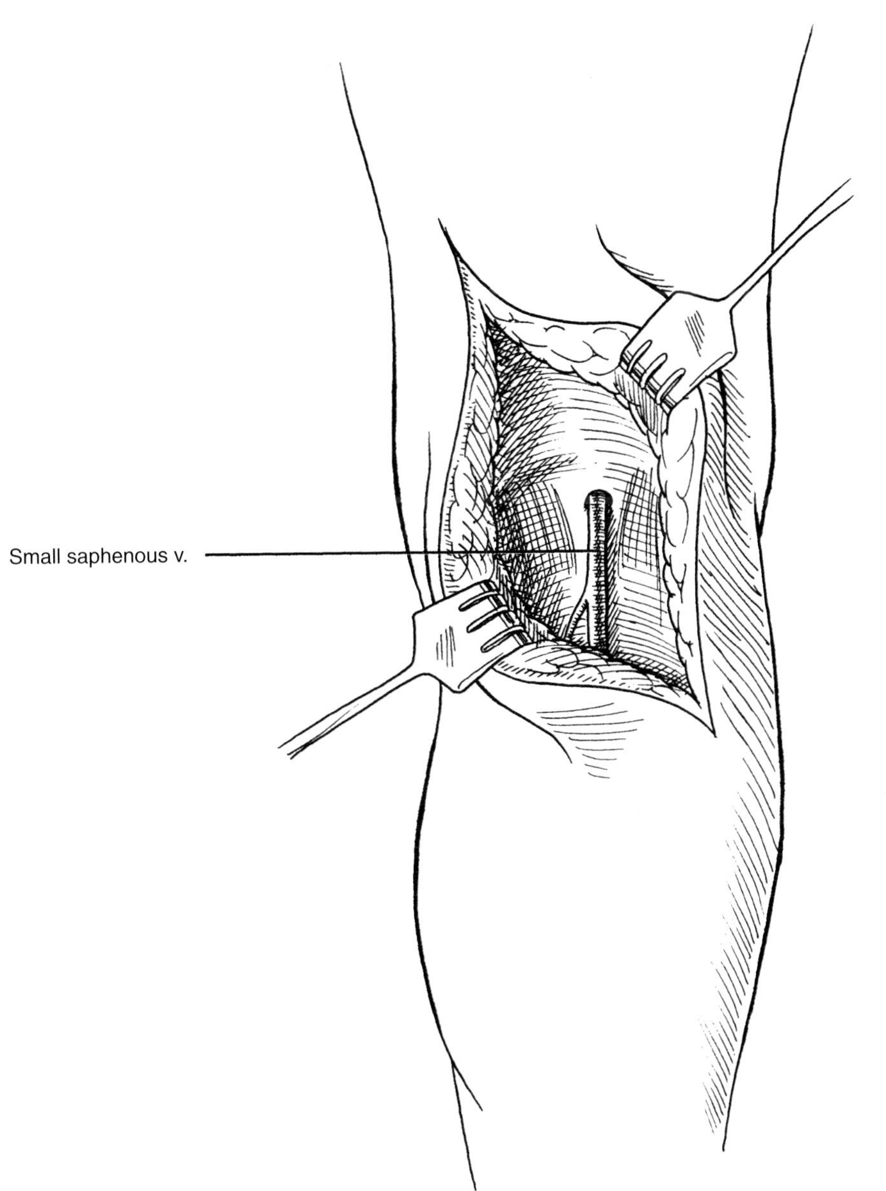

Fig. 17-36 The small saphenous vein is identified in the subcutaneous tissue just superficial to the deep fascia.

medial sural nerve is retracted for clear access to the major neurovascular structures (Fig. 17-37). The tibial nerve is the most superficial major midline structure, and the peroneal nerve follows the biceps femoris tendon obliquely toward the head of the fibula. Distal exposure may be enhanced at this point by retracting the two heads of the gastrocnemius muscle apart; this may require vertical division

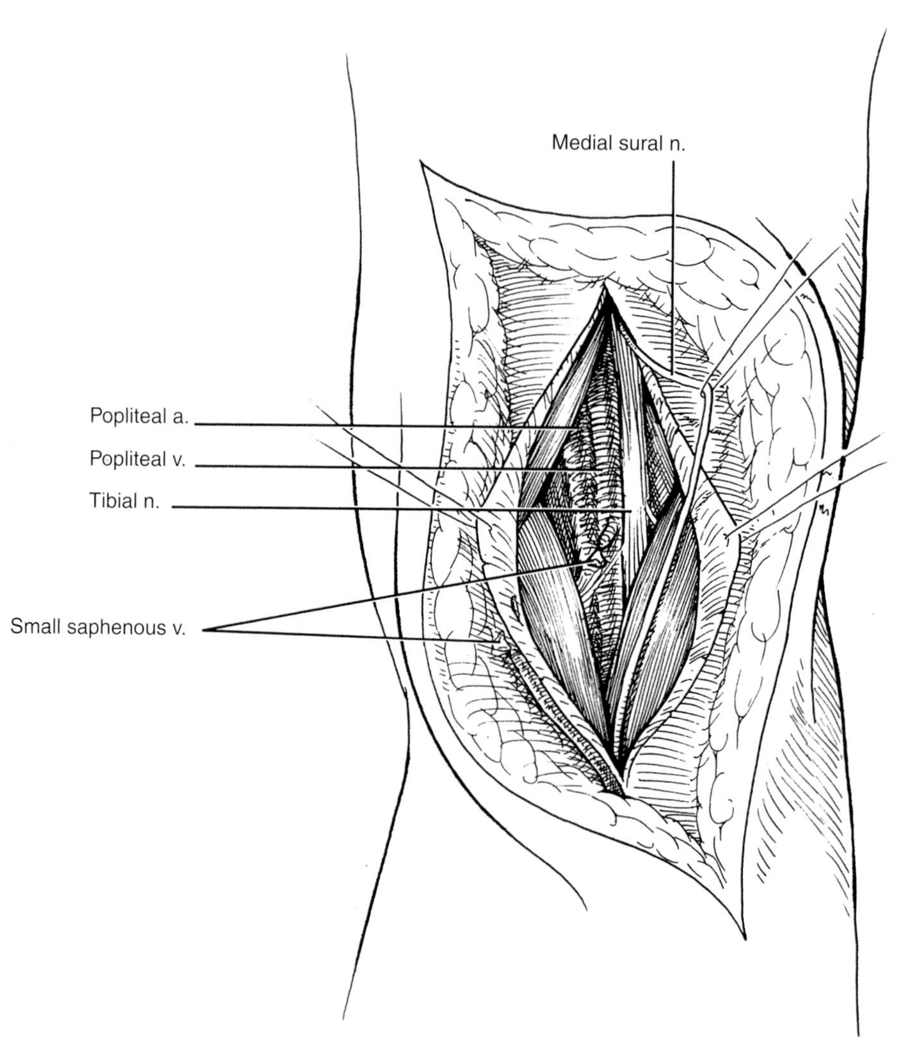

Fig. 17-37 A vertical incision of the deep fascia exposes the contents of the popliteal space. The medial sural cutaneous nerve should be divided for clear access to the major neurovascular structures.

of a fusion seam in some patients[6] (Fig. 17-38). The tibial and peroneal nerves are best retracted laterally, exposing the ensheathed popliteal vessels lying medial to the tibial nerve. The stump of the small saphenous vein is an excellent landmark and can be traced craniad to identify the popliteal vein. The artery lies medially in the sheath and slightly deep to the vein.

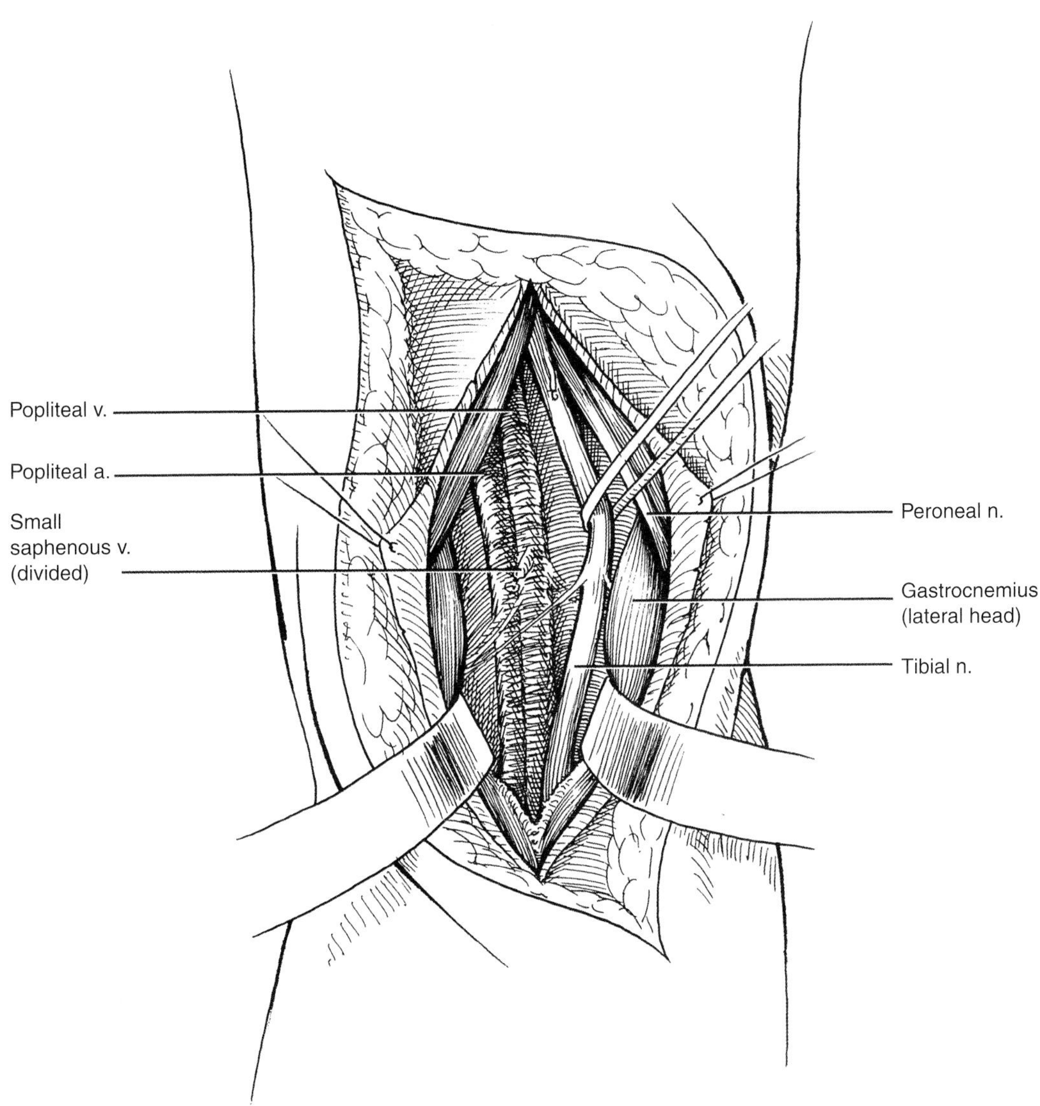

Fig. 17-38 The tibial nerve is the most superficial major midline structure and should be retracted laterally to expose the ensheathed popliteal vessels.

References

1. Takaqi H, Goto SW, Matsui M, et al. A contemporary meta-analysis of dacron versus polytetrafluoroethylene graft for femoropopliteal bypass grafting. *J Vasc Surg.* 2010;52:232–236.
2. Twine CP, McLain AD. Graft type for femoropopliteal bypass surgery. *Cochrane Database Syst Rev.* 2010;12:CD001487.
3. Van Det RJ, Vriens BH, van der Palen J, et al. Dacron or PTFE for femoro-popliteal above-knee bypass grafting: short-and long-term results of a multicentre randomized trial. *Eur J Vasc Endovasc Surg.* 2009;37:457–463.
4. Jackson MR, Belott TP, Dickason T, et al. The consequences of a failed femoropopliteal bypass grafting: comparison of saphenous vein and PTFE grafts. *J Vasc Surg.* 2000;32:498–505.
5. Veith FJ, Aster E, Gupta SK, et al. Lateral approach to the popliteal artery. *J Vasc Surg* 1987;6:119–123.
6. Henry AK. The back of the thigh and the leg. In: Henry AK, ed. *Extensile Exposure,* 2nd ed. Edinburgh, England: Churchill Livingstone; 1973:241–259.
7. The TransAtlantic Inter-Society Consensus (TASC) Working Group. Management of peripheral arterial disease (PAD). *J Vasc Surg.* 2000;31:S217–S225.
8. Parsons RE, Suggs WD, Veith FJ, et al. Polytetrafluoroethylene bypasses to infrapopliteal arteries without cuffs or patches: a better option than amputation in patients without autologous vein. *J Vasc Surg.* 1996;23:347–356.
9. Baril DT, Marone LK, Kim J, et al. Outcomes of endovascular interventions for TASC IIB and C femoropopliteal lesions. *J Vasc Surg.* 2008;48:627–633.
10. Baril DT, Chaer RA, Rhee RY, et al. Endovascular interventions for TASC IID femoropopliteal lesions. *J Vasc Surg.* 2010;51:1406–1412.
11. Ouriel K, Rutherford RB. Femoral infrapopliteal bypass with contralateral saphenous vein. In: Ouriel K, Rutherford RB, eds. *Atlas of Vascular Surgery: Operative Procedures.* Philadelphia, PA: WB Saunders; 1998:34–39.
12. Gelabert HA, Colburn MD, Machleder HI. Posterior exposure of the popliteal artery in reoperative vascular surgery. *Ann Vasc Surg.* 1996;10:53–58.

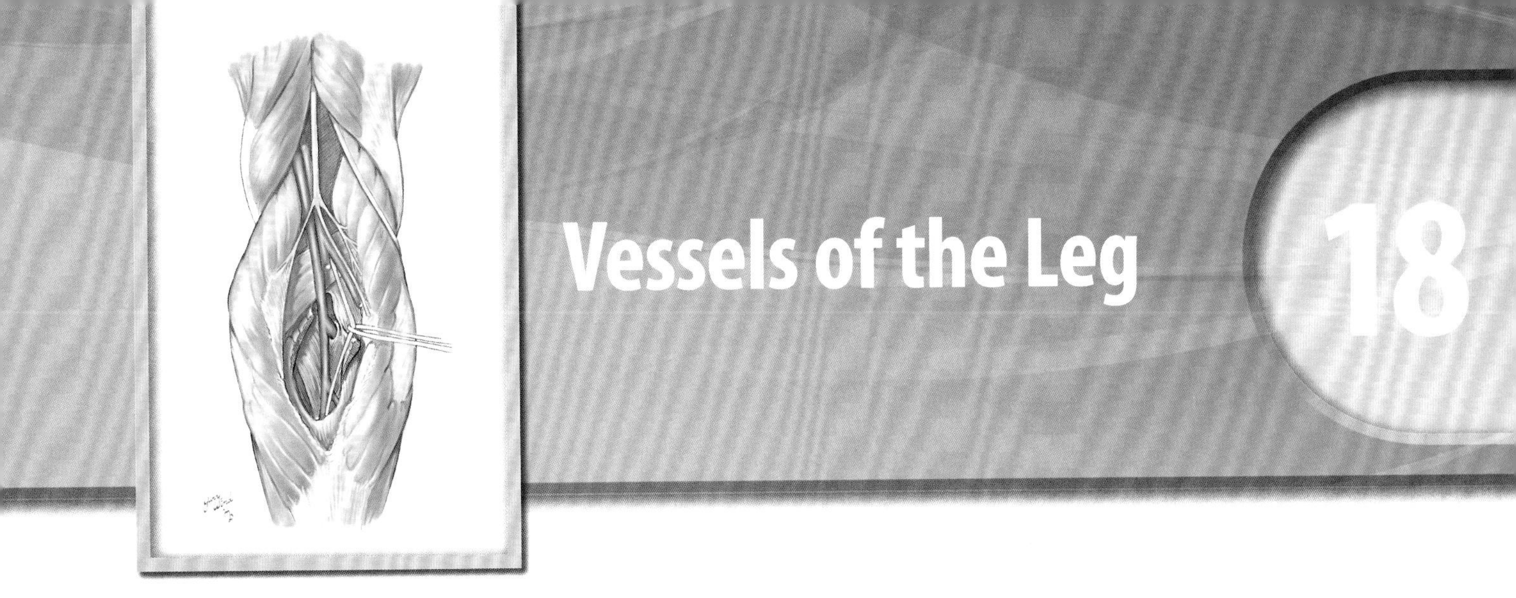

Vessels of the Leg

18

Surgical Anatomy of the Leg

The popliteal artery branches in the proximal leg to ultimately form the anterior tibial, posterior tibial, and peroneal trunks. The older term "trifurcation" is a misnomer because the common tibioperoneal trunk is interposed between the origin of the anterior tibial artery and the bifurcation of the other two vessels some 2 to 3 cm more distally (Fig. 18-1). The popliteal artery terminates in a true trifurcation approximately 3% of the time.[1,2] To understand the relationships of these arteries, it is necessary to review the muscle groups and fascial girdle of the leg. Then the nerves and vessels can be conceptually laid in place.

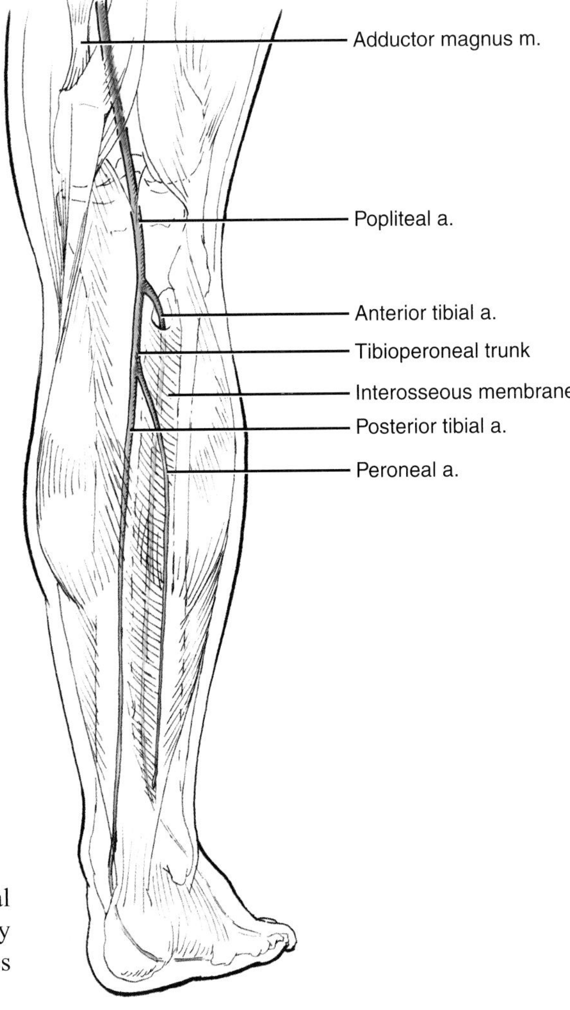

Fig. 18-1 The division of the leg vessels distal to the popliteal artery normally occurs in two stages. The anterior tibial artery arises first, leaving a common tibioperoneal trunk that bifurcates into the posterior tibial and peroneal arteries.

Fascia of the Leg

A dense fascial layer, continuous with the fascia lata of the thigh, encircles the leg. This crural fascia is adherent to underlying structures around the knee joint and ankle joint. Thickened bands of this fascia form retinacula at the ankle that restrain the extensor (dorsiflexor), flexor (plantar flexor), and peroneal (evertor) tendons (Fig. 18-2).

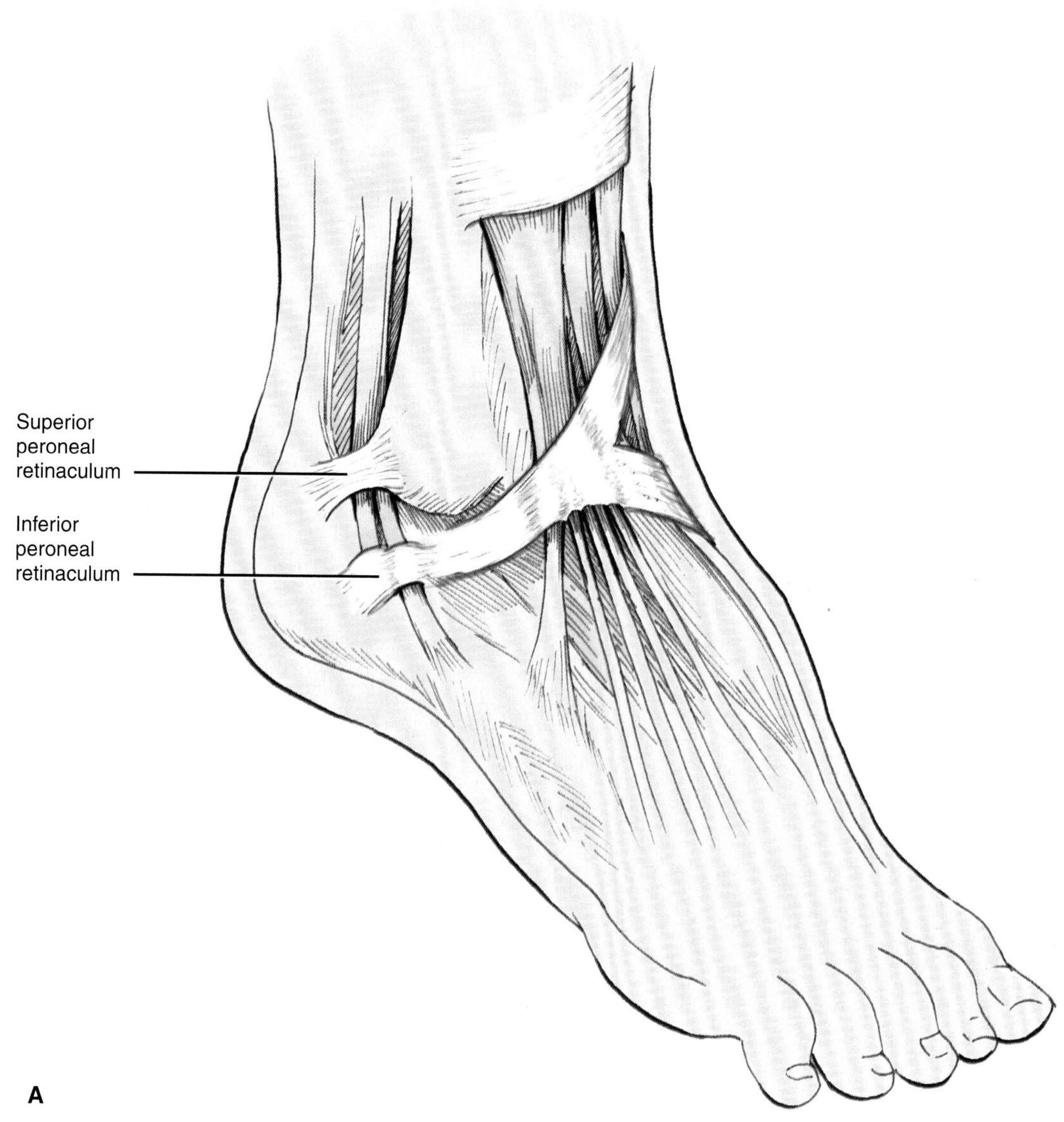

Fig. 18-2 **A, B**: Thickened bands of the dense crural fascia form restraining retinacula at the ankle over the extensor, flexor, and peroneal tendons. The two principal neurovascular bundles lie beneath the extensor and flexor retinacula.

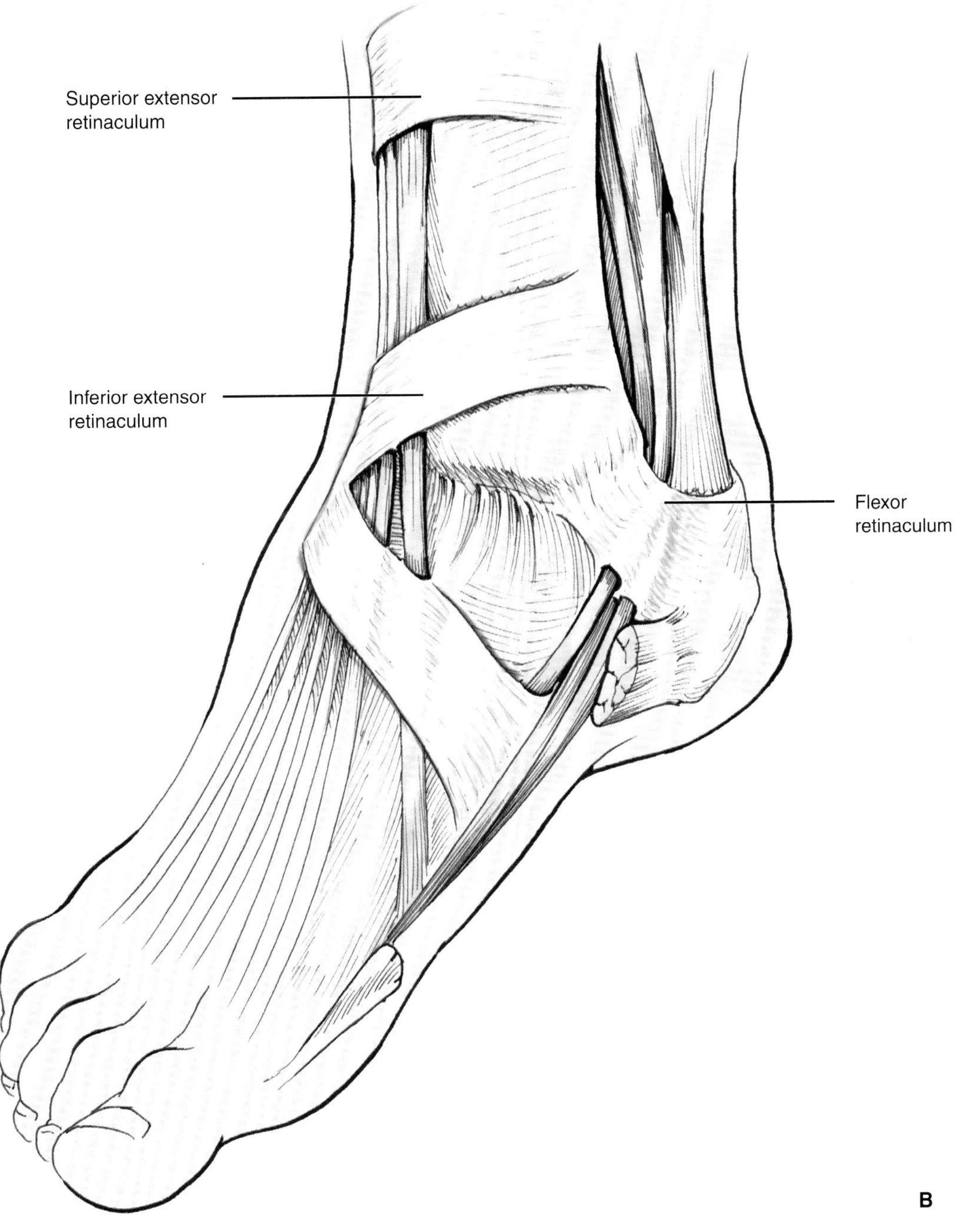
Superior extensor retinaculum
Inferior extensor retinaculum
Flexor retinaculum
B

Strong septa join the crural fascia to the fibula and partition the leg into anterior, posterior, and lateral compartments (Fig. 18-3). The tough interosseous membrane completes the division of the anterior from the posterior space. In addition, a secondary septum arches from the tibia to the fibula posteriorly, creating a deep and superficial posterior compartment.

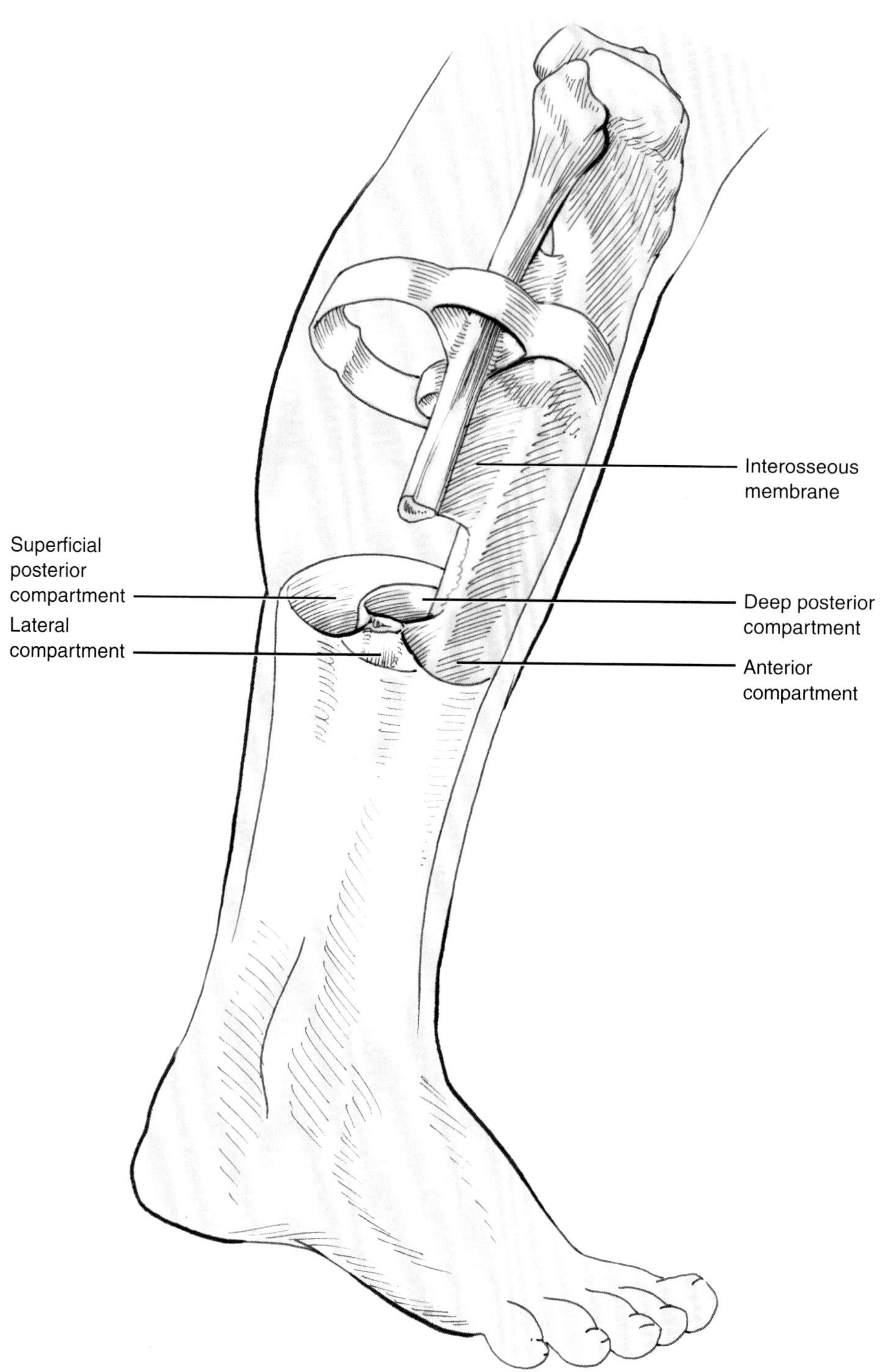

Fig. 18-3 Strong septa between the crural fascia and the bones of the leg separate the leg into discrete compartments.

Interestingly, the three primary arterial trunks of the leg occupy only two of the four spaces (Fig. 18-4). The anterior tibial artery lies in the compartment of the same name. Both the posterior tibial and peroneal arteries lie in the deep posterior compartment and send penetrating branches to the overlying superficial posterior compartment and to the adjacent lateral compartment.

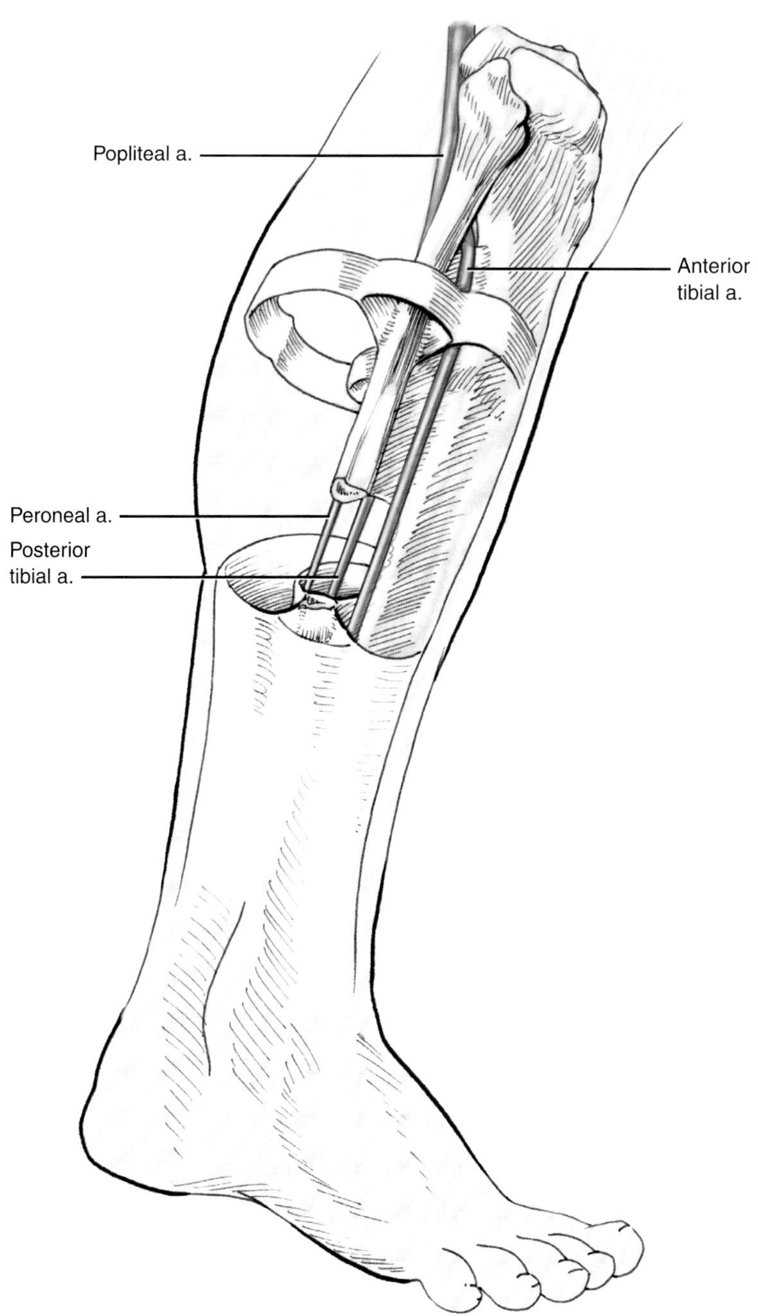

Fig. 18-4 The major arteries of the leg lie in the anterior and deep posterior compartments and supply adjacent compartments through perforating branches.

The nerve distribution differs slightly from the arterial pattern in that a discrete trunk enters each major compartment. The tibial nerve supplies the posterior compartment flexor muscles. The peroneal nerve divides into a superficial branch to the peroneal muscles (peroneus longus and brevis) and a deep branch to the anterior compartment muscles (Fig. 18-5).

The unyielding nature of the crural fascia and its tight adherence at the knee and ankle make the closed compartmental spaces susceptible to buildup of pressure after leg injury. Intramuscular tissue pressure is normally zero. Trauma such as fracture, severe compression, or prolonged ischemia can result in compartmental edema that increases tissue pressure. As the pressure exceeds lymphatic and then venous closing pressure, any egress of fluid from the leg is blocked, and the pressure escalates more quickly. Such compartment syndromes can result in irreversible neuromuscular damage if not relieved by prompt fasciotomy. Four-compartment fasciotomies are usually performed through separate medial and lateral leg incisions (Fig. 18-6).

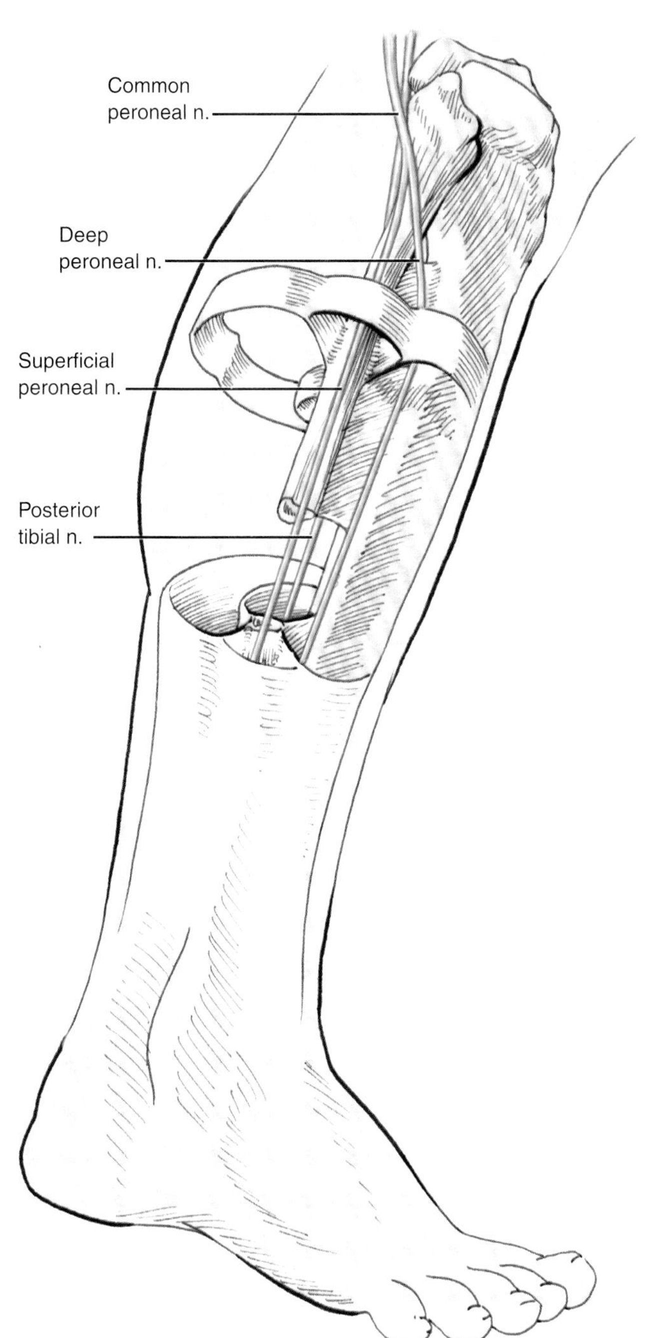

Fig. 18-5 A major nerve trunk runs in each major compartment of the leg.

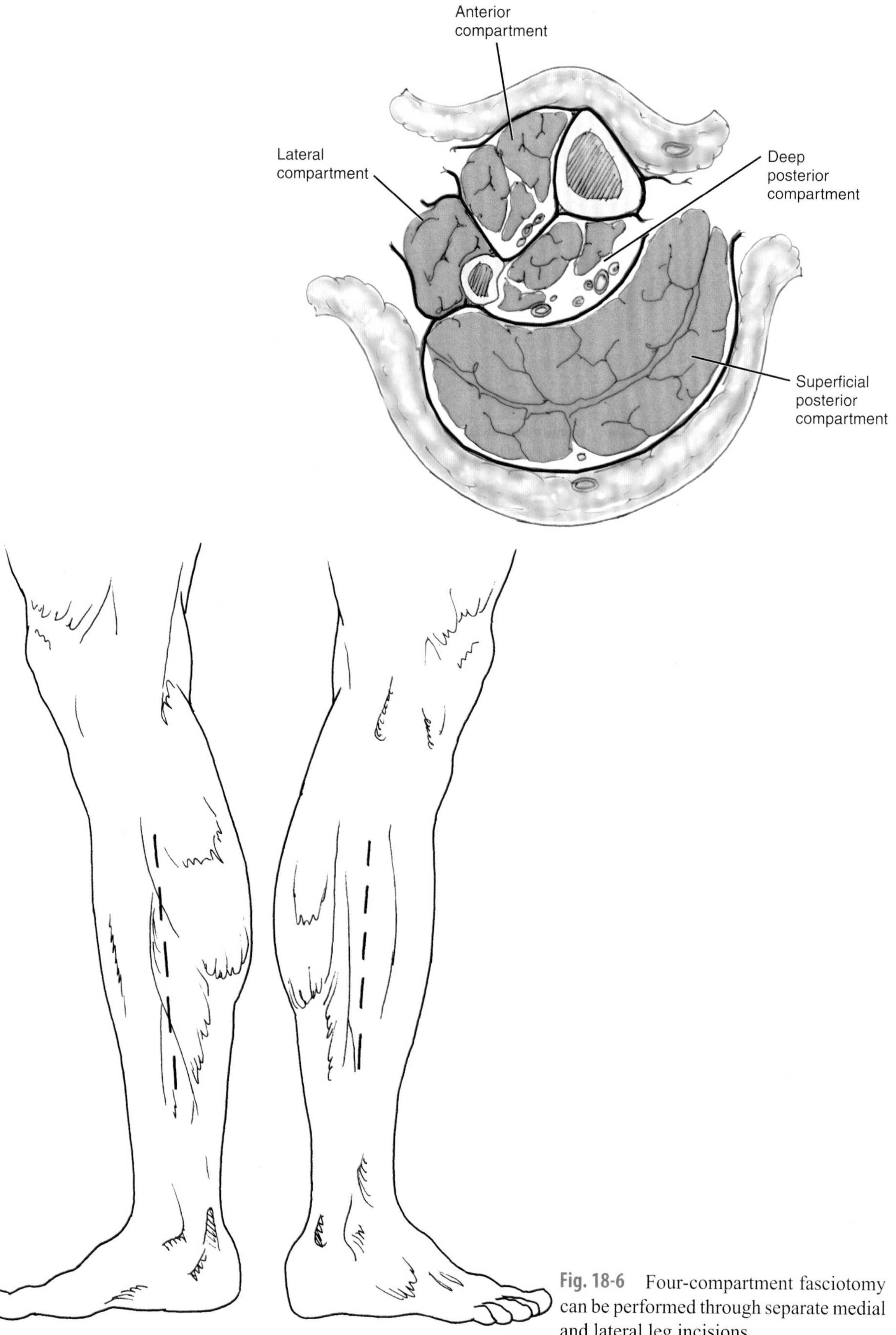

Fig. 18-6 Four-compartment fasciotomy can be performed through separate medial and lateral leg incisions.

Alternatively, all compartments can be simultaneously decompressed through a single lateral incision combined with a fibulectomy (Fig. 18-7).

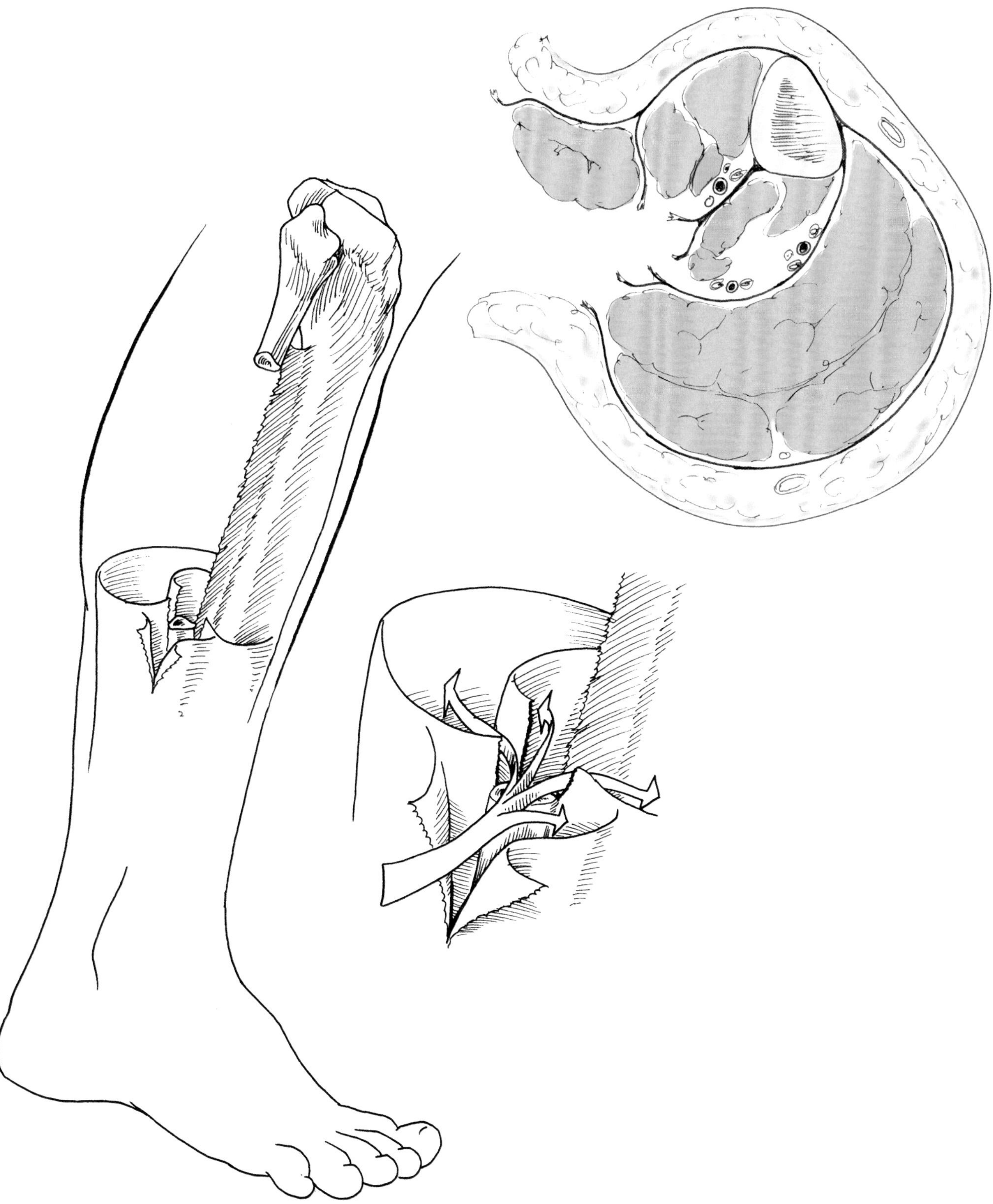

Fig. 18-7 A septum of each compartment attaches to the fibula, allowing universal compartment decompression by fibulectomy.

Musculoskeletal Relationships

The muscle groups of the leg are composed of the large posterior gastrocnemius/soleus complex and three groups of long muscles: the plantar flexors, dorsiflexors, and evertors of the foot. The gastrocnemius muscle group (including the small plantaris muscle) attaches to the calcaneus through the large Achilles tendon (Fig. 18-8).

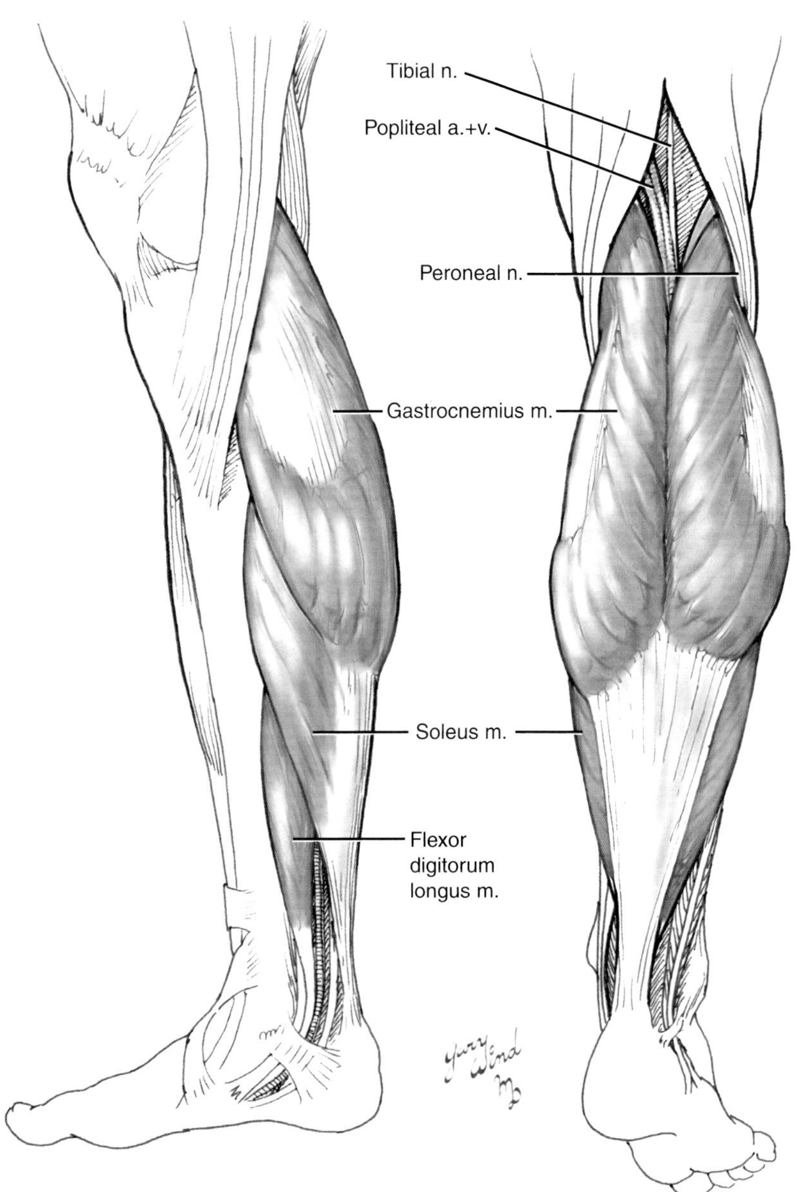

Fig. 18-8 The powerful gastrocnemius and soleus muscles occupy the superficial posterior compartment of the leg.

The other three groups of muscles cross the ankle joint closely applied to bony structures. Their tendons lie beneath thickenings of the deep fascia of the leg that prevent bowstringing of the long tendons at the ankle. The plantar flexors (Fig. 18-9) consist of the tibialis posterior, flexor digitorum longus, and flexor hallucis longus muscles. Their tendons pass behind the medial malleolus under the flexor retinaculum (lacinate ligament) (Fig. 18-10).

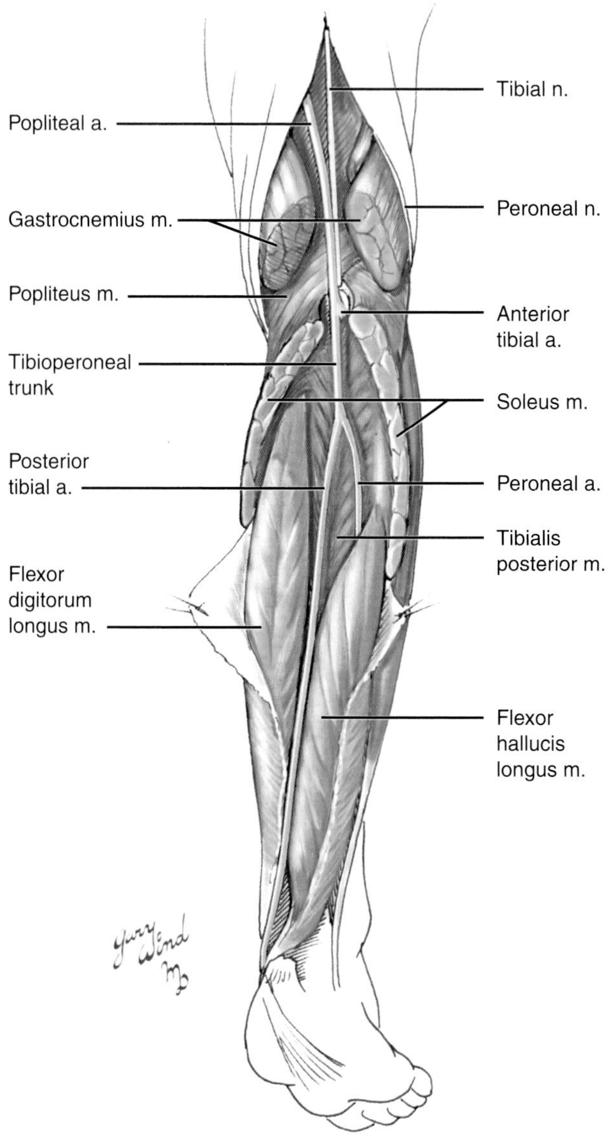

Fig. 18-9 Muscles of the deep posterior compartment are shown.

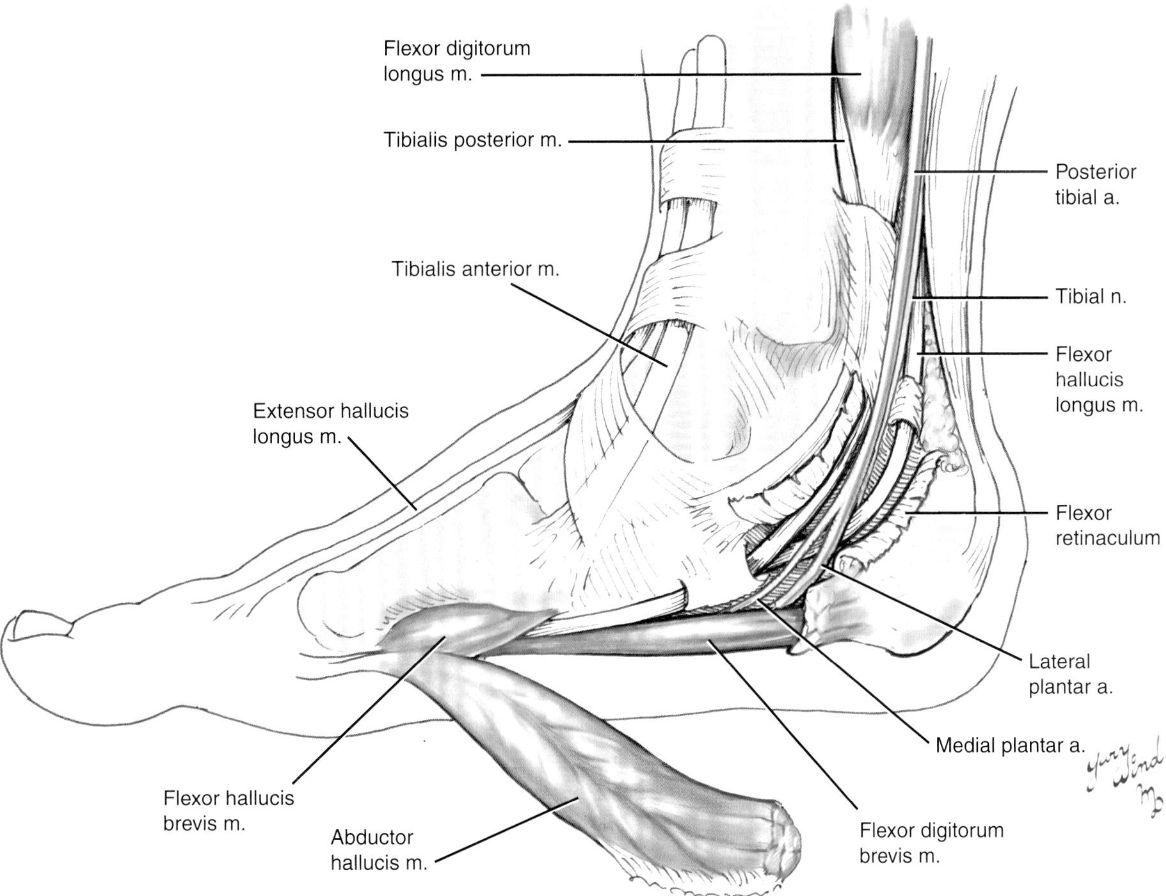

Fig. 18-10 Tendons of the plantar flexor muscles pass behind the medial malleolus under the flexor retinaculum.

The dorsiflexors (Fig. 18-11) consist of the tibialis anterior, extensor digitorum longus, and extensor hallucis longus muscles. Their tendons are held by the superior extensor retinaculum

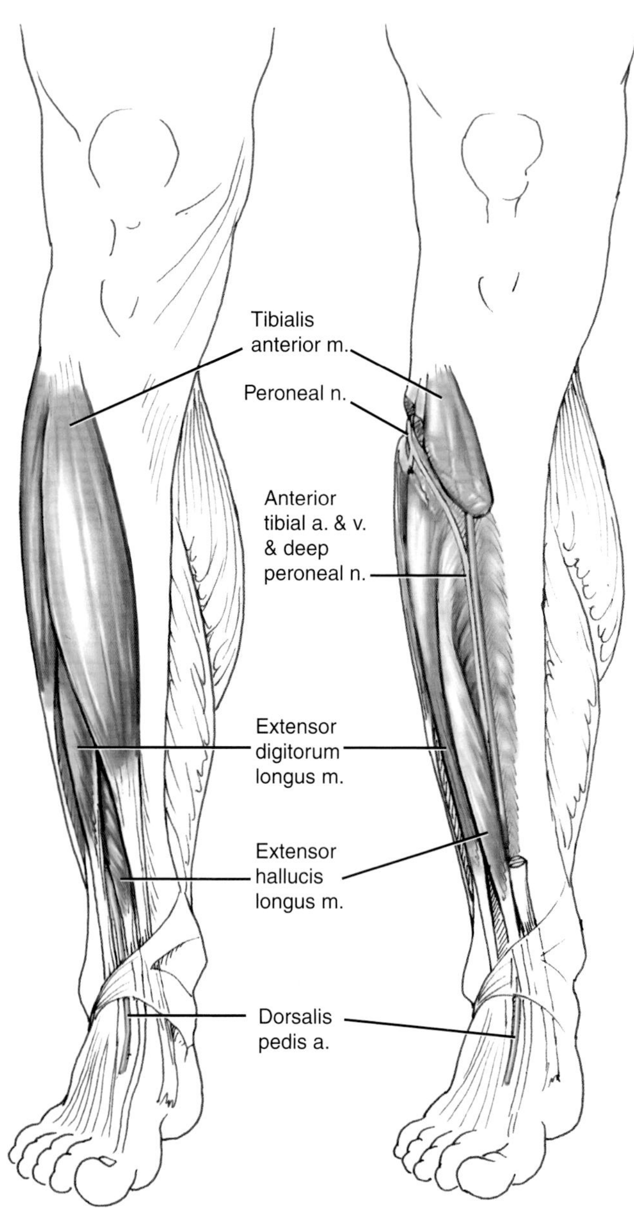

Fig. 18-11 Muscles of the dorsiflexor group are shown.

above the ankle and the inferior extensor retinaculum below the ankle (Fig. 18-12). The tendons of the foot evertors, the peroneus longus and brevis muscles, pass behind the lateral malleolus and are

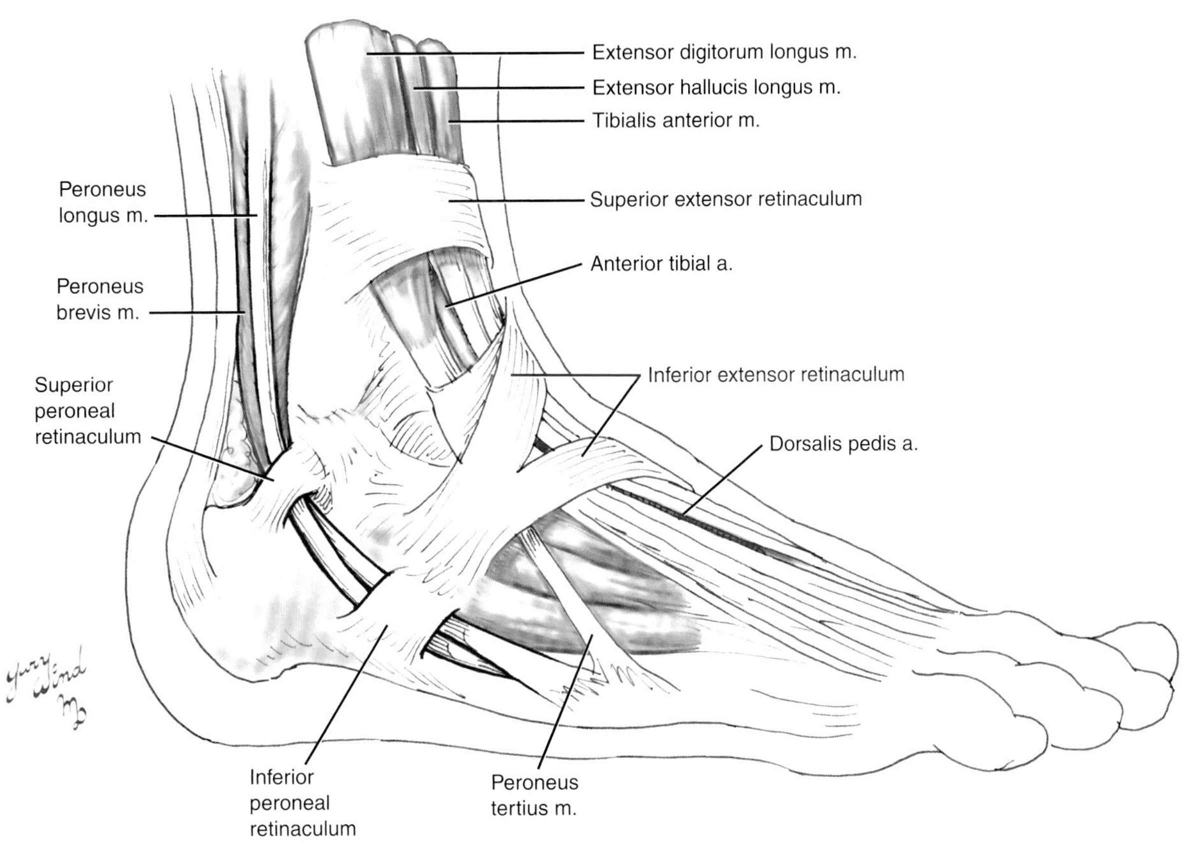

Fig. 18-12 Tendons of the dorsiflexors are held at the ankle and foot by the superior and inferior extensor retinacula.

held by the superior and inferior peroneal retinacula (Fig. 18-13). Deep attachments of the retinacula to the bones of the ankle and foot form sheathlike compartments for the tendons.

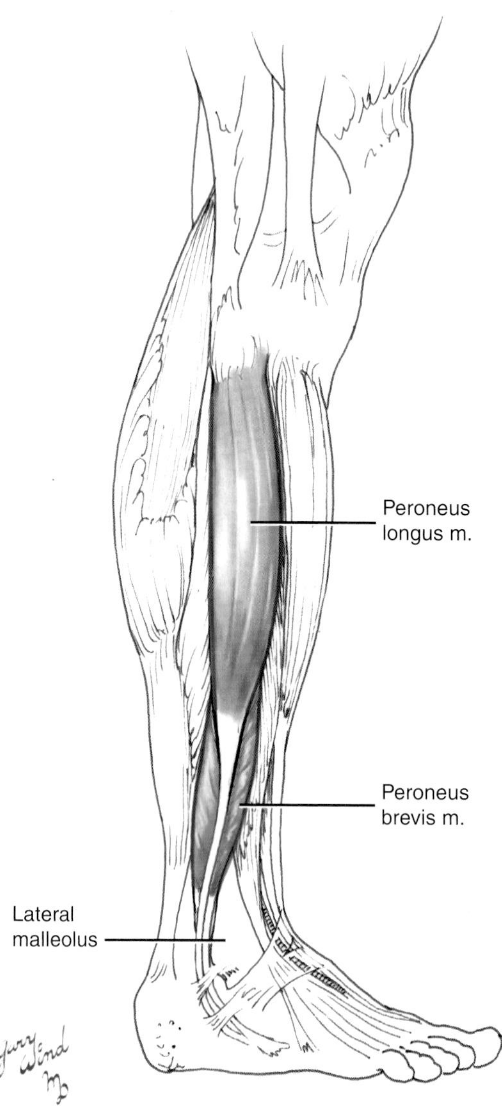

Fig. 18-13 Tendons of the foot evertors pass behind the lateral malleolus.

Anterior Compartment

The anterior, or extensor, compartment is enclosed by the crural fascia attaching to the lateral subcutaneous margin of the tibia and the anterior septum from the fibula to the crural fascia. It contains two parallel muscle masses (Fig. 18-14). The large tibialis anterior muscle lies adjacent to the tibia, arising from that bone and the adjacent interosseous membrane. Lateral to the tibialis anterior is a column of muscles originating sequentially from the fibula and adjacent interosseous membrane. From proximal to distal, these are the extensor digitorum longus, extensor hallucis longus, and peroneus tertius muscles. The anterior tibial vessels and deep peroneal nerve lie between these muscular columns and are directly accessible from an anterior approach. The arched origin of the anterior tibial vessels, passing through the proximal hiatus in the interosseous membrane, can be made more accessible by removing the head of the fibula. The distal anterior tibial artery continues beneath the Y-shaped inferior extensor retinaculum to reach the dorsum of the foot as the dorsalis pedis artery lateral to the tendon of extensor hallucis longus muscle.

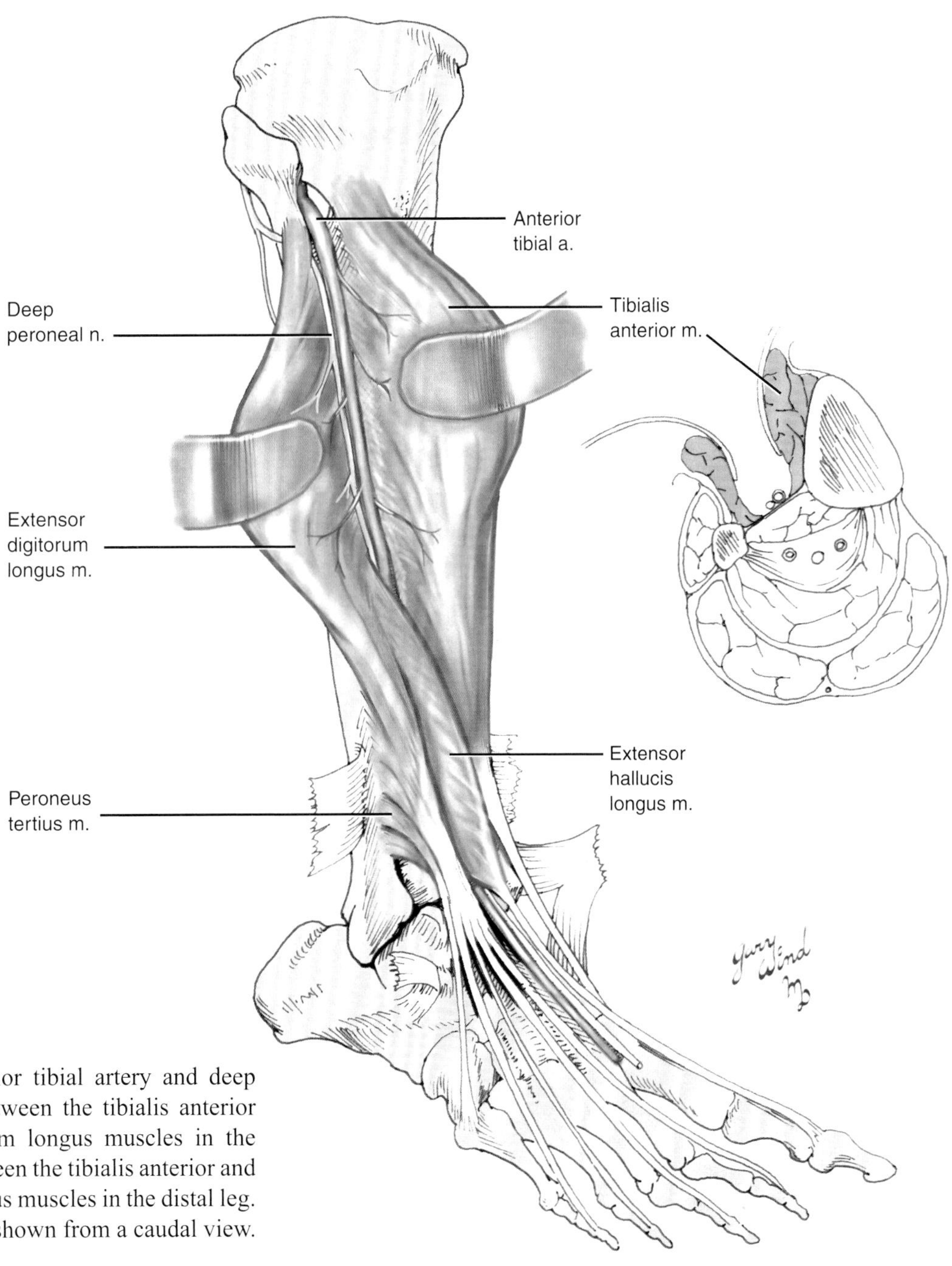

Fig. 18-14 The anterior tibial artery and deep peroneal nerve lie between the tibialis anterior and extensor digitorum longus muscles in the proximal leg and between the tibialis anterior and extensor hallucis longus muscles in the distal leg. All cross sections are shown from a caudal view.

Posterior Compartment

The superficial posterior compartment contains the bulky superficial gastrocnemius/soleus complex that fuses to form a common termination in the calcaneal tendon (Fig. 18-15). The hoodlike origin of the soleus muscle blocks direct access to the underlying posterior tibial and peroneal arteries. From the apex at the fibular head, the shorter lateral fibular origin descends in a straight line down the fibula. The tibial head is in two parts. The proximal diagonal portion originates from the soleal line of the tibia and is interrupted by the hiatus for the popliteal vessels and tibial nerve. On reaching the medial subcutaneous border of the tibia, the tibial origin descends vertically to the midpoint of the tibia. The diagonal muscle fiber disposition of the lateral and medial origins should be used to advantage when stripping the muscle off the bone.

Between the superficial and deep posterior muscle groups, there is a fascial layer that is less dense than the crural fascia and septa. Within and beneath this layer lie the posterior tibial and peroneal vessels. Although the arteries are usually single trunks, the tendency of accompanying veins to be multiple is pronounced in the leg. Exposure of the arteries requires careful dissection of the surrounding veins.

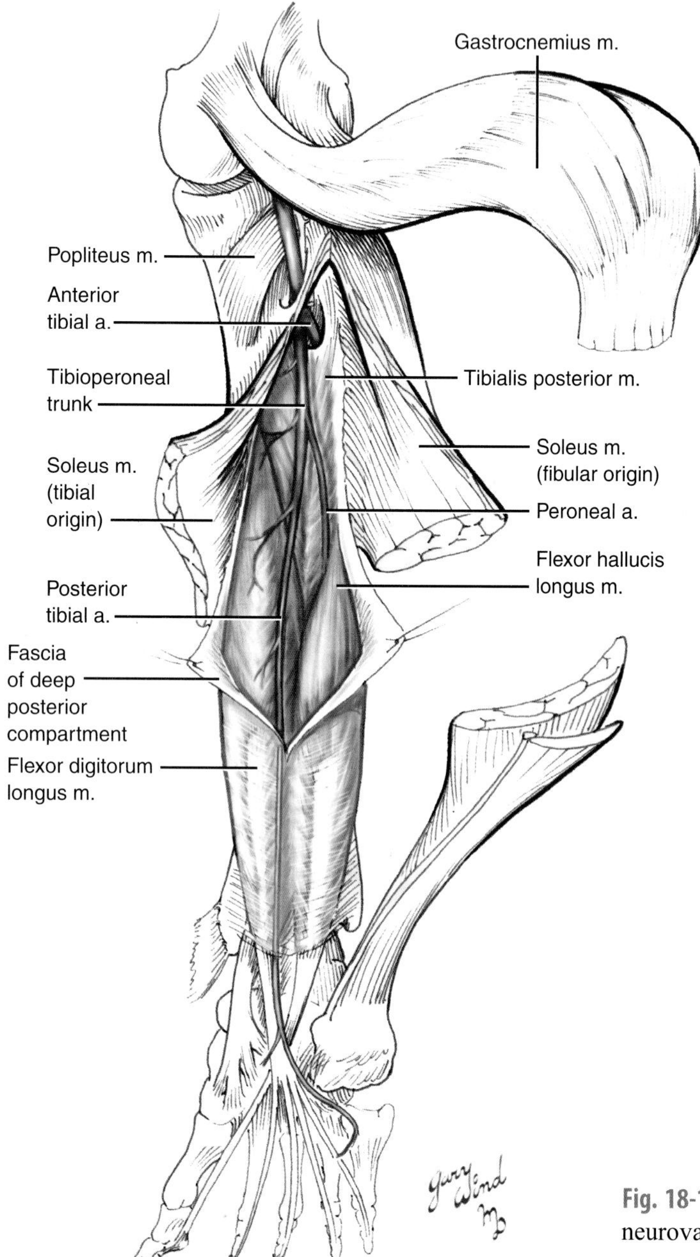

Fig. 18-15 A thin fascial septum covers the muscles and neurovascular structures of the deep posterior compartment.

The deep layer of posterior muscles consists of the central tibialis posterior muscle, running the length of the interosseous membrane and into the foot, flanked by the shorter flexor digitorum longus muscle medially and the short flexor hallucis longus muscle laterally. Both the proximal posterior tibial and peroneal arteries descend on the tibialis posterior muscle. The distal third of the peroneal artery runs within and behind the belly of the flexor hallucis longus muscle. It terminates in a variable branch perforating through the distal interosseous membrane and in calcaneal branches. The posterior tibial neurovascular bundle reaches the ankle posterior to the tendons of tibialis posterior and flexor digitorum longus muscles beneath the flexor retinaculum.

Lateral Compartment

The peroneus longus and brevis muscles originate from the lateral border of the proximal and distal fibula, respectively (Fig. 18-16). Their tendons pass under the superior peroneal retinaculum posterior to the lateral malleolus. The importance of this muscle group in vascular surgery lies in the fact that it must be mobilized from the fibula to resect that bone for lateral access to the posterior compartment vessels and when simultaneous decompression of all compartments through a single incision is necessary.

Henry[3] emphasized fine points for liberating the fibula without damaging adjacent nerves and vessels. Proximal exposure is obtained by gently

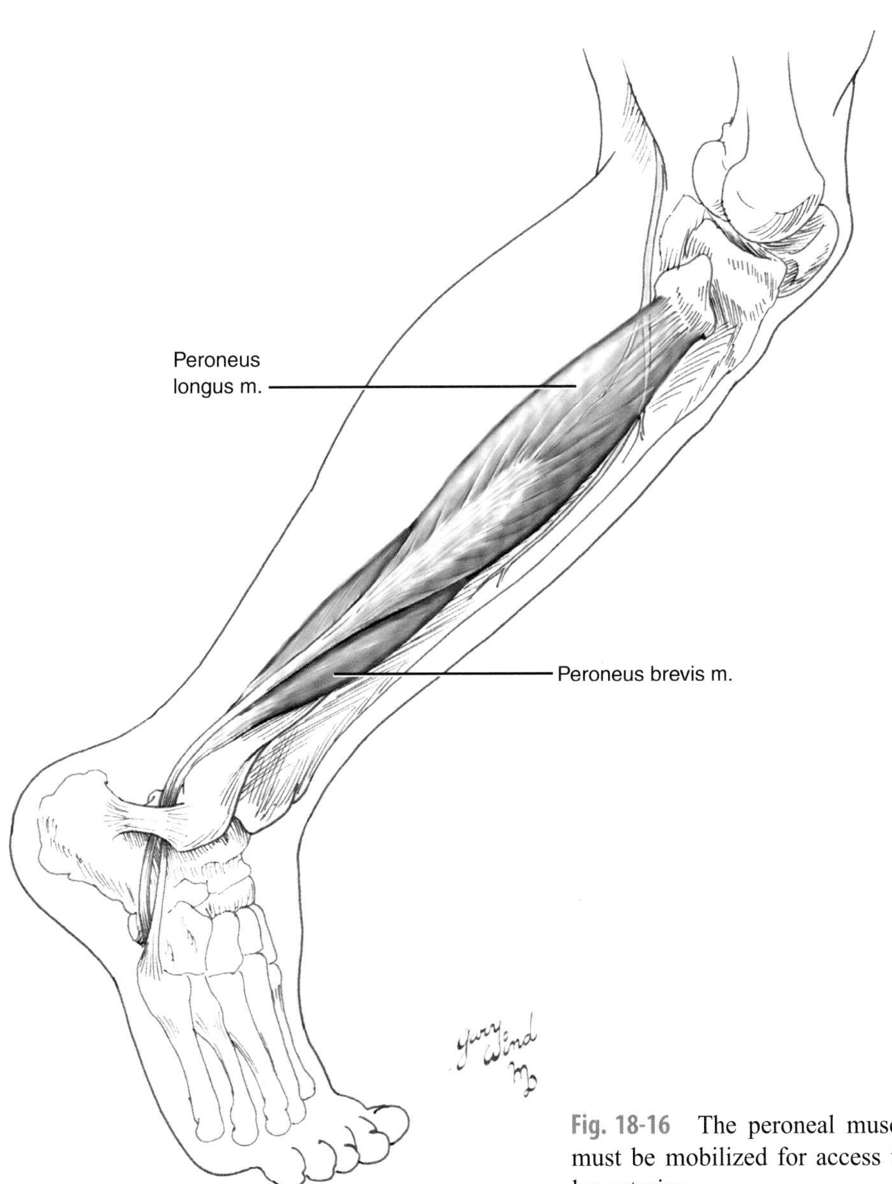

Fig. 18-16 The peroneal muscles of the lateral compartment must be mobilized for access to the fibula and deep posterior leg arteries.

elevating the common peroneal nerve posterior to the biceps femoris tendon. The overlying origin of the peroneus longus is divided to expose the branches (Fig. 18-17). The length of the muscle origins are then elevated laterally to medially, creating a long trapdoor with an intact superficial peroneal nerve

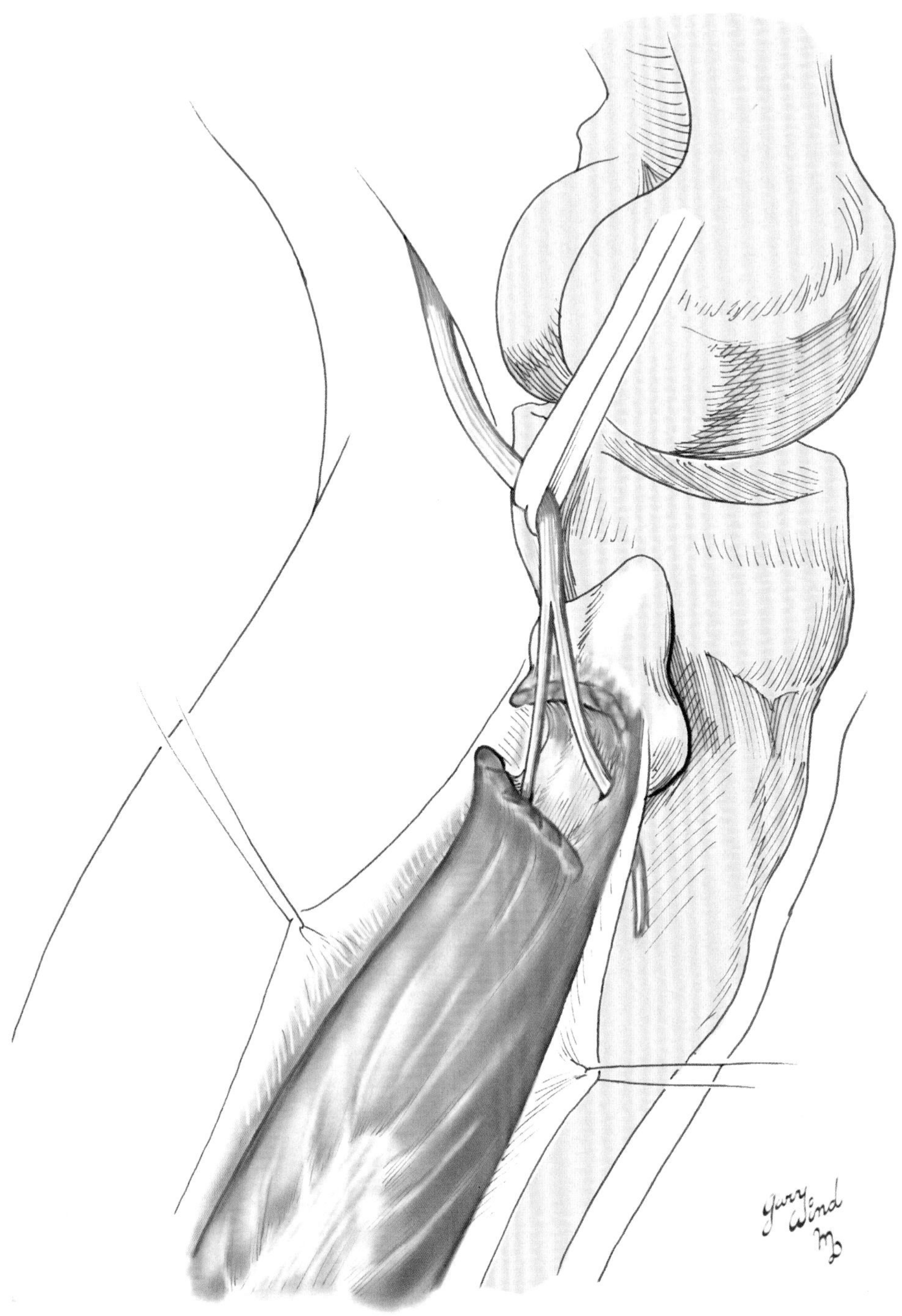

Fig. 18-17 The path of the peroneal nerve and its branches is dissected free of overlying muscles to protect the nerve during mobilization of the fibula.

(Fig. 18-18). The bias of the muscle fibers dictates stripping upward toward the knee, whereas the dominant bias of the interosseous membrane mandates stripping in the opposite direction. Confining dissection to the periosteal plane in the distal leg prevents damage to the nearby peroneal vessels.

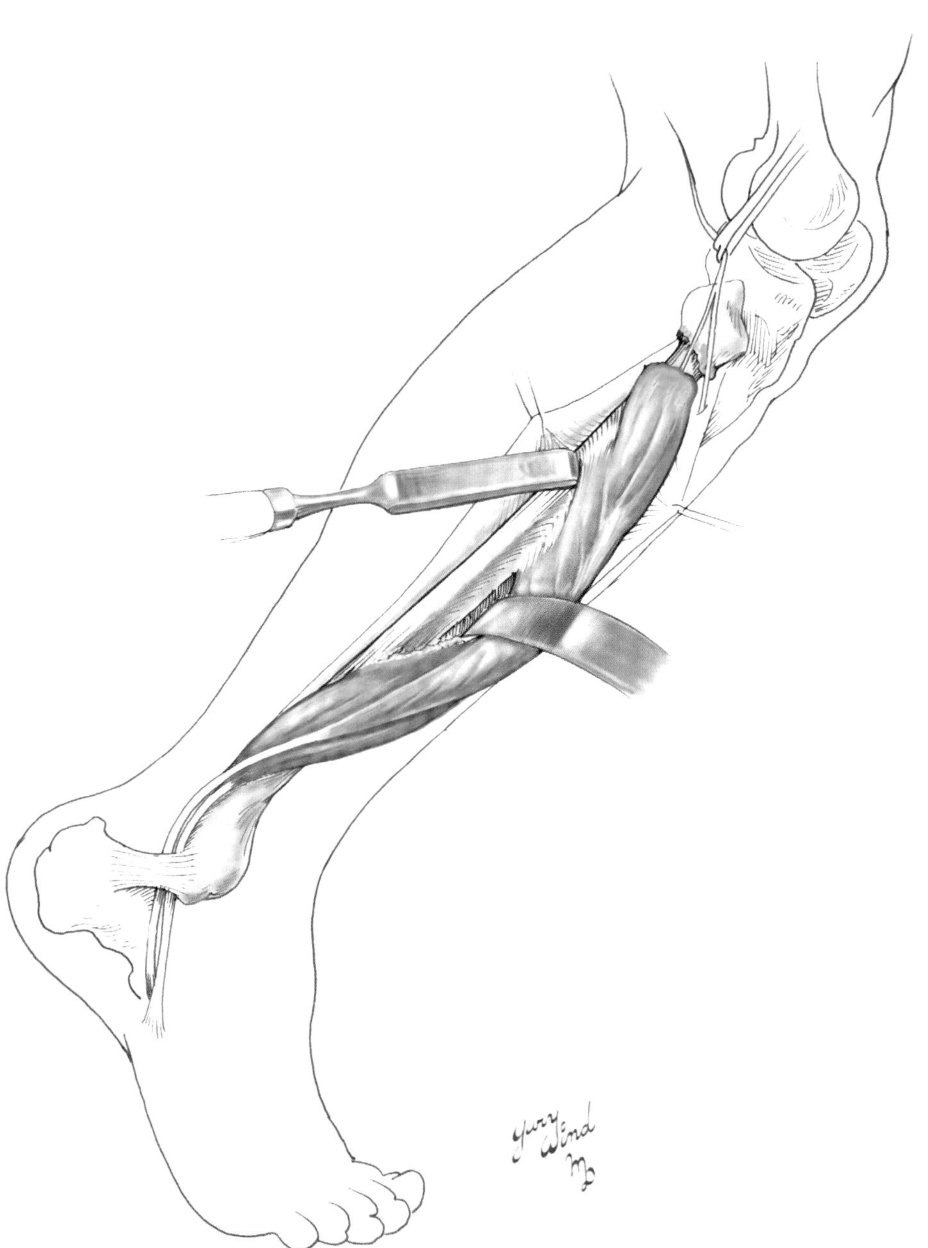

Fig. 18-18 A long flap of peroneal muscles is created by shaving the muscles off the fibula distally to proximally. The interosseous membrane strips best in the opposite direction.

Cross-Sectional Anatomy

The muscle groups are compartmentalized by septa connecting the deep fascia to the tibia and fibula and by the interosseous membrane between the two bones. At the level of the calf (Fig. 18-19), the dorsiflexors lie in the anterior compartment of the leg along with the anterior tibial artery and deep branch of the peroneal nerve. The neurovascular bundle lies on the interosseous membrane. The peroneal compartment is bounded by septa connected to the fibula, and contains the superficial peroneal nerve lying close to the bone at this level. The posterior compartment is bounded externally by the deep fascia running from the lateral peroneal septum to the tibia medially. The superficial compartment containing the gastrocnemius and soleus muscles is separated from the deep posterior compartment containing the plantar flexors by the deep septum spanning from the tibia to the fibula. The posterior tibial and peroneal vessels and the tibial nerve lie between the deep muscles and deep septum at the level of the calf. The long saphenous vein and saphenous nerve lie in the anteromedial subcutaneous tissue. The small saphenous vein lies subcutaneously in the posterior midline, soon to be joined by the sural nerve, seen here deep to the fascia between the gastrocnemius bellies.

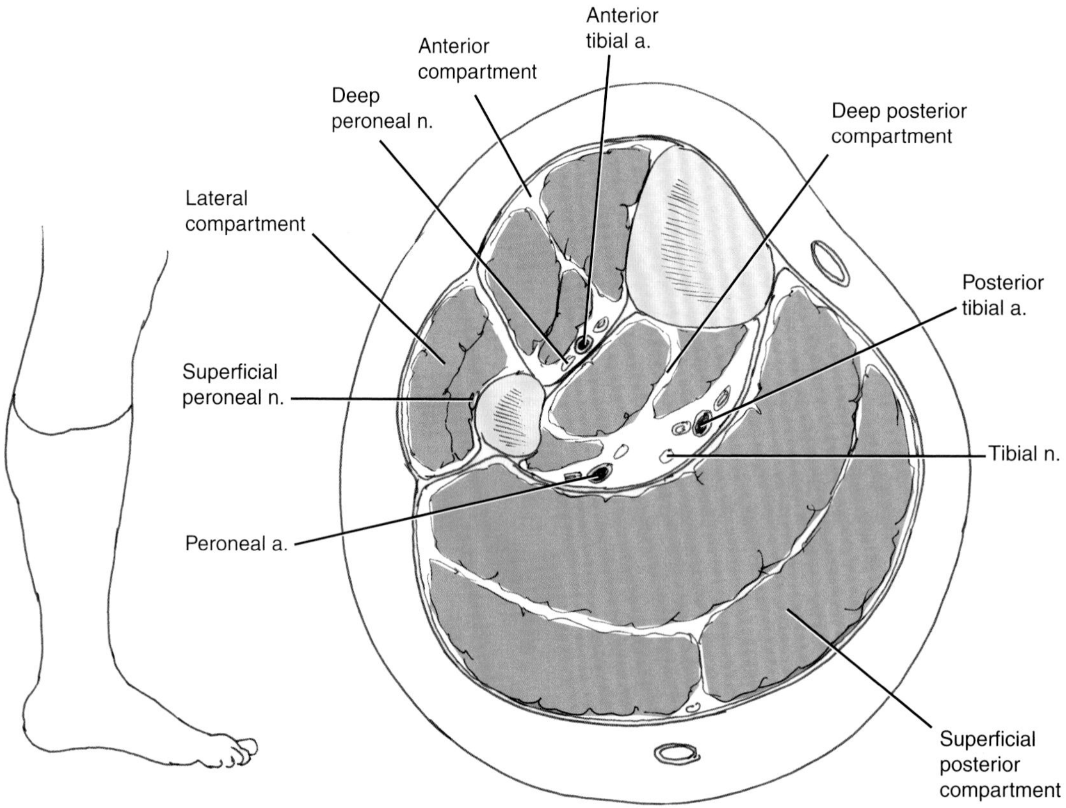

Fig. 18-19 In the midcalf, the neurovascular structures are grouped in the central portion of the leg.

In the lower leg (Fig. 18-20), the unified gastrocnemius/soleus tendon is enclosed by the deep fascia posteriorly and the deep intermuscular septum anteriorly. The narrowed span of the deep fascia over the Achilles tendon puts the medial fusion point posterior to the tibia, allowing direct access to the deep compartment directly over the plantar flexors and posterior tibial neurovascular bundle. The tibialis posterior and flexor digitorum longus muscles are mostly tendinous in the relatively larger deep posterior compartment, whereas the flexor hallucis longus muscle remains fleshy and muscular right down to the ankle. The peroneal artery, which is beginning to diminish above the distal tibiofibular syndesmosis, lies on the interosseous membrane covered by the mass of the flexor hallucis longus muscle. The peroneal tendons lie posterior to the fibula on the lateral side of the Achilles tendon. The deep peroneal nerve remains in the anterior compartment with the anterior tibial artery, whereas branches of the superficial peroneal nerve have penetrated the deep fascia of the lateral compartment to lie in the subcutaneous plane. The anterior tibial artery is moving anteriorly over the flare of the tibia.

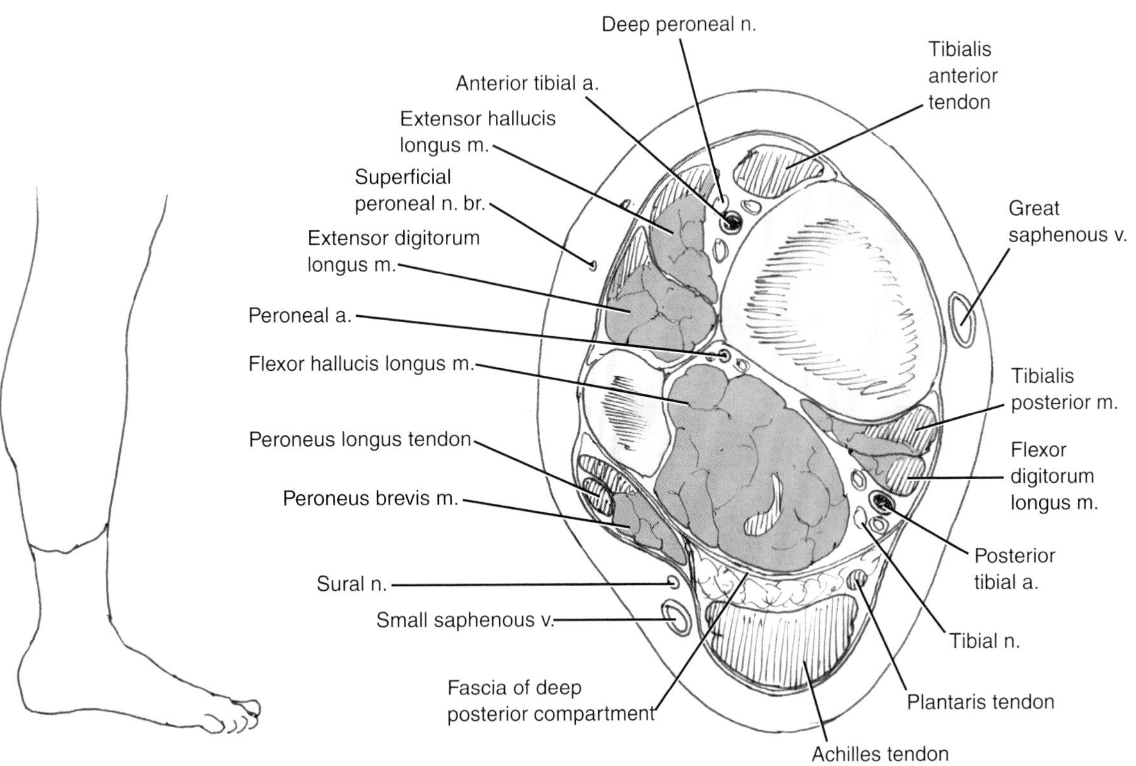

Fig. 18-20 In the distal leg, the anterior and posterior tibial neurovascular structures become more superficial.

Just above the ankle joint (Fig. 18-21), the tendon groups are tightly bound by thickened bands of deep fascia, the inferior extensor retinaculum anteriorly, the flexor retinaculum posteromedially, and the superior peroneal retinaculum posterolaterally. The tendon of the extensor hallucis longus muscle crosses over the anterior tibial neurovascular bundle, and the artery continues onto the dorsum of the foot as the dorsalis pedis artery. The peroneus longus tendon lies posterolateral to the peroneus brevis muscle as they pass behind the medial malleolus. The partially tendinous flexor hallucis longus muscle remains a posterior midline structure right down to the ankle joint. The tibial nerve lies posterior to the posterior tibial artery as the neurovascular bundle enters the foot.

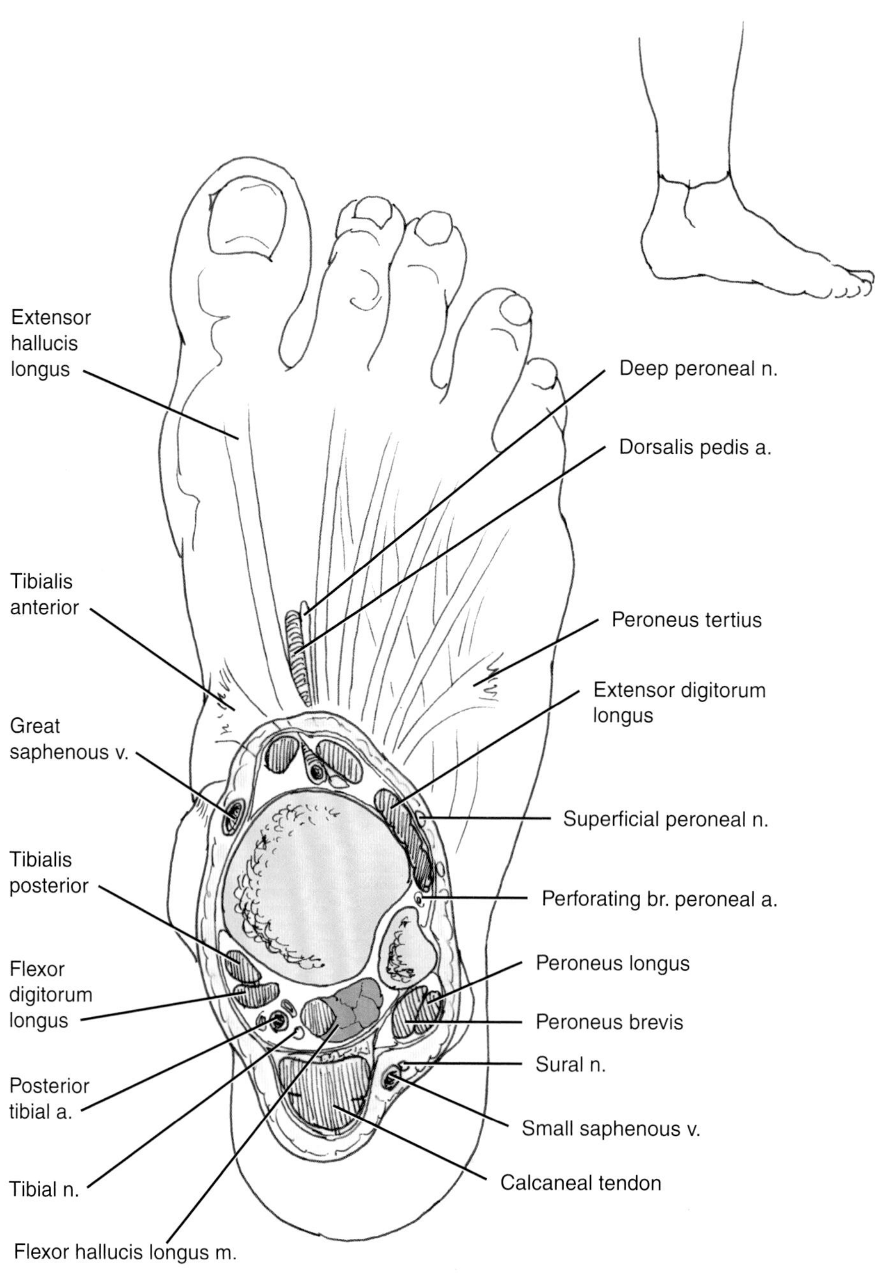

Fig. 18-21 Cross section demonstrates the anatomic relationships at the level of the ankle.

The tibial nerve joins the popliteal vessels in the midpopliteal space (Fig. 18-22) and sural neurovascular bundles splay out to the heads of the gastrocnemius muscles at the junction. Below the gastrocnemius branches, the small saphenous vein joins the popliteal vein, and the median sural nerve branch runs along the course of the vein, tightly bound to it. The continuation of the tibial nerve passes through the hiatus in the tibial attachment of the soleus muscle, along with the popliteal vessels. At the upper end of the interosseous membrane, the anterior tibial artery passes into the anterior compartment. The tibioperoneal trunk lies on the upper part of the tibialis posterior muscle and divides into the smaller peroneal artery laterally and the posterior tibial artery medially. The anterior tibial artery lies on the

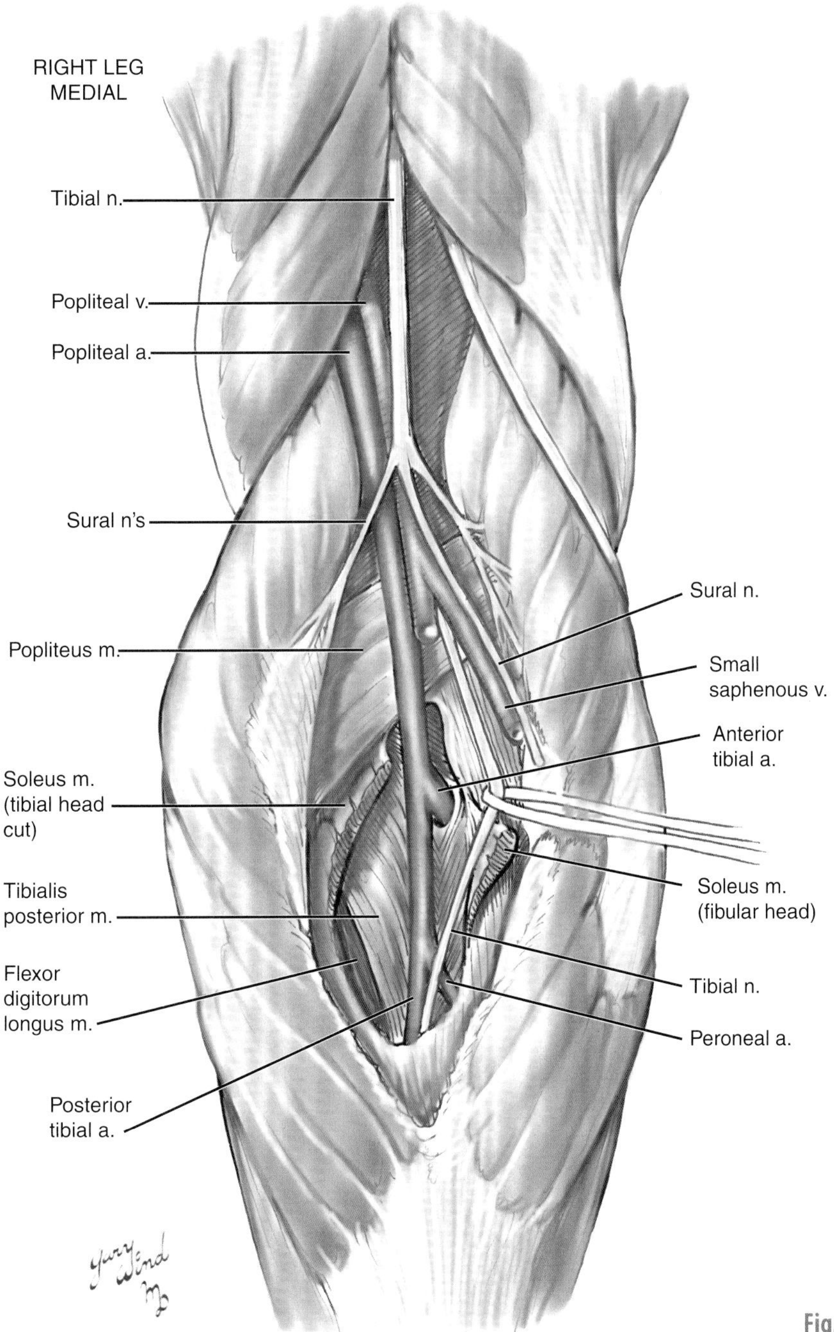

Fig. 18-22 The tibial nerve joins the popliteal vessels in the midpopliteal space.

interosseous membrane, first between tibialis anterior and extensor digitorum longus muscles and then between the tibialis anterior and extensor hallucis longus muscles that arise lower down. The posterior tibial artery lies on tibialis posterior and flexor digitorum longus muscles, medial to flexor hallucis longus muscle, down the length of the leg. The peroneal artery is progressively covered by, and sometimes within, the belly of the flexor hallucis longus muscle as that muscle expands from its low origin.

At the ankle, the anterior tibial artery and deep peroneal nerve emerge between extensor digitorum longus and extensor hallucis tendons after passing under the latter medially to laterally (Fig. 18-23).

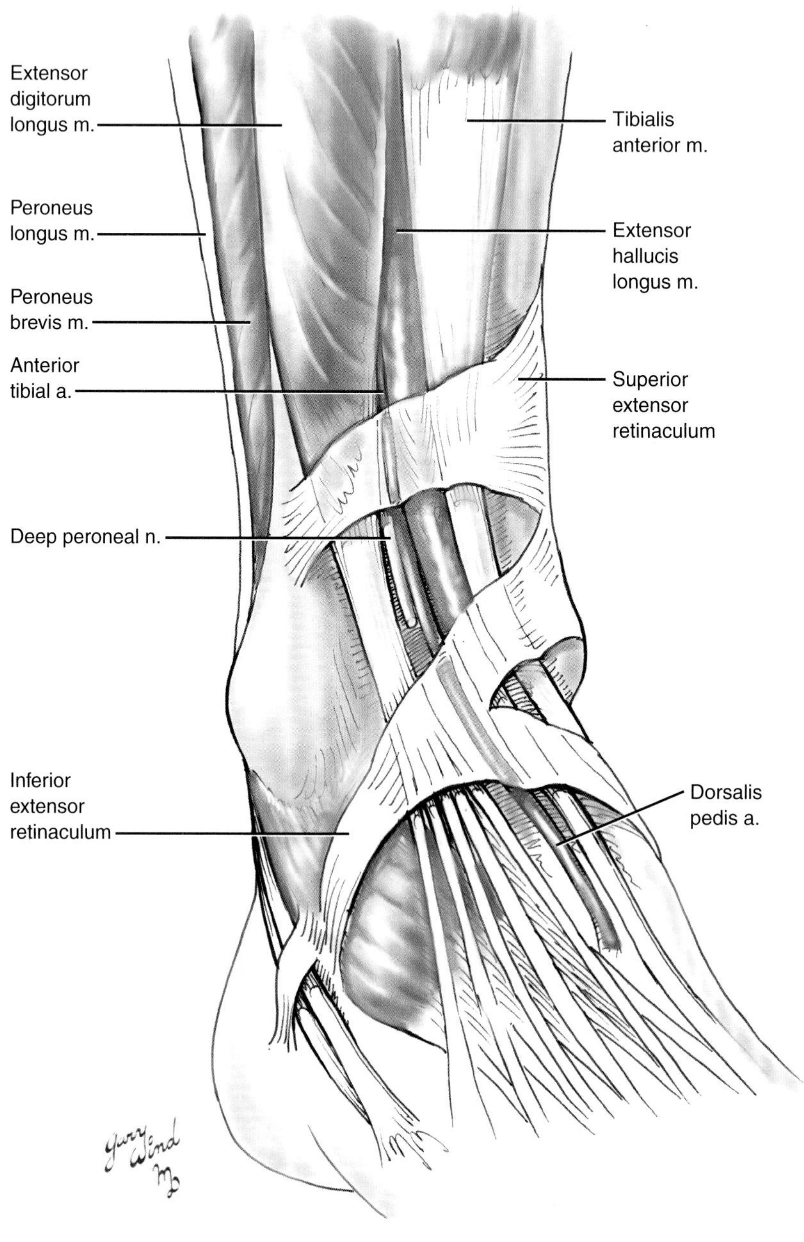

Fig. 18-23 The dorsalis pedis artery and deep peroneal nerve emerge at the ankle between the tendons of the extensor digitorum longus and extensor hallucis longus muscles.

They run along the lateral border of the extensor hallucis muscle beneath the deep fascia of the foot.

Posteromedially, the posterior tibial artery and tibial nerve lie between the flexor digitorum longus and flexor hallucis longus muscles before passing beneath the flexor retinaculum to enter the foot (Fig. 18-24). Posterolaterally, calcaneal branches of the peroneal artery pass down from beneath the lower muscular border of the flexor hallucis longus muscle.

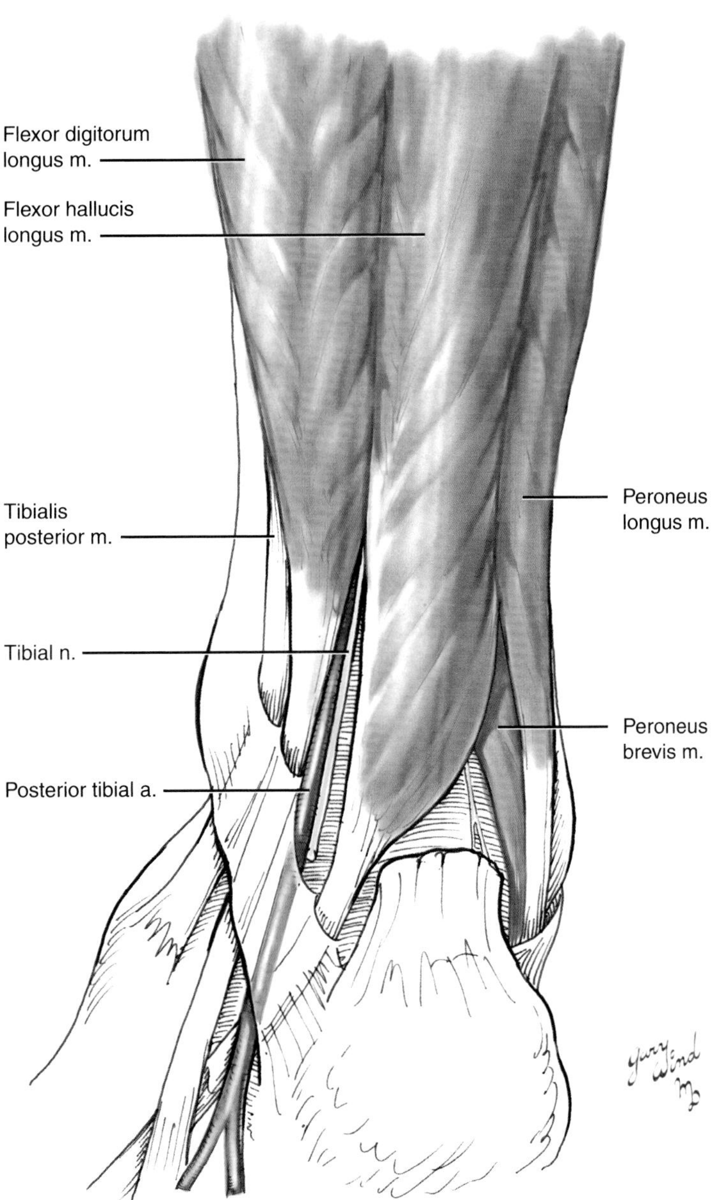

Fig. 18-24 The posterior tibial artery and tibial nerve lie posterior to the medial malleolus in a groove between the flexor digitorum longus and flexor hallucis longus tendons.

With the flexor hallucis longus muscle partially cut away, the course of the peroneal artery can be seen lying on the interosseous membrane just medial to the fibula (Fig. 18-25).

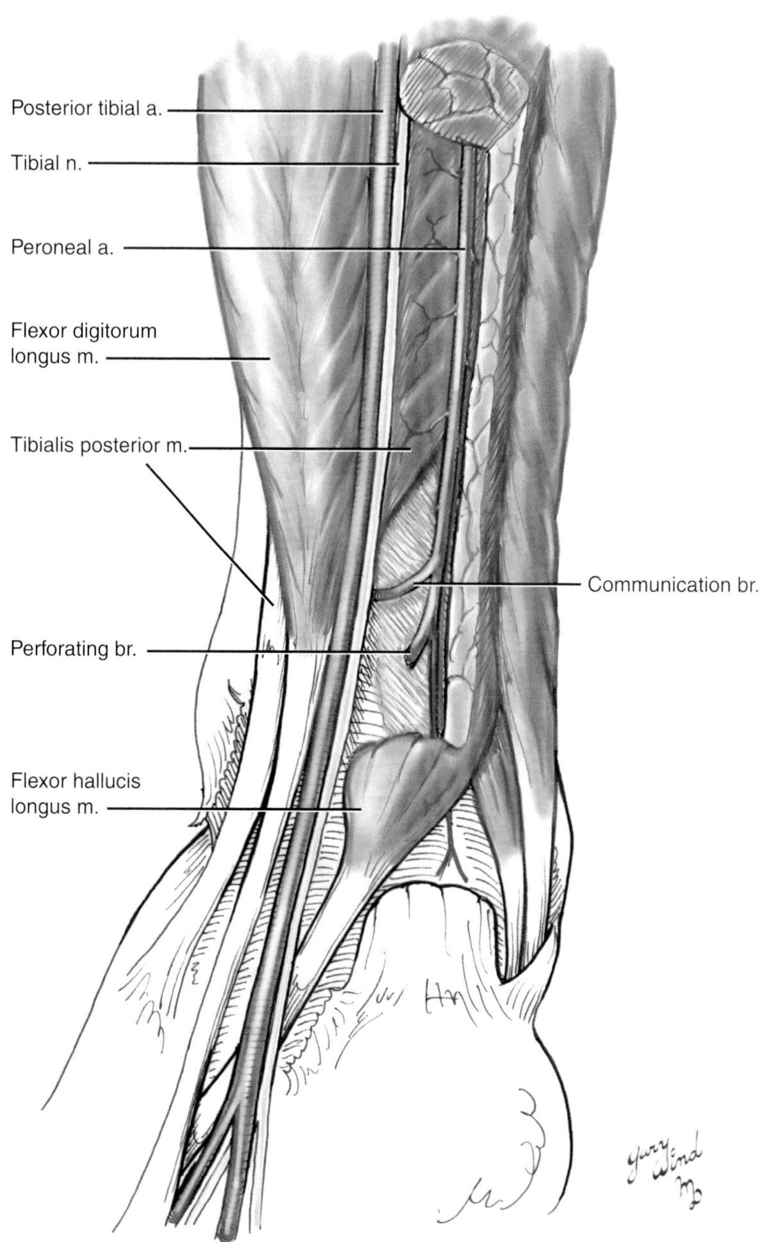

Fig. 18-25 The peroneal artery lies on the interosseous membrane on the medial side of the fibula.

Vessels of the Foot

Two of the leg vessels, the anterior and posterior tibial arteries, enter the foot and form a major anastomotic loop between dorsal and plantar aspects[4] (Fig. 18-26). The anterior tibial artery becomes the dorsalis pedis artery, which runs medial to the extensor hallucis longus tendon down to the proximal space between the first and second metatarsals. There it sends a deep plantar continuation between the heads of the first dorsal interosseous muscle. After passing beneath the flexor retinaculum, the posterior tibial artery divides into a larger lateral plantar artery and a smaller medial plantar branch. The lateral plantar artery bows laterally, crosses beneath the proximal metatarsals, and joins the plantar branch of the dorsalis pedis artery. The anterior tibial artery gives off medial and lateral anterior malleolar branches that anastomose with corresponding branches of the peroneal and posterior tibial arteries. In the midfoot, the dorsalis pedis artery gives off a lateral tarsal artery that anastomoses with branches of the anterior lateral malleolar artery and the more distal arcuate branch of the dorsalis pedis artery, as well as with the lateral plantar artery. Small medial tarsal branches anastomose with the anterior medial malleolar and medial plantar arteries. Calcaneal branches arise from the terminus of the peroneal

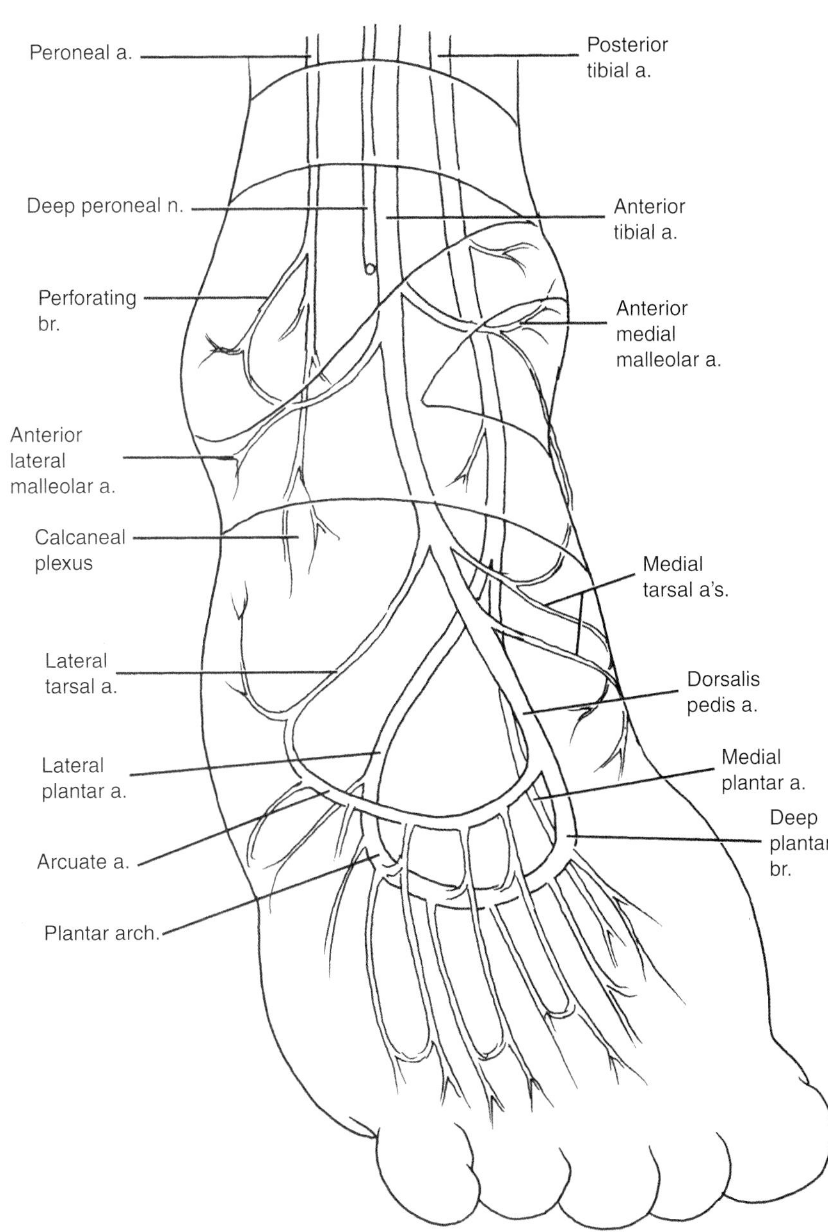

Fig. 18-26 The two arteries of the foot form a major anastomotic loop with interconnecting branches.

artery and the posterior tibial artery and anastomose with plantar branches in the hindfoot as well as with the malleolar plexuses. The peroneal artery sends a perforating branch through the distal interosseous membrane. This branch anastomoses with the anterior lateral malleolar artery and occasionally is the origin of the dorsalis pedis artery in the absence of a dominant anterior tibial artery (see Chapter 19). There is a communicating branch between peroneal and posterior tibial arteries above the ankle. Digital vessels originate from the arcuate artery and plantar arterial arch, the latter being dominant. There are communicating branches between vessels of the two arches, passing between the metatarsals proximally and distally.

The relationships of the vessels of the foot to the bones of the foot are shown in Fig. 18-27. The dominance of the inflow to the plantar arterial arch varies somewhat as do the origins of dorsal and plantar digital vessels.

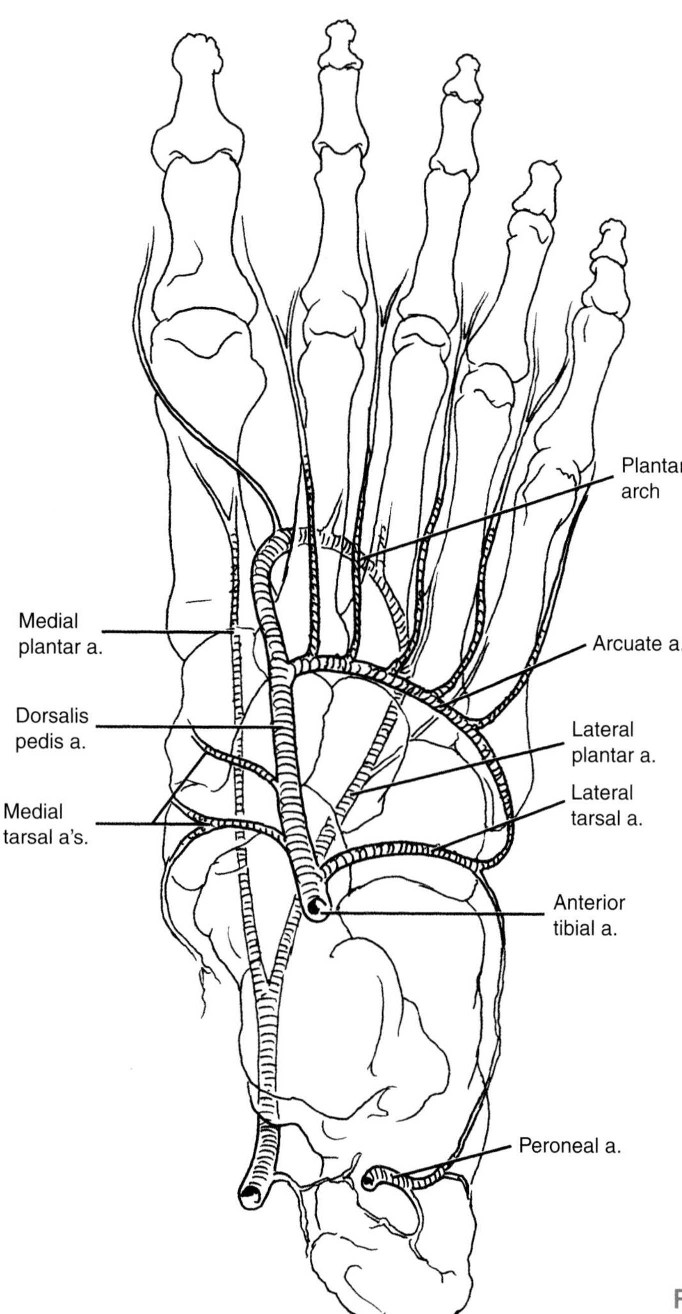

Fig. 18-27 The relationships between the arteries and bones of the foot are shown.

The arteries on the dorsum of the foot lie deep to the long extrinsic and short intrinsic extensor tendons of the toes (Fig. 18-28). The deep peroneal nerve accompanying the dorsalis pedis artery supplies sensation to the web space between the great and second toes. Loss of sensation at this location may be the first indication of increased pressure within the anterior compartment where the proximal portion of this nerve lies. The superficial peroneal nerve branches supply most of the dorsum of the foot, the sural nerve supplies the lateral border of the foot, and the saphenous nerve (the only nerve not of sciatic origin below the knee) supplies the medial ankle and foot. The latter two nerves are bound to the small and great saphenous veins, respectively, and care should be taken to avoid injuring the nerves when harvesting or mobilizing the veins.

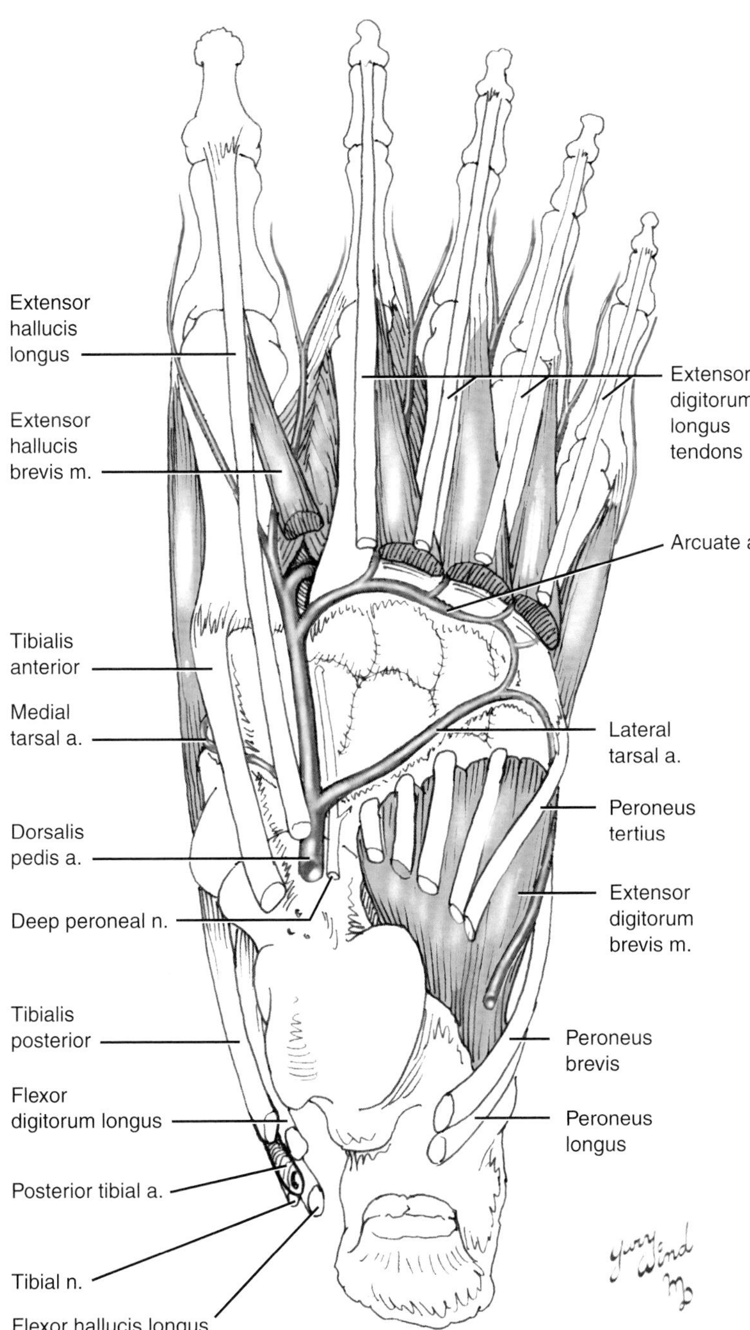

Fig. 18-28 The dorsal foot arteries lie deep to the extensor tendons of the toes.

Plantar Vessels

The posterior tibial neurovascular bundle, consisting of the posterior tibial artery, tibial nerve, and accompanying veins, passes through the tarsal tunnel beneath the flexor retinaculum to enter the foot (Fig. 18-29). The bundle emerges between the flexor digitorum longus and flexor hallucis longus muscles and passes beneath the retinaculum between these two tendons. At the lower end of the retinaculum, the bundle lies posterior to the anterior deflection of the hallucis tendon. The artery and nerve split at the lower border of the retinaculum, just at the upper border of the abductor hallucis muscle. The medial plantar branch passes anteriorly and superficially to the flexor hallucis longus muscle, crossing diagonally and superficially to the flexor digitorum longus tendons. The lateral plantar bows toward the lateral side of the foot before crossing back to the first metatarsal interspace to anastomose with the plantar branch of the dorsalis pedis artery.

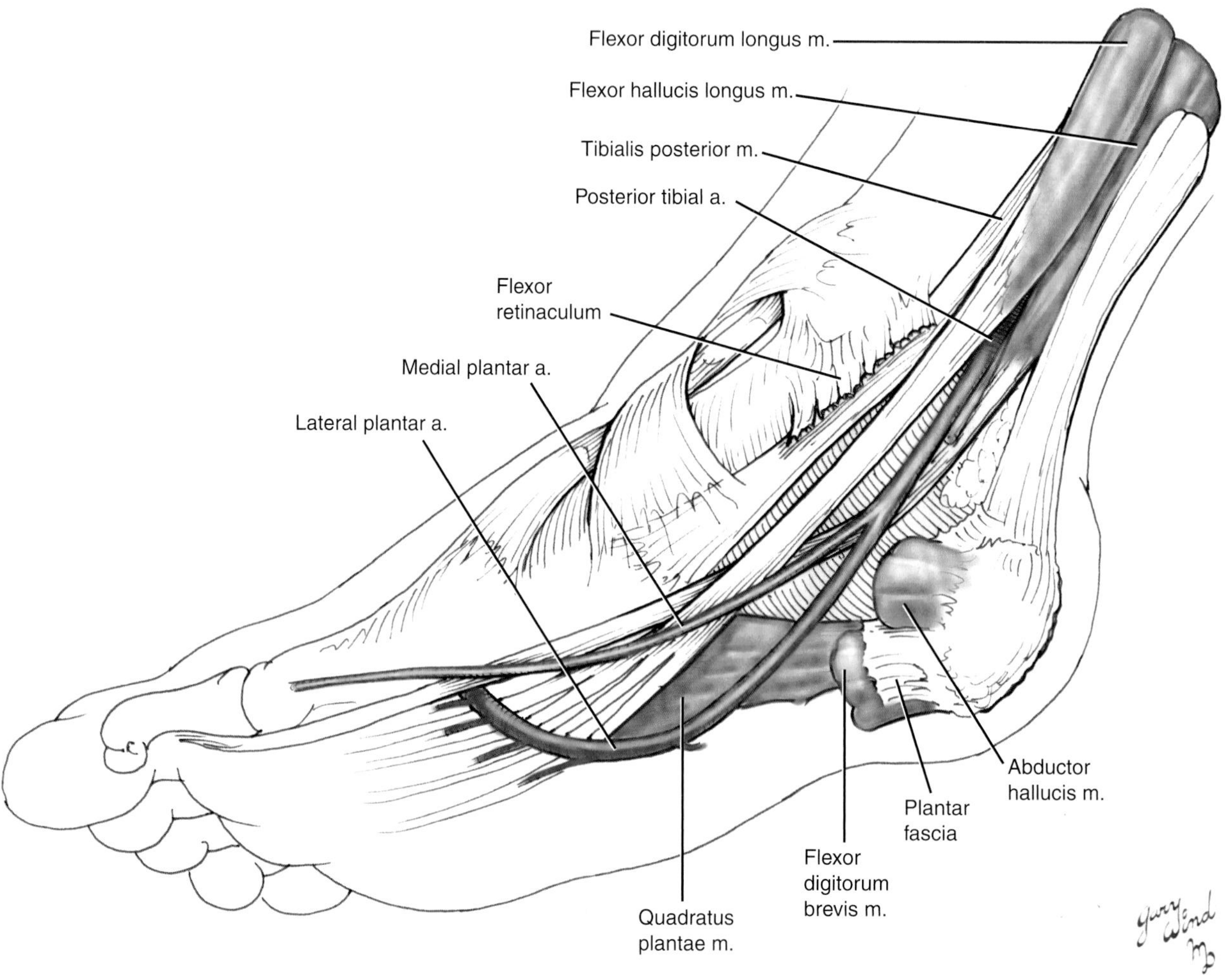

Fig. 18-29 The lateral plantar artery courses deep to the flexor digitorum brevis muscle and pierces the first metatarsal interspace to anastomose with the deep plantar branch of the dorsalis pedis.

With the Achilles tendon removed, the relationships of the posterior tibial neurovascular bundle can be seen (Fig. 18-30). As the Achilles tendon narrows, the attachment of the posterior investing fascia moves posteriorly and fuses with the fascia of the deep posterior compartment rather than extending all the way to the tibia. Thus, the deep posterior compartment fascia can be incised directly behind the medial malleolus to gain access to the posterior tibial artery. The thickened continuation of the deep fascia is the flexor retinaculum. The plantar branches turn beneath the foot deep to the abductor hallucis muscle and run in the plane between the flexor hallucis longus and flexor digitorum longus tendons and the flexor digitorum brevis muscle.

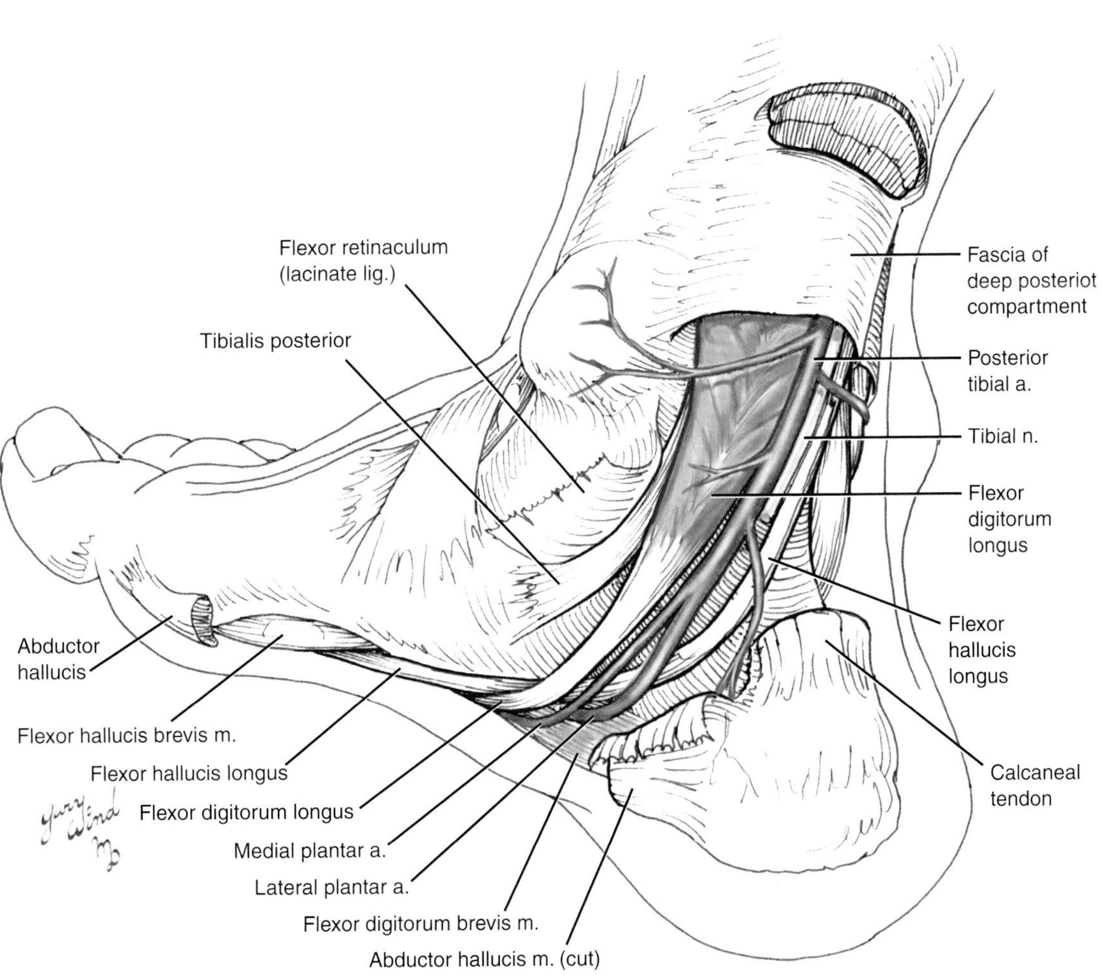

Fig. 18-30 The posterior tibial artery and tibial nerve are located just beneath the deep posterior compartment fascia as they curve posterior to the medial malleolus.

There are three layers of plantar muscles (Fig. 18-31). The deep layer consists of the flexor hallucis brevis, adductor hallucis, and flexor digiti minimi brevis muscles. The flexor hallucis brevis muscle lies between the first metatarsal and the flexor hallucis longus tendon. The adductor hallucis muscle has an oblique head and a transverse head. The second layer consists of the long flexor tendons (the hallucis and digitorum longus muscles and the lumbrical muscles and quadratus plantae of the latter). These tendons maintain the longitudinal arch of the foot. The most superficial layer consists of the abductor hallucis, central flexor digitorum brevis, and abductor digiti minimi muscles. These three muscles are covered on their plantar surface by the plantar fascia, which is thick centrally and thins to the sides. The deep plantar neurovascular structures are the critical elements for the integrity of the forefoot. After the split, the medial and lateral plantar vessels and nerves at first lie in the plane between the superficial muscles and the second group, the long flexors. The plantar arch, as it recurves medially, passes deep to the oblique head of the adductor hallucis muscle, and deep to the lateral part of the flexor hallucis brevis muscle on its course to join with the plantar branch of the dorsalis pedis artery.

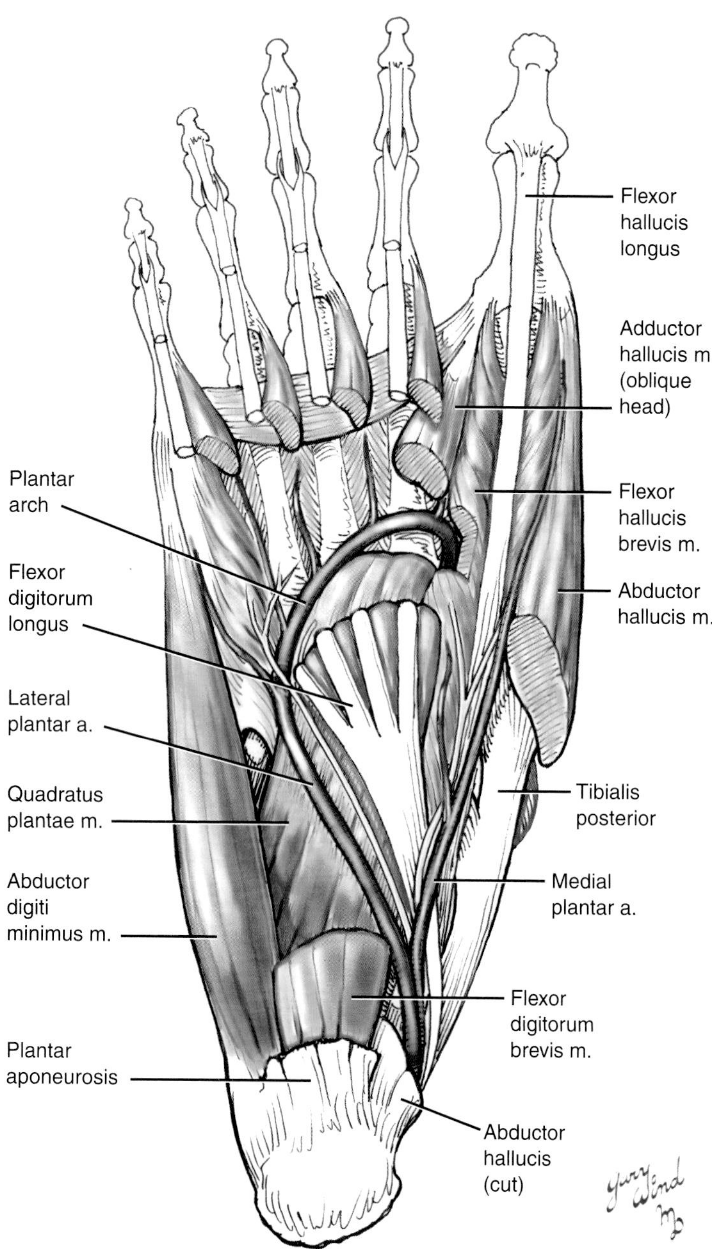

Fig. 18-31 A plantar view demonstrates the relationship of the plantar arch to the three layers of plantar muscles.

Exposure of the Arteries of the Leg

The durability of vein bypasses to infrageniculate arteries has been firmly established. Excellent patency rates can be achieved using a number of autogenous graft alternatives, including in situ great saphenous vein, reversed great saphenous vein, transposed great saphenous vein, spliced small saphenous vein, arm vein, and composite vein from different sources.[5] All three infrageniculate arteries have been shown to be suitable recipient vessels for bypass, provided that there is suitable outflow to the foot.[5–9] The following sections consider exposure of the infrapopliteal arteries at several levels, giving the surgeon access to a suitable vessel in patients with almost any distal occlusive pattern.

Exposure of the Posterior Tibial Artery

The posterior tibial artery is easily accessible through medial leg incisions. Access is particularly convenient when performing a saphenous vein bypass because the posterior tibial artery can be exposed through the same medial skin incision used for vein harvest (Fig. 18-32). The following discussion considers exposure of the posterior tibial artery at the proximal and midleg levels. Exposure of the posterior tibial artery at the ankle is considered in the section dealing with arteries of the foot and ankle.

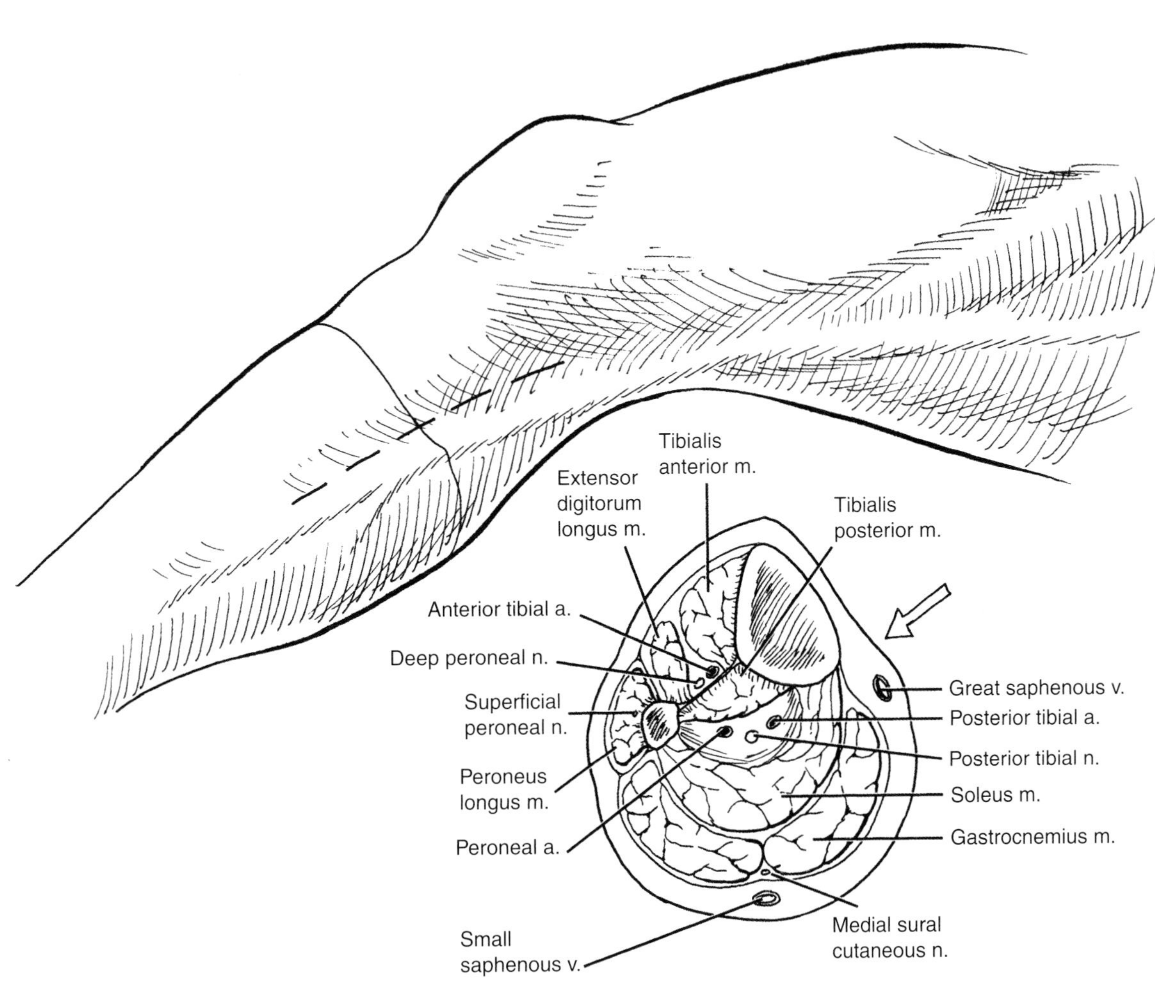

Fig. 18-32 Medial approaches to the posterior tibial artery also provide access to the great saphenous vein when performing an in situ bypass.

Exposure of the Posterior Tibial Artery in the Proximal Leg

This approach provides access to the posterior tibial artery at its most proximal point, the segment just distal to the bifurcation of the tibioperoneal trunk. Bypasses may be brought here preferentially in cases of popliteal artery obstruction, when the proximal posterior tibial artery is patent. This technique is an extension of that used to expose the infrageniculate popliteal artery through a medial incision (see Chapter 17). The patient is placed in the supine position with the leg externally rotated and flexed 60° at the knee. A supporting roll should be placed laterally to hold the knee in position. The entire leg, groin, and foot are prepped and draped. An incision is made 2 cm behind the posterior border of the tibia just below the knee joint and extended distally for 10 to 15 cm. The incision is deepened through subcutaneous tissue, taking care to avoid injury to the saphenous vein that may course through this area (see Chapter 17). The deep fascia is then incised, exposing the underlying fibers of the medial head of the gastrocnemius muscle (Fig. 18-33). Posterior retraction of the gastrocnemius muscle exposes the distal popliteal vessels that penetrate the origin of the soleus muscle. The fibers of the soleus muscle originating on the tibia should be sharply divided to expose the underlying vessels running distally in the leg.

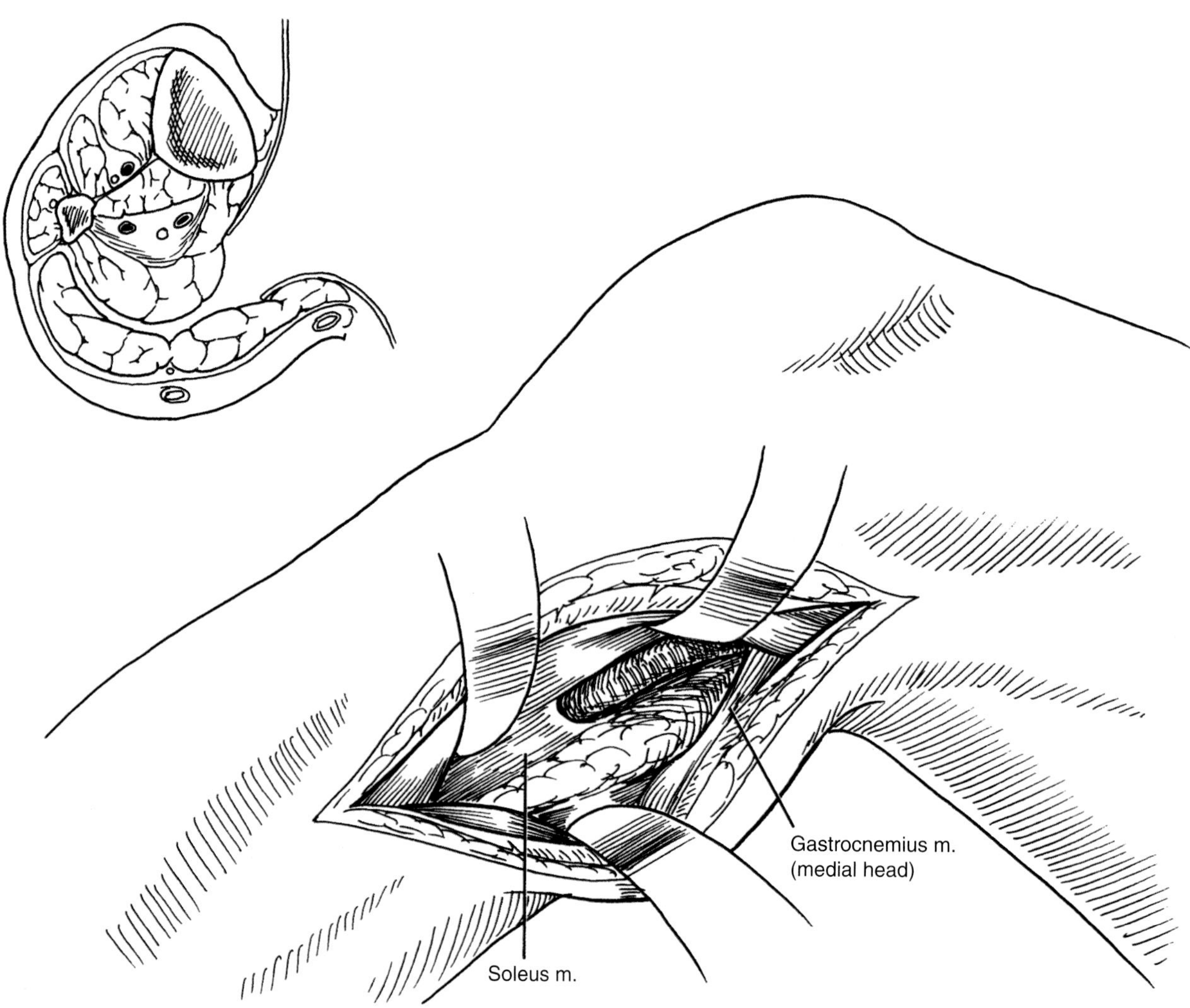

Fig. 18-33 The approach to the proximal posterior tibial artery first requires separation of the gastrocnemius and soleus muscles to expose the distal popliteal artery penetrating the origin of the soleus.

Division over a right-angle clamp placed between the vessels and muscle fibers is invaluable in preventing vessel injury (Fig. 18-34). Immediately beneath the proximal soleus lie the origins of the anterior tibial artery and tibioperoneal trunk. The accompanying veins are paired and sometimes multiple; a complex interconnecting network of venous branches overlies the arteries and must be carefully divided during arterial dissection.

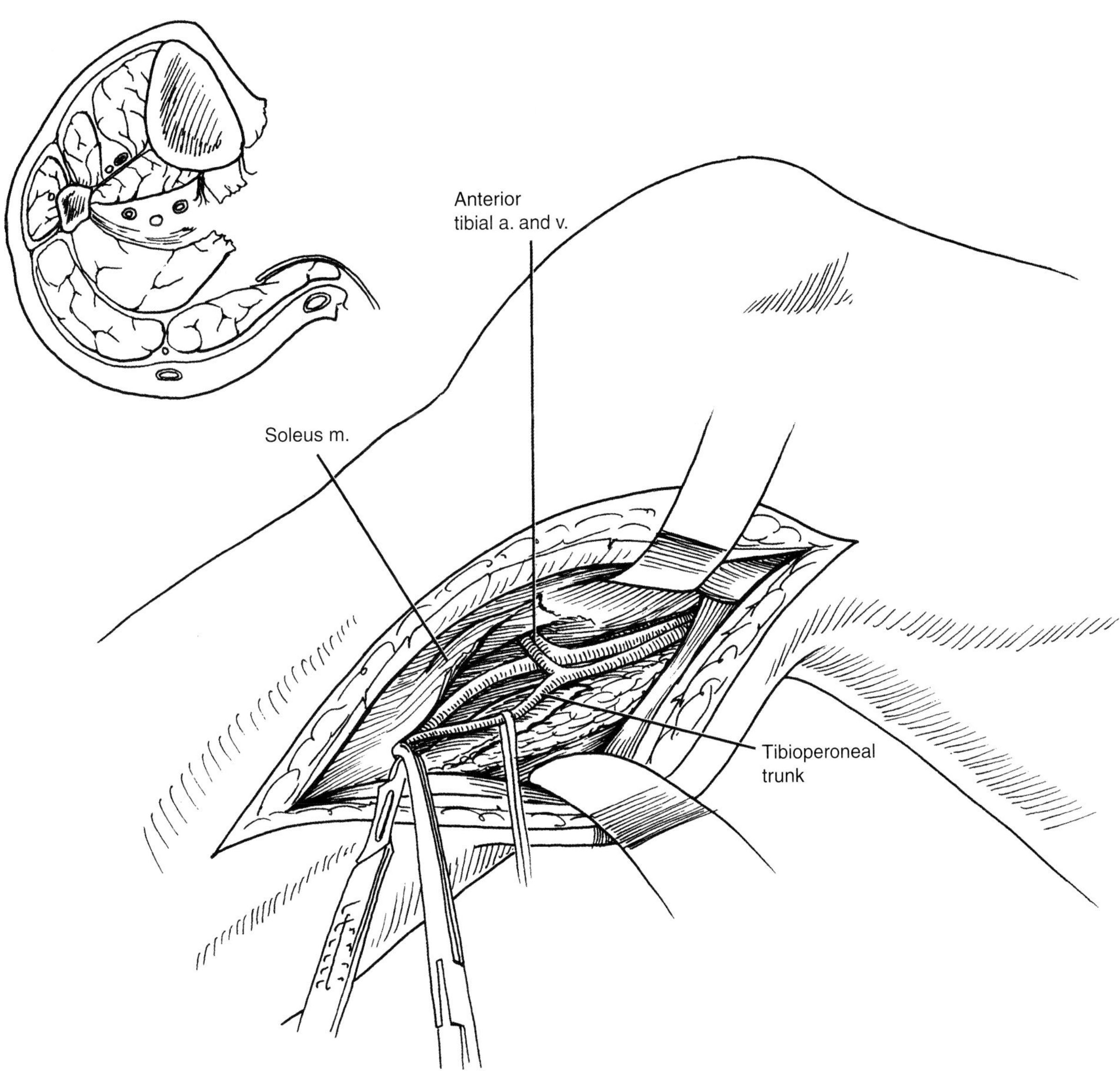

Fig. 18-34 Division of the tibial origin of the soleus exposes the underlying proximal leg vessels.

The tibioperoneal trunk bifurcates approximately 2.5 cm beyond the anterior tibial artery, although this is variable.[1,2] The proximal segment of the posterior tibial artery may be isolated and prepared for bypass at any point distal to the bifurcation (Fig. 18-35).

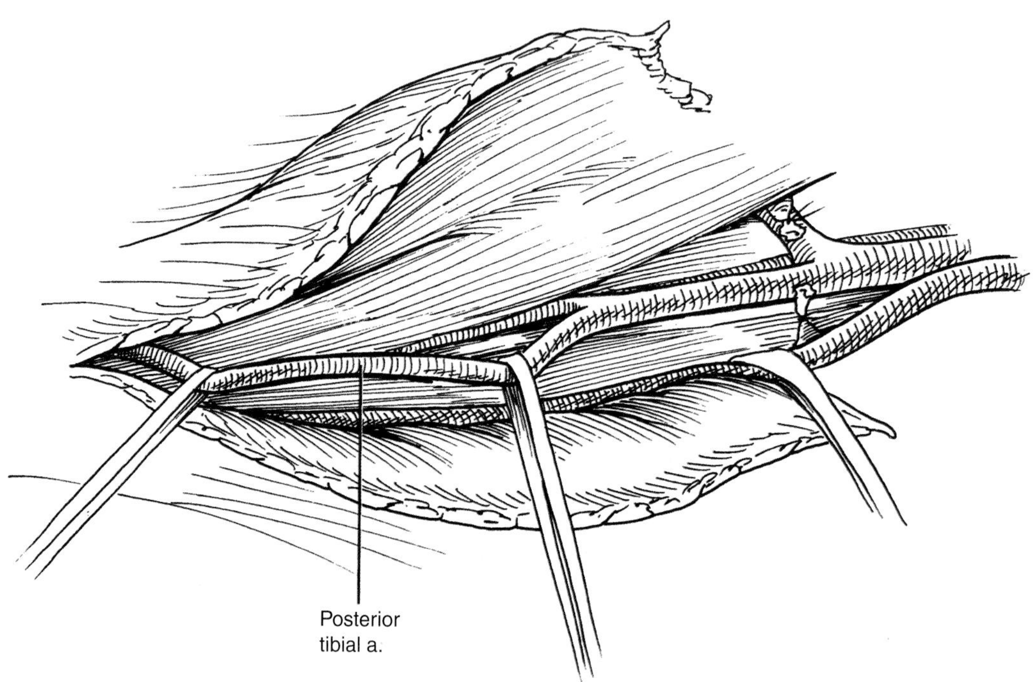

Fig. 18-35 Careful dissection and judicious ligation of surrounding veins allow exposure and isolation of the posterior tibial artery.

Exposure of the Posterior Tibial Artery in the Midleg

The patient is positioned and surgically prepared as above. A medial incision is made 2 cm behind the posterior margin of the tibia and extended for approximately 10 cm (Fig. 18-36). After the incision is deepened through the subcutaneous tissue and crural fascia, the tibial attachments of the soleus muscle are divided.

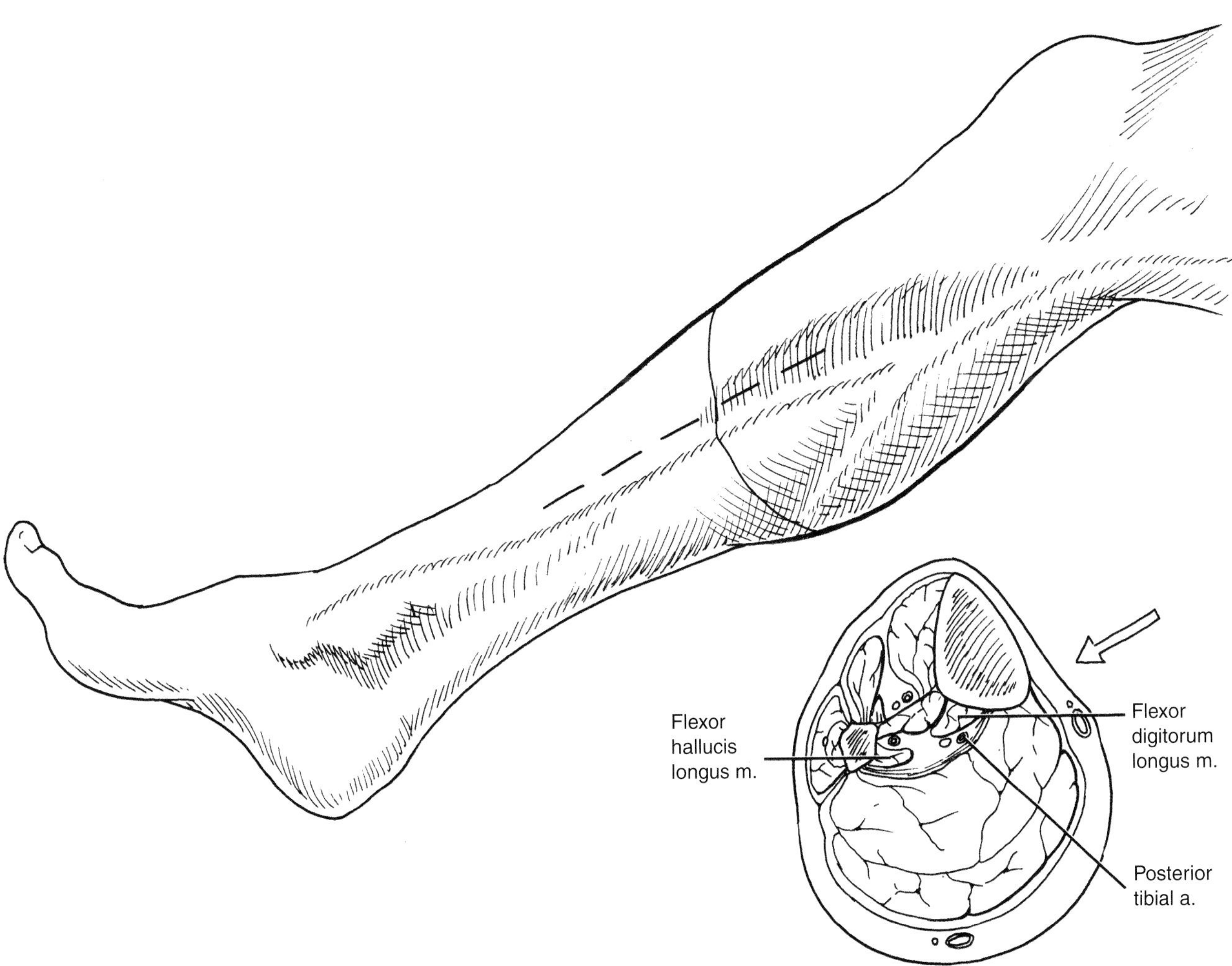

Fig. 18-36 The incision for approaching the posterior tibial artery in the midleg is illustrated.

The soleus muscle is retracted posteriorly, and a plane is developed between the flexor digitorum longus and soleus muscles (Fig. 18-37). The posterior tibial vessels are bound in loose areolar tissue on the posterior surface of the tibialis posterior muscle. The artery is often surrounded by a plexus of vein branches connecting the main venous trunks; several vein branches may require division and ligation to expose an adequate length of the artery for bypass.

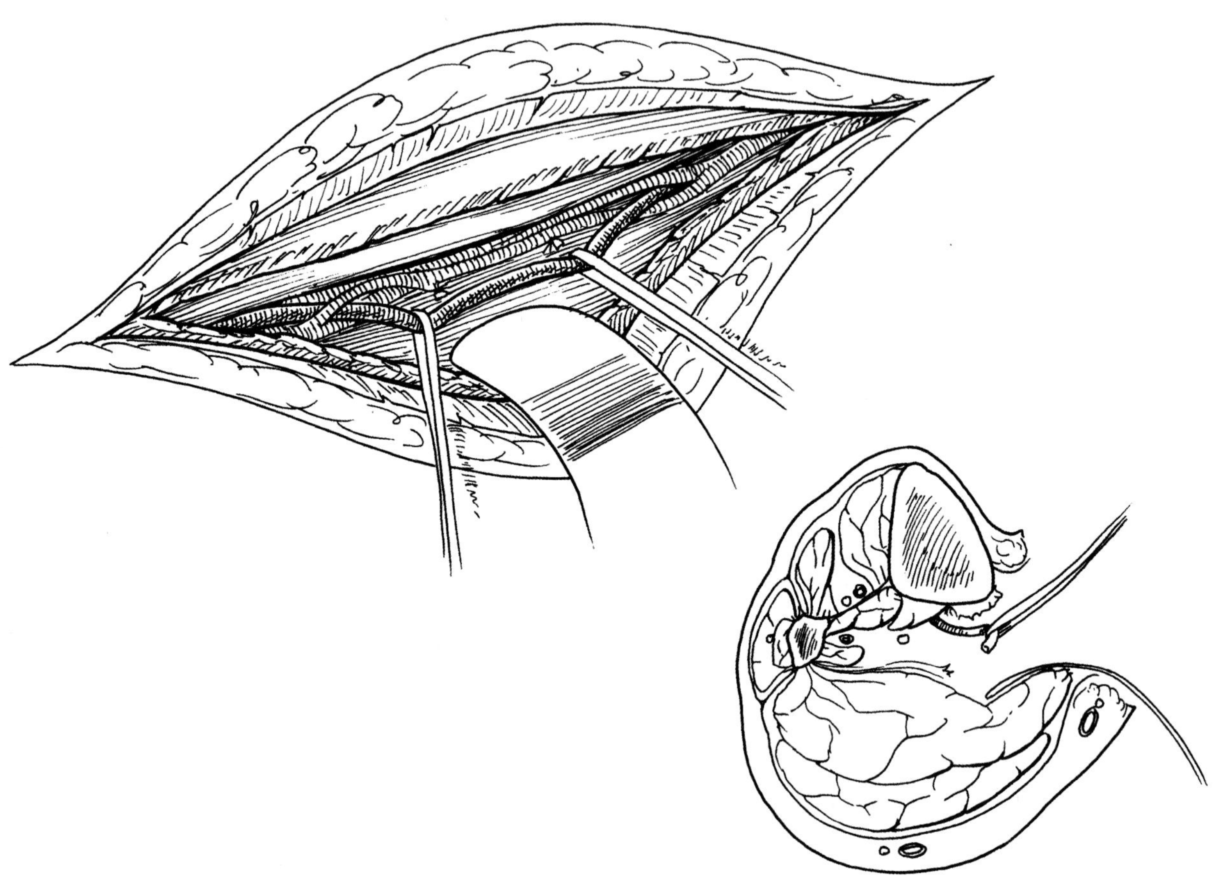

Fig. 18-37 The posterior tibial artery is found on the surface of the flexor digitorum longus muscle beneath the thin fascia enclosing the deep posterior compartment. The extensive mobilization shown in the cross section for purposes of illustration would not be done clinically to preserve important collateral branches.

Exposure of the Posterior Tibial Artery Using a Posterior Approach

Occlusive disease may occasionally be confined to the tibial arteries, with preservation of adequate inflow at the popliteal level. In these select circumstances, popliteal–crural bypass may be desirable, especially if the great saphenous vein can be preserved. Ouriel[10] popularized the posterior approach to the crural vessels, noting that this approach preserves the great saphenous vein and minimizes the required length of the arterial conduit. The approach may also minimize wound-healing problems associated with medial incisions. If one plans to use the small saphenous vein as a conduit, it is important to document the adequacy of the vein during the preoperative period. Patients without adequate small saphenous veins may require preliminary harvest of the great saphenous vein. This is more easily accomplished with the patient in the supine position, before being turned prone.

Posterior exposure requires that the patient be positioned prone, with the knee in full extension. The leg and thigh should be prepped circumferentially and draped to the level of the buttock. A vertical incision is made directly over the small saphenous vein. The vein begins posterior to the lateral malleolus, courses lateral to the calcaneus tendon, and ascends medially toward the midline of the popliteal fossa. It runs on the surface of the crural fascia in the calf and ankle before penetrating through the deep fascia near the popliteal fossa to join the popliteal vein. The incision should be carried to the level of the popliteal fossa, but the distal extent can vary according to the length of vein needed (Fig. 18-38).

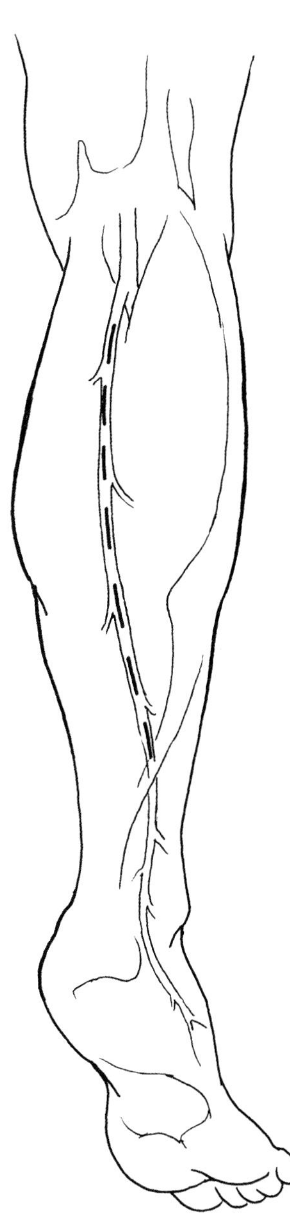

Fig. 18-38 The incision for posterior exposure of the posterior tibial artery should be made directly over the small saphenous vein.

The distal segment of the popliteal artery is exposed first. The proximal incision should be deepened through the crural fascia to expose the popliteal artery between the two heads of the gastrocnemius muscle. The tibial nerve is the most superficial major midline structure and should be reflected laterally to expose the underlying artery and vein. The artery lies medially in the neurovascular sheath and slightly deep to the vein (see Chapter 17). The crural arteries are located by following the popliteal artery to its terminus.[10] Exposure can be enhanced by dividing the fusion seam of the gastrocnemius muscle bellies and incising the tibial insertion of the soleus muscle (Fig. 18-39). The muscular branches of the tibial nerve and associated crossing veins should be carefully avoided during this dissection.[10]

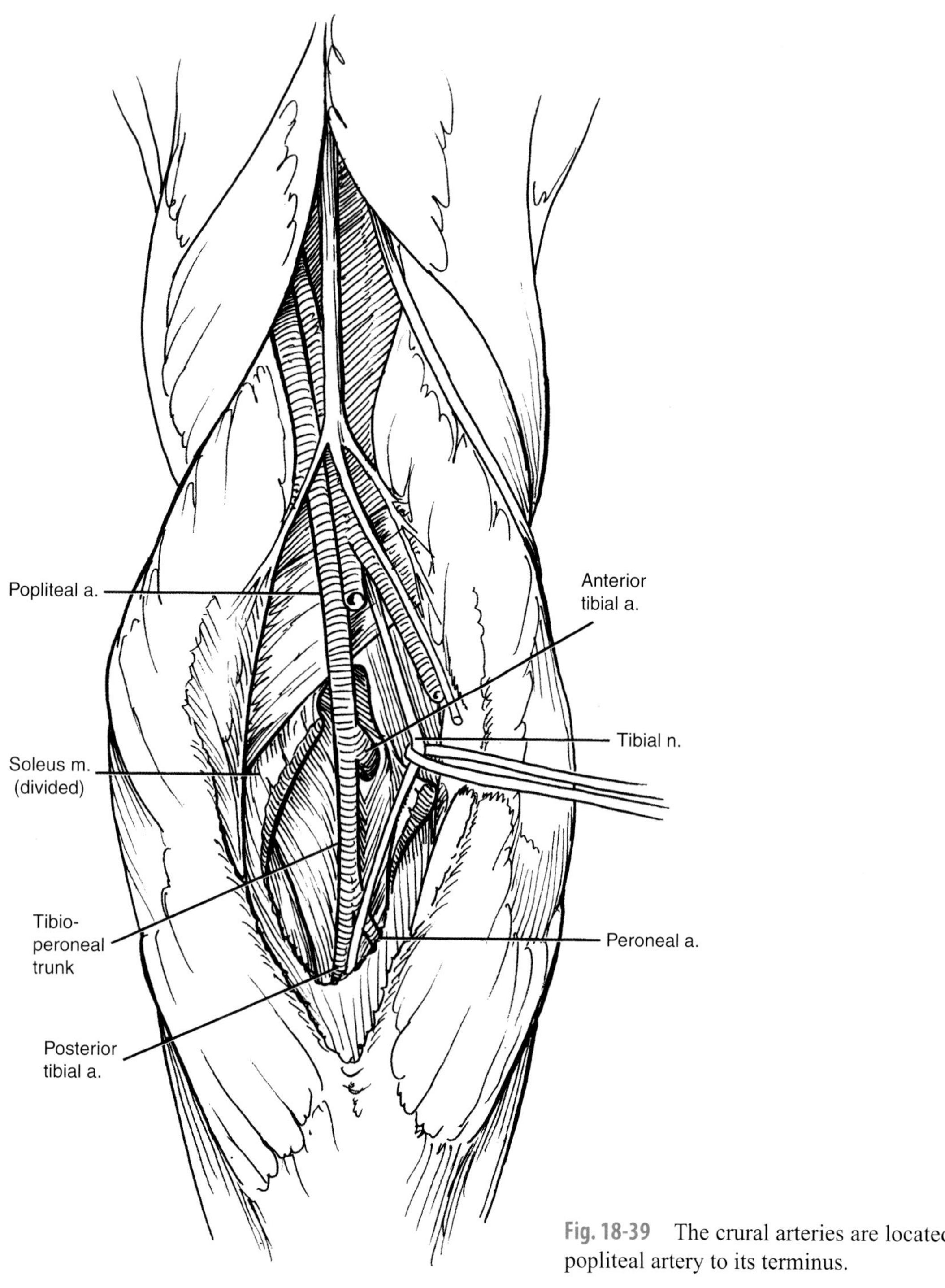

Fig. 18-39 The crural arteries are located by following the popliteal artery to its terminus.

The posterior tibial artery is exposed in the distal third of the calf through a separate vertical incision created medial to the calcaneus tendon (Fig. 18-40). The neurovascular bundle is exposed by incising the crural fascia and a fascial layer separating the deep and superficial posterior muscle compartments at this level. The posterior tibial artery can be located on the medial side of the flexor digitorum longus muscle, just anterior to the tibial nerve.

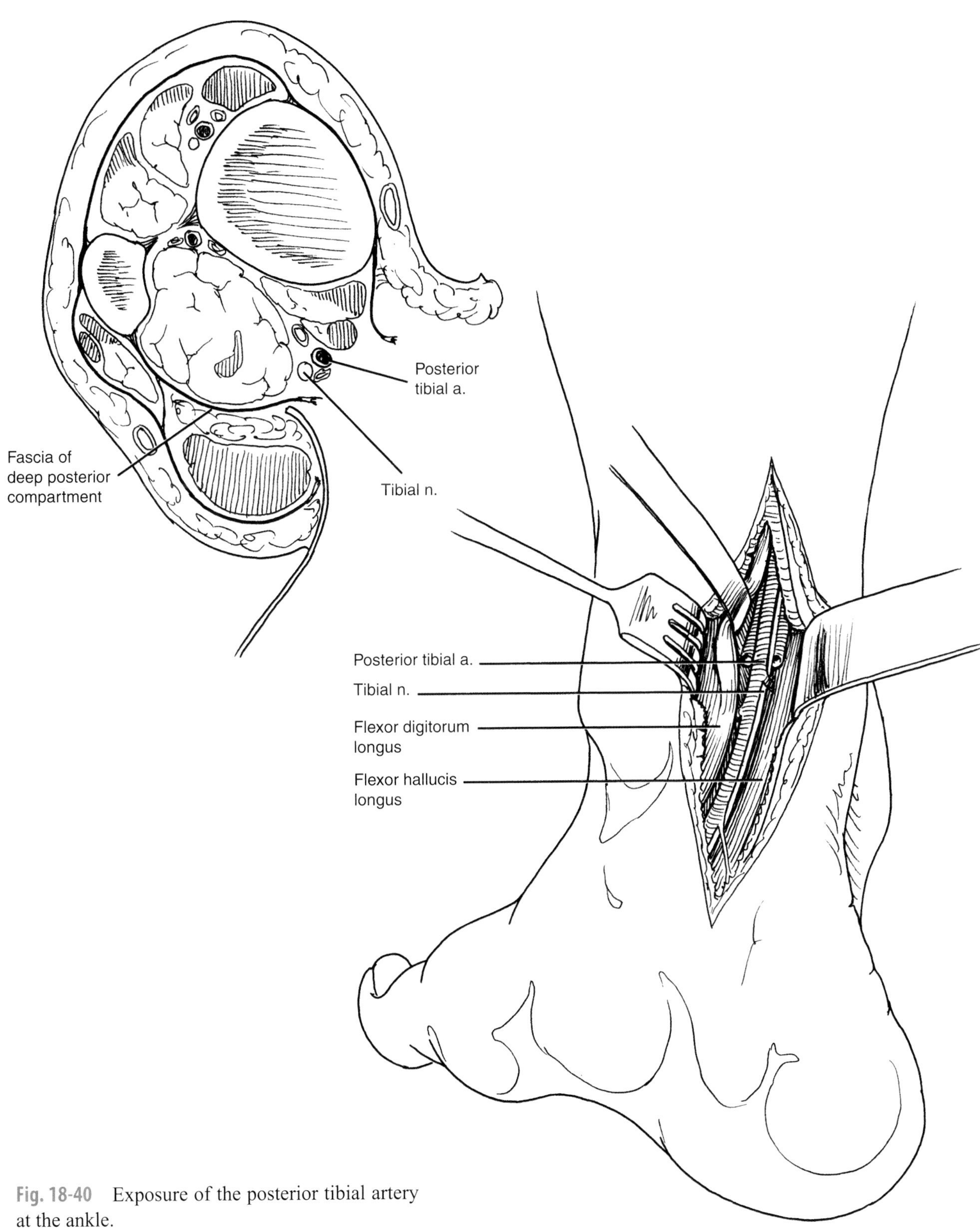

Fig. 18-40 Exposure of the posterior tibial artery at the ankle.

Exposure of the Anterior Tibial Artery

The major portion of the anterior tibial artery courses in the anterior compartment of the leg and is most easily accessible through anterolateral leg incisions. The anterior tibial artery can be isolated at its origin through a medial incision (see above), but constructing bypasses to this section of the artery is awkward and inconvenient compared with other available options. The following discussion considers exposure of the artery in the midleg, distal leg, and foot.

Exposure of the Anterior Tibial Artery in the Midleg

The patient is placed in the supine position with the leg internally rotated and the knee flexed 30°. After surgical preparation of the entire leg and groin, a vertical incision is made in the anterolateral leg midway between the tibia and fibula (Fig. 18-41). The crural fascia is incised along the lateral border of the tibialis anterior muscle. Development of a plane between the tibialis anterior and extensor digitorum longus muscles allows access to the neurovascular bundle lying on the interosseous membrane in the upper third of the leg. Distal to the origin of the

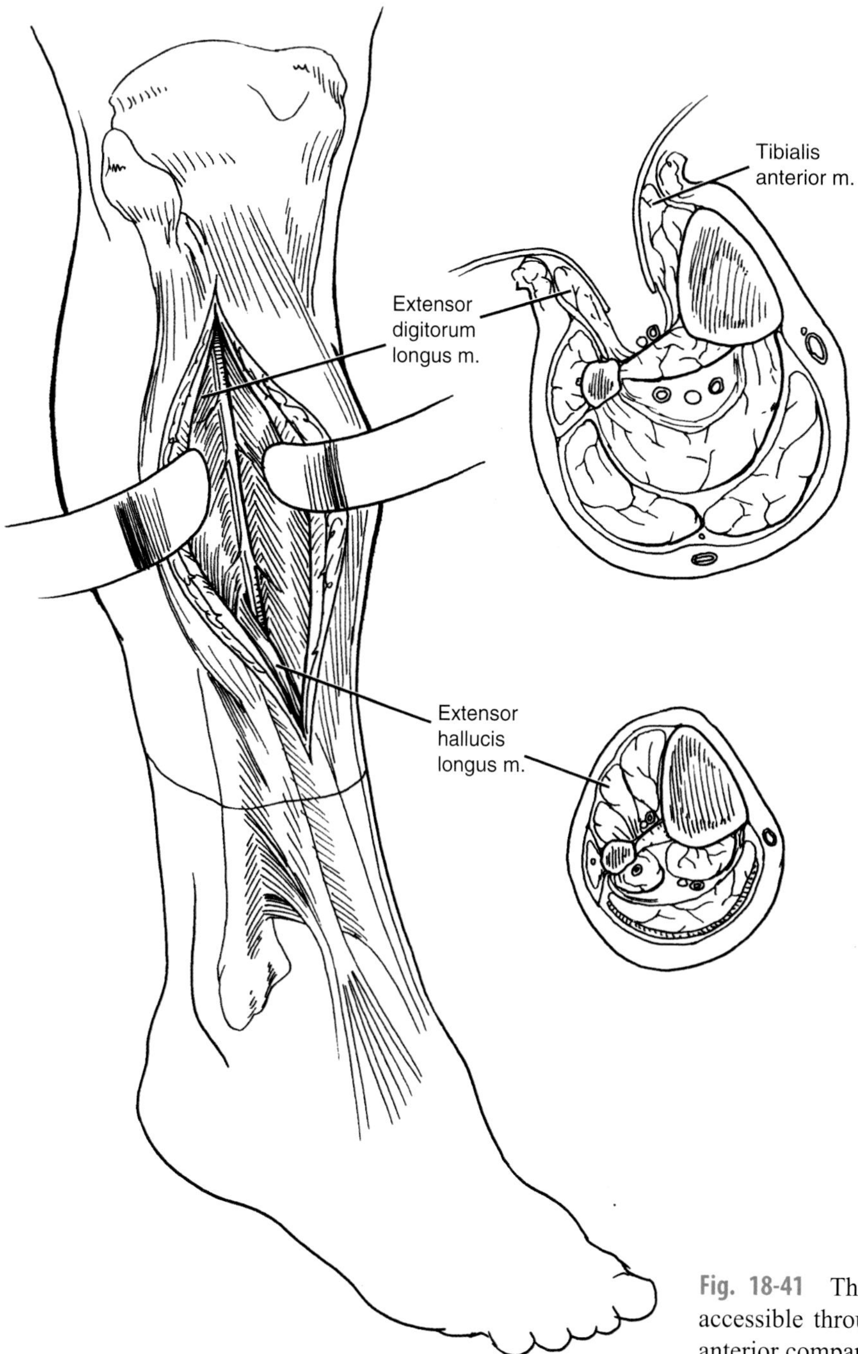

Fig. 18-41 The anterior tibial artery is easily accessible through a longitudinal incision into the anterior compartment.

extensor hallucis longus muscle, the plane between the tibialis anterior and extensor hallucis longus muscles should be developed. The vein is the most anterior structure in the neurovascular bundle, with the artery lying just behind. The deep peroneal nerve lies most posterior. Isolation of the anterior tibial artery requires careful dissection because of the multiple overlying venous branches.

Vein grafts are brought from medial leg incisions to the anterior compartment by creating a tunnel through the interosseous membrane. The interosseous membrane can be penetrated from either direction; we prefer to pass a blunt tunneling instrument from the deep posterior to the anterior compartments. The posterior tibial vessels are exposed through the medial incision and protected by anterior retraction on the tip of the surgeon's index finger (Fig. 18-42). The tunneling instrument is introduced through the interosseous membrane under direct vision in the anterior compartment at the level of the intended anastomosis. The tunneler is directed distally at a 45° angle to meet the index finger in the medial wound. The tunnel will traverse the tibialis posterior muscle, which is broadly attached to the posterior surface of the interosseous membrane. The tunnel should be sufficiently wide to ensure that the graft is not compressed as it courses between the compartments; in most cases, the tunnel should be made wide enough to admit at least two fingers.

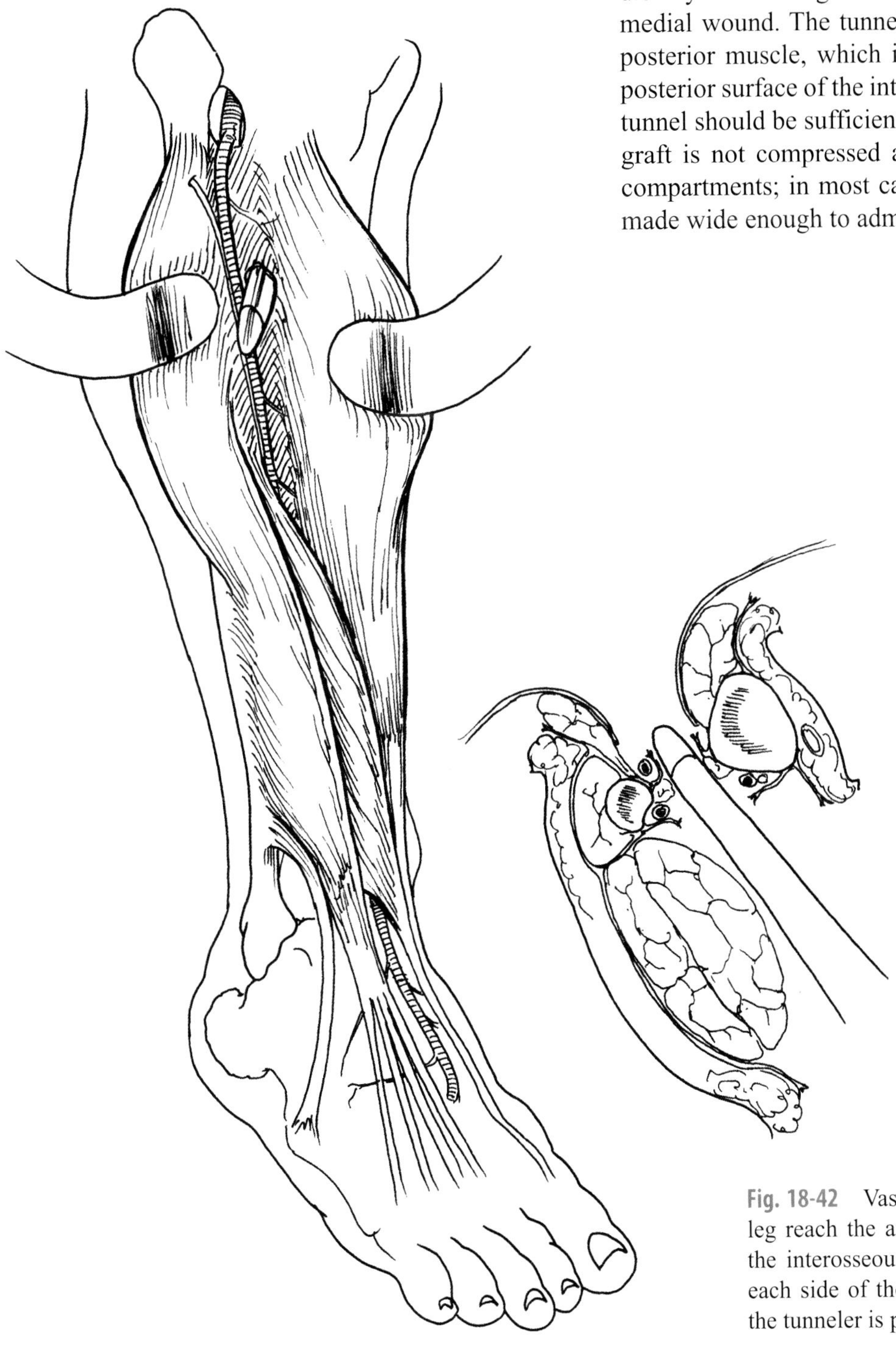

Fig. 18-42 Vascular grafts from the medial leg reach the anterior compartment through the interosseous membrane. The vessels on each side of the membrane are protected as the tunneler is passed.

Exposure of the Anterior Tibial Artery in the Distal Leg

In the distal third of the leg, the anterior tibial artery courses anteriorly, leaving the interosseous membrane to lie on the anterior surface of the lateral tibial flare (Fig. 18-43). It is considered separately because its position on the tibia places vein bypasses at risk of early failure: bypasses brought through the interosseous membrane at this level will kink on the posterolateral border of the tibia as they wind around the bone toward the artery.[11] Veith (personal communication, 1989) prefers to route bypasses through the subcutaneous tissue anterior to the tibia; however, others have found that the vein graft may become compressed against the anterior tibial border.[9] There are three alternatives for routing vein bypasses into the distal anterior compartment. The vein can be routed through the interosseous membrane in the proximal leg and brought to the distal anterior tibial artery through the anterior compartment[11] (Fig. 18-44). It can be routed in a hole drilled

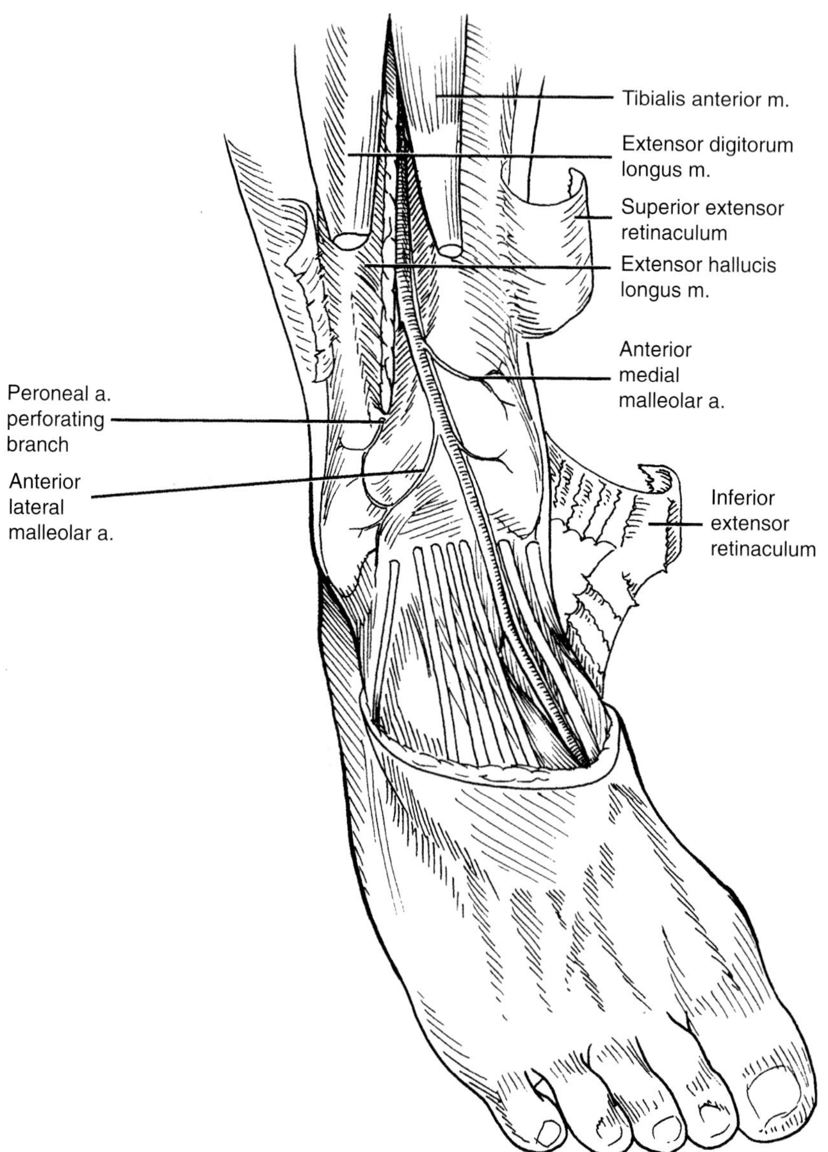

Fig. 18-43 At the ankle, the anterior tibial artery crosses the anterior tibial surface beneath the extensor retinacula.

through the distal tibia to reach the artery directly.[12] The third alternative is to create a superficial gutter in the cortex of the anterior tibial border.[13] Vein grafts can be laid in the gutter and routed anteriorly to the tibia into the anterior compartment for anastomosis with the anterior tibial artery. The anastomosis is protected anteriorly by the tibialis anterior muscle.

The patient is placed in the supine position with the leg internally rotated and flexed 30° at the knee. A vertical incision is made over the anterior compartment in the distal third of the leg and deepened through the crural fascia. The anterior tibial vessels are located by developing a plane between the tibialis anterior and extensor hallucis longus muscle tendons. Division of the superior extensor retinaculum facilitates separation of the tendons. The anterior tibial vessels are isolated deep in the wound on the anterolateral surface of the tibia.

Exposure of the tibia is performed in the lateral wound by mobilizing the tibialis anterior muscle and retracting it anteriorly. Medial exposure of the bone is accomplished in the incision used to expose the saphenous vein. The anterior skin and subcutaneous tissue of the incision are retracted, exposing sufficient bony surface to allow a hole to be drilled to create a tunnel through the bone or a tibial gutter at the anterior bone margin.

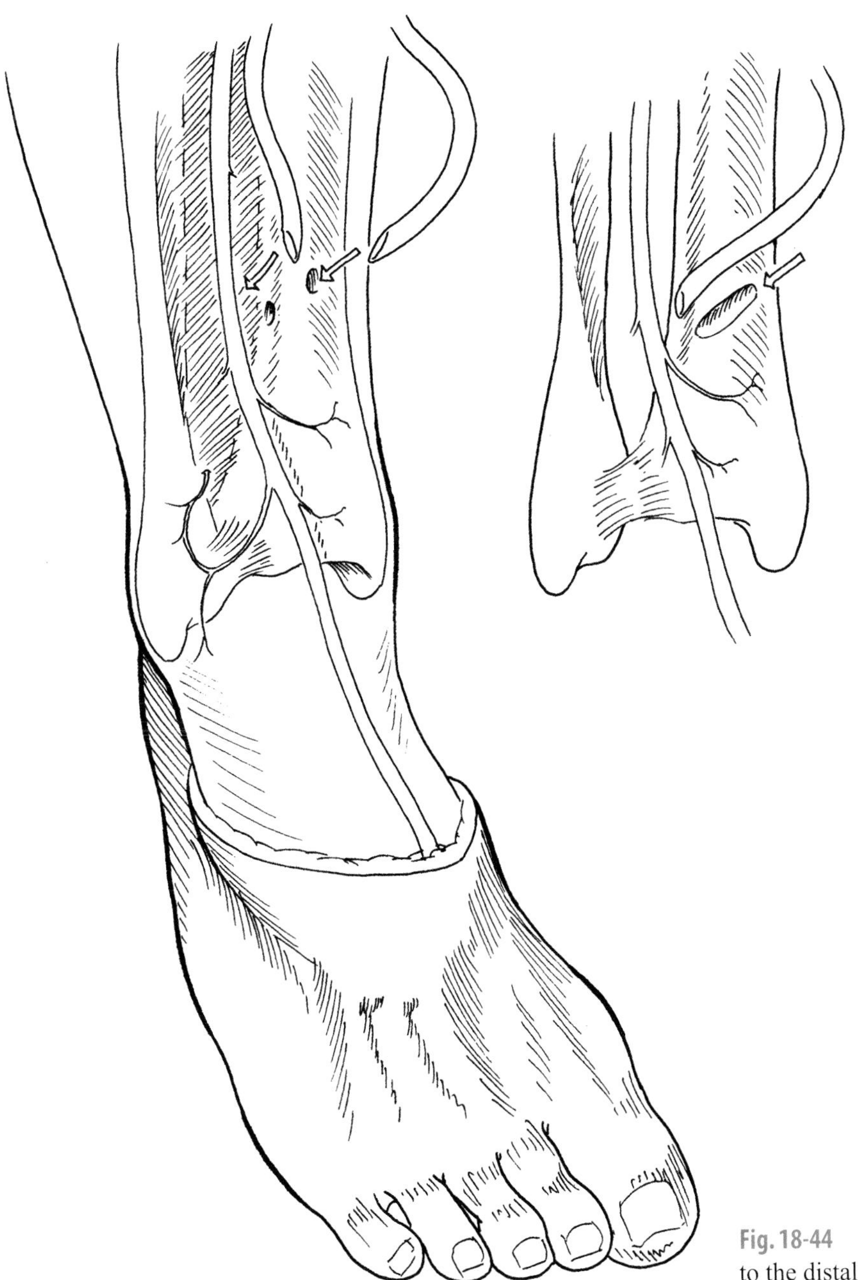

Fig. 18-44 Three options for routing bypass grafts to the distal anterior tibial artery are illustrated.

Exposure of the Peroneal Artery

The suitability of the peroneal artery as a recipient vessel in bypass operations for lower limb salvage has been well documented.[6–8] Patency rates approaching those of bypasses to the anterior and posterior tibial arteries justify its use; however, the peroneal artery is relatively difficult to isolate and has only indirect communications with the arteries of the foot. It should not be used in preference to suitable tibial arteries.[8] The artery lies deep in the lateral leg in apposition to the fibula and may be approached through medial or lateral incisions. Lateral incisions are preferred in obese individuals and in secondary bypass procedures but require resection of the fibula.

Medial Approach to the Peroneal Artery

The patient is placed in the supine position with the leg externally rotated and the knee flexed 30°. The entire leg, thigh, and groin are prepped and draped as before. A vertical incision is made 2 cm behind the posterior border of the tibia in the middle third of the leg and extended for approximately 10 cm (Fig. 18-45). The incision is deepened through the crural fascia, and the tibial attachments of the soleus muscle are divided. Posterior retraction of the soleus muscle exposes the flexor digitorum longus muscle posterior to the tibia. To facilitate dissection, Graham and Hanel[14] recommended entry into the deep posterior compartment of the leg by incising the fascia covering the flexor digitorum longus muscle

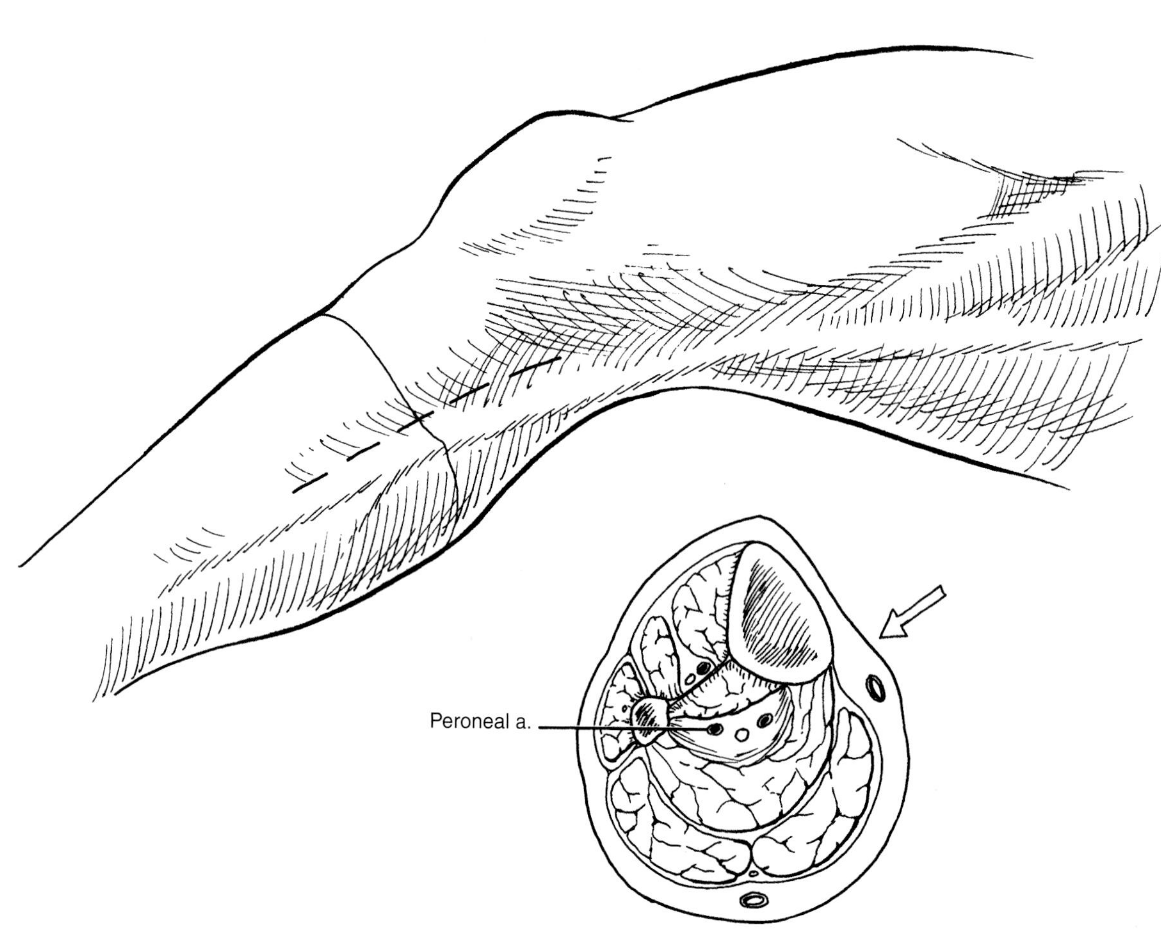

Fig. 18-45 The medial approach to the peroneal artery uses the same incision as the medial approach to the posterior tibial artery.

(Fig. 18-46). The plane of dissection is developed by posterior retraction of the fascia. To prevent injury to muscular branches of the posterior tibial vessels, the neurovascular bundle is best left in the loose areolar tissues overlying the soleus muscle. Deep in the wound, the peroneal vessels are located on the anterior surface of the flexor hallucis longus muscle. Occasionally these vessels are enveloped within the muscle belly, requiring minimal superficial dissection in the muscle fibers for exposure.[14]

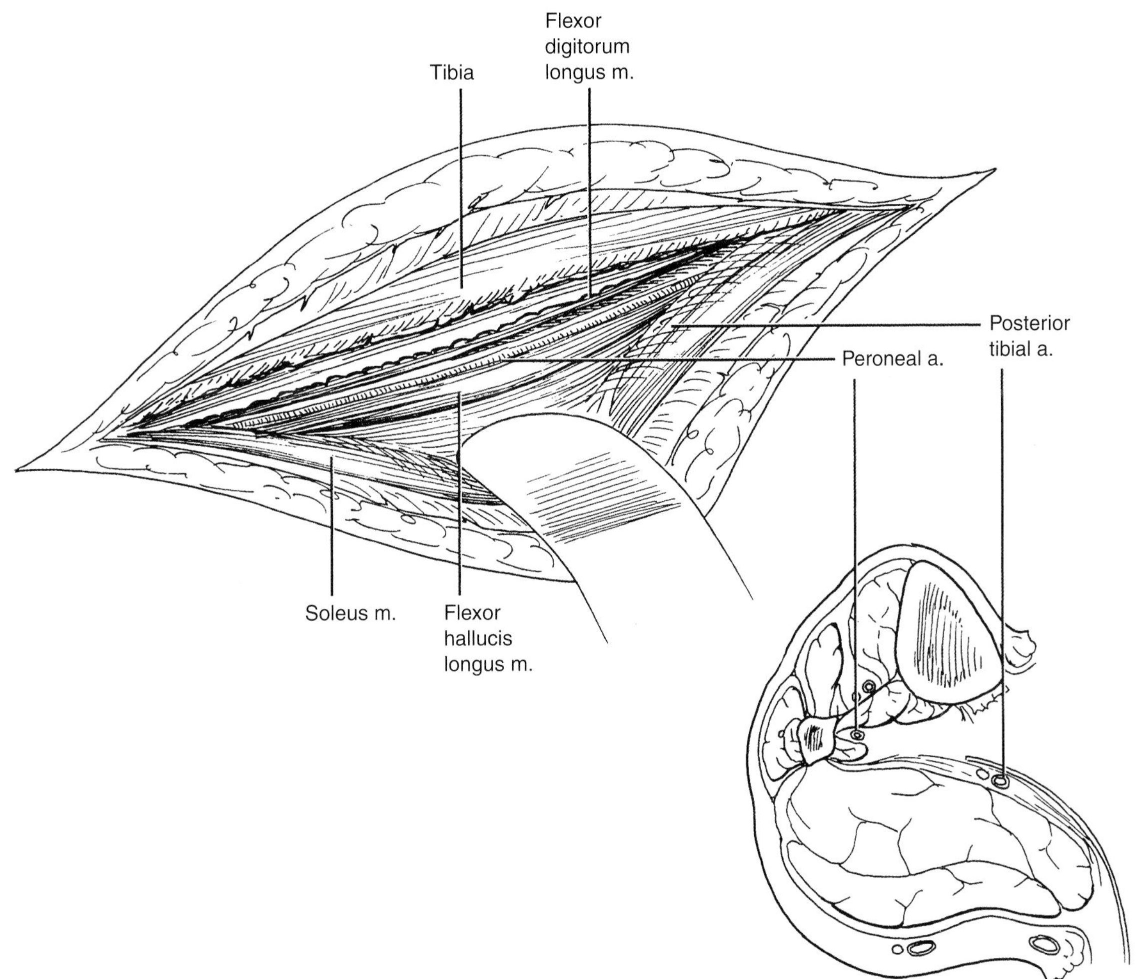

Fig. 18-46 By retracting the posterior tibial vessels and nerve posteriorly with the soleus muscle, the deeper lying peroneal artery anterior to the flexor hallucis longus muscle is exposed.

Lateral Approach to the Peroneal Artery

The patient is placed in the supine position with the leg internally rotated and the knee flexed 60°. An incision is made in the lateral leg over the fibula, centered over the area of intended anastomosis and extending 10 to 15 cm. The incision is continued through the subcutaneous tissue and deep fascia. The common peroneal nerve is identified and carefully protected in the proximal wound, where it winds around the neck of the fibula (Fig. 18-47).

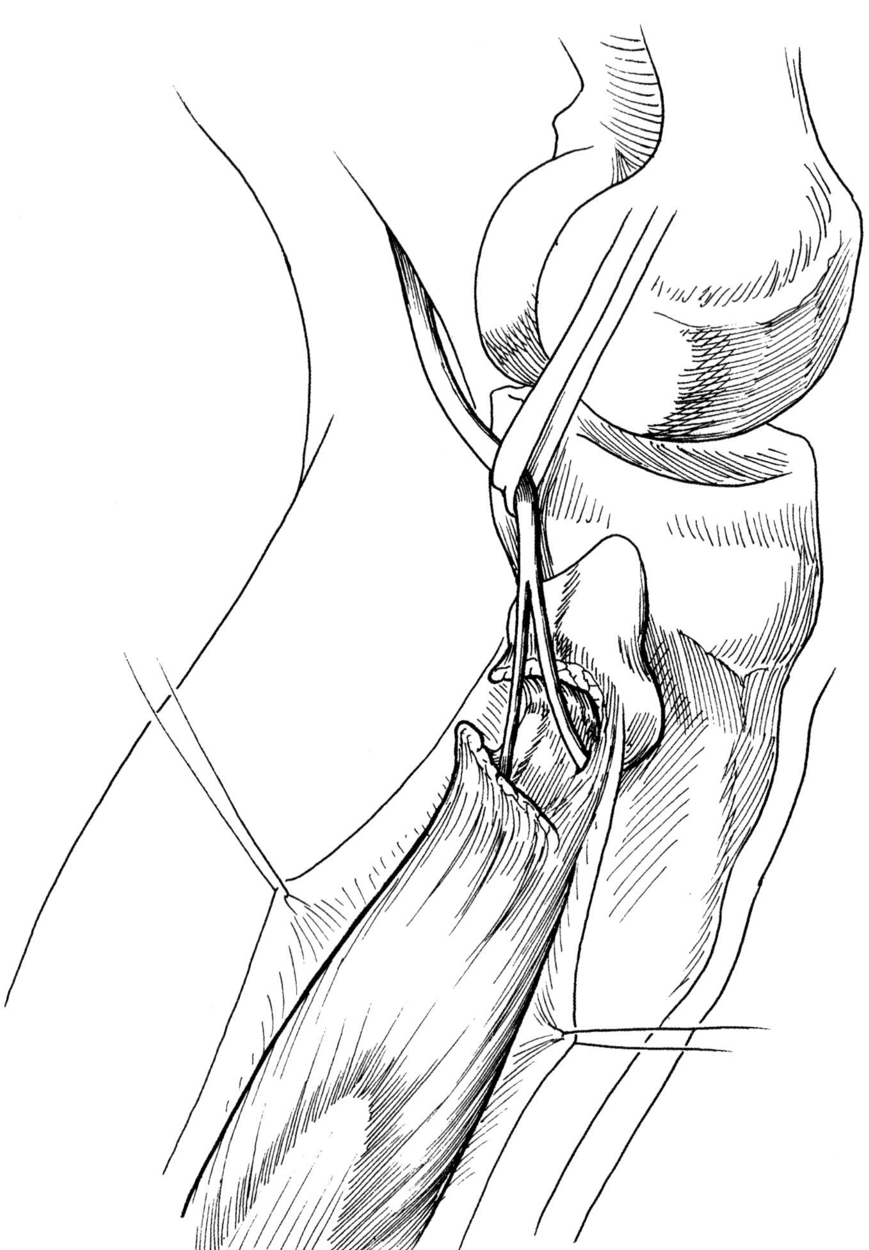

Fig. 18-47 The peroneal nerve is isolated in preparation for the lateral approach to the peroneal artery.

All muscular attachments to the fibula are then separated bluntly, as described above (Fig. 18-48). Some authors advocate a subperiosteal dissection to facilitate this maneuver[15] as opposed to simple stripping of the muscular fibers. Great care should be exercised during dissection on the medial surface of the fibula because the peroneal vessels are in close proximity and therefore prone to injury.

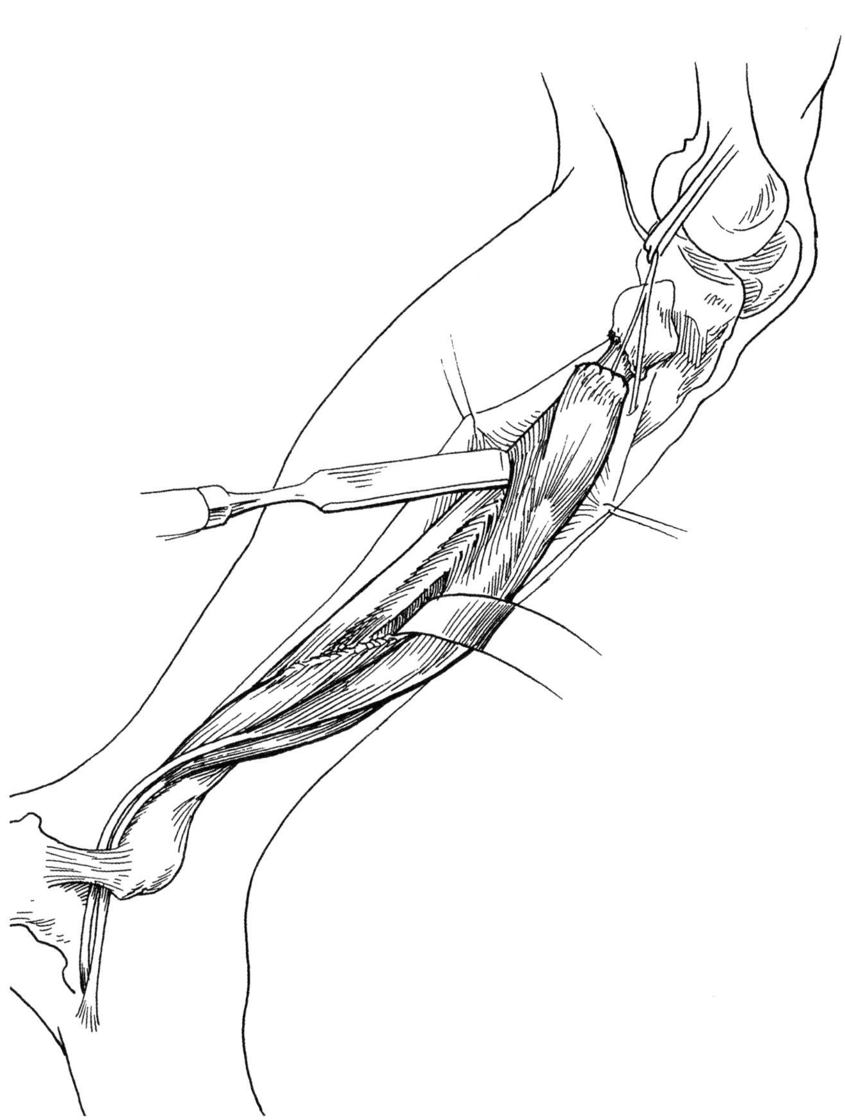

Fig. 18-48 The peroneal muscles are elevated to expose the fibula for excision.

After an adequate segment of fibula has been cleared of surrounding attachments, the bone is resected and removed from its bed. Veith et al.[16] recommended drilling holes through the fibula at the lines of intended division to help gain a clean division of the bone with rib shears. The peroneal vessels are located deep to the fibular bed (Fig. 18-49).

Posterior Approach to the Distal Peroneal Artery

As noted above, a minority of patients with peripheral vascular disease has occlusive lesions confined to the tibial vessels, with preserved inflow to the level of the popliteal artery. In rare cases, the distal peroneal artery may be the only remaining outflow vessel supplying the ankle and foot.[7] Medial approaches to the distal peroneal artery are hampered by the widening flare of the tibia in the distal leg. A posterior approach is desirable because it is more direct and may be associated with fewer wound complications.[10] A popliteal–peroneal bypass may be performed using the small saphenous vein; exposure of the popliteal artery and small saphenous vein are described above.

The patient is placed in the supine position, and the entire leg and thigh are prepped and draped. A vertical incision is made directly over the small saphenous vein. As noted above, the vein begins posterior to the lateral malleolus, courses lateral to the calcaneus tendon, and ascends medially toward the midline of the popliteal fossa. The incision is made in the distal third of the calf along the lateral side of the calcaneus tendon and deepened through the crural fascia (Fig. 18-50). The peroneal artery is identified by retracting the calcaneus tendon medially and the flexor hallucis longus muscle laterally. The artery is located on the medial side of the fibula, which serves as an excellent landmark.[10] The peroneal artery can be isolated as far distally as its bifurcation into perforating and communicating branches.

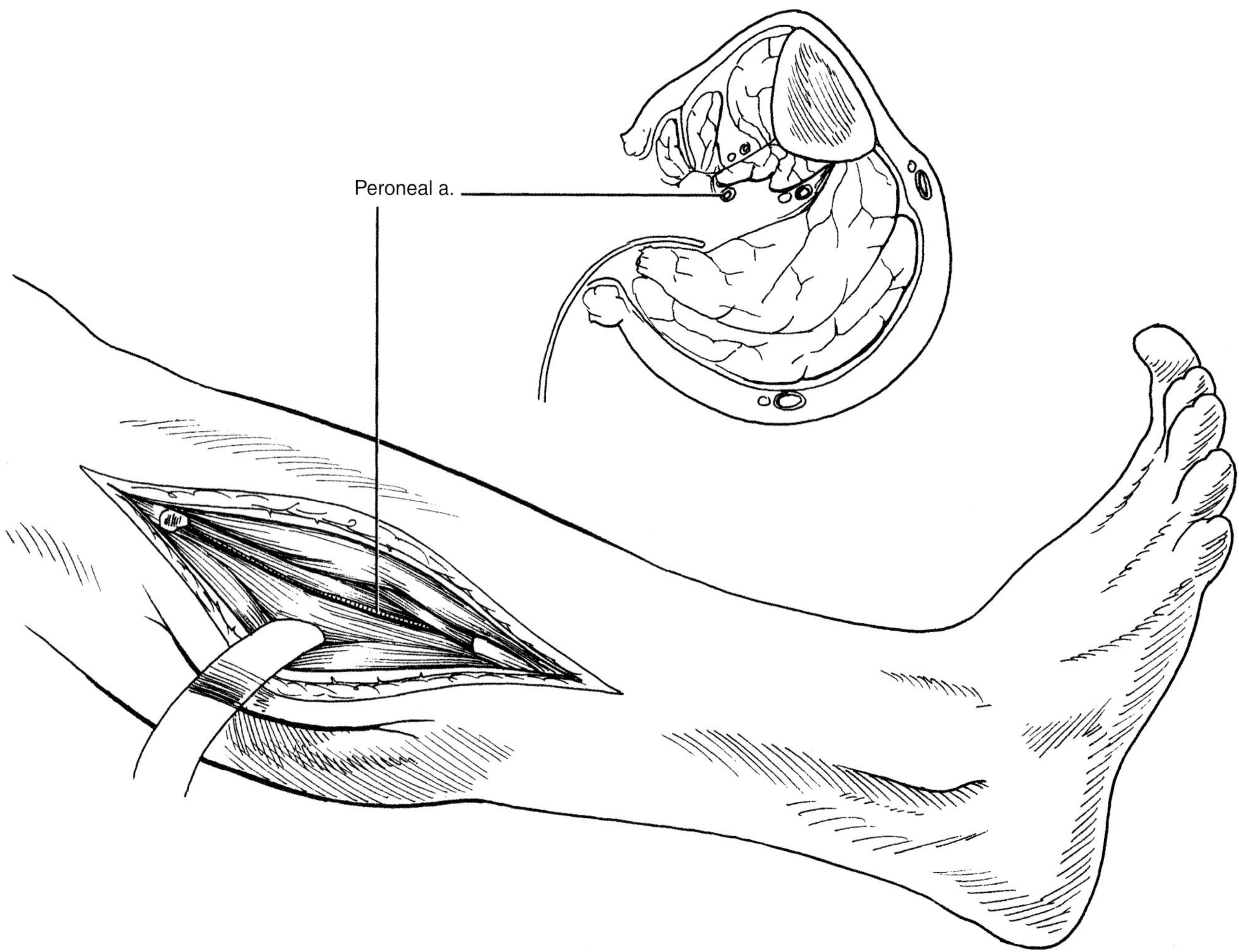

Fig. 18-49 The proximal peroneal artery is located deep to the fibular bed.

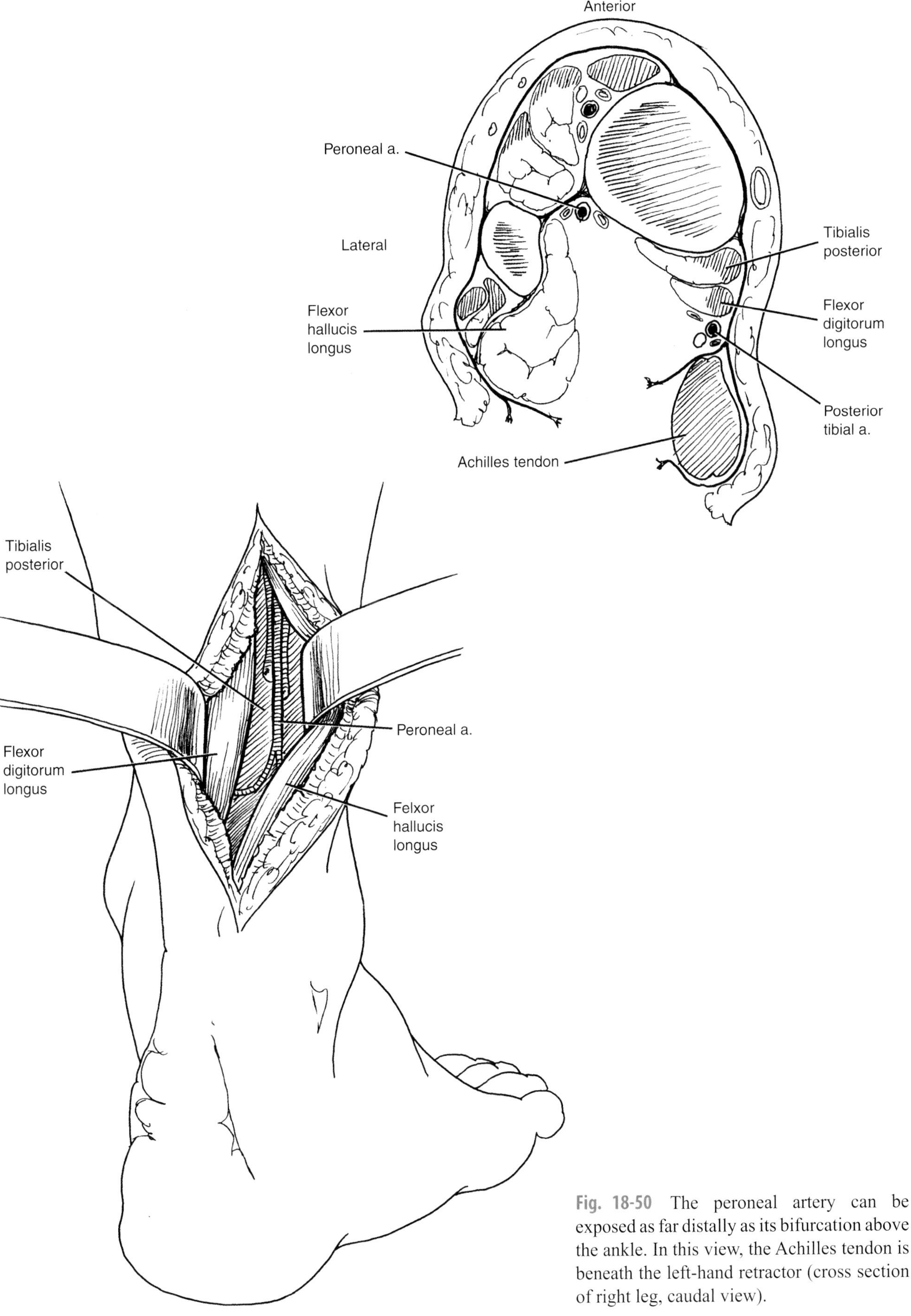

Fig. 18-50 The peroneal artery can be exposed as far distally as its bifurcation above the ankle. In this view, the Achilles tendon is beneath the left-hand retractor (cross section of right leg, caudal view).

Exposure of Arteries of the Foot and Ankle

Exposure of the Posterior Tibial Artery at the Ankle

Long vein bypasses to arteries at the level of the ankle and foot have been shown to have patency rates similar to those of bypasses involving more proximal infrageniculate arteries.[17,18] The superficial location of the posterior tibial artery at the ankle greatly simplifies exposure, making it a very attractive option for bypass (Fig. 18-51).

The patient is placed in the supine position with the leg externally rotated and flexed 60° at the knee. The entire leg, groin, and foot are prepped and draped. A vertical incision is made approximately 1 cm posterior to the distal tibia and curved around the medial malleolus onto the foot. Division of the flexor retinaculum exposes the neurovascular bundle lying in the groove between the tendons of the flexor digitorum longus and flexor hallucis longus muscles (Fig. 18-40). The posterior tibial artery lies anterior to the tibial nerve at this level. Isolation of the artery is aided by mobilization and anterior retraction of the flexor digitorum longus tendon.

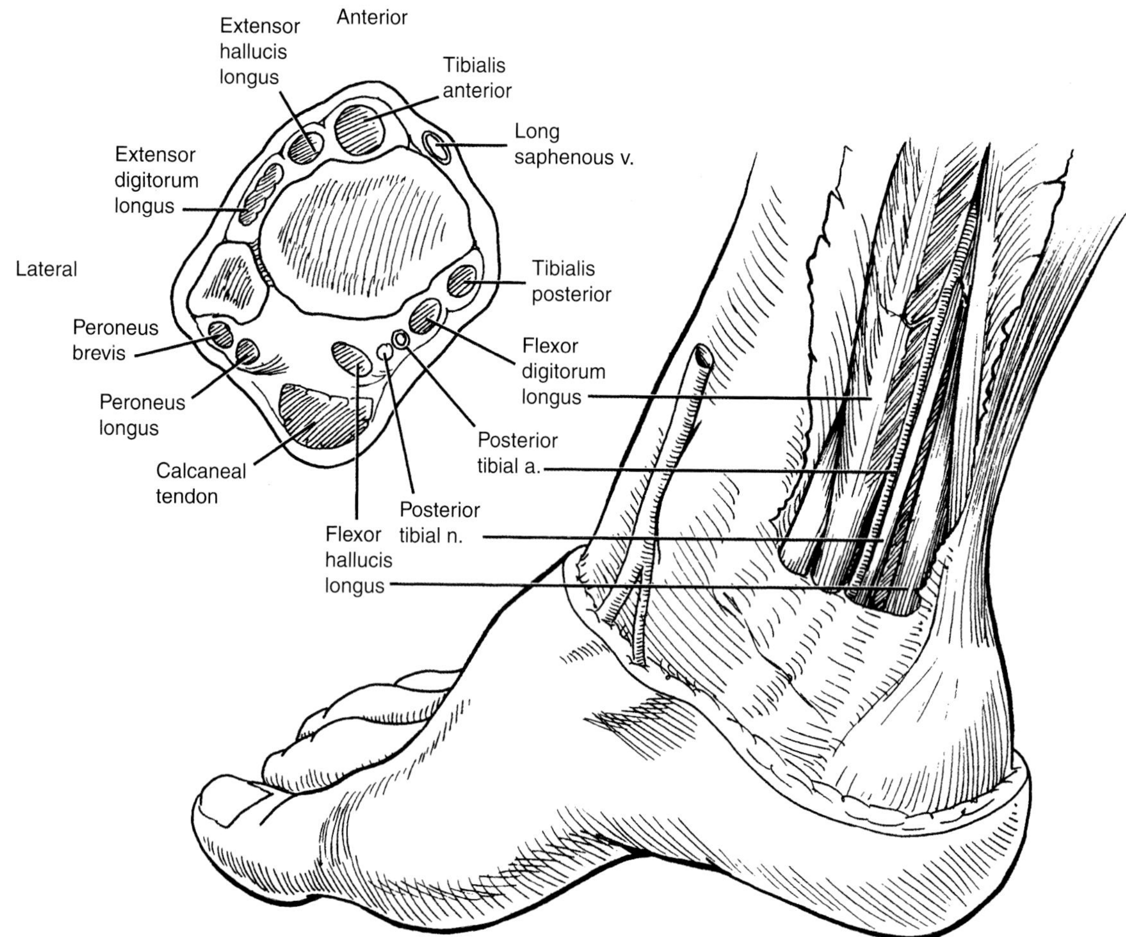

Fig. 18-51 The posterior tibial artery is found just deep to the crural fascia at the ankle and is easily accessible for distal bypass (cross section of right leg, caudal view).

Exposure of the Medial and Lateral Plantar Arteries

Bypasses to the distal branches of the posterior tibial artery are associated with good patency rates and long-term limb salvage, even in patients with gangrene.[19,20] The medial and lateral plantar arteries can be exposed below the level of the medial malleolus. Although either may be used for bypass, the lateral plantar artery is usually the larger of the two.

The leg is positioned as above, with the knee externally rotated and the foot raised on a soft pad behind the lateral malleolus to widen the space between the medial malleolus and the calcaneus bone.[19] A curvilinear incision is made beginning midway between the medial malleolus and the calcaneus tendon, extending longitudinally along the instep for a distance of 4 to 5 cm[16] (Fig. 18-52).

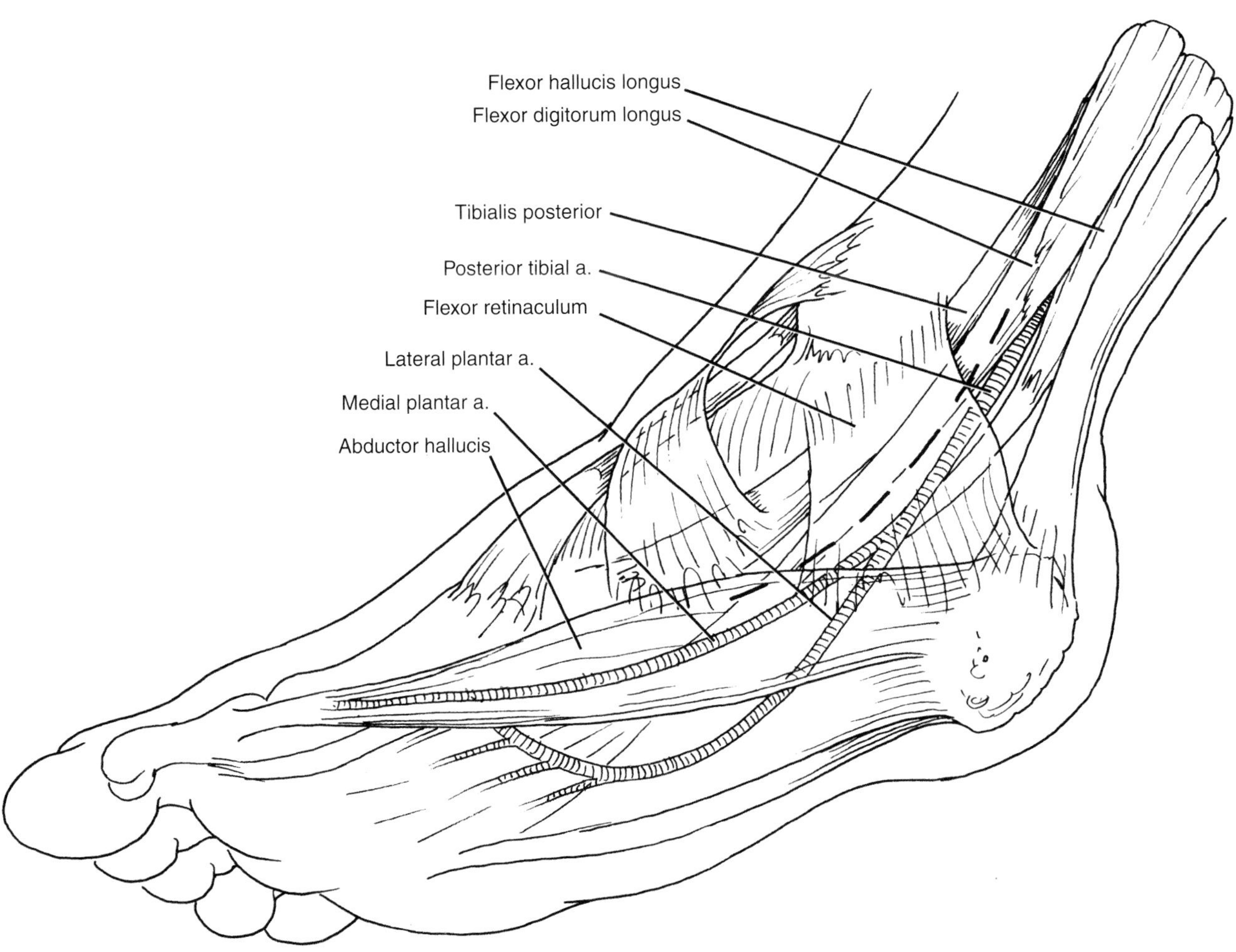

Fig. 18-52 The incision for exposure of the posterior tibial artery branches is shown.

The posterior tibial artery is exposed by dividing the flexor retinaculum. As the artery is traced distally, the bifurcation will be found on the superior border of the abductor hallucis muscle.[19] Exposure of the plantar branches is obtained by incising the abductor hallucis muscle in the direction of the lateral plantar artery (Fig. 18-53).

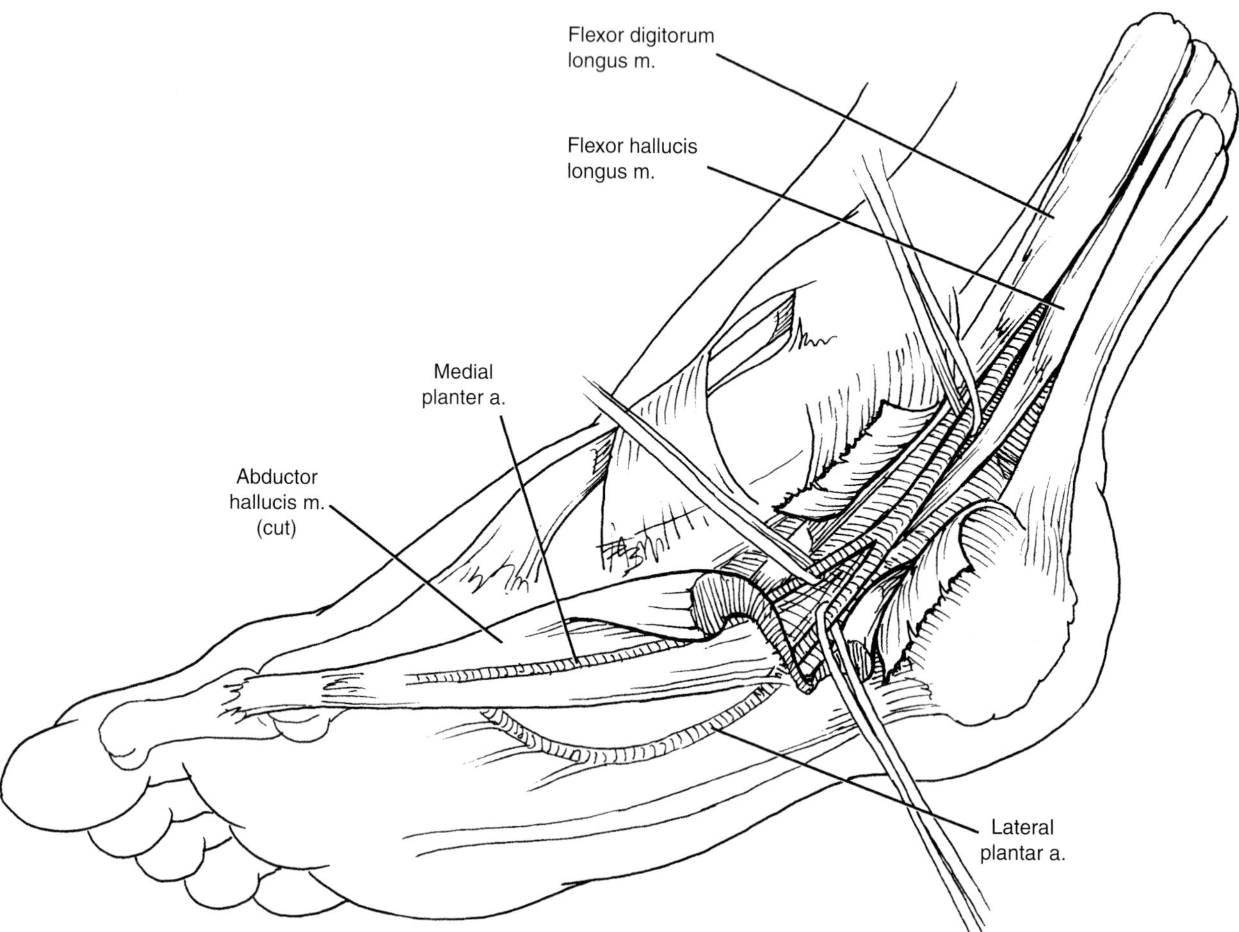

Fig. 18-53 The bifurcation of the posterior tibial artery is located on the superior border of the abductor hallucis muscle.

Exposure of the Dorsalis Pedis Artery

As noted previously, long vein bypasses to arterial segments at the ankle and foot have patency rates similar to bypasses to more proximal leg arteries.[4–7] The dorsalis pedis artery is readily accessible and provides an excellent option for bypass when more proximal arteries are not suitable.

The patient is placed in the supine position, and the leg, foot, and groin are surgically prepared. A vertical incision is made on the dorsal foot lateral to the location of the dorsalis pedis artery midway between the first and second metatarsal bones. This allows creation of a narrow skin flap that will cover the anastomosis if the skin incision fails to heal. The dorsal branch of the superficial peroneal nerve should be identified and retracted laterally. After incising the deep fascia, the neurovascular bundle is exposed by retracting the extensor hallucis longus and brevis muscles apart (Fig. 18-54). The dorsalis pedis artery lies lateral to the deep peroneal nerve. Isolation of the artery may require control of medial and lateral tarsal artery branches, which should be left intact.[21]

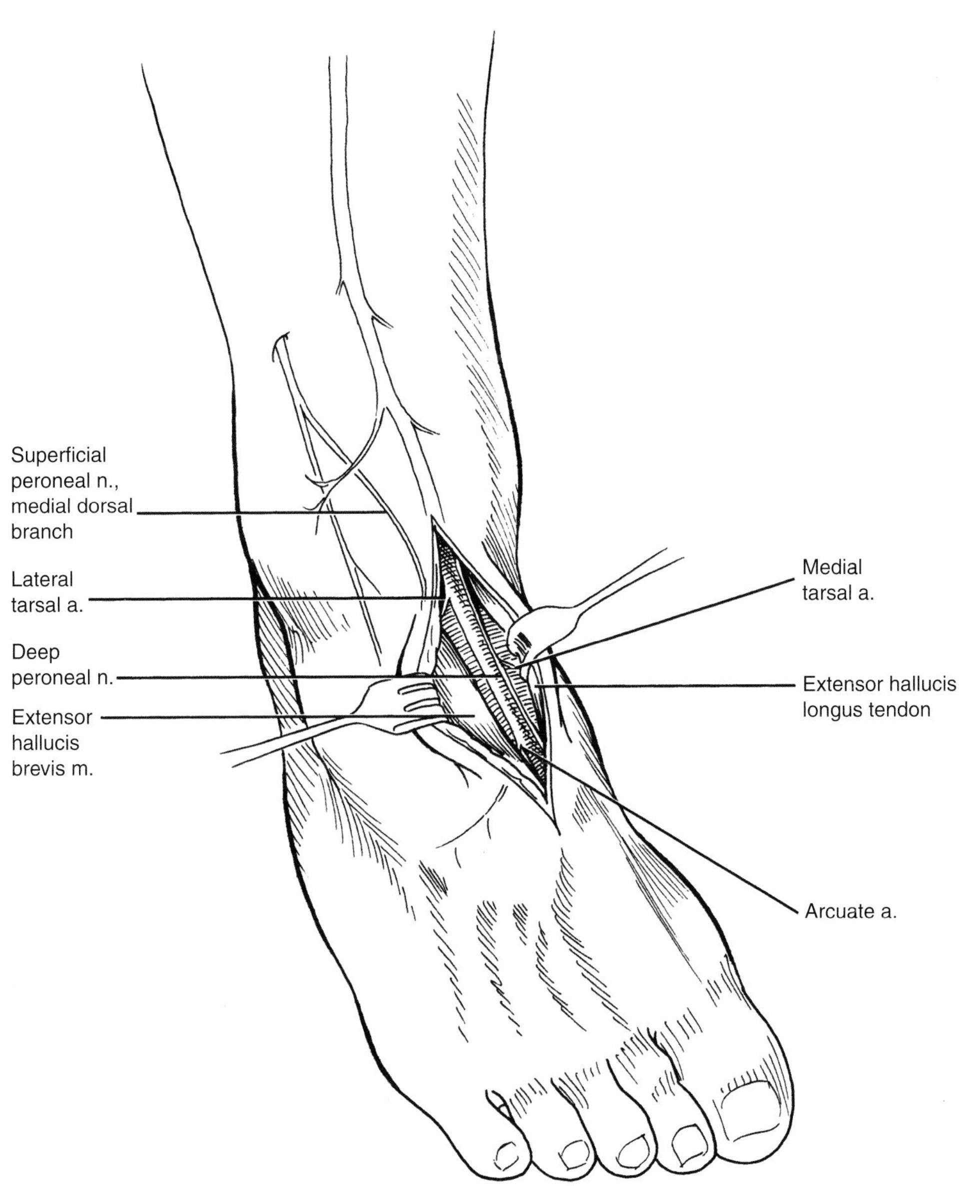

Fig. 18-54 The dorsalis pedis artery is exposed between the extensor hallucis longus tendon and the extensor hallucis brevis muscle.

References

1. Colborn GL, Lumsden AB, Taylor BS, et al. The surgical anatomy of the popliteal artery. *Am Surg*. 1994;60:238–246.
2. Bergman RA, Thompson SA, Afifi AK, et al. *Compendium of Human Anatomic Variation*. Baltimore, MD: Urban & Schwarzenberg; 1988:426–427.
3. Henry AK. Exposure of the fibula and nerves related to it. In: Henry AK, ed. *Extensile Exposure*. Edinburgh, England: Churchill Livingstone; 1973:292–296.
4. Uflacker R. *Atlas of Vascular Anatomy*. Philadelphia, PA: Lippincott Williams & Wilkins; 1997:756–778.
5. Norgen L, Hiatt WR, Dormandy MR, et al. Inter-Society consensus for the management of peripheral arterial disease (TASC II). *J Vasc Surg*. 2007;45(suppl. S):S5–S67.
6. Bergamini TM, George SM Jr, Massey HT, et al. Pedal or peroneal bypass: which is better when both are patent? *J Vasc Surg*. 1994;20:347–356.
7. Ballotta E, Da Giau G, Gruppo M, et al. Infrapopliteal arterial revascularization for critical limb ischemia: is the peroneal artery at the distal third a suitable outflow vessel? *J Vasc Surg*. 2008;47:952–959.
8. Plecha EJ, Seabrook GR, Bandyk DF, et al. Determinants of successful peroneal artery bypass. *J Vasc Surg*. 1993;17:97–106.
9. Shah DM, Paty PSK, Leather RP, et al. Optimal outcome after tibial arterial bypass. *Surg Gynecol Obstet*. 1993;177:283–287.
10. Ouriel K. The posterior approach to popliteal-crural bypass. *J Vasc Surg*. 1994;19:74–80.
11. Tiefenbrun J, Beckerman M, Singer A. Surgical anatomy in bypass of the distal part of the lower limb. *Surg Gynecol Obstet*. 1975;141:528–533.
12. Dardik H. Graft positioning in tunnels. In: Dardik H, ed. *Arterial Reconstruction in the Lower Extremity*. New York, NY: McGraw-Hill; 1986:127–139.
13. Valentine RJ, Blankenship CL, Wind GG. The tibial gutter: a protected route for bypass to the distal anterior tibial artery. *J Vasc Surg*. 1989;10:465–467.
14. Graham JW, Hanel KC. Vein grafts to the peroneal artery. *Surgery*. 1981;89:264–268.
15. Dardik H, Dardik I, With FJ. Exposure of the tibioperoneal arteries by a single lateral approach. *Surgery*. 1974;75:377–382.
16. Veith FJ, Gupta SK, Acer E, et al. Alternative approaches to the deep femoral, the popliteal, and the infrapopliteal arteries in the leg and foot. In: Bergan JJ, Yao JST, eds. *Techniques in Arterial Surgery*. Philadelphia, PA: WB Saunders; 1990:145–156.
17. Gargiulo M, Giovanetti F, Bianchini Massoni C, et al. Bypass to the ankle and foot in the era of endovascular therapy of tibial disease. Results and factors influencing the outcome. *J Cardiovasc Surg (Torino)*. 2012;53(5):617–623.
18. Slim H, Tiwari A, Ahmed A, et al. Distal versus ultradistal bypass grafts: amputation-free survival and patency rates in patients with critical limb ischaemia. *Eur J Vasc Endovasc Surg*. 2011;42:83–88.
19. Andros G, Harris RW, Salles-Cunha SX, et al. Lateral plantar artery bypass grafting: defining the limits of foot revascularization. *J Vasc Surg*. 1989;10:511–521.
20. Brochado-Neto FC, Cury MV, Bonadiman SS, et al. Vein bypass to branches of pedal arteries. *J Vasc Surg*. 2012;55:746–752.
21. Veith FJ. Alternative approaches to the deep femoral, popliteal, and infrapopliteal arteries in the leg and foot: part II. *Ann Vasc Surg*. 1994;8:599–603.

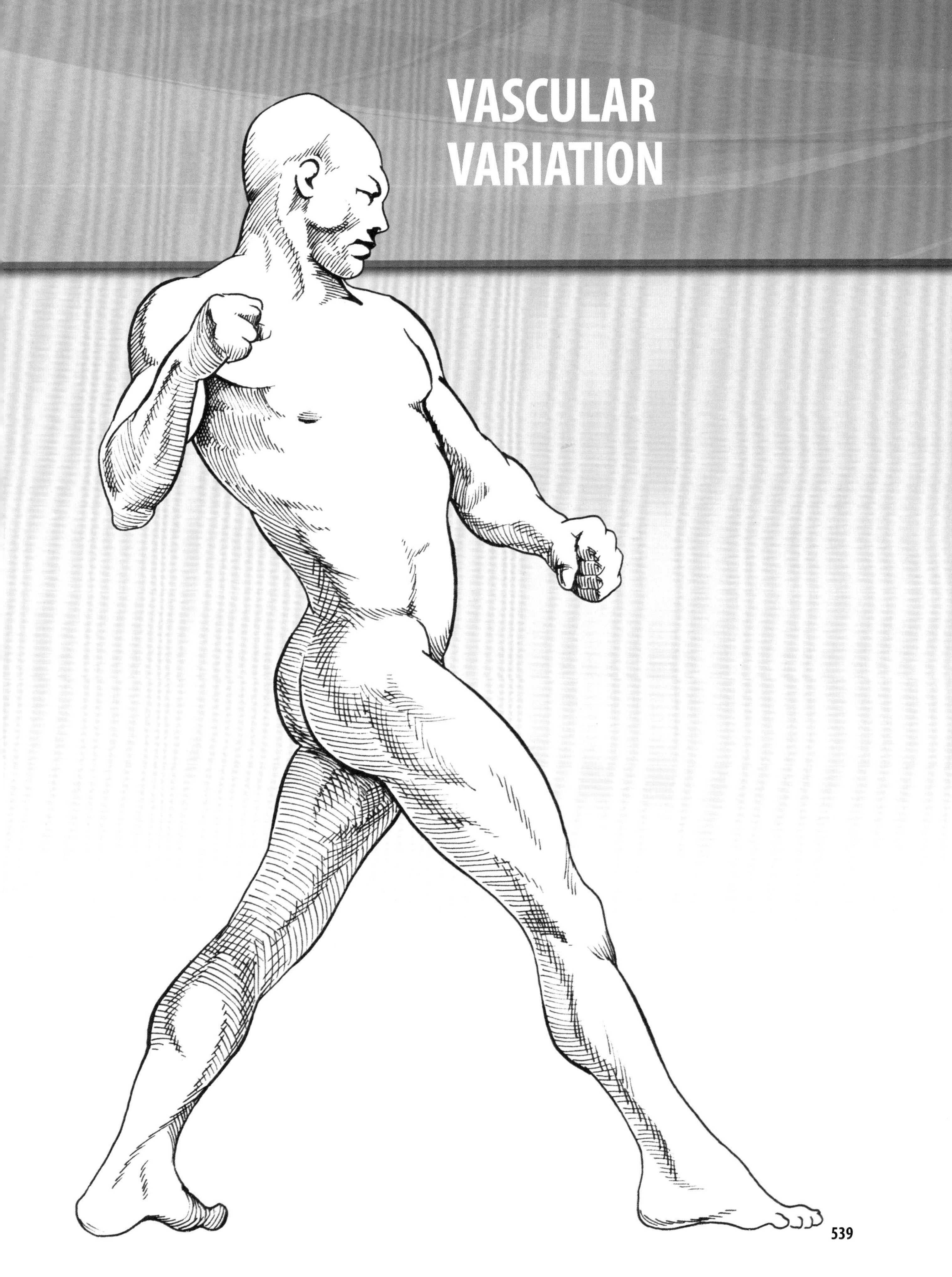

VASCULAR VARIATION

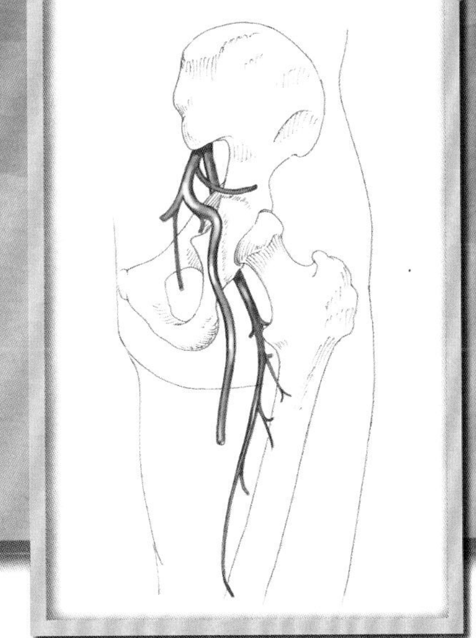

Anatomic Variation of the Blood Vessels

19

Vascular Anatomic Variation

In this book, as in any description of normal anatomy, it is important to recognize that the common vascular patterns depicted will only be encountered 50% to 70% of the time in clinical practice. Some vessels, particularly those supplying the abdominal viscera, are more likely to deviate from the prevalent pattern. Many of these variations can be understood in the context of the vascular embryology described in the Introduction. The variables include the origin and number of vessels supplying particular structures and the course, size, and shape of the vessel. These variations may be as simple as the tortuosity of an internal carotid artery or as drastic as the total deletion of a vessel.

There has been considerable discussion of semantic distinctions in classifying types of variation. The different terms that have been applied basically reflect the degree of atypia and the functional implications of the altered pattern. These terms should be noted in passing, keeping in mind the broad spectrum of patterns that are being differentiated. Terms such as atavism and reversion suggest the persistence of a pattern that occurred in the normal course of embryologic development and the arrest of development short of the mature human pattern.

These deviations frequently resemble the patterns found in lower animals because embryology reflects evolution. The term variation suggests a mild deviation from the typical pattern, whereas the term anomaly implies a more marked deviation from the standard. The terms malformation and abnormal carry a graver connotation, suggesting a dysfunctional pattern that may be injurious to the individual. Such a pattern may divert or disrupt needed blood flow or may impinge on adjacent structures and disrupt their function. The more severe the malformation, the more likely it will be symptomatic and discovered during life. An additional risk exists for even benign variations, such as an aberrant obturator artery that can be easily injured by an unwary surgeon.

There is an almost limitless variety of vascular patterns ranging from the simple to the bizarre. Fortunately for the clinician, 95% to 98% of patterns presented by a particular vessel can be accounted for among two or three variations. To keep this fact in perspective, we focus on the common variations of major vessels and clinically important vessels in the following discussion and briefly note the more obscure patterns.

Thoracic Aorta

Aortic Arch

Anomalies of the aortic arches are rare and are usually the result of atypical segmental regression of the paired arches present at approximately the seventh embryonic week[1] (Fig. 19-1). Many of these anomalies are asymptomatic and are discovered incidentally. Aortic rings, for example, are often totally asymptomatic but may cause dysphagia and dyspnea in the neonatal period.

Aortic arch anomalies have been classified into four groups and 24 subgroups by Stewart et al.[2] The variety of forms seems confusing at first glance but yields to logical analysis when one considers the segments of the paired fourth arches that involute (Fig. 19-2). Regression of the distal segment of the right fourth arch results in the normal pattern of the brachiocephalic, left common carotid, and left subclavian arteries arising from a left-sided arch (Fig. 19-2A). Regression of the right arch segment between the common carotid and right subclavian arteries (Fig. 19-2B) results in an aberrant right subclavian artery arising as the fourth branch of the aortic arch. This vessel most commonly passes posterior to the esophagus and may cause esophageal compression and dysphagia (dysphagia lusoria).[3]

Regression of the distal left arch results in a right-sided aortic arch that is the mirror image of the common pattern (Fig. 19-2C), and regression of the left carotid-subclavian segment results in a right arch with an aberrant left subclavian artery[4] (Fig. 19-2D). Partial persistence of any of the involuted segments as a hypoplastic channel or fibrous band results in a vascular ring surrounding the trachea and esophagus. In addition, connection of the sixth arch to the dorsal continuation of the fourth arch may persist on one or both sides, adding a variety of ductus arteriosus anomalies to the basic aberrant arch patterns. The mirror image variants of each of these patterns accounts for the number of described anomalies. Although some variations of aberrant aortic arch branch patterns are consequences of basic arch anomalies, many others are seen with the common form of a simple left-sided arch.

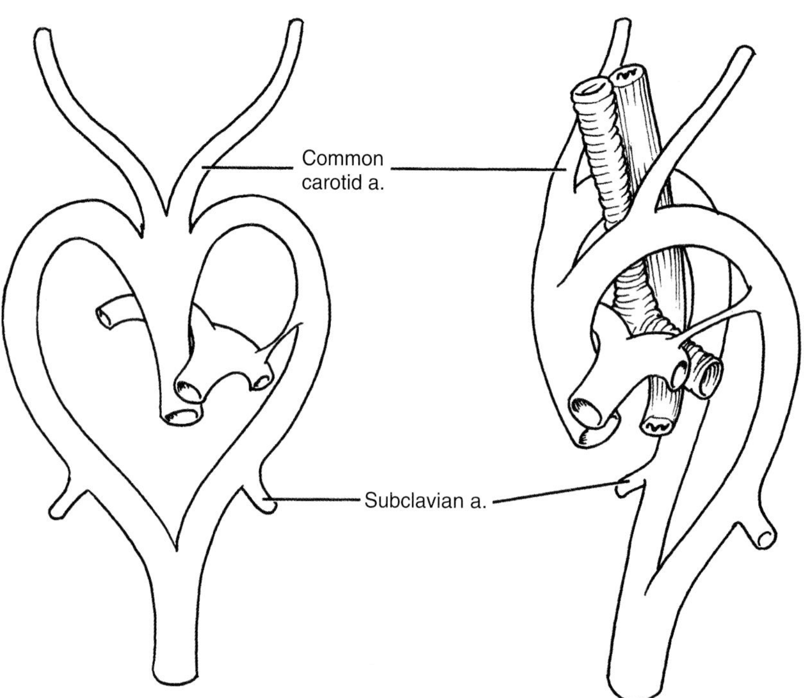

Fig. 19-1 Aortic arch anomalies usually result from disturbances of normal segmental regression of the paired aortic arches in the 7-week embryo.

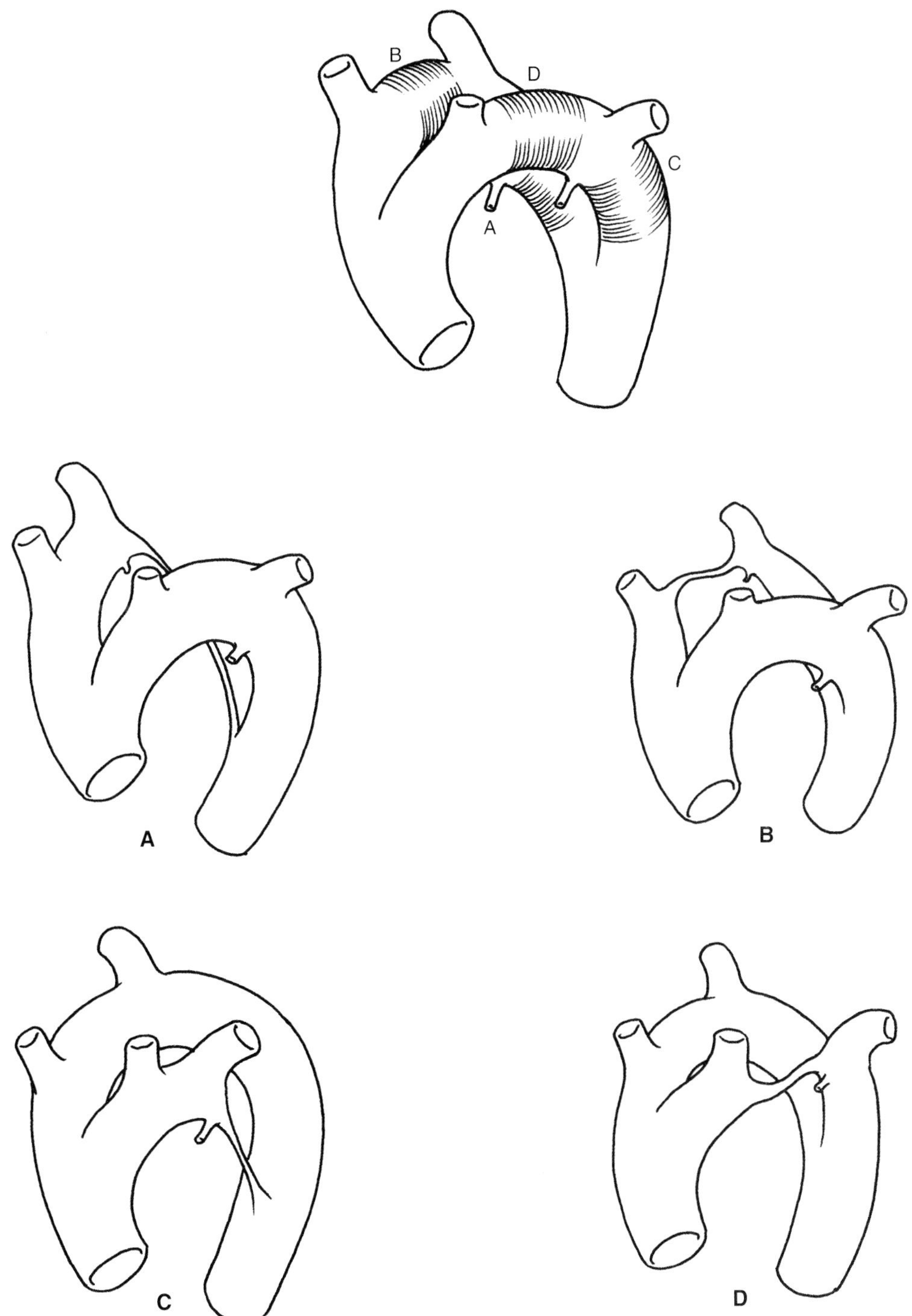

Fig. 19-2 Many aortic arch anomalies are understandable by visualizing the regression of one of four segments **(A–D)**.

Coarctation of the Thoracic Aorta

The transitional segment of thoracic aorta in the region of the ductus arteriosus may be congenitally narrow or even absent.[5] Such narrowing, called coarctation, makes up 6% to 10% of all major cardiovascular malformations and occurs in between one and six per 10,000 live births.[1] The narrowing may also take the form of a fibrotic cord, diaphragm, or complete interruption. Most commonly, coarctation occurs just distal to the left subclavian artery. In rare cases, the narrowing may be found in the arch or anywhere along the distal aorta (coarctation of the abdominal aorta is discussed below).

Coarctation has great clinical significance. It is a common cause of hypertension in children who may be asymptomatic until the overworked ventricles enlarge and ultimately fail. Early correction, however, leads to a normal functional state and life span. The defects have been classified based on the length, position relative to the ductus arteriosus, patency of the ductus, ventricular hypertrophy, and degree of collateral circulation (Fig. 19-3).

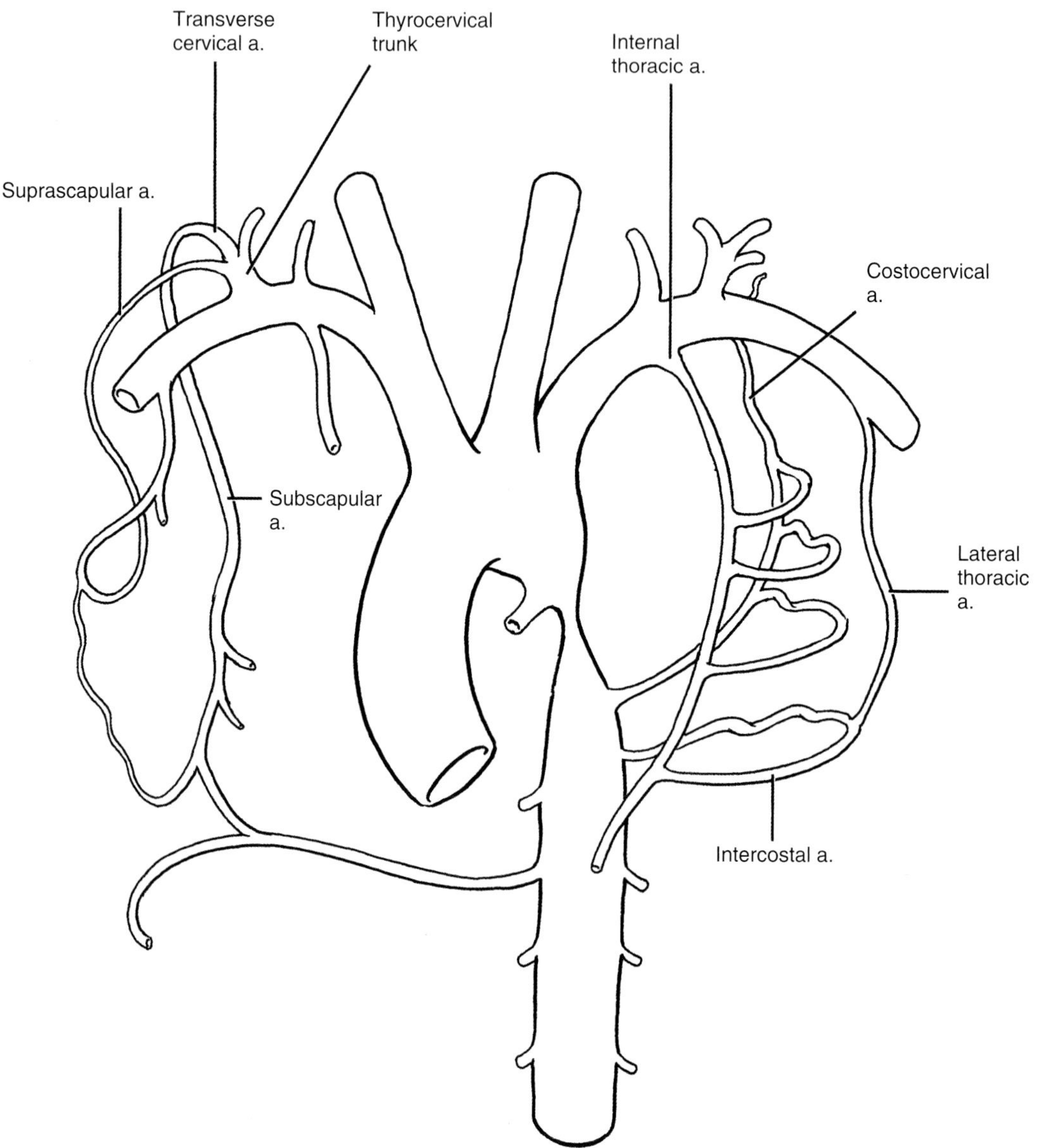

Fig. 19-3 Collateral channels through scapular and chest wall vessels enlarge in response to the pressure gradient created by an aortic coarctation.

Primary Branches of the Aortic Arch

The major branches of the aortic arch vary in their position on the arch, their distance from each other, the number of their primary stems, and their course and tortuosity. In addition, a number of branches that are usually secondary may originate instead directly from the aorta.[6]

Although the common pattern of branching is seen approximately 70% to 80% of the time, as many as one-fourth of the population has a left common carotid originating from or sharing a common root with the brachiocephalic trunk[7] (Fig. 19-4). These two patterns, along with another (the left vertebral artery arising from the arch between the left common carotid and subclavian arteries [2.5% to 5% of cases]), account for 95% to 97% of aortic arch branch patterns. A large variety of other patterns comprise the remaining few percent of aberrations, with the aberrant right subclavian artery mentioned above appearing frequently in combination with other anomalies.

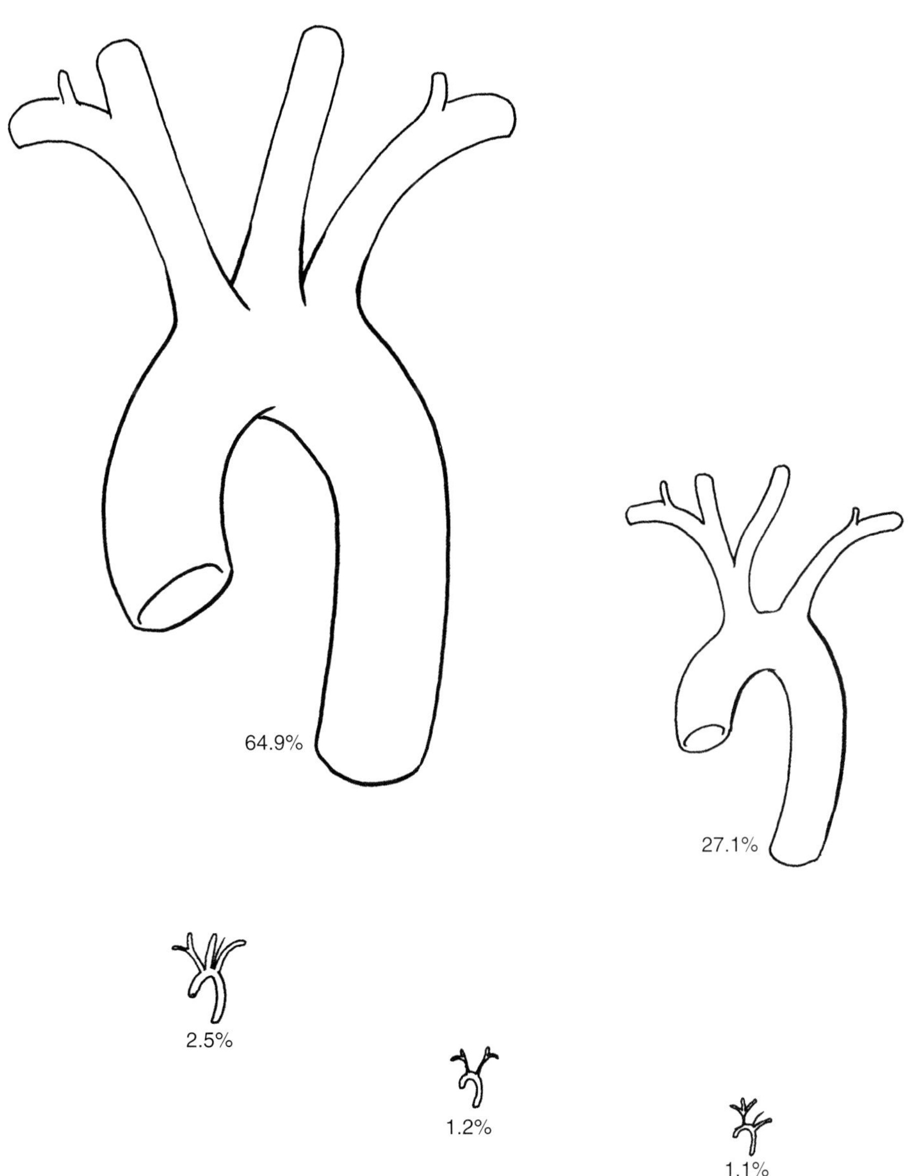

Fig. 19-4 In addition to the common aortic arch branch pattern, origin of the left common carotid from the brachiocephalic and left vertebral artery origin from the arch comprise almost 95% of all arch patterns.

Brachiocephalic Artery

The brachiocephalic artery exhibits some variability in the level at which it bifurcates into right subclavian and right common carotid arteries. When the point of division is high, the brachiocephalic artery can rise above the manubrium of the sternum (12%) and may be medial enough to pose a danger during tracheostomy.[7] A low point of division results in longer subclavian and carotid segments. In the extreme case, the right subclavian and right common carotid may arise directly from the arch with no brachiocephalic trunk (0.5%).

Common Carotid Artery

In addition to the major variations discussed above, the common carotid arteries have variable points of bifurcation, are occasionally tortuous, and occasionally give rise to branches normally originating elsewhere. The variant bifurcation is more commonly found high than low and may be as high as the level of the hyoid bone and more rarely as low as the cricoid cartilage.[6] Tortuosity of the common carotid artery is occasionally found and in rare instances may form a complete loop in the neck. Branches of the external carotid artery sometimes found originating from the normally branchless common carotid include the superior and inferior thyroid, thyroidea ima, and ascending pharyngeal arteries. Rarely, a vertebral artery arises from a common carotid.

Arteries to the Head and Neck

External Carotid Artery

There is great variability in the number and origins of external carotid artery branches. The external carotid artery may occasionally be absent on one or both sides, in which case the branches of the missing vessel arise from the opposite external carotid or the common carotid.[7]

Internal Carotid Artery

In addition to the rare origin directly from the aortic arch, the internal carotid may be absent in approximately 0.1% of individuals.[7] Rare instances of external carotid branches arising from the internal carotid have been reported. The internal carotid may also exhibit tortuosity.

Subclavian Artery

The right subclavian artery is anomalous in approximately 1% of individuals. It may originate in any position from the first to the fourth relative to the other arch vessels, may rise higher or lower in the neck, and may vary in position relative to the scalene muscles.[7] Origin of the right subclavian artery as the first aortic arch branch implies the absence of the brachiocephalic trunk. More commonly, the right subclavian artery originates as the fourth aortic branch and passes behind or between the trachea and esophagus (Fig. 19-5) as discussed previously. In its course, the right subclavian artery may rise as high as 4 cm above the clavicle, depending on the level of brachiocephalic bifurcation. The subclavian artery may rarely be found anterior to the anterior scalene muscle together with the subclavian vein (occasionally the vein is found between the anterior and middle scalene muscles with the artery), may penetrate the middle scalene, or may pass between the middle and posterior scalene muscles. In rare instances, the subclavian artery may divide at the medial border of the scalene muscle into radial and ulnar arteries instead of continuing into the axillary artery.

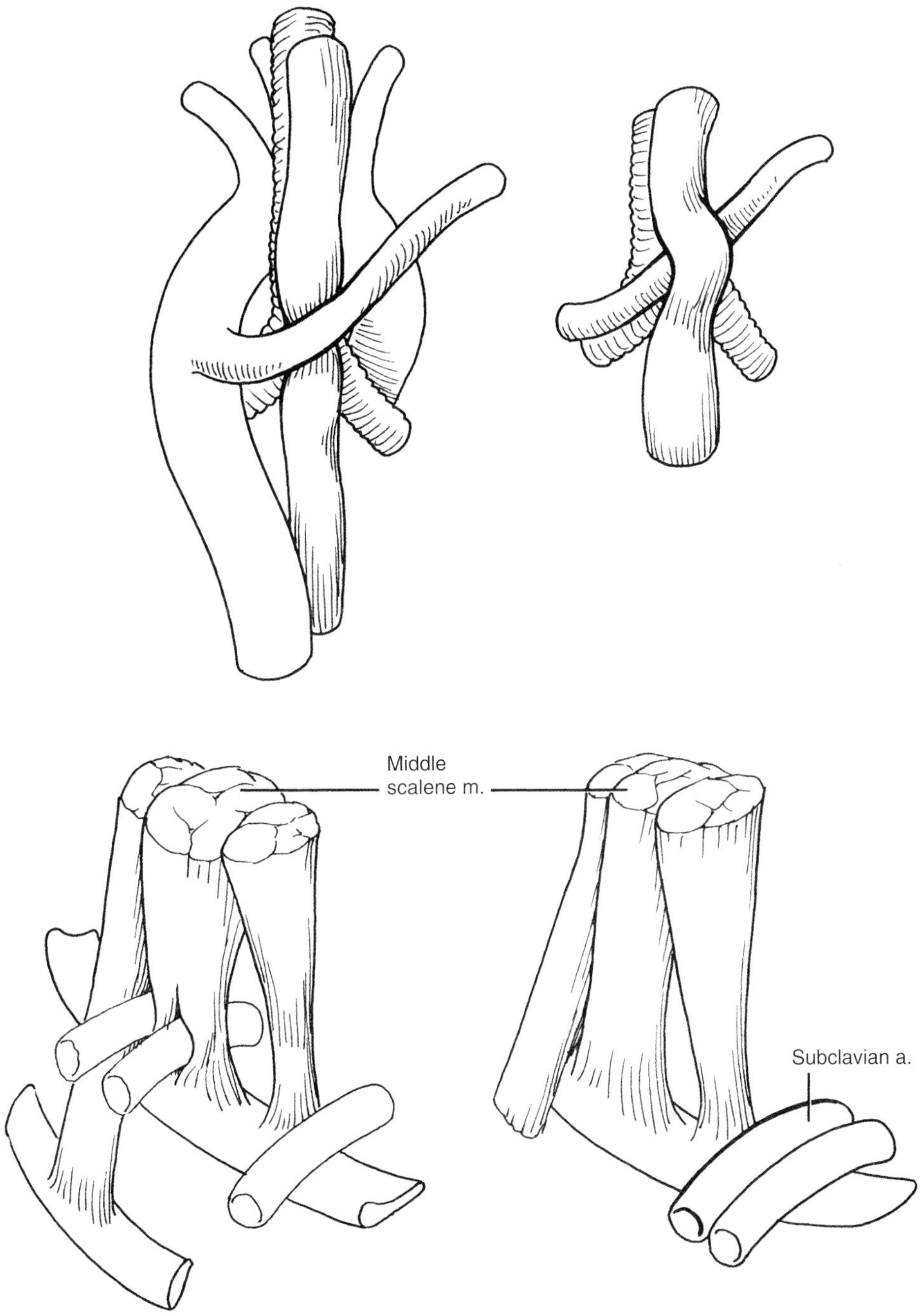

Fig. 19-5 When the right subclavian artery arises distally, it passes behind or between the trachea and esophagus to reach the right side (posterior view). The passage of the subclavian artery through the scalene muscles may vary.

Branches of the Subclavian Artery

The vertebral artery arose from the posterior superior surface of the subclavian artery between 0.5 and 2 cm medial to the thyrocervical trunk 83% of the time in the series of Daseler and Anson.[8] The most common variation of this vessel is an origin greater than 2 cm medial to the thyrocervical trunk, close to the origin of the subclavian artery (Fig. 19-6). In addition, the vertebral artery may arise from the thyrocervical or costocervical trunk, from the left common carotid, or directly from the aorta in rare instances.

The vertebral artery enters the sixth vertebral transverse foramen 88% of the time, the fifth and seventh with equal frequency (7%), and rarely even as high as the second foramen.

The internal thoracic artery, like the vertebral artery, follows the usual pattern in a relatively high percentage of cases (79%). Several common variations include origin as a common trunk with the thyrocervical trunk and origin from the suprascapular, inferior thyroid, transverse cervical, or a combination of these vessels. The point of origin from the subclavian artery also varies from proximal to distal.

The origins and branching patterns of the thyrocervical and costocervical trunks are so highly variable among individuals and between sides that the most common pattern for each is found in less than half of the population.[8]

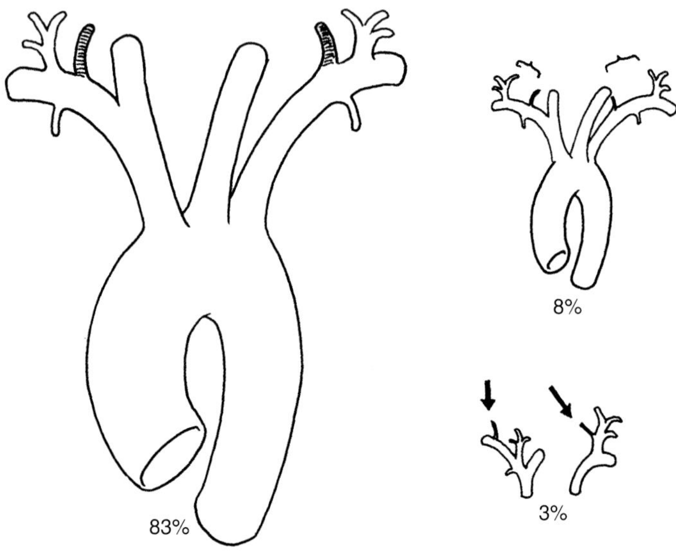

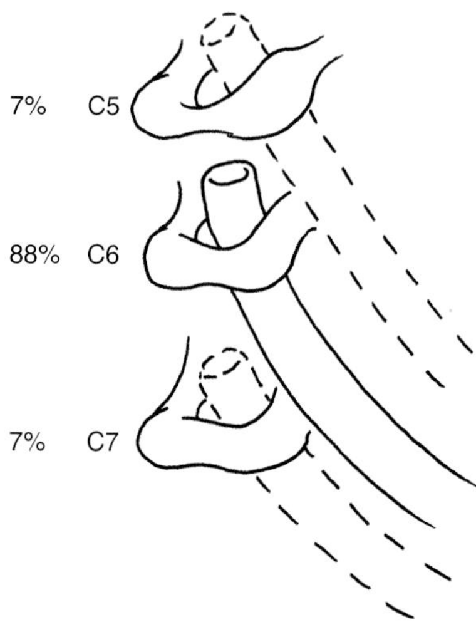

Fig. 19-6 The origins of the vertebral arteries vary somewhat as does that of the transverse foramen entered by the vessel.

Arteries of the Upper Extremity

Axillary Artery

The main trunk of the axillary artery is fairly constant. Significant variations include rare early branching into radial and ulnar arteries and the presence of a latissimus muscle slip over the third part of the vessel. The branches of the axillary artery, conversely, are so variable that the most common pattern occurred in only 20 of 47 bodies studied by Hitzrot.[9] Those contemplating mobilizing a pectoralis musculocutaneous flap based on the pectoral branch of the thoracoacromial artery or a latissimus dorsi flap based on the thoracodorsal branch of the subscapular artery should review this reference.

Brachial Artery

Major variations of the brachial artery have been found in 20% to 25% of individuals.[7] These variations most often take the form of high branching in the proximal third of the arm. Two-thirds of these are unilateral, and most of the remaining bilateral anomalies were different from side to side. Five patterns of early brachial artery branching have been suggested (Fig. 19-7): radial and ulnar common interosseous trunks; ulnar and radial common interosseous trunks; common interosseous or persistent median artery and radioulnar trunk; radial, ulnar, and common interosseous trunks; and a normal brachial artery with a long, thin aberrant branch that runs superficial to the median nerve and ends in the

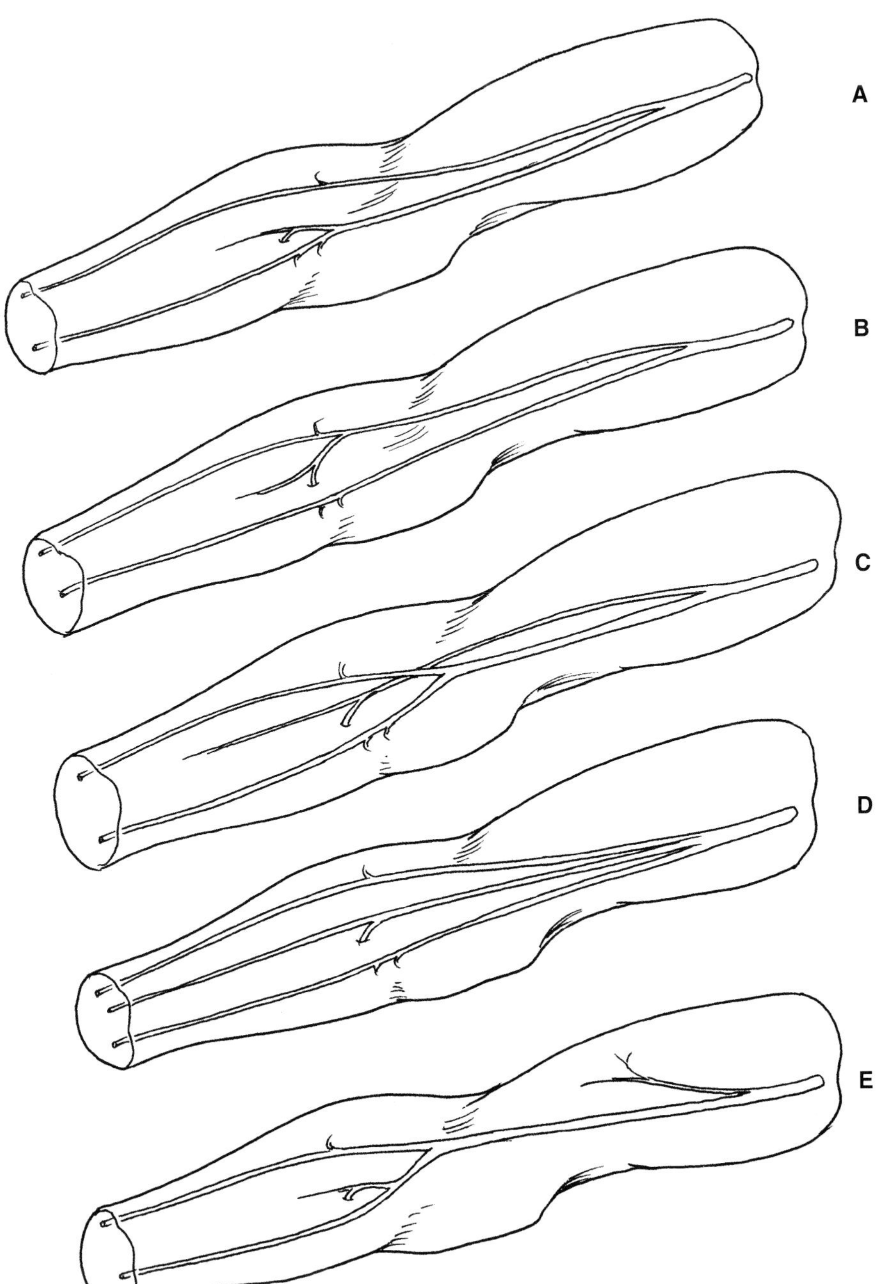

Fig. 19-7 Five patterns of high brachial artery branching: radial and ulnar common interosseous trunks **(A)**; ulnar and radial common interosseous trunks **(B)**; common interosseous or persistent median artery and radioulnar trunk **(C)**; radial, ulnar, and common interosseous trunks **(D)**; and a normal brachial artery with a long, thin aberrant branch that runs superficially to the median nerve and ends in the biceps muscle **(E)**.

biceps muscle. There are minor variations among the profunda, superior, and inferior ulnar collateral branches of the brachial artery in which they may arise from each other, share a common trunk, or replace each other.

Arteries of the Forearm

The radial and ulnar arteries may have high origins, as noted previously. When this occurs, the vessels in the forearm often lie in a more superficial plane than normal, usually just beneath the deep antebrachial fascia and, in rare cases, subcutaneously.[7] A persistent median artery may supplement or replace the radial or ulnar artery. The common interosseous artery and its volar and dorsal branches are variable in their origins, size, and terminations.

Arteries of the Hand

The superficial palmar arch is quite variable in form. Coleman and Anson,[10] in fact, found that an incomplete ulna-based arch is more common than the normal textbook description of a complete arch (Fig. 19-8). In addition, a median artery

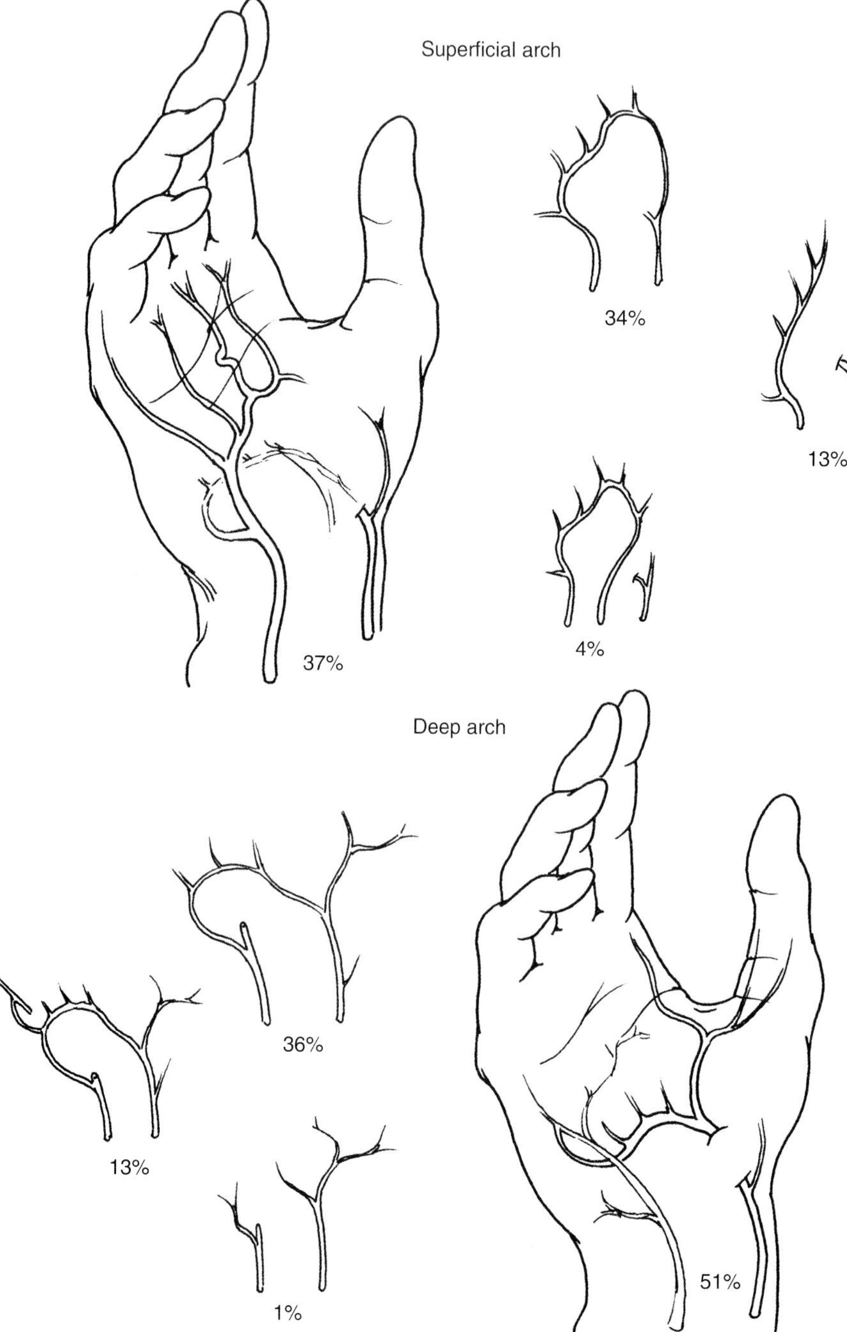

Fig. 19-8 The superficial palmar arch varies more than the deep arch and is most commonly incomplete.

completed or contributed to the arch in 5% of individuals. The deep arch is less variable than the superficial arch. Either arch may supplement small or missing branches of the other. The princeps pollicis and radial indicis arteries, in particular, may arise from either or both arches.

Abdominal Aorta

Variations and anomalies of the abdominal aorta are rare and mostly minor. These include variations in the level of bifurcation, tortuosity, and direct origin of normally secondary visceral branches. The most clinically significant abdominal aortic anomaly is the rare occurrence of coarctation (0.5% to 2% of all coarctations).[11,12] The narrowing is more diffuse than in the thoracic aorta and often involves stenosis of one or both renal arteries, making correction more complex. The secondary branches of the abdominal aorta are among the most variable in the body, in both their origin and course.

Branches of the Abdominal Aorta

Numerous minor variations are found in the paired somatic branches of the abdominal aorta. The inferior phrenic arteries may arise independently or from a common stem, may have supernumerary branches, and may arise from the aorta or from the celiac artery or its branches. The lumbar arteries also vary in their origins and number.

The visceral branches of the abdominal aorta are so highly variable that Nelson et al.[13] found that the celiac, superior mesenteric, and inferior mesenteric arteries followed the classic description in less than one-fourth of cases.

Celiac Trunk and Its Branches

The typical three-branched celiac trunk has been found in 60% to 89% of bodies (Fig. 19-9).

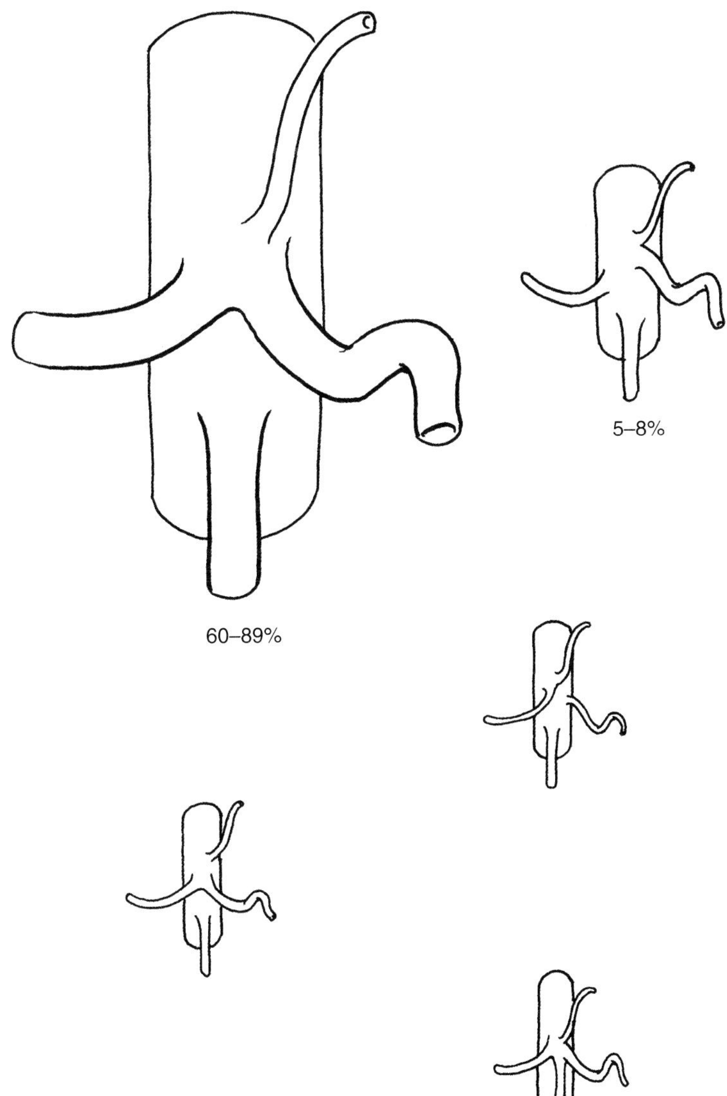

Fig. 19-9 Variations of the celiac trunk vessels are shown.

A gastrosplenic trunk with the hepatic artery arising from the aorta or superior mesenteric artery is the most common variant (5% to 8%). Hepatosplenic and hepatogastric trunks are somewhat less common variants. In rare instances, the superior mesenteric artery is combined with the celiac trunk.

The left gastric artery is relatively constant in its origin from the celiac trunk. The most frequent and significant variation of the left gastric artery is the origin of a branch to the left lobe of the liver in as many as one-fourth of specimens. This may supplement or replace the left hepatic branch of the proper hepatic artery. Inferior phrenic artery branches may also arise from the left gastric artery.

The common hepatic artery arose from the celiac trunk more than 80% of the time in the series of Daseler et al.,[14] but multiple variations in the origins of the right and left hepatic branches result in the classic description being found in only one-third of cases (Fig. 19-10). The most frequent variation of the common hepatic artery in this series was its absence in 12% of cases. In 4.4% of cases, it arose from the superior mesenteric artery. When the common hepatic artery is absent, the right and left hepatic arteries arise independently from the celiac trunk or its branches, the aorta, or the superior mesenteric artery.

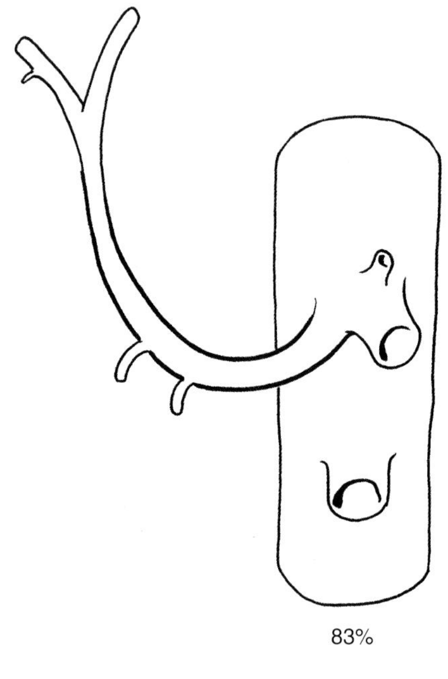

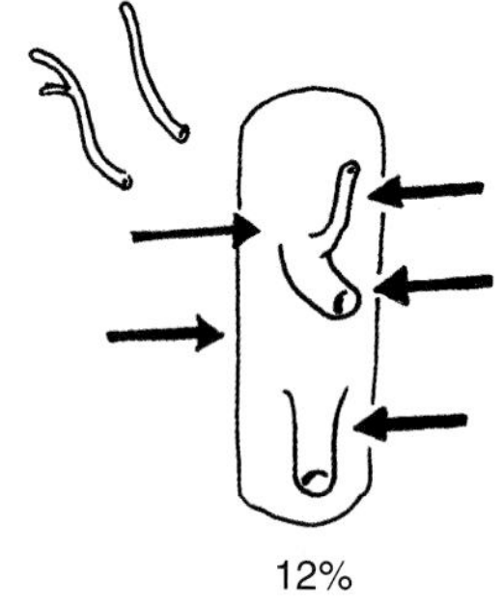

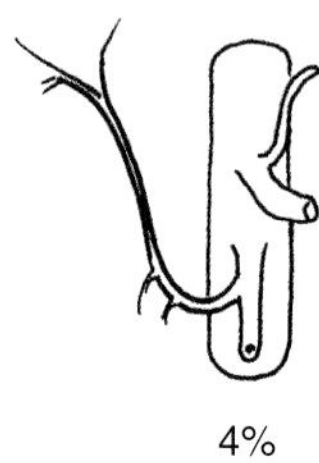

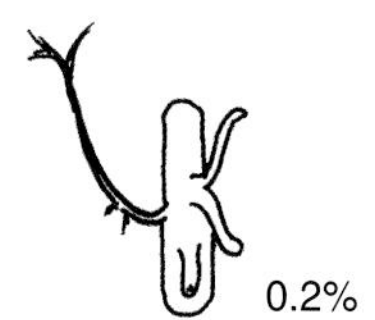

Fig. 19-10 The most frequent anomaly of the common hepatic artery is absence. The right and left hepatic arteries then arise from the aorta, the remaining celiac branches, or the superior mesenteric artery.

The common variations in origins of the right and left hepatic arteries are shown in Figure 19-11. An aberrant vessel is found for each artery one-fourth of the time. Most often the aberrant vessel replaces the standard branch off the proper hepatic artery, and the remaining aberrant vessels are accessory branches.

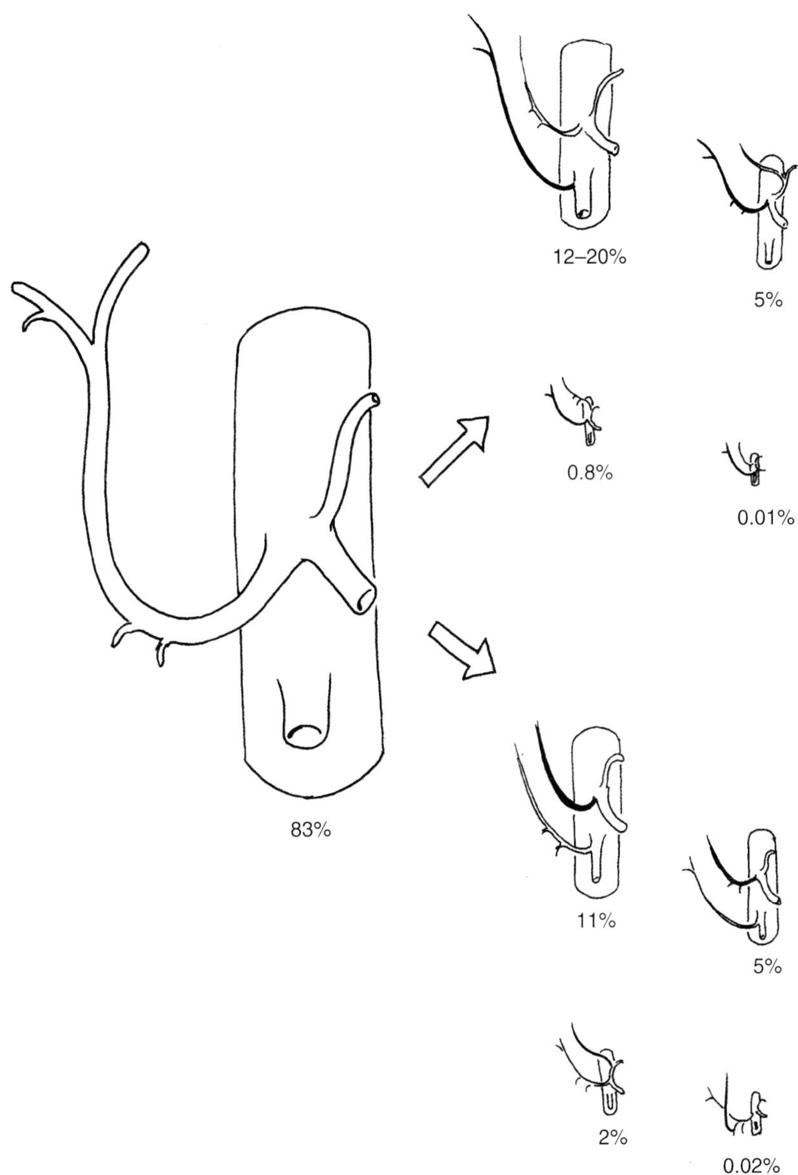

Fig. 19-11 Anomalous origins of the hepatic arteries are shown.

The cystic artery most commonly (70%) arises from a normal right hepatic artery (Fig. 19-12), with the remainder arising from several alternative sources.

In addition, accessory cystic arteries, also arising most often from the right hepatic artery, were found 11% of the time by Daseler et al.

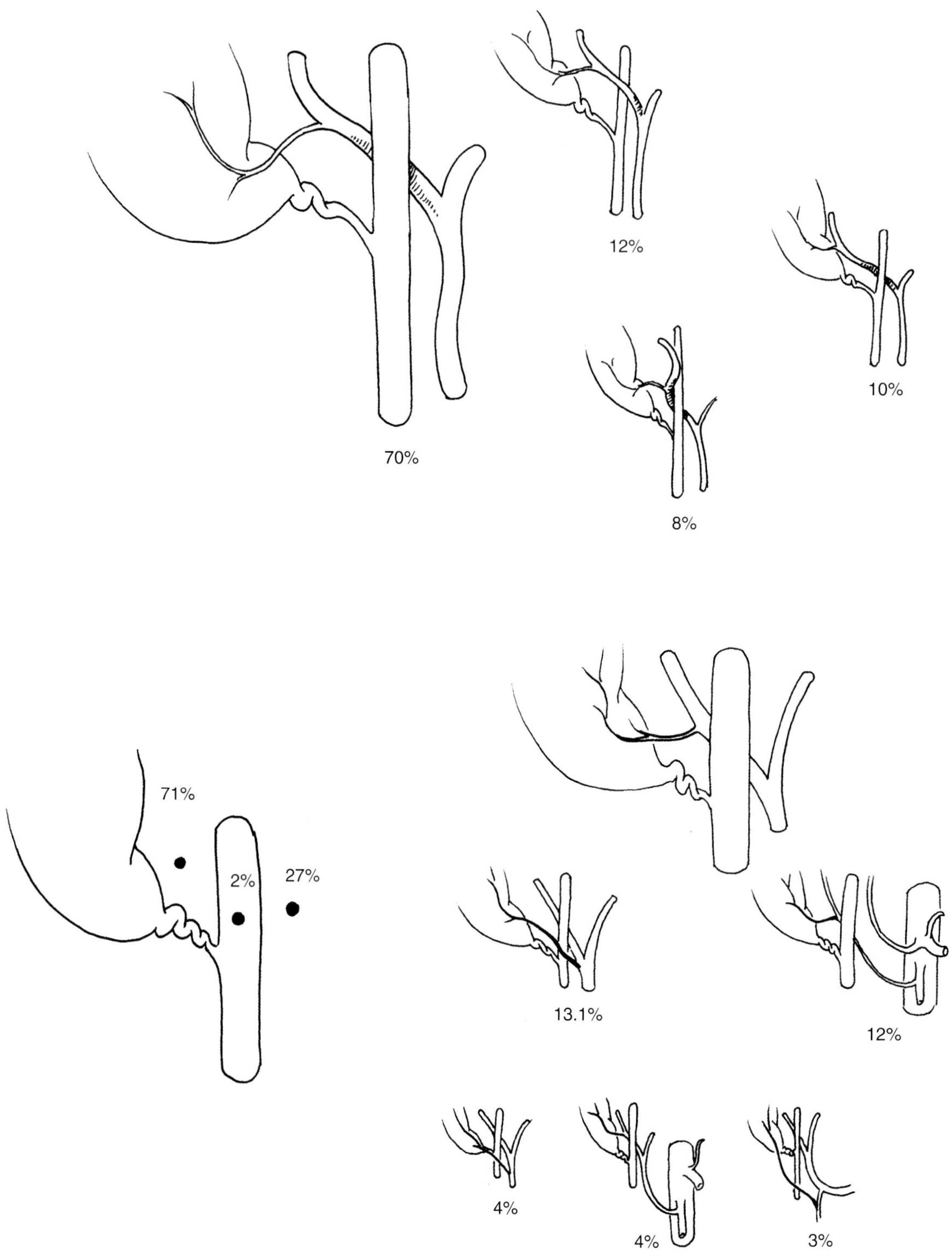

Fig. 19-12 The right hepatic artery varies in position relative to the common hepatic duct (*top*), and the origin and course of the cystic artery vary (*bottom*).

The gastroduodenal artery arises from the common hepatic artery in three-fourths of cases, with three other variations accounting for 94% of instances[14] (Fig. 19-13).

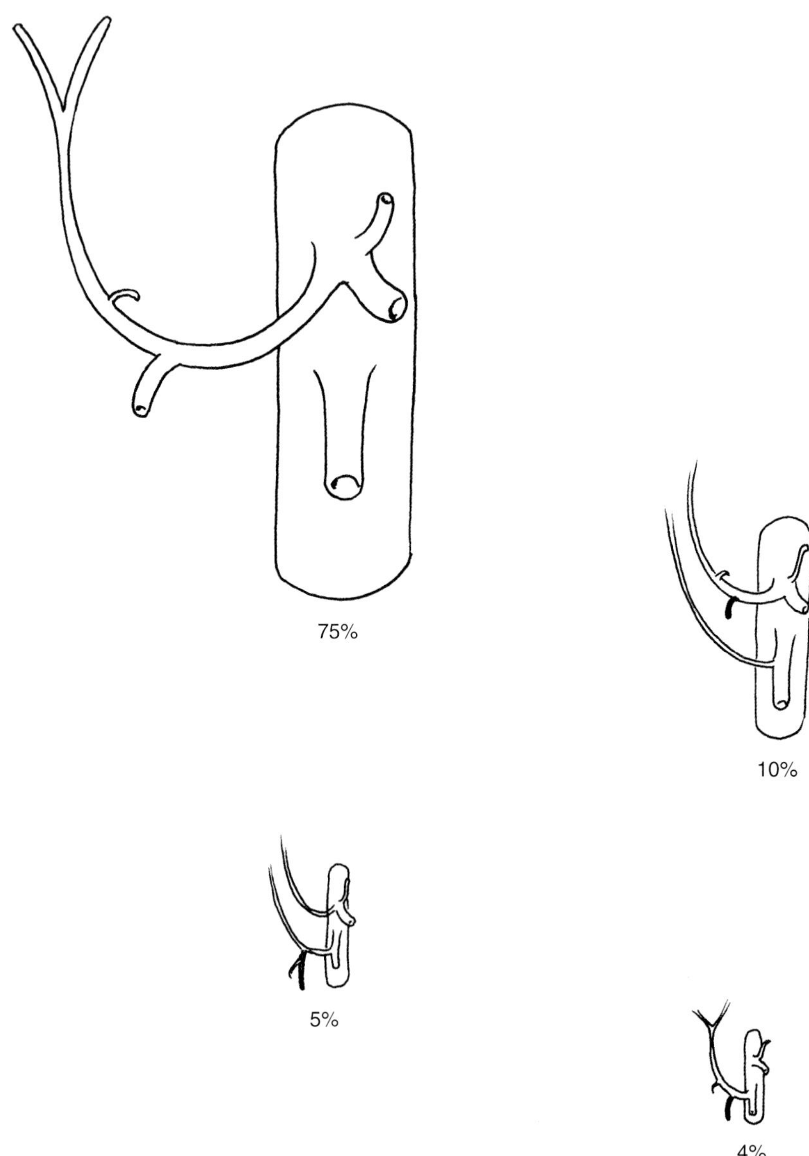

Fig. 19-13 Anomalous gastroduodenal artery origins are often secondary to hepatic artery anomalies.

In the series of Daseler et al., the right gastric artery arose from the common hepatic artery 50% of the time, the left hepatic 32%, the gastroduodenal 9%, and the right hepatic 4% (Fig. 19-14).

The tortuous splenic artery exhibits several variations in addition to the permutations of celiac branching discussed previously. It may arise from the superior mesenteric artery, and it may give rise to the left gastric, middle colic, or left hepatic artery. There may be two splenic arteries, with one or both arising directly from the aorta.

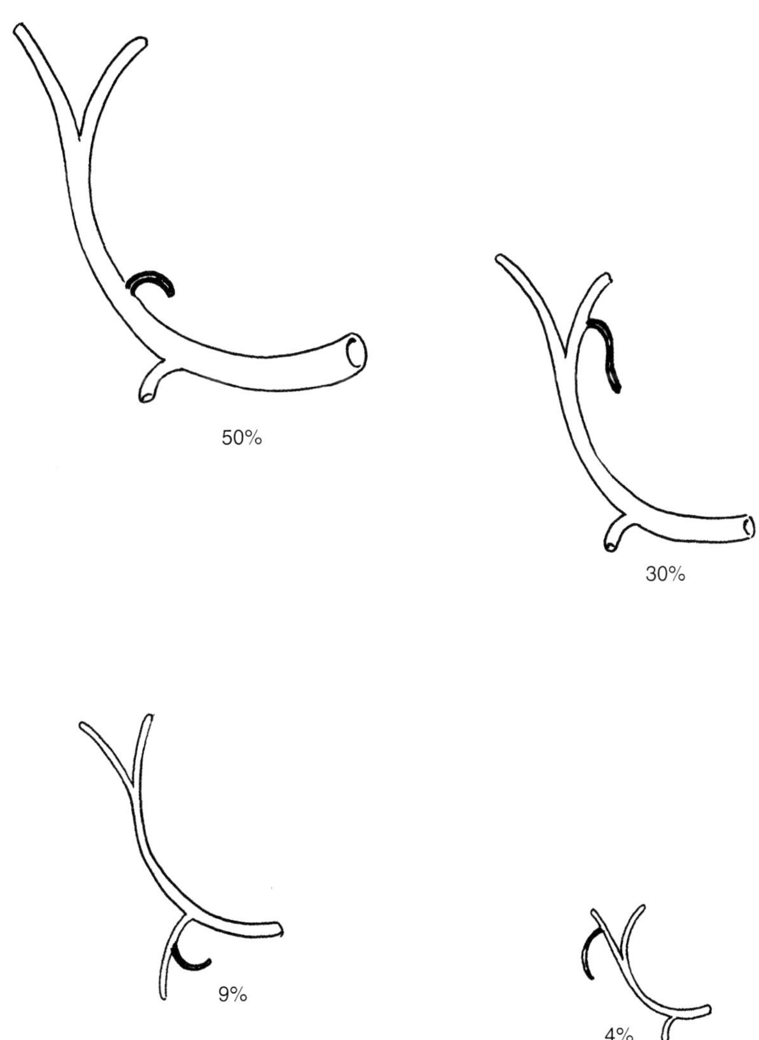

Fig. 19-14 Variations in the origin of the right gastric artery are shown on a single hepatic artery stem for simplicity.

Superior Mesenteric Artery

The superior mesenteric artery, like the other unpaired visceral branches of the abdominal aorta, has many variations. It may originate from the celiac trunk or as two separate trunks from the aorta. It may give rise to the splenic, right, left, or common hepatic artery or a combination of these vessels. A right hepatic artery from the superior mesenteric artery has been found in 12% to 20% of cases and may replace or supplement the usual right hepatic. The superior mesenteric artery may also provide accessory branches to the stomach, pancreas, or spleen. It may also provide left colic and superior rectal branches that replace the inferior mesenteric artery. The greatest variability in the superior mesenteric artery is found in its colic branches. Sonneland et al.[15] divided these variations into seven types (Fig. 19-15).

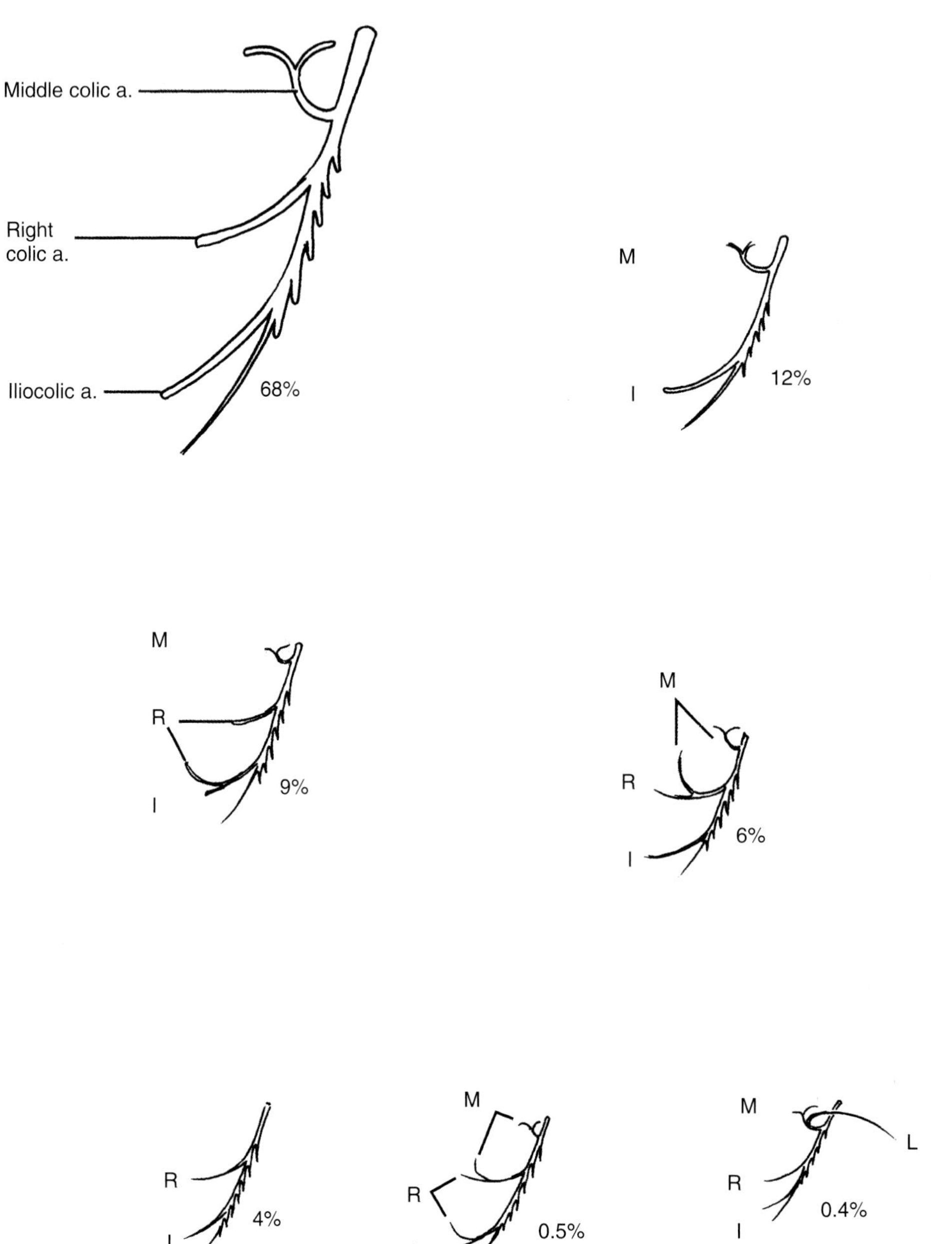

Fig. 19-15 Colic branches of the superior mesenteric artery vary by their absence or duplication.

Inferior Mesenteric Artery

The origin and position of the inferior mesenteric artery vary little.[16] The branching into left colic and superior rectal trunks was also relatively constant. The variability arises in the origins of sigmoidal vessels from the two primary branches and the interconnections between these vessels. Rare anomalies include duplication, absence, origin from the left common iliac, and contribution of accessory branches to the liver or kidneys.[7]

Renal Arteries

The number, source, and course of the renal arteries exhibit a moderate degree of variation. In a review of 45 series documenting vascular patterns in 10,967 kidneys,[7] a single artery to each kidney was found 72% of the time. A single artery having an upper polar branch was found 13% of the time. Two hilar vessels were present in 11% of cases, there was a hilar artery with an upper pole branch arising from the aorta in 6%, and 3% had a hilar and an aortic lower polar branch (Fig. 19-16). In 2.7% of cases, there were two hilar vessels, one of which had an upper polar branch, and in 1.7%, there were three hilar vessels. It is not uncommon to find a single vessel on one side and multiple vessels on the other.

The left renal artery can be located using the left renal vein as a landmark. The artery is most commonly found deep to the cephalad border of the vein.[17] The level of the renal arteries is usually between 2 cm above and below the L1-2 intervertebral disc. The renal artery may divide into anterior and posterior trunks anywhere along its course and has between two and five branches at the renal hilus.

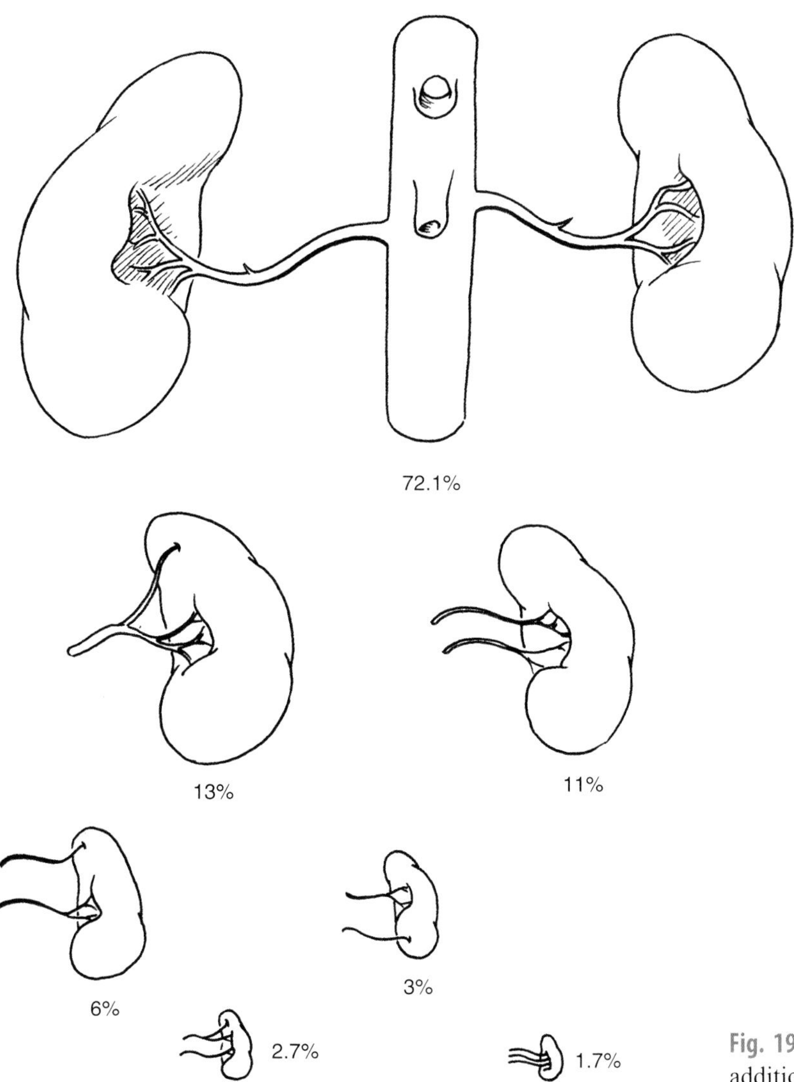

Fig. 19-16 Renal artery anomalies consist of additional hilar and/or polar vessels.

Suprarenal Arteries

A large variety of patterns characterizes the superior, middle, and inferior suprarenal arteries (Fig. 19-17). The superior suprarenal arteries invariably (96%) come from the inferior phrenic arteries (recall the variable origins of the inferior phrenics), and there may be three to 30 branches. The middle suprarenal is single 85% of the time and may arise from the aorta, inferior phrenic, renal, celiac, or superior renal polar vessel. The inferior suprarenal artery may arise from the renal (46%) or aorta (30%) or both (23%), may be absent (12%), and is multiple 11% of the time (average of three).

Gonadal Vessels

The gonadal vessels may be multiple and may originate anywhere along the abdominal aorta and its branches.

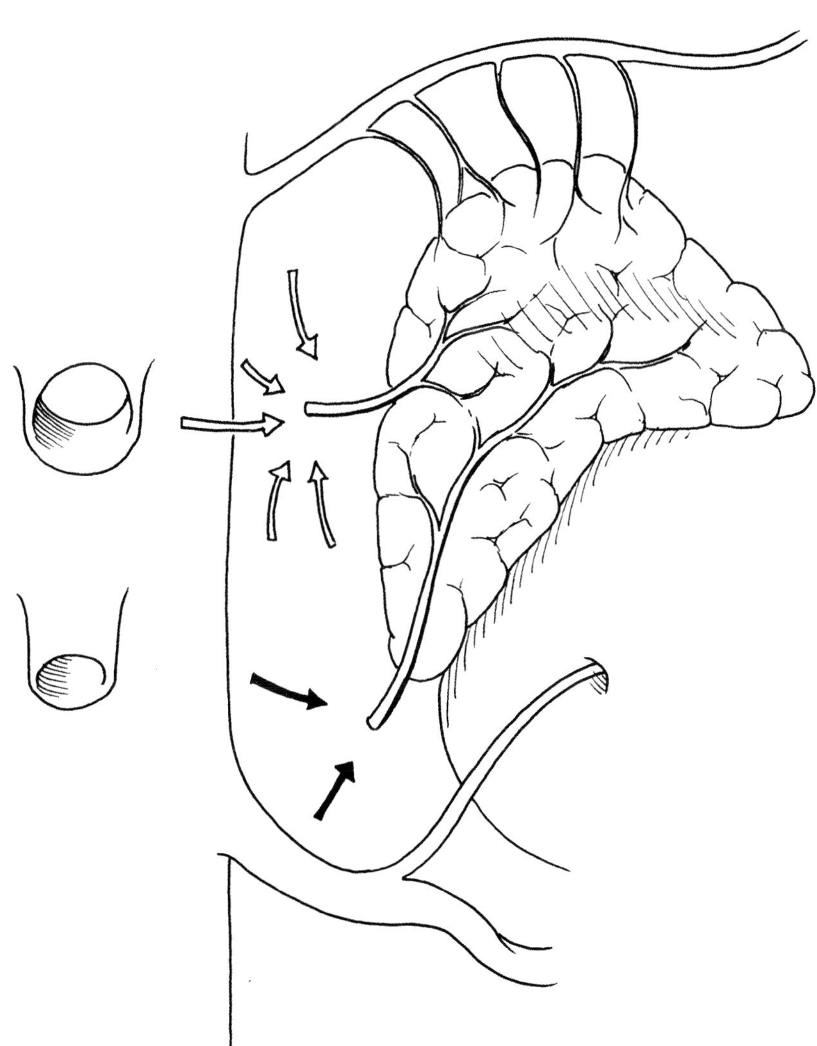

Fig. 19-17 Alternate sites of origin of the middle and inferior suprarenal arteries are shown.

Mesenteric Vascular Compression

Two additional conditions involving aortic visceral branches should be noted: median arcuate ligament syndrome and superior mesenteric artery syndrome.

Compression of the celiac trunk by the median arcuate ligament (Fig. 19-18) may cause a critical reduction of blood flow that is manifested by abdominal pain and an upper abdominal bruit. It is likely that an

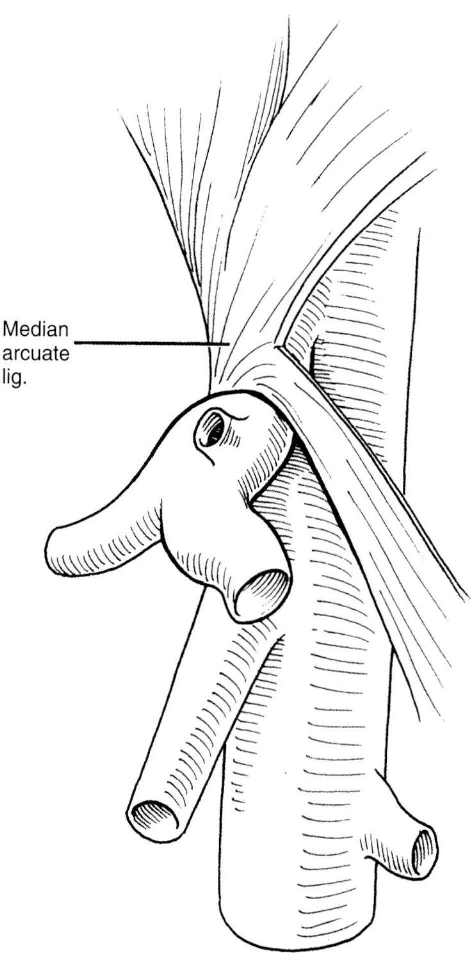

Fig. 19-18 The celiac trunk may be compressed by a low-lying median arcuate ligament.

unusually low placement of the arcuate ligament rather than a high celiac trunk is the primary pathology.[18]

Compression of the third portion of the duodenum by the superior mesenteric artery may cause duodenal obstructive symptoms and weight loss. In some cases, narrowing of the mesenteric-aortic angle (Fig. 19-19) has been attributed to an extrinsic source of compression, such as a body cast or prolonged bed rest in a supine position.[19] Other postulated causes include spinal curvature, rapid weight loss (with loss of the angular fat pad), or a combination of anatomic idiosyncrasies.

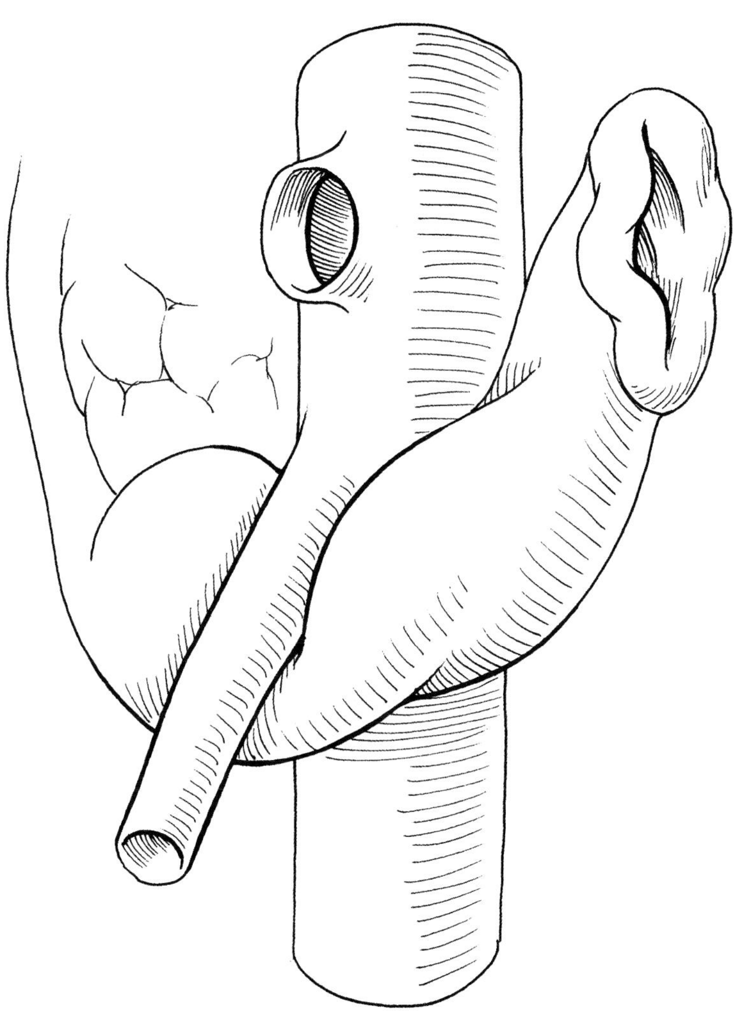

Fig. 19-19 Compression of the duodenum by the superior mesenteric artery is poorly understood.

Arteries of the Pelvis

Common Iliac Arteries

The length of the common iliac arteries depends on the levels at which the aorta and common iliac arteries bifurcate. In the extreme case, both the external and internal iliac arteries may arise directly from the end of the aorta without a common trunk. The common iliac occasionally gives rise to lumbar, sacral, renal, or gonadal branches and rarely to a middle colic, umbilical, obturator, or circumflex iliac branch.

Internal Iliac Artery

The internal iliac artery has a highly variable branching pattern. It may or may not divide into anterior and posterior divisions. Braithwaite[20] documented the branching patterns of the parietal vessels, that is, the internal pudendal and superior and inferior gluteal arteries (Fig. 19-20). The visceral

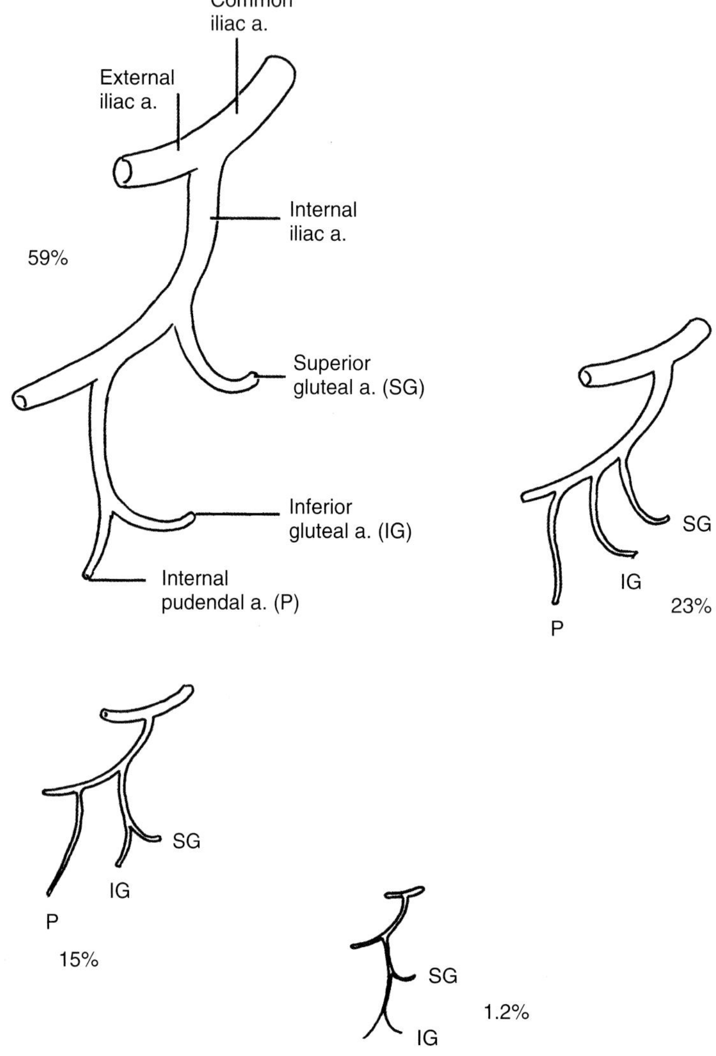

Fig. 19-20 Parietal branch patterns of the internal iliac artery are shown.

branches (vesicle, uterine, and middle rectal) and the obturator artery frequently appear in varying combinations.[6] The most variable branch of the internal iliac is the obturator, which is most often a direct branch of the anterior division.[20] The multiple alternate sites of origin and frequencies are shown in Figure 19-21. The most clinically significant variation is the inferior epigastric origin in one of five individuals, which poses a danger during herniorrhaphy (see Fig. 15-9).

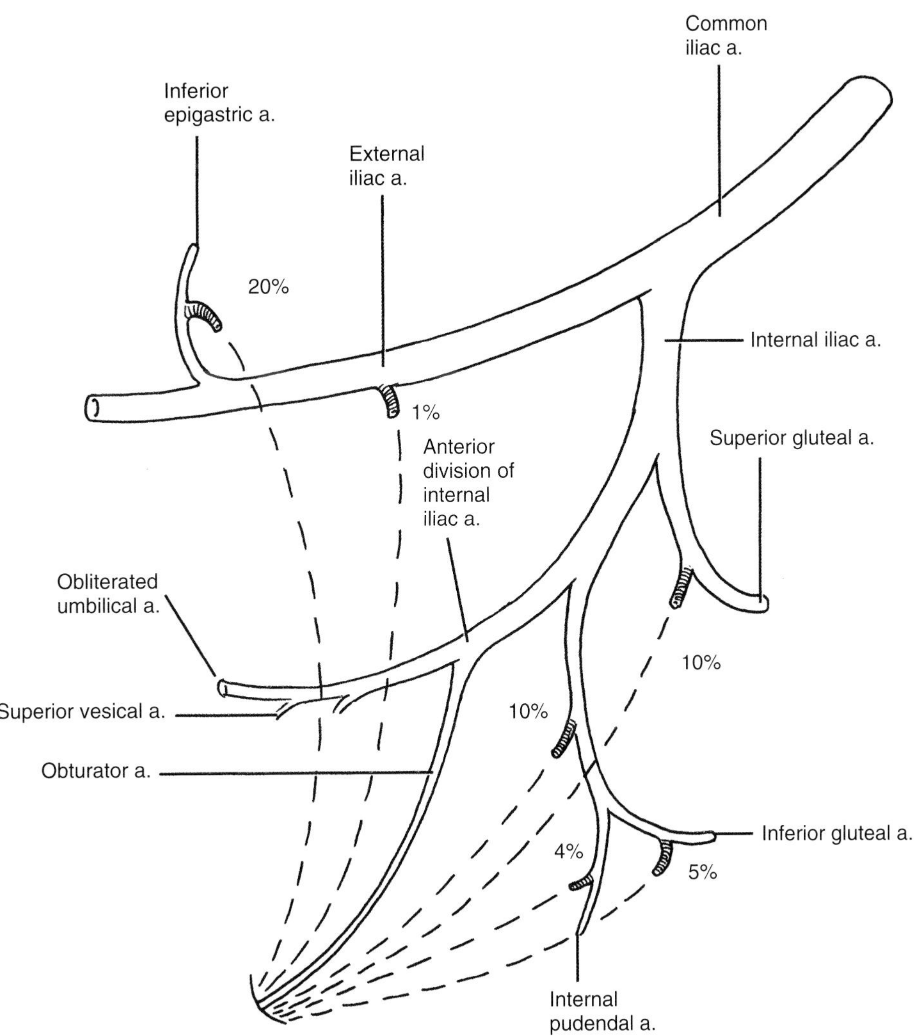

Fig. 19-21 Origins of the highly variable obturator artery include virtually every pelvic vessel.

In rare instances, a persistent sciatic artery from the inferior gluteal may constitute the major arterial supply to the lower extremity, continuing down to the popliteal[21] (Fig. 19-22). In such cases, the external iliac artery ends as the profunda femoris artery in the thigh.

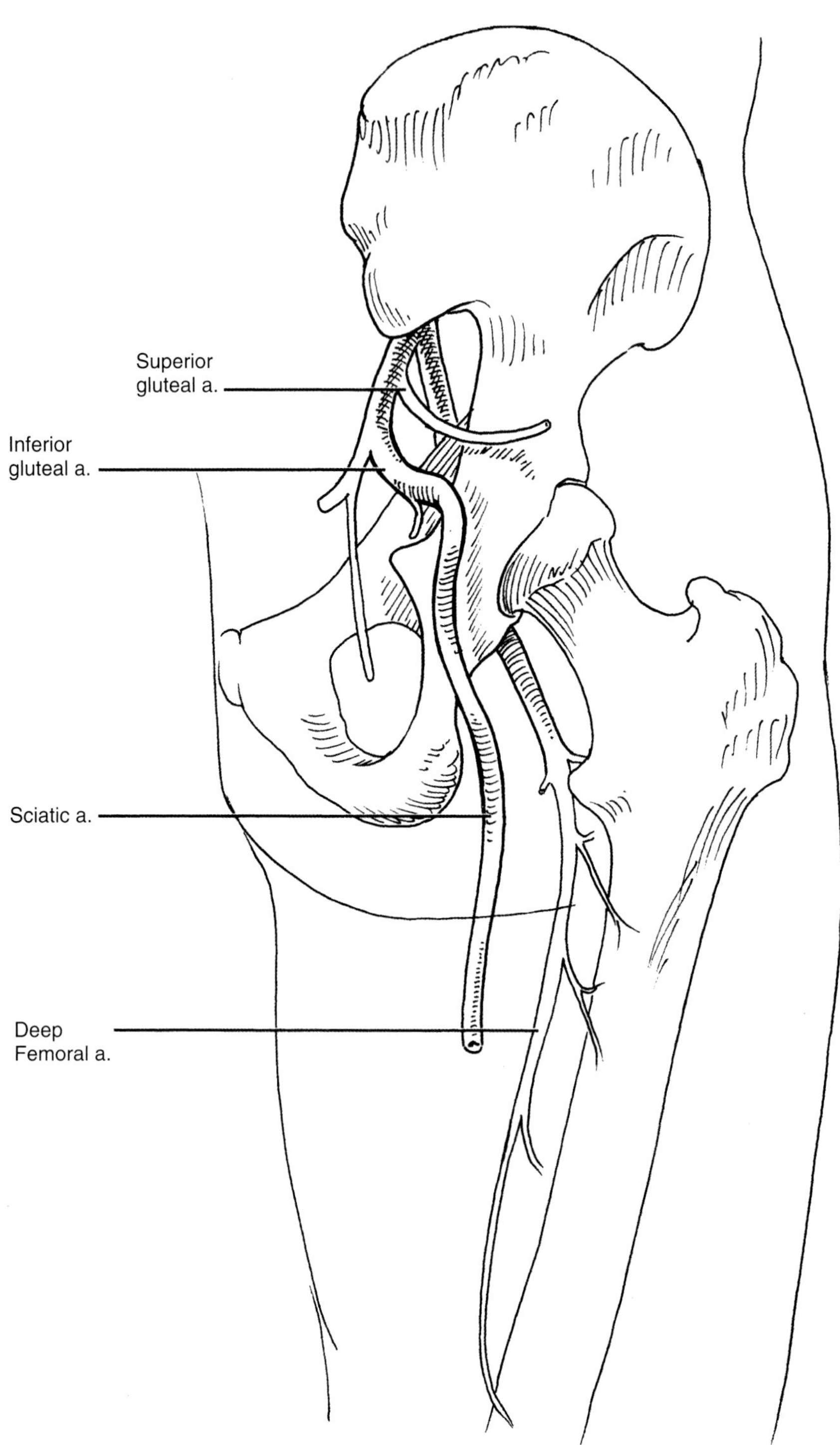

Fig. 19-22 Persistence of the sciatic artery may be associated with absence of the superficial femoral artery.

External Iliac Artery

The external iliac artery exhibits little variability. It may be tortuous or reduced in the presence of the persistent sciatic artery mentioned previously. One of its two usual branches, the inferior epigastric artery, may arise as many as several centimeters proximal to the inguinal ligament. The other branch, the deep circumflex iliac, may be absent, multiple, or arise in common with the inferior epigastric artery and may give rise to the external pudendal, medial, or lateral femoral circumflex artery.

Arteries of the Lower Extremity

Common and Superficial Femoral Arteries

The common femoral artery may give rise to branches more commonly originating from contiguous vessels (e.g., inferior epigastric, deep circumflex iliac, circumflex femoral vessels). Occasionally a greater saphenous artery arises from the superficial femoral artery in the adductor canal and leaves the canal to accompany the great saphenous vein at the knee.[7]

Profunda Femoris Artery

In one-third of individuals, the profunda femoris arises closer than 2.5 or farther than 5.1 cm from the inguinal ligament. In 89% of cases, the profunda arises lateral to the posterior midline of the common femoral and courses laterally. The vessel is directly posterior in 37%, directly lateral in 12%, and posterolateral in 40%.[22] The other 11% of the time, the profunda arises toward the medial side of the common femoral artery.

In 50% to 60% of cases, the medial and lateral femoral circumflex arteries arise from the proximal profunda. The medial and lateral circumflex arteries arise from the common femoral artery 20% and 13% of the time, respectively[23] (Fig. 19-23). The profunda has between two and six perforating branches excluding the termination of the artery.

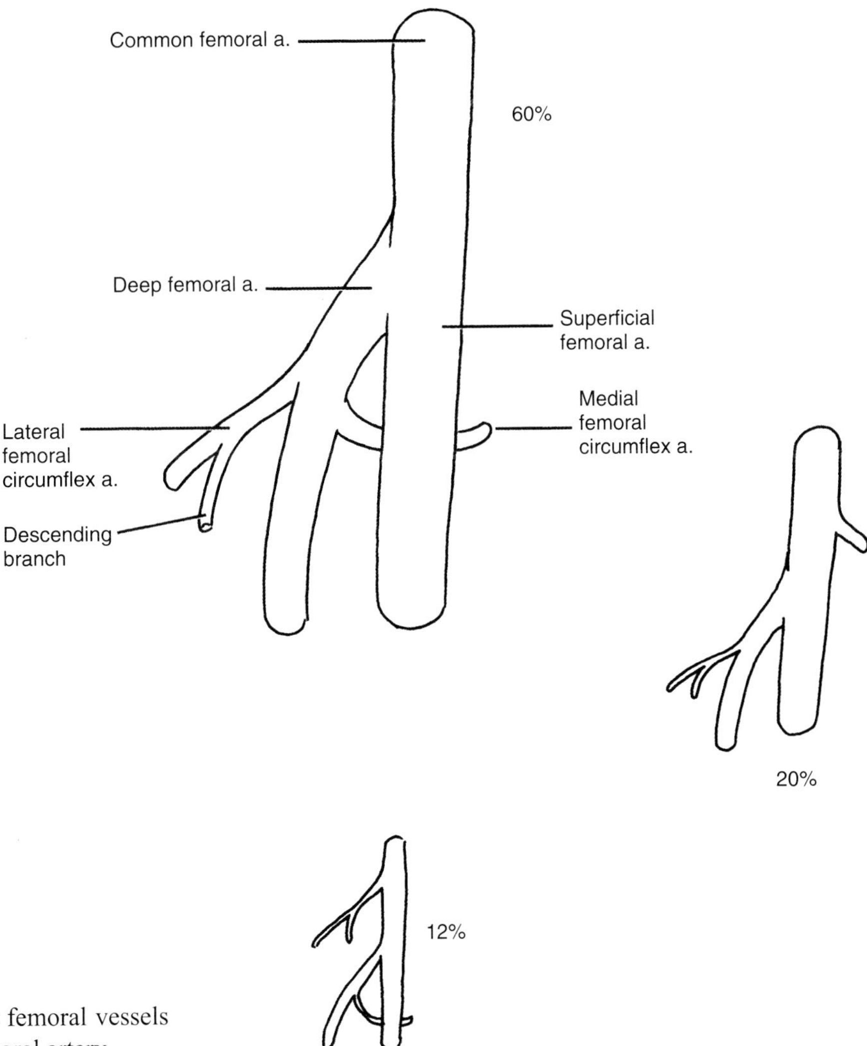

Fig. 19-23 One of the circumflex femoral vessels often arises from the common femoral artery.

Popliteal Artery

Intrinsic variations of the popliteal artery involve its terminal branching pattern. Most often the anterior tibial artery branches off first, leaving a tibioperoneal trunk that divides into posterior tibial and peroneal arteries (Fig. 19-24). When the anterior tibial artery arises abnormally high, it may pass deep to the popliteus muscle and be compressed. Approximately 3% of the time, the popliteal artery may end in a true trifurcation.[7,24] Rarely, the peroneal artery may arise from the anterior tibial artery or have a low origin.

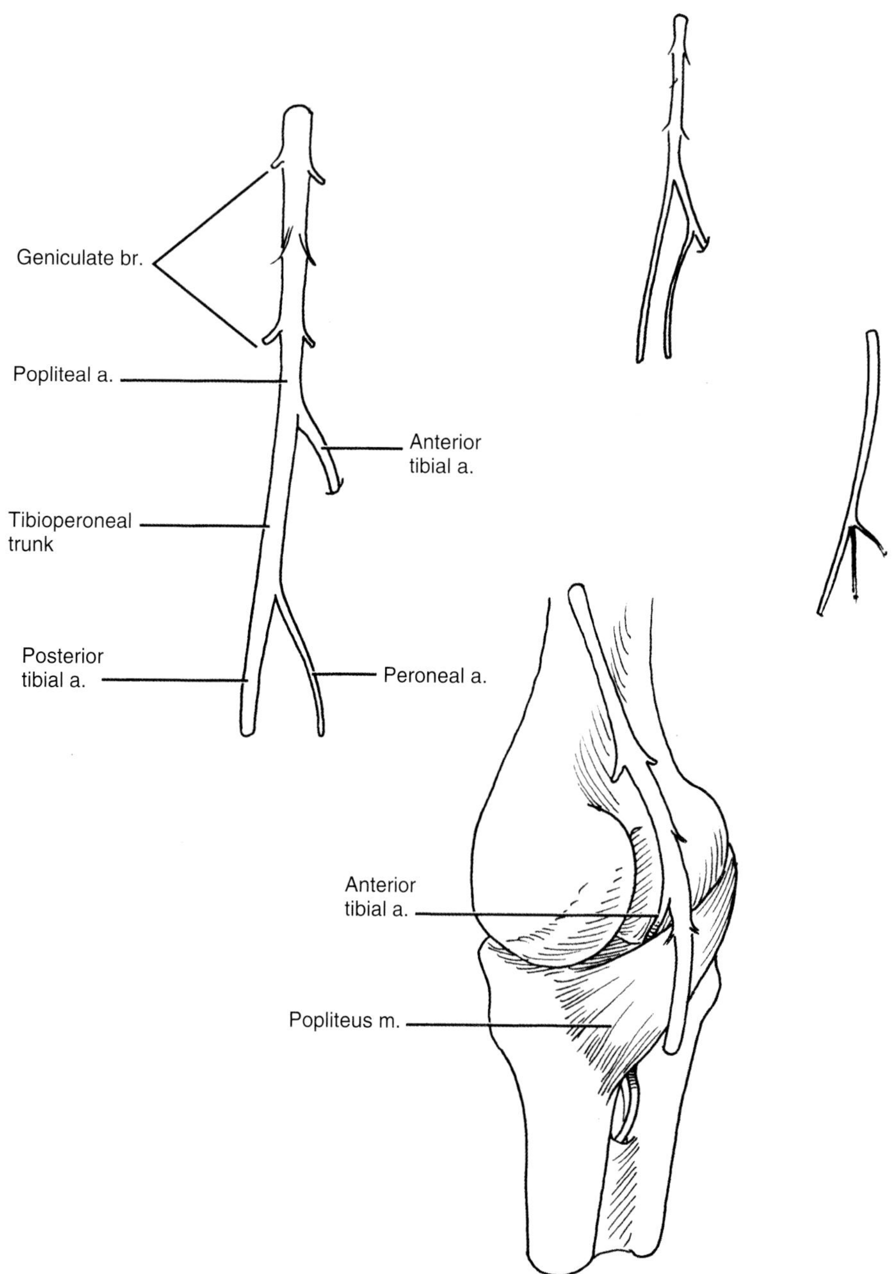

Fig. 19-24 Branch patterns of the leg vessels include a high origin of the anterior tibial artery that then passes deep to the popliteus muscle.

An extrinsic anatomic variant involving the popliteal artery occurs when the vessel follows an aberrant course relative to the calf muscles[25] (Fig. 19-25). The artery may pass medial to a normal or abnormal origin of the medial head of the gastrocnemius (Fig. 19-25B and C), may pass through the muscle (Fig. 19-25D), and in addition may pass deep to the popliteus (Fig. 19-25E). Intermittent compression may cause calf claudication and degenerative changes in the vessel. This condition should be suspected in young patients with calf claudication.

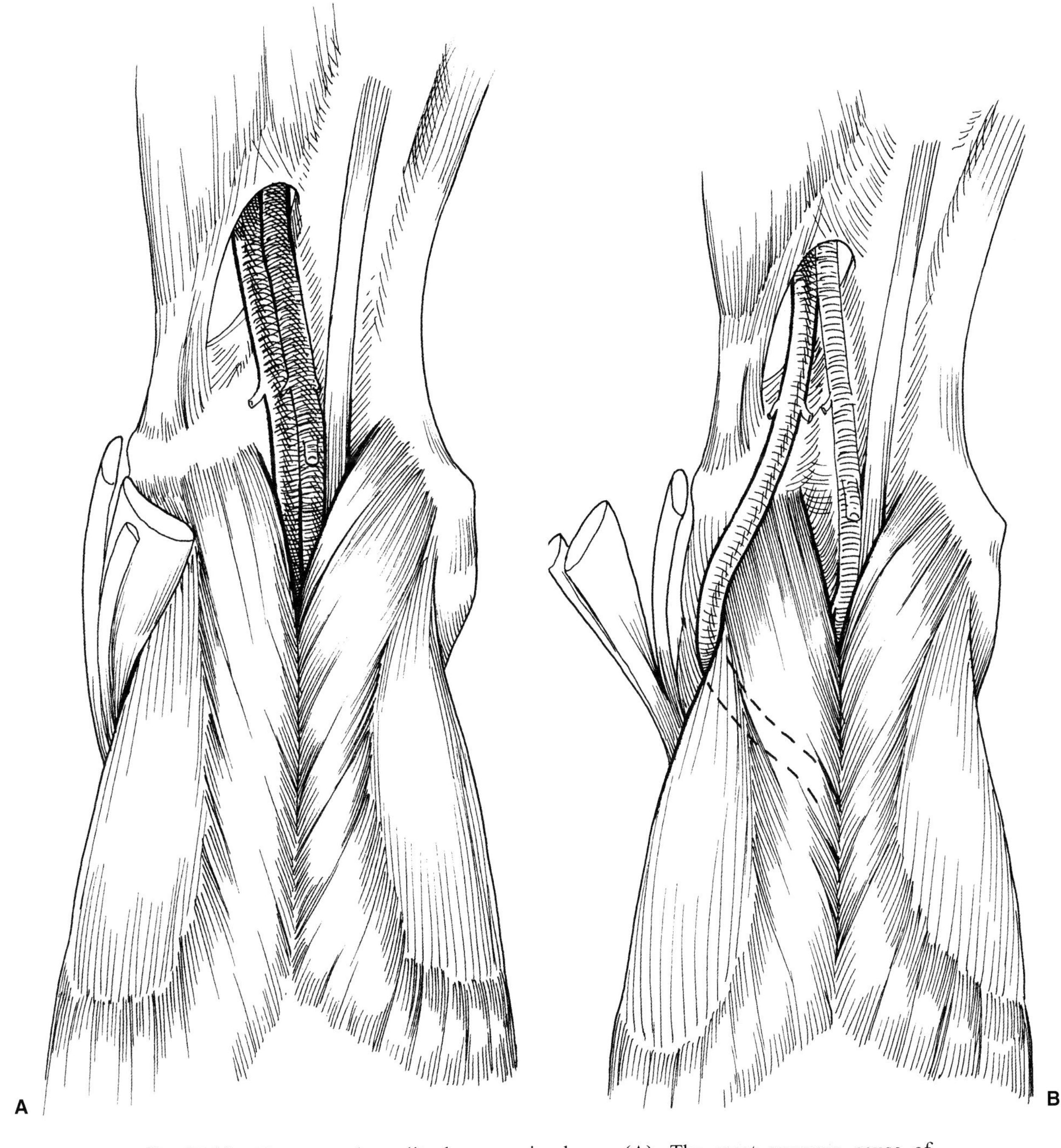

Fig. 19-25 The normal popliteal course is shown **(A)**. The most common cause of popliteal entrapment is medial displacement of the artery around a normal medial head of the gastrocnemius muscle **(B)**.

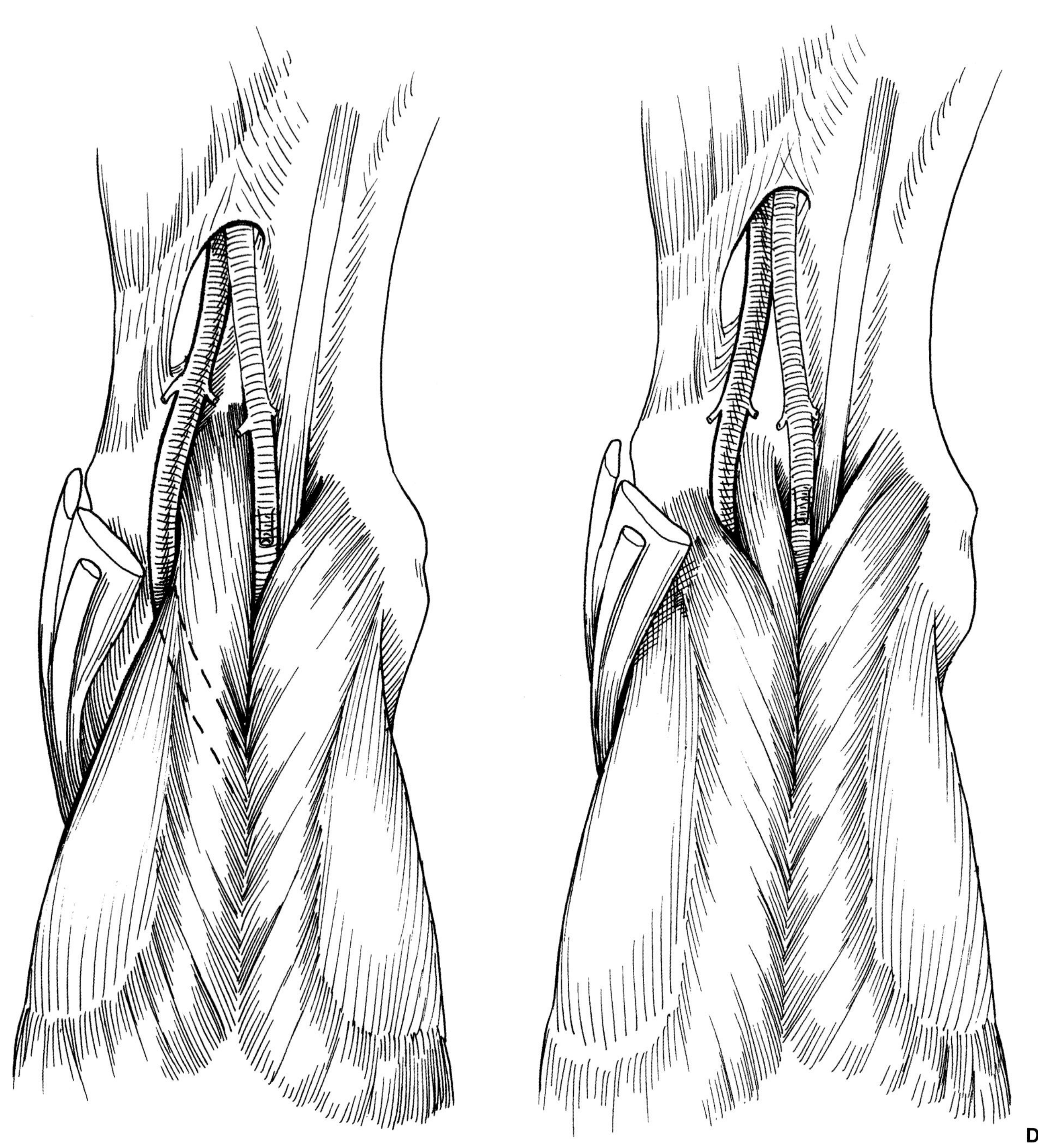

Fig. 19-25 The vessel may be diverted by an abnormal muscle origin **(C)**, pass through the muscle **(D)**, or pass beneath the popliteus muscle **(E)**.

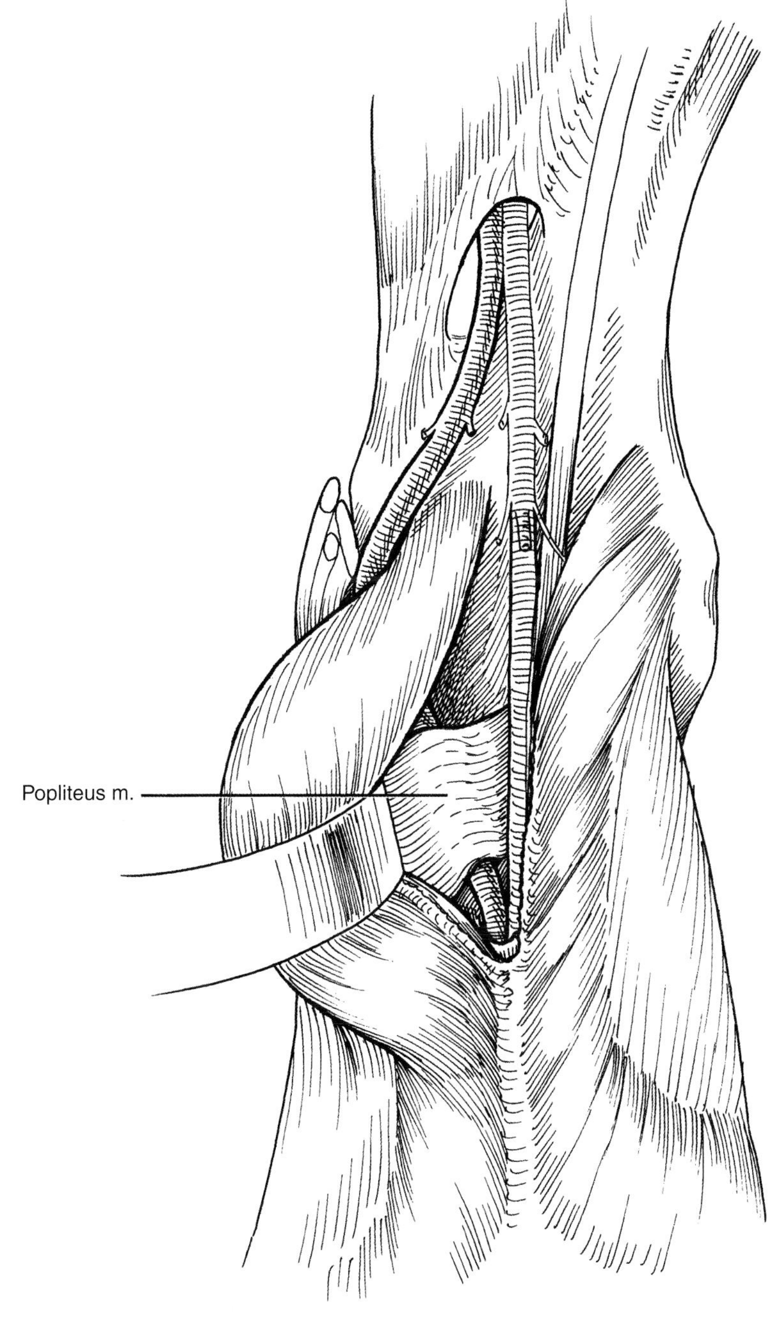

Fig. 19-25 *(continued)*

Arteries of the Leg

In addition to the variations in their origins, each of the three vessels of the leg may be enlarged, reduced, or absent[7] (Fig. 19-26). The most common pattern (Fig. 19-26A) is anterior and posterior tibial arteries continuing into the foot. Approximately 5% of the time, the posterior tibial artery is absent and the plantar vessels are a continuation of the peroneal artery (Fig. 19-26B). Four percent of the time, the anterior tibial may be small or absent

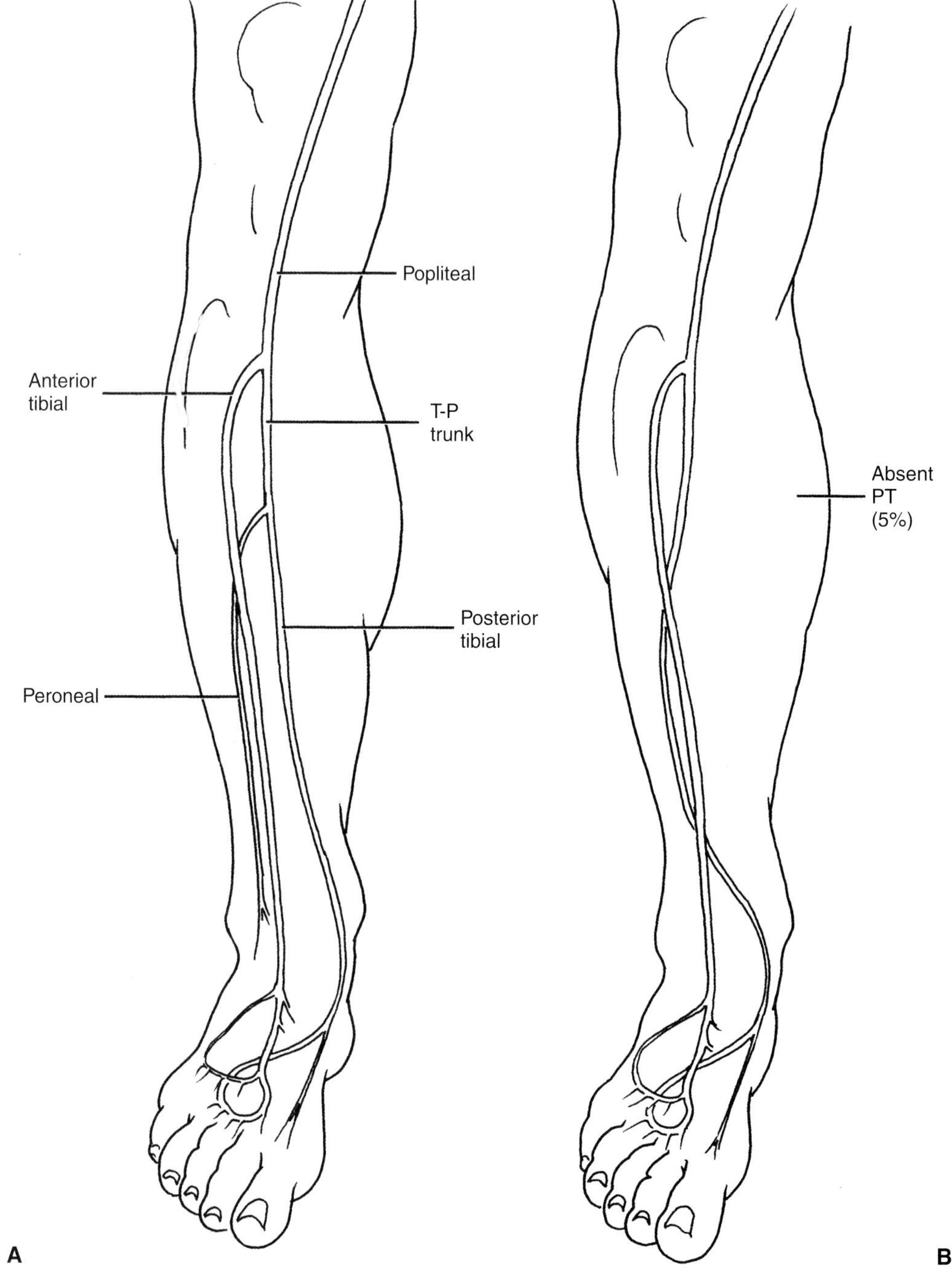

Fig. 19-26 Branch patterns of the leg arteries. In the most common form, the anterior tibial and posterior tibial arteries are continuous to the foot **(A)**. Variations include the absence of the posterior tibial artery with plantar vessels continuing from the peroneal artery **(B)**, absence of the anterior tibial artery with the dorsalis pedis artery continuing from the perforating branch of the peroneal artery **(C)**, and the posterior tibial artery passing through the interosseous membrane to join the anterior tibial artery, with plantar arteries continuing from the peroneal artery **(D)**.

(Fig. 19-26C). The dorsalis pedis artery in such cases is a continuation of the perforating branch of the peroneal artery. Occasionally, the posterior tibial penetrates the interosseous membrane and joins thc anterior tibial artery (Fig. 19-26D). The plantar vessels then arise from the peroneal artery. When one vessel is reduced, its territory is supplied by one or more of the companion vessels.

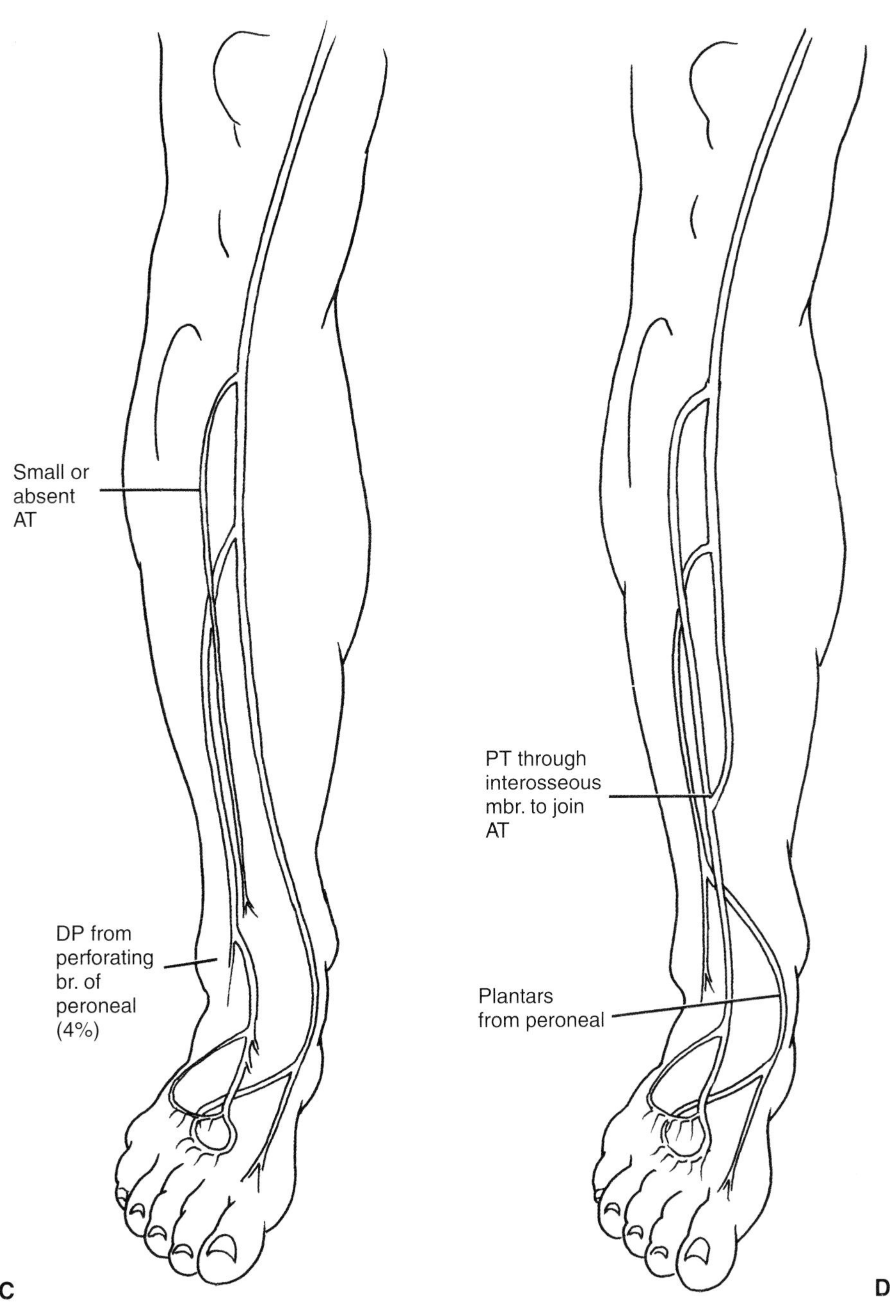

Fig. 19-26 *(continued)*

Arteries of the Foot

The dorsalis pedis artery is usually a continuation of the anterior tibial artery, and the plantar vessels are usually a continuation of the posterior tibial artery with the previously noted exceptions.[7] There is minor variation in the branching of the dorsalis pedis artery. The lateral plantar artery is usually the dominant side of the plantar arch, but there is some variation in relative contributions between the lateral plantar and dorsalis pedis arteries. The extent and size of communications between the dorsal and plantar vessels vary slightly. There are minor variations in the origins of the digital vessels.[26]

Veins

Beyond the secondary branching away from the venae cavae, the normal anatomic condition for the veins accompanying major arteries is to be multiple.

Farther in the periphery, the venous pattern becomes less and less predictable. Major variations in the large veins of the trunk occur and are usually traceable to embryonic events. These major anomalies may have clinical significance.

Superior Vena Cava

Failure of the left anterior and common cardinal veins to regress after the eighth week of embryonic life results in a left-sided superior vena cava. This vessel receives the internal jugular and subclavian veins on that side, descends anterolateral to the aortic arch, and anterior to the hilum of the left lung. It most commonly drains into the coronary sinus (Fig. 19-27). When both superior venae cavae are present (0.16% of individuals), the left brachiocephalic vein may be vestigial or absent.[1] In cases in

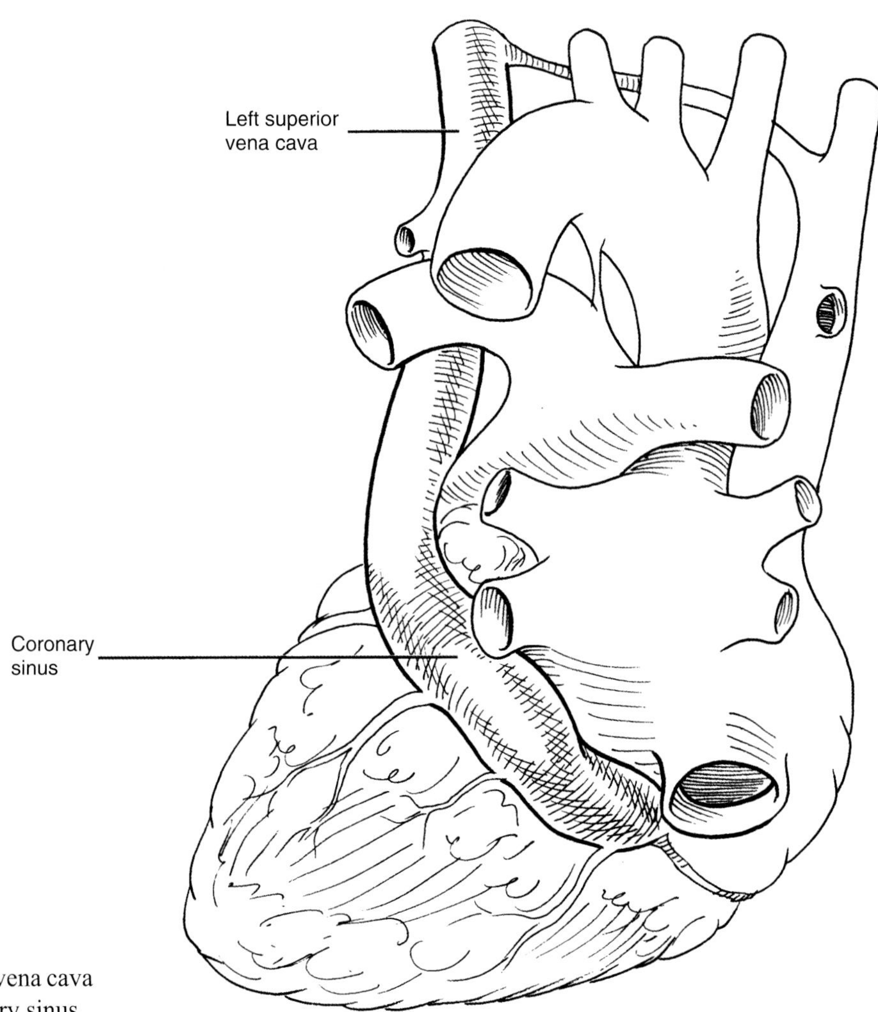

Fig. 19-27 A left-sided superior vena cava most often drains into the coronary sinus.

which the right-sided cardinal vein elements have regressed, only the left superior vena cava remains. In such cases, the right side drains to the left in a mirror image of the normal anatomy, and the azygous veins are also reversed. This condition is not necessarily associated with other visceral transpositions.

Inferior Vena Cava and Renal Veins

Persistence of the left subcardinal vein results in a double inferior vena cava in as many as 2% to 3% of individuals and a single left-sided inferior vena cava in 0.2% to 0.5%.[1] The left vein is commonly smaller than the right and communicates with the right through a preaortic anastomosis at or below the level of the renal veins (Fig. 19-28). The two venae cavae may also be joined by an iliac communication at their caudal end. This latter communication is sometimes preaortic. In addition, there may be a retroaortic left renal vein (2%) with or without a normal anterior left renal vein. In the presence of both, a circumaortic renal collar is formed.

A left-sided inferior vena cava is a component of situs inversus but may be present as an isolated anomaly. In the case of bilateral subcardinal

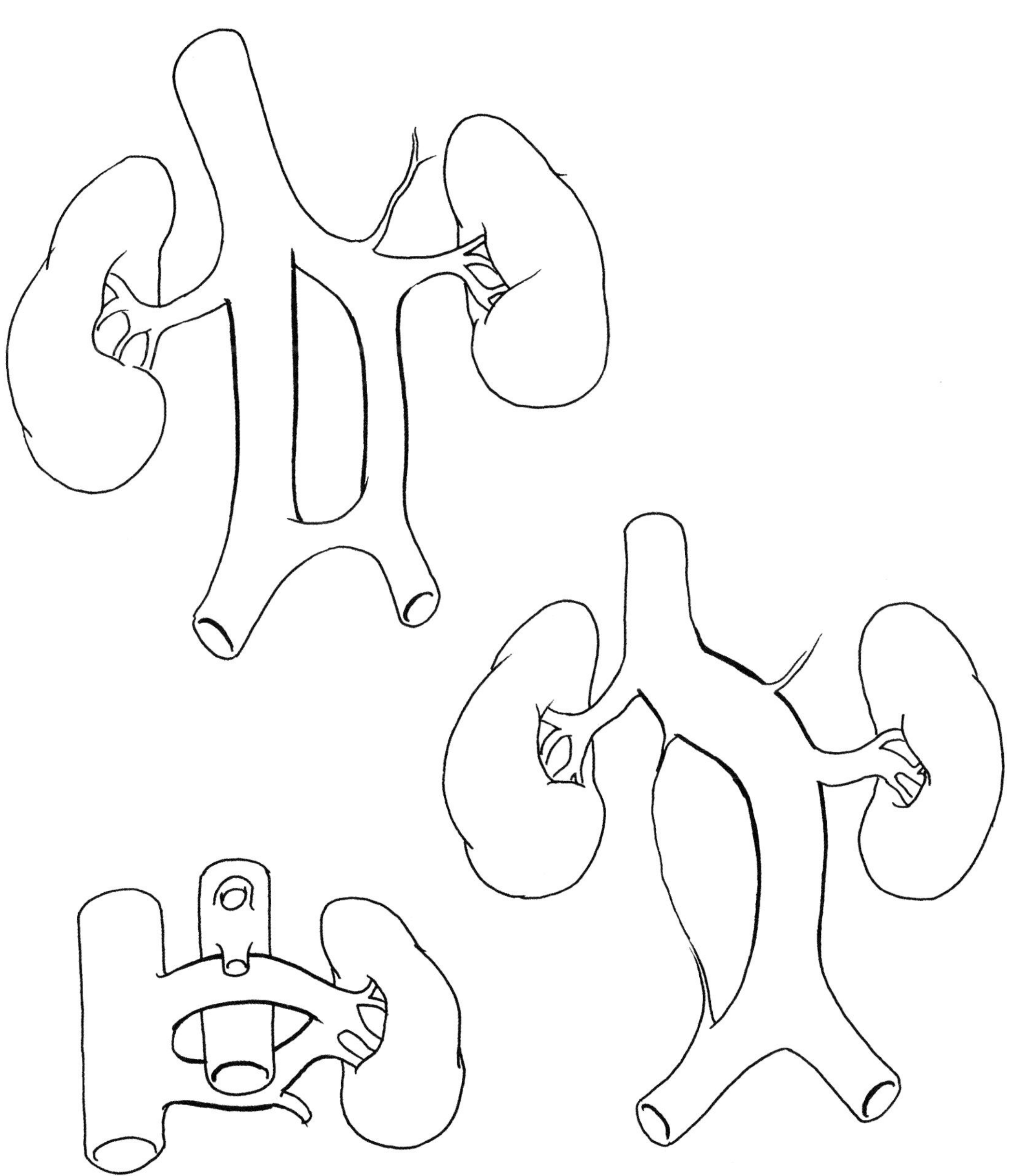

Fig. 19-28 Vena caval anomalies include doubling, left-sided position, and a circumaortic renal venous collar.

involution and absence of the inferior vena cava, blood from the lower half of the body and liver drains through large ascending lumbar veins to the azygous system and into the superior vena cava.

The incidence of clinically discovered inferior vena cava anomalies (0.6% to 2.1%) corresponds almost exactly to the findings in anatomic specimens and complicates surgical procedures, particularly abdominal aortic aneurysm repair.[27,28]

The renal veins may receive lumbar branches, and the left renal vein may communicate with the splenic vein. The right renal vein may be multiple in one-fourth to one-third of individuals, but the left renal vein is usually single. The left suprarenal vein is a constant branch of the left renal vein and may receive the left gonadal vein.

Portal Vein

The portal vein is quite constant, with rare instances of the vein being located anterior to the duodenum, common bile duct, and hepatic artery. Only a few cases of congenital absence of the portal vein have been reported.[7] There is variability in the point at which the inferior mesenteric vein joins the other portal tributaries (Fig. 19-29). In addition, the left gastric vein, whose disconnection is important in selective shunts, drains into the portal vein (54%), splenic vein (29%), or their junction (16%).[7]

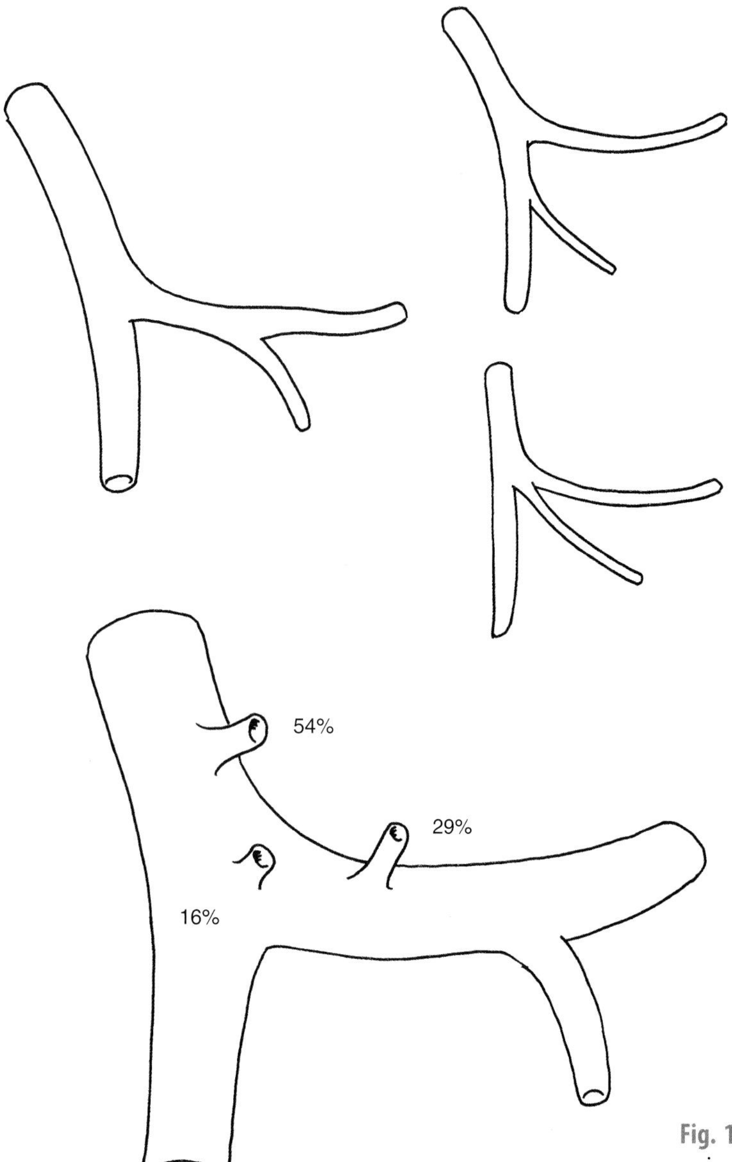

Fig. 19-29 The junction of the inferior mesenteric vein with the other portal tributaries is variable as is the junction of the left gastric vein.

References

1. Gray SW. *Embryology for Surgeons: The Embryological Basis for the Treatment of Congenital Defects*. Philadelphia, PA: WB Saunders; 1972.
2. Stewart JR, Kincaid GW, Edwards JE. *An Atlas of Vascular Rings and Related Malformations of the Aortic Arch System*. Springfield, IL: Charles C Thomas; 1964.
3. Valentine RJ, Carter DJ, Clagett GE. A modified extrathoracic approach to the treatment of dysphagia lusoria. *J Vasc Surg*. 1987;5:498–500.
4. Edwards FH, Wind G, Thompson L, et al. Three-dimensional image reconstruction for planning of a complex cardiovascular procedure. *Ann Thorac Surg*. 1990;49:486–488.
5. Sabiston DC Jr, Spencer FC. *Gibbon's Surgery of the Chest,* 4th ed. Philadelphia, PA: WB Saunders; 1983.
6. Clemente CD, ed. *Gray's Anatomy of the Human Body,* 30th American ed. Philadelphia, PA: Lea & Febiger; 1985.
7. Bergman RA, Thompson SA, Afifi AK, et al. *Compendium of Human Anatomic Variation*. Baltimore, MD: Urban & Schwarzenberg; 1988.
8. Daseler EH, Anson BJ. Surgical anatomy of the subclavian artery and its branches. *Surg Gynecol Obstet*. 1959;108:149–174.
9. Hitzrot JM. A composite study of the axillary artery in man. *Johns Hopkins Hosp Bull*. 1901;12:136–145.
10. Coleman SS, Anson BL. Arterial patterns in the hand based upon a study of 650 specimens. *Surg Gynecol Obstet*. 1961;113:409–424.
11. Scott HW Jr, Dean RH, Boerth R, et al. Coarctation of the abdominal aorta. *Ann Surg*. 1979;189:746–755.
12. Hallet JW, Brewster DC, Darling RC, et al. Coarctation of the abdominal aorta. *Ann Surg*. 1980;191:430–436.
13. Nelson TM, Pollak R, Jonasson O, et al. Anatomic variants of the celiac, superior mesenteric and inferior mesenteric arteries and their clinical relevance. *Clin Anat*. 1988;1:75–91.
14. Daseler EH, Anson BJ, Hambley WC, et al. The cystic artery and constituents of the hepatic pedicle. A study of 500 specimens. *Surg Gynecol Obstet*. 1947;85:47–63.
15. Sonneland J, Anson BJ, Beaton LE. Surgical anatomy of the arterial supply to the colon from the superior mesenteric artery based upon a study of 600 specimens. *Surg Gynecol Obstet*. 1958;106:385–389.
16. Zebrowski W, Augustyniak E, Zajac S. Variation of origin and branches of the inferior mesenteric artery and its anastomoses. *Folia Morphol (Praha)*. 1971;30:510–517.
17. Valentine RJ, Blakenship CL, MacGillivray DC, et al. Variations in the relationship of the left renal vein to the left renal artery. *Clin Anat*. 1990;3:249–255.
18. Stanley JC, Fry WJ. Median arcuate ligament syndrome. *Arch Surg*. 1971;103:252–257.
19. Akin JT, Skandalakis JE, Gray SW. The anatomic basis of vascular compression of the duodenum. *Surg Clin North Am*. 1974;54:1361–1370.
20. Braithwaite JL. Variations in origin of the parietal branches of the internal iliac artery. *J Anat*. 1952;86:423–430.
21. Steele G Jr, Sanders RJ, Riley J, et al. Pulsatile buttock masses: gluteal and persistent sciatic artery aneurysms. *Surgery*. 1977;82:201–204.
22. Uflacker R. *Atlas of Vascular Anatomy*. Philadelphia, PA: Lippincott Williams & Wilkins; 1997:756–778.
23. Williams GD, Martin CH, McIntire LR. Origin of the deep and circumflex group of arteries. *Anat Rec*. 1934;60:189–196.
24. Colborn GL, Lumsden AB, Taylor BS, et al. The surgical anatomy of the popliteal artery. *Am Surg*. 1994;60:238–246.
25. Rich NM, Collins GJ Jr, McDonald PT, et al. Popliteal vascular entrapment. *Arch Surg*. 1979;114:1377–1384.
26. Laterjet A, Testut L. *Traité d'anatomie humaine,* 8th ed. Paris, France: G. Doin a Cie; 1929.
27. Downey RS, Sicard GA, Anderson CB. Major retroperitoneal venous anomalies: surgical considerations. *Surgery*. 1990;107:359–365.
28. Bartle EJ, Pearce WH, Sun JH, et al. Infrarenal venous anomalies and aortic surgery: avoiding vascular injury. *J Vasc Surg*. 1987;6:590–593.

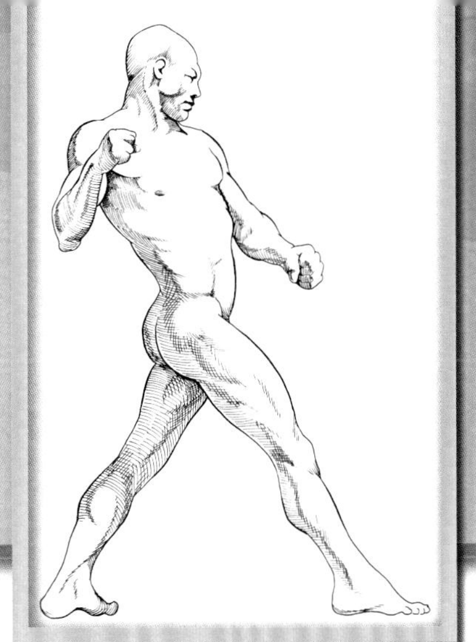

APPENDIX
Selected Anatomic References

General Texts

Hollinshead WH. *Textbook of Anatomy,* 5th ed. Philadelphia, PA: Harper & Row; 1997.

Lockhart RD, Hamilton GF, Fyfe FW. *Anatomy of the Human Body*. Philadelphia, PA: Lippincott Williams & Wilkins; 1974.

Moore KL, Dalley AF, Agur AMR, et al. *Clinically Oriented Anatomy,* 6th ed. Philadelphia, PA: Wolters Kluwer/Lippincott Williams & Wilkins; 2010.

Standring S, ed. *Gray's Anatomy: The Anatomical Basis of Clinical Practice,* 40th ed. Munich, Germany: Churchill Livingstone/Elsevier GmbH; 2008.

Woodburne RT. *Essentials of Human Anatomy,* 9th ed. New York, NY: Oxford University Press; 1994.

Atlases

Abrahams H, Boon J. *McMinn's Clinical Atlas of Human Anatomy,* 6th ed. Munich, Germany: Elsevier GmbH; 2008.

Agur AMR, Dalley AF. *Grant's Atlas of Anatomy,* 13th ed. Baltimore, MD: Wolters Kluwer/Lippincott Williams & Wilkins; 2013.

Bergman RA, Thompson SA, Afifi AK, et al. *Compendium of Human Anatomic Variation*. Baltimore, MD: Urban & Schwarzenberg; 1988.

Clemente CD. *Anatomy, a Regional Atlas of the Human Body,* 6th ed. Philadelphia, PA: Wolters Kluwer/Lippincott Williams & Wilkins; 2010.

Netter FH. *Atlas of Human Anatomy*, 5th ed. Philadelphia, PA: Saunders; 2011.

Pernkopf E. *Atlas of Topographic and Applied Human Anatomy,* 3rd English ed. Baltimore, MD: Urban & Schwarzenberg; 1990.

Putz R, ed. *Sobotta Atlas of Human Anatomy,* 14th ed. Munich, Germany: Elsevier Gmbh; 2008.

Uflacker R. *Atlas of Vascular Anatomy: An Angiographic Approach*. Philadelphia, PA: Lippincott Williams & Wilkins; 1997.

Cross-Sectional Atlases

Cahill D, Orland MJ. *Atlas of Human Cross-sectional Anatomy: With CT and MR Images*. New York, NY: Wiley Liss; 1995.

El-Khoury GY, Bergman RA, Montgomery WJ, et al. *Sectional Anatomy by MRI and CT with Website, 3rd ed*. Edinburgh, England: Churchill Livingstone; 2007.

Eycleshymer AC. *A Cross-section Anatomy*. New York, NY: D. Appleton; 1911.Reprints from the collection of the University of Michigan library.

Kelley LL, Petersen MS. *Sectional Anatomy for Imaging Professionals,* 2nd ed. St. Louis, MO: Mosby/Elsevier; 2007.

Koritke J, Sick H. *Atlas of Sectional Human Anatomy,* 2nd ed. Baltimore, MD: Urban & Schwarzenberg; 1988.

Weir J, Abrahams, P. *Imaging Atlas of Human Anatomy,* St. Louis, MO: Mosby/Elsevier; 2010.

Surgical Anatomy

Anson BJ, McVay CB. *Surgical Anatomy,* 6th ed. Philadelphia, PA: Saunders; 1984.

Henry AK. *Extensile Exposure,* 2nd ed. Edinburgh, England: Churchill Livingstone; 1973.

Scott-Conner CEH, Dawson DL. *Operative Anatomy,* Philadelphia, PA: Wolters Kluwer/Lippincott Williams & Wilkins; 2009.

Skandalakis JE, Skandalakis PN. *Surgical Anatomy and Technique*. New York, NY: Springer Sciences; 2008.

Thorek E. *Anatomy in Surgery*, 2nd ed. Philadelphia, PA: Lippincott Williams & Wilkins; 1962.

Musculoskeletal

Hoppenfeld S. *Surgical Exposures in Orthopedics: The Anatomic Approach*. Philadelphia, PA: Lippincott Williams & Wilkens; 1984.

Virtual Anatomy

http://www.visiblebody.com
http://www.anatronica.com
http://www.interactelsevier.com/netter
http://www.anatomium.com
http://www.primalpictures.com
http://www.anatomy.tv/default.aspx
http://www.nextd.com
http://www.zygotebody.com/no_webgl.html
http://www.3danatomy.co.uk
https://www.biodigitalhuman.com/default.html

Subject index

Page numbers followed by *f* refer to figures

F

G

H

I

J

K

L

M

N

O

P

Q

R

S

T

U

V

W

Y